The Spectrum of Neuro-AIDS Disorders

Pathophysiology, Diagnosis, and Treatment

The Spectrum of Neuro-AIDS Disorders

Pathophysiology, Diagnosis, and Treatment

Edited by

Karl Goodkin, M.D., Ph.D., FAPA
Department of Psychiatry and Behavioral
Neurosciences, Cedars-Sinai Medical Center,
and Department of Psychiatry and Biobehavioral
Sciences, University of California-Los Angeles,
Los Angeles, California

Paul Shapshak, Ph.D.
Ann Lowerey Murphey Laboratory, Department of
Psychiatry and Behavioral Medicine, University of
South Florida College of Medicine, Tampa, Florida

Ashok Verma, M.D., D.M.
Department of Neurology, University of Miami
Miller School of Medicine, Miami, Florida

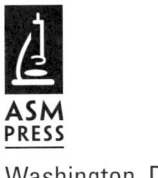

ASM
PRESS

Washington, DC

Copyright © 2009   ASM Press
American Society for Microbiology
1752 N Street, N.W.
Washington, DC 20036-2904

Library of Congress Cataloging-in-Publication Data

The spectrum of neuro-AIDS disorders : pathophysiology, diagnosis, and treatment /
edited by Karl Goodkin, Paul Shapshak, Ashok Verma.
    p. ; cm.
  Includes bibliographical references and index.
  ISBN 978-1-55581-369-7
  1. Brain—Infections. 2. AIDS (Disease) I. Goodkin, Karl. II. Shapshak,
Paul. III. Verma, Ashok.
  [DNLM: 1. HIV Infections—complications. 2. AIDS-Related Opportunistic
Infections. 3. Antiretroviral Therapy, Highly Active—adverse effects. 4. Central
Nervous System Diseases—etiology. 5. Diagnostic Techniques, Neurological.
6. Mental Disorders—etiology. WC 503.5 S741 2009]

  RC359.5.S64 2009
  616.97'92—dc22

      2008039156

ISBN 1-978-1-55581-369-7

All Rights Reserved
Printed in the United States of America

10 9 8 7 6 5 4 3 2 1

Address editorial correspondence to: ASM Press, 1752 N St., N.W., Washington, DC
20036-2904, U.S.A.

Send orders to: ASM Press, P.O. Box 605, Herndon, VA 20172, U.S.A.
Phone: 800-546-2416; 703-661-1593
Fax: 703-661-1501
Email: Books@asmusa.org
Online: estore.asm.org

Contents

v

Contributors

EDWARD ACHEAMPONG
Dept. of Medicine, Thomas Jefferson University, Philadelphia, PA 19107

CAGLA AKAY
Dept. of Pathology, University of Pennsylvania, Philadelphia, PA 19104-6030

ERIC ANDERSON
Laboratory of Neuroregeneration, Dept. of Pharmacology and Experimental Neuroscience, University of Nebraska Medical Center, Omaha, NE 68198-5880

GABRIELE ARENDT
Dept. of Neurology, University Hospital of Duesseldorf (UKD), Duesseldorf, Germany

AARON ARONOW
Dept. of Neurology, Keck School of Medicine, GNH 5641, University of Southern California, Los Angeles, CA 90033

DESHRATN ASTHANA
Laboratory for Clinical and Biological Studies, Dept. of Psychiatry and Behavioral Sciences, Fox Cancer Center, University of Miami, Miami, FL 33136

GAYLE BALDWIN
Dept. of Medicine, David Geffen School of Medicine, and UCLA AIDS Institute, University of California, Los Angeles, Los Angeles, CA 90095

ROGER J. BEDIMO
Infectious Diseases Section, VA North Texas Health Care System, Dallas, TX 75216, and Division of Infectious Diseases, The University of Texas Southwestern Medical Center at Dallas, Dallas, TX 75390-9113

ANITA L. BELMAN
Dept. of Neurology, School of Medicine, Stony Brook University, Stony Brook, NY 11794

JOSEPH R. BERGER
Dept. of Neurology, University of Kentucky College of Medicine, Lexington, KY 40536

AARON J. BERGER
Division of Plastic Surgery, Stanford University, Stanford, CA 94305

JOHN BOOSS
Yale University School of Medicine and Virology Laboratories, VA Connecticut, New Haven, CT 06510

BRUCE BREW
Dept. of Neurology and Dept. of HIV Medicine, Centre for Immunology, and National Centre in HIV Epidemiology and Clinical Research, St. Vincent's Hospital, University of New South Wales, Sydney 2010, Australia

KATIA V. BROWN
Division of Infectious Diseases, The University of Texas Southwestern Medical School, Dallas, TX 75390

ADRIANA CAMPA
Dept. of Dietetics and Nutrition, Florida International University, Stempel School of Public Health, Miami, FL 33199

GLORIA CASTILLO
Dept. of Epidemiology and Public Health, Division of Disease Prevention, University of Miami Miller School of Medicine, Miami, FL 33136

LINDA CHANG
Dept. of Medicine, Division of Neurology, University of Hawaii, John A. Burns School of Medicine, Honolulu, HI 96813

FRANCESCO CHIAPPELLI
Division of Oral Biology and Medicine, Laboratory of Human Oral and Molecular Immunology, UCLA School of Dentistry, University of California at Los Angeles, Los Angeles, CA 90095-1668

PAOLA CINQUE
Clinic of Infectious Diseases, San Raffaele Scientific Institute, Milano, Italy

DAVID B. CLIFFORD
Dept. of Neurology, Washington University School of Medicine, St. Louis, MO 63110

DEBORAH COMMINS
Dept. of Pathology (Neuropathology), University
of Southern California Keck School of Medicine,
Los Angeles, CA 90089

MAURICIO CONCHA
Intercoastal Medical Group, Sarasota, FL 34232

ANNE DE GROOT
EpiVax, Inc., and Biomedical Center, Brown University
School of Medicine, Providence, RI 02912

DAWN EGGERT
Laboratory of Neuroregeneration, Dept. of Pharmacology and
Experimental Neuroscience, University of Nebraska Medical
Center, Omaha, NE 68198-5880

THOMAS ERNST
Dept. of Medicine, Division of Neurology, University of
Hawaii, John A. Burns School of Medicine, Honolulu,
HI 96813

LYDIA ESTANISLAO
Clinical Neurology Specialists, Las Vegas, NV 89146

STEPHEN J. FERRANDO
New York-Presbyterian Hospital, Weill Medical College of
Cornell University, New York, NY 10065

DARREN R. FLOWER
The Jenner Institute, University of Oxford, Compton,
Berkshire, RG20 7NN, United Kingdom

ROY FREEMAN
Dept. of Neurology, Beth Israel Deaconess Medical Center,
Harvard Medical School, Boston, MA 02215

SIMON FROST
Antiviral Research Center, Dept. of Pathology, University of
California San Diego, San Diego, CA 92103

HARRIS A. GELBARD
Center for Aging and Developmental Biology, Kornberg
Medical Research Institute, and Departments of
Neurology, Pediatrics, Microbiology, and Immunology,
University of Rochester Medical Center, Rochester,
NY 14642

HOWARD E. GENDELMAN
Laboratory of Neurotoxicology, Dept. of Pharmacology and
Experimental Neuroscience, Center for Neurovirology and
Neurodegenerative Disorders, University of Nebraska Medical
Center, Omaha, NE 68198-5880

ANTHONY GERACI
St. Luke's-Roosevelt Hospital, New York, NY

MAGNUS GISSLÉN
Dept. of Infectious Diseases, Göteborg University,
Sahlgrenska University Hospital, Göteborg, Sweden

KARL GOODKIN
Dept. of Psychiatry and Behavioral Neurosciences,
Cedars-Sinai Medical Center, and Dept. of Psychiatry and
Biobehavioral Sciences, David Geffen School of Medicine,
UCLA, Los Angeles, CA 90048

LARS HAGBERG
Dept. of Infectious Diseases, Göteborg University,
Sahlgrenska University Hospital, Göteborg, Sweden

W. DAVID HARDY
Division of Infectious Diseases, Dept. of Internal Medicine,
Cedars-Sinai Medical Center, and David Geffen School of
Medicine, UCLA, Los Angeles, CA 90048

Y. JAEGER
Dept. of Surgery, Presbyterian Hospital of Duesseldorf,
Duesseldorf, Germany

BETH D. JAMIESON
UCLA Flow Cytometry Core Facility, Dept. of Medicine/
Hematology-Oncology, UCLA, Los Angeles, CA 90048

KELLY L. JORDAN-SCIUTTO
Dept. of Pathology, University of Pennsylvania, Philadelphia,
PA 19104-6030

PANDJASSARAME KANGUEANE
Biomedical Informatics, 17A Irulan Sundai Annex,
Pondicherry 607402, India

RAJARATHINAM KAYATHRI
Biomedical Informatics, 17A Irulan Sundai Annex,
Pondicherry 607402, India

SERGEI L. KOSAKOVSKY POND
Antiviral Research Center, Dept. of Pathology, University of
California San Diego, San Diego, CA 92103

TOMASZ LASKUS
St. Joseph's Hospital and Medical Center, Phoenix, AZ 85013

TODD LOFTUS
New York-Presbyterian Hospital, Weill Medical College of
Cornell University, New York, NY 10065

ENRIQUE LOPEZ
Dept. of Psychiatry and Behavioral Neurosciences,
Cedars-Sinai Medical Center, and Dept. of Psychiatry and
Biobehavioral Sciences, David Geffen School of Medicine,
UCLA, Los Angeles, CA 90048

CARLOS LUCIANO
Dept. of Physical Medicine and Division of Neurology,
NeuroAIDS Program, UPR, MSC, SNRP, University of
Puerto Rico, Medical Sciences Campus, San Juan,
PR 00936-5067

THOMAS D. MARCOTTE
Dept. of Psychiatry, HIV Neurobehavioral Research Center,
University of California, San Diego, San Diego, CA 92119

RAUL MAYO-SANTANA
Dept. of Physical Medicine and Division of Neurology,
NeuroAIDS Program, UPR, MSC, SNRP, University of
Puerto Rico, Medical Sciences Campus, San Juan,
PR 00936-5067

ROBERT R. McKENDALL
Dept. of Neurology, Dept. of Microbiology and
Immunology, University of Texas Medical Branch, Galveston,
TX 77555

LOYDA M. MELÉNDEZ
Dept. of Microbiology, NeuroAIDS Program, UPR, MSC, SNRP, University of Puerto Rico, Medical Sciences Campus, San Juan, PR 00936-5067

MARIA-JOSE MIGUEZ-BURBANO
Dept. of Psychiatry & Behavioral Sciences, University of Miami Miller School of Medicine, Miami, FL 33136

ALIREZA MINAGAR
Dept. of Neurology and Dept. of Anesthesiology, Louisiana State University Health Sciences Center, Shreveport, LA 71301

ROSA REBECA MOLINA
Sylvester Comprehensive Cancer Center, Fox Cancer Center, University of Miami, Miami, FL 33136

GERALDINE MOREN-BLACK
Dept. of Anthropology, University of Oregon, Eugene, OR 97403

MUHAMMAD MUKHTAR
Dept. of Biochemistry, Pir Mehr Ali Shah Arid Agriculture University Rawalpindi, Murree Road, Rawalpindi 46300, Pakistan

RACHEL NARDIN
Dept. of Neurology, Beth Israel Deaconess Medical Center, Harvard Medical School, Boston, MA 02215

JONATHAN NASSERI
St. Joseph's Hospital and Medical Center, Phoenix, AZ 85013

AVINDRA NATH
Dept. of Neurology, Johns Hopkins University, Baltimore, MD 21287

JUTTA K. NEUENBURG
Immune Tolerance Network, 185 Berry St. Ste. 3515, San Francisco, CA 94107

TH. NOLTING
Dept. of Neurology, University Hospital of Duesseldorf (UKD), Duesseldorf, Germany

JORGE PARDO
Dept. of Neurology, University of Miami Miller School of Medicine, Miami, FL 33136

ZAHIDA PARVEEN
Dept. of Medicine, Thomas Jefferson University, Philadelphia, PA 19107

SETH W. PERRY
Center for Aging and Developmental Biology, Kornberg Medical Research Institute, and Departments of Neurology, Pediatrics, Microbiology, and Immunology, University of Rochester Medical Center, Rochester, NY 14642

ROGER J. POMERANTZ
Tibotec Inc., Yardley, PA 19067

M. JUDITH DONOVAN POST
Dept. of Radiology, Neuroradiology, University of Miami L. Miller School of Medicine, Miami, FL 33136-1094

RICHARD W. PRICE
Dept. of Neurology, University of California San Francisco, and San Francisco General Hospital, San Francisco, CA 94110

MIGUEL QUINONES-MATEU
Life Sciences Division, DIAGNOSTIC HYBRIDS, Athens, OH 45701

ALEJANDRO RABINSTEIN
Mayo Clinic, Rochester, MN 55905

MAREK RADKOWSKI
Institute of Infectious Diseases, Warsaw Medical Academy, Warsaw, Poland

JEFFREY A. RUMBAUGH
Dept. of Neurology, Johns Hopkins University, Baltimore, MD 21287

KRISTEN SADLER
School of Biological Sciences, Nanyang Technological University, Singapore 637551

SOMA SAHAI-SRIVASTAVA
Dept. of Neurology, University of Southern California, 1200 N. State St., Los Angeles, CA 90033

MEENA KISHORE SAKHARKAR
School of Mechanical and Aerospace Engineering, Nanyang Technological University, Singapore 639798

J. COBB SCOTT
Dept. of Psychiatry, HIV Neurobehavioral Research Center, University of California, San Diego, San Diego, CA 92119

DAVID M. SEGAL
Dept. of Health Professions, College of Health & Public Affairs, and Dept. of Medical Education, College of Medicine, University of Central Florida, Orlando, FL 32816-2205

PETER A. SELWYN
Montefiore Medical Center, Albert Einstein College of Medicine, Bronx, NY 10467

PAUL SHAPSHAK
Division of Infectious Diseases and International Medicine, Tampa General Hospital, and Departments of Internal Medicine and Psychiatry-Behavioral Sciences, USF Health, Tampa, FL 33606

GAIL SHOR-POSNER
Dept. of Epidemiology and Public Health, Division of Disease Prevention, University of Miami Miller School of Medicine, Miami, FL 33136

DAVID SIMPSON
Dept. of Neurology, Mount Sinai Medical Center, New York, NY 10029

ELYSE SINGER
Dept. of Neurology, UCLA David Geffen School of Medicine, Los Angeles, CA 90024

DANIEL J. SKIEST
Adult HIV Program, Division of Infectious Diseases, Baystate
Medical Center, Springfield, MA 01119, and Tufts University
School of Medicine

ERNEST TERWILLIGER
Harvard Institute of Medicine, Boston, MA 02115

MAJDA M. THURNHER
Dept. of Radiology, Neuroradiology Section, Medical
University of Vienna, Waehringer Guertel 18-20, 1090-
Vienna, Austria

DARDO TOMASI
Medical Dept., Brookhaven National Laboratory, Upton,
NY 11973

ALEX TSELIS
Dept. of Neurology, UHC-8D, Wayne State University,
Detroit, MI 48201

ASHOK VERMA
University of Miami Miller School of Medicine, Miami,
FL 33136

VALERIE WOJNA
Dept. of Physical Medicine and Division of Neurology,
NeuroAIDS Program, UPR, MSC, SNRP, University of Puerto
Rico, Medical Sciences Campus, San Juan, PR 00936-5067

CONSTANTIN T. YIANNOUTSOS
Dept. of Medicine, Division of Biostatistics, Indiana
University School of Medicine, 410 West 10th Street, Suite
3000, Indianapolis, IN 46202

SELENE ZARATE
Dept. of Genetics, Independent University of Mexico City,
San Lorenzo 290, Col. Del Valle, 03100 México,
D.F., México

JIALIN ZHENG
Laboratory of Neurotoxicology, Dept. of Pharmacology and
Experimental Neuroscience, Center for Neurovirology and
Neurodegenerative Disorders, University of Nebraska Medical
Center, Omaha, NE 68198-5880

WENLI ZHENG
Division of Enrollment Management, Market Research &
Communications, University of Miami, Coral Gables, FL
33146

KAI ZHONG
Dept. of Biomedical Magnetic Resonance, Institute for
Experimental Physics, Otto-von-Guericke-University
Magdeburg, Leipziger Str. 44, Haus 01, D-39120 Magdeburg,
Germany

Preface

The Spectrum of Neuro-AIDS Disorders: Pathophysiology, Diagnosis, and Treatment represents a compendium of knowledge that is unique to the field of neuro-AIDS. At this point in the era of highly active antiretroviral therapy (HAART), we have come to appreciate, more than ever before, the implications of the brain as an organ that becomes a reservoir for resistant HIV, contributing to a deleterious impact of this chronic infection on patient functioning. The book is designed to present a coordinated focus on the integration of knowledge regarding the pathophysiological bases, diagnostic approaches, and clinical treatment strategies specific for neuro-AIDS conditions in the HAART era today. Each chapter bridges the literature in its respective area from the former results in the pre-HAART era to the current knowledge base. Since HAART was introduced in late 1995, it has only recently become possible to present a consensus on changes in clinical outcomes such as those presented in this book. Hence, this book should be useful not only to clinicians but also to students and teachers in many areas.

As the morbidity and mortality of HIV infection have decreased greatly over the HAART era, neuro-AIDS conditions have shifted along with this change. Currently, the most prevalent neuro-AIDS condition is distal sensory polyneuropathy. Primary central nervous system (CNS) lymphoma is now a diagnosis of increased suspicion for mass lesions in the brain with respect to CNS toxoplasmosis, and iatrogenic neurological and neurobehavioral conditions due to prescribed medication toxicities have blossomed. The latter include the toxicities of the antiretroviral medications themselves. Efavirenz is the most widely cited antiretroviral regarding neurological and neurobehavioral outcomes of medication toxicity, including sleep disturbance, vestibular abnormalities, and neurocognitive impairment. However, long-term atherogenic risk, now attributed to HAART toxicity, has also changed the face of neuro-AIDS in the HAART era. A concern for such a vascular risk must now be regularly considered clinically, in addition to the damage to brain tissue caused both by HIV infection directly and by the inflammatory response to the presence of the virus. Thus, the entire neuropathogenic basis for understanding and defining these disorders has been altered. Moreover, in recognition of these changes, the diagnostic approach to several of the neuro-AIDS conditions, in particular the neurocognitive disorders, has evolved. Thus, a book of this magnitude

is timely to integrate the changes noted in HIV-associated neuropathogenesis with associated changes in indicated diagnostic procedures and in treatment decision-making.

Section I of this book covers disorders due to primary HIV pathogenesis. At the outset, HIV-associated neurocognitive disorder (chapter 1, Goodkin et al.) and neuropsychological issues (chapter 2, Marcotte and Scott) are presented. This is followed by a presentation of a rising, long-term, antiretroviral toxicity concern, the risk of cerebrovascular accident (CVA, or stroke) (chapter 3, Concha and Rabinstein). Chapter 4 (Estanislao) presents HIV-associated meningitis, which is particularly frequent in the setting of acute conversion syndrome. Moving down the neuraxis, this chapter also includes HIV-associated myelopathy, radiculopathy, and myopathy. There is a separate presentation in chapter 5 (Freeman and Nardin) of autonomic neuropathies in HIV infection, which are much less frequently noted in clinical pratice than their actual prevalence merits. Peripheral neuropathies are then presented in some detail in chapter 6 (Estanislao et al.), with the most common form, distal sensory polyneuropathy, followed by dideoxynucleoside-induced toxic neuropathy and other toxic neuropathies as well as inflammatory demyelinating polyneuropathy, mononeuropathy multiplex, and progressive polyradiculopathy.

A particularly important area of clinical concern being more closely examined at this point in the HAART era is centered predominantly upon an antiretroviral toxicity, mitochondrial dysfunction with lactic acidosis. Thus, mitochondrial dysfunction is presented in this section, with reference to lactic acidosis as the targeted clinical condition for diagnosis and treatment (chapter 7, Verma and Pardo). In fact, severe lactic acidosis can affect multiple organ systems, particularly the peripheral nerves and muscle (of relevance to neuro-AIDS conditions) as well as the liver, kidneys, and pancreas. Next, chapter 8 (Yiannoutsos) provides an overall view of how neuro-AIDS outcomes are best examined methodologically as clinical events with associated surrogate markers. The latter is a prominent current issue, as the utility of numerous surrogate markers for neuro-AIDS conditions in the pre-HAART era has become eroded or erased over the course of the HAART era. Finally, in chapter 9, Kangueane et al. consider the import of vaccine studies applied to neuro-AIDS conditions, a rapidly evolving area that brings us into the vista for the future.

Section II covers pathophysiological issues. First discussed are the neurovirological aspects of HIV infection in the HAART era (chapter 10, Parveen et al.). This is an area currently experiencing a resurgence of investigative interest compared to the historically greater focus devoted to neuroinflammatory mechanisms. Next, enhancing contrast, neuroimmunology, and neuroinflammation in the pathogenesis of HIV-1 encephalitis in the HAART era are covered, including novel implications for neuroprotective treatments (chapter 11, Perry and Gelbard). A more specific focus is then directed toward the chemokines in the neuropathogenesis of HIV infection (chapter 12, Gendelman and colleagues). A similar level of specific focus is devoted to the cerebrospinal fluid by a contribution representing several groups (chapter 13, Gisslén et al.). Chapter 14 (Neuenburg) examines the changes in the neuropathology of HIV infection, including work demonstrating the surprising increase in incidence of HIV encephalopathy in the HAART era. A specific note is also made therein of recent work supporting the pathophysiological importance of microbial translocation from the gastrointestinal tract.

The next contribution in section II presents a focus on the role of viral genetic variability in HIV-1-associated neurocognitive disorders (chapter 15, Shapshak et al.), acknowledging the growing interest in that area. Further, the role of antioxidants in HIV-associated infection of the brain is considered, together with therapeutic implications including nutritional interventions (chapter 16, Shor-Posner et al.). Section II concludes with a chapter on a novel pathogenic focus in neuro-AIDS that is currently gaining attention: cell cycle proteins (chapter 17, Jordan-Sciutto and Akay).

Section III considers the utility of selected neuroimaging techniques in HIV infection. The first chapter focuses on structural neuroimaging of the brain in HIV-infected patients (chapter 18, Thurnher and Post). This technique has been predominantly utilized for diagnosing and monitoring the treatment response of the complications of HIV infection of the brain (rather than for primary HIV-associated neurocognitive impairment and disorder). The roles of structural neuroimaging in CNS toxoplasmosis and primary CNS lymphoma diagnosis and therapeutic management are discussed in detail. Next in this section is a consideration of functional magnetic resonance imaging (fMRI), which includes a focus on blood oxygenation level-dependent fMRI (BOLD fMRI) (chapter 19, Ernst et al.). This technique can be used to increase the sensitivity with which HIV-associated neurocognitive impairment and disorder may be identified. For example, neuropsychological test challenges can be used with pre- and post-fMRI evaluation of adequacy of performance and identification of the types of abnormalities elicited in response. This neuroimaging technique may be particularly helpful for HIV-infected patients with comorbid psychoactive substance use disorders. The last chapter in this section is devoted to magnetic resonance spectroscopy (MRS) (chapter 20, Chang et al.). MRS provides quantified absolute concentrations of brain tissue metabolites that are region-specific and indicative of tissue damage. It is now recognized to be a useful diagnostic technique for a number of CNS complications of HIV infection as well as for HIV infection itself, the focus of this chapter. MRS is relevant not only to the diagnosis of HIV-associated neurocognitive impairment and disorder but also to the monitoring of treatment response. This noninvasive technique is gaining clinical recognition and is now reimbursable by some third-party payers. Overall, the neuroimaging section of this volume may be considered to provide bridges between section

II on pathophysiological issues and the sections devoted to clinical manifestations (section I on disorders due to primary HIV pathogenesis, and section IV on HIV-associated comorbidities).

Section IV addresses clinically relevant HIV-associated comorbidities. The importance of these comorbidities is reflected by the fact that this section is similar in breadth to both sections I (on clinical manifestations due to primary HIV pathogenesis) and II (on pathophysiological issues). Section IV begins with a contribution on hepatitis C virus (HCV) infection (chapter 21, Radkowski et al.), for which there is mounting evidence of associated neurocognitive impairment that might be synergistic with the neurocognitive effects of HIV itself. Further, these HCV-associated neurocognitive changes do not correlate with the severity of liver disease and are not accounted for by hepatic encephalopathy or by psychoactive substance use disorders, but are indicative, instead, of HCV replication within brain tissue. This chapter is followed by a contribution on CNS toxoplasmosis (chapter 22, Brown and Skiest). Though reduced in incidence, CNS toxoplasmosis remains an important source of morbidity and mortality in the HAART era. The basic and clinical aspects of cytomegalovirus (CMV) infection are then examined (chapter 23, McKendall and Tselis) with regard to CMV encephalitis, polyradiculomyelitis, and mononeuritis multiplex, along with discussion of CMV retinitis. Chapter 24 (Bedimo and Skiest) presents the range of CNS fungal infections, led by cryptococcosis and followed by aspergillosis, coccidioidomycosis, zygomycosis, histoplasmosis, blastomycosis, paracoccidioidomycosis, and candidiasis. The appearance of the "great masquerader" is included, with a chapter on neurosyphilis in the setting of HIV infection (chapter 25, Berger and Berger). Of note, the frequency of asymptomatic neurosyphilis is of special concern in the setting of HIV infection. Chapter 26 (Clifford) examines progressive multifocal leukoencephalopathy (PML) in the HAART era. PML patients now have a longer survival time, although proven JC virus-specific therapy for PML remains lacking. Finally, Epstein-Barr virus infection in HIV infection is presented, with a specific focus on primary CNS lymphoma (chapter 27, Tselis and McKendall).

Section IV continues with another unique aspect of this volume, in that this book focuses not only on the neurological conditions associated with HIV infection, but also upon HIV-associated neurobehavioral conditions. Chapter 28 (Ferrando and Loftus) includes sections on depressive disorders, anxiety disorders, delirium, and psychosis. In addition, this chapter focuses on issues experienced by HIV-infected patients that extend into the normal range of neurobehavioral function: fatigue, lipodystrophy syndrome, sleep abnormalities, and sexual dysfunction. There is also a discussion of drug-drug interactions. The last chapter in section IV focuses on psychoactive substance use in HIV infection (chapter 29, Rumbaugh and Nath). Here, basic and clinical sciences are closely interwoven across sections on the opioids, cocaine, methamphetamine, MDMA, alcohol, cannabinoids, and anabolic steroids. Importantly, interactions between prescribed medications and psychoactive substances are discussed.

Yet another uncharacteristic aspect of this volume on neuro-AIDS is represented by its final two sections: section V on special populations, and section VI on special health care issues. Comparatively little can be found in the published literature on these two critical areas. In section V, the special neuro-AIDS populations represented are ethnic groups (chapter 30, Meléndez et al.), women (chapter 31,

Arendt et al.), children (chapter 32, Belman), and older persons (chapter 33, Goodkin et al.). Each population is reviewed in detail. In section VI on special health care issues and neuro-AIDS conditions, palliative care issues (chapter 34, Selwyn and Booss), medico-legal issues (chapter 35, Sahai-Srivastava), and international/global issues (chapter 36, Brew) are presented.

In summary, this volume on neuro-AIDS is unique in that it inter-relates data from the pre-HAART and HAART eras across a number of areas covering the domains of pathophysiology, diagnosis, and treatment. The book includes coverage in depth of the disorders due primarily to HIV infection as well as to its associated comorbidities. Likewise, pathophysiological mechanisms of multiple types are delineated. Presentation of the published data on the most relevant neuroimaging techniques for clinical purposes is included. This will aid in bridging the gap between research on disease pathophysiology and clinical practice by promoting the translation of research knowledge in neuroimaging to use in the care for the clinical manifestations of neuro-AIDS. Finally, the book provides coverage of neurobehavioral issues, special population issues, and special health care issues.

In short, *The Spectrum of Neuro-AIDS Disorders: Pathophysiology, Diagnosis, and Treatment* is a comprehensive volume that we expect to appeal to many readerships, including infectious disease physicians, internists, and other primary care providers; neurologists, neuropsychiatrists, neuropsychologists, neuroradiologists, and neuropathologists; as well as ethnologists, gynecologists, pediatricians, and geriatricians. Likewise, we expect that virologists, immunologists, epidemiologists, biochemists, and pharmacologists can utilize this book. In addition, from the ancillary professions, this book can be appreciated by registered nurses, nurse practitioners, physician assistants, case managers, and medical and psychiatric social workers. Although the ability of

these different groups to appreciate various aspects of the text may vary, the attraction of the text to all is its comprehensive delivery of current diagnostic issues and treatment recommendations in neuro-AIDS. Thus, the book holds promise for all of the aforementioned groups.

While the literature in this area advances rapidly, we hope that this volume will retain its appeal over time by its structured approach to the epistemology of neuro-AIDS knowledge. We anticipate that this presentation of the conceptual underpinnings of the neuro-AIDS field will allow new data to continue to be added to the organizational tree of knowledge, resulting in a timeless value for its readers.

I would like to acknowledge the much appreciated contributions of my co-editors, Ashok Verma and Paul Shapshak, who endured the long hours of work required to assemble this volume. In addition, I acknowledge the contribution of Walter G. Bradley, a father of this work who was involved with its original conceptualization. My thanks also go to all of the contributors to this volume and the special efforts they made in submitting each of its chapters, without which the sense of "wholeness" of this volume could not have been achieved. I also thank Jeff Holtmeier, Ken April, Ellie Tupper, Elizabeth McGillicuddy, and the rest of the ASM Press staff who pursued the final goal of publication with both diligence and patience. I wish to thank my loving wife, Amity, and my two sons, Devin and Grant (just approaching his first birthday), for reminding me about everything that is important in life and for allowing me the long hours required to produce this text. Finally, I extend my sincere appreciation to all of the patients and research participants afflicted by neuro-AIDS conditions who have contributed to my work as well as that of all of the authors represented, and without whom this work would not have been possible.

KARL GOODKIN

DISORDERS DUE TO PRIMARY HIV-1 PATHOGENESIS AND THEIR TREATMENT

I

The Spectrum of Neuro-AIDS Disorders:
Pathophysiology, Diagnosis, and Treatment
Edited by K. Goodkin et al.
©2008 ASM Press, Washington, DC

1

HIV-1-Associated Neurocognitive Disorders in the HAART Era

KARL GOODKIN, AARON ARONOW, GAYLE BALDWIN,
REBECA MOLINA, WENLI ZHENG, AND W. DAVID HARDY

HISTORY PRIOR TO HIGHLY ACTIVE ANTIRETROVIRAL THERAPY (HAART)

Early in the HIV/AIDS epidemic, the deleterious consequences of HIV-1 infection in the central and peripheral nervous system were described (Snider et al., 1983). They were considered to be due to severe immunosuppression, and encephalitis was considered predominantly attributable to concomitant cytomegalovirus (CMV) infection. In 1986, Navia et al. (1986a, 1986b) first coined the term "AIDS dementia complex (ADC)" and formally described it, documenting motor deficits (including ataxia, leg weakness, tremor, and loss of fine-motor coordination), along with behavioral disturbances (including apathy, withdrawal, and, less frequently, psychosis). The course of the disease was steadily progressive in most patients, with some showing an abrupt acceleration and a minority (20%) showing a protracted, indolent course. This seminal work not only described the manifestations of the disease, but also set the conceptual focus for understanding its pathophysiology. Less than 10% of the brains were histologically normal, with abnormalities being found predominantly in the subcortical grey matter and in the white matter, with relative sparing of the cerebral cortex. Diffuse white-matter pallor was common, with perivascular infiltrates

of lymphocytes and macrophages in mild cases and clusters of foamy macrophages, as well as multinucleated giant cells, in the severe cases. It was concluded that ADC was consistent with the then-emerging concept that direct brain infection by HIV-1 was the cause of the disorder.

ADC was then considered to be a true "complex." That is, it was thought to comprise three types of core manifestations—neurocognitive, motor, and neurobehavioral. The neurocognitive manifestations were thought to be focused upon information-processing speed and attention deficits. The motor manifestations focused upon motor slowing associated with the predilection of HIV-1 for the basal ganglia. Of note, regarding associated Parkinsonian motor symptoms, including the substantia nigra, the neurobehavioral symptoms were less specifically described and were related to emotional blunting and social withdrawal, progressing to psychotic symptoms with mutism, delusions, and hallucinations. The neuropathological data supported the clinical data. This concept of a "complex" would hold sway, overall, in the field for the next 2 decades.

The Centers for Disease Control and Prevention (CDC) published a staging system which differentiated four clinical stages of systemic disease: I, acute infection; II, the asymptomatic stage; III, persistent generalized lymphadenopathy; and IV, the symptomatic stage, including both AIDS-defining and non-AIDS-defining conditions (CDC, 1986). As acute HIV-1 infection was difficult to confirm and had only rarely been detected, the other stages were focused upon. Generally, CDC stages II and III were combined in clinical research studies and were differentiated from the non-AIDS-defining (A and C2) and from the AIDS-defining (C1 and D) substages within stage IV. This yielded three subsequent clinical stages of interest: (i) the asymptomatic stage; (ii) the symptomatic, non-AIDS-defining stage; and (iii) the symptomatic, AIDS-defining stage. These later became clinical stages designated in a revision of this staging system. While only full-blown dementia was denoted by the CDC staging system, neurocognitive manifestations follow the same type of progression by stage: asymptomatic

Karl Goodkin, Dept. of Psychiatry and Behavioral Neurosciences, Cedars-Sinai Medical Center, and Dept. of Psychiatry and Biobehavioral Sciences, University of California–Los Angeles, Los Angeles, CA 90048. **Aaron Aronow,** Dept. of Neurology, Keck School of Medicine, GNH 5641, University of Southern California, Los Angeles, CA 90033. **Gayle Baldwin,** Dept. of Medicine, David Geffen School of Medicine, and UCLA AIDS Institute, University of California–Los Angeles, Los Angeles, CA 90095. **Rebeca Molina,** Sylvester Comprehensive Cancer Center, Clinical Research Services, Miami, FL 33136. **Wenli Zheng,** Division of Enrollment Management, Market Research, and Communications, Coral Gables, FL 33146. **W. David Hardy,** Division of Infectious Diseases, Dept. of Internal Medicine, Cedars-Sinai Medical Center and David Geffen School of Medicine at UCLA, Los Angeles, CA 90048.

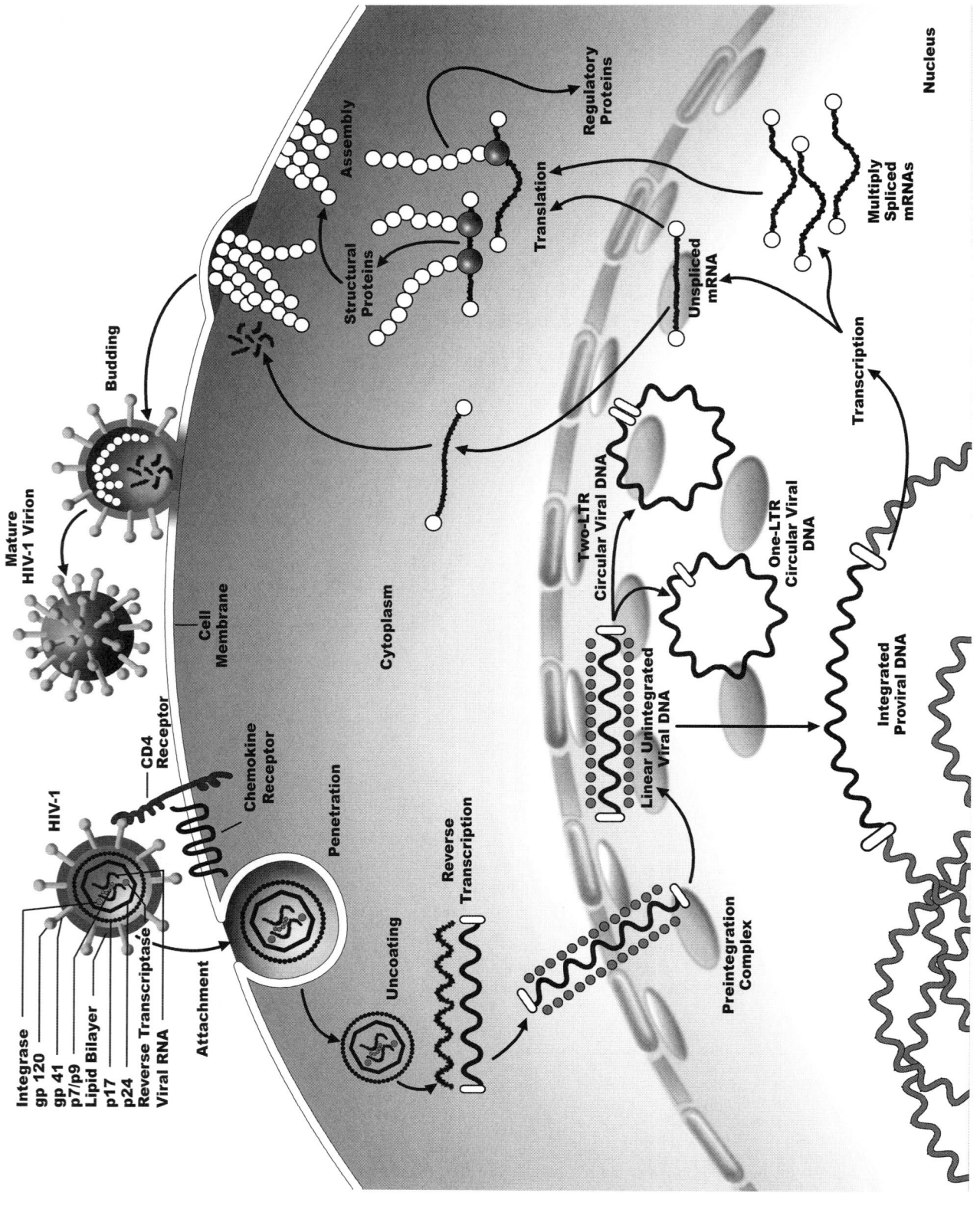

(or "subclinical") neurocognitive impairment (NCI), a less severe form of neurocognitive disorder, and a more severe neurocognitive disorder (ADC).

As the preantiretroviral therapy era continued through 1987, the occurrence of ADC was more widely seen to be common. In fact, two-thirds or more of HIV-1-infected patients were estimated to ultimately manifest ADC prior to death. After the FDA approval of 3'-azido-2',3'-dideoxythymidine (azidothymidine), now referred to as zidovudine (ZDV), in 1987, there was a high level of optimism, not only that systemic HIV-1 disease progression would be significantly deterred, but also that central nervous system (CNS) disease progression would be similarly affected. Suggestions were being made in the literature that ADC had, in fact, been eliminated by the introduction of ZDV (Fig. 1). Two theories were considered: either peripheral viral replication was also controlling replication in the CNS or the penetration of ZDV into the CNS (with a cerebrospinal fluid [CSF]/serum ratio of 0.6) was allowing control of viral replication specific to the CNS compartment. The issue of which of the two processes was occurring, and to what extent, is a controversy that continues to the present day. However, a consensus was established that there was a recrudescence of CNS HIV-1 infection toward the end of the ZDV monotherapy era in late 1991, when didanosine (2',3'-dideoxyinosine [ddI]) was approved by the FDA. By that time, the optimistic hopes for generalized treatment were greatly diminished.

It was recognized at that time that resistance to ZDV could occur as early as 6 months after treatment initiation. In fact, viral isolates from patients who had received ZDV for 6 months or more showed decreased sensitivity, with isolates from 33% of patients showing 100-fold increases in the 50% inhibitory dose (Larder et al., 1989). ZDV resistance was much more common by 2 years postinitiation. Moreover, while the reduction in the viral burden due to ZDV was clinically significant, it remained suboptimal. Hence, it was clear that other antiretroviral agents (ARVs) would need to be developed. It was further noted that patients with HIV-1-associated neurocognitive disorders would initially improve but later progress despite the continued use of ZDV. Similarly, after an initial decrease in the incidence of ADC, its recrudescence was soon noted during the ZDV monotherapy era.

In 1991, the American Academy of Neurology (AAN) introduced a new nomenclature for the neurocognitive disorders associated with HIV-1 infection, as well as specific diagnostic criteria (AAN, 1991). Two specific HIV-1-associated neurocognitive (then referred to as "cognitive-motor") disorders were defined—HIV-1-associated minor cognitive-motor

disorder (MCMD) and HIV-1-associated dementia (HAD) complex, more commonly referred to as HIV-1-associated dementia. The use of the term MCMD represented an addition to the nomenclature, as only the dementia had previously been formally defined. Additionally, the HAD designation was also new, having replaced ADC. The diagnoses of these disorders could be entertained only once the exclusion of other disorders was fully considered. To diagnose MCMD by AAN criteria, at least two of the following six symptoms needed to be present for at least 1 month: impaired attention or concentration, mental slowing, impaired memory, slowed movements, incoordination, or personality change/irritability/emotional lability. In addition to the neurological examination and the neuropsychiatric mental-status examination conducted routinely as part of the medical history and physical examination, it was advocated (but not required) that standardized neuropsychological (NP) testing be employed whenever possible to make the diagnosis of MCMD. No specific recommendations as to defining NP deficits themselves were included in these criteria. A number of research groups agreed on a criterion of two tests at least 1.5 standard deviations (SD) below the relevant normative mean to define significant NP domain-specific impairment (if data on multiple NP tests across neurocognitive domains were available). It should be noted that criteria for MCMD still incorporated the concept of a "complex." That is, only three of the six symptoms of MCMD were explicitly neurocognitive: impaired attention or concentration, memory deficits, and mental slowing. Motor slowing and incoordination referred to the motor sphere, and the single but complex symptom of "personality change/irritability/emotional lability" referred to the neurobehavioral sphere. For the diagnosis of MCMD, minor functional-status impairment must also have been documented in social and occupational activities of daily living. However, this dysfunction could not have been great enough to reach a moderate level, lest the case revert to the more severe diagnosis of HAD. In addition, etiologies other than HIV-1 were to be excluded. Consequently, the diagnosis of MCMD could be made with deficits in motor performance alone or based on one motor symptom and one neurobehavioral symptom without any neurocognitive symptoms. These criteria rendered the diagnosis of MCMD based upon medical symptoms (rather than formal NP testing) and without a specific demand for a core neurocognitive deficit. As a result, this definition would later cause concern about the comparability of the diagnostic criteria for MCMD and HAD.

The diagnosis of HAD was also explicitly defined by AAN criteria: (i) acquired abnormality in at least two of the

---

FIGURE 1 Steps at which ARVs interfere with the replication cycle of HIV-1. Regarding the structure of HIV-1, the glycoprotein coat is comprised of two portions, the outer envelope, gp120, and the transmembrane portion, gp41. The matrix protein, p17, bridges the glycoprotein coat, with the cone-shaped structure forming the viral capsid protein, p24. The viral genomic RNA, the processed nucleocapsid (p7/p9), Pol proteins, the reverse transcriptase enzyme, and the integrase enzyme are located within the capsid core. The life cycle of HIV-1 is depicted from left to right. The first FDA-approved ARVs were the nRTIs, which interfere with the step of reverse transcription, in which the RNA of HIV-1 is reverse transcribed into a complementary DNA copy. Soon afterward, members of two new ARV classes were FDA approved, the NNRTIs and the PIs. The NNRTIs act at the same point as the nRTIs but at a different site of the reverse transcriptase enzyme. The PIs, however, were the first ARVs approved to work at a different step in the viral replicatory cycle, which is a late step in which posttranslational modification of viral preproteins into active proteins occurs prior to virus assembly. Subsequently, the first of the fusion/entry inhibitors (including the CCR5 antagonists) was FDA approved. These drugs act by inhibiting the process of fusion between the viral envelope and the host cell membrane or in the immediately subsequent process of virus entry into the cell. Most recently, another class of ARVs was FDA approved, the integrase inhibitors, which interfere with the process of integration of complementary viral DNA into the host cell DNA in the nucleus. Also shown are several steps of the replicatory cycle that have yet to be targeted by FDA-approved ARVs.

six NP domains of attention/concentration, information-processing speed, abstraction/reasoning, visuospatial skills, memory/learning, and speech/language and (ii) moderate to severe dysfunction in daily activities specific to these NP deficits. In addition, the AAN criteria indicated that there must be either (i) an acquired abnormality in motor function or performance or (ii) a decline in motivation or emotional control or a change in social behavior. The latter was characterized by any of the following: a change in personality with apathy, inertia, irritability, emotional lability, or a new onset of impaired judgment characterized by socially inappropriate behavior or disinhibition. There must also be an absence of clouding of consciousness and the exclusion of other etiologies. As with the AAN definition of MCMD, motor impairment might or might not be present, although evidence of either motor or behavioral impairment was required for the diagnosis. The acquired abnormality in motor function was to be verified by neurological clinical evaluation, justifying the diagnosis of the motor subtype of HAD. However, a standardized assessment of impairment on an NP test from the motor domain (such as the grooved pegboard or the finger-tapping test) would have been preferable for this purpose. The acquired neurobehavioral abnormality in motivation, emotional control, or social behavior was to be verified by neuropsychiatric clinical evaluation, justifying the diagnosis of the behavioral subtype of HAD. Standardized neuropsychiatric testing with distress scales would also have been preferable to neuropsychiatric mental-status examination to define "apathy" (e.g., by the Profile of Mood States [POMS] Vigor-Activity Subscale) (McNair et al., 1971), "inertia" (e.g., by the POMS Fatigue-Inertia Subscale), and/or "irritability" (e.g., by the POMS Anger-Hostility Subscale). If both motor and behavioral abnormalities were present, then the diagnosis of a "mixed" HAD subtype could be made. It never became clear whether these "subtypes" differed in regard to pathogenesis or treatment response; thus, the concept of the "complex" began to erode. Moreover, a basis in NP testing had been adopted in the AAN criteria for HAD, but not for MCMD, laying the groundwork for a non-pathophysiologically based disjunction in the incidences of these two HIV-1-associated neurocognitive disorders.

As mentioned above, in 1991 a second ARV was approved by the FDA, another nucleoside reverse transcriptase inhibitor (nRTI)—ddI. This was soon followed by the introduction of 2',3'-dideoxycytidine (zalcitabine [ddC]) in 1992 and by 2',3'-didehydro-2',3'- dideoxythymidine (stavudine [d4T]) in 1994, ushering in the era of dual-nRTI combination therapy. All combinations of the nRTIs were used, except that of ZDV and d4T, as they had been shown to be antagonistic both in vitro and in vivo. Although these agents inhibited the same mechanism as ZDV, an additional impact in the reduction of viral replication and in clinical disease progression was nonetheless noted during this dual-nRTI era. However, the clinical significance of this gain was not always readily demonstrated, and the search for new ARVs targeting different mechanisms continued. Despite initial enthusiasm for the dual-nRTI therapies, which later included lamivudine, abacavir, emtricitabine, and tenofovir disoproxil fumarate (DF), significant clinical progress waned during this era.

THE HAART AND POST-HAART EXPERIENCE

In December 1995, the HAART era began when the protease inhibitors (PIs) were introduced into practice with the FDA approval of saquinavir. The PIs showed a tremendous advantage over the prior dual-nRTI combination regimens, as evidenced by decreases in the plasma viral load to non-detectable levels. The combination of two nRTIs and one PI was shown to have these effects. Once ritonavir and indinavir were introduced in March 1996, a wider selection of PIs became available. To date there are 10 different PI compounds, with 8 still in regular use, from which to choose. During this period, a new class of RTIs was introduced, the nonnucleoside RTIs (NNRTIs). The introduction of nevirapine and efavirenz (EFV) in 1997 and 1998, respectively, in this class expanded the definition of what could be considered highly effective regimens in combination with two nRTIs. HAART was clearly associated with a marked decrease in progression to AIDS, as well as with reduced mortality. In one retrospective cohort study of 383 consecutive advanced HIV-1-infected patients starting their first PI-containing HAART regimen, 68.1% achieved immune reconstitution. This group of patients also had lower mortality, fewer AIDS-defining events, shorter stays in the hospital, and fewer major infections during the mean follow-up of 808 days (Arici et al., 2001). Moreover, those patients who did not achieve immune reconstitution also experienced salutary changes in all of the foregoing events. These established benefits of HAART are time dependent and may require more than 2 years to occur.

With the introduction of HAART, gains were documented in HIV-1-associated neurocognitive disorders, as well as in systemic disease progression. The incidences of both HAD and MCMD were shown to have decreased. The mean incidence rate of HAD decreased from 21.1 to 10.5/1,000 person-years, a reduction by about half, with HAART (Sacktor et al., 2001). Prior to HAART, MCMD was documented to occur in approximately 15% of early symptomatic individuals and in a range of 20 to 50% of individuals with AIDS (Dana Consortium, 1996). Similarly to HAD, MCMD has decreased post-HAART. Sacktor et al. (2002) reported a post-HAART decrease in MCMD from 44.7% to 33.9%. Although the reduction was less than that of HAD, it was still significant. Despite a higher prevalence, MCMD has been less well studied than HAD. However, given today's treatment focus on maximization of functional status at work and in activities of daily living, MCMD merits increased attention.

Early studies suggested that, similarly to HAD and MCMD, the incidence of HIV-1-associated NCI was reduced post-HAART (Ferrando et al., 1998; Sacktor et al., 1999). However, studies conducted later in the HAART era showed a different trend in which the incidence of NCI was similar to that in the pre-HAART era. Tozzi et al. (2001) reported on a small sample of patients with HIV-1-associated NCI who experienced a positive, sustained neurocognitive improvement on HAART; however, they also reported the presence of NCI and the persistence of significant differences in NP performance between the impaired and nonimpaired groups after more than 3 years of HAART, suggesting that ongoing brain tissue damage was nevertheless occurring. In a similar mode, Sacktor et al. (2002) compared baseline data from 272 HIV-1-seropositive subjects in the Dana Consortium cohort (January 1994 to December 1995) with data from 251 HIV-1-seropositive subjects in the Northeastern AIDS Dementia Consortium cohort (April 1998 to August 1999). These investigators reported no pre-HAART to post-HAART differences in NCI at either 1 SD or 2 SD below the established NP test norms (after adjustment for differences in age, education, gender, race, and CD4 cell count). More recently, Giancola et al. (2006) found

HIV-1-associated NCI in a total of 50.3% of 165 HIV-1-infected patients receiving a stable HAART regimen for at least 6 months. Greater age (odds ratio [OR] = 4.8 for a 10-year age increase) and higher plasma HIV-1 load (OR = 1.90) at the time of testing were independently associated with lower NP performance, and a higher educational level was a protective NP factor (OR = 0.76). Moreover, greater age was correlated negatively with the summary NP performance z score, as shown in other work (see chapter 33, this volume). Thus, it might be concluded, regarding the change of HIV-associated NCI post-HAART, that while initial data were optimistic, data obtained later in the HAART era indicate that HIV-1-associated NCI remains a clinically significant problem and ultimately may not have significantly decreased in incidence post-HAART.

There are several reasons that the data on HIV-1-associated NCI pre-HAART to post-HAART are more variable and difficult to interpret than the data on HAD and MCMD. First, the definitions of the outcome in NCI (or NP performance) vary across studies, with a wide variety in the number of NP tests employed, as well as the sampling of the various NP domains by those tests. Second, the definition of whether criteria are also simultaneously met for MCMD or HAD is frequently not provided in studies in which NCI is being investigated as the primary outcome measure. Thus, one cannot ascertain whether the study refers to asymptomatic (or "subclinical") NCI, a category that would exclude MCMD and HAD, or whether NCI is being studied without reference to the definition of a concomitant neurocognitive disorder. This differentiation will be very helpful to make routinely in future research studies. With reference to this need, a new condition, asymptomatic NCI, was defined by the Frascati Conference to revise the 1991 AAN criteria for the HIV-1-associated neurocognitive disorders (Antinori et al., 2007) (see section V, this volume). Third, different studies use varying methods for establishing impairment with regard to external testing norms versus internal norms defined by a control group. Finally, statistical analyses of effects on NCI use a variety of control variables to define whether an association was present. In order for this research area to progress, a greater uniformity of methods would be propitious.

CHANGES IN HIV-1-ASSOCIATED NEUROCOGNITIVE DISORDER MANIFESTATIONS POST-HAART

A number of changes have occurred across the spectrum of HIV-1-associated neurocognitive disorders since the introduction of HAART (Table 1). The incidence of HAD is widely reported to have decreased following the introduction of HAART; however, the incidence of HIV-1 encephalopathy (as defined neuropathologically) appears to have increased, although interestingly, both the neuropathological and the clinical aspects of the syndrome seem to be less severe than those observed in the pre-HAART era (Gray et al., 2001; Neuenburg et al., 2002). In contrast to the rapidly progressive dementing syndrome commonly seen in the pre-HAART era, the evolution of HAD over time appears to be much more variable in the HAART era. Specifically, chronic forms of HAD (active and inactive), as well as fluctuating forms of HAD, are more common (Brew, 2004). Several studies have confirmed these changes in the manifestations of HIV-1-associated NCI and disorder. For example, a study of a longitudinal cohort including 534 HIV-1-seropositive individuals showed that 47% remained cognitively normal and 11% remained impaired longitudinally. Of note, stable improvement was seen in 18%. Regarding a fluctuating time course, 19% fluctuated between being impaired and being normal across examinations; only 4% were reported to have stably declined.

Whereas HAD was typically related to a low CD4 cell count and a high viral burden (in plasma or CSF) prior to HAART, these relationships seem to be mostly confined to the chronic, active form of HAD post-HAART. While the CD4 cell count remains relevant, it is now the history of the lowest CD4 cell count (i.e., the nadir) that is more predictive of prevalent HAD than the most recent CD4 cell count. Note that the CD4 nadir was associated with an increase in prevalent HIV-1-associated NCI in an analysis of 1,160 participants from the AIDS Clinical Trials Group Longitudinal Linked Randomized Trials study, while there were no significant immunological or virological predictors of incident HIV-1-associated NCI defined in that study (Robertson et al., 2007). With the loss of the current CD4 cell count and viral load as reliable disease predictors, there is a lack of relevant clinical laboratory indicators with which to predict and track the progress of HAD in the post-HAART era, and the search for valid biomarkers continues. While the presentation of HAD may be more commonly identified now at a mild stage with regard to functional status, this is only the case when there is a sufficient index of suspicion for the diagnosis.

The evolution of HAD toward a milder, more variable syndrome has also been associated with a longer survival time (Dore et al., 2003). Consequently, it has been suggested that the prevalence of HAD is increasing despite the fact that the incidence has substantially decreased. In turn, a longer survival time may be related to changes occurring in HAD pathogenesis in the context of HAART, as well as being a documented benefit of therapy. Further, the apparent effect of longstanding infection and associated brain tissue inflammation may parallel the association between older age and HAD (Chiesi et al., 1996; McArthur et al., 1993; Valcour et al., 2004), as well as MCMD (Goodkin et al.,

TABLE 1 The changing manifestations of HAD pre- and post-HAART

Index	Pre-HAART	Post-HAART
Last CD4 cell count	Low (<100 cells/mm³)	High (>200 cells/mm³)
Last plasma viral load	High	Low (or undetectable)
Functional status	Moderate to severe decline	Mild decline
Course of progression	Rapid	Variable
Survival time	Short (6 mo)	Longer (≥2 yr)

2001). As age is also associated with so-called mild cognitive impairment in the general population, the aging process may overlap with the length of HIV-1 infection, thus contributing to the variance of HIV-1-associated neurocognitive disorder. Given the high degree of similarity in patterns of neurocognitive deficits associated with aging and those associated with HIV-1 infection, there is growing concern about a synergism between the two conditions. Nevertheless, it should be noted that the pattern of neurobehavioral deficits associated with HIV-1 infection includes several aspects (e.g., Parkinsonian motor deficits) that appear to be more specific to HIV-1 infection.

The concept of a milder, more variable neurocognitive syndrome with longer survival time has garnered significant support in the literature. Confirming the increase in the incidence of HIV-1 encephalopathy post-HAART, Neuenburg et al. (2002) conducted a postmortem neuropathology study of 436 consecutive HIV-1-seropositive patients who died between 1985 and 1999. This study was conducted in Frankfurt, Germany, where accessibility to HAART was good throughout the period (see chapter 14, this volume). As expected, the total number of autopsies of HIV-1-infected patients declined with the introduction of HAART. Of special note, while the prevalence of CNS opportunistic infections (e.g., CMV encephalitis, toxoplasmosis, and cryptococcosis) decreased over time, the incidence of HIV-1 encephalopathy actually increased. Multivariate statistical analysis showed that antiretroviral therapy itself was the best predictor of HIV-1 encephalopathy (followed by the latest CD4 cell count, the nadir CD4 count, and a proxy estimator of disease duration). This suggests that it may be the toxicity of HAART that is responsible for the increased incidence of HIV-1 encephalopathy.

Since the introduction of HAART, the occurrence of a lipodystrophy syndrome has been closely associated with treatment with the ARVs, both the PIs and the nRTIs, but particularly the PIs. The lipodystrophy syndrome manifests with the metabolic syndrome superimposed by dysmorphic body features. The metabolic abnormalities include elevated total cholesterol, triglyceride, glucose, C peptide, and insulin levels and decreased HDL cholesterol levels (Carr et al., 1999), as well as increased C-reactive protein and homocysteine levels (Vigouroux et al., 1999). The lipodystrophy syndrome may present with three subtypes of dysmorphic body features: lipoatrophy syndrome (fat wasting), lipohypertrophy syndrome (fat accumulation), and a mixed syndrome (with signs of both). The prevalence of the syndrome among HIV-1-infected individuals varies widely, due in part to differences in how it is defined. For our purposes, we shall use the general term "lipodystrophy syndrome." Progression of HIV-1 infection itself has also been associated with the lipodystrophy syndrome. Of note, the HIV Outpatient Study showed that, of 337 patients with no lipoatrophy at baseline, 13.1% developed moderate or severe lipoatrophy 21 months later without an impact of ARV use (Lichtenstein et al., 2003). One etiological hypothesis is that the lipodystrophy syndrome results from selective damage by the ARVs to autonomic nervous system pathways in the CNS innervating subcutaneous and/or visceral fat depots (Fliers et al., 2003). In addition, an independent factor associated with lipoatrophy is tumor necrosis factor (TNF) gene polymorphisms. The PIs show an effect on dyslipidemia by drug and by dose. For example, ritonavir at 500 mg orally (p.o.) twice a day has been associated with a 25% increase in cholesterol and a 200-fold increase in triglycerides (Moyle, 2005). In contrast, the PI atazanavir appears to be associated with very little, if any, dyslipidemia. As for the nRTIs,

both d4T and, to a lesser extent, ZDV have been associated with increases in total cholesterol and triglyceride levels; in contrast, tenofovir DF appears to have little effect on total cholesterol levels. The occurrence of the lipodystrophy syndrome is linked to cerebrovascular risk and NCI. Therefore, these body dysmorphic changes (and the associated laboratory abnormalities) may be considered a part of the changed manifestations associated with the HIV-1-related neurocognitive disorders in the HAART era. However, it should be noted that most of the data currently available, and reviewed above, on the changed manifestations of HIV-1-associated neurocognitive disorders refer to HAD. Future studies should include a greater emphasis on changes in the manifestations of MCMD and subclinical NCI.

HIV-1-ASSOCIATED NEUROCOGNITIVE DISORDER PATHOPHYSIOLOGY

In addition to the above-mentioned changes in clinical manifestations of HIV-1-associated neurocognitive disorders, their underlying pathophysiology has also evolved. Aside from the original focus on virologic (pathogen), inflammatory/immunologic (host response), and comorbid infection factors, there are now three additional categories of pathogenic factors that demand attention. These are the vascular, medication toxicity, and genetic factors (Fig. 2).

Virologic Factors

In considering HIV-1-associated neurocognitive-disorder pathogenesis, it is of historical interest to note that the host response, including both inflammatory and immunologic factors, had originally dominated the research scene, although recently, considerably more attention has been devoted to aspects of the pathogen itself, as well. A thorough discussion of the virological contribution to neuropathogenesis by HIV-1 is beyond the scope of this chapter; however, several relevant aspects related to the neurocognitive disorders should be noted. In the current worldwide pandemic of HIV-1, one must consider the fact that approximately two-thirds of cases derive from sub-Saharan Africa. There are three strains of HIV-1—the "major" group, M; the "outlier" group, O; and the "new" group, N. While group O appears to be restricted to Central and West Africa and group N (discovered in Cameroon) is extremely rare, group M encompasses >90% of HIV-1 infections worldwide. Within group M, there are known to be at least nine genetically distinct subtypes (or clades) of HIV-1 (A, B, C, D, F, G, H, J, and K) with great variability worldwide. Regarding neuro-AIDS in general and neurocognitive disorders in particular, we know little about the relevance of HIV-1 clades to neuropathogenesis. Most research has been conducted on clade B, which has greatest prevalence in the Americas, Western Europe, Japan, and Australia, yet clade C, predominant in southern and East Africa, India, and Nepal, has caused about 50% of infections worldwide. While clade C infections have a rate lower than or similar to that of clade B (Ball et al., 2003; Alaeus et al., 1999), the data on the associated neurocognitive relevance of this clade has been conflicting. One report has suggested a lower incidence of HAD with clade C infection in India (Ranga et al., 2004), while another report suggested a higher incidence (Yepthomi et al., 2006). Clade D is generally limited to East and Central Africa and appears to be more closely associated with rapid disease progression (Baeten et al. 2007), although little is known about neurovirulence. In addition, hybrid viruses may result when two or more different clades infect one person and become

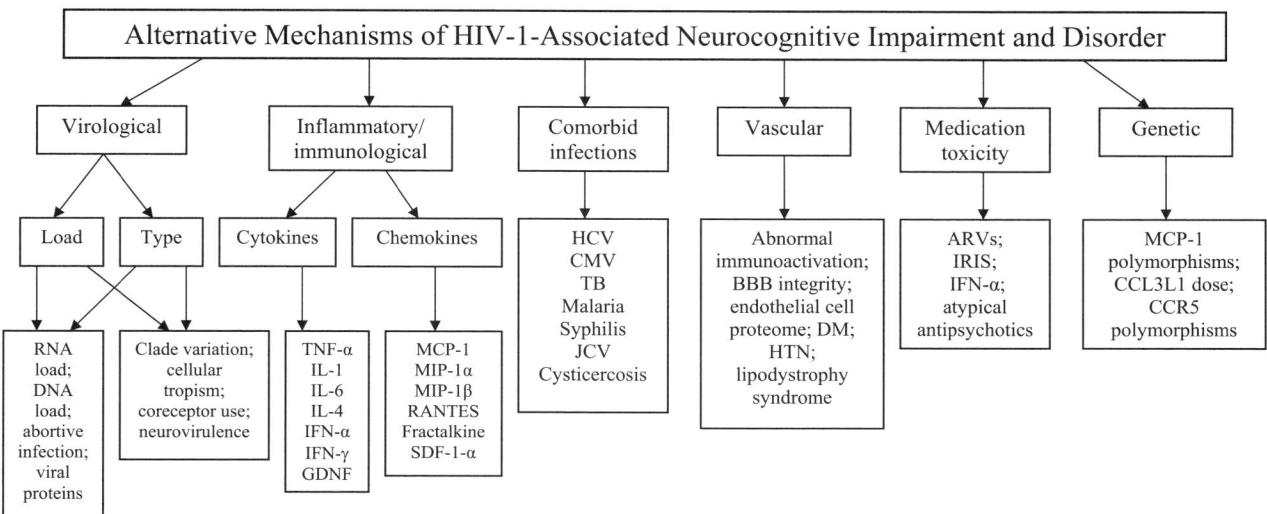

FIGURE 2 Contributory factors to HIV-1-associated neurocognitive-disorder pathogenesis. Studies of HIV-1-associated neurocognitive-disorder pathogenesis have become more complex in the HAART era. Viral and inflammatory/immunologic factors had been the major concerns pre-HAART. In a subset of cases, comorbid infection was also a concern as a contributory factor pre-HAART. A number of additional factors have been identified to be important post-HAART. In particular, a vascular factor is now a routine consideration for pathogenesis. Moreover, newly identified medication toxicity factors (including those due to the ARVs themselves) and host genetic factors have also come to the fore.

"circulating recombinant forms" (CRFs). The HIV-1 CRFs, like the clades, are highly variable in distribution worldwide. The most common CRFs involve clades A and C. It is highly likely that new HIV-1 clades and CRFs will evolve over time. Hence, longitudinal research will be needed to examine the neurocognitive relevance of the current clades (and widespread CRFs), as well as those that newly evolve.

Another important virologic factor regarding HIV-1 infection is cellular tropism. With the discovery of the chemokine coreceptors, a large amount of research has been dedicated to the area of viral tropism. It is now well established that chemokine (C-C motif) receptor 5 (CCR5) is the coreceptor most commonly expressed by monocytes and macrophage, whereas chemokine "CXC" receptor 4 (CXCR4, or fusin) is expressed by CD4+ T lymphocytes. (Note that the two N-terminal cysteines of CXC chemokines are separated by 1 amino acid, represented by the "X.") The fact that CCR5-using viruses are almost exclusively the type of virus transmitted from human to human and, thus, particularly common in the early stages of infection supports the earlier reports of viral penetration of an intact blood-brain barrier (BBB) by HIV-1-infected monocytes (Zhu et al., 1993). This suggests that a specific focus on this subgroup of viruses for NCI and disorder is warranted. Nevertheless, the presence of CXCR4 has been noted in later stages of brain infection and may be responsible, in part, for the progression of early encephalitis to a clinically demonstrable disorder (van der Meer et al., 2000).

In line with the increased information on cellular tropism, the data on the contribution of the viral load to HIV-1-associated neurocognitive disorder have evolved. Pre-HAART, the mean CSF HIV-1 load (adjusting for the CD4 cell count) was significantly higher in patients with dementia, was correlated with the severity of dementia, and was significantly correlated with the plasma load for patients with CD4 cell counts of <200/mm³ (McArthur et al., 1997). In the HAART era, CSF and plasma HIV-1 dynamics became increasingly independent of one another in advanced HIV-1 disease. HIV-1 has been shown to evolve differently in plasma, CSF, and brain tissue. Additionally, variation in gp120 by brain region has been demonstrated (Shapshak et al., 1999), a phenomenon that may be related functionally to neurovirulence and could explain an increased frequency of neurocognitive disorder despite the lower plasma viral loads achieved in the HAART era. The compartmental discrepancy has been widest in HAD (Ellis et al., 2000). One issue related to the utility of quantified RNA in the CNS is that it is a measure that reflects recent genomic viral replication. Of note, it has now been shown that the proviral (DNA) HIV-1 load in the peripheral blood is associated with HAD in the HAART era. Although peripheral in origin, this measure may better reflect the "library" of latent HIV-1 over the course of infection. This may, in turn, be significantly correlated with latent HIV-1 infection of brain tissue, a reservoir that may remain relatively unperturbed in the face of long-term HAART. Thus, this measure may prove to be useful in generating predictors of HAD in the context of HAART and is still being studied. Another aspect of the viral load that is poorly studied is reflected in the potential import of astrocyte infection of brain tissue. While astrocytes are nonproductively and transiently infected, they are present in very high numbers and may be of pathophysiological relevance. Research using a multispliced/unspliced RNA ratio in brain tissue has suggested that this mechanism deserves further study (Fujimura et al., 2004). Thus, new ways of measuring and of conceptualizing the viral burden may be of particular importance in the HAART era.

Independent of the viral load, the neurotoxicity of viral proteins is another area of growing interest in the pathophysiology of HIV-1-associated neurocognitive disorder. Neurons do not appear to be directly infected by HIV-1; however, it is well known that the part of the gp120 glycoprotein coat of HIV-1 that binds to the CD4 receptor and the chemokine coreceptors is associated with dendritic pruning and with neuronal apoptosis (Petito and Roberts, 1995). The regulatory protein Tat is likewise known to be independently associated with neurotoxicity and can be found circulating in the peripheral blood (Khan et al., 2003). Given the fact that the PIs act at a posttranscriptional point in HIV-1 replication, significant amounts of defective, nonreplicating viral remains (or "viral ghosts") containing neurotoxic viral proteins may be left behind. The accumulation of these proteins over years of HAART could also explain a potential divergence from traditional measures of the viral burden (i.e., quantified genomic HIV-1 RNA) and the observed incidence of HIV-1-associated neurocognitive outcomes.

Inflammatory/Immunologic Factors

Over the course of the pandemic, the inflammatory response to the virus in the brain has been held to be of great importance for pathophysiological investigation of neurocognitive disorders. Several studies have shown that the extent of the antiviral inflammatory response in the brain may be more important than any direct measure of the viral burden in predicting and monitoring the progression of HIV-1-associated neurocognitive disorder. Certainly, the proinflammatory cytokines TNF-α, interleukin 1 (IL-1), and IL-6 have long been known to be secreted by HIV-1-infected macrophages in the brain and have been implicated in the eventual development of HIV-1-associated neurocognitive disorder (Table 2). TNF-α has been shown to up-regulate HIV-1 replication, as well as to cause demyelination, thereby causing two deleterious outcomes (Wilt et al., 1995). IL-1, like TNF-α as cited previously, is known to up-regulate HIV-1 replication through activation of the nuclear factor κB (NF-κB) motif binding to the HIV-1 long terminal repeat (Osborn et al., 1989). IL-6 is well known to be associated with polyclonal-B-cell stimulation and with related diseases, such as multiple myeloma; elevated levels of IL-6 and its mRNA have been found in HIV-1-infected individuals (Breen et al. 1990). IL-6 in the CSF may contribute to production of autoimmune, brain-reactive antibodies. Another cytokine, gamma interferon (IFN-γ), a Th1 cytokine, has been shown to stimulate the cellular immune response against HIV-1-infected cells. Of note, in the CNS, macrophages stimulated with IFN-γ in vitro produce large amounts of quinolinic acid, an excitatory neurotoxin, convulsant, and N-methyl-D-aspartate (NMDA) receptor agonist (Heyes et al., 1992). As many as 25% of HAD patients have been reported as having seizures. Increased quinolinic acid concentration in the CSF is associated with the severity of NP impairment and with markers of immune activation. Further, quinolinic acid is increased in brain tissue, as well, particularly in the basal ganglia, which are known to be affected early in HIV-1 infection of the brain (Achim et al., 1993). In addition, IFN-γ appears to regulate the development of demyelination in CNS viral infections and may be associated with toxic effects on both mature oligodendrocytes and oligodendrocyte precursor cells (Popko et al., 1997; Mana et al., 2006). Another type of interferon, IFN-α, appears to exhibit an endogenous neurocognitive toxicity associated

with increased expression in HIV-1 infection of the brain (Sas et al., 2007). Further, it is also commonly used as a therapeutic agent to treat hepatitis C virus (HCV) coinfection in the HIV-1 infected and may cause specific CNS tissue damage related to HAD. Deficits documented with the therapeutic use of IFN-α include decreased information-processing speed, verbal memory, and executive function (Pavol et al., 1995), as well as Parkinsonian motor symptoms (Gomph, 2005).

Interestingly, other cytokines may offset the destructive effects of TNF-α, IFN-γ, and IFN-α on HIV-1-associated neurocognitive disorder. The Th2 cytokine IL-4, known to be deleterious and associated with abnormal humoral immune stimulation in the periphery, appears to be of benefit in the CNS. IL-4 is known to suppress macrophage activation, and a reduction in IL-4 mRNA has been found in the brains of patients with HAD (Wesselingh et al., 1993). Thus, IL-4 secretion in the brain decreases the likelihood of HAD, a disease mediated by macrophage activation rather than by CD4 cell depletion. Another salutary cytokine in the CNS is glial-derived neurotrophic factor (GDNF), with a protective effect specific to dopaminergic neurons that may be damaged due to IFN-α secretion, for example. As GDNF confers protection against 1-methyl 4-phenyl-1,2,3,6-tetrahydropyridine-induced substantia nigra toxicity (Tomac et al., 1995), the possibility that there exists a dynamic equilibrium between GDNF and IFN-α at the level of the substantia nigra should be considered.

More recently, several chemokines have been implicated in HIV-1-associated neurocognitive disorders, with the most evidence favoring monocyte chemotactic protein 1 (MCP-1), although macrophage inflammatory protein 1 alpha (MIP-1α), MIP-1β, and "regulated upon activation, normal T-cell expressed, and presumably secreted" (RANTES) also appear to be involved. The CSF MCP-1 level has been found to predict the occurrence of HAD (Sevigny et al., 2004), to parallel its severity, and to correlate with the CSF viral load (Kelder et al., 1998). RANTES has also been found to be increased in the CSF of HAD patients, although MIP-1α and MIP-1β were not. In fact, some data suggest that MIP-1α is associated with lower CSF levels consistent with decreased macrophage activation (LeTendre et al., 1999) and that MIP-1β inhibits gp120-induced neuronal apoptosis (Kaul and Lipton, 1999). Hence, both may have neuroprotective effects. Fractalkine, the CX3C chemokine, appears to be produced during interactions between astrocytes and HIV-1-infected macrophages and may also play a role in HAD pathogenesis by regulating the trafficking of monocytes into brain tissue (Pereira et al., 2001). Another chemokine possibly participating in HAD neuropathogenesis is stromal-cell-derived factor 1 alpha (SDF-1α), the endogenous ligand for the CXCR4 receptor. SDF-1α is cleaved by matrix metalloproteinase 2 (MMP-2) to yield a highly neurotoxic molecule, SDF(5-67), which does not bind to its cognate receptor and has been detected in brain monocytoid cells of patients with HAD (Vergote et al., 2006). SDF(5-67) activates the expression of proinflammatory cytokine genes and causes neuronal-membrane changes, neurotoxicity, and apoptotic cell death. It is anticipated that the area of research involving chemokine activity and inflammatory control mechanisms of HIV-1 in the brain will continue to evolve, and as a result, it is likely to remain a major focus in HIV-1 brain tissue research.

The light subunit of neurofilament protein (NFL) appears to be a sensitive indicator of CNS axonal injury and, therefore, may be of relevance in the inflammatory response to

TABLE 2 Role of cytokines in the pathogenesis of HIV-1-associated neurocognitive impairment and disorder

Cytokine or factor	Role
Proinflammatory cytokines	Cytokines produced predominantly by activated immune cells (such as microglia) and involved in the amplification of inflammatory reactions.
TNF-α	TNF-α is one of the cytokines most frequently cited as having a destructive effect; related to demyelination seen in HAD; known to cause sphingomyelin hydrolysis and ceramide generation (the latter is an intracellular mediator of apoptosis); also enhances HIV-1 replication.
IL-1	IL-1 stimulates HIV-1 replication; "glial stimulating factor" overlaps activity of IL-1; "glial maturation factor" induces IL-1 production and may be an endogenous signal for reactive astrocytosis; IL-1 is cytotoxic for some cells and is known to stimulate synthesis of β-amyloid precursor proteins (β-APP)
IL-6	IL-6 is known to be involved in the normal inflammatory response to tissue damage and may be elevated as an epiphenomenon in HIV-1-associated neurocognitive impairment and disorder in this respect (see IL-6 under "Th2 cytokines" below).
Th1 cytokines	CD4⁺ T lymphocytes can be divided into two distinct subsets of effector cells based on their functional capabilities and cytokine secretion profile—Th1 and Th2. The Th1 subset secretes cytokines associated with the induction of cell-mediated immune responses.
IFN-γ	IFN-γ enhances expression of surface major histocompatibility complex class II HLA-DR antigens on astrocytes; augments TNF-α and IL-1 production; stimulates macrophage neopterin secretion; causes sphingomyelin hydrolysis, inducing neuronal apoptosis; and increases the production of quinolinic acid, an excitotoxin and convulsant.
Th2 cytokines	The Th2 subset of CD4⁺ T lymphocytes produces cytokines that induce B cells to proliferate and differentiate (such as IL-4 and IL-5) and is associated with humoral-type immune responses.
IL-4	IL-4 is known to suppress macrophage activation; reduction in IL-4 decreases such suppression, increasing the likelihood of HAD, a disease mediated by macrophage activation.
IL-6	IL-6 may contribute to induction of an autoimmune process and brain-reactive antibody formation; however, its role in HAD pathogenesis as a proinflammatory cytokine may oppose this role (see "Proinflammatory cytokines" above).
Neurotrophic factors	Substances responsible for the growth and survival of neurons during development and for maintaining adult neurons that are also capable of inducing regrowth of damaged neurons.
GDNF	GDNF shows a protective effect against neurotoxins specific to dopaminergic neurons in the substantia nigra, which may be damaged or show neuronal-cell loss early in HIV-1 infection of brain.
Chemokines	A subfamily of small size (approximately 8- to 10-kDa) cytokines having 4 cysteine residues in conserved locations that are integral to defining their three-dimensional shapes.
MCP-1	MCP-1 is a chemoattractant for human monocytes that is produced by monocytes and lymphocytes as well as fibroblasts during tissue injury and is involved in HIV-1 Tat-mediated monocyte transmigration across the BBB.
MIP-1α	MIP-1α is a CCR5 receptor ligand that is a member of the C-C subfamily of chemokines. MIP-1α exhibits a variety of proinflammatory activities in vitro. It is a more potent lymphocyte chemoattractant than MIP-1β with a broader range of concentration-dependent chemoattractant specificities, particularly for B cells and CTLs at lower concentrations.
MIP-1β	MIP-1β is a CCR5 ligand that tends to attract CD4⁺ T lymphocytes, with some preference for T cells of the naive (CD45RA) phenotype, compared to MIP-1α.
RANTES	A CCR5 receptor ligand that is a member of the IL-8 superfamily of cytokines, RANTES is a protein that is a selective attractant for memory T lymphocytes and monocytes.
Fractalkine	The only known member of the the CX3C chemokine family; among the chemokines, fractalkine shows the unusual propery of existing as a membrane-bound and as a soluble protein. Together with its receptor, CX3CR1, it is expressed predominantly in the CNS and partially blocks the effects of TNF-α.
SDF-1α	SDF-1α is a chemokine that is the only known ligand for CXCR4 and blocks infection by HIV-1 types using this coreceptor (such as T lymphocytes).

HIV-1. One study retrospectively identified nine subjects participating in a longitudinal cohort study who developed HAD; lumbar puncture performed within 2 years of presentation showed elevated CSF NFL concentrations in seven cases (78%) (Gisslen et al., 2007). In a follow-up study of the response to HAART, NFL concentrations decreased to normal levels in the two subjects with HAD who were followed (Mellgren et al., 2007). As with NFL, levels of soluble Fas (sFas) and sFasL in CSF have been investigated for a relationship with HAD. Significant differences in sFas (median, 116 vs. 30 pg/ml) and sFasL (median, 127 vs. 15 pg/ml), respectively, were found to be associated with the presence or absence of HAD (Sabri et al., 2001). Further, sFasL differed among HIV-1-infected subjects according to the clinical signs of HAD. The CSF load was correlated significantly with levels of CSF sFasL, but not with CSF sFas. These data suggest the potential clinical utility of NFL, sFas, and sFasL as sensitive inflammatory markers in future studies of HIV-1-associated NCI and disorder.

Although research to date has focused upon inflammatory factors, other immunological mediators may play roles in the HIV-1-associated neurocognitive disorders. The CNS is protected by the unique vasculature comprising the BBB, which minimizes the passage of cells and macromolecules into brain tissue. Although it is widely accepted that T cells do survey the resting CNS (Chen et al., 2005), T-cell migration is minimal in the absence of inflammatory signals. Significant inflammatory signals are provided by HIV-1 infection of the brain; however, limited evidence has indicated that T lymphocytes in the HIV-1-infected brain may be involved with specific immunological functions, rather than being simple bystanders. Activated memory (CD45RO$^+$) T lymphocytes have been shown to be significantly increased in the hippocampus in cases of HIV-1 encephalitis, but this increase was not seen in HIV-1-infected cases without encephalitis (Petito et al., 2003). T lymphocytes were present in the perivascular spaces and in microglial nodules in the brains of patients with HIV-1 encephalitis, and some were in direct contact with neurons. Both CD4$^+$ and CD8$^+$ T lymphocytes were found, with the implication that their recruitment required local HIV-1 brain tissue infection. The perineuronal localization of some cells suggests that cytotoxic T lymphocytes (CTLs) could be involved, perhaps through CTL-mediated neuronal killing. Petito et al. (2006) identified the cytotoxic granules (granzyme B and perforin) of CTLs in autopsies of brains of patients with AIDS and HIV-1 encephalitis and confirmed the gene expression profiles of CTL-associated genes in a separate series of cases. CTLs were rare or absent in cases without HIV-1 encephalitis. CD8$^+$ T cells and CTLs could either mediate brain injury in HIV-1 encephalitis or maintain some level of immunological monitoring within the brain. Although little investigated to date, future research focusing upon the potential functions of these cells penetrating HIV-1-infected brain tissue is warranted.

Comorbid Infection Factors

HCV

HCV infection has become a major concern as a comorbidity associated with HIV-1 infection. The major routes of entry are injection drug use (primarily) and sexual transmission (infrequently). Concomitant HIV-1 infection is known to enhance the progression of HCV-associated fibrosis in the liver (Mohsen et al., 2003), eventuating in cirrhosis and death. However, concomitant HCV infection has been

shown to have a variable relationship to the progression of HIV-1 infection, being primarily constrained to the combined effects of HCV and ARVs on hepatic tissue damage and tissue metabolism. However, it is now appreciated that infection with concurrent multiple HCV genotypes accelerates HIV-1 disease progression (van Asten and Prins, 2004) and that HCV-coinfected patients benefit from HAART, including its effect on survival time (Klein et al., 2003). Once liver damage has progressed, HCV infection has been accepted as a cause of metabolic encephalopathy. However, others have shown that HCV infection may have a negative impact on the function of brain tissue independently of its metabolic effect on the liver (see chapter 21, this volume). In addition, the current treatment for HCV infection calls for the use of IFN-α and ribavirin. As previously indicated, the therapeutic use of IFN-α is well known to be associated with deleterious CNS side effects, including neurocognitive deterioration (Poutiainen et al., 1994; Pavol et al., 1995). With the use of the pegylated form, IFN-α toxicity still occurs at a significant frequency, although the effects on mood (depression and anxiety) may be greater than those on cognition (Amodio et al., 2005). Finally, as ribavirin is associated with the side effect of anemia, it can exert a deleterious cognitive impact of its own.

CMV

CMV infection was initially thought to be responsible for the etiology of the encephalopathy seen with HIV-1 disease. While this is not the case, CMV nevertheless is the most common coinfection resident in HIV-1-infected brain tissue found at autopsy (22.7% in one series) (Zelman and Mossakowski, 1998). CMV encephalopathy has decreased to a low frequency in the HAART era, as the immunosuppression associated with reactivation of CMV from the latent state is better controlled and the CMV load has been reduced. As the severity of CMV encephalopathy is related to its viral load, the potential for CMV to exacerbate the effects of HIV-1 infection in the CNS has been reduced in the HAART era. Nonetheless, CMV is known to coinfect cells infected by HIV-1, and each virus can up-regulate the replication and protein synthesis of the other (see chapter 23, this volume). Wohl et al. (2005) longitudinally evaluated a cohort of 190 CMV-seropositive subjects with AIDS who had no history or evidence of CMV disease over a median follow-up interval of 334 days. They found that plasma CMV DNA detectable by PCR was an independent predictor of death, after the plasma HIV-1 load and CD4 cell count. Thus, CMV may still show a clinically significant interaction with HIV-1 in the brain in the context of HAART. This interaction could contribute to HAD pathogenesis, perhaps with greatest frequency in those with the most advanced HIV-1 disease.

Mycobacterium tuberculosis

Tuberculosis (TB) is a much greater concern as a comorbid disease with HIV-1 infection in resource-limited than in resource-rich settings. This also applies to the specific interaction of TB with HIV-1 in the brain. Lanjewar et al. (1998) noted that CNS TB is frequently observed in India and that death due to systemic opportunistic infections may limit the frequency with which the interaction of TB with HIV-1 infection of the brain might be clinically manifested. Although concomitant TB infection requiring treatment has been shown to be associated with a higher level of replication of HIV-1 (Toossi et al., 2007), a clinical correlate of this finding has not yet been substantiated. Regardless of the above-mentioned concern for pathogenic interaction,

TB should be considered a possible (though infrequent) cause of cerebral mass lesions in HIV-1-infected patients, especially when TB is suspected at other sites.

Malaria

Malaria is not an opportunistic infection that has been defined for HIV-1 infection but is a common concern in many resource-limited settings in which HIV-1 is highly prevalent and malaria is endemic. Cerebral malaria, defined by an unarousable state of unconsciousness accompanied by the presence of asexual parasitemia, occurs not uncommonly. While research on this pathogenic interaction is in its early stages and results to date have not been entirely consistent, HIV-1-infected persons with malaria have been found to have a higher prevalence of fever, parasitemia, severe or complicated malaria, and cerebral malaria. Severe malaria has also been shown to be more frequently associated with coma among HIV-1-seropositive persons (16% versus 8%), as well (Grimwade et al., 2004). In one study of pregnant women, malaria was also associated with an increase in CD16$^+$ monocytes in HIV-1-coinfected women; these monocytes expressed higher CCR5 levels and were significantly more likely to harbor HIV-1 (Jaworowski et al., 2007). As HIV-1-infected CD16$^+$ monocytes in the periphery have been linked to HAD pathogenesis through seeding of the bone marrow, this suggests the potential for a neurocognitive synergy between these two infections. Thus, while a specific interaction with HAD pathogenesis has not been determined with systemic or cerebral malaria, a high index of suspicion should be maintained for the neurological and neuropsychiatric manifestations of this coinfection in areas of the world where malaria remains endemic.

Other Comorbid CNS Infections

A number of other comorbid CNS infections could affect HAD pathogenesis. Neurosyphilis represents one such possibility. The manifestations of neurosyphilis are more common than anticipated, more aggressive, and more difficult to treat in the setting of HIV-1 infection (see chapter 25, this volume). Although both infections may manifest with dementia, and the manifestations of neurosyphilis are accelerated by HIV-1-associated immunosuppression, no specific interaction with HAD pathogenesis has been documented. Progressive multifocal leukoencephalopathy (PML), a relatively rare CNS disease due to lytic infection of oligodendrocytes caused by John Cunningham virus (JCV), may be difficult to distinguish from HAD, as PML may also present with dementia (see chapter 26, this volume). HIV-1 and JCV have been established to interact, with results suggesting that the transactivation response element homologue of the JCV late promoter is responsive to HIV-1 Tat induction (Chowdhury et al., 1992). While acceleration of HAD pathogenesis is unlikely to be due to intracellular transactivation, the clinical course of HAD appears to be accelerated in the presence of JCV (Vazeux et al., 1990). It is also possible that HAD pathogenesis may be increased by yet other infections, including cysticercosis (Thornton et al., 1992).

Vascular Factors

In the pre-HAART era, there was little evidence that a vascular factor could have significant relevance for HAD pathogenesis. However, there were reports of abnormal immunological activation related to an increased incidence of cerebrovascular accident (CVA) (Berger et al., 1990). In addition, while initial studies using conventional techniques (the immunoglobulin G-albumin index and gadolin-ium-enhanced magnetic resonance imaging) suggested that the BBB was generally preserved in the HIV-1 infected, as shown by conventional techniques (Wilkinson et al., 1996), there was increased interest in more refined measures of BBB integrity that indicated that minor levels of disruption were actually occurring in the BBB. This was shown by studies of MMPs (particularly, MMP-2 and MMP-9) and their tissue inhibitors, as well as by studies of experimental models of the BBB (Eugenin et al., 2006). Several factors were implicated, including the activation of proinflammatory cytokines, such as TNF-α (Sibson et al., 2002); HIV-1-infected macrophage-induced up-regulation of brain microvascular endothelial-cell proteins (Ricardo-Dukelow et al., 2007); the impact of HIV-1 Tat (Toborek et al., 2005); and the impact of cocaine use (Fiala et al., 2005). Additionally, vascular risk factors for dementia that are present in the general population (e.g., type II diabetes mellitus and hypertension) have also contributed and are associated with the aging of the HIV-1-infected patient population (see chapter 33, this volume).

Most recently, interest has grown in the impact of HAART itself on vascular factors related to HAD pathogenesis. The occurrence of the lipodystrophy syndrome (colloquially referred to as "Crix belly" [for the ARV Crixivan, or indinavir]) was noted with long-term HAART. Dyslipidemia occurs in conjunction with this dysmorphic syndrome, which is characterized by central lipohypertrophy (in the abdomen, breast, and dorsocervical fat pad) and simultaneous lipoatrophy in the face, limbs, and buttocks. The metabolic abnormalities characteristic of this syndrome include persistently elevated total cholesterol, triglyceride, glucose, C peptide, and insulin levels and decreased HDL cholesterol levels (Carr et al., 1999). The mechanism(s) for the occurrence of the dyslipidemia has not been resolved; however, mitochondrial toxicity induced by the ARVs (Stankov et al., 2007), as well as decreased expression of peroxisome proliferator-activated receptor gamma (Lemoine et al., 2006) and decreased GLUT4 (the insulin-regulated glucose transporter found in adipose tissue) (Grigem et al., 2005), has been implicated. Published reports show that the PIs were associated with an increased incidence of myocardial infarction at a younger age in HIV-1-infected patients (Henry et al., 1998). Shortly thereafter, the nRTIs were likewise implicated in these coronary-artery disease effects, albeit to a lesser extent than the PIs. Not surprisingly, similar effects have been documented in the cerebrovascular tree. Increases were noted in abnormal cerebrovascular vasomotor reactivity by transcranial Doppler studies, in carotid intima-media thickness, and in the frequency of internal carotid artery plaques (Concha et al., 2003). Moreover, these effects were shown to be associated with increased clinical events (transient ischemic attack [TIA] and CVA) (Evers et al., 2003) and were found to contribute to HAD pathogenesis, as well (Valcour et al., 2005).

Medication Toxicity Factors

While the overlap of the vascular factors that contribute to HAD pathogenesis and the medication toxicity factors is clinically significant, there are other medication toxicity factors that do not act through the vasculature. One of these is due to the ARV most commonly cited as having CNS side effects: EFV. It has been suggested that EFV is associated with decreased sleep, increased anxiety and depressive disorders, vestibular symptoms, and decreased NP performance (Blanch et al., 2001; Gallego et al., 2004; Lochet et al., 2003). Although CNS toxicity has been reported to be associated with higher blood levels of EFV, the mechanism of toxicity is unknown. Further analysis of EFV has shown higher drug levels and clinical side effects in association with the CYP2B6 haplotype. This haplotype is more common among African Americans, who might benefit from active screening. In one multisite, randomized, controlled trial that prospectively investigated EFV-associated CNS side effects, the investigators reported that transient neurological and neuropsychiatric symptoms are frequent but that they are mild to moderate, time limited, and spontaneously resolving and rarely require drug discontinuation (Clifford et al., 2005). Nevertheless, the implications of a preexisting psychiatric history and the potential for long-term toxicity warrant further study.

In addition to direct toxicity of the ARVs, there is an indirect toxic effect known as immune reconstitution inflammatory syndrome (IRIS). IRIS refers to a "paradoxical" syndrome occurring in HIV-1-infected patients who have recently initiated HAART but experience clinical deterioration despite increasing CD4 cell counts and decreasing plasma viral loads. The pathogens with which IRIS is most frequently associated are *Mycobacterium avium* complex, varicella-zoster virus, and CMV. As one would expect with the latter two pathogens, IRIS is also specifically relevant to the CNS. The observed clinical deterioration is thought to be the result of a robust inflammatory response to both subclinical pathogens and residual antigens posttreatment. The resulting clinical manifestations of IRIS are very diverse and depend on the prior infectious-disease burden of the specific patient population involved. Worsening of PML has been described in this setting (Vendrely et al., 2005), and HAD itself has been associated with IRIS (Miller et al., 2004). The frequency of IRIS is currently unknown, and its mechanism, as yet, is poorly defined. Further research is needed regarding CNS IRIS as a cause of HIV-1-associated NCI and disorder in the HAART era.

As previously indicated, IFN-α, is a frequently prescribed treatment for HIV-1-infected patients with HCV coinfection. Amodio et al. (2005), mentioned above, performed an observational study of IFN-α treatment on a relatively small sample of patients in which depression and anxiety scores significantly increased, along with neurophysiological effects shown by electroencephalogram—increase of alpha power in frontal derivations, reduction of the mean dominant frequency, and increase of theta power in parietal derivations. However, no significant cognitive changes were found. A more rigorously controlled prospective study of chronic hepatitis B virus- or HCV-infected patients who were being treated with only a low dose of IFN-α showed significant decreases in immediate recall and in verbal fluency, both of which are also decreased by HIV-1 infection alone, at 12 weeks of treatment (Lieb et al., 2006). The findings suggest IFN-α-associated damage to the prefrontal cortex and hippocampus, areas known to be damaged in early HIV-1 infection of the brain. Lieb et al. (2006) suggested close monitoring of cognitive function during IFN-α treatment. This seems to be a particular concern for the HIV-1/HCV-coinfected patient population. However, before any conclusions can be drawn about the potential relevance of IFN-α treatment for HAD pathogenesis, more research needs to be conducted on dosing in IFN-α-associated neurocognitive deficits.

Atypical antipsychotic medications (e.g., olanzapine and risperidone) are prescribed in the general population for adjuvant treatment of mood disorders and chronic pain, as well as for primary psychotic symptoms. Thus, this class of medications is not infrequently prescribed to the HIV-1 infected. However, one associated toxicity is a metabolic syndrome that could complicate the HIV-1-associated lipodystrophy syndrome (Henderson et al., 2005; Singh and Goodkin, 2007a, 2007b). To our knowledge, no study has yet examined the interaction of the PIs (or the nRTIs) with the atypical antipsychotic medications to examine the possibility of a synergistic effect on the risk for and sequelae of the HIV-1-associated lipodystrophy syndrome.

Genetic Factors

Genetic factors associated with systemic HIV-1 disease progression have evolved into a significant focus in the later HAART era. On a more limited basis, studies have also extended into HIV-1-associated neurocognitive disorder pathogenesis, where genetic factors have recently been shown to play a role. It is well recognized that the CCR5Δ32 allele is associated with decreased systemic disease progression; it has also been associated with decreased cortical atrophy in HIV-1-infected patients (Barroga et al., 2000). Gonzalez et al. (2002) found that the MCP-1 genotype was associated with accelerated HIV-1 disease progression and with a 4.5-fold-increased risk of HAD. Specifically, the mutant MCP-1-2578G allele conferred greater transcriptional activity via differential DNA-protein interactions, enhancing protein production in vitro and increasing serum MCP-1 levels and macrophage infiltration into tissues. In more recent work, the combination of low versus high CCL3L1 (encoding MIP-1α) copy number and detrimental versus nondetrimental CCR5 haplotypes/genotypes has been used to denote four separate genetic risk groups for HIV-1 disease progression. Gonzalez et al. (2005) used this approach to show that the combination of a low CCL3L1 dose and detrimental CCR5 polymorphisms resulted in the most rapid worsening of immune measures in HIV-1-infected patients and, presumably, HIV-1-associated neurocognitive impairment and disorder risk. Thus, genetic screening for HIV-1-associated neurocognitive disorders may be available in the not-too-distant future.

Other Factors

Other factors may also be related to HAD pathogenesis. As medical treatment may increase the risk for HAD pathogenesis, this may also be true for self-treatment with substances of abuse. The research in this area has yielded variable results. An important issue in the clinical research has been how to focus upon a specific psychoneurotoxic substance when so many other substances have been used over a patient's history. Nevertheless, evidence has associated cocaine use with the development of NCI in the HIV-1 infected (Bagetta et al., 2004), and methamphetamine has been cited as a growing concern (Theodore et al., 2006). In addition, alcohol has received some attention as a possible cofactor in HAD pathogenesis and progression, as well (Tyor and Middaugh, 1999). Studies of cocaine, methamphetamine, and alcohol each target an interaction with HIV-1 Tat (see chapter 29, this volume). Hence, studies directed at the neurocognitive implications of clinical comorbidities of HIV-1 infection with these (as well as other) substances remain to be further pursued in the HAART era. Nutritional deficits of antioxidants (e.g., selenium and green tea) and specific vitamins (e.g., B_6 and B_{12}) may be other factors that merit consideration.

REVISED DIAGNOSTIC CRITERIA POST-HAART

With regard to changes in HIV-1-associated neurocognitive-disorder manifestations (see section III) and to the changes in HIV-1-associated neurocognitive-disorder pathophysiology (see section IV) post-HAART, the need to revise the pre-HAART diagnostic criteria (AAN, 1991) was recognized. Revised criteria were arrived at based upon the Frascati Conference held in 2005, in which a revision of the clinical diagnostic criteria for these disorders was proposed (Antinori et al., 2007). A major change in the newly proposed criteria was the addition of the "condition" of "asymptomatic NP impairment" (ANI) to the disorders of HAD and MCMD. As it has been demonstrated that HIV-1 encephalitis is actually more common, though less severe, in the later HAART era, it followed that the institution of a systematic definition of the previously variably defined condition of subclinical NP impairment would be helpful in order to investigate clinical-pathological correlates.

The condition ANI was defined first by the presence of NP impairment in two or more neurocognitive domains. There also must be no reported or demonstrated functional decline, as a decline in functional status would indicate the presence of a disorder. Further, the NP impairment could not be explained by opportunistic CNS disease, systemic illness, psychiatric disorders (including substance use disorders), or medication toxicity factors. While this condition is referred to as "asymptomatic," a patient may have NP-related complaints that map to NP test deficits with the condition, provided that there is no functional-status decrement. Thus, perhaps a preferable designation for the condition would have been "subclinical NP impairment," which would differentiate it from MCMD and HAD but would not imply the absence of any symptoms. Nevertheless, the addition of this condition to the HIV-1-associated neurocognitive disorders should be helpful in standardizing clinical research in the future so that more powerful relationships might be observed with relevant biomarkers across studies. This would eventually allow the inclusion of biomarkers in the definition of this condition and its associated disorders.

We have previously reported that some discontinuity exists within the AAN (1991) diagnostic criteria for the HIV-1-associated neurocognitive disorders, MCMD and HAD (Goodkin et al., 2000). The diagnosis of MCMD by AAN criteria was made based upon the presence of symptoms rather than the documentation of NCI. For MCMD, by the 1991 criteria, at least two of the following six symptoms must have been present for at least 1 month: impaired attention or concentration, mental slowing, impaired memory, slowed movements, incoordination, and personality change/irritability/emotional lability. Note that the last three criteria do not refer to the neurocognitive sphere. It was only recommended that standardized NP testing be employed whenever possible to support the diagnosis, but it was not required. In fact, the MCMD symptom-based criteria allow symptoms due to deficits in motor performance or neurobehavioral deficits (the presence of personality change, irritability, and/or emotional lability) to define the diagnosis without any symptoms directly referable to neurocognitive deficits. However, reviews of the research have shown that NCI is the primary basis upon which both the MCMD and HAD diagnoses should be based. Motor deficits should be associated only secondarily, with neurobehavioral deficits, in turn, less well identified as contributing to the symptoms of these disorders (Antinori et al., 2007). Clearly, this discrepancy in diagnostic criteria increases the risk for a disjunction to occur in studies of the association of these disorders with other factors of interest (e.g., selected biomarkers and clinical risk factors). As MCMD was not originally required to be based upon documentation of neurocognitive deficits identified by

NP testing and since three of the six MCMD symptoms do not refer to neurocognitive deficits, an important gain could be made by aligning the diagnosis of MCMD with HAD, in conjunction with a requirement for NP testing deficits and the elimination of symptom-based criteria.

The revised criteria for the diagnosis of MCMD address these issues. First, the issue of the prominence of neurocognitive deficits over motor and neurobehavioral symptoms was addressed by a change in the nomenclature for the disorder, as well as a change in its diagnostic criteria. Rather than "minor cognitive-motor disorder," which supports the conception of the "complex" of the triad of neurocognitive, motor, and neurobehavioral spheres, the revised nomenclature proposed is "mild neurocognitive disorder" (MND). The latter term eliminates motor symptoms. Further, the revised criteria for the new term, MND, will require NP-defined deficits (rather than the self-report of symptoms) to show at least a mild level of NP impairment (i.e., ≥ 1 SD below a demographically appropriate normative mean) involving two or more neurocognitive domains. There must also be reported or demonstrated mild functional-status decline, which differentiates MND both from the condition ANI (with no functional-status decline) and from the disorder HAD (with at least moderate functional-status decline). If quantitative tests of functional status are administered, performance must be at least 1 SD below the mean on at least one such task. Finally, as with ANI, MND is a diagnosis of exclusion. Therefore, confounding conditions or disorders must not be able to account for the defining diagnostic criteria.

The diagnosis of HAD was better standardized pre-HAART than those of ANI and MCMD. Nevertheless, an issue had been identified with the former diagnostic criteria for HAD. While the AAN (1991) diagnostic criteria were based upon NP testing that defined neurocognitive deficits, rather than symptoms, there is a mandate for such deficits to be consonant with the severity associated with a dementing syndrome, rather than a milder disorder or a condition. The revised criteria for HAD not only designate the severity level for NP deficits, but also require demonstration of quantified NP deficits that meet a severity level of at least "moderate." This level is defined by deficits greater than 2 SD below demographically appropriate normative means in two or more moderately impaired neurocognitive domains, or alternatively, by a deficit greater than 2.5 SD below the mean in one severely impaired domain and by a deficit greater than 1 SD below the mean in another mildly impaired domain. In addition, reported or demonstrated major functional-status decline is also required, along with the absence of any confounding conditions. If quantitative tests of functional status are administered, performance must be at least 2 SD below the mean on at least one such task or greater than 1 SD below the mean on at least two such tasks. Finally, as with ANI and MND, HAD is also a diagnosis of exclusion.

It has been noted that HIV-1-associated NCI and disorders are diagnoses of exclusion. A deficit in standardization that extends across these diagnoses involves the lack of standardization of the extent to which confounding conditions must be excluded. In the post-HAART era, there has been greater recognition that the number and frequency of conditions that could be confounded with the HIV-1-associated neurocognitive diagnoses are high. Further, the judgment about the presence of confounding factors is not necessarily clear-cut. There may be factors contributory to HIV-1-associated NCI that do not constitute a confound at the time of diagnosis. There may also be secondary factors affecting neurocognitive performance that are present but that do not contribute to the presentation of HIV-1-specific NCI or disorder. In addition, the extent to which the many potentially confounding factors can be feasibly assessed across resource-rich and resource-limited settings is quite variable, incorporating yet another factor that cannot be easily standardized. Hence, while calling for a more precise evaluation of such factors, the revised criteria for HIV-1-associated NCI and disorders cannot explicitly address this aspect of diagnostic variability.

In summary, with regard to the revision of the diagnostic criteria for HIV-1-associated NCI and disorder, it can be stated that several important advances have been made. The addition of the diagnosis of the condition ANI will likely contribute to better agreement on the presence of subclinical HIV-1-associated NCI, which is of special import in the later HAART era. The alignment of all three diagnoses as defined by deficits demonstrated by NP testing and the prominence of the neurocognitive sphere over the motor and neurobehavioral spheres is also of great importance with regard to better standardization of these diagnoses. In addition, the utilization of quantified standards to define levels of NP impairment that differentiate MCMD from HAD is a significant improvement in standardization, as well. However, there remain several areas in which these improvements may be limited. Regarding nomenclature, the term "subclinical NP impairment" may be preferable to ANI, as symptoms may be present in this condition. Similarly, the term "MND" presents issues, as well, since it is also used as a separately defined term by the *Diagnostic and Statistical Manual of Mental Disorders*, 4th ed., text revision in its research appendix, appendix B (pp. 762–764) (American Psychiatric Association, 2000). Therein, "MND" is defined as a general diagnostic term without specific reference to HIV-1 infection. The definition requires that "cognitive deficits cause marked distress or impairment and decline in social, occupational, or other areas of functioning," while "MND," as defined by the Frascati Conference, does not require distress to be present and requires only mild functional-status decline. In addition, while functional-status differences among these diagnostic terms are now stipulated, there is not a requirement for these functional-status differences to be quantified in a standard fashion. This stands in contrast to the quantitative definitions that were adopted for the differentiation of levels of NP impairment. Finally, while the need to be more explicit regarding exclusion criteria was addressed, no specific method for ensuring a standard process in this regard was introduced. Hence, some positive impact upon the diagnoses of these disorders using the revised criteria is expected, although a continued concern about reaching maximal standardization will likely persist. Only future research on the proposed criteria will be able to clarify how well they will perform.

TREATMENT CONSIDERATIONS POST-HAART

ARV Therapies

ARVs reduce the load of HIV-1 in the CSF, as well as in brain tissue, decreasing the direct, pathogenic effects of HIV-1 replication. ZDV, formerly referred to as azidothymidine, was the first ARV approved by the FDA and remains the ARV with the greatest supporting evidence for the treatment of HIV-1-associated neurocognitive disorder. ZDV has been reported to have a CSF/plasma ratio of 0.60. It should be noted that the CSF/plasma ratio may not be the optimal indicator of drug penetration into the CSF (Burger

et al., 1993); the 90% inhibitory concentration (IC_{90}) (the inhibitory concentration of drug needed to reduce HIV-1 replication by 90%) may be a more valuable indicator over the tolerated dosing range. Penetration of ZDV into the CSF appears to be independent of the dose (range, 200 to 1,250 mg daily), which may be an explanation for the efficacy of low doses of ZDV in the prevention and treatment of HIV-1-associated neurological diseases. An early study of ZDV indicated a clinically significant effect on NP performance, although neurological clinical functioning was not improved (Sidtis et al., 1993). Early clinical pharmacotherapy utilized high-dose ZDV therapy (with 1,000 or 2,000 mg/day), doses much above the commonly prescribed total daily dose (600 mg/day) today. Significant toxicity due to neutropenia and anemia has been observed at these higher doses, and lower dosing regimens may be equally effective. A number of other reports have supported the efficacy of ZDV (Azini et al., 1990; Bell et al., 1996; Brew et al., 1992; Schmitt et al., 1988; Vago et al., 1993). However, the issues of ZDV dosing and resistance over time have not yet been fully addressed. Testing for resistance to ZDV, as well as other ARVs, by genotypic or phenotypic methods should be done as a standard of care upon treatment initiation (Sax et al., 2005). This may be particularly true for ZDV, given the current prevalence of ZDV resistance on HIV-1 transmission and the frequency with which ZDV resistance can begin as early as 6 months posttreatment.

Evidence of the impacts of other ARVs on HIV-1-associated NCI and disorder is at a less well-controlled level than that for ZDV. For example, the dideoxynucleoside ddI may have an effect on HIV-1-associated neurocognitive disorder as well, although it has a lower penetration into the CSF than ZDV. In a limited study of five patients with dementia or other cognitive dysfunction, Yarchoan et al. (1990) showed that ddI treatment resulted in improved neurocognitive measurements after 6 to 12 weeks. ddC is rarely included in current ARV regimens, and the neurocognitive results with this medication to date have been mixed. Although the CSF/plasma ratio for d4T is relatively high (0.4), it does not penetrate brain tissue well (Thomas and Segal, 1998). This raises the more general issue of whether the CSF/plasma ratio is necessarily the best predictor of brain tissue penetration. Following its FDA approval, abacavir was shown to inhibit local HIV-1 replication in the CSF (McDowell et al., 1999). The CSF/plasma ratio averaged 0.36, and the value increased throughout the dosing interval (Capparelli et al., 2005). High-dose abacavir was recently evaluated in a limited sample of HIV-1-infected children. The high-dose abacavir-containing regimen showed a safety profile similar to that of the standard abacavir dose, and participants 3 months to 6 years old demonstrated significant NP improvement (whereas those 6 to 18 years old did not) (Saavedra-Lozano et al., 2006). Regarding tenofovir DF, there is negligible transport of the drug across the BBB, although it can cross the blood-CSF barrier, reflecting the differences between the two blood-CNS interfaces (Anthonypillai et al., 2006). Research to date does not suggest clinically significant penetration of other currently FDA-approved nRTIs into brain tissue. The nRTIs are the best-characterized ARV class in regard to CNS distribution. While data support the significant penetration of the CNS by several members of this class, the probenecid efflux transport mechanism limits brain delivery and efficacy in treating neurocognitive impairment and disorder.

Another class of ARVs also inhibits the reverse transcriptase enzyme, the NNRTIs. The most commonly prescribed NNRTIs, nevirapine and EFV, can readily enter the CSF. Nevirapine has one of the best levels of CSF penetration among the ARVs, with a range of CSF/plasma ratios from 0.45 to as high as 0.63 (Antinori et al., 2005), in large part due to its relatively low level of binding to plasma proteins. EFV penetrates to a lesser extent due to its very high level of plasma protein binding. However, in one study, EFV was detected in the CSF at a mean concentration of 35.1 nM, which was above the IC_{95} for wild-type HIV-1, with a mean CSF/plasma ratio of 0.61% (i.e., 0.0061; range, 0.0026 to 0.0099) (Tashima et al., 1999). Thus, EFV is present in CSF at very low levels but is nevertheless effective in suppressing the CSF viral load in HAART regimens, again highlighting the need to use indicators of CNS penetration other than the CSF/plasma (or CSF/serum) ratio. EFV may ultimately prove to have a salutary effect on NP performance, despite its initially deleterious neurocognitive side effects (Clifford et al., 2005). It remains to be seen if a specific transport system is involved in the distribution of the NNRTIs into the brain. A new NNRTI, etravirine (formerly TMC 125), has been approved by the FDA. Etravirine has shown efficacy in a large study of treatment-experienced patients with defined NNRTI resistance in a placebo-controlled trial (Madruga et al., 2007). The safety and tolerability profile of etravirine was comparable to that of a placebo, but no published data yet exist on its possible specific CNS effects.

The third major class of ARVs, the PIs, must be considered as well. In regard to their specific effects within HAART regimens, studies remain very limited. Indinavir (CSF/plasma ratio, 0.16) appears to be the only member of the class with significant CSF penetration, though it is relatively low (Stahle et al., 1997). Nevertheless, similar to EFV, the CSF IC_{95} of indinavir for wild-type HIV-1 can be reached with the currently recommended indinavir dose of 800 mg p.o. three times a day (t.i.d.) (Martin et al., 1999). This dosing of indinavir is rarely, if ever, used in current HAART regimens. However, by combining with low-dose ritonavir, a potent inhibitor of the cytochrome P450 3A4 isoenzyme, the practice known as "ritonavir boosting" significantly increases the CSF concentration of indinavir by exploiting this drug-drug interaction. Although indinavir warrants further investigation as a therapy for HIV-1-associated NCI and disorder, it has a high potential for toxicity. Of particular concern is nephrolithiasis, as well as the lipodystrophy syndrome and dry, brittle hair and nails, among other side effects, limiting the potential utility of indinavir for this indication. As the other PIs have not been shown to penetrate well into brain tissue, for those studied, this class of ARVs has been disappointing in regard to disease control in the CNS despite its great impact on disease control in the periphery. Nevertheless, it is contended that since HAART regimens containing PIs inhibit viral replication with high potency in the periphery and since HIV-1 reaches brain tissue via the peripheral blood, this peripheral control of HIV-1 may extend to the CNS.

New Classes of ARVs

Viral Entry Inhibitors

Fusion Inhibitors

Following the introduction of the nRTIs, PIs, and NNRTIs, the next (fourth) class of ARVs, approved by the FDA in March 2003, was the fusion inhibitors, represented by enfuvirtide (T-20). This 36-amino-acid peptide acts by blocking the conformational change of gp41, the transmembrane portion of the virus-derived envelope protein required for fusion of the viral envelope with the host cell membrane. This fusion allows the core capsid of HIV-1, containing its single strand of RNA, to enter the $CD4^+$ T lymphocyte. Enfuvirtide has demonstrated consistently high levels of antiretroviral activity when used in combination with other ARVs against plasma HIV-1 strains resistant to all three ARV classes approved earlier. Its primary drawback is its unique route of administration by subcutaneous injection twice daily and the associated side effect of injection site reactions. Little or no evidence is yet available on the potential effects of this drug in the CNS. Due to its very large molecular weight, CNS penetration is predicted to be poor.

Chemokine Receptor Antagonists

A fifth FDA-approved class of ARVs, also classified as viral entry inhibitors, comprises the CCR5 antagonists. The first member of this new class, maraviroc, was approved by the FDA in August 2007. Maraviroc is a CCR5 receptor antagonist that selectively and noncompetitively binds to the CCR5 molecules on the surfaces of human cells, rendering them unrecognizable by the viral gp120 envelope protein and thereby interrupting viral attachment and entry. It should be noted that, as a class, CCR5 antagonists are active only against CCR5-tropic strains of HIV-1, which typically infect monocytes and macrophages. They are not active against CXCR4-tropic HIV-1 strains, which typically infect $CD4^+$ T lymphocytes. Since CCR5-tropic strains are thought to be more specific to early CNS HIV-1 infection than CXCR4-tropic strains, this drug is of particular interest in relation to its efficacy for HIV-1-associated neurocognitive impairment and disorders. Data from recent phase III clinical trials have demonstrated excellent antiretroviral activity of maraviroc with twice daily dosing as part of a HAART regimen against highly resistant plasma CCR5-tropic HIV-1 strains in treatment-experienced patients. Moreover, its adverse-event profile has been reported to be similar to that of the comparator placebo. Currently, there is a second CCR5 antagonist, called vicriviroc, in phase III of clinical development.

Of note, prior to the FDA approval of maraviroc, delta-ala_1-peptide T-amide (DAPTA), a drug that was originally thought to block CD4 receptor, was investigated. Recent data, however, indicate that the mechanism of action of DAPTA is that it blocks the binding of gp120 to the CCR5 chemokine coreceptor rather than to the CD4 receptor (Ruff et al., 2001). Pre-HAART, a multi-site, randomized, placebo-controlled clinical trial with intranasal DAPTA, 2 mg, delivered as a nasal spray t.i.d., was conducted with a sample of 215 participants with HIV-1-associated NCI. While no statistically significant difference was found on the global NP battery z score outcome measure compared to placebo, subgroup analyses showed that participants with a CD4 cell count of 201 to 500 cells/mm^3 and with at least moderate NP impairment at baseline did improve significantly on this composite NP outcome measure (Heseltine et al., 1998). In addition, DAPTA was well tolerated, with no clinically significant toxic effects. Recently, a retrospective study was undertaken from the sample repository of that trial to examine possible changes in CSF and peripheral viral load among participants who completed 6 months of treatment (Goodkin et al., 2006). The peripheral viral load (plasma and serum) was significantly reduced in the DAPTA-treated group, but the CSF viral load was not. However, DAPTA is also known to down-regulate the activities of proinflammatory cytokines, which may account for a neurocognitive effect that is independent of its effect on viral load.

Integrase Inhibitors

Long talked about as a potential target against HIV-1 replication, inhibition of viral integrase became clinical reality in September 2007 with the FDA approval of raltegravir, establishing the sixth and most recent class of ARVs. This small-molecule compound selectively inhibits the strand transfer step of the process in which recently reverse transcribed double-stranded viral DNA is spliced into the human genome by the virus-encoded enzyme integrase. This step is critical, not only for the production of new viral particles, but also, more importantly, for embedding the proviral DNA sequences into host CD4 cells and monocytes permanently, establishing viral latency. Given the HAART era focus on the proviral DNA load in HAD risk and HIV-1 as a reservoir of latent infection in the brain (Clements et al., 2005), the integrase inhibitors are of particular interest in the treatment of HIV-1-associated NCI and disorders. However, no published data are yet available describing the CNS penetration of raltegravir or its potential clinical efficacy in this regard. A second integrase inhibitor, elvitegravir, is currently due to enter phase III clinical trials. Further studies of these new agents, as well as the CCR5 antagonists mentioned above, are eagerly anticipated.

Vaccine Treatment Strategies

Most HIV-1 vaccine studies have not addressed the specific need for protection in the CNS. This is a special concern regarding a CNS HIV-1 infection manifesting as a potential late complication of HIV-1 vaccine treatment. Given the wide variability of HIV-1 gp120 across the 10 clades of HIV-1 (as well as the continuously evolving CRFs, as noted above), many feel that a multivalent (and perhaps consensus sequence-derived) vaccine comprised of envelope, *gag*, and selected regulatory-gene sequences will probably prove necessary to achieve some level of protection against HIV-1 infection and control of the HIV/AIDS pandemic. However, at least one study suggests that this might not be the case. This study evaluated the ability of nonpathogenic SIV$_{mac}$ and nonpathogenic chimeric simian/human immunodeficiency virus (SHIV) to induce protection in macaques against superinfection with a pathogenic variant of SHIV (SHIV$_{KU-1}$) originally containing the *tat*, *rev*, *vpu*, and *env* genes of HIV-1 (strain HXB2). Specifically, three macaques inoculated with molecularly cloned, macrophage-tropic SIV$_{mac}$LG1 developed an early systemic infection but recovered and were then inoculated parenterally with pathogenic SHIV$_{KU-1}$. All three resisted infection with SHIV$_{KU-1}$, as indicated by lack of virus recovery and absence of SHIV Env sequences in visceral lymphoid tissues and in multiple CNS regions (Stephens et al., 1997). Five other macaques were inoculated with nonpathogenic SHIV, and similar to the SIV$_{mac}$LG1-inoculated macaques, these animals also resisted the pathogenic SHIV$_{KU-1}$ challenge. Evaluation of similar vaccines in human trials has yet to be undertaken.

Given the prior issues around the independent neurotoxicity of HIV-1 proteins, in particular extracellular Tat, development of a vaccine including a biologically inactivated but immunogenic Tat ("Tat toxoid") would seem to be important to ensure CNS coverage. In humans, Tat toxoid immunization has been shown to be safe and to induce persistently high levels of anti-Tat antibodies in HIV-1-seronegative persons (and in immunodeficient patients, as well) (Le Buanec et al., 1998). In the context of acute HIV-1 exposure, this would be expected to allow an anti-HIV-1 cellular immune response to develop more fully, with the subsequent result of inhibited viral replication and decreased likelihood of eventual progression to AIDS.

While vaccine strategies based on antibodies targeting the viral envelope have been unsuccessful, antibody-based vaccine strategies (to selected cytokines) may still play an important role in therapeutic strategies. Serum TNF-α antibodies have been correlated positively and directly with the plasma HIV-1 load and CD8 cell count and inversely with the CD4 cell count and percentage, as well as the CD4/CD8 ratio (Capini et al., 2001). TNF-α antibodies also correlated positively with antibodies to the CD4 binding site peptides of gp160, the CD4 identity region, and the V3 loop. Thus, TNF-α antibodies may be constitutively produced in response to HIV-1 infection, indicating the potential utility of this particular cytokine antibody-based vaccine at a pharmacological dosing level. Following their development of biologically inactive but immunogenic specific TNF-α peptides, this group has proposed targeting TNF-α by active immunization. This strategy could elicit a high-titer humoral response against endogenous TNF-α, ultimately neutralizing its biological activity.

The development of vaccine strategies for protection against HIV-1 infection continues. However, current findings suggest that vaccines may need to incorporate, among other components, modified virus and/or viral products and antibody-based mechanisms. For example, Vif is an HIV accessory protein with a primary function to negate the action of APOBEC3G, a naturally occurring cellular HIV-1 replication inhibitor. Vif acts by binding APOBEC3G, inducing its protein degradation and reducing its levels in viral progeny (Carr et al., 2006). Vaccine strategies interfering with the Vif-APOBEC3G interaction could raise intracellular levels of APOBEC3G or reduce intracellular levels of Vif and hold clinical promise for enhancing the cell's innate antiviral activity. It is possible that careful vaccine design may reveal a cocktail formulation that is able to prevent HIV-1 infections worldwide, overcoming the political and financial dilemmas associated with clade-specific vaccines. In any case, it must be concluded that coverage of the CNS by vaccines in development has been underinvestigated and this particular area demands greater attention in the future. This is especially true given the current concern that the brain acts as a reservoir for HIV-1 infection despite highly effective ARV therapy in the periphery.

Anti-Inflammatory Therapies and Immunotherapies

The largest number of treatment studies to date on HIV-1-associated NCI and disorder have used anti-inflammatory or immunotherapeutic agents, predominantly the former. The calcium influx associated with neuronal-cell dysfunction preceding cell death has been one treatment focus. Nimodipine, a calcium channel blocker that penetrates the BBB, has been studied with mixed results. Galgani et al. (1997) showed that ZDV and nimodipine at 30 mg p.o. t.i.d. improved NP performance over ZDV alone at 6 months of treatment in a sample across HAD stages 0 to 2, whereas Navia et al. (1998) found no evidence for the efficacy of nimodipine on an eight-NP-test composite score. The latter study used a dose of 60 mg p.o. five times a day and 30 mg p.o. t.i.d. (versus placebo) over 16 weeks of treatment in patients with mild to severe HAD. The calcium channels of particular interest for blocking in brain tissue are those associated with NMDA receptors. To that end, memantine is a noncompetitive, open-channel, low-affinity NMDA receptor modulator that has been used with the aim of reducing glutamate-induced excitotoxicity in HIV-1-infected persons. It was tested in AIDS Clinical Trial Group Protocol 301 at a dose of 10 to 40 mg/day orally. Participants did not show improvement in NP performance over 16 weeks of treatment, although improvements in magnetic resonance spectroscopy measures of the N-acetyl aspartate/creatine ratio in the frontal white matter and parietal cortex were noted, suggesting the need for a future study with a longer treatment period (Schiffito et al., 2007). Overall, the clinical research results published to date with these agents have been disappointing.

In terms of immunomodulation and its relevance to the treatment of HIV-1-associated neurocognitive impairment and disorders, inhibitors of TNF-α have been of interest. One such inhibitor, pentoxifylline, has shown a significant neuroprotective effect in vitro. Pentoxyfylline enhanced the cellular viability of a human neuronal cell line, NT2N, after these cells were exposed to gp120 (Westmoreland et al., 1996). However, no controlled clinical trial with pentoxyfylline has been reported to substantiate this effect in vivo. In contrast, in a randomized, double-blind, placebo-controlled pilot study (n = 15 per group) of lexipafant (500 mg/day), a platelet-activating factor (PAF) antagonist, there was a trend toward improved NP performance (Schifitto et al., 1999). Thalidomide (300 mg/day) has also been shown to suppress expression of TNF-α and has been effective in the treatment of oral aphthous ulcers and wasting syndrome associated with HIV-1 infection. However, there are no data on the effects of thalidomide on HIV-1-associated NCI and disorder. CPI-1189 is a novel compound that has pronounced anti-free-radical effects and protects neurons from TNF-α-induced apoptosis. In a Neurology AIDS Research Consortium-sponsored clinical trial of CPI-1189, 64 participants with mild to moderate HIV-1-associated NCI were randomized to either placebo or 50 or 100 mg daily of the drug, in addition to optimal HIV-1 background ARV therapy. During the 10-week follow-up, no significant treatment effects on the change in the composite NP z score were observed over eight tests (Clifford et al., 2002). Etanercept inhibits TNF-α as a soluble p75 TNF receptor-FC fusion protein and may also hold promise for the treatment of the HIV-1 infected, specifically those with HIV-1-associated NCI and disorder. In regard to another deleterious proinflammatory cytokine in the CNS, IL-1, endogenous IL-1 receptor antagonist in the CSF has been found to be a sensitive measure of inflammation in HIV-1 CNS disease. Thus, it may be of interest to study the possible therapeutic effect of IL-1 receptor antagonist as well, though this has not yet been reported. Finally, MCP-1 antagonists are currently in the experimental phases of development and may prove to be useful once they are moved to the clinical phase of evaluation.

In addition to the prospect of inhibiting potentially neurotoxic cytokines, the activation of other, neuroprotective cytokines/growth factors may also prove helpful. As an example, erythropoietin is generally used clinically with the HIV-1 infected to treat ARV-induced anemia or anemia of chronic disease. Of note regarding CNS implications, a low hemoglobin level has also been shown to be a significant and independent risk factor for the occurrence of HAD (McArthur et al., 1993). Moreover, and of more specific relevance within the CNS, erythropoietin has been found to prevent neuronal death due to inflammation or excitotoxicity. Further, erythropoietin has been found to protect cerebrocortical neurons against apoptosis induced by gp120 (Digicaylioglu et al., 2004). Thus, it merits clinical trial for NCI and disorder in HIV-1 infection. Of note regarding another generally obtained hematological parameter, like the homoglobin level cited above, a decline in platelet count

has been related to increased HAD risk in a recent study (Wachtman et al., 2007). HIV-1-infected individuals with a decline in platelet counts had a twofold-increased risk of HAD on univariate and multivariate analyses; perhaps upregulation of thrombopoietin in response to the peripheral platelet destruction known to potentially occur with HIV-1 infection adversely affects the CNS microenvironment. In fact, thrombopoietin has been noted to induce neuronal apoptosis, in contrast to the neuroprotective effect against gp120-induced neuronal apoptosis conferred by erythropoietin. Thus, it would be of interest in future research to determine whether erythropoietin and thrombopoietin are coordinately regulated vis à vis protection against and risk for this mechanism of cell death, which is thought to have import in HAD pathogenesis.

Activation of GDNF and brain-derived neurotrophic factor is also of clinical interest. Of note, gp120 induces neuronal apoptosis in rats, and microinjection of gp120 into the striata of rats has been used as an experimental model of HAD pathogenesis. GDNF immunoreactivity, but not that of brain-derived neurotrophic factor, has been shown to be decreased in the substantia nigra at 4 days postinjection in gp120-treated rats, suggesting gp120-induced retrograde degeneration of nigrostriatal neurons via a reduction in GDNF expression (Nosheny et al., 2006) and suggesting that GDNF may be a protective factor against such toxicity. Limiting its use therapeutically, however, has been the issue of delivery across the BBB. Addressing this issue, an 11-amino-acid protein transduction domain of HIV-1 Tat is able to cross the BBB, even when coupled with larger peptides. In fact, in a murine model, TAT-GDNF has been shown to be effective in reducing ischemia due to stroke (Kilic et al., 2003), suggesting a potential therapeutic role in HIV-1-associated NCI and disorder in humans. Finally, neuroimmunophilin ligands (NILs) have been shown to have some efficacy in reversing neuronal degeneration and preventing cell death. In a wide range of animal models mimicking different neurological diseases, NILs induce resprouting, are neurotrophic, and prevent nerve damage (Poulter et al., 2004). Their mechanism of action is unknown and may be dependent on the type of neurological damage and genetic variability; nevertheless, NILs may also be of interest to investigate in the context of HIV-1-associated NCI and disorder.

Interestingly, the selective, irreversible monoamine oxidase type B (MAO-B) inhibitor selegiline, typically employed to up-regulate dopamine levels in Parkinson's disease, has been studied as a neurotrophic and antiapoptotic agent in low doses. The Dana Consortium (1998) conducted a randomized, double-blind, placebo-controlled trial evaluating oral selegiline (and an antioxidant, thioctic acid) in a total of 36 patients with HIV-1-associated NCI. Oral selegiline, at 2.5 mg three times a week for 10 weeks, significantly improved verbal memory compared to participants not taking selegiline. Hypothesizing that the selegiline patch would maintain stable blood levels, Sacktor et al. (2000) conducted a double-blind, randomized, placebo-controlled clinical trial using the selegiline patch (a 1.0-mg/cm, 15-cm^2 transdermal patch [delivering 3.1 mg/24 h]). A total of 14 participants with HIV-1-associated NCI on stable ARV therapy were studied. Improvements over 10 weeks of treatment were seen on a delayed verbal-recall measure and a motor measure, as well as on the neurological examination score; however, digit symbol, reaction time, timed-gait, mood, and functional-status measures were not significantly improved. Based on these results, a large, randomized, placebo-controlled clinical trial was conducted with a patch delivering both 3 mg and 6 mg of selegiline over 24 hours for 24 weeks in a total of 128 subjects, most of whom had mild to moderate HAD. No neurocognitive or functional improvement was observed (Schifitto et al., 2007). Despite the use of the higher dose of 6 mg over 24 hours in the latter trial, it might nevertheless be the case that these doses were too low to obtain a therapeutic effect. This interpretation is supported by increased dopaminergic transmission known to occur at a dose of 10 to 20 mg/day, over which selegiline remains selective for MAO-B. Thus, these higher doses of selegiline may still merit formal evaluation.

Glycogen synthase kinase 3 (GSK3) was initially identified more than 2 decades ago and has recently been shown to have a key role in regulating a diverse range of cellular functions, promoting the development of GSK3 inhibitors as therapeutics specifically for neurodegenerative diseases. In addition to being a mood stabilizer, lithium is a neuroprotectant, partly due to its inhibition of GSK3. In vitro investigations have demonstrated that lithium can limit the neuronal injury induced by gp120 (Everall et al., 2002) and Tat (Maggirwar et al., 1999). Recently, lithium was investigated in the treatment of HIV-1-associated NCI in a single-arm, open-label, 12-week pilot study. Participants were on stable ARV therapy and included those having a diagnosis of MCMD or HAD, aged 18 to 65, with a Karnofsky performance scale score of at least 50. Eight patients with lithium levels titrated to maintain a low dose (12-hour trough concentrations between 0.4 and 0.8 mEq/liter) were enrolled. NP performance improved in all participants after 12 weeks of treatment, with clinical ratings indicating improvements specifically in executive functioning and information-processing speed (LeTendre et al., 2006). Similar to lithium, valproic acid (VPA), used as a mood stabilizer, as well as an anticonvulsant, has been shown to inhibit neuronal apoptosis caused by PAF-induced GSK3 activation (Tong et al., 2001). Originally, there was concern about the potential for VPA to increase HIV-1 replication. This was based upon an often-cited in vitro study that showed that VPA stimulated HIV-1 replication in acutely and chronically infected cells and enhanced long-terminal-repeat-driven gene expression (Moog et al., 1996). A subsequent retrospective clinical case-control study, however, examined the effects of VPA on changes in the CSF and plasma HIV-1 loads and did not confirm any deleterious effect of VPA on the viral load, although at follow-up a trend toward a lower CD4 cell count was observed (Ances et al., 2006). These effects were observed over concentrations that are normally reached in the plasma of VPA-treated patients. Despite these concerns, 16 participants with HIV-1-associated NCI were enrolled in a clinical trial employing a randomized block design by impairment strata, which were used to assign treatment to either 250 mg VPA or placebo twice daily for 10 weeks (Schifitto et al., 2006). Changes in NP performance showed no statistically significant differences in the composite z score or in clinical global impression ratings. Nevertheless, the authors reported that all NP measures but two (including the composite z score) favored those in the VPA group, suggesting the need for a larger trial of increased duration specifically designed to assess VPA efficacy. In another study with a similarly small sample size, eight advanced HIV-1-infected participants on VPA (at a somewhat higher mean dose of 850 mg/day) were compared to 32 advanced HIV-1-infected individuals not on VPA (Cysique et al., 2006). This trial was conducted over a much longer period (18 months on average) than the trial by Schifitto et al. (2006) (10 weeks).

Surprisingly, significantly increased NCI was found in the VPA group on the reliable cognitive-change index used to summarize changes in six NP measures. This deleterious effect was maintained after controlling for depressed mood level and viral load. Thus, while considerable enthusiasm has accompanied trials of the GSK3 inhibitors, the data do not yet confirm any therapeutic benefit and, in fact, there is a possibility that VPA may prove to be deleterious. In summary, anti-inflammatory medications and immunotherapies have demonstrated little evidence of clinical efficacy in the treatment of HIV-1-associated NCI and disorders. Although there is suggestive evidence that these approaches may be of benefit in the future, additional studies will need to combine proper dose-finding preliminary work with longer-term controlled treatment intervals.

Neurotransmitter Modulators

While some of the approaches noted above would typically be included in the category of neurotransmitter modulation (see the discussions of memantine and selegiline), they were grouped by mechanisms of action proposed for the studies undertaken. This section will focus on agents explicitly used for the mechanism of neurotransmitter modulation. Given the early demonstration of low CSF homovanillic acid levels (Larsson et al., 1991), followed by the confirmation of decreased dopamine levels in brain tissue (Sardar et al., 1996) in patients with AIDS, enhancement of dopaminergic transmission is prioritized for consideration here. Limited supportive data can be obtained from case studies of carbidopa and L-dopa use for the indication of HIV-1-associated NCI and disorder (Kieburtz et al., 1991). Psychostimulants enhance dopaminergic transmission and have been used widely as palliative treatments for HIV-1-associated NCI and disorder since the early days of the epidemic. These studies indicate efficacy, but they lack well-controlled evaluation. Significant improvement was shown in early symptomatic and in late symptomatic (AIDS) patients in a clinical trial using methylphenidate at 10 mg p.o. t.i.d. (to a maximum of 90 mg/day over 2 weeks) with crossover to dextroamphetamine at 15 mg p.o. twice a day (to a maximum of 60 mg/day) if there was no response (Fernandez et al., 1988). An inpatient, double-blind, placebo-controlled crossover trial was conducted of sustained-release methylphenidate (20 to 40 mg/day) in a small sample of substance abusers with HIV-1-associated NCI. On a composite NP performance measure, improvement from baseline was noted with sustained-release methylphenidate, but not placebo; still, performance on the drug did not differ significantly from placebo performance (van Dyck et al., 1997). Hinkin et al. (2001) enrolled 16 HIV-1-infected participants in a single-blind, placebo-controlled, crossover design of methylphenidate (30 mg/day). Participants with evidence of cognitive slowing at study entry showed greater improvement on methylphenidate than on placebo; thus, decrements in information-processing speed may be a more specific indicator for psychostimulant treatment. Studies of selegiline have been confined to low-dose regimens not expected to increase dopaminergic transmission; thus, higher-dose selegiline treatment does warrant further study. Also, there are few or no controlled data reported on the utility of specific dopamine receptor agonists.

Other neurotransmitters are worthy of consideration in the context of the need for additional treatments for HIV-1-associated NCI and disorders. Serotonin has been shown to have low levels in the CSF of HIV-1-infected individuals

(Kumar et al., 2001). Potentially, then, the selective serotonin reuptake inhibitors may play some role in the treatment of HIV-1-associated NCI and disorder. It has also been suggested that the selective serotonin reuptake inhibitors may reduce the CSF HIV-1 load (LeTendre et al., 2007), though this remains to be convincingly demonstrated. In addition, the question has been raised as to whether the use of acetyl-cholinesterase inhibitors may alleviate HAD (Alisky, 2005) based, in part, on their effects in Alzheimer's disease. However, very little study of cholinergic neurotransmission has been undertaken in HIV-1 CNS disease. Using a SIV-infected rhesus monkey model, Koutsilieri et al. (2000) reported on post-mortem studies showing that choline acetyltransferase activity was significantly reduced in the putamen and hippocampus as early as the asymptomatic stage and further in AIDS. However, these reductions in choline acetyltransferase activity were not related to the brain viral load or to CNS pathological lesions. Hence, there is only minimal evidence to suggest that acetylcholine is decreased in HIV-1 infection of the brain and no controlled evidence to show that this class of drugs might be therapeutically useful.

Nutritional Manipulation

A number of nutritional therapies have been suggested to target HIV-1 infection of the brain (Baldewicz et al., 2000). Treatment of deficiencies of several micronutrients may prove relevant for HIV-1-associated NCI and disorder. However, whether such micronutrients may also be helpful at supernormal levels (i.e., as true "supplements") is a separate question. As a class, the antioxidants have received some attention. However, thioctic acid (as mentioned above) was not found to be significant in improving HIV-associated NCI in a well-controlled clinical trial (Dana Consortium, 1998). Micronutrients that have been studied include, but are not limited to, vitamin B_6, vitamin B_{12}, and selenium. Each has been related to cognitive function in HIV-1-seropositive individuals. Vitamin B_6 deficiency has been related to increased psychological distress overall and to confusion-bewilderment specifically. The latter may be indicative of actual neurocognitive deficits in B_6-deficient subjects (Baldewicz et al., 1998). Likewise, vitamin B_{12} deficiency, which occurs in up to 20% of patients with AIDS, has been associated with HIV-1-associated NCI (Beach et al., 1992). One report of decreased serum vitamin B_{12} level showed that the presence of B_{12} deficiency was associated with symptoms of dementia in an HIV-1-infected patient and that treatment of that deficiency resolved the dementia symptoms over a 2-month period (Herzlich and Schiano, 1993). In addition, the significance of a deficiency in the antioxidant effects of the mineral selenium has also received some attention, as it relates to glutathione deficiency. However, in a recent cross-sectional study of 365 HIV-1-seropositive and HIV-1-sero-negative adolescents and young adults, selenium deficiency (a plasma selenium level of <0.070 µg/ml) was not seen in any subjects and plasma selenium in 244 HIV-1-seropositive subjects did not differ significantly from levels in 121 HIV-1-seronegative subjects (Stephensen et al., 2007). However, a controlled analysis did show that abnormal HIV-1-associated immunological activation (indicated by higher plasma neopterin levels) was associated with lower plasma selenium concentrations. Glutathione peroxidase is a selenoenzyme, the depletion of which eventually may be associated with dementia in HIV-1-infected patients (Foster, 2004); however, deficiency is apparently infrequent, and it is unclear that selenium supplementation above the normal range has any clinical value.

In addition to selenium, green tea may be of value as an antioxidant, as well (Nance and Shearer, 2003). While it has been promulgated for a wide range of diseases, including cancer and cardiovascular disease, there is supportive evidence for its use in HIV-1 infection. The active components of green tea are the polyphenolic catechins, among which epigallocatechin gallate accounts for approximately 50%. One study has shown that epigallocatechin gallate treatment of primary neurons from healthy mice reduced the IFN-γ-associated neurotoxicity of gp120 and Tat by inhibiting activation of the JAK/STAT1 pathway. Although these findings were confirmed in vivo (Giunta et al., 2006), there has been no formal clinical evaluation in humans. In overview, despite the intriguing evidence of the neurocognitive relevance of nutritional deficiencies for HIV-1-infected patients, significant caution must be exercised in the presumption that correction of a deficiency or supplementation above normal levels will have any observable clinical effect on HIV-1-associated NCI or disorder. Nevertheless, future controlled trials of selected micronutrients of interest are warranted in this area, particularly given the larger background setting of polypharmacy and associated toxicities that occur frequently among the HIV-1 infected.

Other Agents of Potential Utility

A number of agents not included in the categories above may prove to have clinical utility. For example, the antibiotic minocycline is now known to significantly inhibit HIV-1 and SIV replication in vitro and also to reduce the incidence and severity of encephalitis in a rigorous SIV_{mac} model of HIV-1 CNS disease (Zink et al., 2005). Minocycline prevents increased expression of MCP-1 in the brain, and, thus, may be considered an anti-inflammatory medication. However, it seems unlikely that it will have true antiretroviral activity. The dose used in macaques was 4 mg/kg of body weight/day, which is within the tolerated range for humans. Given that minocycline is a safe, inexpensive, and readily available antibiotic, it merits investigation for HIV-1-associated NCI and disorders.

There is also a possible role of treatment of the novel vascular pathogenic factor for HIV-1-associated neurocognitive impairment and disorders. This vascular pathogenic factor was introduced by HAART toxicity and is related to the dyslipidemia associated with the lipodystrophy syndrome. To date, few specific treatments for this toxicity have been investigated, and no treatment is established. Rosiglitazone and metformin have been evaluated, with supportive data for both medications on improving the insulin sensitivity seen as an early manifestation of this ARV toxicity (Mulligan et al., 2007). In addition, atypical antipsychotic medications (e.g., olanzapine and risperidone) are known to induce a form of metabolic syndrome very similar to that demonstrated to occur with HAART-associated toxicity in the setting of the lipodystrophy syndrome (Singh and Goodkin, 2007a, 2007b). Thus, those atypical antipsychotic agents with the lowest propensity to cause the metabolic syndrome are recommended, i.e., ziprasidone and aripiprazole. The dyslipidemia linked to the HIV-1-associated lipodystrophy syndrome is a proven risk for TIA and CVA, as well as for HIV-1-associated NCI and disorders. Hence, the development of specific treatments for this new etiological factor must be considered a priority for both prevention and care at this time.

A group of drugs that inhibit cyclin-dependent kinases (CDKs), key regulators of the cell cycle and RNA polymerase II transcription, may also be relevant for treatment in this setting. In the last few years, the antiretroviral effects of pharmacological CDK inhibitors have been observed. Through the inhibition of CDK2 and CDK9, cellular cofactors for HIV-1 Tat transactivation, HIV-1 replication may be blocked by two specific pharmacological CDK inhibitors, CYC202 and flavopiridol (Pumfery et al., 2006). Another example of a novel therapy involves the multidrug resistance (MDR) modulators. Molecular investigations of MDR resulted in the isolation and characterization of genes coding for several associated proteins, including P-glycoprotein and the MDR-associated protein MRP1. These proteins cause MDR either by decreasing the intracellular drug concentration or redistributing accumulation of drugs away from the target organelles. Several MDR modulators are currently in clinical development (Tan et al., 2000). A potential use of these agents may be to increase the penetration of currently FDA-approved PIs into brain tissue.

REFERENCES

Achim, C. L., M. P. Heyes, and C. A. Wiley. 1993. Quantitation of human immunodeficiency virus, immune activation factors, and quinolinic acid in AIDS brains. *J. Clin. Investig.* **91:**2769–2775.

Alaeus, A., K. Lidman, A. Bjorkman, J. Giesecke, and J. Albert. 1999. Similar rate of disease progression among individuals infected with HIV-1 genetic subtypes A–D. *AIDS* **13:**901–907.

Alisky, J. M. 2005. Could cholinesterase inhibitors and memantine alleviate HIV dementia? *J. Acquir. Immun. Defic. Syndr.* **38:**113–114. (Letter.)

American Academy of Neurology. 1991. Nomenclature and research case definitions for neurological manifestations of human immunodeficiency virus type-1 (HIV-1) infection. *Neurology* **41:**778–785.

American Psychiatric Association. 2000. *Diagnostic and Statistical Manual of Mental Disorders*, 4th ed., text revision. American Psychiatric Association, Washington, DC.

Amodio, P., E. N. De Toni, L. Cavalletto, D. Mapelli, E. Bernardinello, F. Del Piccolo, C. Bergamelli, R. Costanzo, F. Bergamaschi, S. Z. Poma, L. Chemello, A. Gatta, and G. Perini. 2005. Mood, cognition and EEG changes during interferon alpha (alpha-IFN) treatment for chronic hepatitis C. *J. Affect. Disord.* **84:**93–98.

Ances, B. M., S. Letendre, M. Buzzell, J. Marquie-Beck, D. Lazaretto, T. D. Marcotte, I. Grant, R. J. Ellis, and the HNRC Group. 2006. Valproic acid does not affect markers of human immunodeficiency virus disease progression. *J. Neurovirol.* **12:**403–406.

Anthonypillai, C., J. E. Gibbs, and S. A. Thomas. 2006. The distribution of the anti-HIV drug, tenofovir (PMPA), into the brain, CSF and choroid plexuses. *Cerebrospinal Fluid Res.* **3:**1–10.

Antinori, A., G. Arendt, J. T. Becker, B. J. Brew, D. A. Byrd, M. Cherner, D. B. Clifford, P. Cinque, L. G. Epstein, K. Goodkin, M. Gisslen, I. Grant, R. K. Heaton, J. Joseph, K. Marder, C. M. Marra, J. C. McArthur, M. Nunn, R. W. Price, L. Pulliam, K. R. Robertson, N. Sacktor, V. Valcour, and V. Wojna. 2007. Updated research nosology for HIV-associated neurocognitive disorders. *Neurology* **69:**1789–1799.

Antinori, A., C. F. Perno, M. L. Giancola, F. Forbici, G. Ippolito, R. M. Hoetelmans, and S. C. Piscitelli. 2005. Efficacy of cerebrospinal fluid (CSF)-penetrating antiretroviral drugs against HIV in the neurological compartment: different patterns of phenotypic resistance in CSF and plasma. *Clin. Infect. Dis.* **41:**1787–1793.

Arici, C., D. Ripamonti, V. Ravasio, F. Maggiolo, M. Rizzi, M. G. Finazzi, and F. Suter. 2001. Long-term clinical benefit after highly active antiretroviral therapy in advanced HIV-1 infection, even in patients without immune reconstitution. *Int. J. STD AIDS* **12:**573–581.

Azini, M., S. Nanni, M. R. Astori, A. Brunetto, and L. Massobrio. 1990. Evaluation of neuropsychiatric parameters in HIV positive subjects treated with zidovudine. *Acta Neurol.* **12:**36–39.

Baeten, J. M., B. Chohan, L. Lavreys, V. Chohan, R. S. McClelland, L. Certain, K. Mandaliya, W. Jaoko, and J. Overbaugh. 2007. HIV-1 subtype D infection is associated with faster disease progression than subtype A in spite of similar plasma HIV-1 loads. *J. Infect. Dis.* **195:**1177–1180.

Bagetta, G., S. Piccirilli, C. Del Duca, L. A. Morrone, L. Rombola, G. Nappi, J. De Alba, R. G. Knowles, and M. T. Corasaniti. 2004. Inducible nitric oxide synthase is involved in the mechanisms of cocaine enhanced neuronal apoptosis induced by HIV-1 gp120 in the neocortex of rat. *Neurosci. Lett.* **356:**183–186.

Baldewicz, T., K. Goodkin, D. J. Feaster, N. T. Blaney, M. Kumar, A. Kumar, G. Shor-Posner, and M. Baum. 1998. Plasma pyridoxine deficiency is related to increased psychological distress in recently bereaved homosexual men. *Psychosom. Med.* **60:**297–308.

Baldewicz, T. T., P. Brouwers, K. Goodkin, A. M. Kumar, and M. Kumar. 2000. Nutritional contributions to the CNS pathophysiology of HIV-1 infection and implications for treatment. *CNS Spectr.* **5:**61–72.

Ball, S. C., A. Abraha, K. R. Collins, A. J. Marozsan, H. Baird, M. E. Quinones-Mateu, A. Penn-Nicholson, M. Murray, N. Richard, M. Lobritz, P. A. Zimmerman, T. Kawamura, A. Blauvelt, and E. J. Arts. 2003. Comparing the ex vivo fitness of CCR5-tropic human immunodeficiency virus type 1 isolates of subtypes B and C. *J. Virol.* **77:**1021–1038.

Barroga, C. F., C. Raskino, M. C. Fangon, P. E. Palumbo, C. J. Baker, J. A. Englund, and S. A. Spector. 2000. The CCR5Δ32 allele slows disease progression of human immunodeficiency virus-1-infected children receiving antiretroviral treatment. *J. Infect. Dis.* **182:**413–419.

Beach, R. S., R. Morgan, F. Wilkie, E. Mantero-Atienza, N. Blaney, G. Shor-Posner, Y. Lu, C. Eisdorfer, and M. K. Baum. 1992. Plasma vitamin B_{12} level as a potential cofactor in studies of human immunodeficiency virus type 1-related cognitive changes. *Arch. Neurol.* **49:**501–506.

Bell, J. E., Y. K. Donaldson, S. Lowrie, C. A. McKenzie, R. A. Elton, A. Chiswick, R. P. Brettle, J. W. Ironside, and P. Simmonds. 1996. Influence of risk group and zidovudine therapy on the development of HIV encephalitis and cognitive impairment in AIDS patients. *AIDS* **10:**493–499.

Berger, J. R., J. O. Harris, J. Gregorios, and M. Norenberg. 1990. Cerebrovascular disease in AIDS: a case control study. *AIDS* **4:**239–244.

Blanch, J., E. Martínez, A. Rousaud, J.-L. Blanco, M.-Á. García-Viejo, J.-M. Peri, et al. 2001. Preliminary data of a prospective study on neuropsychiatric side effects after initiation of efavirenz. *J. Acquir. Immun. Defic. Syndr.* **27:**336–343.

Breen, E. C., A. R. Rezai, K. Nakajima, G. N. Beall, R. T. Mitsuyasu, T. Hirano, T. Kishimoto, and O. Martinez-Maza. 1990. Infection with HIV is associated with elevated IL-6 levels and production. *J. Immunol.* **144:**480–484.

Brew, B. J. 2004. Evidence for a change in AIDS dementia complex in the era of highly active antiretroviral therapy and the possibility of new forms of AIDS dementia complex. *AIDS* **18**(Suppl. 1):S75–S78.

Brew, B. J., R. B. Bhalla, M. Paul, J. J. Sidtis, J. J. Keilp, A. E. Sadler, H. Gallardo, J. C. McArthur, M. K. Schwartz, and R. W. Price. 1992. Cerebrospinal fluid beta 2-microglobulin in patients with AIDS dementia complex: an expanded series including response to zidovudine treatment. *AIDS* **6:**461–465.

Burger, D. M., C. L., Kraaijeveld, P. L. Meenhorst, J. W. Mulder, C. H. Koks, A. Bult, and J. H. Beijnen. 1993. Penetration of zidovudine into the cerebrospinal fluid of patients infected with HIV. *AIDS* **7**:1581–1587.

Capini, C. J., M. W. Richardson, H. Hendel, A. Sverstiuk, J. Mirchandani, E. G. Regulier, K. Khalili, J. F. Zagury, and J. Rappaport. 2001. Autoantibodies to TNFα in HIV-1 infection: prospects for anti-cytokine vaccine therapy. *Biomed. Pharmacother.* **55**:23–31.

Capparelli, E. V., S. L. Letendre, R. J. Ellis, P. Patel, D. Holland, and J. A. McCutchan. 2005. Population pharmacokinetics of abacavir in plasma and cerebrospinal fluid. *Antimicrob. Agents Chemother.* **49**:2504–2506.

Carr, A., K. Samaras, A. Thorisdottir, G. R. Kaufmann, D. J. Chisholm, and D. A. Cooper. 1999. Diagnosis, prediction, and natural course of HIV-1 protease-inhibitor-associated lipodystrophy, hyperlipidaemia, and diabetes mellitus: a cohort study. *Lancet* **353**:2093–2099.

Carr, J. M., A. J. Davis, F. Feng, C. J. Burrell, and P. Li. 2006. Cellular interactions of virion infectivity factor (Vif) as potential therapeutic targets: APOBEC3G and more? *Curr. Drug Targets* **7**:1583–1593.

Centers for Disease Control and Prevention. 1986. Classification system for human T-lymphotropic virus type III/lymphadenopathy-associated virus infections. *MMWR Morb. Mortal. Wkly. Rep.* **35**:34–39.

Chen, A. M., N. Khanna, S. A. Stohlman, and C. C. Bergmann. 2005. Virus-specific and bystander CD8 T cells recruited during virus-induced encephalomyelitis. *J. Virol.* **79**:4700–4708.

Chiesi, A., S. Vella, L. G. Dally, C. Pedersen, S. Danner, A. M. Johnson, S. Schwander, F. D. Goebel, M. Glauser, F. Antunes, and J. D. Lundgren for the AIDS in Europe Study Group. 1996. Epidemiology of AIDS dementia complex in Europe. *J. Acquir. Immun. Syndr. Hum. Retrovirol.* **11**:39–44.

Chowdhury, M., J. P. Taylor, C. F. Chang, J. Rappaport, and K. Khalili. 1992. Evidence that a sequence similar to TAR is important for induction of the JC virus late promoter by human immunodeficiency virus type 1 Tat. *J. Virol.* **66**:7355–7361.

Clements, J. E., M. Li, L. Gama, B. Bullock, L. M. Carruth, J. L. Mankowski, and M. C. Zink. 2005. The central nervous system is a viral reservoir in simian immunodeficiency virus-infected macaques on combined antiretroviral therapy: a model for human immunodeficiency virus patients on highly active antiretroviral therapy. *J. Neurovirol.* **11**:180–189.

Clifford, D. B., S. Evans, Y. Yang, E. P. Acosta, K. Goodkin, K. Tashima, D. Simpson, D. Dorfman, H. Ribaudo, and R. M. Gulick for the A5097s Study Team. 2005. Impact of efavirenz on neuropsychological performance and symptoms in HIV-infected individuals. *Ann. Intern. Med.* **143**:714–721.

Clifford, D. B., J. C. McArthur, G. Schifitto, K. Kieburtz, M. P. McDermott, S. Letendre, B. A. Cohen, K. Marder, R. J. Ellis, C. M. Marra, and the Neurologic AIDS Research Consortium. 2002. A randomized clinical trial of CPI-1189 for HIV-associated cognitive-motor impairment. *Neurology* **59**:1568–1573.

Concha, M., S. Symes, K. Goodkin, S. Nathan, P. Zortea, J. G. Romano, A. M. Forteza, and M. Kolber. 2003. Risk of cerebrovascular disease in HIV-1-infected subjects with lipodystrophy syndrome and long-term exposure to protease inhibitors Presented at the 28th International Stroke Conference, Phoenix, AZ, Feb 13–15, 2003, p. 213.

Cysique, L. A., P. Maruff, and B. J. Brew. 2006. Valproic acid is associated with cognitive decline in HIV-infected individuals: a clinical observational study. *BMC Neurol.* **6**:42.

Dana Consortium. 1998. A randomized, double-blind, placebo-controlled trial of deprenyl and thioctic acid in human immunodeficiency virus-associated cognitive impairment. *Neurology* **50**:645–651.

Dana Consortium. 1996. Clinical confirmation of the American Academy of Neurology algorithm for HIV-associated cognitive/motor disorder. *Neurology* **47**:1247–1253.

Digicaylioglu, M., M. Kaul, L. Fletcher, R. Dowen, and S. A. Lipton. 2004. Erythropoietin protects cerebrocortical neurons from HIV-1/gp120-induced damage. *Neuroreport* **15**:761–763.

Dore, G. J., A. McDonald, Y. Li, J. M. Kaldor, and B. J. Brew. 2003. Marked improvement in survival following AIDS dementia complex in the era of highly active antiretroviral therapy. *AIDS* **17**:1539–1545.

Ellis, R. J., A. C. Gamst, E. Capparelli, S. A. Spector, K. Hsia, T. Wolfson, I. Abramson, I. Grant, and J. A.McCutchan. 2000. Cerebrospinal fluid HIV RNA originates from both local CNS and systemic sources. *Neurology* **54**:927–936.

Eugenin, E. A., K. Osiecki, L. Lopez, H. Goldstein, T. M. Calderon, and J. W. Berman. 2006. CCL2/monocyte chemoattractant protein-1 mediates enhanced transmigration of human immunodeficiency virus (HIV)-infected leukocytes across the blood-brain barrier: a potential mechanism of HIV-CNS invasion and neuroAIDS. *J. Neurosci.* **26**:1098–1106.

Everall, I. P., C. Bell, M. Mallory, D. Langford, A. Adame, E. Rockestein, and E. Masliah. 2002. Lithium ameliorates HIV-gp120-mediated neurotoxicity. *Mol. Cell. Neurosci* **21**:493–501.

Evers, S., D. Nabavi, A. Rahmann, C. Heese, D. Reichelt, and I. W. Husstedt. 2003. Ischemic cerebrovascular events in HIV infection. *Cerebrovasc. Dis.* **15**:199–205.

Fernandez, F., F. Adams, and J. K. Levy. 1988. Cognitive impairment due to AIDS-related complex and its response to psychostimulants *Psychosomatics* **29**:38–46.

Ferrando, S., W. van Gorp, M. McElhiney, K. Goggin, M. Sewell, and J. Rabkin. 1998. Highly active antiretroviral treatment in HIV infection: benefits for neuropsychological function. *AIDS* **12**:F65.

Fiala, M., A. J. Eshleman, J. Cashman, J. Lin, A. S. Lossinsky, V. Suarez, W. Yang, J. Zhang, W. Popik, E. Singer, F. Chiappelli, E. Carro, M. Weinand, M. Witte, and J. Arthos. 2005. Cocaine increases human immunodeficiency virus type 1 neuroinvasion through remodeling brain microvascular endothelial cells. *J. Neurovirol.* **11**:281–291

Fliers, E., H. P. Sauerwein, J. A. Romijn, et al. 2003. HIV-associated adipose redistribution syndrome as a selective autonomic neuropathy. *Lancet* **362**:1758–1760.

Foster, H. D. 2004. How HIV-1 causes AIDS: implications for prevention and treatment. *Med. Hypotheses* **62**:549–553.

Fujimura, R. K., I. Khamis, P. Shapshak, and K. Goodkin. 2004. Regional quantitative comparison of multispliced to unspliced ratios of HIV-1 RNA copy number in infected human brain. *J. Neuro-AIDS* **2**:45–60.

Galgani, S., P. Balestra, P. Narciso, V. Tozzi, P. Sette, F. Pau, and G. Visco. 1997. Nimodipine plus zidovudine versus zidovudine alone in the treatment of HIV-1-associated cognitive deficits. *AIDS* **11**:1520–1521.

Gallego, L., P. Barreiro, R. del Río, D. González de Requena, A. Rodríguez-Albariño, J. González-Lahoz, et al. 2004. Analyzing sleep abnormalities in HIV-infected patients treated with efavirenz. *Clin. Infect. Dis.* **38**:430–432.

Giancola, M. L., P. Lorenzini, P. Balestra, D. Larussa, F. Baldini, A. Corpolongo, P. Narciso, R. Bellagamba, V. Tozzi, and A. Antinori. 2006. Neuroactive antiretroviral drugs do not influence neurocognitive performance in less advanced HIV-infected patients responding to highly active antiretroviral therapy. *J. Acquir. Immun. Defic. Syndr.* **41**:332–337.

Gisslen, M., L. Hagberg, B. J. Brew, P. Cinque, R. W. Price, and L. Rosengren. 2007. Elevated cerebrospinal fluid neurofilament light protein concentrations predict the development of AIDS dementia complex. *J. Infect. Dis.* **195**:1774–1778.

Giunta, B., D. Obregon, H. Hou, J. Zeng, N. Sun, V. Nikolic, J. Ehrhart, D. Shytle, F. Fernandez, and J. Tan. 2006. EGCG mitigates neurotoxicity mediated by HIV-1 proteins gp120 and Tat in the presence of IFN-γ: role of JAK/STAT1 signaling and implications for HIV-associated dementia. *Brain Res.* **1123:**216–225.

Gomph, S. 2005. Side effects in interferon and ribavirin therapy for chronic viral hepatitis. *e-Med. Hepatitis C Newsl.* **2.** http://www.emedicine.com/email/hepc/issue2.htm.

Gonzalez, E., H. Kulkarni, H. Bolivar, A. Mangano, R. Sanchez, G. Catano, R. J. Nibbs, B. I. Freedman, M. P. Quinones, M. J. Bamshad, K. K. Murthy, B. H. Rovin, W. Bradley, R. A. Clark, S. A. Anderson, R. J. O'Connell, B. K. Agan, S. S. Ahuja, R. Bologna, L. Sen, M. J. Dolan, and S. K. Ahuja. 2005. The influence of CCL3L1 gene-containing segmental duplications on HIV-1/AIDS susceptibility. *Science* **307:**1434–1440.

Gonzalez, E., B. H. Rovin, L. Sen, G. Cooke, R. Dhanda, S. Mummidi, H. Kulkarni, M. J. Bamshad, V. Telles, S. A. Anderson, E. A. Walter, K. T. Stephan, M. Deucher, A. Mangano, R. Bologna, S. S. Ahuja, M. J. Dolan, and S. K. Ahuja. 2002. HIV-1 infection and AIDS dementia are influenced by a mutant MCP-1 allele linked to increased monocyte infiltration of tissues and MCP-1 levels. *Proc. Natl. Acad. Sci. USA* **99:**137795–137800.

Goodkin, K., B. Vitiello, W. D. Lyman, D. Asthana, J. H. Atkinson, P. N. R. Heseltine, R. Molina, W. Zheng, I. Khamis, F. L. Wilkie, and P. Shapshak. 2006. Cerebrospinal and peripheral human immunodeficiency virus type1 load in a multi-site, randomized, double blind, placebo-controlled trial of D-ala1-peptide T-amide for associated cognitive-motor impairment. *J. Neurovirol.* **12:**178–189.

Goodkin, K., F. L. Wilkie, T. T. Baldewicz, M. Concha, M. D. Tyll, C. J. LoPiccolo, and P. Shapshak. 2000. HIV-1 associated cognitive-motor disorders: a research-based approach to diagnosis and treatment. *CNS Spectr.* **5:**49–60.

Goodkin, K., F. L. Wilkie, M. Concha, C. H. Hinkin, S. Symes, T. T. Baldewicz, D. Asthana, R. K. Fujimura, D. Lee, M. H. van Zuilen, I. Khamis, P. Shapshak, and C. Eisdorfer. 2001. Aging and neuro-AIDS conditions: a potential interaction with the changing spectrum of HIV-1 associated morbidity and mortality in the era of HAART? *J. Clin. Epidemiol.* **54**(Suppl. 1):S35–S43.

Gray, F., H. Adle-Biassette, F. Chretien, G. Lorin de la Grandmaison, G. Force, and C. Keohane. 2001. Neuropathology and neurodegeneration in human immunodeficiency virus infection. *Clin. Neuropathol.* **20:**146–155.

Grigem, S., P. Fischer-Posovszky, K. M. Debatin, E. Loizon, H. Vidal, and M. Wabitsch. 2005. The effect of the HIV protease inhibitor ritonavir on proliferation, differentiation, lipogenesis, gene expression and apoptosis of human preadipocytes and adipocytes. *Horm. Metab. Res.* **37:**602–609.

Grimwade, K., N. French, D. D. Mbatha, D. D. Zungu, M. Dedicoat, and C. F. Gilks. 2004. HIV infection as a cofactor for severe falciparum malaria in adults living in a region of unstable malaria transmission in South Africa. *AIDS* **18:**547–554.

Henderson, D. C., E. Cagliero, P. M. Copeland, C. P. Borba, E. Evins, D. Hayden, M. T. Weber, E. J. Anderson, D. B. Allison, T. B. Daley, D. Schoenfeld, and D. C. Goff. 2005. Glucose metabolism in patients with schizophrenia treated with atypical antipsychotic agents: a frequently sampled glucose tolerance test and minimal model analysis. *Arch. Gen. Psychiatry* **62:**19–28.

Henry, K., H. Melroe, J. Huebsch, J. Hermundson, C. Levine, L. Swensen, and J. Daly. 1998. Severe premature coronary artery disease with protease inhibitors. *Lancet* **351:**1328.

Herzlich, B. C., and T. D. Schiano. 1993. Reversal of apparent AIDS dementia complex following treatment with vitamin B$_{12}$. *J. Int. Med.* **233:**495–497.

Heseltine, P. N. R., K. Goodkin, J. H. Atkinson, B. Vitiello, J. Rochon, R. K. Heaton, E. Eaton, F. Wilkie, E. Sobel, S. Brown, D. Feaster, L. Schneider, E. Stover, and S. H. Koslow. 1998. Randomized, double-blind placebo-controlled trial of peptide T for HIV-associated cognitive impairment. *Arch. Neurol.* **55:**41–51.

Heyes, M. P., K. Saito, and S. P. Markey. 1992. Human macrophages convert L-tryptophan into the neurotoxin quinolinic acid. *J. Biochem.* **83:**633–635.

Hinkin, C. H., S. A. Castellon, D. J. Hardy, R. Farinpour, T. Newton, and E. Singer. 2001. Methylphenidate improves HIV-1-associated cognitive slowing. *J. Neuropsychiatry Clin. Neurosci.* **13:**248–254.

Ho, W., J. Harouse, R. Rando, E. Gonczol, A. Srinivasan, and S. Plotkin. 1990. Reciprocal enhancement of gene expression and viral replication between human cytomegalovirus and human immunodeficiency virus-1. *J. Gen. Virol.* **71:**97–103.

Jaworowski, A., D. D. Kamwendo, P. Ellery, S. Sonza, V. Mwapasa, E. Tadesse, M. E. Molyneux, S. J. Rogerson, S. R. Meshnick, and S. M. Crowe. 2007. CD16$^+$ monocyte subset preferentially harbors HIV-1 and is expanded in pregnant Malawian women with *Plasmodium falciparum* malaria and HIV-1 infection. *J. Infect. Dis.* **196:**38–42.

Kaul, M., and S. A. Lipton. 1999. Chemokines and activated macrophages in HIV gp120-induced neuronal apoptosis. *Proc. Natl. Acad. Sci. USA* **96:**8212–8216.

Kelder, W., J. C. McArthur, T. Nance-Sproson, D. McClernon, and D. E. Griffin. 1998. Beta-chemokines MCP-1 and RANTES are selectively increased in cerebrospinal fluid of patients with human immunodeficiency virus-associated dementia. *Ann. Neurol.* **44:**831–835.

Khan, N. A., F. Di Cello, A. Nath, and K. S. Kim. 2003. Human immunodeficiency virus type 1 tat-mediated cytotoxicity of human brain microvascular endothelial cells. *J. Neurovirol.* **9:**584–593.

Kieburtz, K. D., L. G. Epstein, H. A. Gelbard, and J. T. Greenamyre. 1991. Excitotoxicity and dopaminergic dysfunction in the acquired immunodeficiency syndrome dementia complex. *Arch. Neurol.* **48:**1281–1284.

Kilic, U., E. Kilic, G. P. Dietz, and M. Bahr. 2003. Intravenous TAT-GDNF is protective after focal cerebral ischemia in mice. *Stroke* **34:**1304–1310.

Klein, M. B., R. G. Lalonde, and S. Suissa. 2003. The impact of hepatitis C virus coinfection on HIV progression before and after highly active antiretroviral therapy. *J. Acquir. Immun. Defic. Syndr.* **33:**365–372.

Koutsilieri, E., S. Czub, C. Scheller, S. Sopper, T. Tatschner, C. Stahl-Hennig, V. ter Meulen, and P. Riederer. 2000. Brain choline acetyltransferase reduction in SIV infection. An index of early dementia? *Neuroreport* **11:**2391–2393.

Kumar, A. M., J. R. Berger, C. Eisdorfer, J. B. Fernandez, K. Goodkin, and M. Kumar. 2001. Cerebrospinal fluid 5-hydroxytryptamine and 5-hydroxyindoleacetic acid in HIV-1 infection. *Neuropsychobiology* **44:**13–18.

Lanjewar, D. N., P. P. Jain, and C. R. Shetty. 1998. Profile of central nervous system pathology in patients with AIDS: an autopsy study from India. *AIDS* **12:**309–313.

Larder, B. A., G. Darby, and D. D. Richman. 1989. HIV with reduced sensitivity to zidovudine (AZT) isolated during prolonged therapy. *Science* **243:**1731–1734.

Larsson, M., L. Hagberg, A. Forsman, and G. Norkrans. 1991. Cerebrospinal fluid catecholamine metabolites in HIV-infected patients. *J. Neurosci. Res.* **28:**406–409.

Le Buanec, H., A. Lachgar, B. Bizzini, J. F. Zagury, J. Rappaport, E. Santagostino, M. Muca-Perja, and A. Gringeri. 1998. A prophylactic and therapeutic AIDS vaccine containing as a component the innocuous Tat toxoid. *Biomed. Pharmacother.* **52:**431–435.

Lemoine, M., V. Barbu, P. M. Girard, M. Kim, J. P. Bastard, D. Wendum, F. Paye, C. Housset, J. Capeau, and L. Serfaty. 2006. Altered hepatic expression of SREBP-1 and PPARγ is associated with liver injury in insulin-resistant lipodystrophic HIV-infected patients. *AIDS* **20:**387–395.

LeTendre, S., B. Ances, S. Gibson, and R. J. Ellis. 2007. Neurologic complications of HIV disease and their treatment. *Topics HIV Med.* **15:**32–39.

LeTendre, S. L., S. P. Woods, R. J. Ellis, J. H. Atkinson, E. Masliah, G. van den Brande, J. Durelle, I. Grant, I. Everall, and the HNRC Group. 2006. Lithium improves HIV-associated neurocognitive impairment. *AIDS* **20:**1885–1888.

LeTendre, S. L., E. R. Lanier, and J. A. McCutchan. 1999. Cerebrospinal fluid beta chemokine concentrations in neurocognitively impaired individuals infected with human immunodeficiency virus type 1. *J. Infect. Dis.* **180:**310–319.

Lichtenstein, K. A., K. M. Delaney, C. Armon, D. J. Ward, A. C. Mourman, K. C. Wood, S. D. Holmberg, and HIV Outpatient Study Investigators. 2003. Incidence of and risk factors for lipoatrophy (abnormal fat loss) in ambulatory HIV-1-infected patients. *J. AIDS* **32:**48–56.

Lieb, K., M. A. Engelbrecht, O. Gut, B. L. Fiebich, J. Bauer, G. Janssen, and M. Schaefer. 2006. Cognitive impairment in patients with chronic hepatitis treated with interferon alpha (IFNα): results from a prospective study. *Eur. Psychiatry* **21:**204–210.

Lochet, P., H. Peyriere, A. Lotthé, J. M. Mauboussin, B. Delmas, and J. Reynes. 2003. Long-term assessment of neuropsychiatric adverse reactions associated with efavirenz. *HIV Med.* **4:**62–66.

Madruga, J. V., P. Cahn, B. Grinsztejn, R. Haubrich, J. Lalezari, A. Mills, G. Pialoux, T. Wilkin, M. Peeters, J. Vingerhoets, G. de Smedt, L. Leopold, R. Trefiglio, B. Woodfall, and the DUET-1 Study Group. 2007. Efficacy and safety of TMC125 (etravirine) in treatment-experienced HIV-1-infected patients in DUET-1: 24-week results from a randomised, double-blind, placebo-controlled trial. *Lancet* **370:**29–38.

Maggirwar, S. B., N. Tong, S. Ramirez, H. A. Gelbard, and S. Dewhurst. 1999. HIV-1 Tat-mediated activation of glycogen synthase kinase-3β contributes to Tat-mediated neurotoxicity. *J. Neurochem.* **73:**578–586.

Mana, P., D. Linares, S. Fordham, M. Staykova, and D. Willenborg. 2006. Deleterious role of IFNγ in a toxic model of central nervous system demyelination. *Am. J. Pathol.* **168:**1464–1473.

Martin, C., A. Sonnerborg, J. O. Svensson, and L. Stahle. 1999. Indinavir-based treatment of HIV-1 infected patients: Efficacy in the central nervous system. *AIDS* **13:**1227–1232.

McArthur, J. C., D. R. McClernon, M. F. Cronin, T. E. Nance-Sproson, A. J. Saah, M. St Clair, and E. R. Lanier. 1997. Relationship between human immunodeficiency virus-associated dementia and viral load in cerebrospinal fluid and brain. *Ann. Neurol.* **42:**689–698.

McArthur, J. C., D. R. Hoover, H. Bacellar, E. N. Miller, B. A. Cohen, J. T. Becker, N. M. Graham, J. H. McArthur, O. A. Selnes, L. P. Jacobson, B. R. Visscher, M. Concha, and A. Saah. 1993. Dementia in AIDS patients: incidence and risk factors. Multicenter AIDS Cohort Study. *Neurology* **43:**2245–2252.

McDowell, J. A., G. E. Chittick, J. R. Ravitch, R. E. Polk, T. M. Kerkering, and D. S. Stein. 1999. Pharmacokinetics of [(14)C]abacavir, a human immunodeficiency virus type 1 (HIV-1) reverse transcriptase inhibitor, administered in a single oral dose to HIV-1-infected adults: a mass balance study. *Antimicrob. Agents. Chemother.* **43:**2855–2861.

McNair, D. M., M. Lorr, and L. F. Droppleman. 1971. *Profile of Mood States Manual.* Educational Industrial Testing Service, San Diego, CA.

Mellgren, A., R. W. Price, L. Hagberg, L. Rosengren, B. J. Brew, and M. Gisslen. 2007. Antiretroviral treatment reduces increased CSF neurofilament protein (NFL) in HIV-1 infection. *Neurology* **69:**1536–1541.

Miller, R. F., P. G. Isaacson, M. Hall-Craggs, S. Lucas, F. Gray, F. Scaravilli, and S. F. An. 2004. Cerebral CD8+ lymphocytosis in HIV-1 infected patients with immune restoration induced by HAART. *Acta Neuropathol.* **108:**17–23.

Mohsen, A. H., P. J. Easterbrook, C. Taylor, B. Portmann, R. Kulasegaram, S. Murad, M. Wiselka, and S. Norris. 2003. Impact of human immunodeficiency virus (HIV) infection on the progression of liver fibrosis in hepatitis C virus infected patients. *Gut* **52:**1035–1040.

Moog, C., G. Kuntz-Simon, C. Caussin-Schwemling, and G. Obert. 1996. Sodium valproate, an anticonvulsant drug, stimulates human immunodeficiency virus type 1 replication independently of glutathione levels. *J. Gen. Virol.* **77:**1993–1999.

Moyle, G. 2005. A review of the aetiology of dyslipidaemia and hyperlipidaemia in patients with HIV. *Int. J. STD AIDS* **16**(Suppl. 1)**:**14–22.

Mulligan, K., Y. Yang, D. A. Wininger, S. L. Koletar, R. A. Parker, B. L. Alston-Smith, J. T. Schouten, R. A. Fielding, M. T. Basar, and S. Grinspoon. 2007. Effects of metformin and rosiglitazone in HIV-infected patients with hyperinsulinemia and elevated waist/hip ratio. *AIDS* **21:**47–57.

Nance, C. L., and W. T. Shearer. 2003. Is green tea good for HIV-1 infection? *J. Allergy Clin. Immunol.* **112:**851–853.

Navia, B. A., U. Dafni, D. Simpson, T. Tucker, E. Singer, J. C. McArthur, C. Yiannoutsos, L. Zaborski, and S. A. Lipton. 1998. A phase I/II trial of nimodipine for HIV-related complications. *Neurology* **51:**221–228.

Navia, B. A., B. D Jordan, and R. W. Price. 1986a. The AIDS dementia complex. I. Clinical features. *Ann. Neurol.* **91:**517–524.

Navia, B. A., E.-S. Cho, C. K. Petito, and R. W. Price. 1986b. The AIDS dementia complex. II. Neuropathology. *Ann. Neurol.* **91:**525–535.

Neuenburg, J. K., H. R. Brodt, B. G. Herndier, M. Bickel, P. Bacchetti, R. W. Price, R. M. Grant, and W. Schlote. 2002. HIV-related neuropathology, 1985 to 1999: rising prevalence of HIV encephalopathy in the era of highly active antiretroviral therapy. *J. Acquir. Immun. Defic. Syndr.* **31:**171–177.

Nosheny, R. L., A. Bachis, S. A. Aden, M. A. De Bernardi, and I. Mocchetti. 2006. Intrastriatal administration of human immunodeficiency virus-1 glycoprotein 120 reduces glial cell-line derived neurotrophic factor levels and causes apoptosis in the substantia nigra. *J. Neurobiol.* **66:**1311–1321.

Osborn, L., S. Kunkel, and G. J. Nabel. 1989. Tumor necrosis factor alpha and interleukin-1 stimulate the human immunodeficiency virus enhancer by activation of the nuclear factor KB. *Proc. Natl. Acad. Sci. USA* **86:**2336–2340.

Pavol, M. A., C. A. Meyers, J. L. Rexer, A. D. Valentine, P. J. Mattis, and M. Talpaz. 1995. Pattern of neurobehavioral deficits with interferon alpha therapy for leukemia. *Neurology* **45:**947–950.

Pereira, C. F., J. Middel, G. Jansen, J. Verhoef, and H. S. Nottet. 2001. Enhanced expression of fractalkine in HIV-1 associated dementia. *J. Neuroimmunol.* **115:**168–175.

Petito, C. K., J. E. Torres-Munoz, F. Zielger, and M. McCarthy. 2006. Brain CD8+ and cytotoxic T lymphocytes are associated with, and may be specific for, human immunodeficiency virus type 1 encephalitis in patients with acquired immunodeficiency syndrome. *J. Neurovirol.* **12:**272–283.

Petito, C. K., B. Adkins, M. McCarthy, and B. Roberts. 2003. Khamis I. CD4+ and CD8+ cells accumulate in the brains of acquired immunodeficiency syndrome patients with human immunodeficiency virus encephalitis. *J. Neurovirol.* **9:**36–44.

Petito, C. K., and B. Roberts. 1995. Evidence of apoptotic cell death in HIV encephalitis. *Am. J. Pathol.* **146:**1121–1130.

Popko, B., J. G. Corbin, K. D. Baerwald, J. Dupree, and A. M. Garcia. 1997. The effects of interferon-gamma on the central nervous system. *Mol.c Neurobiol.* **14:**19–35.

Poulter, M. O., K. B. Payne, and J. P. Steiner. 2004. Neuroimmunophilins: a novel drug therapy for the reversal of neurodegenerative disease? *Neuroscience* **128:**1–6.

Poutiainen, E., L. Hokkanen, M. L. Niemi, and M. Farkkila. 1994. Reversible cognitive decline during high-dose alpha-interferon treatment. *Pharmacol. Biochem. Behavior* **47:**901–905.

Pumfery, A., C. de la Fuente, R. Berro, S. Nekhai, F. Kashanchi, and S. H. Chao. 2006. Potential use of pharmacological cyclin-dependent kinase inhibitors as anti-HIV therapeutics. *Curr. Pharm. Des.* **12:**1949–1961.

Ranga, U., R. Shankarappa, N. B. Siddappa, L. Ramakrishna, R. Nagendran, M. Mahalingam, A. Mahadevan, N. Jayasuryan, P. Satishchandra, S. K. Shankar, and V. R. Prasad. 2004. Tat protein of human immunodeficiency virus type 1 subtype C strains is a defective chemokine. *J. Virol.* **78:**2586–2590.

Ricardo-Dukelow, M., I. Kadiu, W. Rozek, J. Schlautman, Y. Persidsky, P. Ciborowski, G. D. Kanmogne, and H. E. Gendelman. 2007. HIV-1 infected monocyte-derived macrophages affect the human brain microvascular endothelial cell proteome: new insights into blood-brain barrier dysfunction for HIV-1-associated dementia. *J. Neuroimmunol.* **185:**37–46.

Robertson, K. R., M. Smurzynski, T. D. Parsons, K. Wu, R. J. Bosch, J. Wu, J. C. McArthur, A. C. Collier, S. R. Evans, and R. J. Ellis. 2007. The prevalence and incidence of neurocognitive impairment in the HAART era. *AIDS* **21:**1915–1921.

Ruff, M. R., L. M. Melendez-Guerrero, Q. E. Yang, W. Z. Ho, J. W. Mikovits, C. B. Pert, and F. A. Ruscetti. 2001. Peptide T inhibits HIV-1 infection mediated by the chemokine receptor-5 (CCR5). *Antivir. Res.* **52:**63–75.

Saavedra-Lozano, J., J. T. Ramos, F. Sanz, M. L. Navarro, M. I. de Jose, P. Martin-Fontelos, M. J. Mellado, J. A. Leal, C. Rodriguez, I. Luque, S. J. Madison, D. Irlbeck, E. R. Lanier, and O. Ramilo. 2006. Salvage therapy with abacavir and other reverse transcriptase inhibitors for human immunodeficiency-associated encephalopathy. *Pediatr. Infect. Dis. J.* **25:**1142–1152.

Sabri, F., A. De Milito, R. Pirskanen, I. Elovaara, L. Hagberg, P. Cinque, R. Price, and F. Chiodi. 2001. Elevated levels of soluble Fas and Fas ligand in cerebrospinal fluid of patients with AIDS dementia complex. *J. Neuroimmunol.* **114:**197–206.

Sacktor, N., M. P. McDermott, K. Marder, G. Schifitto, O. A. Selnes, J. C. McArthur, Y. Stern, S. Albert, D. Palumbo, K. Kieburtz, J. A. De Marcaida, B. Cohen, and L. Epstein. 2002. HIV-associated cognitive impairment before and after the advent of combination therapy. *J. Neurovirol.* **8:**136–142.

Sacktor, N., R. H. Lyles, R. Skolasky, C. Kleeberger, O. A. Selnes, E. N. Miller, J. T. Becker, B. Cohen, and J. C. McArthur. 2001. HIV-associated neurologic disease incidence changes: Multicenter AIDS Cohort Study, 1990–1998. *Neurology* **56:**257–260.

Sacktor, N., G. Schifitto, M. P. McDermott, K. Marder, J. C. McArthur, and K. Kieburtz. 2000. Transdermal selegiline in HIV-associated cognitive impairment: pilot, placebo-controlled study. *Neurology* **54:**233–235.

Sacktor, N. C., R. H. Lyles, R. L. Skolasky, D. E. Anderson, J. C. McArthur, G. McFarlane, O. A. Selnes, J. T. Becker, B. Cohen, J. Wesch, and E. N. Miller. 1999. Combination antiretroviral therapy improves psychomotor speed performance in HIV-seropositive homosexual men. *Neurology* **52:**1640–1647.

Sardar, A. M., C. Czudek, and G. P. Reynolds. 1996. Dopamine deficits in the brain: the neurochemical basis of parkinsonian symptoms in AIDS. *Neuroreport* **7:**910–912.

Sas, A. R., H. A. Bimonte-Nelson, and W. R. Tyor. 2007. Cognitive dysfunction in HIV encephalitic SCID mice correlates with levels of interferon-alpha in the brain. *AIDS* **21:**2151–2159.

Sax, P. E., R. Islam, R. P. Walensky, E. Losina, M. C. Weinstein, S. J. Goldie, S. N. Sadownik, and K. A. Freedberg. 2005. Should resistance testing be performed for treatment-naive HIV-infected patients? A cost-effectiveness analysis. *Clin. Infect. Dis.* **41:**1316–1323.

Schifitto, G., B. A. Navia, C. T. Yiannoutsos, C. M. Marra, L. Chang, T. Ernst, J. G. Jarvik, E. N. Miller, E. J. Singer, R. J. Ellis, D. L. Kolson, D. Simpson, A. Nath, J. Berger, S. L. Shriver, L. L. Millar, D. Colquhoun, R. Lenkinski, R. G. Gonzalez, S. A. Lipton, and the Adult AIDS Clinical Trial Group (ACTG) 301, 700 Teams, and the HIV MRS Consortium. 2007. Memantine and HIV-associated cognitive impairment: a neuropsychological and proton magnetic resonance spectroscopy study. *AIDS* **21:**1877–1886.

Schifitto, G., D. R. Peterson, J. Zhong, H. Ni, K. Cruttenden, M. Gaugh, H. E. Gendelman, M. Boska, and H. Gelbard. 2006. Valproic acid adjunctive therapy for HIV-associated cognitive impairment: a first report. *Neurology* **66:**919–921.

Schifitto, G., N. Sacktor, K. Marder, M. P. McDermott, J. C. McArthur, K. Kieburtz, S. Small, and L. G. Epstein. 1999. Randomized trial of the platelet-activating factor antagonist lexipafant in HIV-associated cognitive impairment. *Neurology* **53:**391–396.

Schmitt, F. A., J. W. Bigley, R. McKinnis, P. E. Logue, R. W. Evans, and J. L. Drucker. 1988. Neuropsychological outcome of zidovudine (AZT) treatment of patients with AIDS and AIDS-related complex. *N. Engl. J. Med.* **319:**1573–1578.

Sevigny, J. J., S. M. Albert, M. P. McDermott, J. C. McArthur, N. Sacktor, K. Conant, G. Schifitto, O. A. Selnes, Y. Stern, D. R. McClernon, D. Palumbo, K. Kieburtz, G. Riggs, B. Cohen, L. G. Epstein, and K. Marder. 2004. Evaluation of HIV RNA and markers of immune activation as predictors of HIV-associated dementia. *Neurology* **63:**2084–2090.

Shapshak, P., S. M. Segal, K. A. Crandall, R. K. Fujimura, B.-T. Zhang, K.-Q. Xin, K. Okuda, C. K. Petito, C. Eisdorfer, and K. Goodkin. 1999. Independent evolution of HIV type 1 in different brain regions. *AIDS Res. Hum. Retrovir.* **15:**811–820.

Sibson, N. R., A. M. Blamire, V. H. Perry, J. Gauldie, P. Styles, and D. C. Anthony. 2002. TNF-alpha reduces cerebral blood volume and disrupts tissue homeostasis via an endothelin- and TNFR2-dependent pathway. *Brain* **125:**2446–2459.

Sidtis, J. J., C. Gatsonis, R. W. Price, E. J. Singer, A. C. Collier, D. D. Richman, M. S. Hirsch, F. W. Schaerf, M. A. Fischl, K. Kieburtz, et al. 1993. Zidovudine treatment of the AIDS dementia complex: results of a placebo-controlled trial. *Ann. Neurol.* **33:**343–349.

Singh, D., and K. Goodkin. 2007a. Choice of antipsychotic medications in HIV-infected patients. *J. Clin. Psychiatry* **68:**479–480.

Singh, D., and K. Goodkin. 2007b. Psychopharmacologic treatment responses of HIV-infected patients to antipsychotic medications. *J. Clin. Psychiatry* **68:**631–632.

Snider, W. D., D. M. Simpson, S. Nielsen, J. W. Gold, C. E. Metroka, and J. B. Posner. 1983. Neurological complications of acquired immune deficiency syndrome: analysis of 50 patients. *Ann. Neurol.* **14:**403–418.

Stahle, L., C. Martin, J. O. Svensson, and A. Sonnerborg. 1997. Indinavir in cerebrospinal fluid of HIV-1 infected patients. *Lancet* **350:**1823.

Stankov, M. V., T. Lucke, A. M. Das, R. E. Schmidt, and G. M. Behrens. 2007. Relationship of mitochondrial DNA depletion and respiratory chain activity in preadipocytes treated with nucleoside reverse transcriptase inhibitors. *Antivir. Ther.* **12:**205–216.

Stephens, E. B., S. V. Joag, B. Atkinson, M. Sahni, Z. Li, L. Foresman, I. Adany, and O. Narayan. 1997. Infected macaques that controlled replication of SIVmac or nonpathogenic SHIV developed sterilizing resistance against pathogenic SHIV(KU-1). *Virology* **234:**328–339.

Stephensen, C. B., G. S. Marquis, S. D. Douglas, L. A. Kruzich, and C. M. Wilson. 2007. Glutathione, glutathione peroxidase, and selenium status in HIV-positive and HIV-negative adolescents and young adults. *Am. J. Clin. Nutr.* **85:**173–181.

Tan, B., D. Piwnica-Worms, and L. Ratner. 2000. Multidrug resistance transporters and modulation. *Curr. Opin. Oncol.* **12:**450–458.

Tashima, K. T., A. M. Caliendo, M. Ahmad, J. M. Gormley, W. D. Fiske, J. M. Brennan, and T. P. Flanigan. 1999. Cerebrospinal fluid human immunodeficiency virus type 1 (HIV-1) suppression and efavirenz drug concentrations in HIV-1-infected patients receiving combination therapy. *J. Infect. Dis.* **180:**862–864.

Theodore, S., W. A. Cass, A. Nath, J. Steiner, K. Young, and W. F. Maragos. 2006. Inhibition of tumor necrosis factor-alpha signaling prevents human immunodeficiency virus-1 protein Tat and methamphetamine interaction. *Neurobiol. Dis.* **23:**663–668.

Thomas, S. A., and M. B. Segal. 1998. The transport of the anti-HIV drug 2′,3′-didehydro-3′-deoxythymidine (d4T) across the blood-brain and blood-cerebrospinal fluid barriers. *Br. J. Pharmacol.* **125:**49–54.

Thornton, C. A., S. Houston, and A. S. Latif. 1992. Neurocysticercosis and human immunodeficiency virus infection. A possible association. *Arch. Neurol.* **49:**963–965.

Toborek, M., Y. W. Lee, G. Flora, H. Pu, I. E. Andras, E. Wylegala, B. Hennig, and A. Nath. 2005. Mechanisms of the blood-brain barrier disruption in HIV-1 infection. *Cell. Mol. Neurobiol.* **25:**181–199.

Tomac, A., E. Lindqvist, L.-F. H. Lin, S. O. Ogren, D. Young, B. J. Hoffer, and L. Olson. 1995. Protection and repair of the nigrostriatal dopaminergic system by GDNF in vivo. *Nature* **373:**335–339.

Tong, N., J. F. Sanchez, S. B. Maggirwar, S. H. Ramirez, H. Guo, S. Dewhurst, and H. A. Gelbard. 2001. Activation of glycogen synthase kinase 3 beta (GSK-3β) by platelet activating factor mediates migration and cell death in cerebellar granule neurons. *Eur. J. Neurosci.* **13:**1913–1922.

Toossi, Z., H. Mayanja-Kizza, S. D. Lawn, C. S. Hirsch, L. D. Lupo, and S. T. Butera. 2007. Dynamic variation in the cellular origin of HIV type 1 during treatment of tuberculosis in dually infected subjects. *AIDS Res. Hum. Retrovir.* **23:**93–100.

Tozzi, V., P. Balestra, S. Galgani, P. Narciso, A. Sampaolesi, A. Antinori, M. Giulianelli, D. Serraino, and G. Ippolito. 2001. Changes in neurocognitive performance in a cohort of patients treated with HAART for 3 years. *J. Acquir. Immun. Defic. Syndr.* **28:**19–27.

Tyor, W. R., and L. D. Middaugh. 1999. Do alcohol and cocaine abuse alter the course of HIV-associated dementia complex? *J. Leukoc. Biol.* **65:**475–481.

Vago, L., A. Castagna, A. Lazzarin, G. Trabattoni, P. Cinque, and G. Costanzi. 1993. Reduced frequency of HIV-induced brain lesions in AIDS patients treated with zidovudine. *J. Acquir. Immun. Defic. Syndr.* **6:**42–45.

Valcour, V., C. Shikuma, B. Shiramizu, M. Watters, P. Poff, O. Selnes, P. Holck, J. Grove, and N. Sacktor. 2004. Higher frequency of dementia in older HIV-1 individuals: the Hawaii Aging with HIV-1 Cohort. *Neurology* **63:**822–827.

Valcour, V. G., C. M. Shikuma, B. T. Shiramizu, A. E. Williams, M. R. Watters, P. W. Poff, J. S. Grove, O. A. Selnes, and N. C. Sacktor. 2005. Diabetes, insulin resistance, and dementia among HIV-1-infected patients. *J. Acquir. Immun. Defic. Syndr.* **38:**31–36.

van Asten, L., and M. Prins. 2004. Infection with concurrent multiple hepatitis C virus genotypes is associated with faster HIV disease progression. *AIDS* **18:**2319–2324.

van der Meer, P., A. M. Ulrich, F. Gonalez-Scarano, and E. Lavi. 2000. Immunohistochemical analysis of CCR2, CCR3, CCR5, and CXCR4 in the human brain: potential mechanisms for HIV dementia. *Exp. Mol. Pathol.* **69:**192–201.

van Dyck, C. H., T. J. McMahon, M. I. Rosen, S. S. O'Malley, P. G. O'Connor, C. H. Lin, H. R. Pearsall, S. W. Woods, and T. R. Kosten. 1997. Sustained-release methylphenidate for cognitive impairment in HIV-1-infected drug abusers: a pilot study. *J. Neuropsychiatry Clin. Neurosci.* **9:**29–36.

Vazeux, R., M. Cumont, P. M. Girard, X. Nassif, P. Trotot, C. Marche, L. Matthiessen, C. Vedrenne, J. Mikol, D. Henin, et al. 1990. Severe encephalitis resulting from coinfections with HIV and JC virus. *Neurology* **40:**944–948.

Vendrely, A., B. Bienvenu, J. Gasnault, J. B. Thiebault, D. Salmon, and F. Gray. 2005. Fulminant inflammatory leukoencephalopathy associated with HAART-induced immune restoration in AIDS-related progressive multifocal leukoencephalopathy. *Acta Neuropathol.* **109:**449–455.

Vergote, D., G. S. Butler, M. Ooms, J. H. Cox, C. Silva, M. D. Hollenberg, J. H. Jhamandas, C. M. Overall, and C. Power. 2006. Proteolytic processing of SDF-1α reveals a change in receptor specificity mediating HIV-associated neurodegeneration. *Proc. Natl. Acad. Sci. USA* **103:**19182–19187.

Vigouroux, C., S. Gharakhanian, Y. Salhi, et al. 1999. Diabetes, insulin resistance and dyslipidaemia in lipodystrophic HIV-infected patients on highly active antiretroviral therapy (HAART). *Diabetes Metab.* **25:**225–232.

Wachtman, L. M., R. L. Skolasky, P. M. Tarwater, D. Esposito, G. Schifitto, K. Marder, M. P. McDermott, B. A. Cohen, A. Nath, N. Sacktor, L. G. Epstein, J. L. Mankowski, and J. C. McArthur. 2007. Platelet decline: an avenue for investigation into the pathogenesis of human immunodeficiency virus-associated dementia. *Arch. Neurol.* **64:**1264–1272.

Wesselingh, S., C. Power, J. Glass, et al. 1993. Intracerebral cytokine mRNA expression in AIDS dementia. *Ann. Neurol.* **33:**576–582.

Westmoreland, S. V., D. Kolson, and F. Gonzalez-Scarano. 1996. Toxicity of TNF alpha and platelet activating factor for human NT2N neurons: a tissue culture model for human immunodeficiency virus dementia. *J. Neurovirol.* **2:**118–126.

Wilkinson, I. D., W. K. Chong, M. Paley, J. K. Shepherd, R. J. S. Chinn, R. F. Miller, B. Sweeney, B. E. Kendall, M. A. Hall-Craggs, and M. J. G. Harrison. 1996. Blood-brain barrier integrity in HIV infection: Evaluation by contrast-enhanced magnetic resonance imaging. *J. Neuro-AIDS* **1:**17–31.

Wilt, S. G., E. Milward, J. M. Zhou, K. Nagasato, H. Patton, R. Rusten, D. E. Griffin, M. O'Connor, and M. Dubois-Dalcq. 1995. In vitro evidence for a dual role of tumor necrosis factor-α in human immunodeficiency virus type 1 encephalopathy. *Ann. Neurol.* **37:**381–394.

Wohl, D. A., D. Zeng, P. Stewart, N. Glomb, T. Alcorn, S. Jones, J. Handy, S. Fiscus, A. Weinberg, D. Gowda, and C. van der Horst. 2005. Cytomegalovirus viremia, mortality, and end-organ disease among patients with AIDS receiving potent antiretroviral therapies. *J. Acquir. Immun. Defic. Syndr.* **38:**538–544.

Yarchoan, R., J. M. Pluda, R. V. Thomas, et al. 1990. Long-term toxicity/activity profile of 2′,3′-dideoxyinosine in AIDS or AIDS-related complex. *Lancet* **336:**526–529.

Yepthomi, T., R. Paul, S. Vallabhaneni, N. Kumarasamy, D. F. Tate, S. Solomon, and T. Flanigan. 2006. Neurocognitive consequences of HIV in southern India: a preliminary study of clade C virus. *J. Int. Neuropsych. Soc.* **12:**424–430.

Zelman, I. B., and M. J. Mossakowski. 1998. Opportunistic infections of the central nervous system in the course of acquired immune deficiency syndrome (AIDS). Morphological analysis of 172 cases. *Folia Neuropathol.* **36:**129–144.

Zhu, T., H. Mo, N. Wang, D. S. Nam, Y. Cao, R. A. Koup, and D. D. Ho. 1993. Genotypic and phenotypic characterization of HIV-1 patients with primary infection. *Science* **261:**1179–1181.

Zink, M. C., J. Uhrlaub, J. DeWitt, T. Voelker, B. Bullock, J. Mankowski, P. Tarwater, J. Clements, and S. Barber. 2005. Neuroprotective and anti-human immunodeficiency virus activity of minocycline. *JAMA* **293:**2003–2011.

The Spectrum of Neuro-AIDS Disorders:
Pathophysiology, Diagnosis, and Treatment
Edited by K. Goodkin et al.
©2008 ASM Press, Washington, DC

2

Evolution of Neuropsychological Issues in HIV-1 Infection during the HAART Era

THOMAS D. MARCOTTE AND J. COBB SCOTT

Neurocognitive impairment is a common sequela of infection with human immunodeficiency virus type 1 (HIV-1). In the era preceding the introduction of highly active antiretroviral therapy (HAART), approximately 30% of medically asymptomatic individuals exhibited some form of cognitive impairment; that number rose to 55% in individuals with an AIDS-defining illness (Heaton et al., 1995). Since the advent of HAART, there has been a dramatic increase in the time from infection to a diagnosis of AIDS, as well as subsequent death (Detels et al., 1998; Porter et al., 2003). Although HAART has impacted the development of central nervous system (CNS) disorders (Deutsch et al., 2001; Robertson et al., 2004; Sacktor et al., 2001), the benefit from treatment may not equal that seen for other AIDS conditions (Dore et al., 1999; Sacktor et al., 2002). Many new antiretroviral medications have poor blood-brain penetration (Antinori et al., 2002; Letendre et al., 2004) and may leave the CNS as a potential reservoir for HIV-1 replication. HIV-1 encephalopathy still occurs (Neuenburg et al., 2002), and HIV-1-associated cognitive disorders remain a significant clinical concern (Sacktor et al., 2002).

Here, we summarize the neuropsychological (NP) findings from the HAART and pre-HAART eras, including a discussion of the impact that impairment has on "real-world" functioning. We also include findings from the HIV Neurobehavioral Research Center (HNRC), a National Institute of Mental Health-funded center studying the prevalence, features, course, and pathogenesis of HIV-1 involvement in the CNS.

DEFINITION OF HIV-ASSOCIATED NEUROCOGNITIVE DISORDERS

Neurocognitive complications associated with HIV range from subtle, "subsyndromic" or "asymptomatic" deficits to HIV-associated dementia (HAD), a severe and debilitating dementia that significantly affects activities of daily living. Historically, two different, though similar, criteria were proposed by Grant and Atkinson (1995) and the American Academy of Neurology (AAN) AIDS Task Force (1991). Grant and Atkinson proposed the following taxonomy (1995):

Neurocognitive deficit. An individual is impaired on tests of a single ability area (e.g., learning). In this case, the person would be said to have a learning deficit.

Neurocognitive impairment. An individual has impairment in at least *two* cognitive domains. At this point the person is considered to have a true neurocognitive abnormality, since a focal deficit in a single cognitive ability domain does not qualify one for "global" neurocognitive impairment (American Academy of Neurology AIDS Task Force, 1991; American Psychiatric Association, 1994; Grant and Atkinson, 1995).

Neurocognitive disorder. The term "neurocognitive disorder" is applied when the impairment is considered to be "clinically meaningful" (i.e., the patient is experiencing difficulties with everyday functioning).

With respect to HIV-associated neurocognitive disorders, a diagnosis of *minor cognitive motor disorder* (MCMD; AAN AIDS Task Force, 1991) or *minor neurocognitive disorder* (MND; Grant and Atkinson, 1995) requires objective evidence of NP impairments that cause noticeable difficulty in the execution of everyday activities. The criteria for *HIV-associated dementia* (HAD) are similar but require more severe cognitive impairment and marked disruption in everyday functions (AAN AIDS Task Force, 1991; Grant and Atkinson, 1995). In each of these diagnostic categories, the impairment, in the opinion of the diagnosing clinician, cannot be attributable to a comorbid condition and must represent a decline from previous functioning.

In 2006 the National Institute of Mental Health and National Institute of Neurological Diseases and Stroke organized a workgroup to revisit the AAN criteria (Antinori et al., 2007), based in part on the apparent changes in HIV-associated neurocognitive disorders (HAND) seen in

Thomas D. Marcotte, Department of Psychiatry, HIV Neurobehavioral Research Center, University of California, San Diego, San Diego, CA 92103. **J. Cobb Scott,** HIV Neurobehavioral Research Center, University of California, San Diego, San Diego, CA 92103.

the HAART era and on perceived limitations to the AAN criteria. Consistent with the Grant and Atkinson (1995) schema, the new criteria emphasize the neurocognitive complications of these conditions, excluding the motor, social/personality, and emotional abnormalities that were part of the AAN criteria. Preliminary data suggest that this focus may improve the sensitivity to HIV-related brain changes (Cherner et al., 2007).

Another important aspect of the revised nosology is the inclusion of the mildest ("asymptomatic") form of neuropsychological impairment, in which individuals evidence objective cognitive impairment, but it does not significantly affect everyday functioning (Grant and Atkinson, 1995). These impairments may still predict mortality (Ellis et al., 1997) and brain pathology. Individuals with these impairments may warrant close monitoring for possible cognitive worsening, as well as consideration of different treatment regimens.

The revised criteria for HAND are as follows. As with the earlier criteria, for each diagnosis the cognitive impairment cannot be explained by other comorbidities, nor be the result of a delirium.

Asymptomatic neurocognitive impairment (ANI). Performance needs to be at least 1 standard deviation (SD) below the mean of demographically adjusted normative scores in at least two cognitive domains (attention-information processing, language, abstraction-executive, complex perceptual motor skills, memory [including learning and recall], simple motor skills, *or* sensory perceptual abilities). At least five cognitive domains need to be assessed.

Minor neurocognitive disorder (MND). MND meets the ANI criteria above. In addition, the neurocognitive abnormality must result in at least mildly impaired everyday functioning and cannot meet criteria for dementia.

HIV-associated dementia (HAD). HAD requires (i) acquired moderate-to-severe cognitive impairment (at least 2 SD below demographically corrected normative means in at least two different cognitive areas [see above]) and (ii) marked difficulty in everyday functioning due to the cognitive impairment.

In remission was included as a qualifier for ANI, MND, and HAD because of the apparent fluctuating nature of neurocognitive impairment in some individuals (see below). In addition, the workgroup clarified potential confounding conditions and emphasized the importance of using appropriate normative data in determining neurocognitive status.

THE OVERALL IMPACT OF HAART ON COGNITIVE FUNCTIONING

As noted above, in the pre-HAART era, neurobehavioral complications were found in approximately 30% to 50% of individuals infected with HIV-1, with greater proportions of cognitive impairments emerging in late disease stages (Heaton et al., 1995; McArthur and Grant, 1998; White et al., 1995). HAART has provided substantial improvements in the systemic health of HIV-1-infected individuals and may improve cognition as well. For example, in an early study, Deutsch and colleagues (2001) examined 46 participants from the HAART and pre-HAART eras who had undergone extensive NP assessments at the HNRC. Twice as many pre-HAART subjects became impaired as in the HAART group, with a concomitant shorter time to impairment (Fig. 1). A study using data from the Multicenter

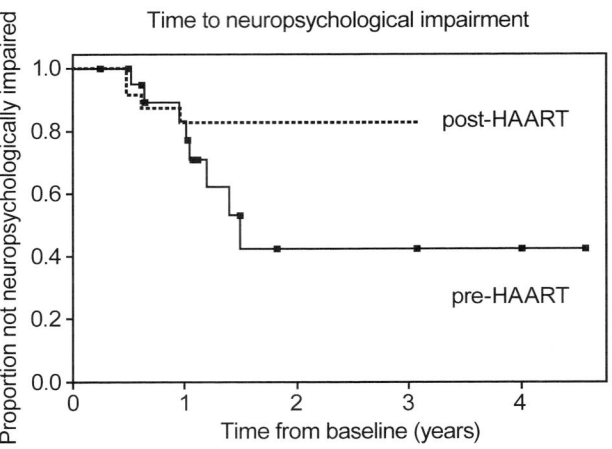

FIGURE 1 Estimate for distribution of time to neurocognitive impairment (in years) on or prior to 31 December 1995 (pre-HAART) versus on or after 1 January 1996 (post-HAART). (From Deutsch et al., 2001.)

AIDS Cohort Study found that the incidence of dementia declined by about 50% compared to the early 1990s (Sacktor et al., 2001).

A number of cross-sectional (e.g., Ferrando et al., 1998) and longitudinal (e.g., Cohen et al., 2001; Letendre et al., 2004; Marra et al., 2003; Robertson et al., 2004) studies have also shown that NP functioning improves with HAART. Medications with greater blood-brain barrier penetration may be more effective at reducing the HIV-1 viral load in the cerebrospinal fluid (CSF) and improving cognition than less-penetrating antiretroviral drugs (Letendre et al., 2004; Letendre et al., 2007), though the importance of penetrability is still uncertain (Cysique et al., 2004a; Robertson et al., 2004). Patients on HAART perform better in many cognitive domains (Ferrando et al., 1998; Tozzi et al., 1999), with the most consistent finding being improvement in psychomotor speed (Ferrando et al., 2003; Suarez et al., 2001). These improvements appear to be generally sustainable, though not universal (Tozzi et al., 1999, 2001), and the continuation of cognitive deficits in some patients suggests that damage may be irreparable or that there is an ongoing process in the CNS (Tozzi et al., 2001).

Although the incidence of dementia has declined, the increased longevity of HIV-1-infected individuals and the possible development of antiretroviral-drug resistance may result in a continued high prevalence of the disorder (Cysique et al., 2004a; Dore et al., 1999; Sacktor et al., 2002; Tozzi et al., 2001).

Course of Impairment

HIV-1 enters the CNS early in the course of infection (Sonnerborg et al., 1988), although the development of severe neurocognitive impairment most often occurs in late-stage disease (Navia et al., 1986b). A matter of controversy at the beginning of the epidemic was whether individuals in the early, asymptomatic (or mildly symptomatic) stages of HIV-1 infection were at increased risk of developing mild neurocognitive impairment. Some studies found an increased risk of at least mild neurocognitive impairment in these medically asymptomatic individuals (Bornstein et al., 1992; Grant et al., 1987; Heaton et al., 1995; Stern et al., 1991), whereas others found no differences between the two groups (McArthur et al., 1989; Selnes et al., 1990). As is unfortunately so often the case, investigators used different NP test batteries, inclusion/exclusion criteria, and methods for determining impairment across studies (see White et al., 1995, for a review). However, in a thorough analysis of 57 studies of medically asymptomatic individuals, White et al. (1995) found that one critical determinant of the study outcome was the length and comprehensiveness of the NP test battery: the more comprehensive the battery, the more likely it was to detect impairment in asymptomatic patients. This finding suggests a "spotty" pattern of impairments in HIV-1 infection (Heaton et al., 1995), in which many different domains might be affected, and that sensitivity can be enhanced by assessing numerous cognitive abilities (Antinori et al., 2007).

In the pre-HAART era, rates of impairment increased in a stair-step fashion (Heaton et al., 1995), with increasing impairment seen across mildly symptomatic and symptomatic patients. While cognitive decline can occur at any disease stage, it is most common in the symptomatic phase of the disease. Reports from a number of cohorts suggest that, in the HAART era, a subset of individuals transition in and out of impairment over time (Antinori et al., 2007), raising the possibility that neurocognitive dysfunction in HIV-1 infection may be neither static nor chronically progressive but in the mildest forms may exhibit a fluctuating, relapsing/remitting course, similar to demyelinating disorders.

It has also been posited that there might be distinct patterns of HIV dementia in the HAART era (Brew, 2004; McArthur, 2004). For example, McArthur (2004) hypothesizes three subtypes: (i) a "subacute progressive" dementia, found in untreated patients with severe, progressive dementia (similar to the pre-HAART era); (ii) a "chronic active" form, in patients with poor adherence or viral resistance and who are at risk for neurocognitive progression; and (iii) a "chronic inactive" dementia, found in persons who suppress the virus with HAART, have recovered from previous neuronal injury, and stay neurologically stable. These subtypes await empirical validation, but suggest that different underlying neuropathogenic mechanisms and responses to treatment may result in varying types of CNS injury.

Profiles of Impairment

HIV-associated NP dysfunction often presents with a "subcortical" pattern of deficits, indicative of preferential disruption of prefrontostriatal circuits. Impairments are frequently seen in the domains of learning, motor skills, attention/working memory, speed of information processing, and executive functioning (Becker et al., 1995; Heaton et al., 1995; Hinkin et al., 2002b; Peavy et al., 1994). Although these are the most common NP domains impaired at a group level, the patterns of NP impairments in HIV-1-infected individuals are quite variable. For example, we (Marcotte et al., 2005) examined impairment patterns in 320 HIV-positive (HIV+) individuals who were classified as having NP impairment (impaired in two or more domains). Learning and attention/working memory were the most frequent individual impairments in this group, yet only 36% of the participants were impaired in both learning and attention/working memory. Given that in order to be in the globally impaired group all participants had to be impaired in at least two domains, there were a potential 247 different impairment patterns. We found 164 distinct impairment patterns across the 322 participants. The most common profiles were one in which there were impairments in attention/working memory

and verbal abilities and one with impairments in attention/working memory and learning. However, these two patterns were seen in only 11 cases each.

At the group level, Lojek et al. (2005) found four primary patterns of neurocognitive deficits by performing cluster analyses in a sample of 217 HIV+ men: (i) a pattern with a primary deficit in psychomotor functioning; (ii) a pattern with primary deficits in memory and learning; (iii) a pattern with almost all neurocognitive ability domains impaired; and (iv) a pattern with unimpaired outcomes similar to the HIV-negative comparison sample. These patterns were mostly stable when participants were tested again a year later, although those in the fourth pattern seemed to have disproportionate decline in executive functions.

It has been proposed that the impairment seen in individuals receiving HAART may be qualitatively different from that in the earlier era (Brew, 2004). The neurocognitive disorders appear to be milder than in the pre-HAART era, with fewer cases of severe dementia (McArthur, 2004). With respect to the cognitive profiles, Cysique et al. (2004b) found that individuals on long-term HAART had worse performance on verbal learning and complex-attention measures than a pre-HAART cohort. There were limitations to the study in that the memory measures differed across the two eras, and the finding of learning impairments is not necessarily new, as it has been found in previous studies with different pre-HAART cohorts. In addition, given the variability of deficits associated with HIV-1, the study will need to be replicated by others. It does, however, raise the possibility of CNS damage persisting despite continued HAART treatment, perhaps even with regionally specific cognitive changes.

While the NP profiles of HIV-1 infection probably lack the specificity to be used as the primary source for a differential diagnosis, NP evaluations nevertheless reliably inform diagnostic hypotheses and can influence treatment planning (Woods et al., 2005).

In addition to commonly used NP measures, investigators have integrated novel experimental paradigms, data interpretation approaches, and findings from cognitive neuropsychology and cognitive science into the study of HIV-associated NP impairment. For example, the n-back paradigm used by Hinkin and colleagues (2002b) was chosen because of the hypothesized sensitivity of working memory to the neurocognitive effects of HIV-1 and the differential brain activation of verbal and spatial memory. This study and other investigations of working memory (e.g., Farinpour et al., 2000; Martin et al., 2001) formed a more specific, cross-modality picture of working memory in HIV-1, and as a result, researchers have postulated that poor working memory might be partially responsible for the deficits seen in other domains in HIV-associated neurocognitive impairment. Moreover, investigators predicted that poor working memory might negatively impact decision-making ability, leading to studies with possible "real-world" implications (e.g., Bechara and Martin, 2004; Martin et al., 2004). Other novel measures, such as action fluency, a verbal-fluency task requiring the spontaneous generation of verbs (Piatt et al., 1999); procedural memory (e.g., motor learning); and prospective memory (remembering one's intentions), may be of particular interest to HIV researchers given the sensitivity of these tasks to frontal-subcortical dysfunction and their possible prediction of everyday functioning, including medication adherence (e.g., Carey et al., 2006; Woods et al., 2005). These approaches may help researchers gain a better conceptual understanding of the cognitive mechanisms underlying the general deficits associated with HIV-1 and provide relevant background for formulating hypotheses. They may also help clinically by improving diagnostic sensitivity to and specificity for impairments and may lead to the development of remedial strategies for those with impairment.

Cognitive Complaints and Cognition

Most commonly, HIV-1-infected individuals complain of difficulty concentrating, fatigability when required to engage in demanding mental tasks, feeling subjectively slowed down, and difficulty in remembering. Data on the concordance between self-reported cognitive problems and objectively measured NP functioning, however, have been equivocal. Many studies have reported that cognitive complaints track with depression rather than neurocognitive impairment (Hinkin et al., 1992; Van Gorp et al., 1991; Wilkins et al., 1991). Subsequent studies have indicated that awareness of one's own cognitive functioning (meta-cognition, or metamemory) may be impacted by both mood disturbances and impairments in executive functioning (Rourke, 1999). Moreover, despite some earlier findings, structural-equation modeling suggests that, in addition to mood, complaints are independently associated with NP performance (Carter et al., 2003). Regardless, it is important to access objective NP testing when cognitive complaints occur, especially when patients also exhibit depressive symptomatology.

THE RELATIONSHIP BETWEEN COGNITION AND BIOLOGICAL MARKERS

Investigations into the relationships between immune function and HIV-1 replication markers and neurocognitive impairment have met with mixed results, depending on the particular markers used as well as the severity of neurocognitive impairment and the disease stage of the individuals under study. Early research suggested that CD4 cell counts were weakly associated with NP performance (Dal Pan et al., 1998); disease stage was often a stronger predictor (Heaton et al., 1995; Podraza et al., 1994). Notably, individuals in the era of HAART are being diagnosed with dementia at higher CD4 levels than those seen prior to the introduction of HAART (Dore et al., 1999), and in the HNRC experience, it now appears that cognitive performance is more closely associated with the nadir (lowest ever) CD4 cell count rather than the current CD4 level.

Pre-HAART studies suggested that the plasma viral load predicted the development of HIV-associated NP impairment (Childs et al., 1999). We examined predictors of future impairment in a group of individuals who were assessed an average of 1 year after seroconversion and found that reductions in CD4 cell counts (<400 cells/μl) or elevated plasma HIV-1 RNA values (>4.5 $\log_{10}$ copies/ml) significantly increased the risk of NP impairment (Marcotte et al., 2003). Using proportional-hazards modeling, the highest-risk subjects had both CD4 counts of <400 cells/mm³ and HIV-1 RNA levels greater than 4.5 $\log_{10}$ copies/ml (risk ratio, 6.0; $P = 0.01$). In most subjects (seven of nine [78%]), NP impairment developed before an AIDS-defining illness.

Viral levels in the CSF, which may serve as a window to the CNS, more closely correspond to neurocognitive impairment (Ellis et al., 1997b; Stankoff et al., 1999). Elevated CSF HIV-1 RNA levels predict progression to NP impairment (Ellis et al., 2002), while a reduction in CSF HIV-1 RNA levels is associated with improvement in cognition (Letendre et al., 2004; Marra et al., 2003). As seen in Fig. 2, in a study of antiretroviral treatment, individuals who suppressed virus in the CSF showed a significant improvement on a global measure of cognitive functioning relative to those who did not suppress the virus (Letendre et al., 2004). Other biomarkers, including markers of macrophage activation (β_2-microglobulin and neopterin), cytokines and chemokines (tumor necrosis factor alpha, macrophage inflammatory protein 1β, and monocyte chemoattractant protein 1), and excitotoxins (quinolinic acid), have been studied in relations to NP impairment, and the potential biomarker candidates continue to grow. While these hold promise with respect to clarifying potential mechanisms of CNS damage, there is some evidence that in an era in which plasma and CSF HIV-1 RNA levels are significantly reduced by treatment, the relationship between biomarkers and neurocognitive functioning has been altered or at least attenuated (MacArthur et al., 2004; Sevigny et al., 2004).

As genetic studies become increasingly feasible and sophisticated, there is burgeoning interest in the effects of "host" (the person) and viral genetics on the development of HIV-related cognitive impairments. Early studies have identified genetic polymorphisms relating to monocyte trafficking (Gonzalez et al., 2002) and positions in and near the V3 loop of HIV *env* as being associated with increased impairment (Pillai et al., 2006).

RELATIONSHIP BETWEEN NP FUNCTIONING AND UNDERLYING NEUROPATHOLOGY

HIV-1 infection of the brain is characterized by HIV encephalitis (HIVE), or the presence of multinucleated giant cells, microglial nodules, astrocytosis, and myelin pallor. HIV-1 has a predilection for subcortical structures. Neurons are not directly infected, but neuronal injury and death occur in the basal ganglia, as well as the cerebral cortex and hippocampus (Masliah et al., 1996; Wiley et al., 1991). The mechanisms underlying the relationship between neurocognitive functioning and HIV-1-related pathophysiological changes

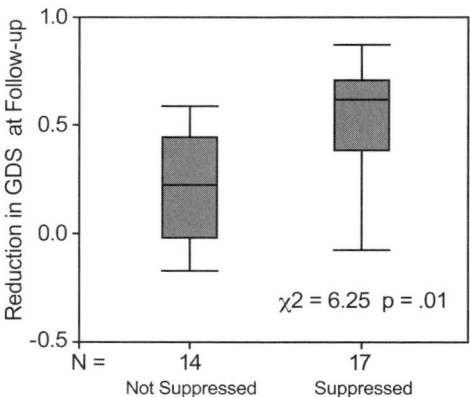

FIGURE 2 Reduction (improvement) in NP performance (GDS) among subjects with and without suppressed CSF HIV RNA viral load at follow-up. The box-and-whisker plots show the median (center line), interquartile range (box), and 5th and 95th percentiles (whiskers). (From Letendre et al., 2004.)

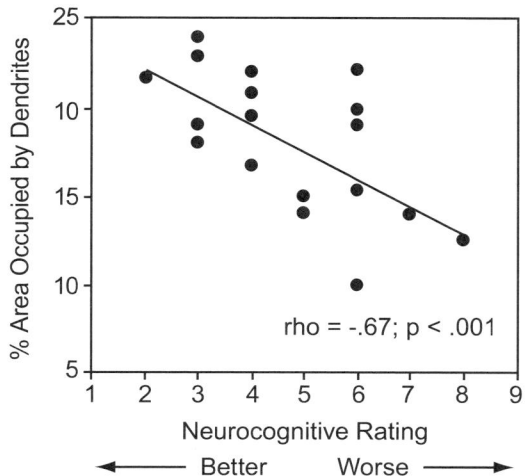

FIGURE 3 Relationship between dendritic complexity in the midfrontal region and blinded clinical rating of global neurocognitive functioning. (From Masliah et al., 1997.)

remain obscure. The brain viral burden increases between the asymptomatic and symptomatic stages of HIV-1 infection, and while it correlates well with brain pathological markers (Achim et al., 1994; Wiley and Achim, 1994), the association with cognitive symptoms has been inconsistent. HIVE was frequently seen in the brains of patients with HAD (Masliah et al., 1992a; Wiley and Achim, 1994), although it may not be present in some cases (Glass et al., 1993; Navia et al., 1986a). Cherner et al. (2002) found that HIV-associated cognitive impairment predicted the presence of HIVE at autopsy, even in cases of milder impairment. This study found a positive predictive power of 95%, with HIVE in 18 of 19 impaired participants. The absence of cognitive deficits did not necessarily indicate an absence of HIVE, however, suggesting that HIVE in some instances occurs as a late event or manifests itself pathologically before doing so clinically. Associations have also been found between cognitive impairment and a decrease in synaptodendritic complexity in both mild and severe neurocognitive disorders (Fig. 3). Damage to structural portions of neurons in both cortical and subcortical brain regions (Moore et al., 2006) may be an important neural substrate of HIV-associated dysfunction, and treatments may have the potential of stopping cognitive decline prior to neuronal death (Everall et al., 1999; Masliah et al., 1992b, 1997).

COFACTORS AND HIV-ASSOCIATED NEUROCOGNITIVE IMPAIRMENT

There is a growing appreciation of the role that comorbid factors may play in the development of cognitive impairment in HIV-1-infected individuals. For example, coinfection with hepatitis C virus may result in psychomotor slowing (von Giesen et al., 2004); poor executive functioning (Ryan et al., 2004); and reduced learning, abstraction, and motor functioning (Cherner et al., 2005). Illicit drugs, such as methamphetamine, which appears to be neurotoxic and may share common pathways of injury with HIV-1 (Langford et al., 2003), may also have additive or synergistic effects on HIV-1 CNS damage (Rippeth et al., 2004).

In the era of HAART, individuals with HIV-1 infection are living much longer, raising the possibility that age may amplify NP impairments associated with HIV-1 (Goodkin et al., 2001). For example, preliminary studies have shown both increased frequency of impairment (Becker et al., 2004; Cherner et al., 2004) and dementia (Valcour et al., 2004) in older HIV-1[+] patients, although at least one study has found no such relationship (Kissel et al., 2005). This will be a growing area of interest as HIV-1[+] individuals live into their 60s and beyond.

THE REAL-WORLD IMPACT OF HIV-ASSOCIATED NEUROCOGNITIVE DISORDERS

HIV-associated cognitive impairment can significantly impact one's quality of life (Kaplan et al., 1995, 1997; Osowiecki et al., 2000; Tozzi et al., 2004). In the age of HAART, when HIV-1 infection is seen as a "chronic" disease, it is of increasing importance to monitor how neurocognitive dysfunction impacts an individual's daily functioning, as it appears to do so even for those who are not suffering a debilitating dementia. Thus, investigators have developed methods of examining this impact on "real-world" functioning (e.g., Albert et al., 1999; Heaton et al., 2004a; Marcotte et al., 2004; van Gorp et al., 1999), as traditional NP tests have, at best, limited validity as measures of daily functioning (Heaton et al., 2004a). Although the literature still leaves much to be explored, there is evidence to suggest that HIV-1-related neurocognitive dysfunction significantly affects both laboratory and real-world measures of everyday functioning, as well as survival time.

Cognition and Mortality

HIV-1-related neurocognitive disorders are associated with increased mortality. In the pre-HAART era, HIV-1[+] individuals diagnosed with dementia had an average survival time of 6 months after diagnosis (McArthur et al., 1993), although a subset of patients remained fairly stable and exhibited a survival period of a year or longer (Bouwman et al., 1998). Even milder forms of impairment put one at increased risk for death, after relevant biological variables were controlled for (Ellis et al., 1997a; Mayeux et al., 1993; Wilkie et al., 1998). One study examined specific NP predictors of mortality, finding that a sustained decline in psychomotor performance was predictive of mortality in the follow-up period (Sacktor et al., 1996). In the HAART era, there has been a dramatic increase in survival time following a diagnosis of dementia, increasing from 1 to 4 years in an Australian cohort (Dore et al., 2003).

Studies have been unable to ascertain the cause of increased mortality in impaired individuals. It may be that individuals who become impaired are suffering from a more virulent strain of the disease, although this virulence is not being captured by standard disease markers, which are normally controlled for in analyses. Tozzi and colleagues (2005) proposed that an increased risk for death may only be seen in neurocognitively impaired patients who also exhibit virological failure on antiretroviral medications. It may also be that impaired individuals have biological features making them more susceptible to the virus. Alternatively, it may be that NP deficits affect patients' abilities to manage their disease or effectively use their available resources, as HIV-1 treatment and maintenance is a complex process.

Activities of Daily Living

Declines in basic activities of daily living, such as grooming, dressing, and bathing, appear to decline only with advanced physical symptoms or in severe HAD (Boccellari and Zeifert, 1994). Instrumental activities of daily living, or more complex everyday activities, such as money management and meal preparation, are affected by subtle HIV-associated neurocognitive impairments.

Heaton and colleagues (2004a) investigated everyday functioning in a cohort of 267 HIV-1+ individuals. The participants completed standardized instruments assessing grocery shopping, financial management, cooking, medication management, and vocational functioning. NP impaired individuals performed significantly worse than NP normal individuals on all functional measures, especially on a global functional-deficit score (a composite score based on the entire functional battery). The largest group differences were reported in vocational skills, followed by finances and medication management. The NP domains that were most predictive of performance on the functional battery included abstraction/executive functioning, learning, verbal abilities, and attention/working memory. Similar results have also been found in a Spanish-speaking sample (Mindt et al., 2003).

Importantly, in the Heaton et al. (2004a) study, both the NP and functional batteries were independent predictors of "real-world" functional status, based on complaints of cognitive difficulties, level of dependence/independence in instrumental activities of daily living, and employment status. Thus, although NP assessments provide information regarding functioning outside of the laboratory, they may not capture all that is involved in successful execution of these tasks in real life. The development and use of more direct assessments and instruments measuring these skills and abilities are therefore warranted.

Medication Management

Of particular importance in the HAART era is the ability of HIV-1+ individuals to effectively manage their antiretroviral medications, as deviations from the prescribed dosing and dietary instructions may increase the risk of developing resistance to the drugs, decrease the drug concentrations, and lower the likelihood of viral suppression (Chesney et al., 2000). Despite reductions in the complexity and restrictions associated with antiretroviral regimens, adherence still remains complicated, partially due to adverse side effects, comorbid psychiatric disorders and substance abuse, and neurocognitive impairments. Preliminary studies suggest that HIV-1+ individuals with impairments in memory, executive function, and psychomotor functioning demonstrate significant difficulties with performance on structured tasks of medication management ability (Albert et al., 1999), as well as adherence to medication regimens in everyday life (Hinkin et al., 2002a). Importantly, the impact of cognitive impairment seems to be most significant in those individuals who have complex medication regimens (three or more doses per day) (Hinkin et al., 2002a). Heaton et al. (2004a) also reported significant differences on a structured task of medication management between those with and without NP impairment, finding that impairments in learning and abstraction/executive functioning were the strongest predictors of failing at the task. Notably, a study using the Disease Management Assistance System (Andrade et al., 2005) suggested that partial remediation of medication management deficits may be possible. This study used simple auditory reminding devices that notified participants of the timing and dosing of their medications. Adherence in the treatment group was 15% higher than in the control group, and the treatment group evidenced significantly lower viral loads and higher CD4 counts, indicating increased efficacy concurrent with improved adherence.

Employment and Vocational Functioning

Unlike most patients with dementing disorders, HIV-1+ individuals tend to be young and have many years of potential work life ahead of them, especially as many patients experience a "second life" (Rabkin and Ferrando, 1997) as result of HAART. Thus, it is important to characterize factors that may lead to a favorable or unfavorable work outcome. Early investigations examined group differences in employment status and job performance in HIV-1+ and HIV-1− groups. Heaton et al. (1994b) found unemployment to be almost three times higher in HIV-1+ NP impaired participants than in HIV-1+ NP normal individuals, even after subjects with potentially disabling medical conditions were removed. Of the participants who were employed, those with NP impairment evidenced a higher rate of difficulty performing their jobs (30% versus 6%). Albert and colleagues (1995) reported a relative risk ratio of work disability of 2.76 for HIV-1+ versus HIV-1− participants during 4.5 years of follow-up. Development of major NP impairment was a significant risk factor for work disability for a subset of participants. In another study of advanced HIV-1 disease, unemployed participants were twice as likely to be NP impaired as employed participants (22% versus 11%) (van Gorp et al., 1999). Physical disabilities and performance on Trails B were significant predictors of employment status in this study.

Objective measures of work performance may help rule out other factors that lead to unemployment, such as physical decline or disability due to an AIDS-defining medical condition. Heaton et al. (1996) utilized a standardized battery of vocational tasks, consisting of both manual and computerized tasks, that provided estimates of 13 job abilities as identified by the U.S. Department of Labor (U.S. Department of Labor, 1991). The HIV+ NP impaired group performed significantly worse on the work sample than an HIV+ cognitively normal group and an HIV− group; furthermore, while the last two groups demonstrated higher current functioning than expected given their work histories, the HIV+ NP impaired group had reduced abilities compared to their prior work histories, suggesting a decline from previous functioning. These results were also replicated in a larger cohort; verbal fluency and attention/working-memory abilities were the strongest predictors of work sample performance (Heaton et al., 2004a).

Automobile Driving

Similar to vocation, driving an automobile is a task that younger persons afflicted with HIV-1 would be expected to undertake frequently, and there is growing evidence that a subset of HIV-1+ individuals with cognitive impairment experience an overall reduction in driving ability. Twenty-nine percent of 146 HIV+ participants surveyed at the HNRC reported a decline in their driving ability since becoming infected and were much less likely to be driving than NP normal individuals (odds ratio = 2.9; $P = 0.02$), even after the CDC stage and employment status were controlled for (Marcotte et al., 2000). Assessment of driving abilities, however, is complex, as there is currently no clear standard for the concept of "impaired driving skills" (Marcotte and Scott, 2004). There are a variety of methodologies for directly assessing driving abilities, each with its own strengths and limitations. Although self-report of crashes and violations provides a valuable sample of behavior over an extended period of time, it is not always reliable, especially with cognitively impaired individuals. In addition, crashes and tickets are rare occurrences and may not show declines, especially given that an accident may be avoided because of the defensive behavior of other drivers or could be the fault of other drivers.

In an attempt to obtain more objective assessments of driving abilities, our group developed driving protocols in order to discern a complete picture of the deficits that might lead to reductions in driving. In the first study, Marcotte and colleagues (1999) examined 68 HIV-1+ individuals at various disease stages on interactive computer-based driving simulations assessing lane tracking, divided attention, driving in traffic, and accident avoidance. Participants with cognitive impairment were approximately five times more likely than cognitively normal participants to fail the lane-tracking task and had a significantly higher number of crashes on a city driving simulation (2.3 accidents versus 1.5 accidents). Impairments in the domains of abstraction/executive functioning and attention/speed of information processing were most often associated with poor performance on the simulations.

To provide a thorough assessment of how individuals function under more "real-world" conditions, we performed a multimodal assessment with 40 HIV+ and 20 HIV− control participants that included a 35-min on-road driving evaluation, city driving and navigation computer-based simulations, and NP testing (Marcotte et al., 2004). HIV− and HIV+ NP normal participants performed similarly on the on-road evaluation, had similar numbers of crashes in the simulated routine and emergency driving tasks, and made a similar number of errors in the navigation task. The NP impaired participants, in contrast to these two groups, were classified as unsafe in the on-road evaluation at a higher rate (36% versus 6%), had more collisions in simulated routine and emergency driving

tasks (mean, 2.0 versus 1.3; $P = 0.03$), and made almost three times the number of navigational errors as the other groups (mean, 3.2 versus 9.2; $P = 0.001$) (Fig. 4). Importantly, performances on the NP tests and simulator tasks were independent predictors of on-road performance, indicating that assessments using seminaturalistic tasks provide information beyond that found using structured neurocognitive tests alone. Impairment in executive functioning was the strongest predictor of failing the on-road driving examination. In addition, some of the individuals who failed the on-road driving test lacked awareness of their performance, indicating that clinicians should be cautious in relying on a patient's self-report of driving ability.

Since one must perceive and identify objects both in the center and on the periphery of the roadway in order to safely drive an automobile, we investigated whether inclusion of visual attentional processing data would improve upon traditional NP tests in identifying individuals who are at risk for poor driving performance (Marcotte et al., 2006). We utilized the useful field of view (UFOV) (Visual Resources, Inc., 1998) task, which has shown particular success in identifying older at-risk drivers (e.g., Ball et al., 1993; Duchek et al., 1998; Myers et al., 2000; Owsley et al., 1998). The UFOV task is a computerized measure that assesses the amount of time it takes one to accurately acquire both central and peripheral visual information without head or eye movements. HIV+ participants evidenced significantly worse performance on the UFOV task than control participants, with the greatest differences seen on divided attention. These declines in visual attention were not solely the result of advancing disease or high levels of general NP impairment, as individuals impaired on the UFOV task covered the spectrum of disease stages and severities of cognitive impairment, suggesting a process occurring at least partially independently of disease progression, as well as a cognitive deficit not entirely captured by common NP tests. Importantly, the UFOV "high-risk" group had a significantly higher number of on-road accidents in the previous year than those who were not at "high risk," and a classification of NP impaired and "high risk" on the UFOV task yielded

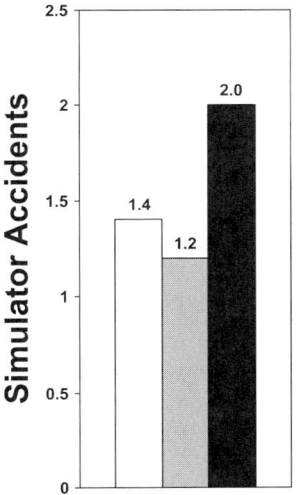 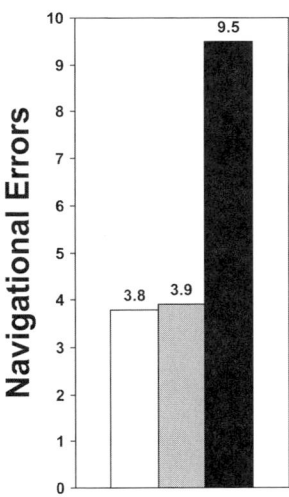 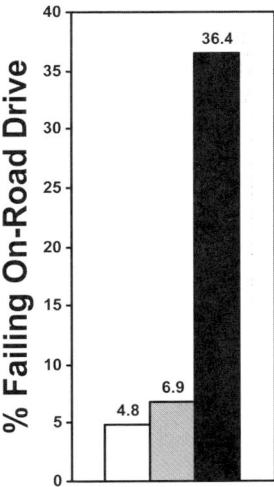

FIGURE 4 Performances of HIV− (open columns), HIV+ NP normal (gray columns), and HIV+ NP impaired (black columns) subjects on driving simulator measures of accidents and navigational errors and an on-road driving evaluation. (Adapted from Marcotte et al., 2004.)

a positive predictive value of 75% and a negative predictive value of 95% for accidents in the past year.

SELECTING AN NP BATTERY

Assessments of NP functioning are important for detection and diagnosis of brain disorder, detection of changes in cognitive functioning longitudinally, and identification of neurocognitive strengths and weaknesses that may impact day-to-day functioning (Heaton and Marcotte, 2000). In HIV-1 disease, an NP evaluation can complement the neurological examination by quantifying the severity of suspected cognitive impairment, and if impairment is detected, it can help determine the individual patterns of involvement. In addition, a more comprehensive NP evaluation may lead to detection of subtle deficits in asymptomatic HIV+ patients (White et al., 1995).

Selection of an appropriate test battery for one's research or clinical question is critical in that one must be able to adequately detect and demarcate the cognitive changes associated with HIV-1 that one is hypothesizing to exist (Woods and Grant, 2005). For example, if the purpose of an assessment is to confirm that a fairly healthy HIV+ individual with cognitive complaints is evidencing mild neurocognitive impairment, then a comprehensive battery of NP tests is warranted, given that the deficits are likely to be mild and spread across ability domains. If an assessment is given for the purposes of measuring change (e.g., in a clinical trial of neuroprotective medications), then one may choose a more focused assessment with NP tests that have proven sensitivity to impairment but show minimal practice effects upon repeat administration. Investigators and clinicians need to weigh the benefits and drawbacks of each approach, along with the specificity of the hypotheses they are testing, to determine the best protocols for their particular purpose.

In 1989, a National Institute of Mental Health workgroup (Butters et al., 1990) recommended that batteries used in HIV-1 research should be comprehensive, covering multiple domains and with enough tests in each domain so that overlapping procedures could cover a broad range of cognitive function and improve classification accuracy. At the HNRC, Heaton and colleagues designed a comprehensive battery with the initial goal of detecting subtle HIV-1-related impairments in individuals who were in the early stages of disease. The battery comprised eight areas of cognitive functioning during the course of an 8-h assessment (detailed in Heaton et al., 1995). After extensive experience, the battery was reduced to 3 to 4 h by using data-driven and theoretical analyses to determine the measures within each domain that were most discriminative of HIV-1-related impairment, both individually and in combination with other measures. The resulting battery consisted of half of the original tests and took half the administration time but still covered all major ability domains and used measures with proven sensitivity and discriminative ability (for a listing of the battery, see Heaton et al., 2004a).

Recently, Heaton and colleagues further refined the test battery to produce an even more focused but still robust assessment of cognitive changes associated with HIV-1 infection. The current battery is reasonably brief (approximately 2 h), addresses cognitive abilities most likely to be impaired in HIV-1-infected individuals, consists of tests with good normative data, and includes a number of tests with alternative forms, thus enhancing its use for repeated assessments (Table 1). (This core battery has also been supplemented by measures facilitating investigation of hypotheses relating to visuospatial functioning [e.g., Hooper Visual Organization Test, Benton Judgment of Line Orientation] and the combined effects of HIV and aging [e.g., Boston Naming Test, Token Test].) In addition to being used at the HNRC, portions of this battery are used in two large national studies:

TABLE 1 Neuropsychological tests in the current HNRC battery

Domain	Neuropsychological test[a]
Premorbid cognitive abilities	WRAT-4 Reading
Verbal fluency	Controlled Oral Word Association Test (FAS)[b]
	Semantic fluency (animals)[b]
	Action fluency[b]
Executive functions	Category Test[b]
	Stroop Color-Word Test[b]
	Trail Making Test, Part B
	Color Trails 2[b,c]
	Wisconsin Card Sorting Test (WCST-64)[b]
Speed of information processing	Trail Making Test, Part A
	Color Trails 1[b,c]
	WAIS-III Digit Symbol[b]
	WAIS-III Symbol Search[b]
Attention and working memory	Paced Auditory Serial Addition Test[b]
	WAIS-III Letter Number Sequencing[b]
	WMS-III Spatial Span[b]
Learning and memory	Hopkins Verbal Learning Test-Revised[b]
	Brief Visuospatial Memory Test-Revised[b]
	Hiscock Forced-Choice Recognition Procedure (SVT)[b]
Motor	Grooved Pegboard Test (dominant and nondominant)[b]

[a]SVT, Symptom Validity Test; WAIS-III, Wechsler Adult Intelligence Scale, 3rd ed; WMS-III, Wechsler Memory Scale, 3rd ed; WRAT-4, Wide Range Achievement Test, revision 4.

[b]Also included in the HNRC International Neuropsychological Test Battery.

[c]Only administered as part of the HNRC International Neuropsychological Test Battery.

CHARTER, a multisite study of the impact of HAART on the CNS, and the National NeuroAIDS Tissue Consortium, a collaborative group of brain banks that are carefully characterizing HIV⁺ individuals who agree to an autopsy and neuropathological studies. Both of these projects make data and samples available to interested investigators. More recently, HNRC investigators have adapted the battery for use in international HIV studies, with some limited modifications (e.g., substituting color trails for the trail-making test; Table 1).

Other batteries in use for large cohort studies include the Northeast AIDS Dementia battery (Rey Auditory Verbal Learning Test, Rey-Osterrieth Complex Figure Test, digit symbol, grooved pegboard, timed gait, a computerized reaction time test [CalCAP], verbal fluency, and the odd-man-out test) and the Macro battery originally designed by the AIDS Clinical Trials Neurology Group to monitor treatment effects in patients with established HAD (Sidtis, 1994). The Macro battery includes vocabulary and digit symbol from the Wechsler Intelligence Scales, timed gait, grooved pegboard, trail-making test parts A and B, finger tapping, Rey Auditory Verbal Learning Test, and the Profile of Mood States (POMS).

Brief Cognitive Screening Measures

Several brief cognitive screening techniques have been developed for situations in which a full or focused NP evaluation is not indicated or not feasible. A common practice is to use screening measures to determine whether cognitive deficits exist, and if so, to then refer the patient for a more comprehensive NP evaluation to better characterize the deficits. Standardized tests in common use, such as the Folstein Mini-Mental State Exam (MMSE) (Folstein, 1983; Folstein et al., 1975), the Mattis Dementia Rating Scale (Gardner et al., 1981; Mattis, 1976), and the Cognitive Capacity Screening Examination (Jacobs et al., 1977), have shown limited utility in screening for HIV-1-related cognitive impairment, given their low ceiling effects and their insensitivity to mild impairment. In addition, most of these traditional screening tests focus on "cortical" cognitive functions, such as language and free recall, and may not adequately assess the "frontal-subcortical" nature of deficits seen in HIV-1-related neurocognitive disorders, such as slowed information-processing speed (Woods and Grant, 2005).

The HIV Dementia Scale (HDS) (Power et al., 1995) is a 5-min instrument intended for use as a rapid screening tool for HAD in outpatient settings. The HDS has shown superior sensitivity to HIV-1-related changes compared to the MMSE (Power et al., 1995). The test includes a measure of mental flexibility, an anti-saccades test, timed alphabet, timed construction, and a memory measure. A number of studies have found the HDS to have excellent specificity, but only modest sensitivity, especially in detecting impairment in nondemented and mildly demented HIV⁺ individuals (Bottiggi et al., 2007; Childers et al., 2002; Smith et al., 2003). Normal performances on the HDS were associated with high rates of false negatives (i.e., NP impaired individuals misclassified as normal on the HDS). Sensitivity may be considerably enhanced by applying demographically adjusted norms (Morgan el al., 2008).

In order to develop a diagnostically accurate but still concise screening battery for HIV-related cognitive impairment, Carey et al. (2004b) examined the classification accuracies of several different test pairs from the HNRC test battery, using global clinical ratings as the "gold standard" of impairment. Pairing the Hopkins Verbal Learning Test-Revised (Brandt and Benedict, 2001) with either the nondominant-hand score from the grooved-pegboard test (Klove, 1963) or the digit symbol subtest of the WAIS-III (Wechsler, 1997) provided the most accurate classification of global NP impairment, providing 78% sensitivity, 85% specificity, and excellent odds ratios. This screening battery was not associated with a high rate of false-negative errors, in contrast to the HDS.

INTERPRETING NP TEST RESULTS

Clinical Ratings

Most research studies of NP function in HIV-1 infection utilize between-group mean comparisons of test scores on individual measures. Although this approach has reliably detected NP impairment in medically symptomatic groups, it has shown less sensitivity in identifying deficits in medically asymptomatic groups with more subtle or "spotty" deficits in functioning (Heaton et al., 1994a). Clinical ratings have been recommended as the "gold standard" approach in interpreting NP test data in HIV-1-infected persons (Butters et al., 1990), due to their sensitivity in detecting subtle HIV-associated NP deficits, as well as their superior classification accuracy compared to mean group difference statistics (Heaton et al., 1995, 1994a). Under the clinical-ratings approach in use at the HNRC, NP tests are grouped into domains; raw scores are converted to t scores, which are standardized scores that have been transformed to fit a normal distribution (mean of 50, standard deviation of 10) and adjust for demographic factors (e.g., age, education, gender, ethnicity) known to be associated with neuropsychological performance. Clinical ratings in each of the domains are assigned using a nine-point scale ranging from 1 (above-average functioning) to 9 (severe impairment). A global NP status rating is then assigned by appropriately weighing the clinical ratings in each domain. Consistent with accepted guidelines (Antinori et al., 2007; Grant and Atkinson, 1995), participants have to exhibit impairment in at least two domains to be classified as NP impaired.

Although clinical ratings are conducted blind to disease status, criticisms exist regarding their possible subjective biases, as well as the expertise and time required to conduct them. However, this approach can be successfully implemented across multiple sites. For example, neuropsychologists in the National NeuroAIDS Tissue Consortium used a manualized approach and, across six sites, achieved an interclass correlation coefficient of 0.94 for ordinal ratings of overall cognitive functioning and 0.96 to 1.00 for individual cognitive domains (Woods et al., 2004). For overall impairment (impaired/unimpaired), the kappa value was 0.87 to 1.0. The group was less successful in agreeing on the cause of the cognitive impairment (e.g., HIV-1 versus substance use).

Actuarial Approaches

Actuarial approaches, such as the Global Deficit Score (GDS) (Carey et al., 2004a; Heaton et al., 1995, 1994a), have been developed as an alternative that can simulate the rating procedures. The GDS is similar to clinical ratings in that it considers both the number and severity of NP deficits. The GDS is computed by converting demographically corrected t scores on the individual NP tests to deficit scores ranging from 0 (no impairment) to 5 (severe impairment) and then averaging these scores to compute the global measure of functioning. Greater weight is thus given to test results showing impairment; above-average performance in one domain does not offset impaired performance in another. Data from the HNRC have shown the GDS to be strongly associated with clinical ratings of global NP functioning and to have excellent classification accuracy (Carey et al., 2004a).

Another approach in common use has been termed NPZ (Clifford et al., 2002; Navia et al., 1998). In this approach, standardized *z* scores (standardized scores representing the distance, in standard deviations, from the group mean) are calculated for each test based upon either norms or the control group, and then a composite score is calculated across all measures. Although useful, it does have the disadvantage of averaging both above- and below-average scores, thus perhaps decreasing the sensitivity to impaired performance.

Demographic Factors

Demographic factors, such as age, education, sex, and ethnicity, have been shown to independently impact test performance. It is therefore important to use norms appropriate for the specific individual being assessed, especially when estimating performance levels before the brain injury (e.g., deciding whether there has been a decline from a previous, unmeasured, level of functioning). Otherwise, abnormal results may simply reflect inadequate adjustment for demographic characteristics. Comprehensive demographic corrections are available for many tests (e.g., Gladsjo et al., 1999; Heaton et al., 2004b; Spreen and Strauss, 1998). If investigators do not use tests with adequate norms and rely on matched control groups, it is important to attend to any group demographic differences, as they can significantly skew results (e.g., attributing higher impairment rates to a group when in fact they may be the result of demographic differences).

Fatigue/Effort

Many HIV-1-infected individuals experience fatigue and various constitutional symptoms, so monitoring for the effects of fatigue and motivation on NP test performance is warranted. When researchers have attempted to investigate fatigue effects on rates of NP impairment, the results have pointed to a lack of systematic association between the two (Hasenauer et al., 1996; Heaton et al., 1995). Nonetheless, suboptimal effort secondary to fatigue or other psychiatric or medical factors may affect NP test performance, and symptom validity testing has been developed for detecting invalid test performance due to lack of effort. Measures such as the Hiscock Forced-Choice Procedure (Hiscock and Hiscock, 1989) and Test of Memory Malingering (Tombaugh, 1997) are designed to detect suboptimal effort by eliciting close to ceiling performance for all but the most severely impaired individuals. In the context of HIV-1, abnormal performance on the Hiscock procedure has been shown to quite rare (Woods et al., 2003), providing some evidence for the specificity of this measure to suboptimal effort.

Mood Disorders and Cognitive Functioning

Some controversy still exists regarding whether affective/mood disorders, such as major depression and anxiety, interact with neurocognitive impairment. These may be especially relevant in HIV-1, given the high prevalence of these disorders in HIV-1 populations (Atkinson and Grant, 1994). Although some studies have found a relationship between mood and NP function (e.g., Vazquez-Justo et al., 2003), most studies have failed to find an association (e.g., Grant et al., 1993; Hinkin et al., 1992). Data from the HNRC indicate that NP impaired individuals are more likely to suffer major depression, but rates of impairment for depressed

versus nondepressed NP impaired participants in this outpatient cohort are similar (Heaton et al., 1995). A subsequent HNRC study found that incident major depression was not associated with a decline in NP performance (Cysique et al., 2007). Thus, it may be that depression is associated with increased complaints of cognitive dysfunction (Van Gorp et al., 1991) but not with any significant decrement in neurocognitive function.

CLINICAL TRIALS AND DETECTING CHANGE

Researchers and clinicians are often interested in determining whether individuals experience a change in cognitive status over time (e.g., in longitudinal studies or treatment monitoring), and NP tests are often used for this purpose, given their standardization and generally adequate reliability (Heaton and Marcotte, 2000). Complicating this task, though, are individual fluctuations in performance from baseline to follow-up testing, despite a lack of significant change in the individuals themselves. Ivnik and colleagues (1995) showed that large positive and negative test score changes were not uncommon for individuals across time, even though test-retest means stay relatively stable across the entire sample.

Given that many factors can impact test performance over time, such as practice effects, poor test-retest reliability, and individual patient characteristics, one must decide among a variety of approaches to ensure that the change on tests represents a true change in the individual's neurocognitive status, especially in measuring the effects of treatment (Temkin et al., 1999). Ideally, an investigator would have appropriate test-retest norms or norms for change for the tests administered. Given that these are not commonly available, a variety of statistical procedures exist to correct for confounding factors of repeated administrations, such as reliable change indices, standard-deviation change scores, and more complicated regression-based procedures (Heaton and Marcotte, 2000). In addition, tests that have alternative or parallel forms can help reduce the effects of practice, especially with regard to the content of a test.

Although it may seem obvious, in clinical trials it is critical that investigators ensure that patients have the disorder of interest at the beginning of the trial. For example, some studies of HIV-1 have used screening measures to identify individuals who might have HIV-1-related neurocognitive disorders and then used a more comprehensive battery for the treatment monitoring. However, in some cases, the more comprehensive battery may demonstrate that the person is in fact not impaired; one is then left looking for a treatment effect in an individual without the problem under study. For example, in one such study, it was discovered that the subset of individuals who were truly impaired at baseline, using a comprehensive battery, showed cognitive improvement with treatment, while the overall treatment group did not (Heseltine et al., 1998).

It is also recommended that treatment trials include NP batteries that assess multiple domains. Even though it is tempting to focus on specific domains (e.g., psychomotor speed), in the era of HAART there remains uncertainty regarding whether CNS damage occurs selectively, and given the spotty nature of HIV-1-related impairments, attending to a limited number of domains may result in missing individuals with other impairments, and likewise, missing improvement in these domains. The GDS is one approach that efficiently captures improvement across multiple domains (Carey et al., 2004b).

SUMMARY

Despite the dramatic impact that HAART has had on disease progression and mortality, HIV-1-related neurocognitive disorders have not been eliminated. These cognitive disorders appear to be milder in the HAART era, however, and it has been hypothesized that they may be qualitatively different in terms of both the types of impairment and their course. These suppositions await additional empirical validation. Biomarkers in the CSF correlate with cognitive performance and may provide insights regarding potential mechanisms for CNS damage, although there is preliminary evidence that HAART may have altered the relationships seen in the pre-HAART era. A number of factors may interact with HIV-1-related CNS damage—aging, hepatitis C virus coinfection, and methamphetamine abuse—and additional research regarding these comorbidities is needed.

NP testing remains a key component in determining the presence or absence of HAND. At the group level, HIV-associated cognitive impairments present with a pattern indicative of frontostriatal damage, although the pattern of impairments is typically "spotty" and can vary between individuals. A comprehensive battery is recommended if one wants to detect subtle impairments. No single test is both sensitive to and specific for HIV-associated impairments; a screening battery composed of a few select tests does show promise, however. Determining whether there has been a decline from previous functioning is best achieved by using norms that adjust for key demographic factors, while tests derived from cognitive neuropsychology can yield insights regarding potential mechanisms for specific impairments.

Even mild levels of impairment affect everyday functioning. As HIV-1 infection is increasingly seen as a chronic illness, the development of additional, validated measures of everyday functioning is needed to further guide clinicians and researchers regarding the types of impairments that put individuals at risk for disability, poor adherence, and impaired real world performance. These would also be applicable to clinical trials, where the impact of medications on quality of life is an important outcome.

We thank Rachel Meyer for her assistance with the research and formatting of this chapter.

REFERENCES

Achim, C. L., R. Wang, D. K. Miners, and C. A. Wiley. 1994. Brain viral burden in HIV infection. *J. Neuropathol. Exp. Neurol.* **53:**284–294.

Albert, S. M., K. Marder, G. Dooneief, K. Bell, M. Sano, G. Todak, and Y. Stern. 1995. Neuropsychologic impairment in early HIV infection. A risk factor for work disability. *Arch. Neurol.* **52:**525–530.

Albert, S. M., C. M. Weber, G. Todak, C. Polanco, R. Clouse, M. McElhiney, J. Rabkin, Y. Stern, and K. Marder. 1999. An observed performance test of medication management ability in HIV: relation to neuropsychological status and medication adherence outcomes. *AIDS Behav.* **3:**121–128.

American Academy of Neurology AIDS Task Force. 1991. Nomenclature and research case definitions for neurologic manifestations of human immunodeficiency virus-type 1 (HIV-1) infection. *Neurology* **41:**778–785.

American Psychiatric Association. 1994. *Diagnostic and Statistical Manual of Mental Disorders,* 4th ed. American Psychiatric Association, Washington, DC.

Andrade, A., H. F. McGruder, A. W. Wu, S. A. Celano, R. L. Skolasky, Jr., O. A. Selnes, I. Huang, and J. C. McArthur. 2005. A programmable prompting device improves adherence to highly active antiretroviral therapy in HIV-infected subjects with memory impairment. *Clin. Infect. Dis.* **41:**875–882.

Antinori, A., G. Arendt, J. T. Becker, B. J. Brew, D. A. Byrd, M. Cherner, D. B. Clifford, P. Cinque, L. G. Epstein, K. Goodkin, M. Gisslen, I. Grant, R. K. Heaton, J. Joseph, K. Marder, C. M. Marra, J. C. McArthur, M. Nunn, R. W. Price, L. Pulliam, K. R. Robertson, N. Sacktor, V. Valcour, and V. E. Wojna. 2007. Updated research nosology for HIV-associated neurocognitive disorders. *Neurology* **69:**1789–1799.

Antinori, A., M. L. Giancola, S. Grisetti, F. Soldani, L. Alba, G. Liuzzi, A. Amendola, M. Capobianchi, V. Tozzi, and C. F. Perno. 2002. Factors influencing virological response to antiretroviral drugs in cerebrospinal fluid of advanced HIV-1-infected patients. *AIDS* **16:**1867–1876.

Atkinson, J. H., and I. Grant. 1994. Natural history of neuropsychiatric manifestations of HIV disease. *Psychiatr. Clin. N. Am.* **17:**17–33.

Ball, K., C. Owsley, M. E. Sloane, D. L. Roenker, and J. R. Bruni. 1993. Visual attention problems as a predictor of vehicle crashes in older drivers. *Investig. Ophthalmol. Vis. Sci.* **34:**3110–3423.

Bechara, A., and E. M. Martin. 2004. Impaired decision making related to working memory deficits in individuals with substance addictions. *Neuropsychology* **18:**152–162.

Becker, J. T., R. Caldararo, O. L. Lopez, M. A. Dew, S. K. Dorst, and G. Banks. 1995. Qualitative features of the memory deficit associated with HIV infection and AIDS: cross-validation of a discriminant function classification scheme. *J. Clin. Exp. Neuropsychol.* **17:**134–142.

Becker, J. T., O. L. Lopez, M. A. Dew, and H. J. Aizenstein. 2004. Prevalence of cognitive disorders differs as a function of age in HIV virus infection. *AIDS* **18**(Suppl 1)**:**S11–S18.

Boccellari, A., and P. Zeifert. 1994. Management of neurobehavioral impairment in HIV-1 infection. *Psychiatr. Clin. N. Am.* **17:**183–203.

Bornstein, R. A., H. A. Nasrallah, M. F. Para, C. C. Whitacre, P. Rosenberger, R. J. Fass, and R. Rice. 1992. Neuropsychological performance in asymptomatic HIV infection. *J. Neuropsychiatry Clin. Neurosci.* **4:**386–394.

Bottiggi, K. A., J. J. Chang, F. A. Schmitt, M. J. Avison, Y. Mootoor, A. Nath, and J. R. Berger. 2007. The HIV Dementia Scale: predicting power in mild dementia and HAART. *J. Neurol. Sci.* **260:**11–15.

Bouwman, F. H., R. L. Skolasky, D. Hes, O. A. Selnes, J. D. Glass, T. E. Nance-Sproson, W. Royal, G. J. Dal Pan, and J. C. McArthur. 1998. Variable progression of HIV-associated dementia. *Neurology* **50:**1814–1820.

Brandt, J., and R. H. B. Benedict. 2001. *Hopkins Verbal Learning Test-Revised. Professional manual.* Psychological Assessment Resources, Inc., Lutz, FL.

Brew, B. J. 2004. Evidence for a change in AIDS dementia complex in the era of highly active antiretroviral therapy and the possibility of new forms of AIDS dementia complex. *AIDS* **18**(Suppl 1)**:**S75–S78.

Butters, N., I. Grant, J. Haxby, L. L. Judd, A. Martin, J. McClelland, W. Pequegnat, D. Schacter, and E. Stover. 1990. Assessment of AIDS-related cognitive changes: recommendations of the NIMH Workshop on Neuropsychological Assessment Approaches. *J. Clin. Exp. Neuropsychol.* **12:**963–978.

Carey, C. L., S. P. Woods, R. Gonzalez, E. Conover, T. D. Marcotte, I. Grant, R. K. Heaton, and the HNRC Group. 2004a. Predictive validity of global deficit scores in detecting neuropsychological impairment in HIV infection. *J. Clin. Exp. Neuropsychol.* **26:**307–319.

Carey, C. L., S. P. Woods, J. D. Rippeth, R. Gonzalez, D. J. Moore, T. D. Marcotte, I. Grant, R. K. Heaton, and the HNRC Group. 2004b. Initial validation of a screening battery for the detection of HIV-associated cognitive impairment. *Clin. Neuropsychol.* **18**:234–248.

Carey, C. L., S. P. Woods, J. D. Rippeth, R. K. Heaton, I. Grant, and the HNRC Group. 2006. Prospective memory in HIV-1 infection. *J. Clin. Exp. Neuropsychol.* **28**:536–548.

Carter, S. L., S. B. Rourke, S. Murji, D. Shore, and B. P. Rourke. 2003. Cognitive complaints, depression, medical symptoms, and their association with neuropsychological functioning in HIV infection: a structural equation model analysis. *Neuropsychology* **17**:410–419.

Cherner, M., R. J. Ellis, D. Lazzaretto, C. Young, M. R. Mindt, J. H. Atkinson, I. Grant, R. K. Heaton, and the HNRC Group. 2004. Effects of HIV-1 infection and aging on neurobehavioral functioning: preliminary findings. *AIDS* **18**(Suppl 1):S27–S34.

Cherner, M., L. Cysique, R. K. Heaton, T. D. Marcotte, R. J. Ellis, E. Masliah, I. Grant, and the HNRC Group. 2007. Neuropathologic confirmation of definitional criteria for human immunodeficiency virus-associated neurocognitive disorders. *J. Neurovirol.* **13**:23–28.

Cherner, M., S. Letendre, R. K. Heaton, J. Durelle, J. Marquie-Beck, B. Gragg, I. Grant, and the HNRC Group. 2005. Hepatitis C augments cognitive deficits associated with HIV infection and methamphetamine. *Neurology* **64**:1343–1347.

Cherner, M., E. Masliah, R. J. Ellis, T. D. Marcotte, D. J. Moore, I. Grant, R. K. Heaton, and the HNRC Group. 2002. Neurocognitive dysfunction predicts postmortem findings of HIV encephalitis. *Neurology* **59**:1563–1567.

Chesney, M. A., J. R. Ickovics, D. B. Chambers, A. L. Gifford, J. Neidig, B. Zwickl, A. W. Wu, et al. 2000. Self-reported adherence to antiretroviral medications among participants in HIV clinical trials: the AACTG adherence instruments. *AIDS Care* **12**:255–266.

Childers, M. E., R. J. Ellis, R. Deutsch, T. Wolfson, I. Grant, and the HNRC Group. 2002. The utility and limitations of the HIV dementia scale. *J. Int. Neuropsychol. Soc.* **8**:160.

Childs, E. A., R. H. Lyles, O. A. Selnes, B. Chen, E. N. Miller, B. A. Cohen, J. T. Becker, J. Mellors, and J. C. McArthur. 1999. Plasma viral load and CD4 lymphocytes predict HIV-associated dementia and sensory neuropathy. *Neurology* **52**:607–613.

Clifford, D. B., J. C. McArthur, G. Schifitto, K. Kieburtz, M. P. McDermott, S. Letendre, B. A. Cohen, K. Marder, R. J. Ellis, and C. M. Marra. 2002. A randomized clinical trial of CPI-1189 for HIV-associated cognitive-motor impairment. *Neurology* **59**:1568–1573.

Cohen, R. A., R. Boland, R. Paul, K. T. Tashima, E. E. Schoenbaum, D. D. Celentano, P. Schuman, D. K. Smith, and C. C. Carpenter. 2001. Neurocognitive performance enhanced by highly active antiretroviral therapy in HIV-infected women. *AIDS* **15**:341–345.

Cysique, L. A., R. Deutsch, J. A. Atkinson, C. Young, T. D. Marcotte, L. Dawson, I. Grant, R. K. Heaton, and the HNRC Group. 2007. Incident major depression does not affect neuropsychological functioning in HIV-infected men. *J. Int. Neuropsychol. Soc.* **13**:1–11.

Cysique, L. A., P. Maruff, and B. J. Brew. 2004a. Antiretroviral therapy in HIV infection: are neurologically active drugs important? *Arch. Neurol.* **61**:1699–1704.

Cysique, L. A., P. Maruff, and B. J. Brew. 2004b. Prevalence and pattern of neuropsychological impairment in human immunodeficiency virus-infected/acquired immunodeficiency syndrome (HIV/AIDS) patients across pre- and post-highly active antiretroviral therapy eras: a combined study of two cohorts. *J. Neurovirol.* **10**:350–357.

Cysique, L. A., P. Maruff, and B. J. Brew. 2006. Variable benefit in neuropsychological function in HIV-infected HAART-treated patients. *Neurology* **66**:1447–1450.

Dal Pan, G. J., H. Farzadegan, O. Selnes, D. R. Hoover, E. N. Miller, R. L. Skolasky, T. E. Nance-Sproson, and J. C. McArthur. 1998. Sustained cognitive decline in HIV infection: relationship to CD4+ cell count, plasma viremia and p24 antigenemia. *J. Neurovirol.* **4**:95–99.

Detels, R., A. Munoz, G. McFarlane, L. A. Kingsley, J. B. Margolick, J. Giorgi, L. K. Schrager, and J. P. Phair. 1998. Effectiveness of potent antiretroviral therapy on time to AIDS and death in men with known HIV infection duration. *JAMA* **280**:1497–1503.

Deutsch, R., R. J. Ellis, J. A. McCutchan, T. D. Marcotte, S. Letendre, I. Grant, and the HNRC Group. 2001. AIDS-associated mild neurocognitive impairment is delayed in the era of highly active antiretroviral therapy. *AIDS* **15**:1898–1899.

Dore, G. J., P. K. Correll, Y. Li, J. M. Kaldor, D. A. Cooper, and B. J. Brew. 1999. Changes to AIDS dementia complex in the era of highly active antiretroviral therapy. *AIDS* **13**:1249–1253.

Dore, G. J., A. McDonald, Y. Li, J. M. Kaldor, and B. J. Brew. 2003. Marked improvement in survival following AIDS dementia complex in the era of highly active antiretroviral therapy. *AIDS* **17**:1539–1545.

Duchek, J. M., L. Hunt, K. Ball, V. Buckles, and J. C. Morris. 1998. Attention and driving performance in Alzheimer's disease. *J. Gerontol.* **53**:P130–P141.

Ellis, R. J., R. Deutsch, R. K. Heaton, T. D. Marcotte, J. A. McCutchan, J. A. Nelson, I. Abramson, L. J. Thal, J. H. Atkinson, M. R. Wallace, I. Grant, et al. 1997a. Neurocognitive impairment is an independent risk factor for death in HIV infection. *Arch. Neurol.* **54**:416–424.

Ellis, R. J., K. Hsia, S. A. Spector, J. A. Nelson, R. K. Heaton, M. R. Wallace, I. Abramson, J. H. Atkinson, I. Grant, J. A. McCutchan, et al. 1997b. Cerebrospinal fluid human immunodeficiency virus type 1 RNA levels are elevated in neurocognitively impaired individuals with acquired immunodeficiency syndrome. *Ann. Neurol.* **42**:679–688.

Ellis, R. J., D. J. Moore, M. E. Childers, S. Letendre, J. A. McCutchan, T. Wolfson, S. A. Spector, K. Hsia, R. K. Heaton, and I. Grant. 2002. Progression to neuropsychological impairment in human immunodeficiency virus infection predicted by elevated cerebrospinal fluid levels of human immunodeficiency virus RNA. *Arch. Neurol.* **59**:923–928.

Everall, I. P., R. K. Heaton, T. D. Marcotte, R. J. Ellis, J. A. McCutchan, J. H. Atkinson, I. Grant, M. Mallory, and E. Masliah. 1999. Cortical synaptic density is reduced in mild to moderate human immunodeficiency virus neurocognitive disorder. *Brain Pathol.* **9**:209–217.

Farinpour, R., E. M. Martin, M. Seidenberg, D. L. Pitrak, K. J. Pursell, K. M. Mullane, R. M. Novak, and M. Harrow. 2000. Verbal working memory in HIV-seropositive drug users. *J. Int. Neuropsychol. Soc.* **6**:548–555.

Ferrando, S., W. van Gorp, M. McElhiney, K. Goggin, M. Sewell, and J. Rabkin. 1998. Highly active antiretroviral treatment in HIV infection: benefits for neuropsychological function. *AIDS* **12**:F65–F70.

Ferrando, S. J., J. G. Rabkin, W. van Gorp, S. H. Lin, and M. McElhiney. 2003. Longitudinal improvement in psychomotor processing speed is associated with potent combination antiretroviral therapy in HIV-1 infection. *J. Neuropsychiatry Clin. Neurosci.* **15**:208–214.

Folstein, M. 1983. The Mini-Mental State Exam, p. 47–51. *In* T. Crook, S. Ferris, and R. Bartus (ed.), *Assessment in Geriatric Psychopharmacology*. Mark Powley, New Canaan, CT.

Folstein, M. F., S. E. Folstein, and P. R. McHugh. 1975. "Mini-Mental State": A practical method for grading the cognitive state of outpatients for the clinician. *J. Psychiatr. Res.* **12:**189–198.

Gardner, R., S. Oliver-Munoz, L. Fisher, and L. Empting. 1981. Mattis Dementia Rating Scale: internal reliability study using a diffusely impaired population. *J. Clin. Neuropsychol.* **3:**271–275.

Giancola, M. L., P. Lorenzini, P. Balestra, D. Larussa, F. Baldini, A. Corpolongo, P. Narciso, R. Bellagamba, V. Tozzi, and A. Antinori. 2006. Neuroactive antiretroviral drugs do not influence neurocognitive performance in less advanced HIV-infected patients responding to highly active antiretroviral therapy. *J. Acquir. Immune Defic. Syndr.* **41:**332–337.

Gladsjo, J. A., C. C. Schuman, J. D. Evans, G. M. Peavy, S. W. Miller, and R. K. Heaton. 1999. Norms for letter and category fluency: demographic corrections for age, education, and ethnicity. *Assessment* **6:**147–178.

Glass, J. D., S. L. Wesselingh, O. A. Selnes, and J. C. McArthur. 1993. Clinical-neuropathologic correlations in HIV-associated dementia. *Neurology* **43:**2230–2237.

Goodkin, K., F. L. Wilkie, M. Concha, C. H. Hinkin, S. Symes, T. T. Baldewicz, D. Asthana, R. K. Fujimura, D. Lee, M. H. van Zuilen, I. Khamis, P. Shapshak, and C. Eisdorfer. 2001. Aging and neuro-AIDS conditions and the changing spectrum of HIV-1-associated morbidity and mortality. *J. Clin. Epidemiol.* **54**(Suppl 1):S35–S43.

Gonzalez, E., B. H. Rovin, L. Sen, G. Cooke, R. Dhanda, S. Mummidi, H. Kulkarni, M. J. Bamshad, V. Telles, S. A. Anderson, E. A. Walter, K. T. Stephan, M. Deucher, A. Mangano, R. Bologna, S. S. Ahuja, M. J. Dolan, and S. K. Ahuja. 2002. HIV-1 infection and AIDS dementia are influenced by a mutant MCP-1 allele linked to increased monocyte infiltration of tissues and MCP-1 levels. *Proc. Natl. Acad. Sci. U.S.A.* **99:**13795–13800.

Grant, I., and J. H. Atkinson. 1995. Psychiatric aspects of acquired immune deficiency syndrome, p. 1644–1669. *In* H. I. Kaplan and B. J. Sadock (ed.), *Comprehensive Textbook of Psychiatry/VI*, vol. 2, section 29.2. Williams and Wilkins, Baltimore, MD.

Grant, I., J. H. Atkinson, J. R. Hesselink, C. J. Kennedy, D. D. Richman, S. A. Spector, and J. A. McCutchan. 1987. Evidence for early central nervous system involvement in the acquired immunodeficiency syndrome (AIDS) and other human immunodeficiency virus (HIV) infections. *Ann. Intern. Med.* **107:**828–836.

Grant, I., R. A. Olshen, J. H. Atkinson, R. K. Heaton, J. Nelson, J. A. McCutchan, and J. D. Weinrich. 1993. Depressed mood does not explain neuropsychological deficits in HIV-infected persons. *Neuropsychology* **7:**53–61.

Hasenauer, D., O. Selnes, T. E. Nance-Sproson, D. Esposito, and J. C. McArthur. 1996. Psychomotor slowing in HIV-associated dementia (HAD): central nervous system (CNS) dysfunction or fatigue? *J. Neurovirol.* **2:**39.

Heaton, R. K., I. Grant, N. Butters, D. A. White, D. Kirson, J. H. Atkinson, J. A. McCutchan, M. J. Taylor, M. D. Kelly, R. J. Ellis, T. Wolfson, R. Velin, T. D. Marcotte, J. R. Hesselink, T. L. Jernigan, J. Chandler, M. Wallace, I. Abramson, and the HNRC Group. 1995. The HNRC 500—Neuropsychology of HIV infection at different disease stages. *J. Int. Neuropsychol. Soc.* **1:**231–251.

Heaton, R. K., D. Kirson, R. A. Velin, I. Grant, and the HNRC Group. 1994a. The utility of clinical ratings for detecting cognitive change in HIV infection, p. 188–206. *In* I. Grant and A. Martin (ed.), *Neuropsychology of HIV Infection.* Oxford University Press, New York, NY.

Heaton, R. K., and T. D. Marcotte. 2000. Clinical neuropsychological tests and assessment techniques, p. 27–52. *In* F. Boller, J. Grafman, and G. Rizzolatti (ed.), *Handbook of Neuropsychology.* Elsevier Science B.V., Amsterdam, The Netherlands.

Heaton, R. K., T. D. Marcotte, M. R. Mindt, J. Sadek, D. J. Moore, H. Bentley, J. A. McCutchan, C. Reicks, I. Grant, and the HNRC Group. 2004a. The impact of HIV-associated neuropsychological impairment on everyday functioning. *J. Int. Neuropsychol. Soc.* **10:**317–331.

Heaton, R. K., T. D. Marcotte, D. A. White, D. Ross, K. Meredith, M. J. Taylor, R. Kaplan, and I. Grant. 1996. Nature and vocational significance of neuropsychological impairment associated with HIV infection. *Clin. Neuropsychol.* **10:**1–14.

Heaton, R. K., S. W. Miller, M. J. Taylor, and I. Grant. 2004b. *Revised Comprehensive Norms for an Expanded Halstead-Reitan Battery: Demographically Adjusted Neuropsychological Norms for African American and Caucasian Adults.* Psychological Assessment Resources, Inc., Lutz, FL.

Heaton, R. K., R. A. Velin, J. A. McCutchan, S. J. Gulevich, J. H. Atkinson, M. R. Wallace, H. P. D. Godfrey, D. A. Kirson, I. Grant, and the HNRC Group. 1994b. Neuropsychological impairment in human immunodeficiency virus-infection: implications for employment. *Psychosom. Med.* **56:**8–17.

Heseltine, P. N., K. Goodkin, J. H. Atkinson, B. Vitiello, J. Rochon, R. K. Heaton, E. M. Eaton, F. L. Wilkie, E. Sobel, S. J. Brown, D. Feaster, L. Schneider, W. L. Goldschmidts, and E. S. Stover. 1998. Randomized double-blind placebo-controlled trial of peptide T for HIV-associated cognitive impairment. *Arch. Neurol.* **55:**41–51.

Hinkin, C. H., S. A. Castellon, R. S. Durvasula, D. J. Hardy, M. N. Lam, K. I. Mason, D. Thrasher, M. B. Goetz, and M. Stefaniak. 2002a. Medication adherence among HIV+ adults: effects of cognitive dysfunction and regimen complexity. *Neurology* **59:**1944–1950.

Hinkin, C. H., D. J. Hardy, K. I. Mason, S. A. Castellon, M. N. Lam, M. Stefaniak, and B. Zolnikov. 2002b. Verbal and spatial working memory performance among HIV-infected adults. *J. Int. Neuropsychol. Soc.* **8:**532–538.

Hinkin, C. H., W. G. van Gorp, P. Satz, J. D. Weisman, J. Thommes, and S. Buckingham. 1992. Depressed mood and its relationship to neuropsychological test performance in HIV-1 seropositive individuals. *J. Clin. Exp. Neuropsychol.* **14:**289–297.

Hiscock, M., and C. K. Hiscock. 1989. Refining the forced-choice method for the detection of malingering. *J. Clin. Exp. Neuropsychol.* **11:**967–974.

Ivnik, R. J., G. E. Smith, J. F. Malec, and R. C. Petersen. 1995. Long term stability and intercorrelations of cognitive abilities in older persons. *Psychol. Assess.* **7:**155–161.

Jacobs, J. W., M. R. Bernhard, A. Delgado, and J. J. Strain. 1977. Screening for organic mental syndromes in the medically ill. *Ann. Intern. Med.* **86:**40–46.

Kaplan, R. M., J. P. Anderson, T. L. Patterson, J. A. McCutchan, J. D. Weinrich, R. K. Heaton, J. H. Atkinson, L. Thal, J. Chandler, I. Grant, and the HNRC Group. 1995. Validity of the Quality of Well-Being Scale for persons with human immunodeficiency virus infection. *Psychosom. Med.* **57:**138–147.

Kaplan, R. M., T. L. Patterson, D. N. Kerner, J. H. Atkinson, R. K. Heaton, I. Grant, et al. 1997. The Quality of Well-Being scale in asymptomatic HIV-infected patients. *Qual. Life Res.* **6:**507–514.

Kissel, E. C., N. D. Pukay-Martin, and R. A. Bornstein. 2005. The relationship between age and cognitive function in HIV-infected men. *J. Neuropsychiatry Clin. Neurosci.* **17:**180–184.

Klove, H. 1963. Clinical neuropsychology, p. 1647–1658 *In* F. M. Forster (ed.), *The Medical Clinics of North America.* Saunders, New York, NY.

Langford, D., A. Adame, A. Grigorian, I. Grant, J. A. McCutchan, R. J. Ellis, T. D. Marcotte, E. Masliah, and the HNRC Group. 2003. Patterns of selective neuronal damage in methamphetamine-user AIDS patients. *J. Acquir. Immune Defic. Syndr.* **34:**467–474.

Letendre, S., J. Marquie-Beck, E. Capparelli, B. Best, D. Clifford, A. Collier, B. B. Gelman, J. C. McArthur, J. A. McCutchan, S. Morgello, D. Simpson, I. Grant, R. J. Ellis, and the CHARTER Group. 2008. Validation of the CNS Penetrati-Effectiveness rank for quantifying antiretroviral penetration into the central nervous system. *Arch. Neurol.* **65:**65–70.

Letendre, S. L., J. A. McCutchan, M. E. Childers, S. P. Woods, D. Lazzaretto, R. K. Heaton, I. Grant, and R. J. Ellis. 2004. Enhancing antiretroviral therapy for human immunodeficiency virus cognitive disorders. *Ann. Neurol.* **56:**416–423.

Lojek, E., and R. A. Bornstein. 2005. The stability of neuro-cognitive patterns in HIV infected men: classification considerations. *J. Clin. Exp. Neuropsychol.* **27:**665–682.

Marcotte, T. D., R. Deutsch, J. A. McCutchan, D. J. Moore, S. Letendre, R. J. Ellis, M. R. Wallace, R. K. Heaton, I. Grant, and the HNRC Group. 2003. Prediction of incident neurocognitive impairment by plasma HIV RNA and CD4 levels early after HIV seroconversion. *Arch. Neurol.* **60:**1406–1412.

Marcotte, T. D., R. K. Heaton, R. J. Ellis, I. Grant, and the HNRC Group. 2005. Neuropsychological impairment in HIV infection: how typical is the "typical profile"? *J. Int. Neuropsychol. Soc.* **11:**21.

Marcotte, T. D., R. K. Heaton, R. Gonzalez, C. Reicks, I. Grant, and the HNRC Group. 2000. HIV-associated neurocognitive deficits impact on-road driving abilities. *J. Neurovirol.* **6:**268.

Marcotte, T. D., R. K. Heaton, T. Wolfson, M. J. Taylor, O. Alhassoon, K. Arfaa, R. J. Ellis, I. Grant, and the HNRC Group. 1999. The impact of HIV-related neuropsychological dysfunction on driving behavior. *J. Int. Neuropsychol. Soc.* **5:**579–592.

Marcotte, T. D., D. Lazzaretto, J. C. Scott, E. Roberts, S. P. Woods, S. Letendre, and the HNRC Group. 2006. Visual attention deficits are associated with driving accidents in cognitively-impaired HIV-infected individuals. *J. Clin. Exp. Neuropsychol.* **28:**13–28.

Marcotte, T. D., and J. C. Scott. 2004. The assessment of driving abilities. *Adv. Transportation Studies* **4**(Suppl.)**:**79–90.

Marcotte, T. D., T. Wolfson, T. J. Rosenthal, R. K. Heaton, R. Gonzalez, R. J. Ellis, I. Grant, and the HNRC Group. 2004. A multimodal assessment of driving performance in HIV infection. *Neurology* **63:**1417–1422.

Marra, C. M., D. Lockhart, J. R. Zunt, M. Perrin, R. W. Coombs, and A. C. Collier. 2003. Changes in CSF and plasma HIV-1 RNA and cognition after starting potent anti-retroviral therapy. *Neurology* **60:**1388–1390.

Martin, E. M., D. L. Pitrak, W. Weddington, N. A. Rains, G. Nunnally, H. Nixon, S. Grbesic, J. Vassileva, and A. Bechara. 2004. Cognitive impulsivity and HIV serostatus in substance dependent males. *J. Int. Neuropsychol. Soc.* **10:**931–938.

Martin, E. M., T. S. Sullivan, R. A. Reed, T. A. Fletcher, D. L. Pitrak, W. Weddington, and M. Harrow. 2001. Auditory working memory in HIV-1 infection. *J. Int. Neuropsychol. Soc.* **7:**20–26.

Masliah, E., C. L. Achim, N. Ge, R. DeTeresa, R. D. Terry, and C. A. Wiley. 1992a. Spectrum of human immunodeficiency virus-associated neocortical damage. *Ann. Neurol.* **32:**321–329.

Masliah, E., N. Ge, C. L. Achim, L. A. Hansen, and C. A. Wiley. 1992b. Selective neuronal vulnerability in HIV encephalitis. *J. Neuropathol. Exp. Neurol.* **51:**585–593.

Masliah, E., N. Ge, C. L. Achim, and C. A. Wiley. 1996. Patterns of neurodegeneration in HIV encephalitis. *J. Neuro-AIDS* **1:**161–173.

Masliah, E., R. K. Heaton, T. D. Marcotte, R. J. Ellis, C. A. Wiley, M. Mallory, C. L. Achim, J. A. McCutchan, J. A. Nelson, J. H. Atkinson, I. Grant, and the HNRC Group. 1997. Dendritic injury is a pathologic substrate for HIV-related cognitive disorders. *Ann. Neurol.* **42:**963–972.

Mattis, S. 1976. Mental status examination for organic mental syndrome in the elderly patient, p. 77–101. *In* L. Bellak and T. E. Karasu (ed.), *Geriatric Psychiatry: a Handbook for Psychiatrists and Primary Care Physicians.* Grune & Stratton, New York, NY.

Mayeux, R., Y. Stern, M.-X. Tang, G. Todak, K. Marder, J. Sano, M. Richards, Z. Stein, A. Ehrhardt, and J. Gorman. 1993. Mortality risks in gay men with human immunodeficiency virus infection and cognitive impairment. *Neurology* **43:**176–182.

McArthur, J. C. 2004. HIV dementia: an evolving disease. *J. Neuroimmunol.* **157:**3–10.

McArthur, J. C., B. A. Cohen, O. A. Selnes, A. J. Kumar, K. Cooper, J. H. McArthur, G. Soucy, D. R. Cornblath, J. S. Chmiel, M. Wang, D. L. Starkey, H. Ginzburg, D. G. Ostrow, R. T. Johnson, J. P. Phair, and B. F. Polk. 1989. Low prevalence of neurological and neuropsychological abnormalities in otherwise healthy HIV-1 infected individuals: results from the Multicenter AIDS Cohort Study. *Ann. Neurol.* **26:**601–611.

McArthur, J. C., and I. Grant. 1998. HIV neurocognitive disorders, p. 499–524. *In* H. E. Gendelman, S. Lipton, L. Epstein, and S. Swindells (ed.), *Neurology of AIDS.* Chapman and Hall Publishers, New York, NY.

McArthur, J. C., D. R. Hoover, H. Bacellar, E. N. Miller, B. A. Cohen, J. T. Becker, N. M. H. Graham, J. H. McArthur, O. A. Selnes, L. P. Jacobson, B. R. Visscher, M. Concha, and A. Saah. 1993. Dementia in AIDS patients: incidence and risk factors. *Neurology* **43:**2245–2252.

McArthur, J. C., M. P. McDermott, D. McClernon, C. St Hillaire, K. Conant, K. Marder, G. Schifitto, O. A. Selnes, N. Sacktor, Y. Stern, S. M. Albert, K. Kieburtz, J. A. deMar-caida, B. Cohen, and L. G. Epstein. 2004. Attenuated central nervous system infection in advanced HIV/AIDS with combination antiretroviral therapy. *Arch. Neurol.* **61:**1687–1696.

McCutchan, J. A., J. W. Wu, S. Robertson, S. L. Koletar, R. J. Ellis, S. Cohn, M. Taylor, S. Woods, R. Heaton, J. Currier, and P. L. Williams. 2007. HIV suppression by HAART preserves cognitive function in advanced, immune-reconstituted AIDS patients. *AIDS* **21:**1109–1117.

Mindt, M., M. Cherner, T. Marcotte, D. Moore, H. Bentley, M. Esquivel, Y. Lopez, I. Grant, and R. Heaton. 2003. The functional impact of HIV-associated neuropsychological impairment in Spanish-speaking adults: a pilot study. *J. Clin. Exp. Neuropsychol.* **25:**122–132.

Morgan, E. E., S. P. Woods, J. C. Scott, M. Childers, J. M. Beck, R. J. Ellis, I. Grant, R. K. Heaton, and the HNRC Group. 2008. Predictive validity of demographically adjusted normative standards for the HIV Dementia Scale. *J. Clin. Exp. Neuropsychol.* **30:**83–90.

Myers, R. S., K. K. Ball, T. D. Kalina, D. L. Roth, and K. T. Goode. 2000. Relation of useful field of view and other screening tests to on-road driving performance. *Percept. Mot. Skills* **91:**279–290.

Navia, B. A., E.-S. Cho, C. K. Petito, and R. W. Price. 1986a. The AIDS dementia complex: II. Neuropathology. *Ann. Neurol.* **19:**525–535.

Navia, B. A., U. Dafni, D. Simpson, T. Tucker, E. Singer, J. C. McArthur, C. Yiannoutsos, L. Zaborski, S. A. Lipton, and the AIDS Clinical Trial Group. 1998. A phase I/II trial of nimodipine for HIV-related neurologic complications. *Neurology* **51:**221–228.

Navia, B. A., B. D. Jordan, and R. W. Price. 1986b. The AIDS dementia complex: I. Clinical features. *Ann. Neurol.* **19:**517–524.

Neuenburg, J. K., H. R. Brodt, B. G. Herndier, M. Bickel, P. Bacchetti, R. W. Price, R. M. Grant, and W. Schlote. 2002. HIV-related neuropathology, 1985 to 1999: rising prevalence of HIV encephalopathy in the era of highly active antiretroviral therapy. *J. Acquir. Immune Defic. Syndr.* **31:**171–177.

Osowiecki, D. M., R. A. Cohen, K. M. Morrow, R. H. Paul, C. C. Carpenter, T. Flanigan, and R. J. Boland. 2000. Neurocognitive and psychological contributions to quality of life in HIV-1-infected women. *AIDS* **14:**1327–1332.

Owsley, C., K. Ball, G. McGwin, Jr., M. E. Sloane, D. L. Roenker, M. White, and T. Overley. 1998. Visual processing impairment and risk of motor vehicle crash among older adults. *JAMA* **279:**1083–1088.

Parsons, T. D., K. A. Tucker, C. D. Hall, W. T. Robertson, J. J. Eron, M. W. Fried, and K. R. Robertson. 2006. Neurocognitive functioning and HAART in HIV and hepatitis C virus co-infection. *AIDS* **20:**1591–1595.

Peavy, G., D. Jacobs, D. P. Salmon, N. Butters, D. C. Delis, M. Taylor, P. Massman, J. C. Stout, W. G. Heindel, D. Kirson, J. H. Atkinson, J. L. Chandler, and I. Grant. 1994. Verbal memory performance of patients with human immunodeficiency virus infection: evidence of subcortical dysfunction. *J. Clin. Exp. Neuropsychol.* **16:**508–523.

Piatt, A. L., J. A. Fields, A. M. Paolo, and A. I. Troster. 1999. Action (verb naming) fluency as an executive function measure: convergent and divergent evidence of validity. *Neuropsychologia* **37:**1499–1503.

Pillai, S. K., S. L. Pond, Y. Liu, B. M. Good, M. C. Strain, R. J. Ellis, S. Letendre, D. M. Smith, H. F. Gunthard, I. Grant, T. D. Marcotte, J. A. McCutchan, D. D. Richman, and J. K. Wong. 2006. Genetic attributes of cerebrospinal fluid-derived HIV-1 env. *Brain* **129:**1872–1883.

Podraza, A. M., R. A. Bornstein, C. C. Whitacre, M. F. Para, R. J. Fass, R. R. Rice, Jr., and H. A. Nasrallah. 1994. Neuropsychological performance and CD4 levels in HIV-1 asymptomatic infection. *J. Clin. Exp. Neuropsychol.* **16:**777–783.

Porter, K., A. Babiker, K. Bhaskaran, J. Darbyshire, P. Pezzotti, and A. S. Walker. 2003. Determinants of survival following HIV-1 seroconversion after the introduction of HAART. *Lancet* **362:**1267–1274.

Power, C., O. A. Selnes, J. A. Grim, and J. C. McArthur. 1995. HIV Dementia Scale: a rapid screening test. *J. Acquir. Immune Defic. Syndr.* **8:**273–278.

Rabkin, J. G., and S. Ferrando. 1997. A 'second life' agenda. Psychiatric research issues raised by protease inhibitor treatments for people with the human immunodeficiency virus or the acquired immunodeficiency syndrome. *Arch. Gen. Psychiatry* **54:**1049–1053.

Rippeth, J. D., R. K. Heaton, C. L. Carey, T. D. Marcotte, D. J. Moore, R. Gonzalez, T. Wolfson, I. Grant, and the HNRC Group. 2004. Methamphetamine dependence increases risk of neuropsychological impairment in HIV infected persons. *J. Int. Neuropsychol. Soc.* **10:**1–14.

Robertson, K. R., W. T. Robertson, S. Ford, D. Watson, S. Fiscus, A. G. Harp, and C. D. Hall. 2004. Highly active antiretroviral therapy improves neurocognitive functioning. *J. Acquir. Immune Defic. Syndr.* **36:**562–566.

Robertson, K. R., M. Smurzynski, T. D. Parsons, K. Wu, R. J. Bosch, J. Wu, J. C. McArthur, A. C. Collier, S. R. Evans, and R. J. Ellis. 2007. The prevalence and incidence of neurocognitive impairment in the HAART era. *AIDS* **21:**1915–1921.

Rourke, S. B., M. H. Halman, and C. Bassel. 1999. Neuropsychiatric correlates of memory-metamemory dissociations in HIV-infection. *J. Clin. Exp. Neuropsychol.* **21:**757–768.

Ryan, E. L., S. Morgello, K. Isaacs, M. Naseer, and P. Gerits. 2004. Neuropsychiatric impact of hepatitis C on advanced HIV. *Neurology* **62:**957–962.

Sacktor, N., R. H. Lyles, R. Skolasky, C. Kleeberger, O. A. Selnes, E. N. Miller, J. T. Becker, B. Cohen, and J. C. McArthur. 2001. HIV-associated neurologic disease incidence changes: Multicenter AIDS Cohort Study, 1990–1998. *Neurology* **56:**257–260.

Sacktor, N., M. P. McDermott, K. Marder, G. Schifitto, O. A. Selnes, J. C. McArthur, Y. Stern, S. Albert, D. Palumbo, K. Kieburtz, J. A. De Marcaida, B. Cohen, and L. Epstein. 2002. HIV-associated cognitive impairment before and after the advent of combination therapy. *J. Neurovirol.* **8:**136–142.

Sacktor, N., N. Nakasujja, R. Skolasky, K. Robertson, M. Wong, S. Musisi, A. Ronald, and E. Katabira. 2006. Antiretroviral therapy improves cognitive impairment in HIV+ individuals in sub-Saharan Africa. *Neurology* **67:**311–314.

Sacktor, N. C., H. Bacellar, D. R. Hoover, T. E. Nance-Sproson, O. A. Selnes, E. N. Miller, G. J. Dal Pan, C. Kleeberger, A. Brown, A. Saah, and J. C. McArthur. 1996. Psychomotor slowing in HIV infection: a predictor of dementia, AIDS and death. *J. Neurovirol.* **2:**404–410.

Selnes, O. A., J. H. McArthur, R. Fox, D. Starkey, E. N. Miller, and J. C. McArthur. 1990. Frontal lobe functioning in asymptomatic HIV-infection. *Neurology* **40**(Suppl. 1)**:**237.

Sevigny, J. J., S. M. Albert, M. P. McDermott, J. C. McArthur, N. Sacktor, K. Conant, G. Schifitto, O. A. Selnes, Y. Stern, D. R. McClernon, D. Palumbo, K. Kieburtz, G. Riggs, B. Cohen, L. G. Epstein, and K. Marder. 2004. Evaluation of HIV RNA and markers of immune activation as predictors of HIV-associated dementia. *Neurology* **63:**2084–2090.

Sidtis, J. J. 1994. Evaluation of the AIDS dementia complex in adults, p. 273–287. *In* R. W. Price and S. W. Perry (ed.), *HIV AIDS and the Brain.* Raven, New York, NY.

Smith, C. A., W. G. van Gorp, E. R. Ryan, S. J. Ferrando, and J. Rabkin. 2003. Screening subtle HIV-related cognitive dysfunction: the clinical utility of the HIV dementia scale. *J. Acquir. Immune Defic. Syndr.* **33:**116–118.

Sonnerborg, A. B., A. C. Ehrnst, S. K. Bergdahl, P. O. Pehrson, B. R. Skoldenberg, and O. O. Strannegard. 1988. HIV isolation from cerebrospinal fluid in relation to immunological deficiency and neurological symptoms. *AIDS* **2:**89–93.

Spreen, O., and E. Strauss. 1998. *A Compendium of Neuropsychological Tests: Administration, Norms, and Commentary*, 2nd ed. Oxford University Press, New York, NY.

Stankoff, B., V. Calvez, S. Suarez, P. Bossi, O. Rosenblum, L. Conquy, E. Turell, T. Dubard, A. Coutellier, L. Baril, F. Bricaire, L. Lacomblez, and C. Lubetzki. 1999. Plasma and cerebrospinal fluid human immunodeficiency virus type-1 (HIV-1) RNA levels in HIV-related cognitive impairment. *Eur. J. Neurol.* **6:**669–675.

Stern, Y., K. Marder, K. Bell, J. Chen, G. Dooneief, S. Goldstein, D. Mindry, M. Richards, M. Sano, J. Williams, J. Gorman, A. Ehrhardt, and R. Mayeux. 1991. Multidisciplinary assessment of homosexual men with and without human immunodeficiency virus infection. III. Neurologic and neuropsychological findings. *Arch. Gen. Psychiatry* **48:**131–138.

Suarez, S., L. Baril, B. Stankoff, M. Khellaf, B. Dubois, C. Lubetzki, F. Bricaire, and J. J. Hauw. 2001. Outcome of patients with HIV-1-related cognitive impairment on highly active antiretroviral therapy. *AIDS* **15:**195–200.

Temkin, N. R., R. K. Heaton, I. Grant, and S. S. Dikmen. 1999. Detecting significant change in neuropsychological test performance: a comparison of four models. *J. Int. Neuropsychol. Soc.* **5:**357–369.

Tombaugh, T. 1997. *TOMM: Test of Memory Malingering Manual.* Multi-Health Systems, Toronto, Canada.

Tozzi, V., P. Balestra, S. Galgani, P. Narciso, F. Ferri, G. Sebastiani, C. D'Amato, C. Affricano, F. Pigorini, F. M.

Pau, A. De Felici, and A. Benedetto. 1999. Positive and sustained effects of highly active antiretroviral therapy on HIV-1-associated neurocognitive impairment. *AIDS* **13**:1889–1897.

Tozzi, V., P. Balestra, S. Galgani, P. Narciso, A. Sampaolesi, A. Antinori, M. Giulianelli, D. Serraino, and G. Ippolito. 2001. Changes in neurocognitive performance in a cohort of patients treated with HAART for 3 years. *J. Acquir. Immune Defic. Syndr.* **28**:19–27.

Tozzi, V., P. Balestra, R. Murri, S. Galgani, R. Bellagamba, P. Narciso, A. Antinori, M. Giulianelli, G. Tosi, M. Fantoni, A. Sampaolesi, P. Noto, G. Ippolito, and A. W. Wu. 2004. Neurocognitive impairment influences quality of life in HIV-infected patients receiving HAART. *Int. J. STD AIDS* **15**:254–259.

Tozzi, V., P. Balestra, D. Serraino, R. Bellagamba, A. Corpolongo, P. Piselli, P. Lorenzini, U. Visco-Comandini, C. Vlassi, M. E. Quartuccio, M. Giulianelli, P. Noto, S. Galgani, G. Ippolito, A. Antinori, and P. Narciso. 2005. Neurocognitive impairment and survival in a cohort of HIV-infected patients treated with HAART. *AIDS Res. Hum. Retrovir.* **21**:706–713.

U.S. Department of Labor. 1991. *Dictionary of Occupational Titles*, 4th ed. U.S. Government Printing Office, Washington, DC.

Valcour, V., C. Shikuma, B. Shiramizu, M. Watters, P. Poff, O. Selnes, P. Holck, J. Grove, and N. Sacktor. 2004. Higher frequency of dementia in older HIV-1 individuals: the Hawaii Aging with HIV-1 Cohort. *Neurology* **63**:822–827.

Van Gorp, W., P. Satz, C. Hinkin, O. Selnes, E. Miller, J. McArthur, B. Cohen, and D. Paz. 1991. Metacognition in HIV-1 seropositive asymptomatic individuals: self-ratings versus objective neuropsychological performance. *J. Clin. Exp. Neuropsychol.* **13**:812–819.

Van Gorp, W. G., J. P. Baerwald, S. J. Ferrando, M. C. McElhiney, and J. G. Rabkin. 1999. The relationship between employment and neuropsychological impairment in HIV infection. *J. Int. Neuropsychol. Soc.* **5**:534–539.

Vaughn, G., and R. Detels. 2007. Protease inhibitors and cardiovascular disease: analysis of the Los Angeles County adult spectrum of disease cohort. *AIDS Care* **19**:492–497.

Vazquez-Justo, E., M. Rodriguez Alvarez, and M. J. Ferraces Otero. 2003. Influence of depressed mood on neuropsychologic performance in HIV-seropositive drug users. *Psychiatry Clin. Neurosci.* **57**:251–258.

Visual Resources, Inc. 1998. *UFOV Useful Field of View Manual*. The Psychological Coporation, Chicago, IL.

von Giesen, H. J., T. Heintges, N. Abbasi-Boroudjeni, S. Kucukkoylu, H. Koller, B. A. Haslinger, M. Oette, and G. Arendt. 2004. Psychomotor slowing in hepatitis C and HIV infection. *J. Acquir. Immune Defic. Syndr.* **35**:131–137.

Wechsler, D. 1997. *WAIS-III: Administration and Scoring Manual*. The Psychological Corporation, San Antonio, TX.

White, D. A., R. K. Heaton, and A. U. Monsch. 1995. Neuropsychological studies of asymptomatic human immunodeficiency virus-type 1-infected individuals. *J. Int. Neuropsychol. Soc.* **1**:304–315.

Wiley, C., E. Masliah, M. Morey, C. Lemere, R. DeTeresa, M. Grafe, L. Hansen, and R. Terry. 1991. Neocortical damage during HIV infection. *Ann. Neurol.* **29**:651–657.

Wiley, C. A., and C. Achim. 1994. Human immunodeficiency virus encephalitis is the pathological correlate of dementia in acquired immunodeficiency syndrome *Ann. Neurol.* **36**:673–676. (Erratum, **37**:140.)

Wilkie, F. L., K. Goodkin, C. Eisdorfer, D. Feaster, R. Morgan, M. A. Fletcher, N. Blaney, M. Baum, and J. Szapocznik. 1998. Mild cognitive impairment and risk of mortality in HIV-1 infection. *J. Neuropsychiatry Clin. Neurosci.* **10**:125–132.

Wilkins, J. W., K. R. Robertson, C. R. Snyder, W. K. Robertson, C. van der Horst, and C. D. Hall. 1991. Implications of self-reported cognitive and motor dysfunction in HIV-positive patients. *Am. J. Psychiatry* **148**:641–643.

Woods, S. P., C. L. Carey, A. I. Troster, I. Grant, and the HNRC Group. 2005. Action (verb) generation in HIV-1 infection. *Neuropsychologia* **43**:1144–1151.

Woods, S. P., and I. Grant. 2005. Neuropsychology of HIV, p. 357–373. *In* H. Gendelman, I. Grant, I. Everall, S. Lipton, and S. Swindells (ed.), *The Neurology of AIDS*, 2nd ed. Oxford University Press, London, United Kingsom.

Woods, S. P., J. D. Rippeth, A. B. Frol, J. K. Levy, E. Ryan, V. M. Soukup, C. H. Hinkin, D. Lazzaretto, M. Cherner, T. D. Marcotte, B. B. Gelman, S. Morgello, E. J. Singer, I. Grant, and R. K. Heaton. 2004. Interrater reliability of clinical ratings and neurocognitive diagnoses in HIV. *J. Clin. Exp. Neuropsychol.* **26**:759–778.

The Spectrum of Neuro-AIDS Disorders:
Pathophysiology, Diagnosis, and Treatment
Edited by K. Goodkin et al.
©2008 ASM Press, Washington, DC

3

HIV Infection and Stroke: the Changing Face of a Rising Problem

MAURICIO CONCHA AND ALEJANDRO RABINSTEIN

Neurological syndromes are frequently described in HIV infection, but cerebrovascular disease is in general poorly characterized and only seldom the focus of comprehensive series of HIV infection (Pinto, 1996; Price et al., 1988; Bacellar et al., 1994). Autopsy studies report neurological pathology in approximately 80% to 90% of AIDS cases, of which the most commonly described lesions include opportunistic infections, tumors, and HIV-associated encephalitis (Anders et al., 1986; Budka et al., 1987; de la Monte et al., 1987; Kato et al., 1987; Navia et al., 1986; Petito et al., 1986). In contrast, the presence of stroke, either ischemic or hemorrhagic, has been reported in several autopsy series of HIV-infected brains, with prevalence rates ranging between 6% and 34% (Pinto, 1996; Berger et al., 1990; Anders et al., 1986; Mizusawa et al., 1988; Moskowitz et al., 1984; Kieburtz et al., 1993; Connor et al., 2000; Rosemberg et al., 1986). However, most of these cerebrovascular pathological findings were clinically asymptomatic, and stroke did not appear to be diagnosed prior to time of death (Pinto, 1996; Kieburtz et al., 1993; Rosemberg et al., 1986). In fact, the prevalence of clinically diagnosed stroke syndrome has ranged between 0.5% and 3.75% in more than 2,000 patients with AIDS or AIDS-related complex (Pinto, 1996; Snider et al., 1983; Koppel et al., 1985; Berger et al., 1987; McArthur, 1987; Levy and Breseden, 1988; Engstrom et al., 1989). Other early epidemiological studies of the neurological complications in HIV-infected subjects did not report radiological or pathological evidence of stroke as one of their findings, but it is unclear whether stroke was absent or ignored in the reporting of findings (Petito et al., 1986; Bursztyn et al., 1984).

The reporting of stroke in HIV-infected subjects has faced several challenges that have limited our ability to determine whether a direct association between cerebrovascular disease and HIV infection exists. Until recently, the poor survival of the young cohorts overwhelmed with virulent opportunistic infections limited the evaluation of other potentially associated illnesses, for example, stroke, which could become evident with a more chronic HIV infection. Second, tumors and opportunistic infections may cause stroke-like manifestations, which can create a diagnostic dilemma if not evaluated thoroughly and can become a source of confounding in epidemiological studies of stroke. Third, stroke risk factors, such as intravenous drug use, can be highly prevalent in HIV study cohorts. Their presence can also act as a confounder in epidemiological studies of stroke and HIV infection. The introduction of highly active antiretroviral therapy (HAART) has changed the dynamics of the HIV epidemic, with a substantial decrease in morbidity and mortality (Mocroft et al., 1998; Palella et al., 1998). With increased survival, aging of the HIV-infected cohorts is accompanied not infrequently by metabolic and lipid disorders, which are observed often in subjects on HAART. Recent evidence for the development of premature atherosclerotic disease in this population calls for a revision of the association between stroke and HIV infection.

CLINICAL AND AUTOPSY SERIES

In a comprehensive review, Pinto summarized six moderately large clinical studies and nine autopsy series reported between 1983 and 1990 (Pinto, 1996). Only three of these six studies were prospective in nature (Snider et al., 1983; Berger et al., 1987; McArthur, 1987), and most of the HIV-infected subjects had advanced stages of the disease, with only 12% of the study subjects in the asymptomatic stage of HIV infection; all studies lacked control groups. Overall, ischemic infarctions were consistently more common than intracranial hemorrhages, and when the data from these clinical series were combined, 68% of strokes were ischemic and 32% hemorrhagic (Pinto, 1996). This ratio is similar to the distribution of strokes in the general population, where about 71% are ischemic and 26% hemorrhagic (Foulkes

Mauricio Concha, University of Miami, Miami, FL, and Intercoastal Medical Group, Sarasota, FL 34232. **Alejandro Rabinstein,** Mayo Clinic, Rochester, MN 55905.

et al., 1988). The majority of strokes reported in these clinical and postmortem series were associated with underlying diseases. Intracranial hemorrhage was usually associated with underlying thrombocytopenia, primary central nervous system (CNS) lymphoma, or metastatic Kaposi's sarcoma. In contrast, ischemic stroke was most commonly associated with infectious or nonbacterial endocarditis, disseminated intravascular coagulopathy, or opportunistic infections in the CNS.

Over a 5-year period, between 1982 and 1987, the largest of these series retrospectively identified 12 cases of ischemic stroke among 1,600 AIDS patients, yielding a prevalence period rate of 0.75%. This rate suggests that AIDS patients have a substantially higher risk for stroke than the general population between the ages of 35 and 45 years, where the annual incidence is 0.025%, or about 0.125% in a 5-year period (Engstrom et al., 1989; Grindal et al., 1978). However, it is important to recognize that while the first statistic is a prevalence rate in a hospital-based inpatient and neuropathologic population, the second is an incidence rate based on estimates from the general population. Moreover, the increased prevalence of stroke in clinical and autopsy series is not unexpected. A more recent study of 772 consecutive admissions of HIV-infected patients observed a prevalence rate of 1.2% strokes, with a trend toward higher rates in later stages of the infection (Evers et al., 2003). The apparent high rate of stroke must be tempered by the fact that the study subjects were limited to hospital admissions. To what extent risk factors for AIDS influence the etiology and frequency of stroke also remains to be determined. Thus, stroke is associated with intravenous drug abuse, and therefore, a higher rate of stroke may be expected among subjects with AIDS and a history of intravenous drug abuse. Additionally, the elevated frequency of concomitant pathologies in AIDS patients further limits our ability to determine a direct association between HIV and stroke. It is reasonable to speculate that large cohort studies have not found an association between HIV infection and stroke because, so far, a strong survival effect has limited such observations. Irrespective of the epidemiological and statistical limitations already mentioned, it appears clear from these clinical reviews that cerebral infarction should nevertheless be an important consideration in the differential diagnosis of stroke- and transient-ischemic-attack-like events of unknown origin in AIDS patients, young or old.

CONTROLLED STUDIES

In an effort to determine an association between HIV and stroke, controlled studies have followed these early clinical reviews. In one of the first case-control studies to evaluate stroke in HIV infection, Berger et al. proposed comparing the frequency of stroke in patients who died from AIDS to that of other young patients who died from other conditions (Berger et al., 1990). The authors reviewed the autopsy records of 154 subjects who died from AIDS between 1983 and 1987 and compared them to those of 111 subjects, aged 20 to 50 years, who died without AIDS between 1986 and 1987. Thirteen subjects (8%) with AIDS had evidence of a stroke within a week of their demise, while 25 (23%) subjects in the control group had strokes. Similar to prior clinical series, ischemic stroke (10/13 [77%]) predominated over hemorrhagic stroke (3/13 [23%]). The suspected mechanisms involved in the ischemic injuries were evenly distributed and included six thrombotic and four embolic strokes.

Though this study did not support an association between AIDS and stroke, it highlighted the fact that cerebrovascular disease was not uncommon in the population. This study also observed a significant amount of heart disease associated with strokes in both the AIDS group (8/13 [62%]) and the non-AIDS control group (22/25 [88%]). Although efforts were made to reduce diagnosis misclassification by excluding AIDS cases with CNS tumors or opportunistic infections, the retrospective nature of this autopsy review increases the likelihood of a selection bias in the reasons for autopsy in both cases and controls and limits generalizations based on these findings.

Qureshi et al. (1997) conducted a retrospective case-control study to evaluate the relationship between HIV infection and stroke in young patients. They reviewed the medical records of 236 patients from 19 to 44 years of age admitted to a large inner-city hospital with diagnosis of stroke between 1990 and 1994. The HIV serostatus was known for only 113 patients, 25 of whom were seropositive while 10 had AIDS. The selected controls were age- and sex-matched patients admitted with diagnosis of status asthmaticus and a known HIV serostatus during the same period. The study found that the likelihood of being HIV positive among stroke cases was twice as high as among nonstroke controls (odds ratio, 2.3 [95% confidence interval, 1.0 to 5.3]). This likelihood was even higher when limited to cases with cerebral infarction (odds ratio, 3.4 [95% confidence interval, 1.1 to 8.9]) after adjustment for cerebrovascular risk factors. Further subgroup analysis showed that among stroke cases, cerebral infarction was more frequent in HIV-seropositive cases (80% versus 56%). In addition, among patients with cerebral infarctions, HIV-seropositive subjects were significantly more likely to have an associated meningitis or protein S deficiency than HIV-seronegative subjects. When cases with meningitis and protein S deficiency were excluded, the association between HIV infection and stroke or cerebral infarction was no longer present, suggesting that most of the excess risk of stroke in HIV patients could be related to these two cofactors. It was noteworthy that "strokes of undetermined cause" were not more common in the HIV-infected group, and somewhat surprisingly, no cardioembolic strokes were observed in HIV-seropositive subjects. Extrapolation of these results is limited by the likely potential for the physicians' selection bias to screen for HIV in the first place, the higher stroke mortality among strokes not evaluated for HIV serostatus and hence not included in the analysis, and the potential bias inherent in obtaining information from medical charts (for example, the authors stated that the "risk factor[s] was presumed to be absent if we found no documentation"). Lastly, it is important to note that 85% of the study population was African-American, further limiting generalization of the conclusions.

In an attempt to control for stroke confounding factors commonly found in the HIV-infected population in United States, Hoffmann et al. performed a retrospective, controlled analysis of 1,298 young stroke patients from the Durban Stroke Data Bank, a registry in a highly HIV-endemic province of South Africa (Hoffmann et al., 2000). None of the patients were drug users, and only five had associated opportunistic infections. An age- and sex-matched seronegative historical control group from the same registry was used for comparison. Although most of the patients in the registry were white (75%) and blacks represented only 11.6% of the population, 24 of the 25 HIV-seropositive individuals were blacks. While the overall prevalence rate of HIV infection for this stroke registry between 1992 and 1998 was

1.9%, the prevalence rate of HIV among the black subgroup was 15%. The latter rate parallels that of the young black population in this African region. A selected group of 10 of the 25 HIV-seropositive patients and 19 of the 22 seronegative historical controls had angiograms as part of their stroke evaluations. There was a nonsignificant trend toward a higher rate of large intracranial vessel abnormalities in the HIV population. The authors raised the possibility of an underlying prothrombotic state being prevalent in HIV infection and, as a consequence, etiologically linked to the vascular abnormalities and strokes observed in this population. Though an intriguing finding, this was a small study, and the highly selected angiographic subgroup analysis significantly limits its conclusions. The study's suggestion of frequent large intracranial vessel pathology is not supported by other studies that found few or no vessel abnormalities in patients with ischemic infarctions (Mizusawa et al., 1988; Engstrom et al., 1989). Specifically, normal vessels were observed in the circle of Willis in 22 of 24 patients with ischemic stroke who died from AIDS complications in the United States (Mizusawa et al., 1988). In an effort to quantify the risk of AIDS-associated stroke, Cole et al. reviewed all incidents of strokes among young adults 15 to 44 years of age in the central Maryland and Washington, DC, area (Cole et al., 2004). Between 1988 and 1991, the incidence of ischemic stroke and intracerebral hemorrhage was 0.21% per year, and the overall adjusted relative risk for stroke was 17.8 (95% confidence interval, 10 to 31.6). The strong association between AIDS and stroke in this population study is tempered by the small number of strokes ($n = 12$) and the fact that the analysis adjusted only for age, race, and gender without including other cardiovascular risk factors. Further, 60% of the AIDS patients with stroke reported current use of illicit drugs.

It is important to note that all these clinical studies were performed prior to the introduction of protease inhibitors (PIs) to the therapeutic armamentarium against HIV infection and the widespread use of HAART. The pronounced lengthening of the disease-free survival achieved with HAART, along with the growing number of new HIV infections in individuals who are middle-aged or older, has created a new population of HIV-infected patients whose age represents a higher risk for cerebrovascular disease. At present, properly treated HIV-infected patients can lead long, healthy, and productive lives. Therefore, long-term health problems, such as accelerated atherosclerosis risk of premature vascular events and the long-term effects of antiretroviral treatment, need to become a major focus of attention.

POTENTIAL MECHANISMS OF ISCHEMIC STROKE IN HIV-INFECTED PATIENTS

Traditionally, most ischemic strokes in HIV-infected patients have been reported as the consequence of cardioembolism or opportunistic CNS diseases (Pinto, 1996; Berger et al., 1990; Berger et al., 1987; McArthur, 1987; Levy and Breseden, 1988; Engstrom et al., 1989), although alterations in hemostatic mechanisms have also been consistently implicated (Qureshi et al., 1997; Brew and Miller, 1996). Surprisingly, intravenous drug abuse has only rarely been associated with strokes in HIV-infected subjects, except in cases with coexistent endocarditis, although this may be the result of survival or classification bias (Pinto, 1996; Berger et al., 1990). A variable proportion of cerebral infarcts were classified as cryptogenic in several clinical series (Pinto, 1996;

Kieburtz et al., 1993; Engstrom et al., 1989; Hoffmann et al., 2000). Other studies have suggested the existence of an HIV-related vasculopathy in the absence of concomitant opportunistic pathology (Connor et al., 2000; Brilla et al., 1999). Additionally, PIs have been associated with an increased risk of vascular events, including stroke (Menge et al., 2000; d'Arminio et al., 2004). The available evidence supporting the different etiologic factors for stroke in the HIV-infected population is summarized in Table 1.

Cardioembolism

Cardiac disease is common among HIV-infected patients (Berger et al., 1990; Roldan et al., 1987; Cardoso et al., 1998). In the pre-HAART era, the estimated prevalence of cardiac morbidity was 6% to 7% (Yunis and Stone, 1998). Traditionally, the heart has been regarded as an important source of embolic strokes, not only in the general population but also among HIV-infected subjects (Berger et al., 1990). Roldan et al. found pathologic changes in the heart in 55% of patients who died from AIDS in their autopsy study (Roldan et al., 1987). The most common and life-threatening cardiac complication in the pre-HAART era was dilated cardiomyopathy, occurring in 8% of 925 asymptomatic HIV-infected subjects, followed by echocardiography for an average of 60 ± 5.3 months. The mean annual incidence rate was 15.9 cases per 1,000 patients, and a histologic diagnosis of myocarditis was made in 63 (83%) of the patients with dilated cardiomyopathy (Barbaro et al., 1998). Other cardiac complications included marantic endocarditis, toxoplasmic endocarditis, and bacterial endocarditis; mural thrombi; myxoid valvular disease; and degeneration of valves (Berger et al., 1990). Specifically, nonbacterial thrombotic (marantic) endocarditis, as well as bacterial

TABLE 1 Proposed causes of ischemic stroke in HIV-infected patients

Cardioembolism
  Infectious endocarditis
  Marantic endocarditis
  Myxoid valvular disease
  Low left-ventricular ejection fraction
    With dilated cardiomyopathy
    Without dilated cardiomyopathy
  HIV myocarditis
  Mural thrombus
Opportunistic vasculitis/vasculopathy
  Opportunistic infections
  Opportunistic tumors
Prothrombotic states
  Protein S deficiency
  Antiphospholipids
  Disseminated intravascular coagulation
Intravenous drug abuse
  Cocaine
  Amphetamines
  Others
HIV-related vasculopathy
Accelerated atherosclerosis associated with HAART or PIs
  Dyslipidemia
  Insulin resistance
  Endothelial dysfunction
  Impaired vasomotor reactivity
Cryptogenic

endocarditis (both with and without a history of intravenous drug abuse), has been reported as a cause of ischemic stroke in HIV-infected patients (Berger et al., 1990; Snider et al., 1983; Levy and Breseden 1988; Engstrom et al., 1989; Mesquita et al., 1996). Initially reported in a male homosexual with Kaposi's sarcoma, nonbacterial thrombotic endocarditis was found in about 10% of autopsies before 1989 but was seldom reported after that time (Garcia et al., 1983; Fisher and Lipshultz, 2001). A more recent prospective case-controlled study evaluated the left-ventricular function of 98 consecutive HIV-infected patients by echocardiography (Cardoso et al., 1998). Among the seropositive patients, diastolic dysfunction was found in 63% and depressed ejection fraction in 32% of the cases. The prevalence of symptomatic congestive heart failure was 8%. Echocardiographic abnormalities were significantly more frequent in HIV-infected patients than in controls, and the difference could not be explained by any other intercurrent factors. Cardiac dysfunction was more common in later stages of the infection, although it was also found in patients during asymptomatic stages of HIV infection (Cardoso et al., 1998; Barbaro et al., 1998).

Since the introduction of PIs in combination with nucleoside analogues for the suppression of HIV, there has been growing concern about side effects, including metabolic abnormalities and their potential association with premature coronary artery disease (Duong et al., 2001). A retrospective analysis of a cohort of 4,993 HIV-infected subjects revealed an incidence of myocardial infarction (MI) of 3.41 per 1,000 patient years after the introduction of HAART in contrast to 0.59 per 1,000 patient years in the 3 years preceding HAART (Rickerts et al., 2000). By simple association with the increased risk of embolic stroke after an acute MI, the occurrence of embolic strokes in young HIV-infected subjects could be expected to increase. From a practical point of view, underlying ischemic heart disease should be considered in the diagnostic work-up of HIV-infected subjects with stroke.

Opportunistic and Immune Vasculopathy

A number of opportunistic infections have been implicated in the development of vascular pathology associated with ischemic strokes. They include tuberculosis (Berger et al., 1990; Engstrom et al., 1989), cytomegalovirus infection (Berger et al., 1990; Kieburtz et al., 1993), varicella-zoster virus infection (Engstrom et al., 1989; Eidelberg et al., 1986), herpes simplex virus infection (Engstrom et al., 1989), syphilis (Johns et al., 1987; Kase et al., 1988), cryptococcosis (Engstrom et al., 1989), candidiasis (Kieburtz et al., 1993), and lymphoma (Kieburtz et al., 1993). Additional potential causes in this category are toxoplasmosis (Berger et al., 1990; Engstrom et al., 1989; Brew and Miller, 1996), mucormycosis (Berger et al., 1990), aspergillosis (Berger et al., 1990), and, more questionably, coccidioidomycosis and trypanosomiasis (Brannagan, 1999).

Of the two most common viral opportunistic infections, cytomegalovirus infection has been associated with a variety of CNS lesions, including vasculitis, or the presence of body inclusions in isolated capillary endothelial cells associated with vascular thrombosis (Koeppen et al., 1981; Morgello et al., 1987). In cerebral toxoplasmosis, vascular changes may be prominent, with fibrinoid necrosis and fibrin thrombi in vessels, as well as intense perivascular cuffing by mononuclear inflammatory cells. This inflammatory change may be prominent and can be seen with very few or no organisms present, the latter especially in non-AIDS toxoplasma

encephalitis (Anders et al., 1986; Best and Finlayson, 1979). An unusual noninflammatory cellular thickening of small- and medium-size vessel walls with effacement of the media and adventitia may also be present (Moskowitz et al., 1994). Zoster ophthalmicus is thought to occur by direct viral invasion of the carotid or middle cerebral artery through the intracranial branches of the trigeminal nerve. This invasion results in arteritis with or without thrombosis or a predominantly thrombotic process without striking arteritis (Gasperetti and Song, 1985). Herpes-like virions have been identified in the media of the walls of the middle cerebral artery (Doyle et al., 1983). In meningovascular syphilis, there is infiltration of vessel walls by lymphocytes and plasma cells, including involvement of the vasa vasorum of large arteries. It is unclear whether this inflammatory process is the result of immune complexes or direct damage by *Treponema pallidum* (Jorizzo et al., 1986). This inflammation goes on to damage the elastic and muscular fibers in the medial layer. *Mycobacterium tuberculosis* may cause a basal meningitis with associated arteritis of the small- and medium-size arteries and veins at the base of the brain as they penetrate the dura. The exudate surrounding these vessels induces a reaction in the adventitia and media, a pathological feature known as Huebner's arteritis (Hsieh et al., 1992). Aspergillosis appears to have a special predilection for posterior circulation vessels, and similar to mucormycosis, the mechanisms of arterial occlusion include thromboangiitis with presence of the fungus in the arterial wall and/or thrombus or embolic occlusion from endocarditis (Walsh et al., 1985). The actual incidence of stroke in HIV-infected patients with these opportunistic diseases involving the CNS is unknown but is most likely low. These causes should generally be considered when the cerebral infarction occurs in an HIV patient with advanced immunodeficiency. Fortunately, the current use of HAART has dramatically decreased the incidence of these conditions.

Vasculitis not related to opportunistic infections but immune mediated and possibly triggered by HIV infection has also been considered a possible mechanism in several stroke cases. In a review of 148 HIV-positive subjects with biopsy of muscle, peripheral nerve, or skin, medium-size and small arteries were affected in 34 (23%) subjects (Gherardi et al., 1993). Neither viral inclusion bodies nor multinucleated giant cells were observed, and arterial lesions at various stages of development were not found. Small arteritis was seen in most of the cases where vasculitis was observed (30/34). Inflammatory changes resembled neutrophilic inflammatory and mononuclear inflammatory vascular disease. The latter was most commonly found and typically affected postcapillary venules. In situ hybridization performed in three patients failed to reveal HIV RNA. Granular immune deposits of complement and immunoglobulin M (IgM) in medium and small vessel walls were also observed. Of the 34 subjects with inflammatory vasculitic changes, 11 could be classified clinicopathologically: 4 as polyarteritis nodosa, 6 as hypersensitivity vasculitis, and 1 as Henoch-Schonlein purpura. The remaining 23 had heterogeneous features, and few had underlying potential causes, like cytomegalovirus, human T-cell leukemia virus type 1, cryoglobulinemia, or hepatitis C.

The complement and IgM immune deposits in these patients with medium-size and small vasculitis suggest a common immune complex-mediated mechanism. Given the common presence of circulating immune complexes detected in HIV-infected subjects, it is conceivable that these vascular deposits trigger an inflammatory vascular disease. Nevertheless, the presence of immune complexes has an uncertain positive predictive value, since they can be detected at no specific time during the clinical course of the infection (Morrow et al., 1986). On the other hand, cytokines, activators of HIV-infected macrophages, are involved at several points in the inflammatory process (Matsuyama et al., 1991). Tumor necrosis factor alpha, for example, specifically enhances HIV replication in vitro and initiates an inflammatory response at the level of endothelial cells of postcapillary venules (Messadi et al., 1987; Matsuyama et al., 1991). Theoretically, cytokines could play a role in the HIV-related vasculitis changes that may predispose a subgroup of this population to stroke. To date, a relationship of such vasculitic changes and immune complex deposits to stroke has not been established.

The association of necrotizing angiitis and viral illness is a well-described phenomenon in humans, but only a few cases have been reported in HIV-infected subjects with predominant CNS involvement (Yanker et al., 1986). One case resembled granulomatous angiitis of CNS, and a second case had evidence of persistent varicella-zoster virus infection (Yanker et al., 1986; Vinters et al., 1988). Schwartz et al. described a 49-year-old male with a predominantly eosinophilic necrotizing vasculitis of the temporal arteries (Schwartz et al., 1986). There was no other feature of allergic granulomatosis or evidence of peripheral target organ involvement other than recurrent amaurosis fugax (Schwartz et al., 1986). Three cases of lymphomatoid granulomatosis involving the brain also showed various changes in other peripheral organs, including evidence of non-Hodgkin's lymphoma with angiocentric features (Anders et al., 1989).

Prothrombotic Mechanism

Different hemostatic abnormalities have been documented in HIV-infected patients with ischemic stroke. Perhaps the most consistently reported prothrombotic state has been protein S deficiency (Qureshi et al., 1997; Brew and Miller, 1996), but antiphospholipid antibodies have also been found in various series (Brew and Miller, 1996; Abuaf et al., 1997). Protein S is a vitamin K-dependent plasma protein that functions as a cofactor for activated protein C. Congenital deficiencies of protein S predispose to thromboembolic complications. Acquired decreases in protein S levels occur in pregnancy, liver disease, and nephrotic syndrome and during oral-contraceptive and warfarin therapy. In addition to several reports of protein S deficiency (Lafeuillade et al., 1991; Stahl et al., 1993) and increase in anticardiolipin antibody levels, studies have shown a linear correlation between IgG anticardiolipin antibody levels and decreased protein S antigen in long-term HIV-infected subjects. In a 3-year prospective study of 27 HIV-infected patients free of opportunistic disease who presented with transient neurological deficits, Brew and Miller found a high prevalence of IgG anticardiolipin antibodies (70%) and protein S deficiency (53%) (Brew and Miller, 1996). Notably, only two of these patients actually developed documented strokes. An earlier case report documented high IgG anticardiolipin titers (112.2 GPL) as the only abnormality in an extensive stroke work-up of a 32-year-old subject who presented with an ischemic stroke as his first and only manifestation of HIV infection (Casado-Naranjo et al., 1992). Other studies have failed to find a link between increased anticardiolipin antibody levels and thrombosis in HIV disease (Taillan et al., 1990). Although these findings may suggest that HIV-infected subjects are prone to thrombosis, the pathogenesis

of these procoagulant proteins and the full clinical implications of these findings, particularly with regard to stroke, remain to be elucidated in the HIV-infected population.

Unrecognized prothrombotic states have been suspected to be responsible for the high prevalence of "cryptogenic strokes," but no proof has been offered to support this hypothesis (Hoffmann et al., 2000). In terminal cases, stroke can be precipitated by disseminated intravascular coagulation or cerebral venous thrombosis as a consequence of dehydration and cachexia (Berger et al., 1990; Anders et al., 1986). Hyperviscosity has been reported at least once in AIDS and could represent a potential cause of cerebral infarction (Martin et al., 1989). New varieties of antiphospholipid antibodies have recently been described and should be studied in HIV patients. Other forms of hypercoagulability have also been seen in HIV-infected patients, but whether their frequency is higher than in the healthy population has not been assessed (Saif and Greenberg, 2001).

Drug Abuse

The abuse of illicit drugs, particularly using the intravenous route, can produce a series of neurological complications that include stroke and that will be discussed briefly. With amphetamine use, hemorrhagic strokes have been more frequently reported than ischemic strokes, and most of these strokes occur within hours of drug ingestion (Goodman and Becker, 1970; Margolis and Newton, 1971; Yarnell, 1977; Delaney and Estes, 1980; Harrington et al., 1983; Yu et al., 1983; Matick et al., 1983; Imanse and Vanneste, 1990; Johnson et al., 1983). As with amphetamines, most cocaine-related strokes occur near the time of use, and about half the strokes are occlusive and half hemorrhagic in nature (Brust, 1993b). Common among cocaine-associated hemorrhagic strokes are the underlying cerebral congenital aneurysms and vascular malformations, found in about 70% of cases (Levine et al., 1990). Acute hypertension, vasoconstriction, and vasculitis are important mechanisms related to these strokes (Citron et al., 1970; Rumbaugh et al., 1976; Glick et al., 1987). MI, cardiomyopathy, and cardiac arrhythmias due to cocaine may contribute to embolic strokes in addicts or sporadic users (Goldfrank and Hoffman, 1991; Chokshi et al., 1989). Coagulation mechanisms may be altered by cocaine, as well as by heroin; these abnormalities may also play roles in causing strokes.

Heroin overdose can cause severe hypoventilation and hypotension, which may result in anoxic brain damage or a stroke if an underlying intracranial stenosis is present (Jensen et al., 1990). Moreover, heroin nephropathy can cause hypertension, which also contributes to strokes in this population. LSD, a derivative of ergot alkaloids, may have vasoconstrictive properties and has been implicated in a few ischemic strokes in young subjects (Sobel et al., 1971; Lieberman et al., 1974).

Intravenous drug abuse increases the risk of infective endocarditis. Besides intravenous injections, the practice of "skin popping" predisposes to cellulites and local abscesses, increasing the risk for sepsis, pneumonia, and seeding of heart valves. Intracerebral hemorrhage occurs in 2 to 7% of subjects and is usually attributed to mycotic aneurysm or septic arteritis causing vessel wall erosion and rupture. This complication carries an increased mortality (Masuda et al., 1992). Mycotic aneurysms complicate endocarditis in 2 to 4% of cases (Salgado et al., 1987). In addition to these complications, embolization of foreign material to the brain has been documented with heroin jugular vein injectors that accidentally inject the carotid. Furthermore, peripheral veins may be injected with solutes of crushed oral tablets, like methylphenidate (Ritalin). These tablets are dissolved in water. The solute is then filtered through a piece of cotton or cigarette filter before it is injected intravenously (Brust, 1993a; Lahmeyer and Steingold 1980). Finally, it is important to note that these drug mixtures, prepared illicitly, may contain heparin, thus increasing the risk for hemorrhagic strokes (Maqbool and Billett, 1982).

NEW INSIGHTS INTO THE MECHANISMS OF STROKE IN HIV-INFECTED PATIENTS

HIV-Related Vasculopathy

Despite the several epidemiological studies and clinical observations summarized above, it is not clear whether HIV infection itself causes stroke or other neurological abnormalities indicative of neurovascular disease. A nonvasculitic arteriopathy unrelated to concomitant opportunistic infections observed by several studies could correspond to an HIV-related neurovascular disease and a potential stroke mechanism. One of the first reports in this regard included four patients who died from AIDS, and their pathological studies revealed intimal proliferative changes with narrowing of the lumen of the small and large leptomeningeal arteries, including arteries of the circle of Willis. Some of the involved arteries exhibited hyperplasia of smooth muscle cells and/or fibroblasts within the intima and no signs of inflammation (Cho et al., 1987).

Through a highly selective process of exclusion from a pool of 183 autopsy cases, the Edinburgh HIV cohort reported pathological findings in 10 cases (5.5%) with presence of cerebral infarction and without evidence of opportunistic infections, lymphoma, traumatic injury, or potential sources of cerebral emboli (Connor et al., 2000). This study revealed the presence of an asymptomatic vasculopathy characterized by small-vessel wall thickening, perivascular space dilatation, rarefaction and pigment deposition with vessel wall mineralization, and occasional perivascular inflammatory cell infiltrates without definitive evidence of vasculitis. The vascular changes were similar to those found in cases of cerebral arteriolosclerosis in elderly hypertensive, diabetic patients, but in contrast, these patients were young (range, 22 to 47 years) and mostly free of traditional vascular risk factors. It is important to note that 5 of the 10 study patients with vasculopathy were intravenous drug abusers and that similar small-vessel pathology has been found in HIV-negative drug abusers (Connor et al., 2000). Although all patients were severely immunosuppressed, neither the degree of the vasculopathy nor the extent of cerebral infarction was associated with the viral load or the distribution of HIV encephalitis. None of these patients had been exposed to PI, and there was no evidence of systemic embolism in other organs.

Earlier immunocytochemical and histological studies showed evidence of blood-brain barrier perturbation with abnormalities in the microcirculation, including mural thickening, increased cellularity, and enlargement and pleomorphism of endothelial cells (Smith et al., 1990; Power et al., 1993). The evidence for altered microcirculation, however, is limited and was found in three cases, two with a background of intravenous drug abuse and one with a history of Ebstein's anomaly with two corrective cardiac surgeries and endocarditis prior to death (Smith et al., 1990).

In a large autopsy series of 83 AIDS cases, Mizusawa et al. observed multiple and usually small subclinical cerebral infarcts involving the cortex, striatum, and brainstem in 23 (29%) cases (Mizusawa et al., 1988). Further, abnormal mural thickening with or without inflammatory changes was observed in small vessels in 12 of the 23 patients with cerebral infarcts: mild to moderate mural thickening was present in 11 cases and severe thickening with occlusion of the vessel lumen was present in 1 case (Mizusawa et al., 1988). Despite these observations and the documented presence of HIV in vascular endothelial cells in AIDS brains in regions with or without inflammatory cells, a definitive role of HIV in the development of a vasculopathy and its clinical implications remain unclear (Pumarola-Sune et al., 1987; Ward et al., 1987; Wiley et al., 1986).

Pathological studies of a different vascular bed provide support for the possibility of an HIV-related vasculopathy inducing endothelial cell disturbance. In a group of HIV-infected patients, the aortic endothelium showed activation and increased leukocyte adhesion, while the coronary arteries of a second group of HIV-infected subjects showed thickening of the intima and media with proliferation of the smooth muscle cells (Zietz et al., 1996; Tabib et al., 2000). Moreover, retinal fluorescein-angiographic documentation of microaneurysms, telangiectasias, focal area of nonperfusion, and capillary loss, as well as the presence of pathologic findings, including periodic acid-Schiff stain-positive thickening of blood vessel walls and pericapillary closure in patients with AIDS, provide a pattern of microvascular retinopathy reminiscent of many changes seen in diabetes mellitus (Newsome et al., 1984). Evidence of an increased resistance index in the central retinal artery was documented in HIV-infected subjects compared to a group of age-matched healthy controls (Dejaco-Ruhswurm et al., 2001). Observations like this suggest that alterations in the flow may play a role in the pathophysiology of HIV-related retinal microvasculopathies. Although the precise pathogenesis of this HIV-related microvasculopathy remains elusive, several mechanisms may contribute, i.e., procoagulant properties from elevated endothelial cell products, alterations in the vascular flow, and chronic inflammation or infections (Zietz et al., 1996).

Despite the lack of controlled studies, the potential role of the microangiopathic findings documented in the aforementioned studies may become more relevant in light of data suggesting that cerebrovascular hemodynamic function may be impaired in HIV-infected patients. Abnormalities of cerebral perfusion have been documented in asymptomatic HIV-infected patients using ^{113}Xe single-photon emission tomography (Tran Dinh et al., 1990). It is important to highlight that these 18 patients were free of diabetes, hypertension, dyslipidemia, history of drug abuse, stroke, or opportunistic infections. In another study, Brilla et al. utilized transcranial Doppler to evaluate the cerebrovascular reserve capacity (CRC) in 31 HIV-positive subjects without evidence of current infection or cardiovascular or respiratory disease (Brilla et al., 1999). Their mean age was 39 ± 11 years (range, 23 to 59 years); the mean time since diagnosis was 4 years; 6 subjects were classified as CDC (Centers for Disease Control and Prevention) stage A, 16 CDC stage B, and 7 CDC stage C; and 7 had AIDS. These patients showed reduced baseline blood flow velocity and significantly diminished CRC after the administration of acetazolamide (31%) compared to noninfected age-matched controls (46%). No correlation was found between reduced CRC and CD4 count, duration of seropositivity, circulating immunocomplexes, anticardiolipins, or antinuclear antibodies. A nonsignificant trend toward worse CRC was observed. The reduced baseline blood flow velocity and, more importantly, the reduced CRC reflect alterations of cerebral resistance at the arteriolar level. These changes support an HIV-related cerebral vascular dysfunction directly related either to HIV infection or to the other coexistent factors, such as infection or medications. This study in particular did not provide information on the antiretroviral regimens administered. Utilizing an alternative methodology to measure CRC, our group used transcranial Doppler with a CO_2 vasomotor reactivity test in a pilot study. In this study, 21 cases with lipodystrophy syndrome and long-term exposure to PIs (>18 months) were compared to 17 controls without lipodystrophy syndrome or exposure to PIs. After adjusting for age, triglycerides, cholesterol/HDL cholesterol ratio, C peptide, and use of lipid-lowering agents, the odds for abnormal cerebral vasomotor reactivity were 1.9 times higher ($P < 0.005$) among cases than among controls (Concha et al., 2003). A potential role of HIV in the endothelium dysfunction was suggested in our study by the finding that the cerebral vasomotor reactivity seemed to be decreased in all HIV-infected subjects. PIs, in association with lipodystrophy syndrome, appeared to enhance this endothelial dysfunction.

Accelerated Atherosclerosis, Cardiovascular Risk, and Use of PIs

With the introduction of HAART, a steep reduction in mortality and morbidity has been observed in HIV-infected subjects in the United States and other Western countries (Mocroft et al., 1998; Palella et al., 1998). Recent studies suggest a shift in the relative cause of death among HIV-infected subjects, with cardiovascular deaths accounting for fewer than 4% of all deaths prior to 1997 and for 7 to 10% in the following years (Louie et al., 2002; Selik et al., 2002). The development and inclusion of PIs in this antiretroviral regimen have been largely responsible for its success. However, treatment with PIs has recently been associated with severe premature atherosclerotic vascular disease (Henry et al., 1998; Behrens et al., 1998; Vittecoq et al., 1998; Laurence, 1998; Passalaris et al., 2000). PIs can induce a variety of metabolic abnormalities, including hypertriglyceridemia, hypercholesterolemia, raised insulin and peptide C levels in serum with proven insulin resistance, and peripheral lipodystrophy (Carr et al., 1998; Periard et al., 1999). Marked lipid abnormalities may be present in 24% to 64% of patients treated with PIs (Henry et al., 1998; Carr et al., 1998; Tsiodras et al., 2000). Less commonly, nonnucleoside reverse transcriptase inhibitors (NNRTIs) may also cause this lipodystrophy syndrome, possibly related to mitochondrial toxicity (Brinkman et al., 1999). Overall, a large published series on the metabolic effects of PIs has shown an average increase in total cholesterol and serum triglyceride levels of 28% and 96%, respectively, compared to either pretreatment values or matched PI-naïve HIV-infected controls (Passalaris et al., 2000). Furthermore, in a cross-sectional analysis of over 17,000 subjects of the multinational Data Collection on Adverse Effects of Anti-HIV Drugs (DAD) Study, PIs were associated with elevated cholesterol levels in serum (Friis-Moller et al., 2003b). Clinically manifest atherosclerotic disease was infrequently documented in HIV-infected patients in the pre-PI era, although this may have been in part related to the reduced life expectancy of these patients before PIs became available (Passalaris et al., 2000). This survival effect could theoretically account for a growing prevalence of atherosclerosis in HIV-infected patients as they get older. It could also potentially unmask underlying proatherosclerotic effects of HIV infection itself, such as endothelial dysfunction (Lafeuillade et al., 1992; Blann et al., 1998) or hypertriglyceridemia (Grunfeld et al., 1991).

The growing number of reported cases of vascular events in patients treated with PIs causes concern, especially since the metabolic side effects associated with this family of drugs are known to increase the risk of atherosclerosis. The clinical relevance of this risk was highlighted by an early report of two HIV-1-infected individuals documented to have sustained premature MIs (Henry et al., 1998). Other, larger anecdotal reports document what appears to be a close association between PIs and the occurrence of severe vascular events (Behrens et al., 1998; Duong et al., 2001). In these reports, the patients were mostly young (<55 years of age) and male, and the majority had no traditional risk factors for the development of coronary heart disease.

An increased prevalence of premature carotid atherosclerosis in HIV-infected individuals treated with PI-containing regimens for at least 12 months has been shown by ultrasound (Maggi et al., 2000). Among 55 PI-treated patients, 29 (53%) acquired lesions of the carotid wall as measured by intimal-media thickness of >1 mm or the presence of atherosclerotic plaque. In contrast, only 7 of 47 (15%) PI-naïve HIV-infected subjects and less than 7% of 104 healthy non-HIV-infected controls displayed carotid wall lesions. A multivariate logistic regression analysis adjusting for vascular risk factors identified the presence of therapy with PIs as the highest-significance risk factor for the carotid wall lesions in his group. Similarly, in a pilot study performed by our group, HIV-infected subjects with lipodystrophy syndrome and long-term exposure to PIs had significantly more atherosclerotic plaques (68%) and thicker (>1-mm) intimal-media layers (90%) in any of the common or extracranial internal carotid arteries than HIV-infected subjects without lipodystrophy syndrome or exposure to PIs (15% and 39%, respectively; $P < 0.05$) (Concha et al., 2003). An intriguing case of symptomatic intracranial stenosis in an HIV-infected patient who had been treated with PIs for 15 months has been reported (Menge et al., 2000). Although this patient had preexisting vascular risk factors (smoking, hypertension, and diabetes mellitus type 2), his already elevated cholesterol and triglyceride levels markedly increased after the initiation of nelfinavir treatment. Cholesterol and triglyceride levels returned rapidly to baseline after nelfinavir was discontinued.

Whether any one PI drug or combination of PI agents may be more atherogenic remains unclear at this point. Different studies have preferentially implicated different PIs, but all available PIs can potentially induce atherogenic metabolic derangements (Graham, 2000; Periard et al., 1999). Additional observational and epidemiological data are limited so far; nonetheless, pending the availability of further data, it is prudent to monitor these patients for hyperlipidemia and diabetes. Recently, studies have documented that the duration of PI exposure is associated with a significant increase in cardiovascular incidence in a dose-dependent relationship; as little as 60 days of PI exposure was associated with a 70% increased risk of cardiovascular disease (Iloeje et al., 2005; Friis-Moller et al., 2003a; Mary-Krause et al., 2003). More specifically, data from the DAD study group, for nearly 20,000 patients, showed an increased relative risk of MI (26%) for every year of combination antiretroviral therapy (Friis-Moller et al., 2003a). Similar follow-up data on 36,145 person years from the DAD study showed a combined incidence of first cerebro- or cardiovascular event of 5.7 per 1,000 person years (MI, 3.5, and stroke, 1.1 per 1,000 person years), again with a 26% relative risk increase per year of exposure to combination antiretroviral therapy (d'Arminio et al., 2004).

TABLE 2 IDSA-AACTG guidelines for evaluating and managing dyslipidemia in HIV-infected adults[a]

Monitor fasting lipid profile prior to starting antiretrovirals, yearly thereafter, and 3 to 6 months after starting a new antiretrovirals regimen.
Assess coronary heart disease risk factors and modify if possible.
If nonlipid interventions are unsuccessful, consider altering antiretrovirals or adding lipid-lowering drugs.
Elevated low-density lipoprotein cholesterol: pravastatin or atorvastatin
Triglycerides (>500 mg/dl): gemfibrozil or fenofibrate

[a]From Dube, 2003.

Data on stroke in the HIV population studies have been scarce compared to MI, and the challenges with its accurate diagnosis and subsequent coding could be a partial explanation. However, the incidence of stroke lags behind coronary disease by about 8 to 15 years, and it is conceivable that we have not seen yet the effects of the PI-induced dyslipidemia and premature atherosclerosis in the brains of HIV-infected individuals. Based on the above-mentioned literature and our pilot study and experience, it is our prediction that the incidence of early strokes in the HIV-infected population under treatment with antiretrovirals will increase unless we manage to control the premature development of underlying cardio- and cerebrovascular risk factors. Moreover, we estimate that strokes due to small-vessel disease will be as common as or more common than strokes secondary to large-vessel disease or cardioembolism. A major concern will also be the long-term sequelae of strokes, particularly cognitive impairment, in this young population.

Although the long-term consequences of dyslipidemia in HIV-infected individuals remain to be completely understood, it is reasonable to recommend that this population undergo evaluation and treatment of dyslipidemia based on the known risks in the non-HIV-infected population. The management of HIV-infected individuals treated with PIs should include close monitoring of lipid and glucose levels. Risk factors for atherosclerosis should be assessed and, if present, aggressively modified. In September 2003, guidelines from the HIV Medicine Association of the Infectious Diseases Society of America (IDSA) and the Adult AIDS Clinical Trials Group (AACTG) reviewed the growing evidence relating antiretroviral therapy to dyslipidemia and recommended measures to reduce cardiovascular risk (Dube et al., 2003). These guidelines took into consideration the recommendation for lipid management by the National Cholesterol Education Program Expert Panel on Detection, Evaluation, and Treatment of High Blood Cholesterol in Adults (ATP III), published in 2001 (Expert Panel on Detection, Evaluation, and Treatment of High Blood Cholesterol in Adults, 2001). The conclusion of the IDSA-AACTG Guidelines panel was that patients should be evaluated for dyslipidemia according to ATP III guidelines, with particular attention to potential drug interactions with antiretroviral medications and maintenance of virologic control of HIV infection (Table 2). One alternative strategy for addressing dyslipidemia is switching the PI component of the antiretroviral therapy, alone or in combination with lipid-lowering agents. Recently, more rapid onset of carotid lesions has been documented in patients treated with PIs than in patients treated with NNRTIs (as well as a more rapid evolution of previous lesions) (Maggi et al., 2007). Although the switching approach appears safe, particularly in respect to NNRTIs, caution is necessary in regard to the possibility of drug resistance in cases of prior exposure to NNRTIs or nucleoside reverse transcriptase inhibitors before the PI-combining regimen. A detailed review of this topic is beyond the scope of this chapter. We encourage the reader to review the guidelines published by the IDSA-AACTG panel and to keep updated with the results of ongoing clinical trials that will help define the safest and most effective therapeutic approach to this problem.

SUMMARY

In the pre-HAART era, medical attention was centered on the dramatic impact of opportunistic infections and neoplasms. The perception that death from AIDS was inevitable shadowed any concerns about cardiovascular risk factors. Fortunately, this situation has profoundly changed thanks to recent advances in antiretroviral therapy. However, as the prognosis for HIV infection continues to improve, the risk of cardiovascular morbidity, including stroke, now represents a serious concern in the HIV-infected population. Older age is associated with an increased risk for stroke, as well as with a number of stroke risk factors that require ongoing monitoring in this patient population. The risk of MI, and probably stroke, represents the most recent sign of a convergence between morbidity and mortality risks for the general population and those of the HIV-infected, a convergence that is likely to increase in the future. Because older HIV-1-infected individuals will also be exposed to an increased risk for stroke based upon the toxicity of currently approved antiretroviral medications, they might be considered candidates for aggressive vascular screening, risk factor control, and primary prophylactic treatment. Future studies will be required to better assess the macrovascular and microvascular complications that may result from HIV infection, the metabolic derangements induced by HAART, or both, as well as to determine the optimal treatment and prevention for this specific patient population.

REFERENCES

Abuaf, N., S. Laperche, B. Rajoely, R. Carsique, A. Deschaps, A. Rouquette, C. Barthet, Z. Khaled, C. Marbot, N. Saab, J. Rozen, P. Girard, and W. Rozenbaum. 1997. Autoantibodies to phospholipids and to the coagulation proteins in AIDS. *Thromb. Haemost.* **77:**856–861.

Anders, K., H. Latta, B. Chang, U. Tomiyasu, A. Quddusi, and H. Vinters. 1989. Lymphomatoid granulomatosis and malignant lymphoma of the central nervous system in the acquired immunodeficiency syndrome. *Hum. Pathol.* **20:**326–334.

Anders, K., W. Guerra, U. Tomiyasu, and H. Vinters. 1986. The neuropathology of AIDS: UCLA experience and review. *Am. J. Pathol.* **124:**537–558.

Bacellar, H., A. Munoz, E. Miller, B. Cohen, D. Besley, O. Selnes, J. Becker, and J. McArthur. 1994. Temporal trends in the incidence of HIV-1-related neurologic diseases:

Multicenter AIDS Cohort Study, 1985–1992. *Neurology* 44:1892–1900.

Barbaro, G., G. Di Lorenzo, B. Grisorio, and G. Barbarini. 1998. Incidence of dilated cardiomyopathy and detection of HIV in myocardial cells of HIV-positive patients. *N. Engl. J. Med.* 15:1093–1099.

Behrens, G., H. Schmidt, D. Meyer, M. Stoll, and R. E. Schmidt. 1998. Vascular complications associated with the use of HIV protease inhibitors. *Lancet* 351:1958.

Berger, J., J. Harris, J. Gragorios, and M. Norenberg. 1990. Cerebrovascular disease in AIDS: a case-control study. *AIDS* 4:239–244.

Berger, J., L. Moskowitz, M. Fischl, and R. Kelley. 1987. Neurological disease as the presenting manifestation of acquired immunodeficiency syndrome. *South. Med. J.* 80:683–686.

Best, T., and M. Finlayson. 1979. Two forms of encephalitis in opportunistic toxoplasmosis. *Arch. Pathol. Lab. Med.* 103:693–696

Blann, A., J. Constans, F. Dignat-George, and M. Seigneur. 1998. The platelet and endothelium in HIV infection. *Br. J. Haematol.* 100:613–614.

Brannagan, T. 1999. Retroviral-associated vasculitis of the nervous system. *Neurol. Clin.* 15:927–944.

Brew, B., and J. Miller. 1996. Human immunodeficiency virus type 1-related transient neurological deficits. *Am. J. Med.* 101:257–261.

Brilla, R., D. Nabavi, G. Schulte-Altedorneburg, V. Kemény, D. Reichelt, S. Evers, U. Schiemann, and I. Husstedt. 1999. Cerebral vasculopathy in HIV infection revealed by transcranial Doppler: a pilot study. *Stroke* 30:811–813.

Brinkman, K., J. Smeitink, J. Romijn, and P. Reiss. 1999. Mitochondrial toxicity induced by nucleoside-analogue reverse-transcriptase inhibitors is a key factor in the pathogenesis of antiretroviral-therapy-related lipodystrophy. *Lancet* 354:1112–1115.

Brust, J. 1993a. Opioids, p. 16–41. *In* J. Brust, *Neurological Aspects of Substance Abuse.* Butterworth-Heinemann, Boston, MA.

Brust, J. C. 1993b. Clinical, radiological, and pathological aspects of cerebrovascular disease associated with drug abuse. *Stroke* 24(Suppl. 12):I129–I135.

Budka, H., G. Costanzi, S. Cristini, A. Lechi, C. Parravicini, R. Trabattoni, and L. Vago. 1987. Brain pathology induced by infection with the human immunodeficiency virus (HIV). A histological, immunocytochemical and electron microscopical study of 100 autopsy cases. *Acta Neuropathol.* 75:185–198.

Bursztyn, E., B. Lee, and J. Bauman. 1984. CT of AIDS. *Am. J. Neuroradiol.* 5:711–714.

Cardoso, J., B. Moura, L. Martins, A. Mota-Miranda, F. Rocha-Goncalves, and H. Lecour. 1998. Left ventricular dysfunction in human immunodeficicency virus (HIV)-infected patients. *Int. J. Cardiol.* 63:37–45.

Carr, A., K. Samaras, S. Burton, J. Freund, D. Chisholm, and D. Cooper. 1998. A syndrome of peripheral lipodystrophy, hyperlipidemia and insulin resistance in patients receiving HIV protease inhibitors. *AIDS* 12:F51–F58.

Casado Naranjo, I., J. Toledo Santos, and M. Antolin Rodriguez. 1992. Ischemic stroke as the sole manifestation of human immunodeficiency virus infection. *Stroke* 23:117–118.

Cho, E., L. Sharer, N. Peress, and B. Little. 1987. Intimal proliferation of leptomeningeal arteries and brain infarcts in subjects with AIDS. *J. Neuropathol. Exp. Neurol.* 43:385.

Chokshi, S. K., R. Moore, N. G. Pandian, and J. M. Isner. 1989. Reversible cardiomyopathy associated with cocaine intoxication. *Ann. Intern. Med.* 111:1039–1040.

Citron, B. P., M. Halpern, M. McCarron, G. D. Lundberg, R. McCormick, I. J. Pincus, D. Tatter, and B. J. Haverback. 1970. Necrotizing angiitis associated with drug abuse. *N. Engl. J. Med.* 283:1003–1011.

Cole, J., A. Pinto, J. Hebel, D. Buchholz, C. Earley, C. Johnson, R. Macko, T. Price, M. Sloan, B. Stern, R. Wityk, M. Wozniak, and S. Kittner. 2004. Acquired immunodeficiency syndrome and the risk of stroke. *Stroke* 35:51–56.

Concha, M., S. Symes, K. Goodkin, S. Nathan, P. Zortea, J. Romano, A. Forteza, and M. Kolber. 2003. Risk of cerebrovascular disease in HIV-1-infected subjects with lipodystrophy syndrome and long-term exposure to protease inhibitors. *Stroke* 34:295.

Connor, M., G. Lammie, J. Bell, C. Warlow, P. Simmonds, and R. Brettle. 2000. Cerebral infarction in adult AIDS patients: observations form the Edimburgh HIV autopsy cohort. *Stroke* 31:2117–2126.

d'Arminio, A., C. Sabin, A. Phillips, P. Reiss, R. Weber, O. Kirk , W. El-Sadr, S. De Wit , K. Mateu, K. Petoumenos, F. Dabis, C. Pradier, L. Morfeldt, J. Lundgren, N. Friis-Møller, and Writing Committee of the D:A:D: Study Group. 2004. Cardio- and cerebrovascular events in HIV-infected persons. *AIDS.* 18:1811–1817.

Dejaco-Ruhswurm, I., B. Kiss, G. Rainer, K. Krepler, A. Wedrich, S. Dallinger, A. Rieger, and L. Schmetterer. 2001. Ocular blood flow in patients infected with human immunodeficiency virus. *Am. J. Ophthalmol.* 132:720–726.

de la Monte, S., D. Ho, R. Schooley, M. Hirsch, and E. Richardson. 1987. Subacute encephalomyelitis of AIDS and its relation to HTVL-III infection. *Neurology* 37:562–569.

Delaney, P., and M. Estes. 1980. Intracranial hemorrhage with amphetamine abuse. *Neurology* 30:1125–1128.

Doyle, P., G. Gibson, and C. Dolman. 1983. Herpes zoster ophthalmicus with contralateral hemiplegia: identification of cause. *Ann. Neurol.* 14:84–85.

Dube, M., J. Stein, J. Aberg, C. Fichtenbaum, J. Gerber, K. Tashima, W. Henry, J. Currier, D. Sprecher, M. Glesby, the Adult AIDS Clinical Trials Group Cardiovascular Subcommittee, and the HIV Medical Association of the Infectious Disease Society of America. 2003. Guidelines for the evaluation and management of dyslipidemia in human immunodeficiency virus (HIV)-infected adults receiving antiretroviral therapy: recommendations of the HIV Medical Association of the Infectious Disease Society of America and the Adult AIDS Clinical Trials Group. *Clin. Infect. Dis.* 37:613–627.

Duong, M., M. Buisson, Y. Cottin, L. Piroth, I. Lhuillier, M. Grappin, P. Chavanet, J. Wolff, and H. Portier. 2001. Coronary heart disease associated with the use of human immunodeficiency virus (HIV)-1 protease inhibitors: report of four cases and review. *Clin. Cardiol.* 24:690–694.

Eidelberg, D., A. Sotrel, D. Horoupian, P. Neumann, T. Pumarola-Sune, and R. Price. 1986. Thrombotic cerebral vasculopathy associated with herpes zoster. *Ann. Neurol.* 19:7–14.

Engstrom, J., D. Lowenstein, and D. Breseden. 1989. Cerebral infarctions and transient neurological deficits associated with acquired immunodeficiency syndrome. *Am. J. Med.* 86:528–532.

Evers, S., D. Navabi, A. Rahmann, C. Heese, D. Reichelt, and I. Husstedt. 2003. Ischaemic cerebrovascular events in HIV infection: a cohort study. *Cerebrovasc. Dis.* 15:199–205.

Expert Panel on Detection, Evaluation, and Treatment of High Blood Cholesterol in Adults. 2001. Executive summary of the third report of the National Cholesterol Education Program (NCEP) Expert Panel on Detection, Evaluation, and Treatment of High Blood Cholesterol in Adults (Adult Treatment Panel III). *JAMA* 285:2486–2497.

Fisher, S., and S. Lipshultz. 2001. Epidemiology of cardiovascular involvement in HIV disease and AIDS. *Ann. N. Y. Acad. Sci.* 946:13–22.

Foulkes, M., P. Wolf, T. Price, J. Mohr, and D. Hier. 1988. The Stroke Data Bank: design, methods, and baseline characteristics. *Stroke* 19:547–554.

Friis-Moller, N., C. Sabin, R. Weber, A. d'Arminio Monforte, W. El-Sadr, P. Reiss, R. Thiebaut, L. Morfeldt, S. De Wit, C. Pradier, G. Calvo, M. Law, O. Kirk, A. Phillips, J. Lundgren, and the Data Collection on Adverse Events of Anti-HIV Drugs (DAD) Study Group. 2003a. Combination antiretroviral therapy and the risk of myocardial infarction. *N. Engl. J. Med.* **349:**1993–2003.

Friis-Moller, N., R. Weber, P. Reiss, R. Thiebaut, O. Kirk, A. d'Arminio Monforte, C. Pradier, L. Morfeldt, S. Mateu, M. Law, W. El-Sadr, S. De Wit, C. Sabin, A. Phillips, J. Lundgren, and the DAD Study Group. 2003b. Cardiovascular disease risk factors in HIV patients—association with antiretroviral therapy. Results from the DAD study. *AIDS* **17:**1179–1193.

Garcia, I., V. Fainstein, A. Rios, M. Luna, P. Mansell, J. Reuben, and E. Hersh. 1983. Nonbacterial thrombotic endocarditis in a male homosexual with Kaposi's sarcoma. *Arch. Intern. Med.* **143:**1243–1244.

Gasperetti, C., and S. Song. 1985. Contralateral hemiparesis following herpes zoster ophthalmicus. *J. Neurol. Neurosurg. Psychiatry* **48:**338–341.

Gherardi, R., L. Belec, C. Mhiri, F. Gray, M. Lescs, A. Sobel, L. Guillevin, and J. Wechsler. 1993. The spectrum of vasculitis in human immunodeficiency virus-infected patients. A clinicopathologic evaluation. *Arthritis Rheum.* **36:**1164–1174.

Glick, R., J. Hoying, L. Cerullo, and S. Perlman. 1987. Phenylpropanolamine: an over-the-counter drug causing central nervous system vasculitis and intracerebral hemorrhage. Case report and review. *Neurosurgery* **20:**969–974.

Goldfrank, L. R., and R. S. Hoffman. 1991. The cardiovascular effects of cocaine. *Ann. Emerg. Med.* **20:**165–175.

Goodman, S. J., and D. P. Becker. 1970. Intracranial hemorrhage associated to amphetamine abuse. *JAMA* **212:**480.

Graham, N. 2000. Metabolic disorders among HIV-infected patients treated with protease inhibitors: a review. *J. Acquir. Immune Defic. Syndr.* **25:**S4–S11.

Grindal, A., R. Cohen, R. Saul, and J. Taylos. 1978. Cerebral infarction in young adults. *Stroke* **9:**39–42.

Grunfeld, C., D. Kotler, J. Shigenaga, W. Doerrler, A. Tierney, J. Wang, R. Pierson, and K. Feingold. 1991. Circulating interferon-alpha levels and hypertriglyceridemia in the acquired immunodeficiency syndrome. *Am. J. Med.* **90:**154–162.

Harrington, H., H.A. Heller, D. Dawson, L. Caplan, and C. Rumbaugh. 1983. Intracerebral hemorrhage and oral amphetamine. *Arch. Neurol.* **40:**503–507.

Henry, K., H. Melroe, J. Huebsch, J. Hermundson, C. Levine, L. Swensen, and J. Daley. 1998. Severe premature coronary artery disease with protease inhibitors. *Lancet* **351:**1328.

Hoffmann, M., J. Berger, A. Nath, and M. Rayens. 2000. Cerebrovascular disease in young, HIV-infected, black Africans in the KwaZulu Natal province of South Africa. *J. Neurovirol.* **6:**229–236.

Hsieh, F., L. Chia, and W. Shen. 1992. Locations of cerebral infarctions in tuberculous meningitis. *Neuroradiology* **34:**197–199.

Iloeje, U., Y. Yuan, G. L'Italien, J. Mauskopf, S. Holmberg, A. Moorman, K. Wood, and R. Moore. 2005. Protease inhibitor exposure and increased risk of cardiovascular disease in HIV-infected patients. *HIV Med.* **6:**37–44.

Imanse, J., and J. Vanneste. 1990. Intraventricular hemorrhage following amphetamine abuse. *Neurology* **40:**1318–1319.

Jensen, R., T. S. Olsen, and B. B. Winther. 1990. Severe non-occlusive ischemic stroke in young heroin addicts. *Acta Neurol. Scand.* **81:**354–357.

Johns, D., M. Tiernet, and D. Felsenstein. 1987. Alteration in the natural history of neurosyphilis by concurrent infection with the human immunodeficiency virus. *N. Engl. J. Med.* **316:**1569–1572.

Johnson, D. A., H. S. Etter, and D. M. Reeves. 1983. Stroke and phenylpropanolamine use. *Lancet* **ii:**970.

Jorizzo, J., M. McNeely, R. Baughn, A. Solomon, T. Cavallo, and E. Smith. 1986. Role of circulating immune complexes in human secondary syphilis. *J. Infect. Dis.* **153:**1014–1022.

Kase, C., S. Levitz, J. Wolinsky, and C. A. Sulis. 1988. Pontine pure motor hemiparesis due to meningovascular syphilis in human immunodeficiency virus-positive patients. *Arch. Neurol.* **45:**832.

Kato, T., A. Hirano, J. Llena, and H. Dembitzer. 1987. Neuropathology of AIDS in 53 autopsy cases with particular emphasis on microglial nodules and multinucleated giant cells. *Acta Neuropathol.* **73:**287–294.

Kieburtz, K., T. Eskin, L. Ketonen, and M. Tuite. 1993. Opportunistic cerebral vasculopathy and stroke in patients with AIDS. *Arch. Neurol.* **50:**430–432.

Koeppen, A., L. Lansing, S. Peng, and R. Smith. 1981. Central nervous system vasculitis in cytomegalovirus infection. *J. Neurol. Sci.* **51:**395–410.

Koppel, B., G. Wormser, A. Tuchman, S. Maayan, D. Hewlett, and M. Daras. 1985. Central nervous system involvement in patients with acquired immunodeficiency syndrome (AIDS). *Acta Neurol. Scand.* **71:**337–353.

Lafeuillade, A., M. Alessi, I. Poizot-Martin, C. Boyer-Neumann, C. Zandotti, J. Gastaut, R. Quilichini, L. Aubert, C. Tamalet, and I. Juhan-Vague. 1992. Endothelial cell dysfunction in HIV infection. *J. Acquir. Immune Defic. Syndr.* **5:**127–131.

Lafeuillade, A., M. Alessi, I. Poizot-Martin, C. Dhiver, R. Quilichini, L. Aubert, J. Gastaut, and I. Juhan-Vague. 1991. Protein S deficiency and HIV infection. *N. Engl. J. Med.* **324:**1220.

Lahmeyer, H., and R. Steingold. 1980. Pentazocine and tripelenamine: a drug abuse epidemic? *Int. J. Addict.* **15:**1219–1232.

Laurence, J. 1998. Vascular complications associated with the use of HIV protease inhibitors. *Lancet* **351:**1960.

Levine, S., J. Brust, N. Futrell, K. Ho, D. Blake, C. Millikan, L. Brass, P. Fayad, L. Schultz, J. Selwa, and K. Welch. 1990. Cerebrovascular complications of the use of the 'crack' form of alkaloidal cocaine. *N. Engl. J. Med.* **323:**699–704.

Levy, R., and D. Breseden. 1988. CNS dysfunction in AIDS. *J. Acquir. Immune Defic. Syndr.* **1:**41–64.

Lieberman, A. N., W. Bloom, P. S. Kishore, and J. P. Lin. 1974. Carotid artery occlusion following ingestion of LSD. *Stroke* **5:**213–215.

Louie, J., L. Hsu, D. Osmond, M. Katz, and S. Schwarcz. 2002. Trends in causes of death among persons with acquired immunodeficiency syndrome in the era of highly active antiretroviral therapy, San Francisco, 1994–1998. *J. Infect. Dis.* **186:**1023–1027.

Maggi, P., F. Perilli. A. Lillo, M. Gargiulo, S. Ferraro, B. Grisorio, S. Ferrara, V. Carito, C. Bellacosa, G. Pastore, A. Chirianni, and G. Regina. 2007. Rapid progression of carotid lesions in HAART-treated HIV-1 patients. *Atherosclerosis* **192:**407–412.

Maggi, P., G. Serio, G. Epifani, G. Fiorentino, A. Saracino, C. Fico, F. Perilli, A. Lillo, S. Ferraro, M. Gargiulo, A. Chirianni, G. Angarano, G. Rehina, and G. Pastore. 2000. Premature lesions of the carotid vessels in HIV-infected patients treated with protease inhibitors. *AIDS* **14:**123–128.

Maqbool, Z., and H. H. Billett. 1982. Unwitting heparin abuse in a drug addict. *Ann. Intern. Med.* **96:**790–791.

Margolis, M. T., and T. H. Newton. 1971. Methamphetamine ("speed") arteritis. *Neuroradiology* **2:**179–182.

Martin, C., A. Matlow, E. Chew, D. Sutton and W. Pruzanski. 1989. Hyperviscosity syndrome in a patient with acquired immunodeficiency syndrome. *Arch. Intern. Med.* **149:**1435–1436.

Mary-Krause, M., L. Cotte, A. Simon, M. Partisani, D. Costagliola, and the Clinical Epidemiology Group from the French Hospital Database. 2003. Increased risk of myocardial infarction with duration of protease inhibitor therapy in HIV-infected men. *AIDS* **17:**2479–2486.

Masuda, J., C. Yutani, R. Waki, J. Ogata, Y. Kuriyama, and T. Yamaguchi. 1992. Histopathological analysis of the mechanisms of intracranial hemorrhage complicating infective endocarditis. *Stroke* **23:**843–850.

Matick, H., D. Anderson, and J. Brumlik. 1983. Cerebral vasculitis associated with oral amphetamine overdose. *Arch. Neurol.* **40:**253–254.

Matsuyama, T., N. Kobayashi, and N. Yamamoto. 1991. Cytokines and HIV infection: is AIDS a tumor necrosis factor disease? *AIDS* **5:**1405–1417.

McArthur, J. 1987. Neurological manifestations of AIDS. *Medicine* **66:**407–437.

Menge, T., T. Neumann-Haefelin, H. von Geisen, and G. Arendt. 2000. Progressive stroke in an HIV-1-positive patient under protease inhibitors. *Eur. Neurol.* **44:**252–254.

Mesquita, E., R. Ramos, A. Ferrari, W. Martins, and G. da Cruz. 1996. Rheumatic heart disease and infective endocarditis in a patient with acquired immunodeficiency syndrome. *Arq. Bras. Cardiol.* **67:**255–257.

Messadi, D., J. Pober, W. Fiers, M. Gimbrone, and G. Murphy. 1987. Induction of an activation antigen on postcapillary venular endothelium in human skin organ culture. *J. Immunol.* **139:**1557–1562.

Mizusawa, H., A. Hirano, J. Llena, and M. Shintaku. 1988. Cerebrovascular lesions of AIDS. *Acta Neuropathol.* **76:**451–457.

Mocroft, A., S. Vella, T. Benfield, A. Chiesi, V. Miller, P. Gargalianos, A. d'Arminio Monforte, I. Yust, J. Bruun, A. Phillips, J. Lundgren, et al. 1998. Changing patterns of mortality across Europe in patients infected with HIV-1. *Lancet* **8:**1725–1730.

Morgello, S., E. Cho, S. Nielsen, O. Devinsky, and C. Petito. 1987. Cytomegalovirus encephalitis in patients with acquired immunodeficiency syndrome: an autopsy study of 30 cases and a review of the literature. *Hum. Pathol.* **18:**289–297.

Morrow, W., M. Wharton, R. Stricker, and J. Levy. 1986. Circulating immune complexes in patients with acquired immune deficiency syndrome contain the AIDS-associated retrovirus. *Clin. Immunol. Immunopathol.* **40:**515–524.

Moskowitz, L., G. Hensley, J. Chan, F. Conley, M. Post, and S. Gonzalez-Arias. 1994. Brain biopsies in patients with acquired immunodeficiency syndrome. *Arch. Pathol. Lab. Med.* **108:**368–371.

Moskowitz, L., G. Hensley, J. Chan, J. Gregorios, and F. Conley. 1984. The neuropathology of acquired immunodeficiency syndrome. *Arch. Pathol. Lab. Med.* **108:**867–872.

Navia, B., E. Cho, C. Petito, and R. Price. 1986. The AIDS dementia complex. II. Neuropathology. *Ann. Neurol.* **19:**525–535.

Newsome, D., W. Green, and E. Miller. 1984. Microvascular aspects of acquired immunodeficiency syndrome retinopathy. *Am. J. Ophthalmol.* **98:**590–601.

Palella, F., K. Delaney, A. Moorman, M. Loveless, J. Fuhrer, G. Satten, D. Aschman, S. Holmberg, et al. 1998. Declining morbidity and mortality among patients with advanced human immunodeficiency virus infection. *N. Engl. J. Med.* **26:**853–860.

Passalaris, J., K. Sepkowitz, and M. Glesby. 2000. Coronary artery disease and human immunodeficiency virus infection. *Clin. Infect. Dis.* **31:**787–797.

Periard, D., A. Telenti, P. Sudre, J. Cheseaux, P. Halfon, M. Reymond, S. Marcovina, M. Glauser, P. Nicod, R. Darioli, and V. Mooser. 1999. Atherogenic dyslipidemia in HIV-infected individuals treated with protease inhibitors. *Circulation* **100:**700–705.

Petito, C., E. Cho, W. Lemann, B. Navia, and R. Price. 1986. Neuropathology of acquired immunodeficiency syndrome (AIDS): an autopsy review. *J. Neuropathol. Exp. Neurol.* **45:**635–646.

Pinto, A. 1996. AIDS and cerebrovascular disease. *Stroke* **27:**538–543.

Power, C., P. Kong, T. Crawford, S. Wesselingh, J. Glass, J. McArthur, and B. Trapp. 1993. Cerebral white matter changes in acquired immunodeficiency syndrome dementia: alterations of the blood-brain barrier. *Ann. Neurol.* **34:**339–350.

Price, R., B. Brew, J. Sidtis, M. Rosenblum, A. Scheck, and P. Cleary. 1988. The brain in AIDS: central nervous system HIV-1 infection and AIDS dementia complex. *Science* **239:**586–592.

Pumarola-Sune, T., B. Navia, C. Cordon-Cardo, E. Cho, and R. Price. 1987. HIV antigen in the brains of patients with the AIDS dementia complex. *Ann. Neurol.* **21:**490–496.

Qureshi, A., R. Janssen, J. Karon, J. Weissman, M. Akbar, K. Safdar, and M. Frankel. 1997. Human immunodeficiency virus infection and stroke in young patients. *Arch. Neurol.* **54:**1150–1153.

Rickerts, V., H. Brodt, S. Staszewski, and W. Stille. 2000. Incidence of myocardial infarctions in HIV-infected patients between 1983 and 1998: the Frankfurt HIV-cohort study. *Eur. J. Med. Res.* **18:**329–333.

Roldan, E., L. Moskowitz, and G. Hensley. 1987. Pathology of the heart in AIDS. *Arch. Pathol. Lab. Med.* **111:**943–946.

Rosemberg, S., M. Lopes, and A. Tsanadis. 1986. Neuropathology of acquired immunodeficiency syndrome (AIDS): analysis of 22 Brazilian cases. *J. Neurol. Sci.* **76:**187–198.

Rumbaugh, C., H. Fang, R. Higgins, R. Bergeron, H. Segall, and J. Teal. 1976. Cerebral microvascular injury in experimental drug abuse. *Investig. Radiol.* **11:**282–294.

Saif, M., and B. Greenberg. 2001. HIV and thrombosis: a review. *AIDS Patient Care STDS* **15:**15–24.

Salgado, A. V., A. J. Furlan, and T. F. Keys. 1987. Mycotic aneurysm, subarachnoid hemorrhage, and indications for cerebral angiography in infective endocarditis. *Stroke* **18:**1057–1060.

Schwartz, N., Y. So, H. Hollander, S. Allen, and K. Fye. 1986. Eosinophilic vasculitis leading to amaurosis fugax in a patient with acquired immunodeficiency syndrome. *Arch. Intern. Med.* **146:**2059–2060.

Selik, R., R. Byers, and M. Dworkin. 2002. Trends in diseases reported on U.S. death certificates that mentioned HIV infection, 1987–1999. *J. Acquir. Immune Defic. Syndr.* **29:**378–387.

Smith, T., U. DeGirolami, D. Henin, F. Bolgert, and J. Hauw. 1990. Human immunodeficiency virus (HIV) leukoencephalopathy and the microcirculation. *J. Neuropathol. Exp. Neurol.* **49:**357–370.

Snider, W., D. Simpson, S. Nielsen, J. Gold, C. Metroka, and J. Posner. 1983. Neurological complications of the acquired immunodeficiency syndrome: analysis of 50 patients. *Ann. Neurol.* **14:**403–418.

Sobel, J., O. Espinas, and S. Friedman. 1971. Carotid artery obstruction following LSD capsule ingestion. *Arch. Intern. Med.* **127:**290.

Stahl, C., C. Wideman, T. Spira, E. Haff, G. Hixon, and B. Evatt. 1993. Protein S deficiency in men with long-term human immunodeficiency virus infection. *Blood* **81:**1801–1807.

Tabib, A., C. Leroux, J. Mornex, and R. Loire. 2000. Accelerated coronary atherosclerosis and arteriosclerosis in young human-immunodeficiency-virus-positive patients. *Cor. Artery Dis.* **11:**41–46.

Taillan, B., C. Roul, J. Fuzibet, H. Vinti, A. Pesce, J. Bayle, P. Cassuto, and P. Dujardin. 1990. Antiphospholipid antibodies associated with human immunodeficiency virus infection. *Arch. Intern. Med.* **150**:1975.

Tran Dinh, Y., H. Mamo, J. Cervoni, C. Caulin, and A. Saimot. 1990. Disturbances in the cerebral perfusion of HIV-1 seropositive asymptomatic subjects: a quantitative tomography study of 18 cases. *J. Nucl. Med.* **31**:1601–1607.

Tsiodras, S., C. Mantzoros, S. Hammer, and M. Samore. 2000. Effects of protease inhibitors on hyperglycemia, hyperlipidemia, and lipodystrophy: a 5-year cohort study. *Arch. Intern. Med.* **160**:2050–2056.

Vinters, H., W. Guerra, L. Eppolito, and P. Keith. 1988. Necrotizing vasculitis of the nervous system in a patient with AIDS-related complex. *Neuropathol. Appl. Neurobiol.* **14**:417–424.

Vittecoq, D., L. Escaut, and J. Monsuez. 1998. Vascular complications associated with the use of HIV protease inhibitors. *Lancet* **351**:1958–1959.

Walsh, T., D. Hier, and L. Caplan. 1985. Fungal infections of the central nervous system: comparative analysis of risk factors and clinical signs in 57 patients. *Neurology* **35**:1654–1657.

Ward, J., T. O'Leary, G. Baskin, R. Benveniste, C. Harris, P. Nara, and R. Rhodes. 1987. Immunohistochemical localization of human and simian immunodeficiency viral antigens in fixed tissue sections. *Am. J. Pathol.* **127**:199–205.

Wiley, C., R. Schrier, J. Nelson, P. Lampert, and M. Oldstone. 1986. Cellular localization of human immunodeficiency virus infection within the brains of acquired immune deficiency syndrome patients. *Proc. Natl. Acad. Sci. USA* **83**:7089–7093.

Yanker, B., P. Skolnik, G. Shoukimas, D. Gabuzda, R. Sobel, and D. Ho. 1986. Cerebral granulomatous angiitis associated with isolation of human T-lymphotropic virus type III from the central nervous system. *Ann. Neurol.* **20**:362–364.

Yarnell, P. 1977. "Speed" headache and hematoma. *Headache* **17**:69–70.

Yu, Y. J., D. R. Cooper, D. E. Wellenstein, and B. Block. 1983. Cerebral angiitis and intracerebral hemorrhage associated with methamphetamine abuse. *J. Neurosurg.* **58**:109–111.

Yunis, N., and V. Stone. 1998. Cardiac manifestations of HIV/AIDS: a review of disease spectrum and clinical management. *J. Acquir. Immune Defic. Syndr. Hum. Retrovirol.* **1**:145–154.

Zietz, C., B. Hotz, M. Sturzl, E. Rauch, R. Penning, and U. Lohrs. 1996. Aortic endothelium in HIV-1 infection: chronic injury, activation, and increased leukocyte adherence. *Am. J. Pathol.* **149**:1887–1898.

The Spectrum of Neuro-AIDS Disorders:
Pathophysiology, Diagnosis, and Treatment
Edited by K. Goodkin et al.
©2008 ASM Press, Washington, DC

4

HIV-Associated Myelopathy, Myopathy, and Meningitis

LYDIA ESTANISLAO

HIV infection may involve all levels of the neuroaxis, from the brain to the muscle. This chapter discusses the complications arising from involvement of the meninges, spinal cord, and muscles by the virus. Clinical features, diagnostic tests, and management of HIV-associated myelopathy, myopathy, and meningitis are discussed.

HIV-ASSOCIATED MYELOPATHY

First described at the beginning of the AIDS epidemic (Snider et al., 1983), the spinal cord disease defined as AIDS-associated vacuolar myelopathy (VM) is one of the most disabling neurologic complications of HIV infection. It is considered the single most common cause of spinal cord disease in HIV infection and is one of the least understood and least studied among the neurologic manifestations. There is a high prevalence of pathological involvement of the spinal cord reported at autopsy. Most AIDS-related postmortem pathological series report a prevalence of 15 to 55% (Petito et al., 1985; Artigas et al., 1990; Dal Pan et al., 1994), although a prevalence as low as 1% has been reported (Lang et al., 1989).

Clinical Features

VM frequently presents in advanced HIV disease and immunosuppression, although it may occasionally occur in the early stages. It develops insidiously over months. Urinary urgency and frequency are often the first symptoms. Erectile dysfunction may be a common early symptom in men, so that even if there are many other reasons for impotence in AIDS, myelopathy should be a consideration, especially in the setting of a normal testosterone level. Lower-extremity weakness may follow. Because VM typically involves thoracic segments initially, the arms are usually spared at presentation. In other cases, lower-extremity stiffness is

more prominent than weakness and results in gait difficulty. Patients may complain of occasional fleeting paresthesias in the lower extremities that are rarely severe.

Examination reveals paraparesis, lower-extremity spasticity, or both. Increased thresholds of vibration and proprioception with a positive Romberg sign resulting from posterior column impairment. Pain and temperature are usually preserved, unless there is superimposed peripheral neuropathy. Muscle stretch reflexes, particularly those of the lower extremities, are hyperactive, with bilateral ankle clonus and extensor plantar responses. Gait ataxia with impaired tandem gait may also be seen. In advanced cases, patients may be unable to ambulate and may eventually be wheelchair bound.

Laboratory Studies

Mild atrophy of the spinal cord and areas of increased signal on magnetic resonance imaging (MRI) T2-weighted images are common (Fig. 1) (Chong et al., 1999). While the MRI may frequently be normal, cerebrospinal fluid (CSF) studies often reveal mild pleocytosis (5 to 10 cells/mm³) and mild protein elevation, which are nonspecific findings in HIV infection. Cell counts of greater than 30 cells/mm³ should raise the suspicion of other etiologies, including neurosyphilis, tuberculous myelitis, and cytomegalovirus myelitis.

Electrophysiological Data

Somatosensory evoked potentials are believed to provide an objective measure of spinal cord dysfunction. Prolongation of the tibial central conduction time has been found to correlate with the clinical diagnosis of myelopathy. Somatosensory evoked potentials have been used to diagnose subclinical or asymptomatic myelopathy (Tagliati et al., 2000), as well as to follow disease progression (Pierelli et al., 1996).

Pathology

Pathological changes are most often seen in mid- to low-thoracic segments and include intramyelinic and periaxonal patchy vacuolization, usually in the lateral and posterior

Lydia Estanislao, Clinical Neurology Specialists, Las Vegas, NV 89146.

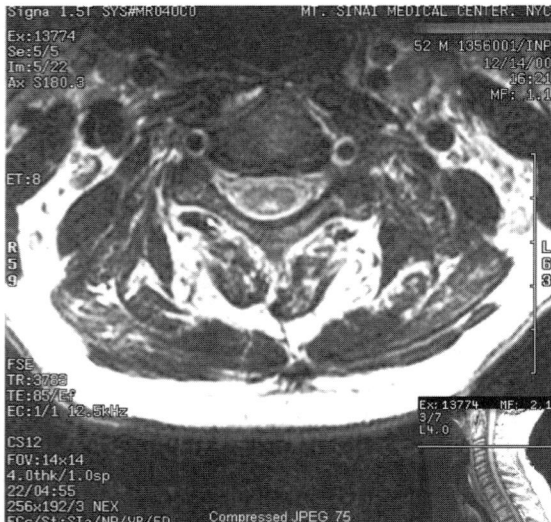 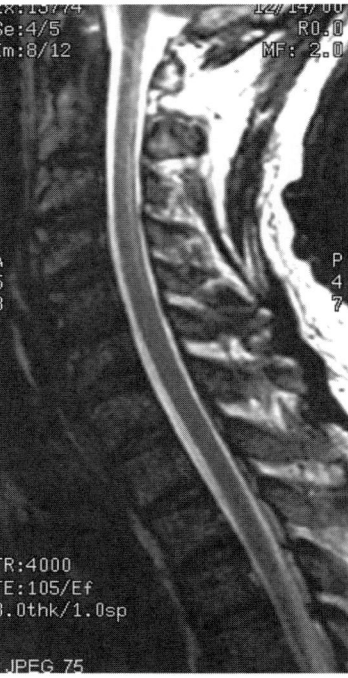

FIGURE 1 Axial and sagittal T2-weighted MRI images of the spinal cord showing increased T2 signal in the posterior columns.

columns. The presence of lipid-laden macrophages within the vacuoles is required to avoid confusion with postmortem artifacts (Petito et al., 1985). Cervical segments may also be involved. Since the first pathological descriptions of VM (Petito et al., 1985; Goldstick et al., 1985), a striking similarity to the myelopathy of vitamin B_{12} deficiency (i.e., subacute combined degeneration) has been noted. These changes are usually observed in adults, while in children, the myelopathy is usually associated with diffuse loss of myelin, axonal loss, the presence of multinucleated giant cells, and prominent inflammatory infiltrates (Tan et al., 1995) (see chapter 14, this volume).

Clinicopathological correlation of spinal cord lesions with myelopathic symptoms and signs has been difficult because of the retrospective nature of the major case series reported in the literature (Petito et al., 1985; Simpson and Tagliati, 1994). Moreover, the neurologic evaluation for myelopathy may be difficult in advanced AIDS patients with severe systemic disease and coexisting peripheral neuropathy and/or dementia. Clear-cut myelopathic signs are infrequent in patients with mild (grade I) VM (Petito et al., 1985), where only a few vacuoles are present. Patients with mild VM rarely have motor signs and may present with fatigue, mild weakness, increased reflexes, and sphincter abnormalities (Petito et al., 1985; Dal Pan et al., 1994; Tan et al., 1995). Symptomatic myelopathy is correlated with moderate and severe VM in several studies, where numerous (grade II) and confluent (grade III) vacuoles involve the posterior and lateral columns of the spinal cord (Petito et al., 1985; Dal Pan et al., 1994; Tan et al., 1995). Approximately 20 to 60% of patients with grade II (moderate) and almost all patients with grade III (severe) VM show symptoms and signs of myelopathy with spastic weakness, ataxia, and incontinence (Petito et al., 1985; Dal Pan et al., 1994; Tan et al., 1995).

Pathogenesis

VM is not believed to be due to direct HIV infection of the spinal cord. With a few exceptions (Budka, 1990), most studies have not found evidence of a direct effect of HIV infection on the spinal cord in subjects with VM. HIV is found within macrophages but not in neuronal cells or microglia, and there is no relationship between the presence of HIV and the development of myelopathy (Eilbott et al., 1989; Kure et al., 1991; Petito et al., 1994; Rosenblum et al., 1989; Tan et al., 1995). There was also no correlation found between the levels of HIV-1 RNA and tumor necrosis factor alpha in CSF and the presence or severity of myelopathy (Geraci et al., 2000).

Because of the similarity of its pathology with that of subacute combined degeneration of the spinal cord (Petito et al., 1985), others have proposed a possible role of vitamin B_{12} deficiency in the pathogenesis of this condition (Kieburtz et al., 1991). A recent proposal has suggested that vitamin B_{12} deficiency is induced by an autoimmune mechanism involving the production of anti-parietal cell antibodies (Misra and Kalita, 2007). However, patients with HIV-associated myelopathy generally have normal serum vitamin B_{12} levels. Vitamin B_{12} treatment has been utilized without clinical improvement, although this replacement therapy could have prevented further neurological dysfunction (Kieburtz et al., 1991). An alternative, indirect mechanism may involve impaired methylation secondary to a deficiency of S-adenosylmethionine (SAMe), a major methyl group donor in the nervous system. SAMe is converted from methionine by methionine synthase. During this process of conversion, vitamin B_{12} acts as a vital coenzyme (Tan and Guiloffe, 1998). SAMe-dependent methylation is essential for myelin formation, stabilization, and repair and in the metabolism of nucleic acids and neurotransmitters. There is evidence linking impaired methylation in the nervous system and neurologic complications of AIDS in adults and children (Surtees et al., 1990; Castagna et al., 1995; Di Rocco et al., 1998). Di Rocco et al. (2002) compared SAMe, methionine, homocysteine, and glutathione in the sera and CSF of 15 patients with HIV-associated myelopathy with those of 13 HIV-infected controls without myelopathy and a non-HIV-infected control group. They found a significant decrease in CSF SAMe in the HIV-associated myelopathy group compared with the group of HIV-infected controls without myelopathy and the non-HIV-infected control group. In line with this finding, the CSF SAMe level in the HIV-infected controls without myelopathy was, in turn, significantly lower than the CSF SAMe level in the non-HIV-infected control group. In addition, the serum methionine level was also significantly lower in the HIV-associated myelopathy group than in the non-HIV-infected control group. The pathogenesis of VM may, therefore, be related to a complex chain of events that is initiated by the viral infection itself with consequent macrophage activation and cytokine release. These events may ultimately lead to transmethylation impairment and myelin vacuolization and destruction (Tan and Guiloff, 1998; Di Rocco et al., 1998).

Diagnosis

VM is a clinical diagnosis based largely on the typical symptoms and findings on neurologic examination, on the slow progression of those symptoms, and on the exclusion of other causes of spinal cord disease. The differential diagnosis of VM is extensive and includes other infections, such as that caused by human T-cell lymphotropic virus type I or II, cytomegalovirus, herpes simplex virus type 2, varicella zoster virus, *Toxoplasma gondii*, *Mycobacterium tuberculosis*, neurosyphilis, and neoplastic diseases, particularly lymphoma. The work-up should include MRI of the spine with contrast studies, serologic studies, and CSF studies. Although the clinical presentation and the evolution of VM are fairly typical, the diagnosis may be difficult in patients with advanced AIDS, severe systemic disease, and/or coexisting peripheral neuropathy and dementia (Di Rocco, 1999; Snider et al., 1983; Petito et al., 1985).

A rapidly progressive myelopathy over days or weeks, the presence of a discrete sensory level, CSF pleocytosis greater than 30 cells/mm³, and back pain are all evidence against the diagnosis of VM and should lead to further diagnostic investigations to disclose the cause of spinal cord disease.

Treatment

There is no definitive treatment for VM. Supplementation with vitamin B_{12} has proven ineffective in improving the symptoms of VM (Kieburtz et al., 1991). Nevertheless, it is commonly administered to patients with clinical evidence of VM. A pilot study using high doses of oral L-methionine led to improvement in clinical and electrophysiological features of the disease in an open-label clinical trial (Di Rocco et al., 1998), as well as improvement in neuropsychological function in these patients (Dorfman et al., 1997). In a subsequent phase II, double-blind, placebo-controlled trial, 56 patients with a clinical diagnosis of HIV-associated myelopathy were randomized to L-methionine (6 g/day in two divided doses) or placebo for 12 weeks. There were no significant clinical effects of treatment on strength, spasticity, or urinary function (Di Rocco et al., 2004). Corticosteroids and intravenous gamma globulin have also been ineffective in uncontrolled

clinical experience (Dal Pan and Berger, 1997). Symptomatic treatment is clearly indicated for patients with spasticity and urinary dysfunction.

To date, there has been no controlled study describing the effects of antiretroviral medications on VM. One study showed a beneficial response to azidothymidine (currently referred to as zidovudine [ZDV]) at a dose of 10 mg/kg of body weight (Oksenhendler et al., 1990), while another study reported no benefit with ZDV treatment (Yarchoan et al., 1987). The effect of highly active antiretroviral therapy (HAART) on the clinical manifestations or electrophysiological measures of VM also has not been systematically studied. A case report described clinical improvement of myelopathy after the introduction of HAART in one patient (Staudinger and Henry, 2000). Although there was a reduction of the plasma viral load, there was no report of CSF viral load measurement and electrophysiological results before and after treatment. Although it may be that HAART had a specific effect on myelopathy, it is also possible that the symptomatic improvement may have been related to general improvement of health without a specific effect on the spinal cord (Di Rocco et al., 2000). Geraci and Di Rocco (2000) reported that the use of different combinations of antiretroviral medications was ineffective in preventing the onset of myelopathy. It is possible, however, that these combination medication regimens are able to delay the progression or alter the course of the disease. It is also not known whether the introduction of these drugs has decreased the incidence of VM.

HIV-ASSOCIATED MYOPATHY

Myopathy may occur at any stage of HIV infection and from a variety of causes, including ZDV therapy, inflammatory myopathy (polymyositis), vasculitis, and infection (*Staphylococcus aureus*, *M. tuberculosis*, cytomegalovirus, and *T. gondii*). The incidence of clinical HIV-associated myopathy has not been established in prospective studies, although on the whole it appears to be relatively uncommon. One series reported two cases of polymyositis out of 101 patients with HIV infection (Berman et al., 1988). In AIDS Clinical Trials Group study 016, a retrospective analysis of a primary antiretroviral protocol, the incidence of myopathy was 0.4% in the placebo group (n = 351) (Simpson et al., 1997). In a report based upon laboratory evidence, 11 of 15 AIDS cases had positive electromyographic evidence of myopathy; four out of seven muscle biopsies were positive for myopathic changes.

Clinical Features

The presentation varies with the underlying cause, but slowly progressive weakness of proximal muscles characterizes most patients. Typical complaints include difficulty in lifting the arms above the head, difficulty in rising from a chair, and difficulty climbing stairs. Myalgias are common and may be present in 25 to 50% of cases.

Neurologic examination reveals symmetric weakness of proximal muscles of the extremities. The neck flexors may be involved as well. Functional tests of muscle strength include having the patient rise up unassisted from a seated position and a squat and having the patient sustain arm extension above the head for 15 seconds. In pure myopathy cases, deep tendon reflexes are normal or preserved. However, in HIV disease, more than one neurologic complication may coexist, such as myelopathy and neuropathy (Jakobsen et al., 1989), yielding a combination of signs. In cases like these, ancillary tests may be necessary to distinguish the different comorbid neurologic conditions.

Laboratory Data

Serum creatine phosphokinase (CPK) levels are usually elevated to a moderate degree, with a median level of approximately 500 IU/liter (Simpson et al., 1993). Levels greater than 1,500 IU/liter have been reported with associated rhabodmyolysis (Chariot et al., 1994). CPK is not a specific marker of myopathy in HIV-positive patients. In AIDS Clinical Trials Group study 016, a majority of the patients with elevated CPK did not have clinical evidence of weakness or myopathy (Simpson et al., 1997). An isolated CPK elevation is not sufficient to make a diagnosis of myopathy without the accompanying clinical features. In contrast, electromyography is sensitive and specific in the diagnosis of myopathy. In a series of 50 patients with myopathy, 94% had myopathic electromyography findings (Simpson et al., 1993) consisting of short, brief motor unit action potentials, recruiting with an early and full interference pattern, with or without irritative activity.

Pathology

Early reports described two histological patterns of HIV-associated myopathy prior to the availability of antiretroviral agents. One was HIV-related polymyositis, characterized by the presence of myofiber necrosis, phagocytosis, and mononuclear cell inflammation in the interstitial and interfascicular areas. Immunohistochemistry revealed HIV in the CD4-positive T cells and macrophages within the infiltrate (Dalakas et al., 1986; Ilia et al., 1991). However, CD8-positive T cells comprised the majority of the cells in the infiltrate (Ilia et al., 1991). Because of the nature of the inflammation, some investigators have proposed an autoimmune process as the pathogenic mechanism, similar to the process occurring in HIV-negative polymyositis.

The second histological pattern is a structural myopathy, characterized by the presence of abnormal myofiber structure, occasionally with rods and cytoplasmic bodies and basophilic granular material (Simpson and Bender, 1988; Gonzales et al., 1988). Inflammatory cell infiltrates were often mild or absent. HIV could not be demonstrated within myofibers by immunohistochemistry and in situ hybridization. With the advent of reverse transcriptase PCR, HIV was demonstrated within endomyseal macrophages and myocyte nuclei (Seidman et al., 1994). This finding raised the possibility of direct infection of myocytes by HIV in ZDV-naïve, HIV-infected patients with myopathy.

ZDV-Associated Myopathy

HIV-associated myopathy was a well-known entity prior to the availability of antiretroviral agents. Following the use of the first available antiretroviral, ZDV, cases of "ZDV myopathy" were reported. In 1988, Bessen et al. reported polymyositis in four HIV-seropositive patients treated with ZDV, three of whom had improvement after ZDV withdrawal (Bessen et al., 1988). Several case reports followed, describing myopathies in ZDV-treated patients, whose symptoms improved after drug withdrawal (Gorard et al., 1988; Helbert et al., 1988; Gertner et al., 1989). Muscle biopsy specimens from ZDV-treated patients with myopathy occasionally revealed ragged red fibers on modified trichrome staining of the muscle, considered to be a pathological hallmark of mitochondrial dysfunction. The percentage of ragged red fibers was reported to be correlated with the severity of clinical myopathy. Other features of inflammatory myopathy were also present. Electron microscopy showed proliferation and enlargement of mitochondria with paracrystalline inclusions. These mitochondrial abnormalities were reportedly not present in the ZDV-naïve group. Another study from the same authors showed that ZDV-treated patients with myopathy had increased numbers of mitochondria with abnormal morphology, while ZDV-naïve patients did not (Dalakas et al., 1990). Myopathy has also been described in some patients exposed to stavudine-containing regimens (Miller et al., 2000; Mokrzycki et al., 2000).

Controversy surrounds the role of mitochondrial dysfunction in HIV-associated and ZDV-associated myopathies and whether there are clear features distinguishing between these disorders (Till and MacDonell, 1991). In 1993, a study of 50 patients with myopathy, diagnosed by clinical, laboratory, and, in some cases, pathological criteria, failed to distinguish ZDV-associated myopathy from HIV-associated myopathy (Simpson et al., 1993). Clinical features did not differ between ZDV-treated and ZDV-naïve patients with myopathy. Muscle biopsy findings, including myofiber degeneration, inflammatory infiltrates, inclusion bodies, and mitochondrial abnormalities (i.e., abnormal mitochondrial morphology and giant double membrane-bounded forms with convoluted tubular cristae) were present in both groups. The conclusion was that mitochondrial abnormalities were not specific to ZDV-associated myopathy. A more detailed pathological characterization of 18 ZDV-treated and 9 ZDV-naïve patients reached similar conclusions. The mitochondrial abnormalities were correlated with the degree of myofiber degeneration present in muscle biopsy specimens, regardless of the ZDV exposure history (Morgello et al., 1995). Further contributing to the question of the relative role of antiretroviral toxicity in myopathy is the observation that some patients with myopathy improve with ZDV withdrawal (Bessen et al., 1988; Gorard et al., 1988; Dalakas et al., 1990; Panegyres et al., 1990), while others do not (Simpson et al., 1993; Espinoza et al., 1991; Manji et al., 1993). Moreover, ZDV rechallenge has failed to reproduce the myopathic symptoms in some patients (Gertner et al., 1989; Panegyres et al., 1990). These findings lead us to believe that HIV itself is associated with myopathy, perhaps mediated by immunological and mitochondrial mechanisms. Antiretroviral therapy may then be superimposed upon a susceptible host, particularly one with preexisting compromise of mitochondrial function, resulting in the manifestation of symptoms or in symptom worsening.

Treatment

Corticosteroids may provide benefit in HIV-associated myopathy (Dalakas et al., 1990; Manji et al., 1993; Mhiri et al., 1991; Chalmers et al., 1991; Simpson et al., 1993). However, they should be used with caution because of their immunosuppressive effects. While intravenous immunoglobulins may be an alternative option without risk of immunosuppression, there is only limited reported experience with their use in HIV-associated myopathy. Recently, two patients with HIV-associated nemaline rod myopathy were documented as responding to intravenous immunoglobulin therapy (de Sanctis et al., 2008).

HIV-ASSOCIATED MENINGITIS

In the early part of the HIV epidemic, CSF mononuclear pleocytosis was reported to occur in 15% to 18% of asymptomatic HIV-infected individuals (McArthur et al., 1988; Marshall et al., 1988). The exact incidence of clinically apparent HIV-associated meningitis is not known. It may be undiagnosed (Hanson et al., 2008), mostly occurring as part of the acute conversion syndrome (ACS) (Kahn and Walker, 1998). In the HAART era, cases of meningitis have been reported in patients with antiretroviral therapy interruptions in medication regimens, which some believe to be "antiretroviral rebound syndrome."

Clinical Features

Like any other virus-induced meningitis, HIV-associated meningitis is self-limited. The symptoms include headache, photophobia, nausea, and neck stiffness. It may be undiagnosed, as it may be overshadowed by concomitant systemic flu-like symptoms during the ACS. Rarely, encephalitis may accompany the meningitis, and alteration of mental status and seizures may occur. In some cases, a subacute increase in intracranial pressure is observed

CSF indices are consistent with an "aseptic meningitis." HIV can be amplified and quantified in the CSF, although its presence does not exclude other coincident causes. Neuroimaging, such as computed tomography scan and MRI, may be normal or may show enhancement of the meninges.

Recently, cases of acute aseptic meningitis have been reported in those who were HAART naïve, those whose HAART treatment was interrupted (Breton et al., 2003; Wendel and McArthur, 2003), and (in one case) a patient who was on poorly CSF-penetrating agents (Wendel and McArthur, 2003). In these cases, the patients presented with severe headaches, photosensitivity, neck rigidity, and (in one case) abnormal brain MRI signal. CSF analysis showed mononuclear pleocytosis, and the viral load of HIV was higher in the CSF than in the plasma. With initiation (or reinitiation) of HAART, or (in one case) a change of the regimen to CSF-penetrating agents, the patients had excellent clinical responses, with complete resolution of meningitis, normalization of CSF inflammatory profiles, and reversal of brain MRI abnormalities. More importantly, there were excellent CSF virologic responses in all cases. Some authors believe that these cases of meningitis occurring with treatment interruption or with lack of a CSF-penetrating agent represent the antiretroviral rebound syndrome, similar to the aseptic meningitis that occurs during the illness during the ACS. Others postulate that it is due to central nervous system escape of HIV replication.

Treatment

There is no specific treatment for HIV-associated meningitis. The immediate initiation or reinitiation of antiretroviral medications, particularly those with more effective CSF penetration (i.e., ZDV, stavudine, abacavir, indinavir, efavirenz, and nevirapine), should be considered. Supportive treatment is the mainstay of management.

SUMMARY

Spinal cord dysfunction, muscle disease, and meningitis may occur associated with HIV infection. The precise pathogenic mechanisms are unclear, but in myelopathy and myopathy, indirect mechanisms are believed to be responsible. The resulting disability from the latter two conditions can be disabling. In HIV-associated myelopathy, symptomatic treatment is the mainstay of management. The effect of HAART in this condition is not well studied. Corticosteroids and intravenous immunoglobulin therapy are used for the treatment of HIV-associated myopathy; the initiation of HAART without myotoxic agents may also provide benefit in those who are untreated. HIV-associated meningitis may

occur as a direct effect of HIV with the ACS, in which case it may be self-limited; with antiretroviral therapy interruption; or with lack of use of CSF-penetrating agents. In the latter two cases, the meningitis may respond to reinitiation of antiretroviral therapy or to a regimen change incorporating a CSF-penetrating agent.

REFERENCES

Artigas, J., G. Grosse, and F. Niedobitek. 1990. Vacuolar myelopathy in AIDS: a morphological analysis. *Pathol. Res. Pract.* **186:**228–237.

Berman, A., L. R. Espinoza, J. D. Diaz, J. L. Aguilar, T. Rolando, F. B. Vasey, B. F. Germain, and R. F. Lockey. 1988. Rheumatic manifestations of human immunodeficiency virus infection. *Am. J. Med.* **85:**59–64.

Bessen, L. J., J. B. Greene, E. Louie, P. Seitzman, and H. Weinberg. 1988. Severe polymyositis-like syndrome associated with zidovudine therapy of AIDS and ARC. *N. Engl. J. Med.* **318:**708. (Letter.)

Breton, G., X. Duval, A. Gervais, P. Longuet, C. Leport, and J. L. Vilde. 2003. Retroviral rebound syndrome with meningoencephalitis after cessation of antiretroviral therapy. *Am. J. Med.* **114:**769–770.

Budka, H. 1990. Human immunodeficiency virus (HIV) envelope and core proteins in CNS tissues of patients with the acquired immune deficiency syndrome (AIDS). *Acta Neuropathol.* **79:**611–619.

Castagna, A., C. Le Grazie, A. Accordini, P. Giulidori, G. Cavalli, T. Bottiglieri, and A. Lazzarin. 1995. Cerebrospinal fluid S-adenosylmethionine (SAMe) and glutathione concentrations in HIV infection: effect of parenteral treatment with SAMe. *Neurology* **45:**1678–1683.

Chalmers, A. C., C. M. Greco, and R. G. Miller. 1991. Prognosis in AZT myopathy. *Neurology* **41:**1181–1184.

Chariot, P., E. Ruet, F. Authier, Y. Levy, and R. Gherardi. 1994. Acute rhabdomyolysis in patients infected with human immunodeficiency virus. *Neurology* **44:**1692–1696.

Chong, J., A. Di Rocco, M. Tagliati, F. Danisi, D. M. Simpson, and S. W. Atlas. 1999. MR findings in AIDS-associated myelopathy. *Am. J. Neuroradiol.* **20:**1412–1416.

Dalakas, M. C., I. Illa, G. H. Pezeshkpour, J. P. Laukaitis, B. Cohen, and J. L. Griffin. 1990. Mitochondrial myopathy caused by long-term zidovudine therapy. *N. Engl. J. Med.* **322:**1098–1105.

Dalakas, M., G. Pezeshkpour, M. Gravell, and J. Sever. 1986. Polymyositis associated with AIDS retrovirus. *JAMA* **256:**2381–2383.

Dal Pan, G., and J. Berger. 1997. Spinal cord disease in human immunodeficiency virus infection, p. 173–187. *In* J. Berger and R. Levy (ed.), *AIDS and the Nervous System*. Lippincott-Raven, Philadelphia, PA.

Dal Pan, G. J., J. D. Glass, and J. C. McArthur. 1994. Clinicopathologic correlations of HIV-1-associated vacuolar myelopathy: an autopsy-based case-control study. *Neurology* **44:**2159–2164.

de Sanctis, J. T., G. Cumbo-Nacheli, D. Dobbie, and D. Baumgartner. 2008. HIV-associated nemaline rod myopathy: role of intravenous immunoglobulin therapy in two persons with HIV/AIDS. *AIDS Reader* **18:**90–94.

Di Rocco, A., P. Werner, T. Bottiglieri, J. Godbold, M. Liu, M. Tagliati, A. Scarano, and D. Simpson. 2004. Treatment of AIDS-associated myelopathy with l-methionine: a placebo-controlled study. *Neurology* **63:**1270–1275.

Di Rocco, A., T. Bottiglieri, P. Werner, A. Geraci, D. Simpson, J. Godbold, and S. Morgello. 2002. Abnormal cobalamin-dependent transmethylation in AIDS-associated myelopathy. *Neurology* **58:**730–735.

Di Rocco, A., A. Geraci, and M. Tagliati. 2000. Remission of HIV myelopathy after highly active antiretroviral therapy. *Neurology* **55:**456. (Letter.)

Di Rocco, A. 1999. Diseases of the spinal cord in human immunodeficiency virus infection. *Semin. Neurol.* **19:**151–155.

Di Rocco, A., M. Tagliati, F. Danisi, D. Dorfman, J. Moise, and D. Simpson. 1998. L-Methionine for AIDS-associated vacuolar myelopathy. *Neurology* **51:**266–268.

Dorfman, D., A. DiRocco, D. Simpson, M. Tagliati, L. Tanners, and J. Moise. 1997. Oral methionine may improve neuropsychological function in patients with AIDS myelopathy: results of an open-label trial. *AIDS* **11:**1066–1067.

Eilbott, D., N. Peress, H. Burger, D. LaNeve, J. Orenstein, H. E. Gendelman, R. Seidman, and B. Weiser. 1989. Human immunodeficiency virus type 1 in spinal cords of acquired immunodeficiency syndrome patients with myelopathy: expression and replication in macrophages. *Proc. Natl. Acad. Sci. USA* **86:**3337–3341.

Espinoza, L. R., J. L. Aguilar, C. G. Espinoza, J. Gresh, J. Jara, L. H. Silveira, P. Martinez-Osuna, and M. Seleznick. 1991. Characteristics and pathogenesis of myositis in human immunodeficiency virus infection. Distinction from azidothymidine-induced myopathy. *Rheum. Dis. Clin. N. Am.* **107:**598–599.

Geraci, A., and A. Di Rocco. 2000. Anti-HIV therapy. *AIDS* **14:**2059–2061.

Geraci, A., A. Di Rocco, M. Liu, P. Werner, M. Tagliati, J. Godbold, D. Simpson, and S. Morgello. 2000. AIDS myelopathy is not associated with elevated HIV viral load in cerebrospinal fluid. *Neurology* **55:**440–442.

Gertner, E., J. Thurn, D. N. Williams, M. Simpson, H. H. Balfour, Jr., F. Rhame, and K. Henry. 1989. Zidovudine-associated myopathy. *Am. J. Med.* **6:**814–818.

Goldstick, L., T. Mandybur, and R. Bode. 1985. Spinal cord degeneration in AIDS. *Neurology* **35:**103–106.

Gonzales, M. F., R. K. Olney, Y. T. So, C. M. Greco, B. A. McQuinn, R. G. Miller, and S. J. DeArmond. 1988. Subacute structural myopathy associated with human immunodeficiency virus infection. *Arch. Neurol.* **45:**585–587.

Gorard, D. A., K. Henry, R. Guiloff, P. K. Panegyres, N. Tan, B. A. Kakulas, J. A. Armstrong, and P. Hollingsworth. 1988. Necrotizing myopathy and zidovudine. *Lancet* **331:**1050–1051.

Helbert, M., T. Fletcher, B. Peddle, J. R. Harris, and A. J. Pinching. 1988. Zidovudine-associated myopathy. *Lancet* **332:**689–690.

Ilia, I., A. Nath, and M. Dalakas. 1991. Immunocytochemical and virological characteristics of HIV-associated inflammatory myopathies: similarities with seronegative patients. *Ann. Neurol.* **29:**474–481.

Jakobsen, J., T. Smith, J. Gaub, S. Helweg-Larsen, and W. Trojaborg. 1989. Progressive neurological dysfunction during latent HIV infection. *Br. Med. J.* **299:**225–228.

Kahn, J. O., and B. D. Walker. 1998. Acute human immunodeficiency virus type 1 infection. *N. Engl. J. Med.* **339:**33–39.

Kieburtz, K., D. Giang, R. Schiffer, and N. Vakil. 1991. Abnormal vitamin B_{12} metabolism in human immunodeficiency virus infection: association with neurologic dysfunction. *Arch. Neurol.* **48:**312–314.

Kure, K., J. Llena, W. Lyman, R. Soreiro, K. Weidenheim, A. Hirano, and D. Dickson. 1991. Human immunodeficiency virus-1 infection of the nervous system: an autopsy study of 268 adult, pediatric and fetal brains. *Hum. Pathol.* **22:**700–710.

Lang, W., J. Miklossy, J. Deruaz, G. Pizzolato, A. Probst, T. Schaffner, E. Gessaga, and E. Kleihues. 1989. Neuropathology of the acquired immunodeficiency syndrome: a report of 135 consecutive autopsy cases from Switzerland. *Acta Neuropathol.* **77:**379–390.

Manji, H., M. J. Harrison, J. M. Round, D. A. Jones, S. Connolly, C. J. Fowler, I. Williams, and I. V. Weller. 1993. Muscle disease, HIV and zidovudine: the spectrum of muscle disease in HIV-infected individuals treated with zidovudine. *J. Neurol.* **240:**479–488.

Marshall, D. W., R. L. Brew, W. T. Cahill, R. W. Houk, R. A. Zajac, and R. N. Boswell. 1988. Spectrum of cerebrospinal fluid findings in various stages of human immunodeficiency virus infection. *Arch. Neurol.* **45:**954–958.

McArthur, J. C., B. A. Cohen, H. Farzedegan, D. R. Cornblath, O. A. Selnes, D. Ostrow, R. T. Johnson, J. Phair, and B. F. Polk. 1988. Cerebrospinal fluid abnormalities in homosexual men with and without neuropsychiatric findings. *Ann. Neurol.* **23**(Suppl)**:**S34–S37.

Mhiri, C., M. Baudrimont, G. Bonne, C. Geny, F. Degoul, C. Marsac, E. Roullet, and R. Gherardi. 1991. Zidovudine myopathy: a distinctive disorder associated with mitochondrial dysfunction. *Ann. Neurol.* **29:**606–614.

Miller, K. D., M. Cameron, L. V. Wood, M. C. Dalakas, and J. A. Kovacs. 2000. Lactic acidosis and hepatic steatosis associated with use of stavudine: report of four cases. *Ann. Intern. Med.* **133:**192–196.

Misra, U. K., and J. Kalita. 2007. Comparison of clinical and electrodiagnostic features in B_{12} deficiency neurological syndromes with and without antiparietal cell antibodies. *Postgrad. Med. J.* **83:**124–127.

Mokrzycki, M. H., C. Harris, H. May, J. Laut, and J. Palmisano. 2000. Lactic acidosis associated with stavudine administration: a report of five cases. *Clin. Infect. Dis.* **30:**198–200.

Morgello, S., D. Wolfe, E. Godfrey, R. Feinstein, M. Tagliati, and D. M. Simpson. 1995. Mitochondrial abnormalities in human immunodeficiency virus-associated myopathy. *Acta Neuropathol.* **90:**366–374.

Oksenhendler, E., F. Ferchal, J. Cadranel, H. Sauvageon-Martre, and J. Clauvel. 1990. Zidovudine for HIV-related myelopathy. *Am. J. Med.* **88:**65–66.

Panegyres, P. K., J. M. Papadimitriou, P. N. Hollingsworth, J. A. Armstrong, and B. A. Kakulas. 1990. Vesicular changes in the myopathies of AIDS. Ultrastructural observations and their relationship to zidovudine treatment. *J. Neurol. Neurosurg. Psychiatry* **53:**649–655.

Petito, C. K., D. Vecchio, and Y. T. Chen. 1994. HIV antigen and DNA in AIDS spinal cords correlate with macrophage infiltration but not with vacuolar myelopathy. *J. Neuropathol. Exp. Neurol.* **53:**86–94.

Petito, C. K., B. A. Navia, E. S. Cho, B. D. Jordan, D. C. George, and R. W. Price. 1985. Vacuolar myelopathy pathologically resembling subacute combined degeneration in patients with the acquired immunodeficiency syndrome. *N. Engl. J. Med.* **312:**874–879.

Pierelli, F., C. Garrubba, G. Tilia, L. Parisi, F. Fattapposta, G. Pozzessere, G. Soldati, P. Stanzione, G. D'Offizi, and I. Mezzaroma. 1996. Multimodal evoked potentials in HIV-1-seropositive patients: relationship between the immune impairment and the neurophysiological function. *Acta Neurol. Scand.* **93:**266–271.

Rosenblum, M., A. C. Scheck, K. Cronin, B. J. Brew, A. Khan, M. Paul, and R. W. Price. 1989. Dissociation of AIDS-related vacuolar myelopathy and productive HIV-1 infection of the spinal cord. *Neurology* **39:**892–896.

Seidman, R., N. Peress, and G. Nuovo. 1994. In situ detection of polymerase chain reaction-amplified HIV-1 nucleic acids in skeletal muscle in patients with myopathy. *Mod. Pathol.* **7:**369–375.

Simpson, D. M., P. Slasor, U. Dafni, J. Berger, M. A. Fischl, and C. Hall. 1997. Analysis of myopathy in a placebo-controlled zidovudine trial. *Muscle Nerve* **20:**382–385.

Simpson, D., and M. Tagliati. 1994. Neurological manifestations of HIV infection. *Ann. Intern. Med.* **121:**769–785.

Simpson, D. M., K. A. Citak, E. Godfrey, J. Godbold, and D. E. Wolfe. 1993. Myopathies associated with human immunodeficiency virus and zidovudine: can their effects be distinguished? *Neurology* **43:**971–976.

Simpson, D. M., and A. N. Bender. 1988. Human immunodeficiency virus-associated myopathy: analysis of 11 patients. *Ann. Neurol.* **24:**79–84.

Snider, W., D. M. Simpson, S. Nielsen, C. Metroka, and J. Posner. 1983. Neurological complications of acquired immunodeficiency syndrome: analysis of 50 patients. *Ann. Neurol.* **14:**403–418.

Staudinger, R., and K. Henry. 2000. Remission of HIV myelopathy after highly active antiretroviral therapy. *Neurology* **54:**267–268.

Surtees, R., K. Hyland, and I. Smith. 1990. Central nervous system methyl group metabolism in children with neurological complications of HIV infection. *Lancet* **335:**619–621.

Tagliati, M., A. Di Rocco, F. Danisi, and D. Simpson. 2000. The role of somatosensory evoked potentials in the diagnosis of AIDS-associated myelopathy. *Neurology* **54:**1477–1482.

Tan, S., R. Guiloff, and F. Scaravilli. 1995. AIDS-associated vacuolar myelopathy. A morphometric study. *Brain* **118:**1247–1261.

Tan, S. V., and R. J. Guiloff. 1998. Hypothesis on the pathogenesis of vacuolar myelopathy, dementia, and peripheral neuropathy in AIDS. *J. Neurol. Neurosurg. Psychiatry* **65:**23–28.

Till, M., and K. MacDonnell. 1991. Myopathy with human immunodeficiency virus type 1 (HIV-1) infection: HIV-1 or zidovudine. *Ann. Intern. Med.* **113:**492–494.

Wendel, K., and J. McArthur. 2003. Acute meningoencephalitis in chronic human immunodeficiency virus (HIV) infection: putative central nervous system escape of HIV replication. *Clin. Infect. Dis.* **37:**1107–1111.

Yarchoan, R., P. Brouwers, A. R. Spitzer, J. Grafman, B. Safai, C. F. Perno, S. M. Larson, G. Berg, M. A. Fischl, A. Wichman, R. V. Thomas, A. Brunetti, P. J. Schmidt, C. E. Myers, and S. Broder. 1987. Response of immunodeficiency virus-associated neurological disease to 3′-azido-3′ deoxythymidine. *Lancet* **329:**132–135.

The Spectrum of Neuro-AIDS Disorders:
Pathophysiology, Diagnosis, and Treatment
Edited by K. Goodkin et al.
©2008 ASM Press, Washington, DC

5

Investigation and Presentation of Autonomic Neuropathies in HIV Infection

ROY FREEMAN AND RACHEL NARDIN

The autonomic nervous system is a complex and widespread neuronal network with multiple functions. It is responsible for controlling homeostatic physiological functions, such as blood pressure, heart rate, and body temperature and is involved in behavioral arousal and emotion. Along with the endocrine system, it regulates the internal bodily milieu and biological rhythms. The autonomic nervous system consists of sympathetic and parasympathetic divisions, both of which have central and peripheral components.

The central autonomic network is composed principally of the insular cortex, anterior cingulate gyrus, ventromedial prefrontal cortex, amygdala, periaqueductal gray matter, hypothalamus, parabrachial nucleus of the pons, nucleus of the tractus solitarius, and ventrolateral medulla. All these regions communicate reciprocally and project to preganglionic autonomic neurons in the spinal cord. The peripheral sympathetic nervous system consists of preganglionic cholinergic neurons with cell bodies in the intermediolateral cell column of the spinal cord from T1 to L2. Most preganglionic sympathetic neurons run with the spinal nerves to the paravertebral sympathetic chain, where they synapse on postganglionic neurons that project to the pupil, face, trunk, limbs, and viscera. Some preganglionic neurons project to prevertebral (autonomic plexus) ganglia that project to the abdominal and pelvic viscera. The sympathetic postganglionic neurotransmitter is norepinephrine in all tissues, except for the sweat glands, which have sympathetic cholinergic innervation. The peripheral parasympathetic nervous system consists of preganglionic neurons with cell bodies in brainstem or sacral spinal cord nuclei, synapsing in ganglia very near their target organs. The parasympathetic neurotransmitter is acetylcholine.

Human immunodeficiency virus (HIV), the causative agent of AIDS, involves the nervous system at every level of the neuraxis, both directly and secondarily to opportunistic infections and neoplasm (McArthur, 1987; Bredesen et al., 1988; Levy et al., 1985). Neurological disease may manifest at any stage of infection, from seroconversion to established AIDS.

It is thus not surprising that the autonomic nervous system is involved in HIV infection. Lin-Greenberg and Taneja-Uppal first drew attention to the association of HIV infection with autonomic dysfunction with their description of a patient with AIDS who had orthostatic hypotension, impotence, and anhidrosis (Lin-Greenberger and Taneja-Uppal, 1987).

Since then, our understanding of the spectrum and nature of autonomic dysfunction in HIV infection has expanded. Autonomic dysfunction appears to be common in HIV-infected individuals, with as many as 76 to 84% of HIV-infected individuals having at least one abnormality on a battery of autonomic tests (Welby et al., 1991; Rogstad et al., 1999).

CLINICAL PRESENTATION

The manifestations of autonomic dysfunction in HIV-infected patients appear to be similar to those in non-HIV-infected patients with autonomic dysfunction. Common symptoms of dysautonomia include orthostatic hypotension, syncope and presyncope, proximal body hyperhidrosis, diminished sweating, diarrhea, bladder dysfunction, and impotence (Craddock et al., 1987; Cornblath et al., 1987; Lin-Greenberger and Taneja-Uppal, 1987; Mulhall and Jennens, 1987; Evenhouse et al., 1987; Rüttimann et al., 1991).

Orthostatic Hypotension

Orthostatic hypotension is defined by a fall in systolic blood pressure of 20 mm Hg or in diastolic blood pressure of 10 mm Hg after standing, resulting in symptoms (Schatz et al., 1996). Mild orthostatic hypotension manifests as occasional postural lightheadedness provoked by sudden standing, a hot environment, or a large meal. Associated symptoms include visual dimming or "tunnel vision," neck pain (caused by ischemia of neck muscles), and ultimately

Roy Freeman and Rachel Nardin, Dept. of Neurology, Beth Israel Deaconess Medical Center, Harvard Medical School, Boston, MA 02215.

syncope. Supine hypertension is a common accompaniment to orthostatic hypotension.

Autonomic dysfunction predisposing to orthostatic hypotension may be quite common in HIV infection, as several studies have shown impaired ability to maintain blood pressure. Brownley et al. documented a disruption of baroreceptor responsiveness and a reduced ability to sustain a blood pressure response during prolonged challenge in 31 symptomatic HIV-infected men (Brownley et al., 2001). Freeman et al. found an excessive fall in mean arterial pressure on tilt table testing in HIV-infected patients (Freeman et al., 1990). Cohen et al. reported five HIV-infected patients with orthostatic hypotension (Cohen et al., 1991). Four patients had AIDS, and one had early symptomatic HIV infection. There was no concurrent infection, severe vomiting, or diarrhea. The patients did not have significant tachycardia with postural change, suggesting parasympathetic dysfunction. They noted a variety of neurological signs, including cognitive abnormalities, extrapyramidal dysfunction, reduced coordination, and peripheral neuropathy. Autonomic evaluation of these patients revealed abnormal heart rate variation with deep breathing in four patients and abnormal quantitative sudomotor axon reflex tests in three patients. All patients improved on therapy with fludrocortisone. Four patients remained asymptomatic once fludrocortisone was discontinued, suggesting that at least some cases of orthostatic hypotension may be transient.

Hypotension in HIV-infected individuals may have other causes. Adrenal insufficiency has been reported in a number of patients with HIV infection and can result in hypotension, often associated with weakness, weight loss, mucocutaneous pigmentation, and hyponatremia (Membreno et al., 1987; Klein et al., 1983). Characteristically, these patients have low plasma cortisol levels with a blunted plasma cortisol response to adrenocorticotropin stimulation, although some patients were reported to have high plasma cortisol values (Membreno et al., 1987; Klein et al., 1983). These high cortisol values have been interpreted as a stress response to illness (Parker et al., 1985), ectopic production of adrenal-cortex-stimulating factors by lymphocytes or monocytes (Whitcomb et al., 1988), or peripheral resistance to glucocorticoids (Norbiato et al., 1992). Dehydration and medications may also play contributing roles.

Hemodynamic Lability

Luginbuhl et al. drew attention to the presence of episodic hypotension in 20%, and episodic hypertension in 19%, of their cohort of HIV-infected children (Luginbuhl et al., 1993). Eleven percent of the patients had episodes of both hypotension and hypertension. Other reports have also documented episodic hypotension, particularly in association with medication administration (Helmick and Green, 1985; Loke et al., 1990; Kelly et al., 1992).

Cardiac Dysfunction

Heart rate and rhythm abnormalities, including resting tachycardia (64%), sinus bradycardia (11%), marked sinus arrhythmia (17%), ventricular tachycardia, and torsades de pointes, have been observed in HIV infection (Luginbuhl et al., 1993). Ventricular tachycardia and torsades de pointes have often been associated with administration of medications (Cohen et al., 1990; Stein et al., 1990; Wharton et al., 1987; Cortese et al., 1992; Eisenhauer et al., 1994). Several medications used frequently in HIV infection can prolong the QT period, including antiretroviral agents, fluconazole, some antibiotics, and methadone; an underlying cardiac autonomic dysfunction may make HIV-infected individuals particularly susceptible to the arrhythmogenic effects of these medications. Palaic et al. reported two patients with AIDS who developed acute pulmonary edema following intravenous fluid administration without evidence for significant left-ventricular dysfunction or flow-limiting coronary lesions or for cardiac uptake of iodine-123 metaiodobenzylguanidine, suggesting a cardiac sympathetic neuropathy (Palaic et al., 1993). The prevalence of cardiovascular autonomic neuropathy has been estimated at 15% in one study of 61 consecutive HIV-infected patients (Gluck et al., 2000) and may be significantly higher in children infected with HIV (Plein et al., 1999). One study of cardiomegaly, seen postmortem in over half of HIV-infected children, showed that postmortem cardiomegaly was associated with increased heart rate, but not hematocrit, HIV viral load, degree of immune suppression, encephalopathy, or myocardial pathology, suggesting that autonomic dysregulation may be pathogenically significant (Kearney et al., 2003a, 2003b).

Gastrointestinal Dysfunction

The gastrointestinal complaints of patients with autonomic dysfunction include nausea, vomiting, early satiety due to gastroparesis, constipation, diarrhea, and incontinence. HIV-infected patients frequently report bowel dysfunction, with diarrhea a particularly troublesome symptom (Ali et al., 1994). Many HIV-infected patients, especially those with more advanced infection, have multiple contributors to gastrointestinal dysfunction, including opportunistic infections and medications; nonetheless, there is supportive evidence that autonomic dysfunction may play a role, as well. Griffin et al. suggested that autonomic denervation of the jejunum might be responsible for noninfectious diarrhea in some patients. They documented structural abnormalities of the axons and Schwann cells of the autonomic nerves of the jejunal mucosa using transmission electron microscopy (Griffin et al., 1988). Batman et al. used the neuron-specific polyclonal antibody PGP 9.5 to quantify the depletion of autonomic axons in the villi and lamina propria of the jejunum. These histological abnormalities were present at all stages of HIV infection, including in asymptomatic patients (Batman et al., 1991). Abnormalities of the rectal autonomic nerves have also been documented on rectal biopsy (Blanshard et al., 1993). Increased gut parasympathetic nervous system activity may be an alternate mechanism for nonpathogen diarrhea (Coker et al., 1992). Although delayed solid gastric emptying, measured by scintigraphy, has been shown in HIV-infected individuals, it did not correlate well with symptoms or autonomic dysfunction, measured by spectral analysis of heart rate variability; this underscores the likelihood of multiple etiologies for many gastrointestinal complaints in HIV-infected patients (Neild et al., 2000).

Genitourinary Dysfunction

The effects of autonomic dysfunction on the bladder are complex. Central autonomic dysfunction usually causes detrusor hyperreflexia, resulting in urinary frequency, urgency, nocturia, and incontinence. Peripheral autonomic dysfunction usually causes detrusor muscle areflexia, resulting in difficulty initiating urination, urinary retention, and overflow incontinence. Impotence, decreased libido, ejaculatory dysfunction, and failure to reach orgasm are all symptoms of autonomic dysfunction. Erectile and bladder dysfunctions are frequent complaints in HIV-infected individuals (Ali et al., 1994).

Erectile dysfunction occurs more frequently in HIV-infected patients than in age- and sex-matched controls and is associated with autonomic dysfunction (Rogstad et al., 1999). Incontinence of the bladder (as well as the bowel) is characteristically a late symptom of AIDS. The incontinence is typically associated with a severe neuropathy, myelopathy, or polyradiculopathy and may be exacerbated by an accompanying dementia; the contribution of autonomic dysfunction is thus difficult to evaluate specifically.

TESTS OF AUTONOMIC FUNCTION

Autonomic testing is used both to confirm that autonomic dysfunction is present and to delineate the anatomical and physiological distribution of the deficit (e.g., parasympathetic versus sympathetic and pre- versus postganglionic). Table 1 lists the major categories of autonomic tests available. Below, we review the ways in which these tests have been used to evaluate autonomic dysfunction in HIV infection.

Autonomic testing of HIV-infected patients has been the subject of several reports and case studies (Cohen and Laudenslager, 1989; Cohen et al., 1991; Correia et al., 2006; Craddock et al., 1987; Evenhouse et al., 1987; Lin-Greenberger and Taneja-Uppal, 1987; Mulhall and Jennens, 1987; Villa et al., 1987, 1990). In a controlled study, Freeman et al. demonstrated significant differences in autonomic function between controls and HIV-infected patients using multiple tests of the autonomic nervous system. A steady decline in autonomic function was noted across diagnostic groups (controls, early symptomatic HIV infection, and AIDS), with the most severe autonomic dysfunction found in the patients with AIDS. The abnormalities in autonomic function correlated with signs of HIV-associated nervous system disease. The three patients with the most severe autonomic dysfunction all had evidence of dementia (see chapter 1), myelopathy (see chapter 4), and distal sensory polyneuropathy (see chapter 6) (Freeman et al., 1990).

The autonomic abnormalities were most prominent in tests of heart rate variation. These tests, which principally assess vagus nerve function, include the expiratory/inspiratory ratio, the standard deviation of heart rate, the heart rate means square successive difference, and the maximum-

minimum heart rate difference on deep respiration. There was a significant difference between the resting heart rate in patients with AIDS and that in control subjects. A resting tachycardia is also commonly observed in diabetic patients with a vagal neuropathy and most likely represents unopposed cardiac sympathetic activity (Freeman, 1997). A similar mechanism may exist in HIV-infected patients. No patient had clinical or laboratory evidence of dehydration or cardiac failure as a cause for the increased resting heart rate. There was also poor correlation between the resting heart rate and the orthostatic fall in blood pressure; this would not be expected if hemodynamic factors were solely responsible for the resting tachycardia. However, the possibility that myocardial dysfunction or myocarditis due to HIV infection might be partially responsible for this resting tachycardia (Anderson et al., 1988; Cohen et al., 1986; Lipshultz et al., 1989) could not be entirely excluded. Comparison of the heart rate response to postural change (30/15 ratio) and the Valsalva ratio between controls and AIDS patients also revealed a trend toward declining autonomic function in the AIDS patients.

Of the tests assessing sympathetic nervous system function, the blood pressure response to isometric exercise and the fall in mean arterial pressure on tilt table testing revealed a statistically significant difference in findings among the study groups. In addition, one patient with AIDS was taking fludrocortisone for the treatment of symptomatic orthostatic hypotension and three patients with early symptomatic HIV infection exhibited pathological falls (greater than 20 mm Hg) in systolic blood pressure in response to standing or passive tilting. None of the controls showed comparable declines in blood pressure. Intergroup comparisons showed that these differences were largely a result of significantly more abnormal test results in the AIDS subgroup. A trend toward declining autonomic function was noted in AIDS patients compared with controls in the systolic blood pressure fall on standing, the systolic blood pressure fall on passive tilting, and the blood pressure response to a cold stimulus.

These test results have been replicated in a number of studies of similar design (Villa et al., 1990, 1992; Rüttimann et al., 1991; Sakhuja et al., 2007; Welby et al., 1991). The HIV-seropositive subjects studied have included homosexual males and drug users. Homosexuals and drug users who were not HIV-seropositive have served as controls in some studies (Rüttimann et al., 1991; Villa et al., 1992). Autonomic test abnormalities were demonstrated in 5.6 to 33.3% of HIV-negative intravenous drug abusers (Villa et al., 1992; Rüttimann et al., 1991).

Spectral analysis has also been used to assess heart rate variability in HIV-infected patients. Two studies have demonstrated that components of heart rate variability, as measured by spectral analysis, are abnormal in subjects with AIDS and no clinical evidence of heart disease (Correia et al., 2006; Neild et al., 2000). A cross-sectional, prospective, longitudinal cohort study of heart rate variability using power spectral analysis showed no differences between asymptomatic HIV-infected individuals and healthy age- and sex-matched controls but significant abnormalities in AIDS patients compared with controls. Measures of heart rate variability worsened progressively with advancing CDC clinical disease stage (Becker et al., 1997). However, a more recent spectral-analysis study of 21 individuals in the early stages of HIV infection showed significantly reduced heart rate variability compared to 18 healthy controls. These subjects had a mean $CD4^+$ count of $426 \pm 166/mm^3$, without clinical

TABLE 1 Tests of autonomic function

Cardiac parasympathetic function
    Heart rate variability at rest or with deep breathing
    High frequency heart rate spectral power
    Heart rate response to Valsalva maneuver
    Heart rate response to postural change
Cardiovascular sympathetic adrenergic function
    Blood pressure response to standing or upright tilt
    Blood pressure response to Valsalva maneuver
    Blood pressure response to isometric exercise or mental stress
    Cold pressor test
    Low frequency heart rate spectral power
Sympathetic cholinergic function
    Thermoregulatory sweat test
    Quantitative sudomotor axon reflex test
    Skin potentials
    Sweat imprint

evidence of autonomic or cardiac dysfunction; echocardiography in these subjects was normal (Mittal et al., 2004).

Villa et al. demonstrated that the corrected QT interval was significantly prolonged in a cohort of HIV-seropositive subjects with autonomic neuropathy (Villa et al., 1995). The corrected QT interval was greater than or equal to 440 ms in 24 out of 37 patients (64.8%) with autonomic neuropathy but only 5 of 20 (25%) HIV-seropositive patients without autonomic neuropathy. There were no clinical signs of cardiac disease in any of these patients, although echocardiographic studies were not performed. Others have observed a prolonged QT interval associated with pentamidine administration (Stein et al., 1991). These observations may underlie the predisposition of HIV-infected patients to cardiac arrhythmias, such as ventricular tachycardia and torsades de pointes (often in association with medication administration), and the observed incidence of unexpected cardiorespiratory arrest (Craddock et al., 1987; Stein et al., 1990; Wharton et al., 1987; Cohen et al., 1990; Luginbuhl et al., 1993; Eisenhauer et al., 1994).

The pupil cycle time provides a noncardiac measure of parasympathetic nervous system function. Maclean and Dhillon reported significant differences in the pupil cycle times between HIV-seropositive patients and controls (Maclean and Dhillon, 1993). The average pupil cycle time in the HIV-seropositive group was 1,370 ms compared to 840 ms in the controls. Approximately half of the AIDS patients developed irregular, jerky pupillary movements or hippus after about 10 pupil cycles. Although patients with cytomegalovirus- and HIV-associated retinopathy were excluded from the study, the authors acknowledged that subclinical optic neuropathy may have influenced their test results. In an earlier uncontrolled report, Scott et al. had noted normal pupil cycle times in 15 of 16 HIV-seropositive subjects in the early stages of infection (Scott et al., 1990). The maximal pupillary area was also shown to be abnormal in 66% of a group of 61 HIV-infected patients (Gluck et al., 2000).

NATURAL HISTORY

Although autonomic dysfunction appears to occur more frequently and with greater severity in AIDS patients, the evidence suggests that asymptomatic HIV-infected patients exhibit evidence of dysautonomia (Mulhall and Jennens, 1987; Villa et al., 1987, 1990, 1992; Rüttimann et al., 1991).

Autonomic dysfunction appears to constitute a continuum across the stages of HIV infection (Freeman et al., 1990; Gastaut et al., 1992; Villa et al., 1992; Rüttimann et al., 1991).

This parallels the data on the natural history of HIV-associated peripheral neuropathy affecting somatic nerves, where subclinical electrophysiologic abnormalities of peripheral nerve function are found to correlate with falling CD4$^+$ counts and where the prevalence of symptomatic peripheral neuropathy increases as the degree of immunocompromise progresses (Ronchi et al., 1992; Brew, 2003; Simpson, 2002). Thus, in most studies, worsening autonomic function appears to correlate with lower CD4$^+$ cell counts (Gluck et al., 2000; Rogstad et al., 1999; Schifitto et al., 2000; Welby et al., 1991). An exception is the prospective study of Scott et al.; however, the fact that the mean CD4$^+$ cell count in their cohort of asymptomatic patients was fairly high at 512 cells/mm^3 when first evaluated and 314 cells/mm^3 at follow-up may have masked the association (Scott et al., 1990).

Although, in general, the severity of autonomic dysfunction correlates with advancing HIV infection, the progression in individual patients is less clear and appears slow. For example, a prospective longitudinal cohort study of heart rate variability using power spectral analysis showed that although measures of heart rate variability worsened progressively with advancing CDC clinical disease stage, follow-up testing after 6 to 16 months did not reveal significant deterioration in measures of heart rate variability in HIV-infected individuals with or without AIDS (Becker et al., 1997). A small longitudinal study of 12 patients with asymptomatic HIV infection who underwent repeated autonomic testing over the course of 9 to 18 months confirmed this, with no patient showing a significant deterioration in autonomic function (Scott et al., 1990). Progression may not invariably be slow, however. In a longitudinal study of 17 patients with more advanced HIV infection, progression of autonomic test abnormalities occurred in 9 patients retested after an average of 11.2 months (Villa et al., 1992). In this period, only two of the patients changed their CDC clinical disease stages.

The progression of autonomic dysfunction may not always be strictly linear. Freeman et al. noted that patients with early symptomatic HIV infection were a heterogeneous group, and several results exhibited a bimodal distribution with a large variance (Freeman et al., 1990). On one hand, some tests of parasympathetic nervous system function (the expiratory/inspiratory ratio, the standard deviation of heart rate, and the means square successive difference) showed a significant difference between the various stages of disease (from controls to early symptomatic HIV infection to AIDS), and there was a trend of declining autonomic function going from the controls to early symptomatic HIV infection to AIDS in the maximum-minimum heart rate difference on deep respiration. On the other hand, several patients in the early symptomatic HIV infection group showed exaggerated normal responses to autonomic testing. These findings in patients with early symptomatic HIV infection are consistent with the demonstration by others that tachycardia, marked heart rate variability, and cardiac arrest are associated with early symptomatic HIV infection (Luginbuhl et al., 1993). The transient appearance of hyperactive autonomic function may occur for a limited period over weeks to months in patients with autonomic nervous system degeneration, probably secondary to denervation supersensitivity. The exaggerated normal response observed in the early stages of HIV infection may reflect this phenomenon.

The effect of highly active antiretroviral therapy (HAART) on the autonomic dysfunction seen in HIV-infected patients is unknown, but there are some encouraging data suggesting that HAART may be protective for the autonomic dysfunction seen in HIV-infected patients not receiving HAART (Correia et al., 2006).

Also of interest is the effect of autonomic dysfunction on the natural history of HIV infection itself. There is increasing evidence that autonomic dysregulation may be an important mechanism by which HIV modulates host immunity to promote its own survival. Cole et al. (2001) have demonstrated that HIV-infected individuals who exhibited constitutively high levels of autonomic activity showed significantly poorer suppression of the viral load and poorer CD4$^+$ cell recovery in response to HAART than subjects with low autonomic activity; however, the measures of autonomic activity were nonstandard and encompassed both sympathetic and parasympathetic functions, raising questions about the conclusions. Using similar nonstandard methodology, these investigators have also suggested that autonomic dysfunction may mediate the known association between socially inhibited temperament and viral pathology.

Cole et al. (2003) studied 54 homosexual men with asymptomatic HIV infection. Following baseline psychological and autonomic assessments, their plasma viral loads and CD4$^+$ T-cell levels were monitored for 12 to 18 months. Plasma viral loads were elevated in socially inhibited individuals, who also showed poorer response to initiation of HAART. Autonomic activity was increased in socially inhibited individuals, and this accounted for a majority of the variance between social inhibition and virologic parameters. Yun et al. (2004a, 2004b) have hypothesized that a shift in the autonomic balance in favor of sympathetic drive by HIV could favor Th2 dominance, an immune state associated with HIV disease progression. These notions remain hypothetical, and further research exploring this concept is warranted.

HIV-associated lipodystrophy may also be mediated by changes in the autonomic nervous system. Chow et al. found decreased heart rate variability in 12 HIV-infected patients with lipodystrophy compared to 20 HIV-infected patients without lipodystrophy and 26 healthy controls. Frequency domain analysis showed a decreased high-frequency power and increased low- to high-frequency power ratio in the lipodystrophy group compared to both of the other groups during rest and to the HIV-infected patients without lipodystrophy during tilt (Chow et al., 2006). Interstitial noradrenaline concentrations have also been found to be increased in the skeletal muscle and subcutaneous adipose tissue of patients with lipodystrophy, consistent with locally increased sympathetic activity. This could promote localized lipolysis in subcutaneous adipose tissue and contribute to the development of lipodystrophy (van Gurp et al., 2006).

PATHOGENESIS

The underlying neuroanatomical cause of the dysautonomia accompanying HIV infection is not established. HIV-1 can involve both the central and peripheral nervous system, and HIV-infected patients are prone to central and peripheral nervous system complications at multiple sites. Autonomic dysfunction can result from impairment of central and/or peripheral autonomic structures. Therefore, in a given patient, there may be more than one cause of dysautonomia. In addition, toxins, medications, vitamin deficiency, and malnutrition may play roles in causing autonomic dysfunction in HIV-infected patients.

The appearance of autonomic dysfunction prior to AIDS implicates HIV or a virus-host interaction in the causation of the dysautonomia. Products of immune activation, such as cytokines and lipid membrane derivatives, have been implicated in the pathogenesis of nervous system damage in HIV infection. A composite measure of autonomic performance (the AZ score) has been shown to be inversely correlated with higher serum β_2-microglobulin and interleukin-4 levels, suggesting that HIV-associated autonomic neuropathy may be due to immune mechanisms (Schifitto et al., 2000).

However, the autonomic nervous system may also be involved as part of a more widespread nervous system dysfunction caused by most of the neurological complications of HIV infection. In the study by Freeman et al., abnormalities revealed by autonomic testing correlated with the presence of neurological signs (Freeman et al., 1990). Although there was no correlation between any specific neurological sign and autonomic abnormalities, the correlation suggests that advancing neurological disease increases the likelihood that the autonomic nervous system will be involved at some level, giving rise to autonomic dysfunction. The

TABLE 2 HIV and the nervous system

Cerebrum
  AIDS dementia complex
  Opportunistic infections
    Viruses
      Cytomegalovirus
      Papovavirus
      Herpes simplex virus I and II
      Adenovirus
      Varicella-zoster virus
    Protozoa
      T. gondii
    Fungi and yeasts
      Cryptococcus neoformans
      Candida albicans
      Aspergillus
      Coccidiomycosis
      Histoplasmosis
    Bacteria
      Mycobacterium tuberculosis var. *hominis*
      Mycobacterium avium-Mycobacterium intracellulare
      Nocardia
  Opportunistic neoplasms
    Primary central nervous system lymphoma
    Metastatic lymphoma
    Metastatic Kaposi's sarcoma
Spinal cord and cauda equina
  Vacuolar myelopathy
  Cytomegalovirus myelitis
  Varicella-zoster virus myelitis
  Herpes simplex I and II myelitis
  Neurosyphilis
  T. gondii
Peripheral nerve
  Distal sensory polyneuropathy
  Acute inflammatory demyelinating polyradiculoneuropathy (AIDP)
  Chronic inflammatory demyelinating polyradiculoneuropathy (CIDP)
  Mononeuritis multiplex

three patients with the most severe autonomic dysfunction all had evidence of dementia, myelopathy, and distal sensory polyneuropathy. The anatomical regions and neurological syndromes discussed below are those most likely to be responsible for autonomic dysfunction in HIV-infected patients (Table 2).

THE NEUROPATHOLOGICAL BASIS OF AUTONOMIC DYSFUNCTION

Cerebrum

HIV-associated dementia is characterized by psychomotor slowing, poor attention, apathy, memory loss, and, less frequently, mania and psychosis. Motor abnormalities that accompany the dementia include pyramidal and extrapyramidal tract dysfunction, tremor, ataxia, incoordination, and frontal-release signs (Navia et al., 1986). The coexistence of these motor system disorders with autonomic dysfunction may rarely result in this disorder being confused with multiple-system atrophy (Miller and Semple, 1987). The anatomical territories involved in this process include the subcortical cerebral regions, such as the basal ganglia, subcortical white matter, thalamus, and other deep brain nuclei. Dysfunction of these structures could constitute a central neuroanatomical basis for the dysautonomia.

The central nervous system may also be affected by opportunistic infections and neoplasms. The clinical manifestations of these disorders will thus depend on the specific sites of involvement. Although these disorders have no predilection for central autonomic structures, the autonomic nervous system may, nevertheless, be involved with these diseases.

Hypothalamus

Purba et al., using immunocytochemical methods to analyze vasopressin and oxytocin neurons in the paraventricular nucleus of the hypothalamus, noted that the number of oxytocin-expressing neurons was 40% lower in AIDS patients than in the controls (Purba et al., 1993). There was no difference between the two groups in the number of vasopressin-expressing neurons in the paraventricular nucleus. Based on animal studies showing that central vasopressin and oxytocin play roles in the expression of autonomic functions, such as eating, cardiovascular regulation, nociception, and thermoregulation, the authors hypothesized that the selective changes in the oxytocin neurons of the paraventricular nucleus may contribute to neuroendocrine and autonomic dysfunction in AIDS.

Spinal Cord and Cauda Equina

HIV-associated vacuolar myelopathy presents as a spastic paraparesis of the lower extremities, although the ankles are often less severely affected than the knees because of a concurrent peripheral neuropathy. Pathologic examination reveals vacuolation of the myelin sheath caused by the enlargement of the periaxonal spaces and splitting of the myelin lamellae due to intramyelinic edema. This process predominantly involves the posterior and lateral columns of the middle and lower thoracic spinal cord. Intravacuolar macrophages that may contain HIV-1 are present in the involved areas (Petito et al., 1985; Tan et al., 1995; Dal Pan et al., 1994).

Symptoms of bladder and bowel dysfunction, including urinary retention and loss of sphincter control causing urinary and fecal incontinence, also occur as a feature of a lumbosacral polyradiculopathy in AIDS patients. The bladder and bowel symptoms are accompanied by progressive, flaccid, areflexic, lower-extremity weakness and paralysis, with pain, paresthesias, and numbness of the legs and perineum. Most cases are due to infection by cytomegalovirus, which can be cultured from the cerebrospinal fluid (CSF). The characteristic CSF profile consists of a mixed pleocytosis with prominent polymorphonuclear leukocytes, hypoglycorhachia, and elevated protein; PCR testing for cytomegalovirus DNA in CSF provides the most rapid diagnosis. Cytomegalovirus inclusions are noted at neuropathological examination of the lumbosacral nerve roots and lower spinal cord (Eidelberg et al., 1986; McArthur, 1987). Therapy with intravenous ganciclovir, foscarnet, or both may result in improvement of this disorder (Miller et al., 1990; So and Olney, 1994; Cohen et al., 1993).

A similar clinical picture may occur with other opportunistic infections of the lumbosacral nerve roots and spinal cord, such as *Toxoplasma gondii* infection (Overhage et al., 1990; Kayser et al., 1990), herpes simplex virus type 2 infection (Wiley et al., 1987), neurosyphilis (Lanska et al., 1988;

Berger, 1992), and leptomeningeal spread of systemic lymphoma (Klein et al., 1990).

Peripheral Neuropathy

The peripheral nervous system is involved in up to 80% of patients with AIDS, with 95% involvement noted postmortem (de la Monte et al., 1988). The most common syndrome is a distal sensory polyneuropathy. Symptoms of this neuropathy include numbness, burning, paresthesias, contact hypersensitivity, and walking difficulties. Although it may present at any stage of HIV infection, the distal sensory polyneuropathy is relatively uncommon early in the course of HIV disease and becomes more prevalent in immunologically compromised HIV-infected persons (Barohn et al., 1993; Leger et al., 1989). The pathological changes include loss of myelinated and unmyelinated fibers and a mononuclear inflammatory infiltrate (de la Monte et al., 1988; Fuller and Jacobs, 1990; Leger et al., 1989; Mah et al., 1988). Pathological examination of the sympathetic and sensory ganglia has revealed a mild ganglionitis consisting of macrophages, T lymphocytes, and an increase in the amount of major histocompatibility complex class II antigen expression. In addition, HIV p24 core protein antigen and HIV gp41 envelope protein antigen were found within macrophages in the ganglia of HIV-infected subjects; these findings were present in HIV-seropositive cases pre-AIDS but were more prominent in cases with clinical AIDS (Esiri et al., 1993).

The prominence of neuropathic pain accompanying this neuropathy is similar to that seen in patients with diabetic neuropathy, a disorder in which pain and autonomic dysfunction may be associated with loss of small myelinated and unmyelinated fibers. Extensive loss of unmyelinated fibers has been described in HIV-infected patients who died shortly after the onset of neuropathic pain. Findings from such morphometric studies suggest that the distal sensory polyneuropathy of AIDS may be a potential cause of autonomic dysfunction.

HIV-infected patients may also develop acute acquired inflammatory demyelinating polyradiculoneuropathy (or the Guillain-Barré syndrome), usually at the time of seroconversion or in asymptomatic HIV infection. HIV-infected patients who have an acute inflammatory demyelinating polyradiculoneuropathy are clinically indistinguishable from non-HIV-infected patients, and therefore, the well-described autonomic symptoms associated with the acute inflammatory demyelinating polyradiculoneuropathy are also likely to exist in HIV-infected patients (Freeman et al., 1990). The laboratory hallmark of acute acquired inflammatory demyelinating polyradiculoneuropathy is an elevated CSF protein; HIV-infected patients usually show spinal fluid pleocytosis as well, with a mean cell count of 25 leukocytes/mm^3 (Cornblath et al., 1987).

Chronic inflammatory demyelinating polyradiculoneuropathy and mononeuritis multiplex, two other neuropathic accompaniments of HIV infection, are not likely to cause autonomic dysfunction (Parry, 1988).

Medications

Several medications commonly used to treat AIDS-related complications have recognized neurological side effects, and new therapies may have unknown neurotoxic effects (Simpson and Tagliati, 1995). Thus, treatment using these agents may produce the symptoms of autonomic dysfunction or may be responsible for some of the abnormalities in autonomic testing. Vincristine, a component of the drug regimen prescribed for Kaposi's sarcoma, is associated with orthostatic hypotension. In a prospective study, however, only 1 of 26 patients treated with vincristine suffered from orthostatic hypotension (Carmichael et al., 1970; DiBella, 1980). Pentamidine (Helmick and Green, 1985; Siddiqui and Ford, 1995), zidovudine (Loke et al., 1990), and trimethoprim-sulfamethoxazole (Kelly et al., 1992) have also been associated with orthostatic hypotension.

Although the antiretroviral nucleoside analogues 2′3′-dideoxyinosine (didanosine) (Cooley et al., 1990; Lambert et al., 1990), 2′3′-dideoxycytidine (zalcitabine) (Dubinsky et al., 1989; Berger et al., 1993), and 2′3′-dihydro 3′-deoxythymidine (stavudine) (Skowron, 1995; Sommadossi, 1995; Simpson, 2002) are associated with peripheral neuropathy, they are not correlated with pupillary or cardiovascular autonomic neuropathy (Gluck et al., 2000). Dapsone and isoniazid are other recognized neurotoxic agents that are used to treat opportunistic infections in HIV-seropositive patients. In the study by Freeman et al., there was no correlation between the use of any therapeutic agent and autonomic dysfunction; however, the relatively small number of subjects may have limited the predictive ability of that study (Freeman et al., 1990).

TREATMENT

There is no prospective study of the effect of treatment on autonomic function. There is at present only anecdotal evidence that treatment with zidovudine results in improved autonomic function (Scott et al., 1990; Confalonieri and Villa, 1993). Preliminary data suggest that HAART may be protective for the autonomic dysfunction seen in AIDS patients not receiving HAART (Correia et al., 2006). Treatment, however, is largely focused on symptomatic management.

Orthostatic symptoms typically respond to standard therapies, such as fludrocortisone, sympathomimetic agents, and other pressors, although the patients in the above-mentioned series responded to fludrocortisone alone. Because autonomic dysfunction is often accompanied by a painful peripheral neuropathy and symptoms of motor dysfunction, supportive stockings are poorly tolerated. Orthostatic hypotension frequently occurs when a tricyclic antidepressant is introduced as therapy for a painful neuropathy or depression. Nortriptyline and desipramine are tricyclic agents with a relatively low incidence of postural hypotension, and their use may minimize this problem (Roose et al., 1981). If orthostatic symptoms persist, the addition of fludrocortisone or a pressor agent, such as midodrine, is usually sufficient to control them.

CONCLUSIONS

Autonomic dysfunction is a common and disabling complication of AIDS. This manifestation of HIV infection has been the subject of several controlled studies and case reports. Characteristic features include syncope and presyncope, blood pressure and heart rate lability, cardiac arrhythmias, impotence, bowel dysfunction, bladder dysfunction, incontinence, and anhidrosis. HIV-infected patients are sensitive to the autonomic side effects of antidepressant and antihypertensive agents. To date, there has been no large prospective study of autonomic failure in patients with AIDS. Our knowledge of the prevalence of this disorder, its association with other neurological and nonneurological complications of AIDS, and its relationship to therapeutic interventions using potentially neurotoxic agents is still

limited. The impact of this disorder on the natural history of HIV infection is unknown, but there is some evidence that autonomic dysfunction may predispose individuals to disease progression. These questions represent areas for further study.

REFERENCES

Ali, S., R. Shaikh, and A. Siddiqi. 1994. HIV-1 associated neuropathies in males; impotence and penile electrodiagnosis. *Acta Neurol. Belg.* **94:**194–199.

Anderson, D., R. Virmani, J. Riely, T. O'Leary, R. Cunnion, M. Robinowitz, A. Macher, U. Punja, S. Villafor, J. Parrillo, and W. Roberts. 1988. Prevalent myocarditis at necropsy in the acquired immunodeficiency syndrome. *J. Am. Coll. Cardiol.* **11:**792–799.

Barohn, R., G. Gronseth, B. LeForce, A. McVey, S. McGuire, C. Butzin, and R. King. 1993. Peripheral nervous system involvement in a large cohort of human immunodeficiency virus-infected individuals. *Arch. Neurol.* **50:**167–171. (Erratum, **50:**388.)

Batman, P., A. Miller, P. Sedgwick, and G. Griffin. 1991. Autonomic denervation in jejunal mucosa of homosexual men infected with HIV. *AIDS* **5:**1247–1252.

Becker, K., I. Gorlach, T. Frieling, and D. Haussinger. 1997. Characterization and natural course of cardiac autonomic nervous dysfunction in HIV-infected patients. *AIDS* **11:**751–757.

Berger, A., J. Arezzo, H. Schaumburg, G. Skowron, T. Merigan, S. Bozzette, D. Richman, and W. Soo. 1993. 2′,3′-dideoxycytidine (ddC) toxic neuropathy: a study of 52 patients. *Neurology* **43:**358–362.

Berger, J. 1992. Spinal cord syphilis associated with human immunodeficiency virus infection: a treatable myelopathy. *Am. J. Med.* **92:**101–103.

Blanshard, C., D. Ellis, G. Tovey, and B. Gazzard. 1993. Electron microscopy of rectal biopsies in HIV-positive individuals. *J. Pathol.* **169:**79–87.

Bredesen, D., R. Levy, and M. Rosenblum. 1988. The neurology of human immunodeficiency virus infection. *Q. J. Med.* **68:**665–677.

Brew, B. 2003. The peripheral nerve complications of human immunodeficiency virus (HIV) infection. *Muscle Nerve* **28:**542–552.

Brownley, K., J. Milanovich, S. Motivala, N. Schneiderman, L. Fillion, J. Graves, N. Klimas, M. Fletcher, and B. Hurwitz. 2001. Autonomic and cardiovascular function in HIV spectrum disease: early indications of cardiac pathophysiology. *Clin. Auton. Res.* **11:**319–326.

Carmichael, S., L. Eagleton, C. Ayers, and D. Mohler. 1970. Orthostatic hypotension during vincristine therapy. *Arch. Intern. Med.* **126:**290–293.

Chow, D., R. Wood, A. Grandinetti, C. Shikuma, I. Schatz, and P. Low. 2006 Cardiovagal autonomic dysfunction in relation to HIV-associated lipodystrophy. *HIV Clin. Trials* **7:**16–23.

Cohen, A., B. Weiser, Q. Afzal, and J. Fuhrer. 1990. Ventricular tachycardia in two patients with AIDS receiving ganciclovir (DHPG). *AIDS* **4:**807–809.

Cohen, B., J. McArthur, S. Grohman, B. Patterson, and J. Glass. 1993. Neurologic prognosis of cytomegalovirus polyradiculomyelopathy in AIDS. *Neurology* **43:**493–499.

Cohen, I., D. Anderson, R. Virmani, B. Reen, A. Macher, J. Sennesh, P. DiLorenzo, and R. Redfield. 1986. Congestive cardiomyopathy in association with the acquired immunodeficiency syndrome. *N. Engl. J. Med.* **315:**628–630.

Cohen, J., and M. Laudenslager. 1989. Autonomic nervous system involvement in patients with human immunodeficiency virus infection. *Neurology* **39:**1111–1112.

Cohen, J., L. Miller, and L. Polish. 1991. Orthostatic hypotension in human immunodeficiency virus infection may be the result of generalized autonomic nervous system dysfunction. *J. Acquir. Immune Defic. Syndr.* **4**:31–33.

Coker, R., P. Horner, K. Bleasdale-Barr, J. Harris, and C. Mathias. 1992. Increased gut parasympathetic activity and chronic diarrhoea in a patient with the acquired immunodeficiency syndrome. *Clin. Auton. Res.* **2**:295–298.

Cole, S., M. Kemeny, J. Fahey, J. Zack, and B. Naliboff. 2003. Psychological risk factors for HIV pathogenesis: mediation by the autonomic nervous system. *Biol. Psychiatry* **54**:1444–1456.

Cole, S., B. Naliboff, M. Kemeny, M. Griswold, J. Fahey, and J. Zack. 2001. Impaired response to HAART in HIV-infected individuals with high autonomic nervous system activity. *Proc. Natl. Acad. Sci. USA* **98**:12695–12700.

Confalonieri, F., and A. Villa. 1993. Human immunodeficiency virus-associated autonomic neuropathy, drug addiction, and zidovudine treatment. *Arch. Intern. Med.* **153**:400–401. (Letter.)

Cooley, T., L. Kunches, C. Saunders, J. Ritter, C. Perkins, C. McLaren, R. McCaffrey, and H. Liebman. 1990. Once-daily administration of 2′3′-dideoxyinosine (ddI) in patients with the acquired immunodeficiency syndrome or AIDS-related complex. Results of a phase I trial. *N. Engl. J. Med.* **322**:1340–1345.

Cornblath, D., J. McArthur, P. Kennedy, A. Witte, and J. Griffin. 1987. Inflammatory demyelinating peripheral neuropathies associated with human-cell lymphotropic virus type III infection. *Ann. Neurol.* **21**:32–40.

Correia, D., L. Rodrigues De Resende, R. Molina, B. Ferreira, F. Colombari, C. Barbosa, V. Da Silva, and A. Prata. 2006. Power spectral analysis of heart rate variability in HIV-infected and AIDS patients. *Pacing Clin. Electrophysiol.* **29**:53–58.

Cortese, L., R. Gasser, D. Bjornson, M. Dacey, and C. Oster. 1992. Prolonged recurrence of pentamidine-induced torsades de pointes. *Ann. Pharmacother.* **26**:1365–1369.

Craddock, C., G. Pasvol, R. Bull, A. Protheroe, and J. Hopkin. 1987. Cardiorespiratory arrest and autonomic neuropathy in AIDS. *Lancet* **ii**:16–18.

Dal Pan, G., J. Glass, and J. McArthur. 1994. Clinicopathologic correlations of HIV-1-associated vacuolar myelopathy: an autopsy-based case-control study. *Neurology* **44**:2159–2164.

de la Monte, S., D. Gabuzda, D. Ho, R. Brown, E. Hedley-White, R. Schooley, M. Hirsch, and A. Bhan. 1988. Peripheral neuropathy in the acquired immunodeficiency syndrome. *Ann. Neurol.* **23**:485–492.

DiBella, N. 1980. Vincristine-induced orthostatic hypotension: a prospective clinical study. *Cancer Treat. Rep.* **62**:359–360.

Dubinsky, R., R. Yarchoan, and M. Dalakas. 1989. Reversible axonal neuropathy from the treatment of AIDS and related disorders with 2′3′-didcoxycytidine (ddC). *Muscle Nerve* **12**:856–860.

Eidelberg, D., A. Sotrel, H. Vogel, P. Walker, J. Kleefield, and I. Crumpacker. 1986. Progressive polyradiculopathy in acquired immune deficiency syndrome. *Neurology* **36**:912–916.

Eisenhauer, M., A. Eliasson, A. Taylor, P. Coyne, and D. Wortham. 1994. Incidence of cardiac arrhythmias during intravenous pentamidine therapy in HIV-infected patients. *Chest* **105**:389–395.

Esiri, M., C. Morris, and P. Millard. 1993. Sensory and sympathetic ganglia in HIV-1 infection: immunocytochemical demonstration of HIV-1 viral antigens, increased MHC class II antigen expression and mild reactive inflammation. *J. Neurol. Sci.* **114**:178–187.

Evenhouse, M., E. Haas, E. Snell, J. Visser, L. Paul, and R. Gonzalez. 1987. Hypotension infection with the human immunodeficiency virus. *Ann. Intern. Med.* **107**:598–599. (Letter.)

Freeman, R. 1997. Noninvasive evaluation of heart rate variability—the time domain, p. 297–308. *In* P. Low (ed.), *Clinical Autonomic Disorders*, 2nd ed. Lippincott-Raven Publishers, Philadelphia, PA.

Freeman, R., M. Roberts, L. Friedman, and C. Broadbridge. 1990. Autonomic function and human immunodeficiency virus infection. *Neurology* **40**:575–580.

Fuller, G., and J. Jacobs. 1990. Axonal atrophy in the painful peripheral neuropathy in AIDS. *Acta Neuropathol.* **81**:198–203.

Gastaut, J., J. Pouget, P. Valentin, A. Lafeuillade, C. Dhiver, and J. Gastaut. 1992. Study of sensory involvement and dysautonomia in HIV infected patients. A prospective study of 55 cases. *Neurophysiol. Clin.* **22**:417–430. (In French.)

Gluck, T., E. Degenhardt, J. Scholmerich, B. Lang, J. Grossmann, and R. Straub. 2000. Autonomic neuropathy in patients with HIV: course, impact of disease stage, and medication. *Clin. Auton. Res.* **10**:17–22.

Griffin, G., A. Miller, P. Batman, S. Forster, A. Pinching, J. Harris, and M. Mathan. 1988. Damage to jejunal intrinsic autonomic nerves in HIV infection. *AIDS* **2**:379–382.

Helmick, C., and J. Green. 1985. Pentamidine-associated hypotension and route of adminstration. *Ann. Intern. Med.* **103**:480.

Kayser, C., R. Campbell, C. Sartorious, and M. Bartlett. 1990. Toxoplasmosis of the conus medullaris in a patient with hemophilia A-associated AIDS. Case report. *J. Neurosurg.* **73**:951–953.

Kearney, D., A. Perez-Atayde, K. Easley, N. Bowles, J. Bricker, S. Colan, S. Kaplan, W. Lai, S. Lipshultz, D. Moodie, G. Sopko, T. Starc, and J. Towbin. 2003a. Postmortem cardiomegaly and echocardiographic measurements of left ventricular size and function in children infected with the human immunodeficiency virus. The Prospective P2C2 HIV Multicenter Study. *Cardiovasc. Pathol.* **12**:140–148.

Kearney, M., A. Zaman, D. Eckberg, A. Lee, K. Fox, A. Shah, R. Prescott, W. Shell, E. Charuvastra, T. Callahan, W. Brooksby, D. Wright, N. Gall, and J. Nolan. 2003b. Cardiac size, autonomic function, and 5-year follow-up of chronic heart failure patients with severe prolongation of ventricular activation. *J. Card. Fail.* **9**:93–99.

Kelly, J., D. Dooley, C. Lattuada, and C. Smith. 1992. A severe, unusual reaction to trimethoprim-sulfamethoxazole in patients infected with human immunodeficiency virus. *Clin. Infect. Dis.* **14**:1034–1039.

Klein, P., G. Zientek, S. VandenBerg, and E. Lothman. 1990. Primary CNS lymphoma: lymphomatous meningitis presenting as a cauda equina lesion in an AIDS patient. *Can. J. Neurol. Sci.* **17**:329–331.

Klein, R., D. Mann, G. Friedland, and M. Surks. 1983. Adrenocortical function in the acquired immunodeficiency syndrome. *Ann. Intern. Med.* **99**:566.

Kumar, M., R. Morgan, J. Szapocznik, and C. Eisdorfer. 1991. Norepinephrine response in early HIV infection. *J. Acquir. Immune Defic. Syndr.* **4**:782–786.

Lambert, J., M. Seidlin, R. Reichman, C. Plank, M. Laverty, G. Morse, C. Knupp, C. McLaren, C. Petinelli, and F. Valentine. 1990. 2′3′-dideoxyinosine (ddI) in patients with the acquired immunodeficiency syndrome or AIDS-related complex. A phase I trial. *N. Engl. J. Med.* **322**:1333–1340.

Lanska, M., D. Lanska, and J. Schmidley. 1988. Syphilitic polyradiculopathy in an HIV-positive man. *Neurology* **38**:1297–1301.

Leger, J., P. Bouche, F. Bolgert, M. Chaunu, M. Rosenheim, H. Cathala, M. Gentilini, J. Hauw, and P. Brunet. 1989. The spectrum of polyneuropathies in patients infected with HIV. *J. Neurol. Neurosurg. Psychiatry* **52**:1369–1374.

Levy, R., D. Bredesen, and M. Rosenblum. 1985. Neurological manifestations of the acquired immunodeficiency syndrome

(AIDS): experience at UCSF and review of the literature. *J. Neurosurg.* **62**:475–795.

Lin-Greenberger, A., and N. Taneja-Uppal. 1987. Dysautonomia and infection with the human immunodeficiency virus. *Ann. Intern. Med.* **106**:167.

Lipshultz, S., S. Chanock, S. Sanders, S. Colan, A. Perez-Atayde, and K. McIntosh. 1989. Cardiovascular manifestations of human immunodeficiency virus infection in infants and children. *Am. J. Cardiol.* **63**:1489–1497.

Loke, R., I. Murray-Lyon, and G. Carter. 1990. Postural hypotension related to zidovudine in a patient infected with HIV. *BMJ* **300**:163–164.

Luginbuhl, L., E. Orav, K. McIntosh, and S. Lipshultz. 1993. Cardiac morbidity and related mortality in children with HIV infection. *JAMA* **269**:2869–2875.

Maclean, H., and B. Dhillon. 1993. Pupil cycle time and human immunodeficiency virus (HIV) infection. *Eye* **7**:785–786.

Mah, V., L. Vartavarian, M. Akers, and H. Vinters. 1988. Abnormalities of peripheral nerve in patients with human immunodeficiency virus infection. *Ann. Neurol.* **24**:713–717.

McArthur, J. 1987. Neurologic manifestations of AIDS. *Medicine* **66**:407–437.

Membreno, L., I. Irony, W. Dere, R. Klein, E. Biglieri, and E. Cobb. 1987. Adrenocortical function in acquired immunodeficiency syndrome. *J. Clin. Endocrinol. Metab.* **65**:482–487.

Miller, R., and S. Semple. 1987. Autonomic neuropathy in AIDS. *Lancet* **ii**:343–344.

Miller, R., J. Storey, and C. Greco. 1990. Ganciclovir in the treatment of progressive AIDS related polyradiculopathy. *Neurology* **40**:569–574.

Mittal, C., N. Wig, S. Mishra, and K. Deepak. 2004. Heart rate variability in human immunodeficiency virus-positive individuals. *Int. J. Cardiol.* **94**:1–6.

Mulhall, B., and I. Jennens. 1987. Testing for neurological involvement in HIV infection. *Lancet* **ii**:1531–1532.

Navia, B., B. Jordan, and R. Price. 1986. The AIDS dementia complex. I. Clinical features. *Ann. Neurol.* **19**:517–524.

Neild, P., A. Amadi, P. Ponikowski, A. Coats, and B. Gazzard. 2000. Cardiac autonomic dysfunction in AIDS is not secondary to heart failure. *Int. J. Cardiol.* **74**:133–137.

Norbiato, G., M. Bevilacqua, T. Vago, G. Baldi, E. Chebat, P. Bertora, M. Moroni, M. Galli, and N. Oldenburg. 1992. Cortisol resistance in acquired immunodeficiency syndrome. *J. Clin. Endocrinol. Metab.* **74**:608–613.

Overhage, J., A. Greist, and D. Brown. 1990. Conus medullaris syndrome resulting from *Toxoplasma gondii* infection in a patient with the acquired immunodeficiency syndrome. *Am. J. Med.* **89**:814–815.

Palaic, M., R. Lisbona, and A. Sniderman. 1993. Pulmonary edema induced by fluid administration in acquired immune deficiency syndrome patients with cardiac autonomic dysfunction. *Can. J. Cardiol.* **9**:115–117.

Parker, L., E. Levin, and E. Lifrak. 1985. Evidence for adrenocortical adaptation to severe illness. *J. Clin. Endocrinol. Metab.* **60**:947–952.

Parry, G. 1988. Peripheral neuropathies associated with human immunodeficiency virus infection. *Ann. Neurol.* **23**(Suppl.):S49–S53.

Petito, C., B. Navia, E. Cho, B. Jordan, D. George, and R. Price. 1985. Vacuolar myelopathy pathologically resembling subacute combined degeneration in patients with the acquired immunodeficiency syndrome. *N. Engl. J. Med.* **312**:874–879.

Plein, D., G. Van Camp, B. Cosyns, A. Alimenti, J. Levy, and J. Vandenbossche. 1999. Cardiac and autonomic evaluation in a pediatric population with human immunodeficiency virus. *Clin. Cardiol.* **22**:33–36.

Purba, J., M. Hofman, P. Portegies, D. Troost, and D. Swaab. 1993. Decreased number of oxytocin neurons in the paraventricular nucleus of the human hypothalamus in AIDS. *Brain* **116**:795–809.

Rogstad, K., R. Shah, G. Tesfaladet, M. Abdullah, and I. Ahmed-Jushuf. 1999. Cardiovascular autonomic neuropathy in HIV infected patients. *Sex. Transm. Infect.* **75**:264–267.

Ronchi, O., A. Grippo, P. Ghidini, F. Lolli, M. Lorenzo, M. Di Pietro, and F. Mazzotta. 1992. Electrophysiologic study of HIV-1+ patients without signs of peripheral neuropathy. *J. Neurol. Sci.* **113**:209–213.

Roose, S., A. Glassman, S. Siris, T. Walsh, R. Bruno, and L. Wright. 1981. Comparisons of imipramine and nortriptyline induced orthostatic hypotension: a meaningful difference. *J. Clin. Pathol.* **1**:316–319.

Rüttimann, S., P. Hilti, G. Spinas, and U. Dubach. 1991. High frequency of human immunodeficiency virus-associated autonomic neuropathy and more severe involvement in advanced stages of human immunodeficiency virus disease. *Arch. Intern. Med.* **151**:2441–2443.

Sakhuja, A., A. Goyal, A. Jaryal, N. Wig, M. Vajpayee, A. Kumar, and K. Deepak. 2007. Heart rate variability and autonomic function tests in HIV positive individuals in India. *Clin. Auton. Res.* **17**:193–196.

Schatz, I., R. Bannister, R. Freeman, C. Goetz, J. Jankovic, H. Kaufmann, W. Koller, P. Low, C. Mathias, R. Polinsky, N. Quinn, D. Robertson, and D. Streeten. 1996. Consensus statement: the definition of orthostatic hypotension, pure autonomic failure, and multiple system atrophy. *J. Auton. Nerv. Syst.* **58**:123–124.

Schifitto, G., M. McDermott, T. Evans, T. Fitzgerald, J. Schwimmer, L. Demeter, and K. Kieburtz. 2000. Autonomic performance and dehydroepiandrosterone sulfate levels in HIV-1-infected individuals: relationship to TH1 and TH2 cytokine profile. *Arch. Neurol.* **57**:1027–1032.

Scott, G., A. Piaggesi, and D. Ewing. 1990. Sequential autonomic function tests in HIV infection. *AIDS* **4**:1279–1281.

Siddiqui, M., and P. Ford. 1995. Acute severe autonomic insufficiency during pentamidine therapy. *South. Med. J.* **88**:1087–1088.

Simpson, D. 2002. Selected peripheral neuropathies associated with human immunodeficiency virus infection and antiretroviral therapy. *J. Neurovirol.* **8**:33–41.

Simpson, D., and M. Tagliati. 1995. Nucleoside analogue-associated peripheral neuropathy in human immunodeficiency virus infection. *J. AIDS Hum. Retrovirol.* **9**:153–161.

Skowron, G. 1995. Biologic effects and safety of stavudine: overview of phase I and II clinical trials. *J. Infect. Dis.* **171**: S113–S117.

So, Y., and R. Olney. 1994. Acute lumbosacral polyradiculopathy in acquired immunodeficiency syndrome: experience in 23 patients. *Ann. Neurol.* **35**:53–58.

Sommadossi, J. 1995. Comparison of metabolism and in vitro antiviral activity of stavudine versus other 2′,3′-dideoxynucleoside analogues. *J. Infect. Dis.* **171**(Suppl. 2):S88–S92.

Stein, K., C. Fenton, A. Lehany, P. Okin, and P. Kligfield. 1991. Incidence of QT interval prolongation during pentamidine therapy of *Pneumocystis carinii* pneumonia. *Am. J. Cardiol.* **68**:1091–1094.

Stein, K., H. Haronian, G. Mensah, A. Acosta, J. Jacobs, and P. Kligfield. 1990. Ventricular tachycardia and torsades de pointes complicating pentamidine therapy of *Pneumocystis carinii* pneumonia in the acquired immunodeficiency syndrome. *Am. J. Cardiol.* **66**:888–889.

Tan, S., R. Guiloff, and F. Scaravilli. 1995. AIDS-associated vacuolar myelopathy. A morphometric study. *Brain* **118**:1247–1261.

van Gurp, P., C. Tack, M. van der Valk, P. Reiss, J. Lenders, F. Sweep, and H. Sauerwein. 2006. Sympathetic nervous system function in HIV-associated adipose redistribution syndrome. *AIDS* **21**:773–775.

Villa, A., V. Cruccu, V. Foresti, G. Guareschi, M. Tronchi, and F. Confalonieri. 1990. HIV related functional involvement of autonomic nervous system. *Acta Neurol.* **12:** 14–18.

Villa, A., V. Foresti, and F. Confalonieri. 1987. Autonomic neuropathy and HIV infection. *Lancet* **ii:**915.

Villa, A., V. Foresti, and F. Confalonieri. 1992. Autonomic nervous system dysfunction associated with HIV infection in intravenous heroin users. *AIDS* **6:**85–89.

Villa, A., V. Foresti, and F. Confalonieri. 1995. Autonomic neuropathy and prolongation of QT interval in human immunodeficiency virus infection. *Clin. Auton. Res.* **5:**48–52.

Welby, S., S. Rogerson, and N. Beeching. 1991. Autonomic neuropathy is common in human immunodeficiency virus infection. *J. Infect.* **23:**123–128.

Wharton, J., P. Demopulos, and N. Goldschlager. 1987. Torsade de pointes during administration of pentamidine isethionate. *Am. J. Med.* **83:**571–576.

Whitcomb, R., W. Linehan, L. Wahl, and R. Knazek. 1988. Monocytes stimulate cortisol production by cultured human adrenocortical cells. *J. Clin. Endocrinol. Metab.* **66:**33–38.

Wiley, C., P. VanPatten, P. Carpenter, H. Powell, and L. Thal. 1987. Acute ascending necrotizing myelopathy caused by herpes simplex virus type 2. *Neurology* **37:**1791–1794.

Yun, A., P. Lee, and K. Bazar. 2004a. Modulation of autonomic balance by tumors and viruses. *Med. Hypotheses* **63:**344–351.

Yun, A., P. Lee, and K. Bazar. 2004b. Modulation of host immunity by HIV may be partly achieved through usurping host autonomic functions. *Med. Hypotheses* **63:**362–366.

The Spectrum of Neuro-AIDS Disorders:
Pathophysiology, Diagnosis, and Treatment
Edited by K. Goodkin et al.
©2008 ASM Press, Washington, DC

6

Distal Sensory Polyneuropathy and Other Selected Neuropathies in HIV Infection

LYDIA ESTANISLAO, ANTHONY GERACI, AND DAVID SIMPSON

Peripheral neuropathy is a common neurologic complication of both HIV infection and its treatment. It is often difficult to distinguish peripheral neuropathy caused by the infection from that due to medication. However, it is crucial to discriminate between the two, as it may impact the therapeutic management of HIV-infected individuals. This chapter discusses the clinical features, diagnosis, and management of HIV distal sensory polyneuropathy (DSP); toxic neuropathies, with emphasis on the antiretroviral (ARV)-associated neuropathies; and other neuropathies found in HIV-infected individuals (Table 1).

DISTAL SENSORY POLYNEUROPATHY IN HIV INFECTION

DSP is the most common neuro-AIDS condition in the HAART era. The clinical features of DSP are characteristic. The principal symptoms of DSP include numbness, paresthesias, and burning sensations in the feet in a symmetrical stocking distribution. The fingertips and hands (glove distribution) may be affected later and to a milder degree. The peripheral nerve manifestations occur in a length-dependent fashion, with a proximal-to-distal gradient (Snider et al., 1983). Dysesthesias first appear in the soles and gradually ascend. The sensory symptoms can be painful and disabling, while motor deficits are minimal and generally confined to the intrinsic muscles of the foot. After initial progression, the sensory symptoms may plateau and cease to progress further but remain despite attempts at treatment. DSP is characterized by the following signs: (i) absent or depressed ankle reflexes relative to the knees, (ii) an elevated vibration threshold in the feet, (iii) decreased distal sensation to

pinprick and temperature, and (iv) relatively normal joint position sensation and muscle strength. Electrophysiologic studies reveal abnormal sensory nerve amplitudes and conduction velocities, particularly of the sural nerve (Tagliati et al., 1999). Motor nerve conduction velocities are usually normal or only mildly diminished in proportion to reduced compound muscle action potentials. Electromyography may reveal evidence of denervation in distal muscles, related to the extent of axonal loss.

In studies of patients with AIDS prior to the use of ARV medications (Snider et al., 1983; Cornblath and McArthur, 1988; So et al., 1988; Leger et al., 1989), approximately 35% of patients had signs and symptoms of DSP. As CD4 cell counts declined, the incidence of DSP increased (Bacellar et al., 1994; Tagliati et al., 1999). A risk of DSP has also been associated with a plasma viral load greater than 30,000 copies/ml and a CD4 cell count less than 500 cells/mm^3 (Childs et al., 1999). An age-associated risk for DSP in HIV-1-infected individuals has been demonstrated clinically (Simpson et al., 1998). Peripheral neuropathy is recognized as a true risk factor for falls in the elderly (Richardson and Hurvitz, 1995), and the pain associated with DSP has been noted to be a significant cause of decreased adherence to HAART. Hence, DSP may be associated with additional health risks and an increased likelihood of subsequent systemic HIV disease progression.

In the highly active ARV therapy (HAART) era, studies have shown that the relationship between the CD4 cell count and the incidence of DSP is no longer apparent (Schifitto et al., 2002; Morgello et al., 2004). One study suggested that the toxicity of the dideoxynucleoside analogues (d-drugs) may have decreased as a current risk factor for the occurrence of HIV-associated DSP (Schifitto et al., 2002). The study followed 272 subjects twice a year for up to 30 months. The criteria for DSP diagnosis were decreased or absent ankle jerks, decreased or absent vibratory perception at the toes, or decreased pinprick or temperature in a stocking distribution. Subjects were classified as having asymptomatic DSP if they

Lydia Estanislao, Clinical Neurology Specialists, Las Vegas, NV 89146.
Anthony Geraci, St. Luke's Roosevelt Hospital, New York, NY 10025.
David Simpson, Mount Sinai Medical Center, New York, NY 10029.

TABLE 1. Comparative summary of neuropathies in HIV infection

Neuropathy type	Clinical manifestations	Neurological signs	Diagnostic studies[a]	Treatment
Distal sensory polyneuropathy; toxic neuropathies	Paresthesias; dysesthesias; distal weakness in severe cases (and in dapsone neuropathy)	Sensory (pinprick and vibration) deficits; stocking and glove distribution; depressed distal reflexes	EMG/NCV: abnormal sensory nerve amplitudes; distal axonopathy	Analgesics (opioid and adjuvant); antidepressants (mixed noradrenergic and serotonergic); anticonvulsants (particularly lamotrigine); neurotoxic drug withdrawal or dose-reduction for toxic neuropathies
Inflammatory demyelinating polyneuropathy (IDP)	Progressive weakness; paresthesias	Weakness; mild sensory deficits; areflexia	CSF lymphocytic pleocytosis (10–50 cells/μl)	Immunomodulating therapy; consider anti-CMV therapy in late-onset IDP (see text)
Mononeuropathy multiplex (MM)	Foot or wrist drop; facial weakness; focal pain	Multifocal cranial and peripheral neuropathy	EMG/NCV: demyelination	Immunomodulating therapy; consider anti-CMV therapy in late-onset MM
Progressive polyradiculopathy (PP)	Lower extremity weakness; paresthesias; sphincter dysfunction	Flaccid paraparesis; saddle distribution anesthesia; depressed reflexes	EMG/NCV: multifocal axonal neuropathy	Anti-CMV therapy (particularly if CSF CMV PCR +)
Autonomic neuropathy	Orthostatic dizziness; syncope; diarrhea; anhydrosis; palpitations; impotence; urinary dysfunction	Orthostatic hypotension; pupillary abnormalities; sweating dysfunction; resting tachycardia	CSF: polymorphonuclear pleocytosis EMG/NCV: polyradiculopathy ECG: arrhythmia Autonomic function studies: abnormal	Fluid and electrolyte replacement; fludricortisone; midodrine; anti-arrhythmic agents; neurotoxic drug withdrawal for toxic causes

[a]EMG, electromyogram; NCV, nerve conduction velocity; ECG, electrocardiogram.

only had neurologic signs or as having symptomatic DSP if they also had paresthesias or pain. While the dideoxynucleosides are associated with a toxic neuropathy (clinically indistinguishable from HIV-associated DSP), these drugs remain an important subclass, although they are less frequently used in current HAART regimens. Schifitto et al. (2002) showed that use of these drugs was not a significant risk factor for incident symptomatic DSP. Such an effect may be related to preservation of immune function, forestalling the potential occurrence of neurotoxicity. This study also addressed the important issue of whether the presence of asymptomatic DSP is a risk factor for incident symptomatic DSP. Surprisingly, the results suggested that asymptomatic DSP was not a significant predictor of incident symptomatic DSP. More recently, Simpson et al. (2006) evaluated 101 subjects with advanced HIV infection over a 48-week period by neurological examination, nerve conduction studies, quantitative sensory testing, and skin biopsies for quantitation of epidermal nerve fiber density (ENFD), with data summed into a total neuropathy score (TNS). The factors associated with progression in the TNS were lower current TNS, low ENFD, and Caucasian race. The previously established DSP risk factors of CD4 cell count, plasma HIV load, and the use of the dideoxynucleoside ARV medications were not predictive of DSP progression. ENFD quantification from skin biopsy as the distal leg has been shown to be related to the severity of DSP as assessed by the TNS and measures of pain (Zhou et al., 2007). ENFD is currently being recommended for use in monitoring the prevention of DSP and to assess response to treatment.

Treatment of DSP in HIV Infection

The pathogenesis of HIV-1-associated DSP is not completely understood. Indirect nerve damage by the proinflammatory cytokine cascade has been a favored explanation. Attempts at therapeutic intervention have been largely palliative so far. HAART itself may delay or improve DSP (Markus and Brew, 1998), but this has not been systematically studied. An attempt should be made to aggressively control pain. Antidepressants, anticonvulsants, and topical agents, alone or in combination, may alleviate pain and functional disability. These agents are preferred to the long-term use of opioid analgesics. The choice of antidepressants in the setting of painful peripheral neuropathy would generally be considered to be those associated with enhancing both noradrenergic and serotonergic transmission. However, the effect of antidepressants has not always been borne out in this area; for example, amitriptyline was found not to be efficacious in one trial (Kieburtz et al., 1998). Among the anticonvulsants, lamotrigine has been reported to be well tolerated and effective for HIV-associated neuropathic pain in patients receiving ARV therapy with neurotoxic agents (Simpson et al., 2000, 2003). Nerve growth factor, a pathophysiologically based treatment, has shown a therapeutic effect (McArthur et al., 2000), although memantine, an N-methyl-D-aspartate receptor antagonist, has not (Schifitto et al., 2006). More pathophysiologically based treatments are needed in the future.

Toxic Neuropathies in HIV Infection

Toxic neuropathy in HIV-infected individuals may arise from the ARVs, as well as from the medications used for concomitant conditions that may occur in this population.

ARV-Associated Neuropathy

ARV-associated neuropathy is clinically and electrophysiologically indistinguishable from HIV-associated DSP. The former, however, tends to be more painful, abrupt in onset, and rapidly progressive (Moyle and Sadler, 1998). Most importantly, it bears a temporal relationship to the drug. However, in clinical practice, with retrospective histories, it is often difficult to determine the precise date of onset of symptoms relative to the frequent changes in a patient's ARV regimen. Among the approved ARVs used in HIV infection, only the d-drugs from the nucleoside reverse transcriptase inhibitor (NRTI) group have been found to be neurotoxic. The neurotoxic ARV d-drugs include didanosine (ddI), zalcitabine (ddC), and stavudine (d4T) (Yarchoan et al., 1988; Merigan et al., 1989; Cooley et al., 1990; Lambert et al., 1990; Browne et al., 1993). An accurate determination of the incidence of nucleoside analogue-induced DSP is difficult. The presence of other contributing factors that may cause or aggravate the neuropathy should be considered. These include alcohol use (Fichtenbaum et al., 1995), nutritional status (Fichtenbaum et al., 1995), concomitant use of other neurotoxic agents (e.g., vincristine), and the increasing incidence of diabetes mellitus in HIV infection (Dube, 2000).

In the pre-HAART era, the reported incidence of peripheral neuropathy varied greatly and closely with CD4 cell count and HIV disease stage. Advanced HIV infection and low CD4 cell counts (especially below 100 cells/μl) increase the risk of peripheral neuropathy (Tagliati et al., 1999). Data from the Multicenter AIDS Cohort Study indicate that the lower the CD4 count, the higher the incidence of peripheral neuropathy (Bacellar et al., 1994). One study showed that the incidence of HIV-associated DSP decreased in the HAART era, while the incidence of ARV-associated neuropathy increased (Maschke et al., 2000). Thus, it is not surprising that patients with advanced HIV infection and severe immunosuppression remain at the greatest risk of neurotoxicity due to ARV agents. Early studies of nucleoside analogue-associated peripheral neuropathy employed dosage schedules that were above the presently approved dosages. Thus, in the analysis of incidence data, it is important to take into consideration the dosages of the drug administered and the stage of disease of the patient cohort under study.

ddC Neuropathy

Data from phase I and II studies of ddC report a DSP incidence of 25% to 66% (Yarchoan et al., 1988; Merigan et al., 1989; A. R. Berger et al., 1993; Fischl et al., 1993; Meng et al., 1992; Skowron et al., 1993; Kieburtz et al., 1992). The incidence, severity, progression, and reversibility of peripheral neuropathy from ddC, as with other toxic neuropathies, are dose dependent. Yarchoan et al. (1988) reported that the period of onset of peripheral neuropathy ranged from 9 to 13 weeks at different ddC doses. Dubinsky and coworkers reported that the total dose of ddC at the onset of neuropathy ranged from 5.67 mg/kg of body weight to 34.02 mg/kg (Dubinsky et al., 1989). In the AIDS Clinical Trials Group (ACTG) 012 substudy, all 29 patients randomized to receive the highest doses of ddC—0.03 mg/kg/4 h and 0.06 mg/kg/4 h—developed peripheral neuropathy with onset at 2 weeks. In the low-dose group—0.01 and 0.005 mg/kg/4 h—the incidence of neuropathy was lower and the onset was delayed: 25% did not develop peripheral neuropathy until they had been on therapy for 9 months. In the group taking the current recommended daily dosage (but at 0.005 mg/kg every 4 h, rather than three times a day), only 2 out of 15 patients developed peripheral neuropathy after >17 weeks of treatment. Also, symptoms were milder and the onset of recovery was earlier—at 11 weeks in the low-dose group compared to the high-dose groups, where onset of recovery was at 19 weeks. Following drug cessation, there may be an associated prolonged intensification of symptoms, termed a "coasting period," lasting for 3 to 6 weeks. Data from the ACTG 106 trial showed that ddC at dosages of 0.005 mg/kg and 0.01 mg/kg given every 8 h and combined with zidovudine (ZDV) resulted in a lower incidence of peripheral neuropathy (Meng et al., 1992).

There is an inverse relationship between the CD4 count and the incidence of ddC neuropathy. In ACTG 119, there was a 26% incidence of peripheral neuropathy in patients with CD4 counts of <50/mm³ as opposed to 15% in those with CD4 counts of >50/mm³. In ACTG 155, 27 to 28% of those with CD4 counts of <150/mm³ had peripheral neuropathy compared to 16% in those with CD4 counts of >150/mm³. In the European expanded-access program, the incidence of neuropathy in those with CD4 counts of <50/mm³ was 13.7%, whereas for those with counts of >50/mm³ it was 11.1%; 16.7% of patients with peripheral neuropathy had a diagnosis of AIDS, while 7.8% had early symptomatic HIV infection.

ddI Neuropathy

Data from phase I and II and open-label studies of ddI showed an incidence of DSP of 12% to 34%. Daily dosages of >12.5 mg/kg (Cooley et al., 1990; Lambert et al., 1990; Kieburtz et al., 1992) or cumulative doses of 1.5 g/kg (Rozencweig et al., 1990; Yarchoan et al., 1990) or 1.16 g/kg in patients with low CD4 cell counts (Rathbun and Martin, 1992) are generally associated with signs and symptoms of peripheral neuropathy. The mean time to onset of peripheral neuropathy is 20 weeks (Steiberg et al., 1991). Symptoms usually resolve within 3 to 5 weeks after withdrawal of the drug. If no resolution of symptoms occurs after 8 weeks, HIV itself or other alternative causes of neuropathy should be considered. As with other neurotoxic neuropathies, a period of coasting may be observed after drug withdrawal. Reintroduction at lower doses and after resolution of symptoms is tolerated in some patients (Kieburtz et al., 1992).

The recommended daily dosage of ddI is 200 mg twice a day (BID) orally or 2.5 mg/kg every 12 h intravenously. At this dosage, some studies have shown that the incidence of peripheral neuropathy is similar to that which occurs with ZDV, a drug that is not considered to be neurotoxic. In ACTG 116b/117, the annualized incidence of grade 2 neuropathy in subjects given ddI at dosages of 750 and 500 mg/day was compared to that of ZDV-experienced patients given ZDV monotherapy. The results were 13, 14, and 14%, respectively (Kahn et al., 1992). In a neurological substudy of ACTG 175, in which patients had entry CD4 count of 200 to 500 cells/mm³, the incidences of DSP were similar in groups that received ZDV monotherapy (4%), ddI monotherapy (3%), and ZDV/ddI combination therapy (4%). The ZDV/ddC combination therapy arm had an increased incidence of peripheral neuropathy (6%) (Simpson et al., 1998).

d4T Neuropathy

The reported incidence of neuropathy due to d4T varies widely from 6% to 55%. In a phase I study, Browne and coworkers (1993) reported sensory peripheral neuropathy as a dose-limiting side effect in 55% of patients with the maximum tolerable dose of 2.0 mg/kg/day. In this dose escalation study, an increase in the dose by 1 mg/kg increased the relative risk of neuropathy by a factor of 2 ($P = 0.001$), supporting the relationship to ARV dose.

The inverse relationship between the CD4 count and the incidence of peripheral neuropathy is also evident in the different studies. In a randomized open trial comparing different doses of d4T—0.5, 1.0, and 2.0 mg/kg/day—in patients with mean CD4 counts of 246 cells/mm³, the incidences of peripheral neuropathy were 6%, 15%, and 31%, respectively. A clinical trial comparing d4T (40 mg/day BID, the current recommended dose) with ZDV (600 mg/day) in 800 HIV-infected patients with a median CD4 count of 250 cells/mm³ revealed an incidence of peripheral neuropathy of 12% at 1 year in the d4T-treated group compared to 6% in those treated with ZDV. A large comparison study of subjects who failed or were intolerant of ZDV, with a median CD4 count of 44 cells/mm³, revealed a neuropathy incidence of 23% in patients on d4T at 40 mg BID (approximately 1 mg/kg/day) and 17% in those on 20 mg BID (0.5 mg/kg/day).

Mechanism of Neurotoxicity by Nucleoside Analogues

Early hypotheses held that ddC, which contains a cytosine base, interfered with the production of sphingomyelin via the formation of a ddC-diphosphocholine metabolite (Cooney et al., 1986). However, similar toxicities are observed with d4T and ddI, which do not have a cytosine base. In vitro and animal experiments suggest inhibition of mitochondrial DNA (mtDNA) synthesis, particularly the potent inhibition of DNA polymerase gamma, as the mechanism for neurotoxicity (see chapter 7, this volume) (Pezeshkpour et al., 1987; Balzarini et al., 1989; Chen and Cheng, 1989; Martin et al., 1994; Cui et al., 1997).

The nucleoside analogues, when phosphorylated to their active triphosphate forms, are incorporated into target viral DNA, resulting in inhibition of the reverse transcriptase or chain termination. This is the mechanism responsible for the antiretroviral activity. However, the same phosphorylated analogues may be used by mammalian mtDNA polymerase gamma. The resultant mtDNA toxicity is the proposed mechanism of ARV-associated neuropathy from NRTIs. In cell culture assays, NRTIs have varying degrees of mtDNA inhibition, as follows (in descending order): ddC > d4T > ddI > lamivudine > ZDV > abacavir.

Keswani et al. (2003) have reported on an in vitro model of ARV-associated neuropathy. They have shown a dose-dependent inhibition of dorsal root ganglion cells by d-drugs in a graded fashion, similar to their toxicities as noted in the clinical setting, i.e., ddC > ddI > d4T. Depending on the dosage of these drugs, the changes noted in dorsal root ganglion neurons ranged from varicosities in the most distal parts of the neurites to frank neuritic degeneration. This neurotoxicity was associated with loss of mitochondrion membrane potential noted 4 h after exposure to d-drugs. Importantly, there were no appreciable morphological neuritic changes or mitochondrial depolarization noted with ZDV.

Animal experiments have provided data on the mitochondrial toxicities of these agents. Patterson et al. (2000) demonstrated the development of a dose-dependent painful myelinopathy in a rat model of exposure to ddI. Sciatic nerve studies after 15 weeks of ddI treatment revealed myelin splitting and edema within the axons, with affected areas appearing shrunken and displaced (Patterson et al., 2000). Anderson et al. observed myelin splitting and intramyelinic edema, axonal demyelination and remyelination, and axonal loss in peripheral nerves and ventral roots of rabbits given ddC by oral intubation (Anderson et al., 1992, 1994). These animal findings, however, do not precisely mirror findings in HIV-seropositive humans. Furthermore, there were several studies that could not reproduce ARV-associated neuropathy in animals, despite administration of neurotoxic ARVs (Warner et al., 1995; Keswani et al., 2002). These findings led some investigators to speculate that there may be a synergistic role of HIV infection in the development of ARV-associated DSP (Keswani et al., 2002). A similar argument has been put forward for cardiomyopathy induced by ARVs in HIV-transgenic mice, but not in wild-type mice (Lewis et al., 2001). Cote and coworkers reported that while subjects with d-drug-associated lactic acidosis had the greatest depletion of mtDNA in peripheral blood mononuclear cells, ARV-naïve patients with HIV also had evidence of mitochondrial dysfunction (Cote et al., 2002).

Several studies have reported in vivo data on mitochondrial toxicity of the d-drugs. Cases of biopsy-proven mitochondrial damage in patients with nucleoside analogue-associated peripheral neuropathy have been reported (Gasnault et al., 1999). Dalakas and companions studied nerve biopsy specimens from HIV-infected patients treated with ddC (Dalakas et al., 2001). They found both structurally abnormal mitochondria in axons and Schwann cells and reduced mtDNA copy numbers in the subjects treated with ddC. Brew and coworkers showed that elevated serum lactate levels (as evidence of mitochondrial impairment) differentiated ARV-associated neuropathy from HIV-associated DSP with 90% specificity and 90% sensitivity (Brew et al., 2003).

Some authors attribute the delayed onset of symptoms of ARV-associated neuropathy to the possible gradual decline of mtDNA levels in the cell and the coasting phenomenon to abnormal signaling that may occur as mtDNA is gradually restored during recovery (Moyle and Sadler, 1998). Other investigators have suggested that the neurotoxicity of nucleoside analogues is due to depletion of acetyl-L-carnitine. Acetyl-L-carnitine may promote peripheral nerve regeneration following injury by causing the release of nerve growth factor (Angelucci et al., 1988). Carnitine depletion causes a disruption of mitochondrial metabolism with resultant toxic accumulation of fatty acids (Colucci and Gandour, 1988). Lower levels of acetyl-L-carnitine were found in HIV-infected patients with peripheral neuropathy taking dideoxynucleosides than in those without neuropathy (Famularo et al., 1997). However, data from ACTG 291 do not support this hypothesis. There was no difference in carnitine levels in those with differing degrees of severity of peripheral neuropathy.

The occurrence of dyslipidemia and frank diabetes mellitus as a long-term toxicity of the protease inhibitors may also contribute to this condition.

Thalidomide Neuropathy

Thalidomide was first used as a sedative and antiemetic agent for pregnant women during the late 1950s and early 1960s. Teratogenicity, which eventually led to its withdrawal from the market, overshadowed its neurotoxic effects. Almost 40 years later, thalidomide is attracting interest due to its effects on immune function (Calabrese and Fleischer, 2000). Thalidomide has recently been approved for erythema nodosum leprosum, an inflammatory complication of leprosy (Calabrese and Fleischer, 2000). Its efficacy has also been shown in the treatment of dermatologic diseases, such as aphthous stomatitis (Grinspan, 1985), cutaneous lesions of Behcet's disease (Hamuryudan et al., 1998), chronic cutaneous lupus erythematosus (Knop et al., 1983), and prurigo nodularis (van den Broek, 1980), and in nondermatologic diseases, such as graft-versus-host disease (Vogelsang et al., 1992). In HIV-infected patients, thalidomide is effective in the treatment of oral and esophageal aphthous ulcers (Jacobson et al., 1997; Alexander and Wilcox, 1997), chronic diarrhea (Quinones et al., 1997; Sharpstone et al., 1995), and wasting syndrome (Reyes-Teran et al., 1996; Kaplan et al., 1998).

Due to the increasing use of thalidomide, there are renewed concerns about its neurotoxicity. The incidence of neuropathy associated with thalidomide varies from 1% to 70% (Tseng et al., 1996). The clinical manifestations of thalidomide neuropathy are mainly sensory and include painful paresthesias of the feet and hands, hyperesthesia, and numbness. Nerve conduction studies have shown a reduction in amplitude of sensory nerve action potentials without an increase in latency. Conduction velocities were normal or only mildly reduced, indicating an axonal neuropathy. Pathologic examination revealed axonal degeneration without evidence of demyelination (Fullerton and O'Sullivan, 1968). Quantitative studies have demonstrated selective loss of large-diameter nerve fibers with relative preservation of the small-fiber population. Others have found pathological changes in the dorsal root ganglion and posterior columns. Thalidomide neuropathy may not be reversible after dose reduction or drug withdrawal. Possible effects on the dorsal root ganglia and posterior columns have been cited as a reason for the incomplete reversibility of symptoms. While the neurotoxicity of thalidomide is a concern with its use in HIV-infected patients, placebo-controlled studies of HIV-associated aphthous ulcers have not demonstrated an increased incidence of peripheral neuropathy (Jacobson et al., 1997).

INH Neuropathy

Isoniazid (INH) is a principal component of antimicrobial therapy for tuberculosis. The neuropathy caused by INH in the absence of pyridoxine supplementation is a predominantly sensory, axonal neuropathy. Motor nerves are severely affected in rats (Blakemore, 1980), while sensory nerves are more affected in humans (Cavanagh, 1979).

INH produces a predominantly sensory neuropathy (Biehl and Skavlem, 1953; Gammon et al., 1953; Jones and Jones, 1953). Symptoms include paresthesias and numbness in a stocking-and-glove distribution, more severe in the distal lower extremities than in the upper extremities. INH neuropathy is dose dependent (Biehl and Nimitz , 1954) and, if untreated, may progress to include decreased proprioception, vibration sensation, and weakness.

INH neuropathy is due to its interference with pyridoxine metabolism. INH competitively inhibits the coenzymes derived from pyridoxine (Biehl and Vilter, 1954; Wiegand, 1956; Price et al., 1957), which in turn reduces the synthesis of several neurotransmitters, including serotonin and γ-aminobutyrate (Girling, 1982). Supplementation with pyridoxine prevents INH neuropathy. A low dose is recommended (10 to 50 mg/day), as pyridoxine may interfere with the antimicrobial activity of INH (Snider, 1980) and in high doses may in itself cause a neuropathy, as discussed below (Schaumburg et al., 1983; Nisar et al., 1990; A. R. Berger et al., 1992).

Pyridoxine Neuropathy

Pyridoxine is neurotoxic when given in doses above 200 mg/day. Clinical manifestations of pyridoxine neuropathy include sensory abnormalities, such as numbness and tingling in the toes, with similar but less intense sensations in the fingertips. These symptoms are often reversible, although a coasting period, during which they may intensify, can occur 2 to 3 weeks after discontinuation of the vitamin (A. R. Berger et al., 1992).

Pyridoxine has three interconvertible forms: pyridoxal phosphate, pyridoxine, and pyridoxamine. The sensory peripheral neuropathy that results from excess pyridoxine is thought to result from competitive inhibition of the more active form, pyridoxal phosphate, by the least active form, pyridoxine. The saturation of the activating enzymes results in paradoxical deficiency of pyridoxine (Nisar et al., 1990).

Ethambutol Neuropathy

Ethambutol is a bacteriostatic drug that is used as part of chemotherapy for tuberculosis. The distal, predominantly sensory neuropathy due to ethambutol is less common than optic neuropathy. Peripheral neuropathy has been reported in patients receiving ethambutol doses of 20 mg/kg or more. This complication, while rare, can be disabling (Tugwell and James, 1972) and may herald the onset of optic neuropathy (Nair et al., 1980). Ethambutol can aggravate or unmask the neurotoxicities of other drugs commonly used in combination (e.g., INH). Discontinuation of ethambutol in patients with peripheral neuropathy is generally followed by prompt improvement of symptoms.

Metronidazole Neuropathy

Metronidazole is used in the treatment of infections caused by anaerobes and protozoans. In animal experiments, metronidazole has mutagenic and teratogenic properties (Bradley et al., 1977). In humans, metronidazole is relatively safe. However, with prolonged use of metronidazole, peripheral neuropathy may occur (Coxon and Pallis, 1976; Dreger et al., 1998). Neuropathy has been reported with doses of 1.5 g/day or use of the drug for longer than 1 month (Duffy et al., 1985; Boyce et al., 1990; Learned-Coughlin, 1994). Symptoms include numbness and painful paresthesias and dysesthesias in a stocking-and-glove distribution. Examination reveals distal hypoalgesia or hypoesthesia, with normal muscle strength. Electrophysiologic findings include abnormal sural nerve action potential amplitude, with relatively normal motor conduction velocities.

Metronidazole neuropathy is generally reversible after withdrawal of the drug or dose reduction. The reported time course of improvement following drug withdrawal varies widely and ranges from 4 weeks to 2 years. Some patients have worsening of symptoms before improvement (Coxon and Pallis, 1976). Metronidazole binds to RNA in nerve cells (Bradley et al., 1977). Neuronal protein synthesis may be inhibited, and peripheral axonal degeneration may then result.

Dapsone Neuropathy

Dapsone is a sulfone antimicrobial agent used in prophylaxis for malaria and in the treatment of leprosy and other dermatologic disorders. In HIV-infected individuals, dapsone is used for prophylaxis for *Pneumocystis carinii* pneumonia in patients with sulfonamide intolerance (Medina et al., 1990). Its use can be limited by an infrequent occurrence of peripheral neuropathy. Unlike other toxic neuropathies, dapsone-induced peripheral neuropathy involves primarily motor nerves (Saqueton et al., 1969; Rapoport and Guss, 1972; Epstein and Bohm, 1976; Fredericks et al., 1976; Guttman et al., 1976; Koller et al., 1977; Navarro et al., 1989). It is manifested by progressive muscle weakness involving proximal and distal muscles of both upper and lower extremities, with less prominent sensory symptoms. The reported onset of symptoms ranges from 6 weeks to several years

after initiation of the drug, with total doses ranging from 4 g to 600 g. Electrophysiologic findings have demonstrated a motor axonopathy. Like most toxic neuropathies, withdrawal of the drug results in improvement of symptoms.

While the neurotoxicity of dapsone in humans appears to be dose dependent, high doses do not cause neuropathy in guinea pigs (Williams and Bradley, 1972). The mechanism of dapsone neurotoxicity is not known. While some believe it to be an idiosyncratic reaction, others have proposed a metabolic alteration, such as slow acetylation (Koller et al., 1977).

Vincristine Neuropathy

Vinca alkaloids are used as chemotherapy for AIDS-related lymphoma and Kaposi's sarcoma. Peripheral neurotoxicity is a major dose-limiting effect that occurs with a cumulative dose of 15 mg to 20 mg (Tuxen and Hansen, 1994). Of the three alkaloids vincristine, vinblastine, and vindesine, vincristine is the most neurotoxic. Manifestations include distal paresthesias, with reduced or absent ankle reflexes in early stages and objective sensory findings and motor weakness developing later. Cranial neuropathies and autonomic dysfunction may also occur (Legha, 1986; Macdonald, 1991; Tuxen and Hansen, 1994).

The mechanism of vincristine neurotoxicity has been linked to its antineoplastic activity. Vinca alkaloids bind to tubulin, which prevents their polymerization into microtubules, important components of the mitotic spindle. Interference with microtubules accounts for vincristine's antineoplastic activity. Since microtubules are essential for the maintenance of cell shape and axoplasmic transport, their disruption by vincristine may explain its neurotoxic effect (Sahen et al., 1987).

Treatment of Toxic Neuropathies

The first step in the management of neurotoxic neuropathy is identification of the offending drug and, if possible, its discontinuation. However, the decision to discontinue the drug should not be automatic. This is especially true with ARVs, for which this decision should be made only after careful weighing of benefits versus risks. At times, dose reduction without sacrificing virologic control is enough to alleviate symptoms. In cases where the choice of an ARV or an alternative drug is limited and substitution is not possible, symptomatic treatment with adequate pain control is necessary. Effective analgesia can usually be attained by following the World Health Organization's suggested ladder of stepwise pain control (Fig. 1). In step 1, patients receive nonopioid analgesics, such as acetaminophen or a nonsteroidal anti-inflammatory drug. If pain remains uncontrolled, the patient is advanced to step 2, in which a weak opioid, such as codeine, is used. Step 3 is for patients whose pain is not controlled by step 1 or 2 drugs. They are treated with a strong opioid, such as morphine. In each step, adjuvant medications are employed, together with the major analgesics. The adjuvant agents consist of tricyclic antidepressants (e.g., amytriptyline, nortriptyline) and anticonvulsants (e.g., lamotrigine, gabapentin). Desipramine and amitriptyline at doses of up to 150 mg/day can be used (Simpson and Tagliati, 1994, 1995). Carbamazepine and phenytoin have been reported to reduce neuropathic pain (Simpson and Tagliati, 1994, 1995). Lamotrigine provided significantly greater reduction in average pain than placebo particularly in those with d-drug neuropathy (Simpson et al., 2000, 2003). Gabapentin is an attractive therapy for painful

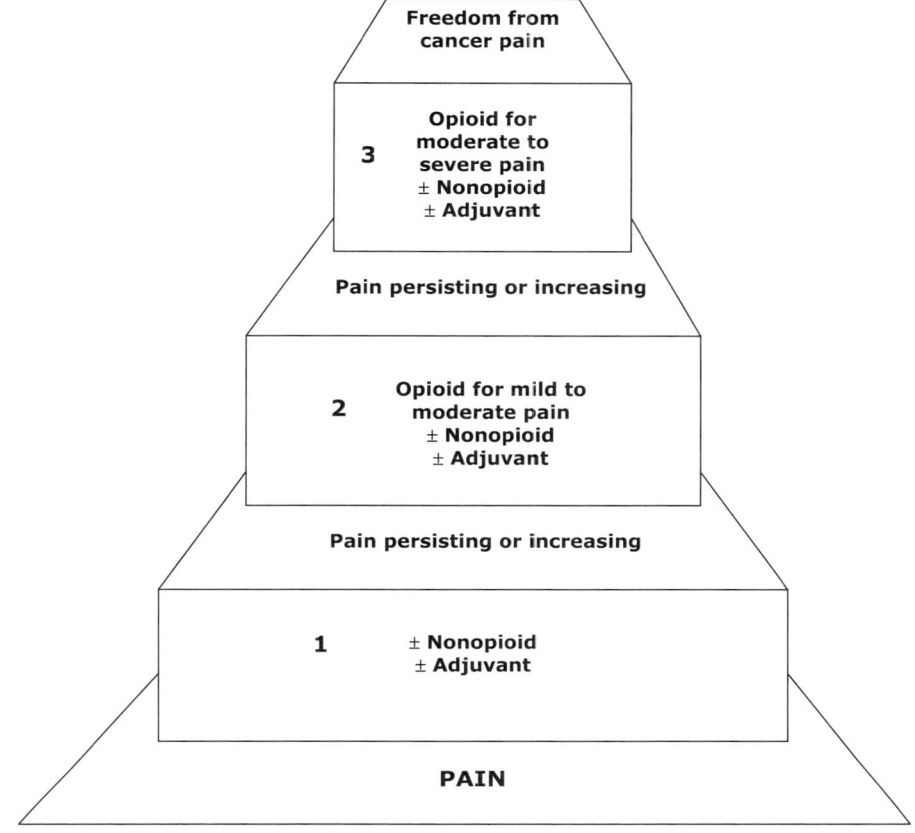

FIGURE 1   The WHO analgesic ladder (adapted from Simpson et al., 2000, with permission).

neuropathy due to its favorable pharmacokinetic profile and sparse drug-drug interactions (Mellick and Mellick, 1997; Rosner et al., 1996).

Non-DSP HIV Neuropathies

Inflammatory Demyelinating Polyneuropathy

In HIV-positive individuals, as in seronegative individuals, two major forms of inflammatory demyelinating polyneuropathy (IDP) occur. The acute type, with rapidly progressive ascending weakness, minor sensory symptoms, and generalized areflexia, is referred to as acute IDP (also called Guillain-Barré syndrome). The chronic, more slowly progressive monophasic or relapsing form is chronic IDP. A lymphocytic pleocytosis (10 to 50 cells/mm³) in the cerebrospinal fluid (CSF) in HIV-seropositive patients with IDP (Cornblath et al., 1987) helps to distinguish them from seronegative individuals. The presence of CSF lymphocytes at >5/mm³ in this setting should raise suspicion of undiagnosed HIV infection.

Electrophysiologic findings in HIV-related IDP are similar to those in non-HIV-infected patients. They include markedly decreased motor and sensory-nerve conduction velocity, conduction block, prolonged distal latencies, reduced compound muscle action potential amplitudes, reduced sensory-nerve action potential amplitudes, and reduced motor unit recruitment proportional to the degree of weakness.

The pathogenesis of IDP is likely immune mediated, particularly in patients early in the course of HIV infection with relatively high CD4 lymphocyte counts. In advanced patients with CD4 counts at <100/mm³, cytomegalovirus (CMV) infection may cause IDP. Other laboratory abnormalities in IDP include increased levels of soluble CD8 and neopterin in the CSF (Griffin et al., 1990) and anti-peripheral-nerve myelin antibody titers that parallel the course of the disease (Misha et al., 1985).

Nerve biopsy in patients with chronic IDP reveals inflammatory cell infiltrates and internodal demyelination (Cornblath et al., 1987). In mildly affected nerves, there is moderate subperineurial edema and small numbers of lymphocytes near endoneurial vessels. Within the endoneurial space, there is significant demyelination. In more severe cases, there is phagocyte-mediated myelin stripping (Cornblath et al., 1987) and axonal degeneration. In two cases of AIDS-associated IDP, CMV inclusions were detected in Schwann cells, implying a direct role of the virus (Morgello and Simpson, 1994).

Case series have shown a positive response of IDP to immunomodulating therapy, such as high-dose intravenous immunoglobulin infusion (0.5 mg to 1.0 mg/kg for 2 days) and plasmapheresis (four or five exchanges). However, rigorous controlled studies have not confirmed a therapeutic effect. In advanced HIV infection, antiviral therapy against CMV, such as ganciclovir, cidofovir, or foscarnet, may be indicated.

Mononeuropathy Multiplex

Mononeuropathy multiplex (MM) is an infrequent manifestation of HIV infection. MM is characterized clinically by the rapid onset of multifocal nerve abnormalities.

Distinguishing features include asymmetric distribution, with involvement of cutaneous nerves, mixed nerves, nerve roots, and cranial nerves. Tendon reflexes are preserved in uninvolved areas. The incidence of MM seems to be bimodal. The first peak occurs early in the course of HIV infection, when CD4 cell counts are above 200/mm^3, with a limited distribution of deficits. Facial nerve palsy is a common presentation of this form of MM. These deficits in early MM commonly resolve within several months with or without immunomodulating treatment. Pathological findings reveal axonal degeneration with epineural and endoneural perivascular inflammatory infiltrates. MM may also occur in advanced immunosuppression, with CD4 counts of 50/mm^3 or less. Extensive nerve involvement may rapidly progress to include multiple cranial nerves. This form of MM may appear similar to IDP or progressive polyradiculopathy (PP). Nerve biopsy revealed numerous polymorphonuclear infiltrates with mixed axonal and demyelinative lesions. In several patients with HIV-associated MM, CMV has been identified in peripheral nerve specimens with various assays (Said, 1991). Nerve biopsy has revealed evidence for necrotizing arteritis (Gherardi et al., 1989) and vasculitis in some patients with HIV-associated MM.

As in IDP, an autoimmune phenomenon is the proposed pathogenesis underlying MM that occurs early in HIV infection. Additional mechanisms may be involved in the late onset of MM, including herpes zoster (Engstrom et al., 1991; J. R. Berger et al., 1993), cryoglobulinemia (Stricker et al., 1992), cryptococcal meningitis (particularly in cranial neuropathies) (Engstrom et al., 1991), and CMV infection (Roullet et al., 1994).

Early MM may resolve spontaneously within several months (So and Olney, 1991). In cases of delayed or incomplete recovery, corticosteroids, plasmapheresis, or high-dose intravenous immunoglobulins may be indicated. In late-onset MM occurring in advanced HIV infection, empiric therapy for CMV should be considered.

Progressive Polyradiculopathy

PP occurs most commonly in advanced HIV infection, when CD4 cell counts drop below 50 cells/mm^3. PP is characterized clinically by the rapid onset of radicular pain and paresthesias in a cauda equina distribution, followed by signs of progressive involvement of multiple nerve roots, usually lumbar and sacral. Clinical signs include flaccid paraparesis, sphincter dysfunction, and lower-extremity areflexia. Occasional patients have associated myelopathic features (see chapter 4, this volume), leading to its occasional description as polyradiculomyelopathy or myeloradiculitis (Cohen et al., 1993; Anders and Goebel, 1998). While PP is usually a late manifestation of AIDS, it may be the presenting manifestation in rare cases (Anders and Goebel, 1998).

CSF findings in PP include marked polymorphonuclear neutrophilic pleocytosis (white blood cell count mean, 651 × 10^6 cells/liter, with 68% polymorphonuclear neutrophils), elevated protein (mean, 2.28 ± 1.78 g/dl), and hypoglycorrhachia (mean CSF glucose ratio, 0.48 ± 0.17) (Anders and Goebel, 1998). Electromyography reveals reduced numbers of motor units and abnormal spontaneous activity in weak muscles. Nerve conduction velocities are only mildly abnormal. The severe and widespread proximal axonal pathology in lumbar nerve root segments helps differentiate PP from MM or IDP.

PP is an inflammatory, necrotizing polyradiculitis most commonly involving the lumbosacral ventral and dorsal nerve roots, with less frequent thoracic cervical- and cranial-nerve pathology. Most reported autopsied cases of patients with PP have revealed nuclear and cytoplasmic cytomegalic inclusions within endothelial, Schwann, and ependymal cells that stained positively for CMV by immunohistochemistry and in situ hybridization (Eidelberg et al., 1986; de Gans et al., 1990; Miller et al., 1990). CMV detection by PCR analysis of CSF in PP has a sensitivity of 92% and a specificity of 94% (Gozlan et al., 1995; Shinkai and Spector, 1995; Vogel et al., 1996).

CMV is the major cause of PP in patients with AIDS, although less common causes include neurosyphilis (Lanska et al., 1988) and lymphomatous meningitis (Leger et al., 1992). Case series have reported improvement of CMV-associated PP with antiviral therapy for CMV. A prospective study evaluating treatment of AIDS-associated PP was suspended due to the marked reduction in the incidence of CMV disease in the current HAART era.

Autonomic Neuropathy

Early case studies reported clinical and laboratory evidence of autonomic impairment in HIV-infected patients (Freeman et al., 1990; Shahmanesh et al., 1991) (see chapter 5, this volume). Clinical findings include syncope, dizziness, orthostatic hypotension, diarrhea, decreased sweating, impotence, bladder dysfunction, resting tachycardia, and fatal arrhythmias (Craddock et al., 1987).

Autonomic neuropathy may be due to numerous causes, including drugs, such as tricyclic antidepressants, vincristine, and pentamidine. Malnutrition and dehydration may be contributory in later stages of disease. Rarely, patients with severe DSP may develop autonomic dysfunction.

Pathologic examination reveals abnormalities in several sites of the autonomic nervous system. Autonomic axons are depleted in small-bowel mucosa of HIV-infected patients (Batman et al., 1991). T-lymphocyte inflammatory infiltrates, ganglion nerve cell loss, and macrophages were noted in the sympathetic ganglia of autopsied cases (Chimelli and Scaravilli, 1991). Another study showed HIV antigens detected in macrophages in 50% of cases (Chimelli and Martins, 2002). A reduced number of oxytocin neurons in the paraventricular nucleus of the hypothalamus have also been described, although the clinical significance of this is unclear (Purba et al., 1993). This work suggested that the pathophysiological mechanism may be due to HIV infection itself as well as an autoimmune mechanism.

The management of autonomic neuropathy is mainly supportive. It includes recognition and discontinuation of offending medications, correction of fluid and electrolyte imbalance, use of compressive stockings and abdominal binders, liberal salt intake, and reconditioning exercises, as well as maneuvers such as squatting and standing with crossed legs. In severe cases, pharmacologic agents, such as fludricortisone, midodrine, and antiarrhythmic agents, may be needed.

SUMMARY

Peripheral neuropathy is the most common neurologic complication in HIV-infected individuals. It may arise from HIV itself or from medications used to treat HIV infection and other concomitant infections. Different forms of neuropathy may occur, such as MM, PP, and IDP. The most common, however, is DSP. Adequate pain control remains the mainstay in the management of neuropathy. Future studies need to address medications aimed at pathophysiological mechanisms.

REFERENCES

Alexander, L., and C. Wilcox. 1997. A prospective trial of thalidomide for the treatment of HIV-associated idiopathic esophageal ulcers. *AIDS Res. Hum. Retrovir.* **13:**301–304.

Anders, H, and F. Goebel. 1998. Cytomegalovirus polyradiculopathy in patients with AIDS. *Clin. Infect. Dis.* **27:**345–352.

Anderson, T., A. Davidoch, D. Feldman, T. Sprinkle, J. Arezzo, C. Brosnan, R. O. Calderon, L. H. Fossom, J. DeVries, and G. DeVries. 1994. Mitochondrial schwannopathy and peripheral myelinopathy in a rabbit model of dideoxycytidine neurotoxicity. *Lab. Investig.* **70:**724–739.

Anderson, T. D., A. Davidovich, R. Arceo, C. Brosnan, J. Arezzo, and H. Schaumburg. 1992. Peripheral neuropathy induced by 2′,3′-dideoxycytidine. A rabbit model of 2′,3′-dideoxycytidine neurotoxicity. *Lab. Investig.* **66:**63–74.

Angelucci, L., M. Ramacci, G. Taglialatela, C. Hulsebosch, B. Morgan, K. Werrbach-Perez, and R. Perez-Polo. 1988. Nerve growth factor binding in aged rat central nervous system: effect of acetyl-L-carnitine. *J. Neurosci. Res.* **20:**491–496.

Bacellar, H., A. Munoz, E. N. Miller, B. A. Cohen, D. Besley, O. A. Selnes, J. T. Becker, and J. C. McArthur. 1994. Temporal trends in the incidence of HIV-1-related neurologic diseases: multicenter AIDS cohort study, 1985–1992. *Neurology* **44:**1892–1900.

Balzarini, J., P. Herdewlin, and E. De Clercq. 1989. Differential patterns of intracellular metabolism of 2′3′-dideoxythymidine and 3′-azido-2′3′-dideoxythymidine, two potent anti-human immunodeficiency virus compounds. *J. Biol. Chem.* **264:**6127–6133.

Batman, P. A., A. R. Miller, P. M. Sedgwick, and G. E. Griffin. 1991. Autonomic denervation in jejunal mucosa of homosexual men infected with HIV. *AIDS* **5:**1247–1252.

Berger, A. R., J. C. Arezzo, H. H. Schaumburg, G. Skowron, T. Merigan, S. Bozzette, D. Richman, and W. Soo. 1993. Dideoxycytidine (ddC) toxic neuropathy: a study of 52 patients. *Neurology* **43:**358–362.

Berger, A. R., H. H. Schaumburg, C. Schroeder, S. Apfel, and R. Reynolds. 1992. Dose response, coasting, and differential fiber vulnerability in human toxic neuropathy: a prospective study of pyridoxine neurotoxicity. *Neurology* **42:**1367–1370.

Berger, J. R., M. Flaster, N. Schatz, D. Droller, P. Benedetto, R. Poblete, and M. J. Post. 1993. Cranial neuropathy heralding otherwise occult AIDS-related large cell lymphoma. *J. Clin. Neurophysiol.* **13:**113–118.

Biehl, J., and H. Nimitz. 1954. Studies on the use of a high dose of isoniazid. *Am. Rev. Tuberc.* **70:**430–444.

Biehl, J., and J. Skavlem. 1953. Toxicity of isoniazid. *Am. Rev. Tuberc.* **68:**296–297.

Biehl, J., and R. Vilter. 1954. Effect of isonazid on vitamin B_{12} metabolism, its possible significance in producing isoniazid neuritis. *Proc. Soc. Exp. Biol. Med.* **85:**389–395.

Blakemore, W. 1980. Isoniazid, p. 476–489. *In* P. Spencer, and H. Schaumburg (ed.), *Experimental and Clinical Neurotoxicology.* Williams & Wilkins, Baltimore, MD.

Boyce, E., E. Cookson, and W. Bond. 1990. Persistent metronidazole-induced peripheral neuropathy. *Ann. Pharmacother.* **24:**19–21.

Bradley, W., I. Karlsson, and C. Rassol. 1977. Metronidazole neuropathy. *Br. Med. J.* **2:**610–611.

Brew, B., S. Tisch, and M. Law. 2003. Lactate concentrations distinguish between nucleoside neuropathy and HIV neuropathy. *AIDS* **17:**1094–1096.

Browne, M., K. Mayer, and S. Chafee. 1993. Didehydro-3′-deoxythymidine (d4T) in patients with AIDS or AIDS-related complex: a phase I trial. *J. Infect. Dis.* **167:**21–29.

Calabrese, L., and A. Fleischer, Jr. 2000. Thalidomide: current and potential clinical applications. *Am. J. Med.* **108:**487–495.

Cavanagh, J. 1979. The "dying back" process, a common denominator in many naturally occurring and toxic neuropathies. *Arch. Pathol. Lab. Med.* **193:**659–664.

Chen, C. H., and Y. C. Cheng. 1989. Delayed cytotoxicity and selective loss of mitochondrial DNA in cells treated with the anti-human immunodeficiency virus compound 2′3′-dideoxycytidine. *J. Biol. Chem.* **264:**11934–11937.

Childs, E. A., R. H. Lyles, O. A. Selnes, B. Chen, E. N. Miller, B. A. Cohen, J. T. Becker, J. Mellors, and J. C. McArthur. 1999. Plasma viral load and CD4 lymphocytes predict HIV-associated peripheral neuropathy. *Neurology* **52:**607–613.

Chimelli, L., and A. R. Martins. 2002. Degenerative and inflammatory lesions in sympathetic ganglia: further morphologic evidence for an autonomic neuropathy in AIDS. *J. Neuro-AIDS* **2:**67–82.

Chimelli, L., and F. Scaravilli. 1991. Morphological changes in the autonomic nervous system of patients with AIDS, p. 89. *Proc. Seventh Int. Conf. Neurosci. HIV Infect.* Padova, Italy.

Cohen, B. A., J. C. McArthur, S. Grohman, B. Patterson, and J. D. Glass. 1993. Neurologic prognosis of cytomegalovirus polyradiculomyelopathy in AIDS. *Neurology* **43:**493–499.

Colucci, W., and R. Gandour. 1988. Carnitine acetyltransferase: a review of its biology, enzymology and bioorganic chemistry. *Bioorg. Chem.* **16:**307–334.

Cooley, T. P., L. M. Kunche, C. A. Saunders, J. K. Ritter, C. J. Perkins, C. McLaren, R. P. McCaffrey, and H. A. Liebman. 1990. Once-daily administration of 2′3′ dideoxyinosine (ddI) in patients with the acquired immunodeficiency syndrome or AIDS-related complex. *N. Engl. J. Med.* **322:**1340–1345.

Cooney, D. A., M. Dalal, H. Mitsuya, J. B. McMahon, M. Nadkarni, J. Balzarini, S. Broder, and D. G. Johns. 1986. Initial studies on the cellular pharmacology of 2′3′-dideoxycytidine, an inhibitor of HTLV-III infectivity. *Biochem. Pharmacol.* **35:**2065–2068.

Cornblath, D., and J. McArthur. 1988. Predominantly sensory neuropathy in patients with AIDS and AIDS-related complex. *Neurology* **38:**794–796.

Cornblath, D. R., J. C. McArthur, P. G. Kennedy, A. S. Witte, and J. W. Griffin. 1987. Inflammatory demyelinating peripheral neuropathies associated with human T-cell lymphotropic virus type III infection. *Ann. Neurol.* **21:**32–40.

Cote, H., B. Brumme, K. Craib, M. Math, C. Alexander, B. Wynhoven, L. Ting, H. Wong, M. Harris, R. Harrigan, M. O'Shaughnessy, and J. Montaner. 2002. Changes in mitochondrial DNA as a marker of nucleoside toxicity in HIV-infected patients. *N. Engl. J. Med.* **346:**811–820.

Coxon, A., and C. Pallis. 1976. Metronidazole neuropathy. *J. Neurol. Neurosurg. Psychiatry* **39:**403–405.

Craddock, C., G. Pasvol, R. Bull, A. Protheroe, and J. Hopkin. 1987. Cardiorespiratory arrest and autonomic neuropathy in acquired immunodeficiency syndrome. *Lancet* **ii:**16–18.

Cui, L., L. Locatelli, M. Y. Xie, and J. P. Sommadossi. 1997. Effect of nucleoside analogs on neurite regeneration and mitochondrial DNA synthesis in PC-12 cells. *J. Pharmacol. Exp. Ther.* **280:**1228–1234.

Dalakas, M., C. Semino-Mora, and M. Leon-Monzon. 2001. Mitochondrial alterations with mitochondrial DNA depetion in the nerves of AIDS patients with peripheral neuropathy induced by 2′3′-dideoxycytidine (ddC). *Lab. Investig.* **81:**1537–1544.

de Gans, J., P. Portegies, G. Tiessens, D. Troost, S. A. Danner, and J. M. Lange. 1990. Therapy for cytomegalovirus polyradiculopathy in patients with AIDS: treatment with ganciclovir. *AIDS* **4:**421–425.

Dreger, L. M., P. P. Gleason, T. K. Chowdhry, and D. J. Gazzuolo. 1998. Intermittent-dose metronidazole-induced peripheral neuropathy. Ann. Pharmacother. 32:267–268.

Dube, M. 2000. Disorders of glucose metabolism in patients infected with human immunodeficiency virus. Clin. Infect. Dis. 31:1467–1475.

Dubinsky, R. M., R. Yarchoan, M. Dalakas, and S. Broder. 1989. Reversible axonal neuropathy from the treatment of AIDS and related disorders with 2'3'-dideoxycytidine (ddC). Muscle Nerve 12:856–860.

Duffy, L. F., F. Daum, S. E. Fisher, J. Selman, S. M. Vishnubhakat, H. W. Aiges, J. F. Markowitz, and M. Silverberg. 1985. Peripheral neuropathy in Crohn's disease. Patients treated with metronidazole. Gastroenterology 88:681–684.

Eidelberg, D., A. Sotrel, H. Vogel, P. Walker, J. Kleefield, and C. S. Crumpacker III. 1986. Progressive polyradiculopathy in acquired immune deficiency syndrome. Neurology 36:912–916.

Engstrom, J., E. Lewis, and D. McGuire. 1991. Cranial neuropathy and the acquired immunodeficiency syndrome. Neurology 41(Suppl. 1):S374.

Epstein, F., and M. Bohm. 1976. Dapsone-induced peripheral neuropathy. Arch. Dermatol. 112:1761–1762.

Famularo, G., S. Moretti, S. Marcellini, V. Trinchieri, S. Tzantzoglou, G. Santini, A. Longo, and C. De Simone. 1997. Acetyl-carnitine deficiency in AIDS patients with neurotoxicity on treatment with antiretroviral nucleoside analogues. AIDS 11:185–190.

Fichtenbaum, C., D. Clifford, and W. Powderly. 1995. Risk factors for dideoxynucleoside-induced toxic neuropathy in patients with the human immunodeficiency virus infection. J. Acquir. Immune Defic. Syndr. Hum Retrovirol. 10:169–174.

Fischl, M., R. Olson, and S. Follansbee. 1993. Zalcitabine compared with zidovudine in patients with advanced HIV-1 infection who received previous zidovudine therapy. Ann. Intern. Med. 118:762–769.

Fredericks, E., R. Kugelman, and N. Kirsch. 1976. Dapsone-induced motor polyneuropathy. Arch. Dermatol. 112:1158–1160.

Freeman, R., M. S. Roberts, L. S. Friedman, and C. Broadbridge. 1990. Autonomic function and human immunodeficiency virus infection. Neurology 40:575–80.

Fullerton, P., and D. O'Sullivan. 1968. Thalidomide neuropathy: a clinical, electrophysiological, and histological follow-up study. J. Neurol. Neurosurg. Psychiatry 31:543–551.

Gammon, G., F. Burge, and G. King. 1953. Neural toxicity in tuberculous patients treated with isoniazid (isonicotinic acid hydrazide). Am. Med. Assoc. Arch. Neurol. Psychiatry 70:64–69.

Gasnault, J., C. Pinganaud, and P. Kousignian. 1999. Subacute ascendant neuropathy revealing a nucleoside-induced mitochondrial cytopathy. Presented at the Seventh European Conference on Clinical Aspects and Treatment of HIV Infection, 23–27 October 1999, Lisbon, Portugal.

Gherardi, R., F. Lebargy, P. Gaulard, C. Mhiri, J. F. Bernaudin, and F. Gray. 1989. Necrotizing vasculitis and HIV replication in peripheral nerves. N. Engl. J. Med. 321:685–686.

Girling, D. 1982. Adverse effects of antituberculosis drugs. Drugs 23:56–74.

Gozlan, J., M. el Amrani, M. Baudrimont, D. Costagliola, J. M. Salord, C. Duvivier, O. Picard, M. C. Meyohas, C. Jacomet, V. Schneider-Fauveau, J.-C. Petit, and E. Roullet. 1995. A prospective evaluation of clinical criteria and polymerase chain reaction assay of cerebrospinal fluid for the diagnosis of cytomeglovirus-related neurological diseases during AIDS. AIDS 9:253–260.

Griffin, D., J. McArthur, and D. Cornblath. 1990. Soluble interleukin-2 receptor and soluble CD8 in serum and cerebrospinal fluid during human immunodeficiency virus-associated neurologic disease. J. Neuroimmunol. 28:97–109.

Grinspan, D. 1985. Significant response of oral aphthosis to thalidomide treatment. J. Am. Acad. Dermatol. 12:85–90.

Guttman, L., J. Martin, and W. Welton. 1976. Dapsone motor neuropathy—an axonal disease. Neurology 26:514–516.

Hamuryudan, V., C. Mat, S. Saip, Y. Ozyazgan, A. Siva, S. Yurdakul, K. Zwingenberger, and H. Yazici. 1998. Thalidomide in the treatment of the mucocutaneous lesions of Behcet's syndrome: a randomized, double-blind, placebo controlled trial. Ann. Intern. Med. 128:443–459.

Jacobson, J. M., J. S. Greenspan, J. Spritzler, N. Ketter, J. L. Fahey, J. B. Jackson, L. Fox, M. Chernoff, A. W. Wu, L. A. MacPhail, G. J. Vasquez, and D. A. Wohl. 1997. Thalidomide for the treatment of oral aphthous ulcers in patients with human immunodeficiency virus infection. N. Engl. J. Med. 336:1487–1493.

Jones, W., and G. Jones. 1953. Peripheral neuropathy due to isoniazid. Report of two cases. Lancet i:1073–1074.

Kahn, J. O., S. W. Lagakos, D. D. Richman, A. Cross, C. Pettinelli, S. H. Liou, M. Brown, P. A. Volberding, C. S. Crumpacker, and G. Beall. 1992. A controlled trial comparing continued zidovudine with didanosine in human immunodeficiency virus infection. N. Engl. J. Med. 327:581–587.

Kaplan, G., M. Schambelan, M. Gottlieb, et al. 1998. Thalidomide reverses cachexia in HIV-wasting syndrome, abstr. 476, p. 59. Program and Abstracts of the 5th Conf. Retrovir. Opportunistic Infect. (Chicago). Foundation for Retrovirology and Human Health, Alexandria, VA.

Keswani, S., B. Chander, C. Hasan, J. Griffin, J. McArthur, and A. Hoke. 2003. FK506 is neuroprotective in a model of antiretroviral toxic neuropathy. Ann. Neurol. 53:57–64.

Keswani, S. C., C. A. Pardo, C. L. Cherry, A. Hoke, and J. C. McArthur. 2002. HIV-associated sensory neuropathies. AIDS 16:2105–2117.

Kieburtz, K., M. Seidlin, and J. Lambert. 1992. Extended follow-up of peripheral neuropathy in patients with AIDS and AIDS-related complex treated with dideoxyinosine. J. Acquir. Immune Defic. Syndr. 5:60–64.

Kieburtz, K., D. Simpson, C. Yiannoutsos, M. B. Max, C. D. Hall, R. J. Ellis, C. M. Marra, R. McKendall, E. Singer, G. J. Dal Pan, D. B. Clifford, T. Tucker, B. Cohen, and the AIDS Clinical Trials Group 242 Protocol Team. 1998. A randomized trial of amitriptyline and mexiletine for painful neuropathy in HIV infection. Neurology 51:1682–1688.

Knop, J., G. Bonsmann, R. Happle, A. Ludolph, D. R. Matz, E. J. Mifsud, and E. Macher. 1983. Thalidomide in the treatment of sixty cases of chronic discoid lupus erythematosus. Br. J. Dermatol. 108:461–466.

Koller, W. C., L. K. Gehlmann, F. D. Malkinson, and F. A. Davis. 1977. Dapsone-induced peripheral neuropathy. Arch. Neurol. 34:644–646.

Lambert, J. S., M. Seidlin, R. C. Reichman, C. S. Plank, M. Laverty, G. D. Morse, C. Knupp, C. McLaren, and C. Pettinelli. 1990. Dideoxyinosine (ddI) in patients with the acquired immunodeficiency syndrome or AIDS-related complex. N. Engl. J. Med. 322:1333–1340.

Lanska, M., D. Lanska, and J. Schmidley. 1988. Syphilitic polyradiculopathy in an HIV-positive man. Neurology 38:1297–1301.

Learned-Coughlin, S. 1994. Peripheral neuropathy induced by metronidazole. Ann. Pharmacother. 28:536. (Letter.)

Leger, J. M., P. Bouche, F. Bolgert, M. P. Chaunu, M. Rosenheim, H. P. Cathala, M. Gentilini, J. J. Hauw, and P. Brunet. 1989. The spectrum of polyneuropathies in patients infected with HIV. J. Neurol. Neurosurg. Psychiatry 52:1369–1374.

Leger, J. M., D. Henin, L. Belec, B. Mercier, L. Cohen, P. Bouche, J. J. Hauw, and P. Brunet. 1992. Lymphoma-induced polyradiculopathy in AIDS: 2 cases. *J. Neurol.* **239:** 132–134.

Legha, S. 1986. Vincristine neurotoxicity: pathophysiology and management. *Med. Toxicol.* **1:**421–427.

Lewis, W., C. Haase, S. Raidel, R. Russ, R. Sutliff, B. Hoit, and A. Samarel. 2001. Combined antiretroviral therapy causes cardiomyopathy and elevates plasma lactate in transgenic AIDS mice. *Lab. Investig.* **81:**1527–1536.

Macdonald, D. 1991. Neurologic complications of chemotherapy. *Neurol. Clin.* **9:**955–967.

Markus, R., and B. J. Brew. 1998. HIV-1 peripheral neuropathy and combination antiretroviral therapy. *Lancet* **352:**1906–1907. (Letter.)

Martin, J. L., C. E. Brown, N. Matthews-Davis, and J. E. Reardon. 1994. Effects of antiviral nucleoside analogs on human DNA polymerases and mitochondrial DNA synthesis. *Antimicrob. Agents Chemother.* **38:**2743–2749.

McArthur, J. C., C. Yiannoutsos, D. Simpson, B. T. Adornato, E. J. Singer, H. Hollander, C. Marra, M. Rubin, B. A. Cohen, T. Trucker, B. A. Navia, G. Schifitto, D. Katzenstein, C. Rask, L. Zaborski, M. E. Smith, S. Shriver, L. Millar, D. B. Clifford, and the AIDS Clinical Trials Group Team 291. 2000. A phase II trial of nerve growth factor for sensory neuropathy associated with HIV infection. *Neurology* **54:**1080–1088.

Medina, I., J. Mills, and G. Leoung. 1990. Oral therapy for *Pneumocystis carinii* pneumonia in the acquired immunodeficiency syndrome: a controlled trial of trimethoprim-sulfamethoxazole versus trimethoprim-dapsone. *N. Engl. J. Med.* **323:**776–782.

Mellick, G., and L. Mellick. 1997. Reflex sympathetic dystrophy treated with gabapentin. *Arch. Phys. Med. Rehab.* **78:**89–105.

Meng, T., M. Fischl, and A. Boota. 1992. Combination therapy with zidovudine and dieoxycytidine in patients with advanced human immunodeficiency virus infection: a phase I/II study. *Ann. Intern. Med.* **116:**13–20.

Merigan, T. C., G. Skowron, S. A. Bozzette, D. Richman, R. Uttamchandani, M. Fischl, R. Schooley, M. Hirsch, W. Soo, and C. Pettinelli. 1989. Circulating p24 antigen levels and responses to dideoxycytidine in human immunodeficinecy virus (HIV) infections. *Ann. Intern. Med.* **110:**189–194.

Miller, R., J. Storey, and C. Greco. 1990. Ganciclovir in the treatment of progressive AIDS-related polyradiculopathy. *Neurology* **1990:**569–574.

Misha, B., W. Sommers, C. Koski, et al. 1985. Acute inflammatory demyelinating polyneuropathy in the acquired immunodeficiency syndrome. (Abstract.) *Ann. Neurol.* **18:**131–132.

Morgello, S., and D. Simpson. 1994. Multifocal cytomegalovirus demyelinative polyneuropathy associated with AIDS. *Muscle Nerve* **17:**176–182.

Morgello, S., L. Estanislao, D. Simpson, A. Geraci, A. DiRocco, P. Gerits, E. Ryan, T. Yakoushina, S. Khan, R. Mahboob, M. Naseer, D. Dorfman, V. Sharp, and the Manhattan HIV Brain Bank. 2004. HIV-associated distal sensory polyneuropathy in the era of highly active antiretroviral therapy: *Arch. Neurol.* **61:**546–551.

Moyle, G. J., and M. Sadler. 1998. Peripheral neuropathy with nucleoside antiretrovirals: risk factors, incidence and management. *Drug Saf.* **19:**481–494.

Nair, V., M. LeBrun, and I. Kass. 1980. Peripheral neuropathy associated with ethambutol. *Chest* **77:**98–100.

Navarro, J. C., R. L. Rosales, A. T. Ordinario, S. Izumo, and M. Osame. 1989. Acute dapsone-induced peripheral neuropathy. *Muscle Nerve* **12:**604–606.

Nisar, M., S. W. Watkin, R. C. Bucknall, and R. A. Agnew. 1990. Exacerbation of isoniazid induced peripheral neuropathy by pyridoxine. *Thorax* **45:**419–420.

Patterson, T., L. Schmued, J. Sandberg, and J. W. Slikker. 2000. Temporal development of 2',3'-dideoxyinosine (ddI)-induced peripheral myelinopathy. *Neurotoxicol. Teratol.* **22:** 429–434.

Pezeshkpour, G., C. Krarup, F. Buchthal, S. DiMauro, N. Bresolin, and J. McBurney. 1987. Peripheral neuropathy in mitochondrial disease. *J. Neurol. Sci.* **77:**285–304.

Price, J., R. Brown, and F. Larson. 1957. Quantitative studies on human urinary metabolites of tryptophan as affected by isoniazid and deoxypyridoxine. *J. Clin. Investig.* **36:**1600–1607.

Purba, J. S., M. A. Hofman, P. Portegies, D. Troost, and D. F. Swaab. 1993. Decreased number of oxytocin neurons in the paraventricular nucleus of the human hypothalamus in AIDS. *Brain* **116:**795–805.

Quinones, F., J. Sierra-Madero, J. J. Calva-Mercado, G. M. Ruiz-Palacios, and Instituto Nacional de Nutricion, Mexico City. 1997. Thalidomide in patients with HIV infection, and chronic diarrhea: double-blind placebo controlled clinical trial, abstr. 682. *Fourth Conf. Retrovir. Opportunistic Infect.*, Washington, DC.

Rapoport, A., and S. Guss. 1972. Dapsone-induced peripheral neuropathy. *Arch. Neurol.* **27:**184–185.

Rathburn, R., and E. I. Martin. 1992. Didanosine therapy in patients intolerant of or failing zidovudine therapy. *Ann. Pharmacother.* **2:**1347–1351.

Reyes-Teran, G., J. G. Sierra-Madero, V. Martinez del Cerro, H. Arroyo-Figueroa, A. Pasquetti, J. J. Calva, and G. M. Ruiz-Palacios. 1996. Effects of thalidomide on HIV-associated wasting syndrome: a randomized, double-blind, placebo-controlled clinical trial. *AIDS* **10:**1501–1507.

Richardson, J. K., and E. A. Hurvitz. 1995. Peripheral neuropathy: a true risk factor for falls. *J. Gerontol.* **50:**M211–M215.

Rosner, H., L. Rubin, and A. Kestenbaum. 1996. Gabapentin adjunctive therapy in neuropathic pain states. *Clin. J. Pain* **12:**56–58.

Roullet, E., V. Assuerus, J. Gozlan, A. Ropert, G. Said, M. Baudrimont, M. el Amrani, C. Jacomet, C. Duvivier, G. Gonzales-Canali, M. Kirstetter, M.-C. Meyohas, O. Picard, and W. Rozenbaum. 1994. Cytomegalovirus multifocal neuropathy in AIDS: analysis of 15 consecutive cases. *Neurology* **44:**2174–2182.

Rozencweig, M., C. McLaren, M. Beltangady, J. Ritter, R. Canetta, L. Schacter, S. Kelley, C. Nicaise, L. Smaldone, L. Dunkle, C. Barbhaiya, C. Knupp, A. Cross, M. Tsianco, and R. R. Martin. 1990. Overview of phase I trials of 2'3'-dideoxyinosine (ddI) conducted on adult patients. *Rev. Infect. Dis.* **12**(Suppl5):S570–S575.

Sahen, S., S. Brady, and J. Mendell. 1987. Studies on the pathogenesis of vincristine-induced neuropathy. *Muscle Nerve* **10:**80–84.

Said, C. 1991. Multifocal neuropathy in HIV infection, p. 89. *Proc. Seventh Int. Conf. HIV Infect*, Padova, Italy.

Saqueton, A. C., A. L. Lorincz, N. A. Vick, and R. D. Hamer. 1969. Dapsone and peripheral motor neuropathy. *Arch. Dermatol.* **100:**214–217.

Schaumburg, H., J. Kaplan, and A. Windebank. 1983. Sensory neuropathy from pyridoxine abuse. *N. Engl. J. Med.* **309:**445–448.

Schifitto, G., M. McDermott, J. McArthur, K. Marder, N. Sacktor, L. Epstein, and K. Kieburtz. 2002. Incidence of and risk factors for HIV-associated distal sensory polyneuropathy. *Neurology* **58:**1764–1768.

Shahmanesh, M., C. S. Bradbeer, A. Edwards, and S. E. Smith. 1991. Autonomic dysfunction in patients with human immunodeficiency virus infection. *Int. J. STD AIDS* **2:**419–423.

Sharpstone, D., A. Rowbottom, M. Nelson, and B. Gazzard. 1995. The treatment of microsporidial diarrhea with thalidomide. *AIDS* **9:**658–659.

Shinkai, M., and S. Spector. 1995. Quantitation of human cytomegalovirus (HCMV) DNA in cerebrospinal fluid by competitive PCR in AIDS patiets with different HCMV central nervous system diseases. *Scand. J. Infect. Dis.* **27:** 559–561.

Simpson, D., and M. Tagliati. 1994. Neurological manifestations of HIV infection. *Ann. Intern. Med.* **121:**769–785.

Simpson, D., and M. Tagliati. 1995. Nucleoside analogue-associated peripheral neuropathy in HIV infection. *J. Acquir. Immune Defic. Syndr.* **9:**153–161.

Simpson, D. M., D. A. Katzenstein, M. D. Hughes, S. M. Hammer, D. L. Williamson, Q. Jiang, and J. T. Pi. 1998. Neuromuscular function in HIV infection: analysis of a placebo-controlled combination antiretroviral trial. *AIDS* **12:**2425–2432.

Simpson, D. M., R. Olney, J. C. McArthur, A. Khan, J. Godbold, and K. Ebel-Frommer. 2000. A placebo-controlled trial of lamotrigine for painful HIV-associated neuropathy. *Neurology* **54:**2115–2119.

Simpson, D. M., D. Kitch, S. R. Evans, J. C. McArthur, D. M. Asmuth, B. Cohen, K. Goodkin, M. Gerschenson, Y. So, C. M. Marra, R. Diaz-Arrastia, S. Shriver, L. Millar, D. B. Clifford, and the ACTG A5117 Study Group. 2006. HIV neuropathy natural history cohort study: assessment measures and risk factors. *Neurology* **66:**1679–1687.

Simpson, D. M., J. C. McArthur, R. Olney, D. Clifford, Y. So, D. Ross, B. J. Baird, P. Barrett, A. E. Hammer, and the Lamotrigine HIV Neuropathy Study Team. 2003. Lamotrigine for HIV-associated painful sensory neuropathies: a placebo-controlled trial. *Neurology* **60:**1508–1514.

Skowron, G., S. A. Bozzette, L. Lim, C. B. Pettinelli, H. H. Schaumburg, J. Arezzo, M. A. Fischl, W. G. Powderly, D. J. Gocke, D. D. Richman, J. C. Pottage, D. Antoniskis, G. F. McKinley, N. E. Hyslop, G. Ray, G. Simon, N. Reed, M. L. LoFaro, R. B. Uttamchandani, L. D. Gelb, S. J. Sperber, R. L. Murphy, J. M. Leedom, M. H. Grieco, J. Zachary, M. S. Hirsch, S. A. Spector, J. Bigley, W. Soo, and T. C. Merigan. 1993. Alternating and intermittent regimens of zidovudine and dideoxycytidine in patients with AIDS or AIDS-related complex. *Ann. Intern. Med.* **118:**321–330.

Snider, D. 1980. Pyridoxine supplementation during isoniazid therapy. *Tubercle* **61:**191–196.

Snider, W. D., D. M. Simpson, S. Nielsen, J. W. Gold, C. E. Metroka, and J. B. Posner. 1983. Neurological complications of acquired immunodeficiency syndrome: analysis of 50 patients. *Ann. Neurol.* **14:**403–418.

So, Y., D. Holtzman, and D. Abrams. 1988. Peripheral neuropathy associated with acquired immunodeficiency syndrome: prevalence and clinical features from a population-based survey. *Arch. Neurol.* **45:**945–948.

So, Y., and R. Olney. 1991. The natural history of mononeuritis multiplex and simplex in HIV infection. *Neurology* **41**(Suppl. 1):375.

Steiberg, J., G. C. J., R. White, A. M. Morris, and the AIDS Research Consortium of Atlanta. 1991. Outcomes and toxicities on 2'3'-dideoxyinosine (ddI) in the expanded access program, abstr. 707. *Proc. 31st Intersci. Conf. Antimicrob. Agents Chemother.* American Society for Microbiology, Washington, DC.

Stricker, R. B., K. A. Sanders, W. F. Owen, D. D. Kiprov, and R. G. Miller. 1992. Mononeuritis multiplex associated with cryoglobulinemia in HIV infection. *Neurology* **42:**2103–2105.

Tagliati, M., J. Grinnell, J. Godbold, and D. M. Simpson. 1999. Peripheral nerve function in HIV infection. Clinical, elctrophysiologic and laboratory findings. *Arch. Neurol.* **56:**84–89.

Tseng, S., G. Pak, K. Washenik, M. K. Pomeranz, and J. L. Shupack. 1996. Rediscovering thalidomide: a review of its mechanism of action, side effects, and potential uses. *J. Am. Acad. Dermatol.* **35:**969–979.

Tugwell, P., and S. James. 1972. Peripheral neuropathy with ethambutol. *Postgrad. Med. J.* **48:**667–670.

Tuxen, M., and S. Hansen. 1994. Neurotoxicity secondary to antineoplastic drugs. *Cancer Treat. Rev.* **20:**191–214.

van den Broek, H. 1980. Treatment of prurigo nodularis with thalidomide. *Arch. Dermatol.* **116:**571–572.

Vogel, J. U., J. Cinatl, A. Lux, B. Weber, A. J. Driesel, and H. W. Doerr. 1996. New PCR assay for rapid and quantitative detection of human cytomegalovirus in cerebrospinal fluid. *J. Clin. Microbiol.* **34:**482–483.

Vogelsang, G. B., E. R. Farmer, A. D. Hess, V. Altamonte, W. E. Beschorner, D. A. Jabs, R. L. Corio, L. S. Levin, O. M. Colvin, and J. R. Wingard. 1992. Thalidomide for the treatment of chronic graft-versus-host disease. *N. Engl. J. Med.* **326:**1055–1058.

Warner, W., C. Bregman, C. Comereski, J. Arezzo, T. Davidson, C. Knupp, S. Kaul, S. Durham, A. Wasserman, and J. Frantz. 1995. Didanosine (ddI) and stavudine (d4T): absence of peripheral neurotoxicity in rabbits. *Food Chem. Toxicol.* **33:**1047–1050.

Wiegand, R. 1956. The formation of pyridoxal and pyridoxal 5-phosphate hydrazones. *J. Am. Chem. Soc.* **78:**5307–5309.

Williams, M., and W. Bradley. 1972. An assessment of dapsone toxicity in the guinea pig. *Br. J. Dermatol.* **86:**650.

Yarchoan, R., C. F. Perno, R. V. Thomas, R. W. Klecker, J. P. Allain, R. J. Wills, N. McAtee, M. A. Fischl, R. Dubinsky, M. C. McNeely, H. Mitsuya, J. M. Pluda, T. J. Lawley, M. Leuther, B. Satai, J. M. Collins, C. E. Myers, and S. Broder. 1988. Phase I studies of 2'3'-deoxycytidine in severe human immunodeficiency virus infection as a single agent and alternating with zidovudine. *Lancet* **i:** 76–81.

Yarchoan, R., J. Pluda, and R. Thomas. 1990. Long term toxicity/activity profile of 2'3'-dideoxyinosine in AIDS or AIDS-related complex. *Lancet* **336:**526–529.

Zhou, L., D. W. Kitch, S. R. Evans, P. Hauer, S. Raman, G. J. Ebenezer, M. Gerschenson, C. M. Marra, V. Valcour, R. Diaz-Arrastia, K. Goodkin, L. Millar, S. Shriver, D. M. Asmuth, D. B. Clifford, D. M. Simpson, and J. C. McArthur. 2007. Correlates of epidermal nerve fiber densities in HIV-associated distal sensory polyneuropathy. *Neurology* **68:**2113–2119.

The Spectrum of Neuro-AIDS Disorders:
Pathophysiology, Diagnosis, and Treatment
Edited by K. Goodkin et al.
©2008 ASM Press, Washington, DC

7

Mitochondrial Dysfunction and Lactic Acidosis in HIV Disease

ASHOK VERMA AND JORGE PARDO

Mitochondria are the chief source of energy in cells. They are critical for the function of tissues that are highly dependent on aerobic metabolism, such as brain and muscle. Mitochondria also play a crucial role in programmed cell death, known as apoptosis (Susin et al., 1998). Apoptosis is important in embryonic development, immune cell regulation, and several other physiological functions.

Mitochondria differ from other subcellular organelles in that they contain their own DNA (mitochondrial DNA [mtDNA]). The human mitochondrial genome is a 16.5-kb circular, double-stranded, maternally inherited DNA (Attardi and Schatz, 1988). It contains genes encoding 13 subunits of the respiratory chain, as well as 2 rRNAs and 22 tRNAs. Of the 13 mtDNA-encoded respiratory-chain subunits, 7 belong to complex I (NADH-coenzyme Q oxidoreductase), 1 belongs to complex III (coenzyme Q-cytochrome c oxidoreductase), 3 belong to complex IV (cytochrome c oxidase [COX]), and 2 belong to complex V (ATP synthase). The mitochondrial genome does not encode any complex II subunits; all complex II subunits are encoded by the nuclear genome. The 13 mtDNA-encoded peptide subunits are synthesized within the mitochondrion and are assembled with other subunits encoded by the nuclear genome, which are synthesized in the cytoplasm and then transported into the mitochondrion. The term "mitochondrial disorder" encompasses a group of clinical disorders associated with structurally or functionally abnormal mitochondria in virtually all tissues, although brain and muscle, which are highly dependent on aerobic metabolism, are generally affected earlier and to a greater extent.

The oxidation of major nutrients in mitochondria leads to the generation of reducing equivalents, H^+ (Attardi and Schatz, 1988). These are transported through the mitochondrial respiratory chain in a process known as oxidative phosphorylation. The energy generated by the oxidation-reduction reactions of the respiratory chain is stored in an electrochemical gradient, which is coupled to ATP synthesis. In mitochondrial disorders, not only does energy failure in tissues and organs result, with a variety of clinical symptoms, but the metabolic block at the end of the anaerobic glycolysis can also lead to excessive pyruvate and lactate accumulation. Lactic acidosis, therefore, can be a manifestation of mitochondrial dysfunction.

In the past 20 years, pathogenic mtDNA mutations have been identified in many brain and muscle diseases. They include mtDNA rearrangements, mtDNA point mutations, and quantitative mtDNA alterations (DiMauro et al., 1998; Schapira, 2002; Verma et al., 2008). Additionally, because the majority of mitochondrial structural proteins are encoded by the nuclear genome, many nuclear genomic mutations can also manifest as primary mitochondrial disorders (Schapira, 2002; Verma et al., 2008). Further, several therapeutic agents, such as nucleoside analog antiviral and anticancer drugs, can interfere with mtDNA replication or transcription and cause secondary mitochondrial dysfunction (Lewis and Dalakas, 1995; Brinkman et al., 1998; Martin et al., 1994; Gérard et al., 2000; Pan-Zhou et al., 2000; Chariot et al., 2000; Lim and Copeland, 2001). Symptomatic hyperlactatemia associated with antiretroviral therapy is linked to the mitochondrial respiratory-chain impairment in HIV disease (Miró et al., 2003). Whether high kinetic states of the immune system and apoptosis in HIV disease (Plymale et al., 1999; Ferri et al., 2000) are associated with alteration in mitochondrial function remains unexplored.

ANTIRETROVIRAL THERAPY, MITOCHONDRIA, AND HYPERLACTATEMIA

The recent availability of antiretroviral drugs has substantially reduced HIV-associated mortality and morbidity through decreased viral burden and immune restoration (Palella et al., 1998; Carpenter et al., 2000). Among

Ashok Verma and Jorge Pardo, Department of Neurology, University of Miami Miller School of Medicine, Miami, FL 33136.

antiretroviral drugs, nucleoside analog reverse transcriptase inhibitors (NRTI) constitute a major group, and as the terminology suggests, they act by inhibiting the key retroviral enzyme, reverse transcriptase (RT). To obviate drug resistance, combinations of NRTI and protease inhibitors (PI) are currently included in highly active antiretroviral therapy (HAART) regimens. While addition of PI to NRTI has changed the management of HIV disease drastically, the cerebral penetration of NRTI makes them the cornerstone of most HAART regimens.

All eukaryotic cells normally use triphosphorylated nucleosides (deoxynucleoside triphosphates [dNTPs]: dATP, dCTP, dGTP, and dTTP) as substrates for DNA synthesis. The reaction is catabolized by a group of five DNA polymerase enzymes (DNA polymerases α, β, γ, δ, and ϵ). HIV encodes a polymerase (RT) that synthesizes a DNA strand from the RNA template. Currently used antiviral NRTI differ from natural dNTPs in that the former lack the hydroxyl group at the 3' position in their sugar moieties. Incorporation of NRTI (instead of dNTPs) into the new DNA strand terminates strand prolongation and the subsequent DNA replication (Lewis and Dalakas, 1995; Brinkman et al., 1998; Kakuda, 2000).

Antiretroviral NRTI are designed to selectively inhibit viral RT, but most of them also inhibit other DNA polymerases, though variably and at very low levels (Martin et al., 1994; Gérard et al., 2000; Pan-Zhou et al., 2000; Chariot et al., 2000; Lim and Copeland, 2001; Kakuda, 2000). NRTI-induced mitochondrial toxicity may occur for a number of reasons (Attardi and Schatz, 1988; Lewis and Dalakas, 1995; Brinkman et al., 1998; Kakuda, 2000). First, the substrate affinity and kinetics of DNA polymerase λ show greater similarity to the viral RT (Brinkman et al., 1998; Martin et al., 1994; Gérard et al., 2000; Pan-Zhou

et al., 2000; Chariot et al., 2000; Lim and Copeland, 2001; Kakuda, 2000); mitochondria exclusively use DNA polymerase λ for mtDNA synthesis. Second, mtDNA replication levels are generally higher than those of nuclear DNA in tissues. Third, mtDNA lacks introns and protective histones; mutations in mtDNA would occur in coding exons. Finally, a new mtDNA mutation is likely to persist, as the mitochondrion is devoid of DNA repair mechanisms, while the nuclear genome is provided with DNA polymerase β and DNA ligase, the repair enzymes.

Mitochondria are the site of generation of most of the cellular ATP pool. The conversion of one molecule of glucose to pyruvate or lactate is associated with the net formation of two molecules of ATP. The subsequent aerobic oxidation of pyruvate takes place within the mitochondria, and it generates 36 additional molecules of ATP, for a total of 38 molecules per completely oxidized molecule of glucose (Medias, 1986). The glycolytic pathway, which is common to both aerobic and anaerobic glucose metabolism, ends with the production of pyruvate. Pyruvate then becomes the substrate of either cytosolic lactate dehydrogenase for the production of lactic acid, the substrate of mitochondrial enzymes (pyruvate dehydrogenase and pyruvate decarboxylase) for entry into the Krebs cycle, or the substrate for gluconeogenesis (Fig. 1). Lactate is a metabolic end product; its only fate is oxidation back to pyruvate or, to some extent, excretion in urine. The equilibrium of the pyruvate-lactate equation normally favors the formation of lactate (Medias, 1986). Thus, under normal conditions, the concentration of lactate (1.0 meq/liter) is approximately 10- to 20-fold greater than that of pyruvate (0.05 to 0.1 meq/liter). The lactate production increases substantially when for any reason the pyruvate oxidative (mitochondrial) pathway is unavailable

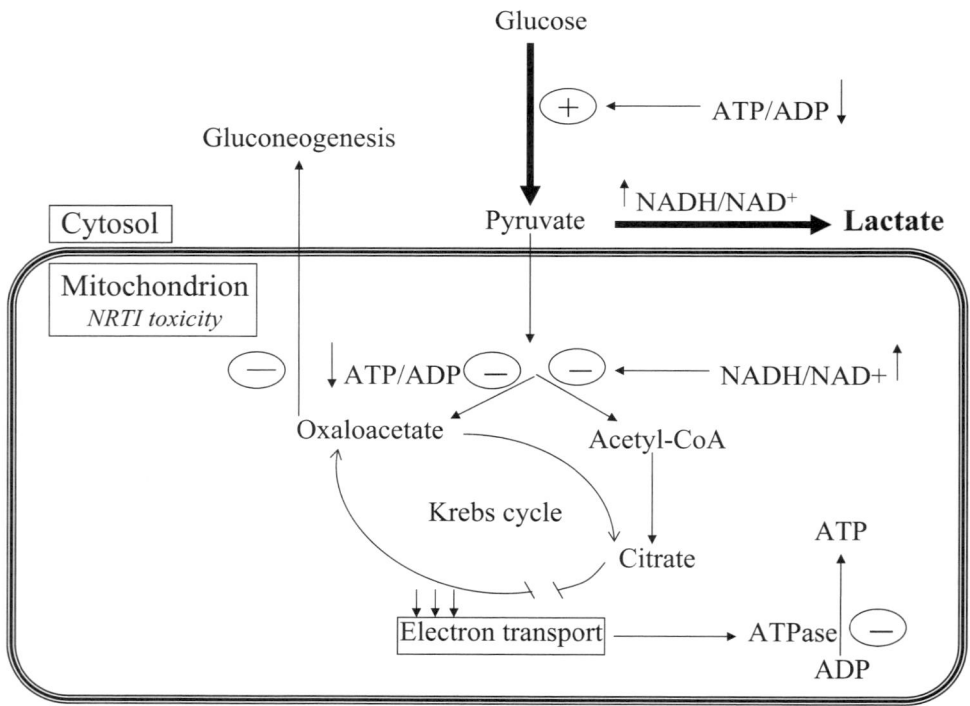

FIGURE 1 Mechanism of NRTI-induced mitochondrial toxicity and lactate accumulation. $-$, inhibition; $+$, potentiation.

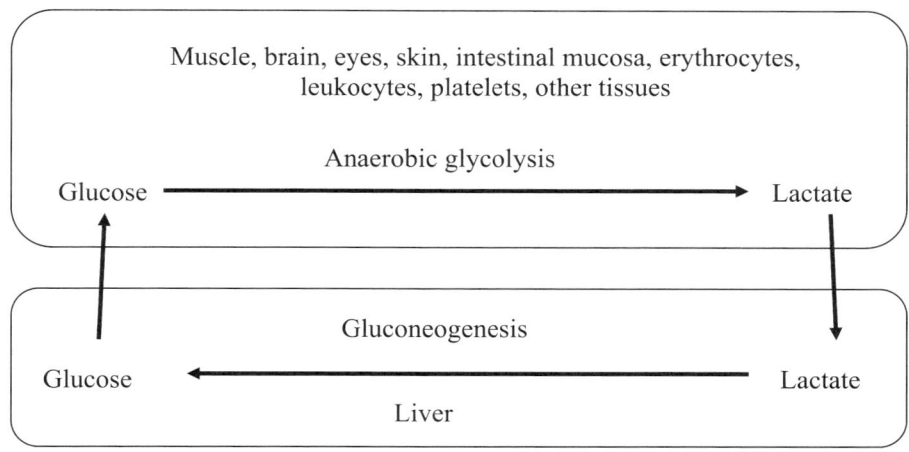

FIGURE 2 The Cori cycle.

or impaired. With a mitochondrial oxidation block, glycolysis becomes the main source of energy for the tissues; increased lactate production represents the toll paid by the organism to maintain energy during anaerobiosis. Thus, in NRTI-induced mitochondrial dysfunction, the lactate accumulation generally reflects both the overproduction of pyruvate and the underutilization of pyruvate through its mitochondrion-dependent pathways (Fig. 1).

While lactate is normally produced in all tissues, the liver is the chief lactate-consuming organ under normal conditions (the Cori cycle) (Fig. 2). Lactate (via pyruvate) constitutes a substrate for gluconeogenesis in the liver, besides being a substrate for conversion (in mitochondria) to CO_2 and water in the liver and other tissues. Animal studies indicate that gluconeogenesis is the primary mode of lactate processing in the liver (Plymale et al., 1999). Lactic acidosis, therefore, may become particularly severe or life threatening when mitochondrial dysfunction is coupled with a liver disorder. Mitochondrion-associated toxicity might be particularly severe with concomitant liver disease, such as in HIV- and hepatitis C-coinfected individuals (de Mendoza and Soriano, 2005). Virtually all cases of severe NRTI-associated lactic acidosis (NALA) in HIV disease are associated with liver impairment, mostly hepatic microsteatosis (Gérard et al., 2000; Chariot et al., 2000; Lenzo et al., 1997; Sundar et al., 1997; John et al., 2001; Fortgang et al., 1995; Carr et al., 2000). Hepatic steatosis represents impaired β-oxidation of fatty acids in mitochondria. Thus, mitochondrial impairment in liver tissue causes hepatic steatosis and contributes to systemic lactic acidosis (Miró et al., 2003).

LACTATE HOMEOSTASIS AND LACTIC ACIDOSIS IN HIV DISEASE

The average basal turnover rate of lactate in healthy humans has been estimated at about 25 meq/kg/day with a range of 15 to 35 meq/kg/day (Medias, 1986). This amount is approximately 1 meq/min, or 1,400 meq/day for a 70-kg subject. Unfortunately, available information on quantitative aspects of lactate production and utilization by humans in different physiological conditions and disease states is quite limited. However, under conditions of lactate excess, hepatic clearance of lactate can be augmented; organs, such as the

kidney, may utilize more lactate, and other tissues, such as muscle, that are mostly lactate producers can also become lactate consumers (Medias, 1986). Hence, the large (up to 100-fold) acute elevation in lactate after vigorous exercise is rapidly reequilibrated in a healthy person, indicating the efficiency of lactate regulation. This is thought to be a part of a generalized homeostatic system regulating organic acids via systemic pH. This homeostatic mechanism may be in jeopardy when lactate is overproduced or when the liver, the major lactate-consuming organ, is unavailable or impaired, or both.

Increased Lactate Production in HIV Disease

NRTI-related mitochondrial toxicity appears to be the major factor responsible for hyperlactatemia and lactic acidosis in patients with HIV disease (Brinkman et al., 1998; Gérard et al., 2000; Chariot et al., 2000; Miró et al., 2003; Fortgang et al., 1995; Delgado et al., 2001; Falco et al., 2002). As indicated above, NRTI inhibit HIV replication but can also inhibit human mtDNA polymerase λ and thereby replication of mtDNA, leading to depletion of mtDNA (Falco et al., 2002; Côté et al., 2002). The decrease in mtDNA precedes the rise in venous lactate levels in HIV-infected patients receiving NRTI therapy (Côté et al., 2002). Mitochondrial dysfunction impairs pyruvate utilization and promotes its conversion to lactate, which is then released into the plasma. Although initially believed to be a rare event, recent studies have demonstrated elevated serum lactate levels in asymptomatic patients receiving NRTI with an estimated incidence between 15% and 35% (John et al., 2001; Falco et al., 2002; Brinkman, 2001; Brinkman et al., 2000). Symptomatic NRTI-induced lactic acidosis is less common, with an incidence of approximately 1.4% (John et al., 2001; Brinkman, 2001; Lonergan et al., 2003).

The risk profile for NALA in an individual is less clear. The specific NRTI in the HAART regimen, the combination of NRTI, duration of therapy with NRTI, and concomitant liver disease seem to play roles (de Mendoza and Soriano, 2005; John et al., 2001; Falco et al., 2002) and to determine the risk of NALA. Among the different NRTI, stavudine has been particularly incriminated as a dominant risk factor for developing chronic hyperlactatemia (John et al., 2001; Falco et al., 2002; Côté et al., 2002). In in vitro studies, the triphosphorylated form of stavudine has been shown to be incorporated into DNA more readily than other currently used NRTI (Martin et al., 1994). Stavudine exerts greater inhibition of the human mtDNA polymerase λ (Martin et al., 1994; Falco et al., 2002; Côté et al., 2002). The relative potencies of other NRTI with regard to their inhibitory effects on mtDNA polymerase λ in vitro, from most potent to least potent, are as follows: zalcitabine > didanosine > lamivudine > zidovudine > abacavir (Martin et al., 1994; Falco et al., 2002). Host factors, such as mtDNA polymorphisms, tissue-specific kinase kinetics involved in the production of the active triphosphorylated metabolites of NRTI, and tissue-specific energy thresholds for organ dysfunction, may also determine the NRTI toxicity. Female gender (Falco et al., 2002), high body mass index (Falco et al., 2002), riboflavin and thiamine deficiencies (Fouty et al., 1998), and viral hepatitis (de Mendoza and Soriano, 2005) have also been linked to NRTI-induced hyperlactatemia. Finally, the risk profile for hyperlactatemia seems to mirror features of the "lipodystrophy syndrome" of AIDS in some patients (Carr et al., 2000; Mallal et al., 2000). The mitochondrial contribution to lipodystrophy in HIV disease has been speculated (Brinkman et al., 1999; Miro et al., 2005; Moyle, 2004).

A recent report describing significantly lower mtDNA than nuclear-DNA levels in HIV-infected asymptomatic patients who had never received NRTI is intriguing (Côté et al., 2002). Also unexplained are the reports of mild elevation of lactate levels in some treatment-naïve HIV-infected patients (John et al., 2001). These differences cannot be explained by the lower CD4 lymphocyte counts in these patients (John et al., 2001; Côté et al., 2002). A mitochondrion-controlled mechanism of apoptotic and necrotic cell death has been postulated in HIV infection (Plymale et al., 1999), and high levels of daily CD4 lymphocyte turnover (in the range of a billion cells a day) and high viral kinetics continue to occur during asymptomatic HIV disease (Palella et al., 1998; Carpenter et al., 2000). Whether mtDNA levels and low-level asymptomatic hyperlactatemia in HIV infection suggest mitochondrial involvement is unknown.

Impaired Lactate Clearance in HIV Disease

Chronic mild hyperlactatemia with a lactate concentration of 1 to 2 meq/liter, maintained over many months, is the most common pattern of hyperlactatemia in HIV-infected patients with NRTI therapy (John et al., 2001; Falco et al., 2002). Presumably, homeostatic mechanisms are preserved enough to compensate (see above) at least partially for lactate excess in these patients. Asymptomatic hyperlactatemia (<5 meq/liter) is perhaps the next most common pattern in HIV patients with NRTI therapy. Reversible asymptomatic hyperlactatemia is associated with mitochondrial respiratory-chain impairment and liver dysfunction, and the liver function improves and lactate levels regress following discontinuation of antiretroviral therapy in patients with HIV infection (Miró et al., 2003). The reason why asymptomatic hyperlactatemia in some patients later progresses to the syndrome of lactic acidosis (lactate at >5 meq/liter) is not completely understood. Progressive mtDNA depletion with mitochondrial dysfunction could be one reason. It is also conceivable that the impaired consumption of lactate contributes to NALA in HIV disease. A study of exercise physiology in HIV-infected healthy persons has shown that basal lactate production, lactate/pyruvate metabolism, and lactate clearance in skeletal muscle were not significantly different from those in matched controls (Roge et al., 2000).

The liver is almost invariably affected in NALA (Chariot et al., 2000; Miró et al., 2003; Lenzo et al., 1997; Sundar

et al., 1997; John et al., 2001; Fortgang et al., 1995; Carr et al., 2000; Verma et al., 1999). Liver enzyme abnormalities preceding frank NALA suggest that liver dysfunction (related to NRTI toxicity, HIV, or other factors) may play an important role in disrupting lactic acidosis metabolism in patients with NALA. Lactic acidosis has been described in HIV-infected pregnant women with liver dysfunction (Sarner and Fakoya, 2002) and HIV-infected neonates (Giaquinto et al., 2001). It is conceivable that impaired lactate clearance secondary to liver impairment plays a significant role in lactate accumulation in HIV disease.

DIAGNOSIS AND MANAGEMENT OF LACTIC ACIDOSIS IN HIV DISEASE

NRTI-associated hyperlactatemia can develop at any stage of HIV disease. Cases of NALA have been reported as early as 1 month and as late as 20 months after the initiation of NRTI therapy (Falco et al., 2002). The key to the diagnosis of lactic acidosis in HIV disease is the index of suspicion. If it is suspected, a simple laboratory test confirms the clinical diagnosis and reduction or removal of NRTI improves the plasma lactate levels. If it is not suspected and the toxic NRTI agent is continued, NALA can progress to a fatal outcome (Gérard et al., 2000; Pan-Zhou et al., 2000; Chariot et al., 2000; Lenzo et al., 1997; Carr et al., 2000; Falco et al., 2002; Verma et al., 1999; Sarner and Fakoya, 2002).

Lactic acidosis is primarily an acid-base disorder. In acid-base disorder evaluations, a simple calculation of the anion gap (AG) is helpful; the AG represents unmeasured anion in plasma (normally 10 to 12 meq/liter) and is calculated as follows: $AG = [Na^+] - ([Cl^-] + [HCO_3^-])$. When lactic acid, an unmeasured anion, accumulates in extracellular fluid, it typically causes high-AG acidosis. Other common causes of high-AG acidosis are diabetic ketoacidosis, acute and chronic renal failure, and methanol and salicylate poisoning. Unrecognized bowel ischemia, sepsis, and shock also can cause lactic acidosis in hospitalized sick AIDS patients.

All metabolic acidoses have profound effects on the respiratory, cardiac, and nervous systems (Lenzo et al., 1997; Sundar et al., 1997; John et al., 2001; Falco et al., 2002; Brinkman, 2001; Verma et al., 1999). Isolated symptoms of lactic acidosis, such as malaise, fatigue, weakness, paresthesia, abdominal pain, vomiting, weight loss, and cardiopulmonary symptoms, are very common in AIDS. However, combinations of several symptoms or, more specifically, exercise-induced dyspnea seems sufficient to justify the measurement of arterial blood gases and lactate levels. Tachycardia and tachypnea, especially in an afebrile patient, may also be suggestive of hyperlactatemia. It is important to recognize that more than one clinical condition can coexist in HIV-infected individuals, especially in late-stage HIV disease. Blood tests should be carefully conducted, and measurements of lactate must be performed under a basal resting condition on samples immediately put on ice and shipped to the laboratory.

Treatment of NALA is discontinuation of the offending agent(s) and supportive therapy. Sick patients with systemic lactic acidosis require hospitalization for monitoring and therapy. Supportive therapy of lactic acidosis includes fluid and electrolyte balance, bicarbonate administration, and respiratory support when needed. Alkali therapy is generally advocated for acute, severe acidemia (pH <7.1) to improve cardiac function and lactate utilization (Medias, 1986). However, $NaHCO_3$ therapy may paradoxically depress cardiac performance and exacerbate acidosis by enhancing lactate production (HCO_3^- stimulates phosphofructokinase, a rate-limiting enzyme in glycolysis). $NaHCO_3$ therapy can also cause fluid overload, hypertension, and overshoot alkalosis if it is not carefully monitored. Frequent metabolic monitoring is therefore necessary to manage such patients. The algorithm in Fig. 3 summarizes the management of HIV-associated hyperlactatemia.

It seems essential to discontinue all antiretroviral drugs at the time of NALA diagnosis; however, surviving patients often need to continue antiretroviral therapy. Careful switching to alternative NRTI with less mitochondrial toxicity can be an option for some patients for effective HAART. Nonnucleoside RT inhibitors lack affinity for mtDNA polymerase λ (John et al., 2001; Falco et al., 2002; Brinkman et al., 2000), and a combination of nonnucleoside RT inhibitors with PI could be a safe regimen for those patients (Khouri and Cushing, 2000). Although some patients have subsequently tolerated challenge with a new NRTI-containing regimen (Lenzo et al., 1997; Falco et al., 2002; Lonergan et al., 2000; Miller et al., 2000), it is not without risk, and clearly, such patients would require close clinical and laboratory monitoring. Among NRTI, abacavir and tenofovir appear to have lower affinities for mtDNA polymerase λ (John et al., 2001; Cihlar and Chen, 1996). In one recent report, replacement of stavudine and didanosine by another combination of NRTI in HAART regimen was found to be relatively safe and effective (Lonergan et al., 2003).

Administration of essential cofactors and supplements, such as thiamine, riboflavin, L-carnitine, vitamin C, and antioxidants, has been used empirically for genetic mitochondrial diseases with little and variable success (Verma et al., 2008). A few published case reports have suggested that this "mitochondrial cocktail" can enhance recovery from NALA (John et al., 2001; Falco et al., 2002; Brinkman, 2001; Khouri and Cushing, 2000; Dalton and Rahimi, 2001; Schramm et al., 1999). Dicloroacetate (DeStefano et al., 1995), a pyruvate dehydrogenase enzyme enhancer, and idebenone (Napolitano et al., 2000), an artificial electron transport coenzyme equivalent, have been reported to be useful in genetic mitochondrial diseases, but their use in NALA has not been studied.

Asymptomatic, mild, and stable hyperlactatemia (<2 meq/liter) is relatively common in long-term NRTI-treated individuals (Falco et al., 2002; Lonergan et al., 2000). It is unclear whether periodic serum lactate estimation (Brinkman, 2001) or quantitative mtDNA assays (Côté et al., 2002) are useful tools to monitor and evaluate NRTI toxicity in such asymptomatic patients. Severe NALA (>5 meq/liter) is almost always associated with the syndrome of metabolic acidosis and often with hepatopathy, myopathy, neuropathy, renal failure, or pancreatitis (Lenzo et al., 1997; Sundar et al., 1997; John et al., 2001; Falco et al., 2002; Verma et al., 1999; Sarner and Fakoya, 2002; Giaquinto et al., 2001; Allaouchiche et al., 1999). The prognosis in lactic acidosis with liver failure and other target organ dysfunction is poor, with a mortality of up to 60% (John et al., 2001; Falco et al., 2002; Brinkman, 2001; Brinkman et al., 2000), even after the NRTI therapy is discontinued.

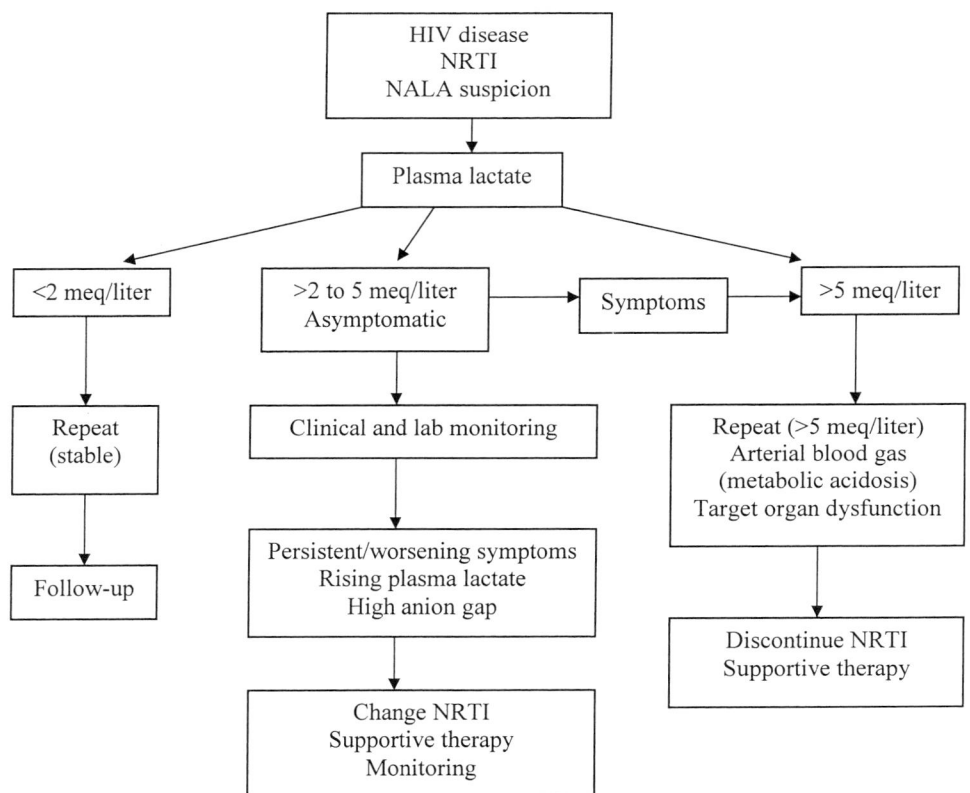

FIGURE 3   Management of NRTI-associated hyperlactatemia.

CONCLUSION

The prognosis of patients with HIV infection has improved dramatically since the introduction of HAART in 1996. However, the increase in life expectancy and the need for permanent antiretroviral therapy for HIV suppression have led to the recognition of new problems. NRTI are linchpins of HAART regimens in HIV disease. Among the newly recognized HAART-related adverse effects, NALA is a rare but serious complication. Lactic acidosis occurs from NRTI-associated mitochondrial toxicity that results in inhibition of mtDNA polymerase λ, which in turn impairs oxidative metabolism. In published reports, stavudine-containing HAART regimens are particularly incriminated in NALA. It is important to recognize hyperlactatemia in HIV disease, as early diagnosis of hyperlactatemia and change in the HAART regimen leads to reversal of lactic acidosis and complete recovery. Severe lactic acidosis carries high mortality. Several issues concerning NALA remain unresolved, especially with regard to prevention and treatment. The question of whether routine lactate measurements in asymptomatic patients provide predictive information or lead to unnecessary treatment alterations needs to be addressed. Discovery of safer antiretroviral agents would help obviate this potentially fatal complication.

REFERENCES

Allaouchiche, B., F. Duflo, L. Cotte, L. Mathon, and D. Chassard. 1999. Acute pancreatitis with severe lactic acidosis in an HIV-infected patient on didanosine therapy. *J. Antimicrob. Chemother.* **44:**137–138.

Attardi, G., and G. Schatz. 1988. Biogenesis of mitochondria. *Annu. Rev. Cell Biol.* **4:**289–333.

Brinkman, K. 2001. Management of hyperlactatemia: no need for routine lactate measurements. *AIDS* **15:**795–797.

Brinkman, K., H. ter Hofstede, D. Burger, J. Smeitink, and P. Koopmans. 1998. Adverse effects of reverse transcriptase inhibitors: mitochondrial toxicity as common pathway. *AIDS* **12:**1735–1744.

Brinkman, K., J. Smeitink, J. Romijn, and P. Reiss. 1999. Mitochondrial toxicity induced by nucleoside-analogue reverse-transcriptase inhibitors is a key factor in the pathogenesis of antiretroviral-therapy-related lipodystrophy. *Lancet* **354:**1112–1115.

Brinkman, K., S. Vrouenraets, R. Kauffmann, H. Weigel, and J. Frissen. 2000. Treatment of nucleoside reverse transcriptase inhibitor-induced lactic acidosis. *AIDS* **14:**2801–2802.

Carpenter, C., D. Cooper, M. Fischl, J. Gatell, B. Gazzard, S. Hammer, M. Hirsch, D. Jacobsen, D. Katzenstein, J. Montaner, D. Richman, M. Saag, M. Schechter, R. Schooley, M. Thompson, S. Vella, P. Yeni, and P. Volberding. 2000. Antiretroviral therapy in adults: updated recommendations of the International AIDS Society-USA Panel. *JAMA* **283:** 381–390.

Carr, A., J. Miller, M. Law, and D. Cooper. 2000. A syndrome of lipoatrophy, lactic acidaemia and liver dysfunction associated with HIV nucleoside analogue therapy: contribution to protease inhibitor-related lipodystrophy syndrome. *AIDS* **14:**F25–F32.

Chariot, P., I. Drogou, I. de Lacroix-Szmania, M. C. Eliezer-Vanerot, B. Chazaud, A. Lombès, A. Schaeffer, and E. S. Zafrani. 2000. Zidovudine-induced mitochondrial disorder with massive liver steatosis, myopathy, lactic acidosis, and mitochondrial DNA depletion. *J. Hepatol.* **30:**156–160.

Cihlar, T., and M. Chen. 1996. Identification of enzymes catalyzing two-step phosphorylation of cidofovir and the effect of cytomegalovirus infection on their activities in host cells. *Mol. Pharmacol.* **50:**1502–1510.

Côté, H. C., Z. L. Brumme, K. J. Craib, C. S. Alexander, B. Wynhoven, L. Ting, H. Wong, M. Harris, P. R. Harrigan, M. V. O'Shaughnessy, and J. S. Montaner. 2002. Changes in mitochondrial DNA as a marker of nucleoside toxicity in HIV-infected patients. *N. Engl. J. Med.* **346:**811–820.

Dalton, S., and A. Rahimi. 2001. Emerging role of riboflavin in the treatment of nucleoside analogue induced type B lactic acidosis. *AIDS Patient Care STDS* **15:**611–614.

Delgado, J., M. Harris, A. Tesiorowski, and J. Montaner. 2001. Symptomatic elevations of lactic acid and their response to treatment manipulation in human immunodeficiency virus-infected persons: a case series. *Clin. Infect. Dis.* **33:**2072–2074.

de Mendoza, C., and V. Soriano. 2005. The role of hepatitis C virus (HCV) in mitochondrial DNA damage in HIV/HCV-coinfected individuals. *Antivir. Ther.* **10:**M109–M115.

DeStefano, N., P. Mathews, B. Ford, A. Genge, G. Karpati, and D. Arnold. 1995. Short-term dichloroacetate treatment improves indices of cerebral metabolism in patients with mitochondrial disorders. *Neurology* **45:**1193–1198.

DiMauro, S., E. Bonilla, M. Davidson, M. Hirano, and E. Scchon. 1998. Mitochondria in neuromuscular disorders. *Biochim. Biophys Acta* **1366:**199–210.

Falco, V., R. Rodrigues, E. Ribera, E. Martinez, J. Miro, P. Domingo, R. Diazarague, J. Arribas, J. Gonzalez-Garcia, F. Montero, L. Sanchez, and A. Pahissa. 2002. Severe nucleoside-associated lactic acidosis in human immunodeficiency virus-infected patients: report of 12 cases and review of literature. *HIV/AIDS* **34:**838–846.

Ferri, K., E. Jacotot, J. Blanco, J. Este, and G. Kroeer. 2000. Mitochondrial control of cell death induced by HIV-1-encoded proteins. *Ann. N. Y. Acad. Sci.* **926:**149–164.

Fortgang, I., P. Belitsos, R. Chaisson, and R. Moore. 1995. Hepatomegaly and steatosis in HIV-infected patients receiving nucleoside analog antiretroviral therapy. *Am. J. Gastroenterol.* **90:**1433–1436.

Fouty, B., F. Frerman, and R. Reves. 1998. Riboflavin to treat nucleoside analogue-induced lactic acidosis. *Lancet* **352:**291–292.

Gérard, Y., L. Maulin, Y. Yazdanpanah, X. De La Tribonnière, C. Amiel, C. A. Maurage, S. Robin, B. Sablonnière, C. Dhennain, and Y. Mouton. 2000. Symptomatic hyperlactataemia: an emerging complication of antiretroviral therapy. *AIDS* **14:**2723–2730.

Giaquinto, C., A. De Romeo, V. Giacomet, O. Rampon, E. Ragu, A. Burlina, A. De Rossi, M. Sturkenboom, and R. D'Elia. 2001. Lactic acid levels in children perinatally treated with antiretroviral agents to prevent HIV transmission. *AIDS* **15:**1074–1075.

John, M., C. Moore, I. James, D. Nolan, R. Upton, E. McKinnon, and S. Mallal. 2001. Chronic hyperlactatemia in HIV-infected patients taking antiretroviral therapy. *AIDS* **15:**717–723.

Kakuda, T. 2000. Pharmacology of nucleoside and nucleotide reverse transcriptase inhibitor-induced mitochondrial toxicity. *Clin. Ther.* **22:**685–708.

Khouri, S. and H. Cushing. 2000. Lactic acidosis secondary to nucleoside analogue antiretroviral therapy. *AIDS Read.* **10:**602–606.

Lenzo, N., B. Garas, and M. French. 1997. Hepatic steatosis and lactic acidosis associated with stavudine treatment in an HIV patient: a case report. *AIDS* **11:**1294–1296.

Lewis, W., and M. Dalakas. 1995. Mitochondrial toxicity of antiviral drugs. *Nat. Med.* **1:**417–422.

Lim, S., and W. Copeland. 2001. Differential incorporation and removal of antiviral deoxynucleotides by human DNA polymerase gamma. *J. Biol. Chem.* **276:**23616–23623.

Lonergan, J., C. Behling, H. Pfander, T. Hassanein, and W. Mathews. 2000. Hyperlactatemia and hepatic abnormalities in 10 human immunodeficiency virus-infected patients receiving nucleoside analogue combination regimens. *Clin. Infect. Dis.* **31:**162–166.

Lonergan, J., R. Barber, and W. Mathews. 2003. Safety and efficacy of switching to alternative nucleoside analogues following symptomatic hyperlactatemia and lactic acidosis. *AIDS* **17:**2495–2499.

Mallal, S., M. John, C. Moore, I. James, and E. McKinnon. 2000. Contribution of nucleoside analogue reverse transcriptase inhibitors to subcutaneous fat wasting in patients with HIV infection. *AIDS* **14:**1309–1316.

Martin, J., C. Brown, N. Matthews-Davis, and J. Reardon. 1994. Effects of antiviral nucleoside analogs on human DNA polymerases and mitochondrial DNA synthesis. *Antimicrob. Agents Chemother.* **38:**2743–2749.

Medias, M. 1986. Lactic acidosis. *Kidney Int.* **29:**752–774.

Miller, K., M. Cameron, L. Wood, M. Dalakas, and J. Kovacs. 2000. Lactic acidosis and hepatic steatosis associated with use of stavudine: report of four cases. *Ann. Intern. Med.* **133:**192–196.

Miró, O., S. López, E. Martínez, B. Rodríguez-Santiago, J. L. Blanco, A. Milinkovic, J. M. Miró, V. Nunes, J. Casademont, J. M. Gatell, and F. Cardellach. 2003. Reversible mitochondrial respiratory chain impairment during symptomatic hyperlactatemia associated with antiretroviral therapy. *AIDS Res. Hum. Retrovir.* **19:**1027–1032.

Miro, O., S. Lopez, F. Cardellach, and J. Casademont. 2005. Mitochondrial studies in HAART-related lipodystrophy: from experimental hypothesis to clinical findings. *Antivir. Ther.* **10:**M73–M81.

Moyle, G. 2004. Mitochondrial toxicity: myths and facts. *J. HIV Ther.* **9:**45–47.

Napolitano, A., S. Salvetti, M. Vista, V. Lombardi, G. Siciliano, and C. Giraldi. 2000. Long-term treatment with idebenone and riboflavin in a patient with MELAS. *Neurol. Sci.* **21:**S981–S982.

Palella, F. J., Jr., K. M. Delaney, A. C. Moorman, M. O. Loveless, J. Fuhrer, G. A. Satten, D. J. Aschman, S. D.

Holmberg, et al. 1998. Declining morbidity and mortality among patients with advanced human immunodeficiency virus infection. *N. Engl. J. Med.* **338:**853–860.

Pan-Zhou, X., L. Cui, X. Zhou, J. Sommadossi, and V. Darley-Usmar. 2000. Differential effects of antiretroviral nucleoside analogs on mitochondrial function in HepG2 cells. *Antimicrob. Agents Chemother.* **44:**496–503.

Plymale, D., D. Tang, A. Comardelle, C. Fermin, D. Lewis, and R. Garry. 1999. Both necrosis and apoptosis contribute to HIV-1-induced killing of CD4 cells. *AIDS* **13:**1827–1839.

Roge, B., J. Calbet, K. Moller, H. Ullum, H. Hendel, J. Gerstoft, and B. Pederson. 2000. Mitochondrial function and exercise capacity in HIV infected patients with lipodystrophy, p. 1232. Geneva, Switzerland. *XII Int. AIDS Conf.*

Sarner, L., and A. Fakoya. 2002. Acute onset lactic acidosis and pancreatitis in the third trimester of pregnancy in HIV-1 positive women taking antiretroviral medication. *Sex. Transm. Infect.* **78:**58–59.

Schapira, A. H. 2002. The "new" mitochondrial disorders. *J. Neurol. Neurosurg. Psychiatry* **72:**144–149.

Schramm, C., R. Wanitschke, and P. Galle. 1999. Thiamine for the treatment of nucleoside analogue-induced severe lactic acidosis. *Eur. J. Anaesthesiol.* **16:**733–735.

Sundar, K., M. Suarez, P. Banogon, and J. Shapiro. 1997. Zidovudine-induced fatal lactic acidosis and hepatic failure in patients with acquired immunodeficiency syndrome: report of two patients and review of the literature. *Crit. Care Med.* **25:**1425–1430.

Susin, S., N. Zamzami, and G. Kroemer. 1998. Mitochondria as regulators of apoptosis: doubt no more. *Biochim. Biophys. Acta* **1366:**151–165.

Verma, A., M. Hirano, and C. T. Moraes. 2008. Mitochondrial disorders, p. 1785–1798. *In* W. G. Bradley, R. B. Daroff, G. M. Fenichel, and J. Jankovic (ed.), *Neurology in Clinical Practice*, 5th ed. Elsevier Butterworth-Heinemann, Philadelphia, PA.

Verma, A., R. Schein, D. Jayaweera, and D. Kett. 1999. Fulminant neuropathy and lactic acidosis associated with nucleoside analog therapy. *Neurology* **53:**1365–1367.

The Spectrum of Neuro-AIDS Disorders:
Pathophysiology, Diagnosis, and Treatment
Edited by K. Goodkin et al.
©2008 ASM Press, Washington, DC

8

Neurologic Outcomes in HIV Infection: Clinical Events and Surrogate Markers

CONSTANTIN T. YIANNOUTSOS

HIV infection is associated with multifactorial neurological complications. Direct central nervous system infection results in encephalopathies and HIV-associated dementia (HAD), while peripheral nervous system damage is associated with distal neuropathies. The attendant immunosuppression also leaves patients vulnerable to secondary opportunistic infections, such as toxoplasmosis and progressive multifocal leukoencephalopathy. A marked decrease in the incidence of neurological complications has been observed with advances in antiviral treatment (Albrecht et al., 1998; Miralles et al., 1998; Moore et al., 1998; McArthur, 1999; Neuenburg et al., 2002; Sacktor, 2002; Dore et al., 2003), collectively referred to as highly active antiretroviral therapy. Nevertheless, the long-term prevalence of neurological opportunistic infections, cognitive disorders, and peripheral neuropathies may be increasing as patients live longer (Dal Pan and McArthur, 1996; Dore et al., 1999; Neuenburg et al., 2002; Sacktor, 2002), and neurotoxic medications, such as nucleoside analogs, are increasingly part of highly active antiretroviral therapy regimens (Simpson and Tagliati, 1995; Williams et al., 2001; Sacktor, 2002; Nolan and Mallal, 2004), suggesting that antiretroviral therapy alone does not confer complete protection from the neurological sequelae of HIV (Bouwman et al., 1998; McArthur, 2004). Thus, HIV-related neurological disorders will likely remain a challenge in the treatment of HIV-infected patients.

Increasing evidence suggests that neurological perturbation in HIV-infected individuals may increase mortality and morbidity independently from the severity of systemic disease, as this is reflected by CD4 counts and levels of virus in the plasma (Ellis et al., 1997a; Price et al., 1999). Despite this, current therapeutic strategies remain focused primarily on plasma virologic suppression, even though it is unclear whether virologic control in the periphery is sufficient to avert neurocognitive impairment (Sacktor et al., 2002) and peripheral disease (Sacktor, 2002; Lichtenstein et al., 2005). As a result, there are limited data on the neurological benefits of widely prescribed antiretroviral medications. Moreover, there are limited and sometimes conflicting data concerning the efficacies of a number of symptomatic therapies for HIV-associated neurological injury and opportunistic infections. As a result, there is neither a clear standard for antiretroviral therapy optimization in patients with cognitive deterioration or peripheral neuropathy nor a well-established criterion for the timing of initiation of symptomatic therapy. Apart from frank scientific debate and controversy about these issues, lack of progress in this area is due, at least in part, to a lack of measures assessing the neurological benefit of antiviral and symptomatic therapy. Thus, the development and validation of markers of HIV-related neurological diseases are urgently needed.

Below, I provide a review of the methodology and selection criteria that might be employed in order to identify and validate candidate measures as surrogates of clinical outcome. The analytical procedures outlined here are applicable to a wide range of HIV neurological research but are broad enough to be helpful in general medical investigation. The subsequent discussion is organized as follows. First, the operational definition of a "surrogate marker" is given, followed by practical criteria for identifying such candidate markers. The statistical methodology for testing and validating these candidate surrogate markers, along with the related problem of diagnostic testing, is reviewed next, followed by a number of examples that illustrate a variety of these approaches in the context of neuro-AIDS.

CLINICAL EVENTS VERSUS SURROGATE MARKERS: DEFINITION AND OPERATIONAL CRITERIA

In clinical trials, as well as patient care, it is often desirable to use a measure as a surrogate for the clinical event of interest. In HIV infection, monitoring of CD4+ T-lymphocyte counts

Constantin T. Yiannoutsos, Division of Biostatistics, Department of Medicine, Indiana University School of Medicine, Indianapolis, IN 46202.

and plasma HIV RNA levels (viral load) is routinely used, rather than observing the occurrence of new opportunistic infections or death (Jacobson et al., 1995; Katzenstein et al., 1996; Welles et al., 1996; Mellors et al., 1997; Kaplan et al., 2001). A decrease in the plasma HIV viral load is a criterion of treatment efficacy (Marschner et al., 1998). Conversely, lack of virus suppression may be used as a criterion for change of therapy (Elashoff and Lagakos, 1996; Gazzard, 1996; DeGruttola et al., 1998; Dybul et al., 2002). Both levels of CD4 counts and plasma HIV RNA have also been employed as entry criteria in HIV clinical trials or for initiation or delay of therapy (Dybul et al., 2002). Use of surrogate markers in place of a clinical endpoint dramatically decreases the size and duration of clinical trials, especially if the clinical event is rare or slow to manifest. Furthermore, observing the marker in advance of the clinical event allows treatment initiation or change in order to ultimately prevent its occurrence.

In general, surrogate markers must have a strong biological link and statistical correlation with the occurrence of the clinical event. A frequently overlooked fact, however, is that biological relevance and adequate prognostic ability are insufficient to justify the use of the marker in place of the clinical event. Consider the CD4 count, for example. There is a strong biological rationale for the use of the CD4 count as a surrogate marker of disease progression or death, the usual events of interest (see Fauci et al., 1984, for a review of early evidence in this area). Both baseline levels of CD4 counts and change over time have been associated with the rate of clinical progression (Cooper and Lacey, 1988). Therefore, the first criterion is satisfied. However, the second criterion, which states that the effect of treatment on the clinical outcome is fully manifested by its effect on CD4 counts, is at best only partially fulfilled (Choi et al., 1993; Lin et al., 1993; Fleming and DeMets, 1996; Goldman et al., 1996; Hughes et al., 1998).

The following criteria are necessary for a measure to be defined as a surrogate marker for the endpoint of interest (Prentice, 1989; Freedman et al., 1992; Lin et al., 1993; Mildvan et al., 1997).

1. The marker is predictive of the clinical event.
2. The treatment effect on the clinical outcome manifests entirely through its effect on the marker (Fig. 1).

Criterion 1 is fundamental for identifying candidate markers. It implies that there is a strong, biologically plausible relationship between fluctuations in the marker and the likelihood or risk of the clinical event. As I mentioned, however, this is a necessary but not a sufficient condition for surrogacy. Criterion 2 is more difficult to assess. It means that when the level of the marker is known, knowledge of the specific treatment does not confer any additional information about the risk of the clinical outcome. In other words, two patients with identical marker histories will have the same prognosis, regardless of treatment (Freedman et al., 1992; Lin et al., 1993)! This was not the case, for example, in a large placebo-controlled study of zidovudine (ZDV) in which subjects assigned to ZDV had better prognosis at every level of CD4 cell count (Volberding et al., 1990). An additional criterion, not essential in the definition but crucial in the validation of a candidate measure as a true surrogate marker, is the following:

3. The treatment produces discernible changes on the marker.

This principle requires that the underlying treatment must have a measurable (clinically meaningful) effect on the

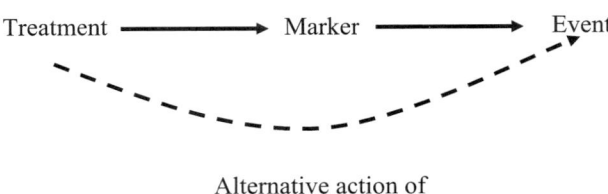

FIGURE 1 Valid surrogate marker (solid arrows), in which the treatment effect is manifested through the marker, and incomplete marker (dashed line), in which treatment affects a clinical event through a mechanism that does not involve the marker.

disease and, at the same time, be able to change the marker under investigation. If treatment is ineffective, an inadequate marker may seem to capture all of the (rather weak) treatment effect. On the other hand, a treatment that is effective against the clinical event but does not affect the marker may be thought ineffective if it is assessed solely by its effect on the marker. For example, *Pneumocystis carinii* pneumonia therapy may decrease patient mortality without affecting CD4 counts.

Complete adherence to the strict definition outlined above would exclude the majority of useful measures from consideration. No single marker can possibly account for all the biological aspects of disease or of the total clinical effect of treatment (Albert et al., 1998). Even if several markers combined could capture the effect of a particular treatment, they might not be valid in predicting the effects of therapies with different biological mechanisms of action (Lagakos and Hoth, 1992). Thus, a more realistic strategy involves the use of biologically relevant measures that are prognostic for the clinical event of interest and that individually or jointly account for a substantial proportion of the treatment effect (Freedman et al., 1992; Lagakos, 1993; Lin et al., 1997).

STATISTICAL VALIDATION OF SURROGATE MARKERS

In a validation study, the changes in both the surrogate marker and the occurrence of the clinical event must be recorded. The three criteria in the definition of a surrogate marker can then be assessed by statistical modeling. Discussed below are some of the methods that have been proposed for the validation of markers as surrogates of clinical outcomes.

PTE

Surrogate marker fluctuations should account for a large proportion (50% to 75% or higher) of the treatment effect on the clinical event. In a validation study of a surrogate marker, the proportion of treatment effect (PTE) is estimated by the following equation: $p = [(\beta - \beta^*) / \beta]$. Here p is the PTE, β^* is the estimate of the treatment effect obtained from a statistical model that includes both the treatment and marker effects, and β is the estimate of the treatment effect produced by a statistical model that includes the treatment effect but not the marker effect. In general, β* and β would be estimates of the slope of a regression line (e.g., in linear regression, logistic regression, analyses of covariance, or survival analysis models). The estimates β* and β can also be produced by analyses involving additional explanatory variables, as long as the two models are "nested," that is, one contains all ancillary explanatory factors, along with the treatment effect, while the other is comprised of the same factors and the treatment effect plus the marker effect. If the candidate marker is a perfect surrogate for the clinical outcome, then inclusion of the marker effect in the model will render the treatment effect nonsignificant, i.e., β* ≈ 0, and thus the PTE explained by the marker will be $p ≈ 100\%$. Statistical methods for estimating the PTE have been proposed by Freedman and colleagues and Lin and colleagues (Freedman et al., 1992; Lin et al., 1997). Confidence intervals around a PTE estimate can be constructed. A marker will be considered adequate if the confidence interval of the PTE excludes (i.e., its lower bound lies above) a PTE of 50% or higher.

PTE estimation has two serious drawbacks. First, to ensure that the confidence interval excludes a meaningful proportion (e.g., 50% or higher) with sufficient probability (power), the estimate of the treatment difference must be at least four times its standard error. In practical terms, this means that the statistical test resulting from the treatment comparison must yield a P value below 0.0001. To obtain such highly significant P values, either treatment differences must be spectacular or the standard error of estimation must be very small. Studies that indicate a definitive superiority of one treatment over another are often interrupted prior to completion in order to bring a promising medication to patients as soon as possible. Thus, differences of the required magnitude are unlikely to materialize (even in cases of strong treatment superiority). Therefore, only large validation studies will produce the requisite small standard errors and thus the required precision of PTE estimates. Another conceptual problem is that the PTE can be larger than 1 (i.e., higher than 100%). This might occur if the therapy has a mechanism of action that is not mediated through the marker (Fig. 1), and this mechanism results in an adverse reaction (Hughes et al., 1995). For these reasons, PTE estimates are often more useful in disproving the utility of a marker than in confirming it.

Meta-Analysis

In the absence of a single large validation study, the utility of a surrogate marker can be assessed by meta-analysis of several smaller studies. Meta-analysis methods are applicable both in instances where the treatments in the reviewed studies are the same and when a class of treatments is being considered (e.g., nucleoside reverse transcriptase inhibitors). Because estimates of the validity of the marker can vary widely from one study to another, meta-analysis with random effects (DerSimonian and Laird, 1986; Daniels and Hughes, 1997) is one of the best ways in which to appropriately account for differences among studies.

Meta-analysis of related studies can be used to produce a weighted PTE estimate. The weights are inversely proportional to the PTE variability within each study, so that studies with less variability provide more information than studies with higher variability. This weighted estimate is significantly more accurate than estimates derived from individual studies (Hughes et al., 1998).

Another approach is to fit a regression line through the points defined by the effect of the treatment on the marker levels and the effect of treatment on the clinical outcome (Daniels and Hughes, 1997; Hughes et al., 1998). Figure 2 presents two alternative scenarios from a meta-analysis of a surrogate marker. The horizontal error bars enclose a 95% confidence interval of the marker level, while the vertical error bars enclose a 95% confidence interval of the treatment effect, both estimated from each study. In Fig. 2A, there is a strong association between marker levels and treatment effects, shown by a tight linear relationship. By contrast, in Fig. 2B, the opposite situation is presented, in which there is substantial variability in the treatment effect at each marker level.

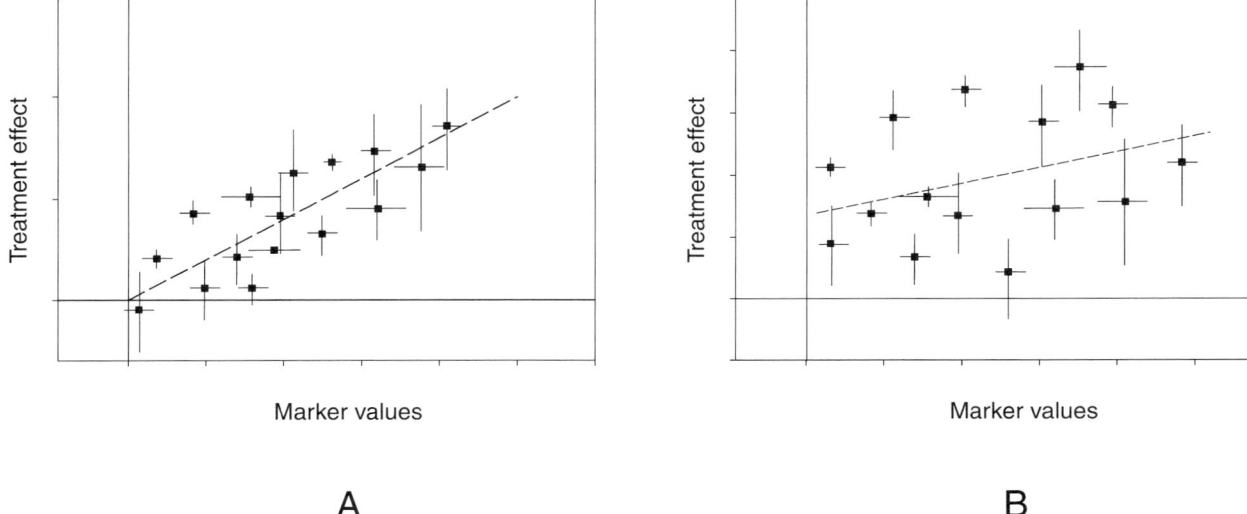

FIGURE 2 Two alternative meta-analysis situations. (A) Meta-analysis supporting marker surrogacy. (B) Meta-analysis that does not support marker surrogacy, both with regard to the variability among the studies and with respect to the regression line not going through the origin.

The strength of the association can be statistically verified by testing whether the slope of the regression line is different from zero, that is, by assessing whether changes in the marker are strongly associated with the treatment effect. A perfect surrogate marker would require that all points fall on a straight line. A further requirement is that the regression line pass through the origin (point [0, 0]) so that if the treatment has zero effect on the marker, the treatment effect on the clinical outcome will also be zero (Daniels and Hughes, 1997; Hughes et al., 1997). This methodology can be extended to include both controlled (comparative) and uncontrolled (single-treatment) studies (Li and Begg, 1994). The ability to include uncontrolled studies in meta-analyses evaluating surrogate markers is extremely significant, especially in neuro-AIDS, because the majority of studies that have assessed neurological surrogate markers in HIV have included only a single treatment regimen.

Case-Cohort Studies

If measuring the clinical event and the surrogate marker is difficult because of cost or other considerations, a case-cohort design can be implemented. This design does not require that the surrogate marker and the clinical event be observed for all subjects. In the case-cohort formulation, a number of subjects (the "subcohort") are selected at random out of all subjects involved in a study. Both the clinical event and the surrogate marker are recorded for subcohort subjects. In addition, the surrogate marker is measured for all subjects who have experienced the clinical event (the "cases"), some of whom may already be members of the subcohort (Prentice, 1986; Barlow et al., 1999).

The case-cohort design is particularly useful in situations where large numbers of specimens are being collected as part of a study but have not been processed. With this design, processing is required only for a small subset of subjects, thus dramatically decreasing cost. For example, viral-load specimens that have been collected and stored as part of a clinical study can be retrieved and analyzed based on membership in the subcohort and information on the clinical event. A case-cohort design can easily be applied to both prospective and retrospective studies. A variant of the case-cohort design can also be used when validating a marker-based "screening" test versus a more complicated diagnostic procedure. The case-cohort design can be adapted so that the "cases" are selected based on a positive screening-test value. Then, the diagnosis is confirmed by the "gold standard" method in members of the random subcohort, as well as subjects who test positive on the screening test. Thus, the administration of a potentially time-consuming, invasive, or costly procedure to the entire cohort is unnecessary (Miller et al., 2002).

SURROGATE MARKERS IN NEURO-AIDS

Example 1. Creation of a Composite Surrogate Factor for Survival of HIV-Infected Patients: a PTE Validation Approach

CD4 counts and the HIV viral load in plasma have been extensively studied as predictive markers of progression and survival for HIV-infected patients, both individually (Jacobson et al., 1991; Coombs et al., 1996; Katzenstein et al., 1996; Daniels and Hughes, 1997; Mellors, 1997) and combined (Hughes et al., 1997; Mellors et al., 1997; Marschner et al., 1998). Nevertheless, it has been reported that the CD4 count is an incomplete marker of patient survival (Choi et al., 1993; Lin et al., 1993; Hughes et al., 1998). It is useful, therefore, to explore additional markers of disease progression in an attempt to derive a composite surrogate marker.

Cognitive impairment has been recognized as a risk factor for survival (Mayeux et al., 1993; Neaton et al., 1994; Sacktor et al., 1996; Bouwman et al., 1998; Wilkie et al., 1998). In addition, neurological dysfunction has been observed to be an additional dimension of disease, along with systemic (immunologic/virologic) considerations (Mayeux et al., 1993; Ellis et al., 1997a; Price et al., 1999). Characteristic symptoms of HAD include impaired concentration, psychomotor slowing, and difficulty with sequential mental tasks (Navia et al., 1986b; Price et al., 1988). The neuropsychological profile generally agrees with the clinical picture, as deficits are typically found in areas of sustained attention, mental flexibility, and motor speed (Tross et al., 1988). Tests that have been found to be sensitive to HAD-associated deficits include trail making B, digit symbol, grooved pegboard, and the computerized reaction time test (Tross et al., 1988; Miller et al., 1991; Selnes and Miller, 1994; Carey et al., 2004). An aggregate eight-test battery based on these tests has been correlated with regional brain metabolism (measured by proton magnetic resonance spectroscopy) in the subcortical areas of the brain (Paul et al., 2007). This finding is consistent with the definition of HAD as a subcortical disease (Navia et al., 1986a; Benson, 1987).

In a study undertaken by the AIDS Clinical Trials Group (Henry et al., 1998), an aggregate neuropsychological testing battery based on four of the above-mentioned tests (namely, timed gait, digit symbol, grooved pegboard performed with the dominant hand, and finger tapping performed with the nondominant hand) was observed to be prognostic of survival even after the prognostic abilities of CD4 counts (baseline and change from baseline to week 8) and the HIV viral load (baseline viral load, as well as change from baseline to week 24) had been accounted for (Price et al., 1999). This observation replicates the findings of an earlier study by Ellis and colleagues (Ellis et al. 1997b), which suggested that neurological deterioration is a strong prognostic factor of clinical outcome, in addition to immunologic (CD4 count) and virologic (HIV plasma viral load) measures. Combined, these data highlight the relevance of neuropsychological testing as a useful measure of neurological performance in HIV-infected patients.

We illustrate here the methodology for estimating the PTE represented by a composite marker comprised of three measures: the CD4 count (baseline and change from baseline to week 8), the HIV plasma viral load (baseline and change from baseline to week 24), and a four-test neuropsychological test battery administered to a subset of HIV-infected patients enrolled in the trial reported by Price and colleagues (Price et al., 1999).

In the parent study (Henry et al., 1998), 1,313 patients were treated with four antiretroviral-drug combinations: ZDV alternated monthly with didanosine (ddI) and in combination with zalcitabine (ddC), ddI, or ddI and nevirapine (NVP). Survival advantages were observed in the ZDV-plus-ddI and ZDV-plus-ddI-plus-NVP arms compared to the alternating-monotherapy and ZDV-plus-ddC arms, while improvements in neuropsychological performance were observed over the first 52 weeks of the study (Price et al., 1999) in the same groups. In the subsequent analyses, the ZDV/ddI monotherapy and ZDV-plus-ddC treatment groups and ZDV-plus-ddI and ZDV-plus-ddI-plus-NVP treatment groups were combined.

The cohort considered here was comprised of 177 subjects with available vital status, CD4 cell count, HIV RNA, and neuropsychological data. The last was a composite index made up of four neuropsychological test scores: timed gait, digit symbol, grooved pegboard performed with the dominant hand, and finger-tapping performed with the nondominant hand. All subjects included in this analysis survived at least 20 weeks on the study.

Table 1 shows estimates of the regression slope associated with the treatment effect. First, the slope estimate was produced by a model that included the treatment as the sole predictor of patient survival. Three markers were then sequentially considered: a marker based jointly on baseline CD4 counts and CD4 change from baseline to week 8, a second marker that was comprised of the combined CD4-based marker plus baseline HIV RNA and RNA change from baseline to week 24, and a third marker that was made up of the elements of the second marker plus change in an aggregate score made up of four age-adjusted neuropsychological test scores (NPZ-4) from baseline to week 20. The PTE in each of these three cases, along with a 95% confidence interval, are also listed in the table (Lin et al., 1997). The P value of the statistical test assessing the significance of each factor is also presented, based on the Cox proportional-hazards model.

The PTE estimates were very low when the CD4 count and HIV viral load were considered and increased only slightly with the addition of NPZ-4 in the model, despite the highly significant nature of neuropsychological performance in subsequent survival (an important finding in itself that suggests that CD4 counts and the HIV viral load do not adequately summarize the disease risk without knowledge of neurological function). Clearly, these data are insufficient for obtaining a precise estimate of the PTE. The confidence intervals all encompass zero percent, which means that we cannot be certain that the combination marker explains a meaningful proportion of the effect of treatment on patient survival. This is due to a combination of high variability in all measurements, suboptimal antiviral treatment, and the small number of subjects.

Example 2. Case-Cohort Validation of a Diagnostic Test: Validation of a Neuropathy and a Neuropsychological Screening Questionnaire

HIV-associated distal sensory polyneuropathy (DSP) is a frequent complication in patients with advanced immune suppression (Bacellar et al., 1994; Sacktor, 2002; Lichtenstein et al., 2005) and has been previously reported to affect as many as 35% of patients with AIDS (So et al., 1988). Its pathogenesis remains poorly understood, although it is suspected to be a consequence of HIV-associated immune activation (Tyor et al., 1995) and to be exacerbated by the use of certain antiviral compounds (Simpson and Tagliati, 1995; Williams et al., 2001; Sacktor, 2002; Nolan and Mallal, 2004). The clinical manifestations indicate that DSP is predominantly a small-fiber sensory neuropathy (American Academy of Neurology, 1991; McCarthy et al., 1995; Holland et al., 1998). The diagnosis of DSP relies on symptoms of symmetrical pain, burning, or tingling discomfort in the feet; diminished or absent ankle reflexes; and distal diminution sensation in the legs. The diagnosis of peripheral neuropathy, however, is not standardized, and no method exists that can be universally administered in clinical studies. In fact, peripheral neuropathy has been significantly underdiagnosed or misdiagnosed, even in large clinical trials (D. Simpson, personal communication). A simple screening test has been proposed that can be administered by non-neurologists and that may be useful in identifying subjects with DSP (Marra et al., 1998). A validation study for this screening instrument has just been completed in the AIDS Clinical Trials Group. The diagnostic gold standard is based on an adaptation of the total neuropathy score (Cornblath et al., 1999), which has been studied in the context of diabetic peripheral neuropathy.

In a validation study, the gold standard diagnostic procedure and the new experimental procedure are applied to the same subjects. As a simple example, consider the diagnosis of DSP as a binary (yes/no) decision. Then, the subject cohort is distributed in a 2-by-2 table, like Fig. 3. Two routinely estimated indices of test accuracy are the sensitivity and the specificity of the diagnostic test. In the usual estimation procedure, the estimate of the sensitivity is $\hat{\eta} = N_{11}/N_1$ and that of specificity is $\hat{\theta} = N_{12}/N_2$. This estimation procedure is adequate when the diagnosis of interest is not rare and when administration of the gold standard test is not invasive, time-consuming, or expensive. When this is the case, because either a large number of subjects or expensive and invasive assessments are required to ensure adequate precision of the estimates, an alternative design

TABLE 1 PTE explained by three alternative markers

Model	Treatment slope (β)	P value[a]	PTE	95% CI[b]
Treatment	−0.55	0.011		
Treatment	−0.46	0.039	0.174	−0.463 to −0.810
Baseline CD4	−0.02	0.001		
Week 8 CD4 change	−0.02	0.003		
Treatment	−0.44	0.046	0.203	−0.410 to −0.816
Baseline CD4	−0.02	0.001		
Week 8 CD4 change	−0.02	0.009		
Baseline HIV RNA	0.80	<0.001		
Week 24 RNA change	0.64	0.038		
Treatment	−0.44	0.047	0.204	−0.409 to −0.817
Baseline CD4	−0.02	0.001		
Week 8 CD4 change	−0.02	0.009		
Baseline HIV RNA	0.80	<0.001		
Week 24 RNA change	0.53	0.087		
Week 20 NPZ-4 change	−0.44	0.008		

[a]Wald test in proportional-hazards regression.
[b]Lin et al., 1997.

T_1	T_2		Total
	+	-	
+	N_{11}	N_{12}	$N_{1.}$
-	N_{21}	N_{22}	$N_{2.}$
Total	$N_{.1}$	$N_{.2}$	N

Conventional study design

T_1	T_2		Total
	+	-	
+	N_{11}	N_{12}	$N_{1.}$
-			$N_{2.}$
Total			N

Total cohort

T_1	T_2		Total
	+	-	
+	M_{11}	M_{12}	$M_{1.}$
-	M_{21}	M_{22}	$M_{2.}$
Total	$M_{.1}$	$M_{.2}$	M

Subcohort

Case cohort design

FIGURE 3 Numbers of subjects classified by two tests. T_1 is the gold standard, and T_2 is the diagnostic test under assessment in a conventional validation study (top) and the case-cohort design (bottom). Notice that all subjects who test positive by the screening test (T_2) are tested by the gold standard test (T_1), along with a small number (M) of randomly selected subjects (the subcohort). Thus, it is not known which of the subjects in the overall cohort who tested negative by the gold standard were misclassified by the new test (false positives). Only known group sizes are included in the tables. The numbers of correctly classified subjects are shown in boldface.

based on the case-cohort design (Prentice, 1986) may be used (Miller et al., 2002). This modified case-cohort design proceeds as follows. All N subjects are administered the screening test. Then, a subcohort of size M < N is randomly selected from the study population (with M much smaller than N). All members of the subcohort are administered a gold standard diagnostic procedure. In the case of validation for a DSP screening test, the standard diagnostic procedure would involve the total neuropathy score, nerve conduction velocity studies, and skin biopsies, in addition to clinical evaluation in order to determine the true disease status. The gold standard method is also administered to all subjects who have screening-test scores suggestive of neuropathy. The numbers of groups involved in the case-cohort study are presented in Table 2.

The estimates of the sensitivity and specificity in the case-cohort design are given by the following equations (Miller et al., 2002):

$$\hat{\eta} = \frac{N_{11}}{N_{11} + N_{2.}\left[M_{21} / M_{2.}\right]}$$

$$\hat{\theta} = \frac{N_{2.}\left[M_{22} / M_{2.}\right]}{N_{2.}\left[M_{22} / M_{2.}\right] + N_{12}}$$

We simulated a validation study of the screening test evaluated by Marra and colleagues (Marra et al., 1998). In this study, we assumed that the true sensitivity and specificity of the screening instrument were at the midpoints of the reported intervals (i.e., 93% and 77%). We also assumed an overall prevalence of 30% for HIV-associated peripheral neuropathy in the patient population. We simulated 1,000 validation studies of 300 to 500 subjects each, 100 of whom were randomly enrolled in the subcohort. Out of the remaining subjects, everyone with a positive screening test was administered the gold standard diagnostic procedure to determine the presence of peripheral neuropathy. The case-cohort-derived estimates of sensitivity and specificity are listed, along with their estimated standard errors, in Table 2. They are contrasted with the conventional estimates described above, which are based on a full evaluation of the complete study cohort (Fig. 3). The numbers of subjects administered the complete neuropathy

TABLE 2 Comparison of case-cohort and conventional estimates of sensitivity and specificity

Parameter	Estimates[a]	
	Simulated case-cohort design [mean (SD)]	Conventional approach
Sensitivity	0.492 (0.057)	0.485
Specificity	0.876 (0.004)	0.876
Total number of subjects tested by the gold standard	127.9 (3.19)	292

[a]Based on 1,000 simulated studies of (n = 292) subjects such as the validation study of the brief peripheral neuropathy screening (Marra et al., 1998) performed by Ellis et al. (2005). The size of the subcohort in all simulated studies (M) was 100. By contrast to the 292 subjects that would be evaluated by the conventional design, on average only 127.9 subjects were administered the standard test.

examination in the case-cohort validation study are listed in the last row.

The case-cohort estimates of the sensitivity and specificity (the true parameters were 77% and 93%, respectively) are very close to the conventional estimates and have slightly less accuracy. The mean number of subjects evaluated was 127.9 (standard deviation, 4.73). By contrast, all 300 subjects would have to be tested in a conventional study design, resulting in 57% savings in cost or study complexity. The savings of the case-cohort design become even more dramatic in validation studies, where the prevalence of the disease is low. An example of this would be a similar test validation procedure applied in the context of cognitive impairment, where the prevalence of neurological symptoms is low, even among patients with advanced HIV disease. In that case, a smaller number of subjects not belonging to the subcohort would have to be tested.

DISCUSSION

Increasing availability of treatment options in HIV infection has improved the prognosis of many patients infected with HIV. Nevertheless, neurological complications, such as HAD, progressive multifocal leukoencephalopathy, and, in particular, DSP, will likely remain a major challenge in patient management. Investigation into measures that can be used as surrogates of neurological complications has seriously lagged behind research on immunologic and virologic markers. Neurological markers will aid in the quantification of the effect of the virus on the nervous system and will serve as instruments for screening patients and comparing treatments in clinical trials.

Several neurological markers have been proposed in the literature, but their utility as surrogates has not been validated. Here, I have presented the essential elements for identification and validation of a candidate measure as a surrogate marker. These are distilled into two criteria related to the prognostic ability of the marker for the event of interest and its ability to adequately summarize the treatment effect on the clinical event.

Traditional validation studies are complicated to design, time-consuming, and expensive. Repeated measurements of the candidate surrogate markers for a large number of subjects are required, and observation must continue until a sufficiently large number of them have experienced the clinical event of interest (e.g., cognitive deterioration or peripheral nerve damage). However with improved prognosis for a large proportion of patients, large clinical studies that are based

on invasive measures or that follow patients until the occurrence of a clinical endpoint are difficult to implement and are undertaken with diminishing frequency. Creative study designs that do not require large patient samples, such as the case-cohort design, which does not necessitate the administration of an invasive or expensive procedure to all subjects, or meta-analysis, which synthesizes the experiences in several smaller trials, should be considered viable alternatives to the traditional large validation trials.

With increasing evidence that the neurological aspect of HIV infection constitutes a separate part of the disease, acting synergistically with its immunologic and virologic dimensions (Ellis et al., 1997b; Price et al., 1999), research into HIV neurological outcomes should proceed on par with immunologic and virologic investigations. Identification and validation of appropriate measures that assess the evolution of neurologic disease will be critical in this endeavor.

The research was supported by NIH grants AI-38855 (NIAID), NS3228 and NS36524 (NINDS), and MH60565 (NIMH). I thank Karl Kieburtz and Steve Lagakos for incisive discussions and guidance during the development of this chapter, Soyeon Kim for supplying the software for the calculation of PTE confidence intervals, and Sherri Bucher for sharpening the focus of its content.

REFERENCES

Albert, J. M., J. P. Ioannidis, P. Reichelderfer, B. Conway, R. W. Coombs, L. Crane, R. Demasi, D. O. Dixon, P. Flandre, M. D. Hughes, L. A. Kalish, K. Larntz, D. Lin, I. C. Marschner, A. Muñoz, J. Murray, J. Neaton, C. Pettinelli, W. Rida, J. M. Taylor, and S. L. Welles. 1998. Statistical issues for HIV surrogate endpoints: point/counterpoint. An NIAID workshop. *Stat. Med.* 17:2435–2462.

Albrecht, H., C. Hoffmann, O. Degen, A. Stoehr, A. Plettenberg, T. Mertenskötter, C. Eggers, and H. J. Stellbrink. 1998. Highly active antiretroviral therapy significantly improves the prognosis of patients with HIV-associated progressive multifocal leukoencephalopathy. *AIDS* 12:1149–1154.

American Academy of Neurology. 1991. Nomenclature and research case definitions for neurologic manifestations of human immunodeficiency virus-type 1 (HIV-1) infection. Report of a working group of the American Academy of Neurology AIDS Task Force. *Neurology* 41:778–785.

Bacellar, H., A. Muñoz, E. N. Miller, B. A. Cohen, D. Besley, O. A. Selnes, J. T. Becker, and J. C. McArthur. 1994. Temporal trends in the incidence of HIV-1-related neurologic diseases: Multicenter AIDS Cohort Study, 1985–1992. *Neurology* 44:1892–1900.

Barlow, W. E., L. Ichikawa, D. Rosner, and S. Izumi. 1999. Analysis of case-cohort designs. *J. Clin. Epidemiol.* 52:1165–1172.

Benson, D. F. 1987. The spectrum of dementia: a comparison of the clinical features of AIDS/dementia and dementia of the Alzheimer type. *Alzheimer Dis. Assoc. Disord.* 1:217–220.

Bouwman, F. H., R. L. Skolasky, D. Hes, O. A. Selnes, J. D. Glass, T. E. Nance-Sproson, W. Royal, G. J. Dal Pan, and J. C. McArthur. 1998. Variable progression of HIV-associated dementia. *Neurology* 50:1814–1820.

Carey, C. L., S. P. Woods, J. D. Rippeth, R. Gonzalez, D. J. Moore, T. D. Marcotte, I. Grant, and R. K. Heaton. 2004. Initial validation of a screening battery for the detection of HIV-associated cognitive impairment. *Clin. Neuropsychol.* 18:234–248.

Choi, S., S. W. Lagakos, R. T. Schooley, and P. A. Volberding. 1993. CD4+ lymphocytes are an incomplete surrogate marker for clinical progression in persons with asymptomatic HIV infection taking zidovudine. *Ann. Intern. Med.* 118:674–680.

Coombs, R. W., S. L. Welles, C. Hooper, P. S. Reichelderfer, R. T. D'Aquila, A. J. Japour, V. A. Johnson, D. R. Kuritzkes, D. D. Richman, S. Kwok, J. Todd, J. B. Jackson, V. DeGruttola, C. S. Crumpacker, and J. Kahn. 1996. Association of plasma human immunodeficiency virus type 1 RNA level with risk of clinical progression in patients with advanced infection. AIDS Clinical Trials Group (ACTG) 116B/117 Study Team. ACTG Virology Committee Resistance and HIV-1 RNA Working Groups. *J. Infect. Dis.* **174:**704–712.

Cooper, E. H., and C. J. Lacey. 1988. Laboratory indices of prognosis in HIV infection. *Biomed. Pharmacother.* **42:**539–545.

Cornblath, D. R., V. Chaudhry, K. Carter, D. Lee, M. Seysedadr, M. Miernicki, and T. Joh. 1999. Total neuropathy score: validation and reliability study. *Neurology* **53:**1660.

Dal Pan, G. J., and J. C. McArthur. 1996. Neuroepidemiology of HIV infection. *Neurol. Clin.* **14:**359–382.

Daniels, M. J., and M. D. Hughes. 1997. Meta-analysis for the evaluation of potential surrogate markers. *Stat. Med.* **16:**1965–1982.

DeGruttola, V., M. Hughes, P. Gilbert, and A. Phillips. 1998. Trial design in the era of highly effective antiviral drug combinations for HIV infection. *AIDS* **12**(Suppl. A)**:**S149–S156.

DerSimonian, R., and N. Laird. 1986. Meta-analysis in clinical trials. *Control. Clin. Trials* **7:**177–186.

Dore, G. J., P. K. Correll, Y. Li, J. M. Kaldor, D. A. Cooper, and B. J. Brew. 1999. Changes to AIDS dementia complex in the era of highly active antiretroviral therapy. *AIDS* **13:**1249–1253.

Dore, G. J., A. McDonald, Y. Li, J. M. Kaldor, and B. J. Brew. 2003. Marked improvement in survival following AIDS dementia complex in the era of highly active antiretroviral therapy. *AIDS* **17:**1539–1545.

Dybul, M., A. S. Fauci, J. G. Bartlett, J. E. Kaplan, and A. K. Pau. 2002. Guidelines for using antiretroviral agents among HIV-infected adults and adolescents. *Ann. Intern. Med.* **137:**381–433.

Elashoff, M., and S. Lagakos. 1996. HIV treatment strategies utilizing virologic and immunologic markers as criteria for changing treatments. *Stat. Med.* **15:**2425–2443.

Ellis, R. J., R. Deutsch, R. K. Heaton, T. D. Marcotte, J. A. McCutchan, J. A. Nelson, I. Abramson, L. J. Thal, J. H. Atkinson, M. R. Wallace, I. Grant, et al. 1997a. Neurocognitive impairment is an independent risk factor for death in HIV infection. *Arch. Neurol.* **54:**416–424.

Ellis, R. J., S. R. Evans, D. B. Clifford, L. R. Moo, J. C. McArthur, A. C. Collier, C. Benson, R. Bosch, D. Simpson, C. T. Yiannoutsos, Y. Yang, K. Robertson, and Neurological AIDS Research Consortium AIDS Clinical Trials Group Study Teams A5001 and A362. 2005. Clinical validation of the neuroscreen. *J. Neurovirol.* **11:**503–511.

Ellis, R. J., K. Hsia, S. A. Spector, J. A. Nelson, R. K. Heaton, M. R. Wallace, I. Abramson, J. H. Atkinson, I. Grant, J. A. McCutchan, et al. 1997b. Cerebrospinal fluid human immunodeficiency virus type 1 RNA levels are elevated in neurocognitively impaired individuals with acquired immunodeficiency syndrome. *Ann. Neurol.* **42:**679–688.

Fauci, A. S., A. M. Macher, D. L. Longo, H. C. Lane, A. H. Rook, H. Masur, and E. P. Gelmann. 1984. NIH conference. Acquired immunodeficiency syndrome: epidemiologic, clinical, immunologic, and therapeutic considerations. *Ann. Intern. Med.* **100:**92–106.

Fleming, T. R., and D. L. DeMets. 1996. Surrogate end points in clinical trials: are we being misled? *Ann. Intern. Med.* **125:**605–613.

Freedman, L. S., A. Schatzkin, and M. H. Schiffman. 1992. Statistical validation of intermediate markers of precancer for use as endpoints in chemoprevention trials. *J. Cell. Biochem. Suppl.* **16G:**27–32.

Gazzard, B. 1996. HIV treatment strategies utilizing virologic and immunologic markers as criteria for changing treatments. *Stat. Med.* **15:**2425–2443, 2455–2458.

Goldman, A. I., B. P. Carlin, L. R. Crane, C. Launer, J. A. Korvick, L. Deyton, and D. I. Abrams. 1996. Response of CD4 lymphocytes and clinical consequences of treatment using ddI or ddC in patients with advanced HIV infection. *J. Acquir. Immune Defic. Syndr. Hum. Retrovirol.* **11:**161–169.

Henry, K., A. Erice, C. Tierney, H. H. Balfour, Jr., M. A. Fischl, A. Kmack, S. H. Liou, A. Kenton, M. S. Hirsch, J. Phair, A. Martinez, J. O. Kahn, et al. 1998. A randomized, controlled, double-blind study comparing the survival benefit of four different reverse transcriptase inhibitor therapies (three-drug, two-drug, and alternating drug) for the treatment of advanced AIDS. *J. Acquir. Immune Defic. Syndr. Hum. Retrovirol.* **19:**339–349.

Holland, N. R., T. O. Crawford, P. Hauer, D. R. Cornblath, J. W. Griffin, and J. C. McArthur. 1998. Small fiber sensory neuropathies: clinical course and neuropathology of idiopathic cases. *Ann. Neurol.* **44:**47–59.

Hughes, M. D., M. J. Daniels, M. A. Fischl, S. Kim, and R. T. Schooley. 1998. CD4 cell count as a surrogate endpoint in HIV clinical trials: a meta-analysis of studies of the AIDS Clinical Trials Group. *AIDS* **12:**1823–1832.

Hughes, M. D., V. DeGruttola, and S. L. Welles. 1995. Evaluating surrogate markers. *J. Acquir. Immune Defic. Syndr. Hum. Retrovirol.* **10**(Suppl 2)**:**S1–S8.

Hughes, M. D., V. A. Johnson, M. S. Hirsch, J. W. Bremer, T. Elbeik, A. Erice, D. R. Kuritzkes, W. A. Scott, S. A. Spector, N. Basgoz, M. A. Fischl, R. T. D'Aquila, et al. 1997. Monitoring plasma HIV-1 RNA levels in addition to CD4+ lymphocyte count improves assessment of antiretroviral therapeutic response. *Ann. Intern. Med.* **126:**929–938.

Jacobson, M. A., P. Bacchetti, A. Kolokathis, R. E. Chaisson, S. Szabo, B. Polsky, G. T. Valainis, D. Mildvan, D. Abrams, J. Wilber, et al. 1991. Surrogate markers for survival in patients with AIDS and AIDS related complex treated with zidovudine. *BMJ* **302:**73–78.

Jacobson, M. A., V. De Gruttola, M. Reddy, J. M. Arduino, S. Strickland, R. C. Reichman, J. A. Bartlett, J. P. Phair, M. S. Hirsch, A. C. Collier, et al. 1995. The predictive value of changes in serologic and cell markers of HIV activity for subsequent clinical outcome in patients with asymptomatic HIV disease treated with zidovudine. *AIDS* **9:**727–734.

Kaplan, J. E., D. L. Hanson, J. L. Jones, and M. S. Dworkin. 2001. Viral load as an independent risk factor for opportunistic infections in HIV-infected adults and adolescents. *AIDS* **15:**1831–1836.

Katzenstein, D. A., S. M. Hammer, M. D. Hughes, H. Gundacker, J. B. Jackson, S. Fiscus, S. Rasheed, T. Elbeik, R. Reichman, A. Japour, T. C. Merigan, M. S. Hirsch, et al. 1996. The relation of virologic and immunologic markers to clinical outcomes after nucleoside therapy in HIV-infected adults with 200 to 500 CD4 cells per cubic millimeter. *N. Engl. J. Med.* **335:**1091–1098.

Lagakos, S. W. 1993. Surrogate markers in AIDS clinical trials: conceptual basis, validation, and uncertainties. *Clin. Infect. Dis.* **16**(Suppl 1)**:**S22–S25.

Lagakos, S. W., and D. F. Hoth. 1992. Surrogate markers in AIDS: where are we? Where are we going? *Ann. Intern. Med.* **116:**599–601.

Li, Z., and C. Begg. 1994. Random effects models for combining results from controlled and uncontrolled studies in a meta-analysis. *J. Am. Stat. Assoc.* **89:**1523–1527.

Lichtenstein, K. A., C. Armon, A. Baron, A. C. Moorman, K. C. Wood, and S. D. Holmberg. 2005. Modification of the incidence of drug-associated symmetrical peripheral neuropathy by host and disease factors in the HIV outpatient study cohort. *Clin. Infect. Dis.* **40:**148–157.

Lin, D., M. Fischl, and D. Schoenfeld. 1993. Evaluating the role of CD4-lymphocyte counts as surrogate endpoints in human immunodeficiency virus clinical trials. Stat. Med. 12:835–842.

Lin, D. Y., T. R. Fleming, and V. De Gruttola. 1997. Estimating the proportion of treatment effect explained by a surrogate marker. Stat. Med. 16:1515–1527.

Marra, C. M., P. Boutin, and A. C. Collier. 1998. Screening for distal sensory peripheral neuropathy in HIV-infected persons in research and clinical settings. Neurology 51:1678–1681.

Marschner, I. C., A. C. Collier, R. W. Coombs, R. T. D'Aquila, V. DeGruttola, M. A. Fischl, S. M. Hammer, M. D. Hughes, V. A. Johnson, D. A. Katzenstein, D. D. Richman, L. M. Smeaton, S. A. Spector, and M. S. Saag. 1998. Use of changes in plasma levels of human immunodeficiency virus type 1 RNA to assess the clinical benefit of antiretroviral therapy. J. Infect. Dis. 177:40–47.

Mayeux, R., Y. Stern, M. X. Tang, G. Todak, K. Marder, M. Sano, M. Richards, Z. Stein, A. A. Ehrhardt, and J. M. Gorman. 1993. Mortality risks in gay men with human immunodeficiency virus infection and cognitive impairment. Neurology 43:176–182.

McArthur, J. 1999. Neurology update. Hopkins HIV Rep. 11:8.

McArthur, J. C. 2004. HIV dementia: an evolving disease. J. Neuroimmunol. 157:3–10.

McCarthy, B. G., S. T. Hsieh, A. Stocks, P. Hauer, C. Macko, D. R. Cornblath, J. W. Griffin, and J. C. McArthur. 1995. Cutaneous innervation in sensory neuropathies: evaluation by skin biopsy. Neurology 45:1848–1855.

Mellors, J. W. 1997. Prognosis depends on viral load. AIDS: frequently too much time is wasted. Fortschr. Med. 115:14.

Mellors, J. W., A. Muñoz, J. V. Giorgi, J. B. Margolick, C. J. Tassoni, P. Gupta, L. A. Kingsley, J. A. Todd, A. J. Saah, R. Detels, J. P. Phair, and C. R. Rinaldo, Jr. 1997. Plasma viral load and CD4+ lymphocytes as prognostic markers of HIV-1 infection. Ann. Intern. Med. 126:946–954.

Mildvan, D., A. Landay, V. De Gruttola, S. G. Machado, and J. Kagan. 1997. An approach to the validation of markers for use in AIDS clinical trials. Clin. Infect. Dis. 24:764–774.

Miller, E. N., P. Satz, and B. R. Visscher. 1991. Computerized and conventional neuropsychological assessment of HIV-1 infected homosexual men. Neurology 41:1608–1616.

Miller, L. C., C. T. Yiannoutsos, and M. D. Hughes. 2002. Diagnostic test validation: optimal designs, p. 463–470. In Proc. 17th Int. Workshop Statistical Modeling, Chania, Greece.

Miralles, P., J. Berenguer, D. G. de Viedma, B. Padilla, J. Cosin, J. C. López-Bernaldo de Quirós, L. Muñoz, S. Moreno, and J. Bouza. 1998. Treatment of AIDS-associated progressive multifocal leukoencephalopathy with highly active antiretroviral therapy. AIDS 12:2467–2472.

Moore, R., J. Keruly, J. Gallant, and R. Chaisson. 1998. Decline in mortality rates and opportunistic disease with combination antiretroviral therapy. 12th World AIDS Conference, Geneva, Switzerland.

Navia, B. A., E. S. Cho, C. K. Petito, and R. W. Price. 1986a. The AIDS dementia complex: II. Neuropathology. Ann. Neurol. 19:525–535.

Navia, B. A., B. D. Jordan, and R. W. Price. 1986b. The AIDS dementia complex: I. Clinical features. Ann. Neurol. 19:517–524.

Neaton, J. D., D. N. Wentworth, F. Rhame, C. Hogan, D. I. Abrams, and L. Deyton. 1994. Considerations in choice of a clinical endpoint for AIDS clinical trials. Terry Beirn Community Programs for Clinical Research on AIDS (CPCRA). Stat. Med. 13:2107–2125.

Neuenburg, J. K., H. R. Brodt, B. G. Herndier, M. Bickel, P. Bacchetti, R. W. Price, R. M. Grant, and W. Schlote. 2002. HIV-related neuropathology, 1985 to 1999: rising prevalence of HIV encephalopathy in the era of highly active antiretroviral therapy. J. Acquir. Immune Defic. Syndr. 31:171–177.

Nolan, D., and S. Mallal. 2004. Complications associated with NRTI therapy: update on clinical features and possible pathogenic mechanisms. Antivir. Ther. 9:849–863.

Paul, R. H., C. T. Yiannoutsos, E. N. Miller, L. Chang, C. M. Marra, G. Schifitto, T. Ernst, E. Singer, T. Richards, G. J. Jarvik, R. Price, D. J. Meyerhoff, D. Kolson, R. J. Ellis, G. Gonzalez, R. E. Lenkinski, R. A. Cohen, and B. A. Navia. 2007. Proton MRS and neuropsychological correlates in AIDS dementia complex: evidence of subcortical specificity. J. Neuropsych. Clin. Neurosci. 19:283–292.

Prentice, R. L. 1986. A case-cohort design for epidemiologic cohort studies and disease prevention trials. Biometrika 73:1–11.

Prentice, R. L. 1989. Surrogate endpoints in clinical trials: definition and operational criteria. Stat. Med. 8:431–440.

Price, R. W., B. Brew, J. Sidtis, M. Rosenblum, A. C. Scheck, and P. Cleary. 1988. The brain in AIDS: central nervous system HIV-1 infection and AIDS dementia complex. Science 239:586–592.

Price, R. W., C. T. Yiannoutsos, D. B. Clifford, L. Zaborski, A. Tselis, J. J. Sidtis, B. A. Cohen, C. D. Hall, A. Erice, and K. Henry. 1999. Neurological outcomes in late-stage HIV-1 infection: adverse influence of neurological impairment on survival and protective effect of antiviral therapy. AIDS 13:1677–1686.

Sacktor, N. 2002. The epidemiology of human immunodeficiency virus-associated neurological disease in the era of highly active antiretroviral therapy. J. Neurovirol. 8(Suppl 2):115–121.

Sacktor, N., M. P. McDermott, K. Marder, G. Schifitto, O. A. Selnes, J. C. McArthur, Y. Stern, S. Albert, D. Palumbo, K. Kieburtz, J. A. De Marcaida, B. Cohen, and L. Epstein. 2002. HIV-associated cognitive impairment before and after the advent of combination therapy. J. Neurovirol. 8:136–142.

Sacktor, N. C., H. Bacellar, D. R. Hoover, T. E. Nance Sproson, O. A. Selnes, E. N. Miller, G. J. Dal Pan, C. Kleeberger, A. Brown, A. Saah, and J. C. McArthur. 1996. Psychomotor slowing in HIV infection: a predictor of dementia, AIDS and death. J. Neurovirol. 2:404–410.

Selnes, O. A., and E. N. Miller. 1994. Development of a screening battery for HIV-related cognitive impairment: the MACS experience, p. 176–187. In I. Grant and E. Martin (ed.), Neuropsychology of HIV Infection: Current Research and New Directions. Oxford University Press, New York, NY.

Simpson, D. M., and M. Tagliati. 1995. Nucleoside analogue-associated peripheral neuropathy in human immunodeficiency virus infection. J. Acquir. Immune Defic. Syndr. Hum. Retrovirol. 9:153–161.

So, Y., D. Holtzman, D. Abrams, and R. Olney. 1988. Peripheral neuropathy associated with acquired immunodeficiency syndrome. Prevalence and clinical features from a population-based survey. Arch. Neurol. 45:945–948.

Tross, S., R. W. Price, B. Navia, H. T. Thaler, J. Gold, D. A. Hirsch, and J. J. Sidtis. 1988. Neuropsychological characterization of the AIDS dementia complex: a preliminary report. AIDS 2:81–88.

Tyor, W., S. Wesselingh, J. Griffin, J. McArthur, and D. Griffin. 1995. Unifying hypothesis for the pathogenesis of HIV-associated dementia complex, vacuolar myelopathy, and sensory neuropathy. J. Acquir. Immune Defic. Syndr. Hum. Retrovirol. 9:379–388.

Volberding, P., S. Lagakos, M. Koch, et al. 1990. The efficacy of AZT in patients with asymptomatic HIV infection having less than 500 CD4 cells. N. Engl. J. Med. 322:941–949.

Welles, S. L., J. B. Jackson, B. Yen Lieberman, L. Demeter, A. J. Japour, L. M. Smeaton, V. A. Johnson, D. R. Kuritzkes,

R. T. D'Aquila, P. A. Reichelderfer, D. D. Richman, R. Reichman, M. Fischl, R. Dolin, R. W. Coombs, J. O. Kahn, C. McLaren, J. Todd, S. Kwok, C. S. Crumpacker, et al. 1996. Prognostic value of plasma human immunodeficiency virus type 1 (HIV-1) RNA levels in patients with advanced HIV-1 disease and with little or no prior zidovudine therapy. *J. Infect. Dis.* **174:**696–703.

Wilkie, F. L., K. Goodkin, C. Eisdorfer, D. Feaster, R. Morgan, M. A. Fletcher, N. Blaney, M. Baum, and J. Szapocznik. 1998. Mild cognitive impairment and risk of mortality in HIV-1 infection. *J. Neuropsychiatry Clin. Neurosci.* **10:**125–132.

Williams, D., A. Geraci, and D. M. Simpson. 2001. AIDS and AIDS-treatment neuropathies. *Curr. Neurol. Neurosci. Rep.* **1:**533–538.

The Spectrum of Neuro-AIDS Disorders:
Pathophysiology, Diagnosis, and Treatment
Edited by K. Goodkin et al.
©2008 ASM Press, Washington, DC

9

Designing HIV gp120 Peptide Vaccines: Rhetoric or Reality for Neuro-AIDS

PANDJASSARAME KANGUEANE, RAJARATHINAM KAYATHRI, MEENA KISHORE SAKHARKAR, DARREN R. FLOWER, KRISTEN SADLER, FRANCESCO CHIAPPELLI, DAVID M. SEGAL, AND PAUL SHAPSHAK

PAST HIV VACCINES

Antiretroviral drugs have dramatically improved the health and extended the lives of people with HIV/AIDS. However, the high cost of these pharmaceutical modes of implementation and their associated demanding clinical requirements put them out of reach for the majority of HIV-infected people in developing countries, where HIV infection levels are high. The potential value of a preventative and cost-effective vaccine strategy to protect against HIV is indisputable. The development of vaccines as HIV prevention tools has gained momentum in recent years (Cohen, 2005a, 2005b), and the general principles for the selection of HIV vaccine candidates were recently described by the AIDS Vaccine Integrated Project (Ensoli, 2005). The classical first-generation approaches for vaccine preparation, in which whole inactivated and live attenuated viruses are utilized, are not considered feasible for a human HIV vaccine due to safety concerns (http://hiv-web.lanl.gov/; Osborn, 1995). Therefore, the majority of candidate vaccines under development are so-called "second-generation" subunit recombinant vaccines.

Pandjassarame Kangueane and Rajarathinam Kayathri, Biomedical Informatics, 17A Irulan Sundai Annex, Pondicherry 607402, India. **Meena Kishore Sakharkar,** School of Mechanical and Aerospace Engineering, Nanyang Technological University, Singapore 639798. **Darren R. Flower,** The Jenner Institute, University of Oxford, Compton, Berkshire, United Kingdom RG20 7NN. **Kristen Sadler,** School of Biological Sciences, Nanyang Technological University, Singapore 637551. **Francesco Chiappelli,** Laboratory of Human Oral and Molecular Immunology, Division of Oral Biology and Medicine, UCLA School of Dentistry, CHS 63-090, University of California at Los Angeles, Los Angeles, CA 90095-1668. **David M. Segal,** Department of Health Professions, College of Health and Public Affairs, and Department of Medical Education, College of Medicine, University of Central Florida, Orlando, FL 32816-2205. **Paul Shapshak,** Division of Infectious Diseases and International Medicine, Tampa General Hospital, and Departments of Internal Medicine and Psychiatry-Behavioral Medicine, USF Health, Tampa, FL 33606.

However, there are also safety and regulatory concerns associated with such subunit candidates. A prime example of a subunit vaccine inducing undesirable effects is that of the NEF (negative factor) protein, which induced pathogenesis in a simian immunodeficiency virus vaccine model (Whatmore et al., 1995). The majority of HIV subunit vaccines are based on the envelope proteins of HIV, namely, gp120 and gp41, which form the gp160 glycoprotein complex, or on selected epitopes (immunogenic peptides) identified within these proteins (Bond et al., 2001). These vaccines are generally aimed at generating a humoral response with induction of neutralizing antibodies that bind to the viral proteins and effectively inhibit host cell receptor interaction and/or membrane fusion events. In the most infamous of HIV vaccine trials, the monomeric form of gp120 protein failed to induce protective immunity in phase III trials (Cohen, 2003). Nevertheless, gp120 remains a major target for the development of protective vaccines due to its surface exposure. The unfortunate failure of an initial generation of gp120-based subunit vaccines to induce protective immunity warranted the development of novel constructs based on gp120 for the induction of a neutralizing antibody response of appropriate quality and quantity. Vaccine candidate selection has proven to be a significant challenge, with many relatively small peptide-based constructs ineffective at inducing an appropriate response. One of the major limitations is the ability to effectively mimic structurally significant and highly conserved regions using synthetic vaccine candidates.

In combination with the antibody response, the advantages of inducing a cellular immune response using T-cell epitope-based vaccines have been identified and investigated (De Groot et al., 2001; Sbai et al., 2001). Candidate vaccines designed to induce cell-mediated immunity (CMI) have focused on the use of naked DNA inserted into different bacterial or viral vectors, including poxvirus, adenovirus, and retroviral vectors. In this instance, the target proteins are the buried conserved proteins of the HIV core (Letvin, 1998). Brave et al. (2006) reported that the multigene approach was successfully used to produce a cellular immune response in a mouse model. For this, the DNA coding for several different HIV proteins was included in a single vaccine candidate: gp160 envelope (env subtypes A, B, and C), p37gag (gag subtypes A and B), rev (subtype B), and reverse transcriptase (subtype B). In contrast to the protective responses observed using naked-DNA vaccines, peptide-based vaccines containing known T-cell epitopes induce only low levels of immunity and for short durations. The technological exploitation of peptide binding to HLA molecules as a component of the T-cell-mediated immune response for the development of peptide vaccines has been more seriously considered in recent years (De Groot et al., 2001). The identification of peptides capable of degenerate binding in a supertype-like manner (multiple HLA alleles capable of binding the same peptide exhibiting overlapping functional repertoires) could also alleviate the limitations imposed by HIV restriction of the cellular responses (Kangueane et al., 2005). The conventional approach (overlapping peptides 8 to 10 residues long) for screening short linear peptides from viral antigens to bind allele (variant form of a gene)-specific HLA molecules is laborious and expensive. This is because HLA molecules are highly polymorphic among various ethnic groups covering different populations, and about 2,000 alleles are known today (http://www.ebi.ac.uk/imgt/hla). The use of prediction models for selecting potential HLA-binding peptides prior to experimental validation has been realized in recent years (De Groot et al., 2001; Sbai et al., 2001; Zhao et al., 2003). The focus of this chapter is to describe a novel strategy using comparative genomics to select a potential HIV-1 antigen (gp120). This novel approach has proven most promising for the subsequent screening of short peptides from HIV-1 gp120 antigen that are predicted to bind to a wide array of HLA alleles with a view toward the design of cocktail peptide vaccines.

ISSUES IN DEFINING HLA SUPERTYPES

All supertypes are theoretically derived, even the "experimental" supertypes defined by Sette and coworkers (Sidney et al., 1996). His supertypes were based on "binding motifs," which are, as we have seen, an inadequate description of peptide specificity. While they possess a certain verisimilitude, they are at best only a partial definition of supertypes, limited by the lack of available data for most major histocompatibility complex (MHC) molecules. Structural supertypes, based on sequences and/or three-dimensional (3D) structural data, represent an encouraging potential solution to this problem, unencumbered by limitations imposed by existing binding data. Modern approaches, such as those proposed by Doytchinova et al. (2004) and Kangueane et al. (2005), allow us to propose supertype definitions based solely on sequence and structural data.

Polymorphism confounds studies of the peptide specificities of MHC molecules. Indeed, HLA is arguably the best studied of all human polymorphic proteins. The international ImMunoGeneTics information system/HLA database stores over 1,700 different HLA class I and II alleles. Such allelic variants have arisen through a process of mutation, filtered and constrained by evolutionary processes operating in the face of host-pathogen interactions, which are themselves constrained by geography and time. Since MHCs exhibit such extensive polymorphic amino acid variation, small alterations in the identities of binding-site residues will give rise to differences in peptide selectivity exhibited during peptide binding.

Since HLA alleles have been demonstrated to bind peptides with similar anchor residues, the concept of MHC supertypes has emerged: the idea that sequence-distinct MHCs can be grouped into distinct classes that exhibit equivalent, if not necessarily identical, peptide specificities. The veracity and celerity of vaccine discovery would be increased if one could identify effective rules able to group together HLA alleles with similar specificities. Such a classification, if accurate and extensive, would significantly diminish experimental work, since it would not be necessary to study every allele, thus allowing more efficient discovery of epitope-based vaccines targeting multiple alleles.

One approach to the classification of HLA has been evolutionary analysis. McKenzie et al. (1999) constructed phylogenetic trees for MHC using three methods: maximum parsimony, distance-based minimum evolution, and maximum likelihood. Different classifications were conducted, based on either the whole protein/nucleotide sequence, the sequence of the binding site, or sequence excluding the binding site. Two clusters were found for HLA-A: one with A1, A3, A9, A11, A36, A8001, and some A19 members and the other with A2, A10, A28, A4301, and the other A19 members. While neither HLA-B nor HLA-C produced consistent clusters, Cano et al. clustered the HLA-A and HLA-B alleles by constructing similarity matrices (Cano et al., 1998). MHC molecules were compared in a geometric space in which each amino acid occupied one dimension. The similarity among MHC alleles was measured using experimental peptide elution data and by comparing the alleles using the similarity matrix. The method identified three clusters. Cluster 1 included HLA-A3, HLA-A11, HLA-31, and HLA-33. Cluster 2 included HLA-B7, HLA-B35, HLA-B51, HLA-B53, and HLA-B54. Cluster 3 included HLA-A29, HLA-B44, and HLA-B61.

Arguably the best-known supertype classification is the motif-based approach of Sette and coworkers; they even coined the term MHC "supertype" (Sidney et al., 1996). Four supertypes were defined by examining reported cross-reactive epitopes, from which they identified MHC alleles that might be grouped into one supertype. They then compared anchor residue binding pockets B and F. Experimentally confirmed binding motifs of the alleles were also examined, and those with similar motifs were grouped into one supertype. The supertypes identified in the paper were A2, A3, B7, and B44. Later, A*0207 was added to the A2 supertype and B*1508 and B*5602 were added to the B7 supertype (Sette and Sidney, 1998). Sette and Sidney later defined a total of nine supertypes, including the four previously defined supertypes (Sette and Sidney, 1999). These nine supertypes cover about 99% of the world population.

Based on the work of Sette and coworkers, Lund et al. (2004) classified HLA-A and -B molecules using specificity matrices. The nonamer ligands of all HLA-A and -B molecules were collected from the SYFPEITHI and MHCPEP databases and aligned. The frequencies of each amino acid at each position were summarized in matrices. The matrices were used as the input for a clustering analysis, and the HLA superfamilies were organized in a consensus tree. In their results, the A26 alleles were separated from the A1 cluster and a new B8 superfamily was defined.

In contrast to data-driven models, which rely on accumulated binding data, an important alternative approach seeks a structural understanding of peptide binding through a thorough analysis of the structures of MHC receptor binding sites. Such studies provide important information about underlying binding interactions. This allows links to be drawn between different MHC alleles, but at the peptide binding level rather than the phylogenetic level. Any significant propinquity apparent between binding sites should also be mirrored in the overall peptide selectivities exhibited by these variant MHCs.

Over the years, and for class I in particular, several studies have examined binding pockets in MHC molecules. Chelvanayagam has attempted to define so-called "road maps" for both class I (Chelvanayagam et al., 1996; Chelvanayagam, 1996) and class II (Chelvanayagam, 1997; Baas et al., 1999). In Chelvanayagam's work, new, less restrictive descriptions, largely based on sequence composition within pockets, of the peptide binding sites of MHC molecules were developed and were referred to as peptide binding environments. Such environments are defined by a set of amino acid residues within crystal structures of peptide-MHC complexes, which lie within a preset neighborhood of individual residues. Combining this information with sequence alignments of class I MHCs, Chelvanayagam made predictions for those MHC molecules that share similar profiles of environments. Chelvanayagam found that the whole site contributes to the definition of antigen binding.

Recently, Doytchinova et al. (2004) have used a computational-chemistry approach to address the problem of supertype definition. This extends the GRID/consensus principal component analysis (CPCA) technique to encompass comparative molecular similarity indices analysis and hierarchical clustering to generate a robust, consensus clustering of human class I MHC alleles. GRID/CPCA is a well-established methodology allowing one to analyze and classify sets of related molecules, including proteins that exhibit significant polymorphism. Molecular interaction fields are computed for each protein model and are then analyzed using a chemometrical method, such as CPCA. Classification does not rely on sequence similarities but on descriptors derived from 3D binding site information computed using molecular interaction fields. The method is based on information that is obtained solely from 3D protein structures generated automatically from sequence data. Binding data are not required. This allows one to examine peptide specificities for large numbers of allelic variants of MHCs. Two chemometric techniques, hierarchical clustering and principal-component analysis, were used independently on a set of 783 HLA class I molecules to identify supertypes based on structural similarities of their binding sites. The two techniques gave a 77% consensus: 605 HLA class I alleles were classified in the same supertype by both methods. Overall, eight supertypes were defined: A2, A3, A24, B7, B27, B44, C1, and C4.

HLA-B is the most polymorphic locus in the human HLA genes, and most attempts to derive HLA-B supertypes have encountered significant problems in properly classifying alleles. For example, recent work (I. A. Doytchinova and D. R. Flower, unpublished data) has shown that no HLA-B supertype classification is able to correctly rationalize sets of discriminant models of allele-dependent peptide specificity. When learning to use both experimental and theoretical methods, one must be aware of both the strengths and weaknesses inherent in them and use any method in an appropriate way.

IDENTIFICATION OF HIV-1 PROTEINS SIMILAR TO HUMAN PROTEINS

We specifically describe the model of choice in our laboratory, which compares the nine HIV-1 protein sequences (nef, rev, tat, env, pol, vif, vpr, vpu, and gag) with the 27,675 human protein sequences from the human genome project described at NCBI (ftp://ftp.ncbi.nih.gov/ genomes/ H_sapiens) using the sequence comparison program BLASTP (Basic Local Alignment Search Tool) at an E (expect value) cutoff of $<1 \times 10^{-2}$ (Fig. 1). This undertaking, while complex and laborious, led to the identification of human proteins matching HIV-1 proteins by sequence comparison. The human proteins that matched segments of the HIV proteins were thereafter referred to as human homologs of the HIV-1 proteins. Our research team then mapped different sequence segments of these HIV-1 proteins to their matching segments of the human homologs. The matching regions are schematically represented in Color Plate 1. We also mapped the matching HIV-1–human segments to the known structures of HIV-1 proteins available at the Protein Data Bank (PDB), as shown in Color Plate 1.

Selection of Antigen Protein

The HIV-1 protein selected for vaccine development should induce protective levels of an immune response. As immunity is directed against nonself viral antigens, the selected antigen protein should exhibit little or no sequence similarity to the host (human) protein sequences. Color Plate 1 shows the human homologs matching segments of HIV-1 proteins forming the viral core. Among the nine HIV-1 proteins, the ENV protein shows the least sequence homology with the human protein sequences. Hence, we discuss gp120 as the target antigen for further analysis and investigation below.

RECOGNITION OF VIRAL ANTIGENS BY CMI

Immunity confers protection of the organism against pathogens. Innate immunity concerns humoral (e.g., proinflammatory cytokines and complement) and cellular (e.g., myeloid cells and natural killer cells) events that do not require priming by antigens. Antigen-specific immunity addresses that branch of cellular (e.g., cytotoxic T lymphocytes) and humoral (e.g., TH1 and TH2 patterns of cytokines) immune surveillance that depends upon the phenotypic (e.g., naïve and memory T cells and regulatory T cells [Tregs]) and functional-stage maturation of lymphocytes following presentation of the antigen by MHC molecules (Romagnani, 1992; Chiappelli, 2007).

Viruses, bacteria, and classical parasites all probe the limits of immunity and of the three basic parameters of immunology: specificity, tolerance, and memory. In the case of viral antigens, the practical specificity repertoire of T cells is probably on the order of 10^4 to 10^5 specificities. Tolerance, which is the state acquired following successful vaccination, represents rules of reactivity to eliminate infections while avoiding destruction of normal cells by complete elimination of T cells that are specific for antigens persisting in the blood and lymphohematopoietic system locally and systemically, as well as in putative "immune-privileged" (see below) organs (Chiappelli, 2007).

Induction of a T-cell response, such as following a vaccination event, is typically the result of antigens newly entering the lymph nodes or the spleen, initially in a local fashion and exhibiting optimal distribution kinetics within the lymphohematopoietic system. Antigens that stay outside lymphatic tissues are generally immunologically ignored. Immunity is regulated by the antigen dose, time, and rela-

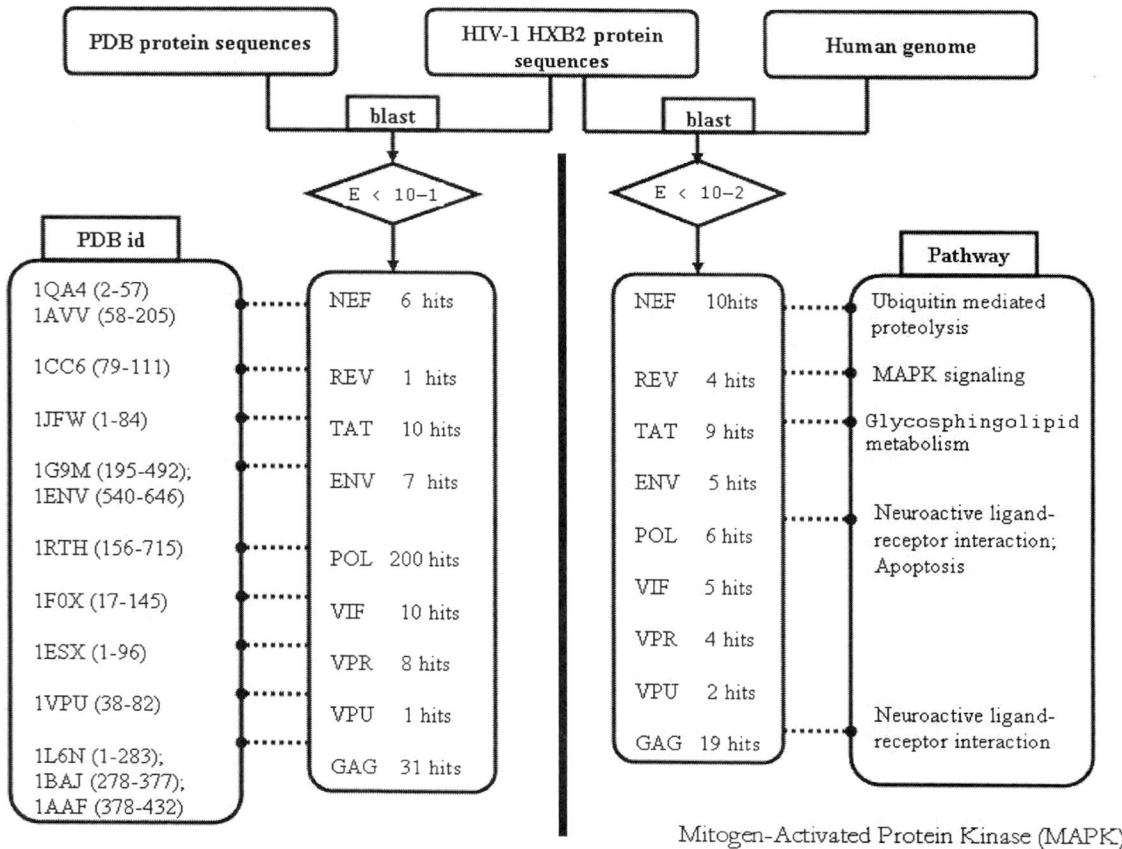

FIGURE 1 Flowchart describing the comparison of HIV-1 proteins (NEF, REV, TAT, ENV, POL, VIF, VPR, VPU, and GAG) with the human proteins from genome projects and known structures from the PDB using BLASTP. NEF, REV, TAT, POL, and GAG have matching human HOMOLOGS in several pathways. This implies potential interference by HIV-1 proteins with the host pathways in infected individuals.

tive distribution kinetics. There is some debate about the mechanism of neutralization. The identification of specific neutralizing epitopes indicates that the site of antibody binding is as important as the threshold level of the virion surface covered by antibody that binds the native envelope oligomer regardless of specificity (Parren and Burton, 2001).

T cells recognize virus-infected cells by specific interactions between the T-cell receptor and 8 to 10 amino acid peptides processed from viral antigens and presented in the context of MHC molecules. T cells can recognize and clear virus only after exposure has occurred, either via infection or via vaccination. The recognition is restricted by the MHC molecule, which recognizes particular viral epitopes, depending on the set of inherited alleles encoding the MHC molecules. Therefore, the multiplicity of epitope dominance varies among individuals, which implies that the epitope repertoire in a vaccine needs to have substantial breadth to encompass the principal relevant MHC haplotypes. Another caveat to the development of viral vaccines is that they must be designed to induce a broad response in every individual against several viral antigens in order to prevent the possibility of immune escape and host selection of merely the dominant viral epitopes.

Memory relates to the host's resistance following a second exposure to the same agent, which corresponds to successful vaccination, and it correlates with antigen-dependent maintenance of circulating antibody titers and with T-cell responses (Chiappelli, 2007). CD4[+] T lymphocytes initiate the immune response and also represent the major targets for HIV infection. Therefore, concerted efforts at developing anti-HIV vaccines have consistently faced the significant hurdle of how to effectively induce protective immunity against HIV while minimizing the risk of infecting HIV-specific CD4[+] T cells at risk of infection. In addition, CD4[+] T cells have some capacity for lysis of HIV-infected cells (Stanhope et al., 1993; Cecilia et al., 1998).

CD8[+] T cells are the principal effector mechanism of the adaptive immune response to clear virus-infected cells (Walker et al., 1986). The appearance of HIV-specific CD8[+] T cells is involved with reducing the viral load in acute infections (Koup et al., 1994). HIV-1 escape mutants, which can elude recognition by CD8[+] T cells, may play an important role in HIV pathogenesis. These escape mutants have been found to occur in both acute and chronic infections with rapid progression to AIDS (Borrow et al., 1997). It is important for any vaccine approach to induce as many CD8[+] T-lymphocytic responses as possible against HIV epitopes that are recognized during the acute phase of infection, when viral replication is controlled, or to force the selection of nonviable viral mutants (Gray et al., 2001). Together, CD4-mediated and CD8-mediated anti-HIV responses cause cytopathology, not only of the virus-infected cell, but also to various degrees in bystander cells. When these events occur in the brain, serious toxicity to surrounding astroglias, oligodendroglias, microglias, and neurons may occur as a consequence of cell death, as well as proximal cytokine concentration, which, in concert, may contribute to precipitating neuro-AIDS.

The question then is whether these CMI responses can occur in the brain parenchyma, or in other words, what is the nature and extent of the putative "immune privilege" of the central nervous system? It is unquestionable that systemic inflammation and related immune responses are associated with sickness behavior, and signals pass from the blood to the brain via myeloid cells (e.g., macrophages and microglias) (Lassmann et al., 1991; Weller et al., 1996; Pachter et al., 2003). The amplitude of this transduction process is directly dependent on the state of activation of these cell populations. Therefore, systemic inflammation may impact local inflammation in the brain, leading to exaggerated synthesis of inflammatory cytokines and other mediators in the brain, including adenosine (Hasko et al., 2005), which in turn influence brain cytopathology, brain function, and behavior (van Marle and Power, 2005; Speth et al., 2005). In brief, it is now generally well accepted that systemic infections also contribute to the outcome or progression of chronic neurodegenerative disease (Perry, 2004).

HIV penetrates the infected individual either systemically via the blood port or by infecting the genital or colonic mucosa. In a large proportion of cases, mucosal immunity establishes the first line of defense against HIV (Bivas-Benita et al., 2005), which has opened conceptual avenues for cutting-edge cellular-immunity-based mucosa-directed anti-HIV vaccines. It has been shown that mucosal anti-HIV vaccines can induce a much broader CD8$^+$ response in both mucosal and systemic immunocompetent tissues than systemic vaccines (Belyakov et al., 1998; Kozlowski and Neutra, 2003). Mucosal cellular immune responses eventually impinge upon the brain. An attractive class of such vaccines targets the pulmonary mucosal immune system (Bivas-Benita et al., 2005).

In brief, the minimal requirement to start brain inflammation is the presence of activated circulating T cells, which migrate into the brain. In addition, other local and systemic immunological factors (e.g., cytokines) profoundly alter the threshold for the induction of brain inflammation (Lassmann et al., 1991). HIV penetration into the brain via infected T cells is frequent (Speth et al., 2005). Together, these events contribute to the cytopathology associated with neuro-AIDS.

There is considerable evidence suggesting that the brain acts as a separate reservoir of HIV infection (as does the cerebrospinal fluid [CSF] to an extent), and evolutionary studies have demonstrated independent evolution of HIV in different body compartments. There are significant differences in viral molecular heterogeneity between body compartments within an infected individual. The blood shows much more HIV-1 genetic variability and expanded tropism than the central nervous system (Di Stefano et al., 1996; Korber et al., 1994; Power et al., 1994). The V3 (variable 3) region of the *env* gene exhibits considerable genetic variability even within the same individual. Numerous studies have shown unique region-specific evolution, drug resistance,

replication, and macrophage activation, which led to the formation of distinct HIV strains in the brain compartment. A significant amount of viral evolution occurs in different body compartments as the virus phenotypes select different cell types (Korber et al., 1994). This selective evolution between brain regions has been demonstrated, resulting in distinct clusters of HIV-1 variants within each brain region (Salemi et al., 2005; Shapshak et al., 1999). Hence, vaccines against brain and CSF compartments need investigation as well (Chang et al., 1998; Elovaara et al., 1993; van Marle and Power, 2005; Power et al., 1994; Resnick et al., 1988; Shapshak et al., 1999; Singer et al., 1994). Therefore, the dogma that the central nervous system may be immunologically privileged now appears to be a fallacy. It is evident that activated T cells migrate and cross the intact blood-brain barrier and initiate and propagate CMI responses within the brain parenchyma (Toda, 2003).

Cell migration is critical to immune surveillance and is brought about by the concerted actions of specialized factors and receptors, and it is regulated by chemokines. Chemokines belong to three groups, C-X-C, C-C, and C, depending on the number and position of cysteine residues. CXCR4 favors X4 HIV-1 strain tropism, and CCR5 favors tropism of the R5 strain. Recruitment of immune cells generally occurs by upregulating cell surface adhesion molecule expression, such as ELAM-1 (endothelial leukocyte adhesion molecule 1) and increased ICAM-1, thereby enhancing cell adherence to the endothelial surface and facilitating cell diapedesis through endothelial vessel walls. Interleukin 8, a C-X-C representative, mediates the recruitment and activation of immune T cells (Chiappelli, 2007). The CD4 and CD8 moieties are complexed with lck, but are significantly divergent in their structures: CD4 is a monomer, while CD8 consists of two chains and occurs as a homodimer (α/α) or heterodimer (α/β). lck interacts with CD4 and CD8, but active lck kinase is released in the cytoplasmic environment only following CD4$^+$ cell activation (Chiappelli, 2007).

lck and related molecular events involved in the regulation of T-cell stimulation include AkT (phosphoinositide 3-kinase; protein kinase B); the tumor suppressor PTEN (phosphatase and tensin homologue deleted on chromosome 10); and tyrosine kinase inhibitor peptide (Tkip), a mimetic of SOCS-1 that binds to the autophosphorylation site of JAK2 and inhibits phosphorylation of STAT1β. Tkip could serve as a potentially important therapeutic target for constitutive and interleukin 6-induced STAT3 activation (Chiappelli, 2007), as well as, putatively, for a new generation of HIV vaccines aimed at regulating CD4 T-cell responses.

Suppressors of cytokine signaling (SOCS) constitute a family of seven known cytoplasmic proteins that regulate the stimulation of T cells and induce signaling via JAK/STAT. In certain experimental models, SOCS inhibit focal adhesion kinase (FAK) activity and tyrosine phosphorylation of FAK, thus blunting an essential regulatory step in T-cell migration (Liu et al., 2003).

Another important pathway related to SOCS is the P3 member of the first forkhead box (FOX) transcription factor (FoxP3), which is a transcriptional repressor targeting composite NF-AT/AP-1 sites in cytokine gene promoters. Introduction of FoxP3 into conventional mouse T cells converts these cells to Tregs (Yagi et al., 2004; Chiappelli, 2007).

Since depletion of Tregs significantly ($P < 0.05$) enhances the activation and proliferation of CD4$^+$ T cells, it is possible, and even probable, that Tregs could become the target of novel molecular/cellular immunity-based anti-HIV vaccines.

This is particularly relevant when one considers that different subsets of Tregs have been identified: Tregs can be divided into subsets according to cell surface expression of the migration and homing receptor CD62L. The suppressive function of the CD62L$^+$ subset is far more potent on a per-cell basis than the CD62L$^-$ Treg population (Fu et al., 2004). Tregs can also be differentiated based on expression of the chemokine receptors that direct their migration properties, specifically, the CXCR4 and CXCL12 moieties (Zou et al., 2004; Chiappelli, 2007).

Identification of HIV-1 gp120 Peptide Cocktail Vaccine Candidates

As discussed above, CMI occurs through the binding of short antigen peptides to host HLA molecules. The binding of short peptides to HLA molecules is allele specific because HLA alleles are highly polymorphic and about 2,000 HLA alleles are known today (http://www.ebi.ac.uk/imgt/hla). Screening all possible combinations of overlapping peptides against known HLA alleles using the competitive binding assay is time-consuming. Alternatively, the use of HLA peptide prediction is highly helpful in selecting potential peptide candidates for further investigation or validation. In the experimental model we describe here, we chopped the 510-residue segments of the gp120 envelope protein sequence into overlapping 9-residue-long peptides and then predicted the binding of all the peptides to 295 HLA-A alleles and 540 HLA-B alleles using T-Epitope Designer (http://www. bioinformation.net/ted/; Kangueane and Sakharkar, 2005; Zhao et al., 2003). T-Epitope Designer is a web server for HLA peptide prediction using a model that is superior to many existing methods because of its potential application to any given HLA allele whose sequence is clearly defined. This process identified 28 peptides binding to HLA-A alleles and 29 peptides binding to HLA-B alleles in a supertype-like manner (with overlapping functional repertoires), as shown in Fig. 2. Examples of HLA supertypes are given in Table 1.

B-Cell Epitopes in HIV

Humoral immunogenicity, mediated by soluble or membrane-bound cell surface antibodies through recognition of B-cell epitopes, can be measured in several ways. Methods such as enzyme-linked immunosorbent assay or competitive-inhibition assays yield values for the antibody titer, the concentration at which the ability of antibodies in the blood to bind an antigen has reached its half-maximal value. This is a well-used measure of antibody-mediated immunity, and it is also possible to measure directly the affinity of antibody and antigen using, for example, equilibrium dialysis. HIV has been extensively mapped for B-cell epitopes. B-cell epitopes are classified as linear and conformational. Linear epitopes are typically short subsequences, excised from full-length protein sequences, that are deemed to be cross-reactive with antibodies raised against whole protein. Conformational B-cell epitopes are regions on the surface of a protein, or other biomacromolecule, that are recognized by soluble or membrane-bound antibody molecules. Usually such epitopes are comprised of a set of discontinuous amino acids well separated within the linear sequence but intimately juxtaposed within the 3D structure. It is the recognition of epitopes by T cells, B cells, and soluble antibodies that lies at the heart of the immune response, which in turn leads to activation of the cellular and humoral immune systems and, ultimately, to the effective destruction of pathogenic organisms. The accurate prediction of B-cell and T-cell epitopes is thus the pivotal challenge for immunoinformatics. The

prediction of B-cell epitopes remains primitive (Pellequer and Westoff, 1993; Alix, 1999) or is contingent upon an often elusive knowledge of 3D protein structure. A decade or two ago, both T- and B-cell epitope prediction methods were based on looking for maximally valued regions in antigen sequences—essentially, looking for peaks in some form of propensity plot. While prediction of T-cell epitopes has progressed significantly, such techniques are still the only ones in common use for predicting B-cell epitopes.

Blythe and Flower (2005) have demonstrated that methods that are based on finding peaks in propensity plots fail completely in correctly identifying experimentally defined polyclonal linear B-cell epitopes. Systematic studies using more sophisticated machine learning techniques, such as support vector machines and hidden Markov models, have proven equally unsuccessful in prediction. The underlying issue is with the quality, quantity, and interpretation of extant linear B-cell data. Despite a significant growth in B-cell epitopes identified by overlapping peptide mappings of different proteins, there is a relative dearth of such studies. They have also been conducted using a wide variety of different techniques with different levels of accuracy and precision. While such worrying characteristics are common to many biological data, arguably the greatest problem with B-cell data is the way they are interpreted. Biologically active linear epitopes are cross-reactive with the whole proteins they are derived from, at least in terms of antibodies raised against the folded full-length proteins. With vaccine studies, the goal of identifying B-cell epitopes is the reverse of this: isolated epitopes should induce antibodies that are able to recognize the whole protein. If one visualizes mapped linear epitopes back onto the structure of the full protein, only certain linear epitopes exhibit sufficient numbers of amino acid residues accessible to inspection by the antibody for them to be recognized by the immune system using this mechanism. However they are recognized, linear epitopes are not simple mimics of conformational epitopes. Conformational epitopes have been identified experimentally using either X-ray crystallography or mutagenesis studies. Compared to linear epitopes, attempts to predict conformational epitopes show promise, particularly using methods based on in silico approaches to dock antigen and antibody structures together.

It is often assumed that a successful polyepitope vaccine will contain one or more T-cell epitopes and one or more B-cell epitopes and possibly include de facto generic adjuvant properties. Such self-adjuvanting vaccines are under development, with lipopeptides proving to possess adequate adjuvanting capabilities (BenMohamed et al., 2002; Zeng et al., 2000). Likewise, when attempting to identify subunit vaccines, it would be desirable to account for both T-cell and B-cell epitopes using in silico techniques. However, with current technology, the B-cell aspect of this remains eclipsed by the proven success of T-cell epitope prediction. The prediction of HIV epitopes and antigens using an in silico technique for B-cell epitopes awaits the development of an effective approach to this problem.

Induction of a Humoral Response Using the HIV gp120 Bridging Sheet

The HIV surface envelope protein gp160 is a glycoprotein comprised of two subunit proteins: gp120, which contains receptor binding sites, and gp41, a supporting stem structure involved in virus membrane fusion. The gp160 glycoprotein exists in trimeric complexes on the viral surface and binds to the host cell receptor (CD4) and coreceptor (CCR5 or CXCR4) to trigger membrane fusion events and eventual

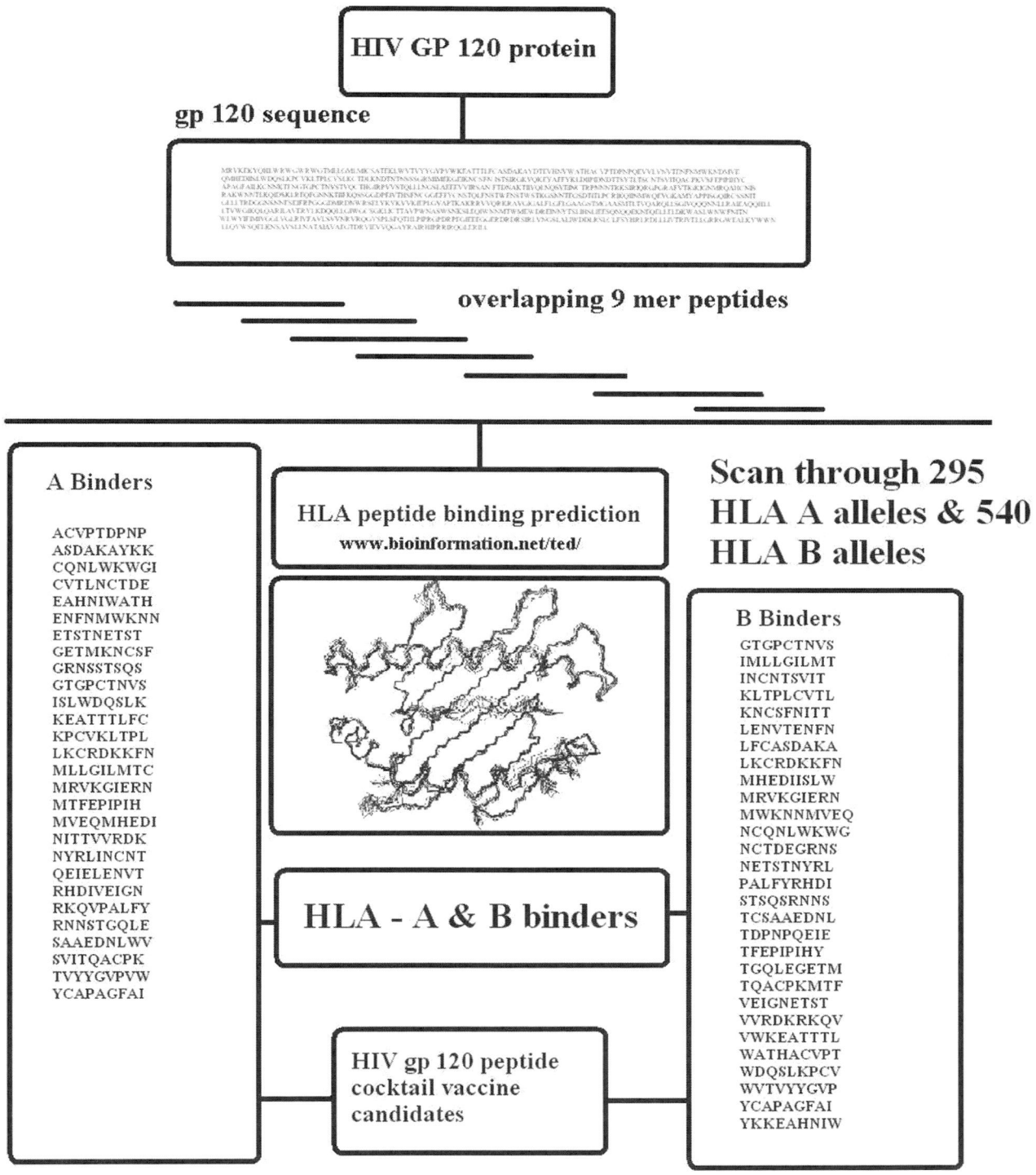

FIGURE 2 The HIV-1 gp120 envelope protein was chopped into overlapping 9-mer peptides, and their binding with 296 A alleles and 540 B alleles was estimated using T-Epitope Designer. This procedure generated 28 peptide binders for 295 A alleles and 29 peptide binders for 540 B alleles in a combinatorial manner.

virus entry (Wyatt and Sodroski, 1998). This entry process can be inhibited by antibodies that bind to critical regions on either gp120 or gp41, effectively neutralizing HIV-1. Induction of neutralizing antibodies during infection is not

a simple matter, as the virus mutates during infection to escape antibody recognition and persist in the host. As well as mutating surface amino acid residues within known variable regions to evade antibody recognition, the virus also

TABLE 1 Examples of HLA supertypes[a]

Peptide	Supertypes	Binding for HLA-A allele[b]:					Reference
		A*0201	A*0202	A*0203	A*0206	A*6802	
LLFNILGGWV	A2	B	B	B	B	B	S[c]
YLVAYQATV	A2	B	B	B	B	B	S
KVAELVHFL	A2	B	B	B	B	B	K[d]
FLWGPRALV	A2	B	B	B	B	B	K
FLLLADARV	A2	B	B	B	B	B	S
IMIGVLVGV	A2	B	B	B	B	B	K
KIFGSLAFL	A2	B	B	B	B	NB	K
CLTSTVQLV	A2	B	B	B	B	NB	K
RLIVFPDLGV	A2	B	B	B	B	NB	S
YLQLVFGIEV	A2	B	B	B	B	NB	K
LLTFWNPPV	A2	B	B	B	B	NB	K
VLVGGVLAA	A2	B	B	B	B	NB	S
WMNRLIAFA	A2	B	B	B	NB	B	S
DLMGYIPLV	A2	B	NB	B	B	B	S
ILHNGAYSL	A2	B	B	B	NB	NB	K
YLSGANLNL	A2	B	B	B	NB	NB	K
VMAGVGSPYV	A2	B	B	B	NB	NB	K
ILAGYGAGV	A2	B	B	B	NB	NB	S
LMTFWNPPV	A2	B	NB	B	B	NB	K
YLVTRHADV	A2	B	NB	B	B	NB	S
HMWNFISGI	A2	B	NB	B	B	NB	K
YLLPRRGPRL	A2	B	NB	B	B	NB	S
LLFLLLADA	A2	B	B	NB	NB	NB	S
LLTFWNPPT	A2	B	NB	B	NB	NB	K
ALCRWGLLL	A2	B	NB	B	NB	NB	S

[a]Known HLA supertypes are shown.
[b]Binding information is available for five HLA-A alleles. B, binder; NB, nonbinder.
[c]S, Scognamiglio et al., 1999.
[d]K, Kawashima et al., 1998.

undergoes specific genetic changes, resulting in the acquisition and rearrangement of surface glycans, specifically on gp120. Such changes in the glycan shield are an effective method for constantly evading immune surveillance and increasing viral infectivity through the generation of variants (Richman et al., 2003; Wei et al., 2003). Therefore, any vaccine aimed at inducing broad cross-clade protection must be directed toward highly conserved regions of the surface glycoprotein complex to combat in situ genetic variation.

Over 65 different potential vaccine products have been evaluated in clinical trials worldwide, many aimed at eliciting anti-gp120 neutralizing antibodies. However, success has been limited, with antisera (sera from inoculated individuals) displaying little neutralizing capacity (Bolognesi and Matthews, 1998; Letvin, 1998; McMichael and Hanke, 2003). This has been partly attributed to the failure of monomeric gp120 and gp160 to induce antibodies that recognize the native quaternary trimeric state, or the antibodies are directed to variable regions and are not cross-reactive among HIV isolates (Graham et al., 1998; Schonning et al., 1998; Van Cott et al., 1999). A plausible strategy for designing an HIV vaccine based on envelope proteins is to focus on conserved regions of gp120 essential to receptor binding and viral entry. A prime vaccine target is the conserved gp120 "bridging-sheet" region that connects the inner and outer domains of gp120 and consists of four discontinuous antiparallel β-strands (Kwong et al., 1998). Furthermore,

66% of bridging-sheet residues are conserved among all HIV-1 isolates (Kwong et al., 1998).

Studies with monoclonal antibodies (MAbs) against the bridging-sheet domain support its validity as a vaccine target by highlighting its role in both CD4 and coreceptor binding (Kwong et al., 2002). Two types of B-cell epitopes exist in this domain: CD4 binding site epitopes, which compete with and block CD4 binding, and CD4-induced epitopes, which are formed or exposed by CD4 binding (Poignard et al., 2001). A single CD4 binding site MAb, immunoglobulin Gb12, has been identified that efficiently neutralizes about 75% of clade B primary viruses (Burton et al., 1994; Moore et al., 1995) and also protects against viral challenge in vivo (Parren et al., 2001). The crystal structure has shown that the epitope recognized by the broadly neutralizing CD4-induced MAb 17b is located within the bridging sheet. Since 17b mimics coreceptor binding, this binding site is also thought to be near or within the domain (Moore, 1997). Thus, a vaccine strategy targeting the bridging-sheet domain holds promise to elicit broadly neutralizing antibodies by inhibiting both CD4 and coreceptor binding.

A strategy that focuses only on the relevant and conserved sequences of the gp120 bridging sheet requires the removal of other immunological decoys, such as prominent variable loops and carbohydrates that conceal the bridging sheet (Reitter et al., 1998; Sattentau and Moore, 1995). In addition, it is essential that synthetic forms of the domain mimetic conformationally represent active gp120 intermediate states during the entry and fusion process. To achieve this without having defined structures on which to model critical intermediate or transition states, several groups have used chemical synthesis for preparing mimetics. Incorporation of small segments of the bridging sheet into peptide immunogens has been achieved with antibodies neutralizing a limited range of HIV isolates (Haynes et al., 1993; Javaherian et al., 1990; Letvin et al., 2001). The most frequently used segment is the C4 region, which covers the bridging-sheet strands known as β20 and β21; this peptide is generally included in linear V3-C4 peptides solely as a T-helper cell determinant for V3 loop B-cell epitopes (Letvin et al., 2001; Zinckgraf et al., 1999). Peptide C4 has been examined as an immunogen, with a multivalent C4 peptide and a cyclic C4 peptide tested; both were immunogenic yet failed to induce neutralizing antibodies (Patterson et al., 2001; Robey and Robert-Guroff, 2001).

Tam and colleagues (School of Biological Sciences, Nanyang Technological University) have recently made significant progress in the development of a bridging-sheet-based vaccine candidate. The results (unpublished data) demonstrate that a series of bridging-sheet mimetics induce antibodies in animals that are capable of binding to native protein (Table 2). Antisera elicited by selected mimetics were also observed to inhibit gp120 from interacting with the receptor protein CD4 in vitro. Furthermore, antisera were found to inhibit HIV infection in vitro. The most effective vaccine candidate induced antisera that inhibited 88% ± 7% of infection with TCLA (T-cell line-adapted) ($n = 8$) virus and 73% ± 10% of infection with primary isolates ($n = 7$), as tested using the standard multinuclear-activation galactosidase indicator (MAGI) assay.

There is much to learn about gp120 conformation, particularly after receptor interaction, and the associated activation states. By continuing with a strategy of antigen design and antiserum analysis through several rounds of refinement, an improved structural mimic of the bridging sheet may emerge as a viable vaccine candidate. Given that HIV nucleotide sequences may differ by up to 25% between clades and 15% within clades (Johnston, 1997) and that up to 30% of gp120 residues are subject to mutation in variable regions (Klein and Ho, 2000), a vaccine preparation

against a conserved region, such as the bridging sheet, holds significant promise for producing a vaccine against HIV isolates from various clades.

Generation of Electrostatic Distribution Maps for HLA Molecules

HLA structures corresponding to alleles A*0201, A*6801, B*0801, B*2701, B*3501, B*5301, B*2705, B*2709, B*5101, C*w3, and C*w4 were downloaded from the PDB (http://www.rcsb.org/pdb/). The electrostatic distribution maps were calculated for each structure using Coulomb's law (which states that the force between two point charges is directly proportional to the product of the charges and inversely proportional to the square of the distance between them) as implemented in Deep View (Swiss PDB Viewer version 3.7), which is available for download (http://www.expasy.org/spdbv/). The electrostatic differences in the peptide binding groove between HLA alleles (A*0201, A*6801, B*0801, B*2701, B*3501, B*5301, B*2705, B*2709, B*5101, C*w3, and C*w4) are shown in Color Plate 2.

Possible Future HIV Vaccines

The study model presented here allowed the comparison of nine HIV-1 protein sequences with the protein sequences from the human genome, which showed that almost all HIV-1 proteins have some degree of sequence similarity to one or more human proteins (Fig. 1). It also showed that a number of human proteins mimic human proteins involved in several signaling pathways (Fig. 1), which could actualize certain cutting-edge molecular immunity-based approaches to HIV vaccines discussed above. Specifically, the similarity between human and HIV-1 proteins is locally segmented and discontinuous (Color Plate 1). Examination of Color Plate 1 shows further that the env protein has the least sequence similarity to human proteins. Consequently, these observations led us to select the env protein sequence for further epitope screening. The env protein consists of a 510-residue-long N-terminal gp120 domain, and we used the gp120 protein domain for the identification of potential T-cell epitopes using T-Epitope Designer (Kangueane and Sakharkar, 2005).

Figure 2 shows the prediction of gp120 peptide binding to HLA molecules using T-Epitope Designer. The prediction of binding of all overlapping peptides of the gp120 sequence to all known HLA alleles is combinatorial and computationally intensive. This is because HLA alleles are polymorphic, and peptide binding to HLA alleles is determined by the chemical property of the binding groove. The differences in the electrostatic potential distributions of HLA alleles A*0201, A*6801, B*0801, B*2701, B*3501, B*5301, B*2705, B*2709, B*5101, C*w3, and C*w4 are shown in Color Plate 2, which provides visual discrimination of HLA alleles using the electrostatic differences between them. Thus, HLA peptide binding prediction is nontrivial.

The robustness of the T-epitope prediction algorithm led to scanning through all the overlapping peptides in the gp120 sequence for all known HLA alleles in a combinatorial manner. The predicted binders with high scores were sorted in supertype-like fashion for known HLA alleles. Examples of HLA-A2 supertypes, where different A2 alleles bind peptides in an overlapping fashion, are given in Table 1. By this process, our model generated 28 peptides binding to 295 A alleles and 29 peptides binding to 540 B alleles, with overlapping binding functions to HLA alleles, as shown in Fig. 2.

TABLE 2 Immunogenicity and antigenicity of gp120 bridging-sheet mimetics

Mimetic antisera	ELISA titer		
	Antimimetic	Anti-gp120	Anti-gp160
A	3.0[a]	2.1	<2
B	4.0	<2	2.1
C	4.7	<2	3.0
D	4.1	<2	<2
E	4.9	3.5	3.8
F	4.8	3.7	3.9
G	1.3	<2	ND[b]
H	2.9	2.3	ND
I	5.4	2.4	2.2

[a]The titer is the reciprocal of the $\log_{10}$ dilution corresponding to four times the absorbance of the background.

[b]ND, not determined. Limiting volume precluded use.

HIV/AIDS Vaccine Development

The development of a novel approach to HIV/AIDS vaccine design is imperative due to the limited success of subunit vaccines and DNA vaccines against HIV/AIDS (Mortara et al., 1998; Nickle et al., 2003; Wyatt and Sodrowski, 1998; Xin et al., 1998). The criteria used for the selection of HIV vaccine candidates have been described by the AIDS Vaccine Integrated Project (Ensoli, 2005). The challenge is to identify antigen proteins that can trigger effective antibodies against the surface protein of the virus to prevent the virus from getting to first base (entering cells in the first place). Hence, the fundamental problem in vaccine design is selection of a vaccine antigen candidate. Furthermore, direct entry of vaccine components into the brain is essential so that reliance on immune cells to enter the brain is not the rate-limiting step in the vaccine response process. The reasons for this are several. The brain and CSF in patients with HIV-associated dementia are immunologically separate reservoirs and show a more TH1 pattern of cytokine response rather than the TH2 pattern found in blood (Perrella et al., 2003; Wesselingh et al., 1993). This reservoir effect is apparent even at early stages of HIV-associated neuropsychological deficits (Resnick et al., 1988; Singer et al., 1994). Indeed, neuroanatomically, the brain for the most part is sequestered from the CSF and blood by tight junctions in the endothelial cell lining of the vasculature that are disrupted in HIV encephalitis (Dallasta et al., 1999). The brain, CSF, and blood also show separation as reservoirs virologically (van Marle and Power, 2005; Shapshak et al., 1995, 1996). This view is supported both pre- and post-highly active antiretroviral therapy (Clements et al., 2005). Thus, the brain, which may not be "immune privileged" as once thought (see above), may actually, by contrast, reveal itself to be "vaccine privileged." Indeed, there are concerns about the types of vaccines developed and the targets within the host against which they may effectively function.

Selection of a Nonself HIV Protein as a Target Antigen

Earlier studies suggested the possibility of molecular mimicry of virus proteins and the human host. Oldstone first predicted problems in immunity due to virus-host molecular mimicry (Oldstone, 1987, 1989), especially autoimmunity (Barnett and Fujinami, 1992). Other early studies showed, for example, gp41 potential molecular mimicry with HLA proteins and elicited autoantibodies (Golding et al., 1989; Young, 1988). Furthermore, HIV-related neurological disease was at one point suggested to be due to HIV neurorleukin molecular mimicry (Lee et al., 1987). Furthermore, Pert et al. (1986) first suggested that an HIV gp120 tetrapeptide (peptide T) may be related to HIV neurological disease through homologies with VIP (vasoactive intestinal peptide). With these caveats in mind, we performed a systematic comparative-genomics experiment between the host human proteins (27,675 sequences) and the viral HIV-1 proteins (nef, rev, tat, env, pol, vif, vpr, vpu, and gag), as shown in Fig. 1. This analysis, using BLASTP, detected a number of human proteins that showed sequence homology with HIV-1 proteins. Some of these human proteins have similarity to the HIV-1 proteins and are known to be involved in several signaling pathways (ubiquitin-mediated proteolysis, MAPK signaling, glycosphingolipid metabolism, neuroactive ligand

receptor interaction, and apoptosis), as shown in Fig. 1 (Minagar et al., 2004; Shapshak et al., 2004). This observation was confirmed using microarray expression data in HIV-1 gp120/tat-induced neurons. The gene expression in cultured human neurons exposed to cocaine and the HIV-1 proteins gp120 and tat using microarray technologies led to the development of the pathways regulated by HIV-associated dementia (Shapshak et al., 2006). These results are expected to shed light on the understanding of HIV molecular mimicry in the human host, which would confirm the feasibility of vaccines directed at the molecular pathways and/or constituents of immune cells that fall victim to infection with HIV (e.g., CD4 T cells) and, more specifically, as noted above, Tregs. Specifically, one could conceive of a vaccine based on molecular mimicry, or an analog of CXCR4, which could act by luring HIV to bind to it rather than to Tregs, thus preserving the cellular integrity of the cellular immune response until a highly active antiretroviral therapy cocktail takes effect and reaches its maximal potency in the patient.

The data from our experiments indicate that the segments of HIV-1 proteins that have sequence similarity to the host proteins are those shown in Color Plate 1. All of the HIV-1 proteins showed some degree of sequence similarity to one or more of the human proteins. The sequence level similarity of HIV-1 proteins with the human proteins is perplexing, and these matching proteins may have a role in explaining the phenomenon of HIV molecular mimicry in the human host. The matching regions are linearly discontinuous, and these regions are highlighted in the known 3D structures of HIV-1 proteins. Nonetheless, examination of Color Plate 1 and comparison of all of the HIV proteins to each other show that the HIV ENV protein has the least sequence match with the host proteins. This suggests the potential for minimum interference by gp120 with the host system and provides insight into antigenic peptide selection, degeneration, and discrimination during T-cell-mediated immune response by the host system. Hence, we selected the 510-residue-long HIV-1 gp120 protein domain (part of the HIV ENV protein) for the subsequent identification of potential T-cell epitopes.

Prediction of gp120 Peptide Binding to HLA Alleles

A recombinant live attenuated measles vaccine vector primes effective HLA-A0201-restricted cytotoxic T lymphocytes and broadly neutralizing antibodies against HIV-1 conserved epitopes (Lorin et al., 2005). The development of SAVINE (synthetic antigen vaccine) using overlapping peptides from HIV-1 proteins designed in the global context has also been described (Thomson et al., 2005). Thus, the relationship between HLA restriction and HIV-1 antigen is already well established (De Groot et al., 2001, 2005). HIV vaccine development based on computer-assisted design using HLA peptide prediction models has been described in recent years (De Groot et al., 2001, 2005). Taken together, these data confirm the complexity of searching for an epitope-based HIV vaccine, as noted above. In our experimental model, the predicted binding of gp120 peptides to different class I HLA alleles was obtained. The 510-residue-long HIV-1 gp120 protein sequence was cut into 502 short overlapping peptides that were 9 residues in length. The host HLA molecules in the T-cell-mediated immune system bound to short antigen peptides. However, HLA molecules are highly polymorphic among different populations (http://www.ebi.ac.uk/imgt/hla/), and peptide binding specificities vary for different HLA alleles. The current update of the international ImMunoGeneTics information system/HLA database contains about 2,000 HLA alleles, and more than 1,000 of them are class I alleles. These alleles were found to be polymorphic, and they show sequence level variations among themselves. The sequence level variations in HLA alleles affect the type of residues forming the peptide binding groove. The residue level variation determines the chemical and physical properties of the groove for specific selection of antigen peptides for restriction (Kangueane et al., 2001; Adrian et al., 2002). The varying chemical characteristics of the peptide binding groove, as shown in Color Plate 2, are determinants of specific and differential binding. In Color Plate 2, the electrostatic distribution of the HLA alleles A*0201, A*6801, B*0801, B*2701, B*3501, B*5301, B*2705, B*2709, B*5101, C*w3, and C*w4 is shown to differ in the binding groove. Some alleles are predominately electronegative, and others are either electropositive or neutral. This provides visual insight into the HLA function in selecting peptides. The difference in the electrostatic distributions of HLA alleles with known structures is a direct demonstration of HLA specificity in peptide binding. Because the peptide vaccine for HIV/AIDS should have a global application with effective immunity in the entire population, a "cocktail" vaccine should be explored. The peptide mixture considered for vaccine development should accommodate the subtle chemical properties of more than 1,000 class I HLA alleles in binding. Therefore, the cocktail peptide vaccine should contain a mixture of short peptides from gp120 capable of binding to all or most HLA alleles. However, this is a challenging task given the number of known HLA alleles and overlapping peptide diversities generated from antigen protein sequences. For example, we used the HLA-binding peptide prediction server T-EPITOPE. The overlapping gp120 peptides for HLA binding were scanned using T-Epitope Designer (Fig. 2). T-Epitope Designer is based on a model that defines peptide binding pockets using information gleaned from X-ray crystal structures of HLA-peptide complexes, followed by the estimation of peptide binding to pockets in the HLA proteins. This model is superior to many existing methods because of its potential application to any given HLA allele whose sequence is clearly defined. This experiment identified 28 peptides binding to 295 HLA-A alleles and 29 short peptides binding to 540 HLA-B alleles in a supertype manner, as shown in Fig. 2. The peptide cocktail serves as a framework for the design and development of a HIV-1 peptide vaccine.

Nonetheless, these predicted peptides require extensive experimental validation using a competitive binding assay with HLA proteins and peptide or tetramer staining in HIV-infected patients. Interestingly, most of these peptides have already been verified experimentally for peptide binding with some of the known HLA alleles in the HIV molecular immunology database (http://hiv-web.lanl.gov/content/immunology/tables/ctl_summary.html).

In brief, the HIV molecular immunology database contains data for 289 peptides derived from HIV-1 gp160 envelope protein with known HLA restriction elements of CD8[+] epitopes. The database is a valuable resource for comparing predicted peptides generated in this study. The availability of peptides with known HLA restrictions provides optimism and encouragement for designing HIV-1 peptide vaccine components. It should also be noted that the HLA restricted-epitope data available in the database are a community effort made available through extensive collaborations and manual curation (process of refining data) of published HIV anti-

gen peptides. Thus, development of a peptide epitope-based cocktail vaccine for HIV/AIDS is a highly feasible approach for prevention of the disease pandemic.

CONCLUSIONS

Development of an effective HIV/AIDS vaccine is challenging due to complex host-virus pathogenesis. The inadequate success of subunit and DNA vaccines for HIV/AIDS warrants the development of T-cell-based, as well as rationally designed B-cell epitope-based, peptide vaccines. These can be conceived of as epitope based or molecule/cell based (e.g., Treg constituents). We have discussed a model approach that pertains to the latter. We have noted that the first obstacle to the design of a global HIV vaccine is viral diversity. The second impediment in the context of peptide vaccine design is HLA polymorphism among host genomes. The viral diversity, together with host HLA variation in ethnic groups, sets the limit for peptide vaccine progress. Here, we have outlined possible solutions to these issues using methods to predict appropriate T-cell epitopes and the rational design and synthesis of a highly conserved antigenic region of gp120. Yet another dimension added to HIV vaccine development complexity is the molecular mimicry of HIV due to extensive sequence similarity with the human host protein sequences. Results have shown that the gp120 (envelope) protein showed minimum sequence similarity with the human proteins. However, the gp120 surface is comprised of several variable loops, as well as a glycan shield that effectively protects the viral machinery from the immune system. Despite these concerns, we demonstrated the use of T-Epitope Designer (a computational model for the prediction of HLA-peptide binding) for the identification of potential peptide candidates from HIV gp120. The computational approach identified 28 peptides binding to 295 HLA-A alleles and 29 short peptides binding to 540 HLA-B alleles in a supertype manner. Some of these peptide candidates are already documented in the HIV molecular immunology database with experimentally known allele-specific HLA restriction. Nonetheless, comprehensive information on HLA allele restriction for all the peptides presented in this chapter is not available for verification. Hence, the experimental model we have described here serves as a framework for HIV-1 peptide vaccine design.

REFERENCES

Adrian, P. E. H., G. Rajaseger, V. Mathura, M. K. Sakharkar, and P. Kangueane. 2002. Types of inter-atomic interactions at the MHC-peptide interface: identifying commonality from accumulated data. *BMC Struct. Biol.* **2**:1–14.

Alix, A. J. 1999. Predictive estimation of protein linear epitopes by using the program PEOPLE. *Vaccine* **18**:311–314.

Baas, A., X. Gao, G. Chelvanayagam. 1999. Peptide binding motifs and specificities for HLA-DQ molecules. *Immunogenetics* **50**:8–15.

Barnett, L. A., and R. S. Fujinami. 1992. Molecular mimicry: a mechanism for autoimmune injury. *FASEB J.* **6**:840–844.

Belyakov, I. M., M. A. Derby, J. D. Ahlers, B. L. Kelsall, P. Earl, B. Moss, W. Strober, and J. A. Berzoksky. 1998. Mucosal immunization with HIV-1 peptide vaccine induces mucosal and systemic cytotoxic T lymphocytes and protective immunity in mice against intrarectal recombinant HIV-vaccinia challenge. *Proc. Natl. Acad. Sci. USA* **95**:1709–1714.

BenMohamed, L., S. L. Wechsler, and A. B. Nesburn. 2002. Lipopeptide vaccines—yesterday, today, and tomorrow. *Lancet Infect Dis.* **ii:**425–431.

Bivas-Benita, M., T. H. Ottenhoff, H. E. Junginger, and G. Borchard. 2005. Pulmonary DNA vaccination: concepts, possibilities and perspectives. *J. Control Release.* **20:**1–29.

Blythe, M. J., and D. R. Flower. 2005. Benchmarking B cell epitope prediction: underperformance of existing methods. *Protein Sci.* **14:**246–248.

Bolognesi, D. P., and T. J. Matthews. 1998. HIV vaccines. Viral envelope fails to deliver? *Nature* **391:**638–639.

Bond, K. B., B. Sriwanthana, T. W. Hodge, A. S. De Groot, T. D. Mastro, N. L. Young, N. Promadej, J. D. Altman, K. Limpakarnjanarat, and J. M. McNicholl. 2001. An HLA-directed molecular and bioinformatics approach identifies new HLA-A11 HIV-1 subtype E cytotoxic T lymphocyte epitopes in HIV-1 infected Thais. *AIDS Res. Hum. Retrovir.* **17:**703–718.

Borrow, P., H. Lewicki, X. Wei, M. S. Horwitz, N. Peffer, H. Meyers, J. A. Nelson, J. E. Gairin, B. H. Hahn, M. B. Oldstone, and G. M. Shaw. 1997. Antiviral pressure exerted by HIV-1-specific cytotoxic T lymphocytes (CTLs) during primary infection demonstrated by rapid selection of CTL escape virus. *Nat. Med.* **3:**205–211.

Brave, A., K. Ljungberg, A. Boberg, E. Rollman, G. Engstrom, J. Hinkula, and B. Wahren. 2006. Reduced cellular immune responses following immunization with a multigene HIV-1 vaccine. *Vaccine* **24:**4524–4526.

Burton, D. R., J. Pyati, R. Koduri, S. J. Sharp, G. B. Thornton, P. W. Parren, L. S. Sawyer, R. M. Hendry, N. Dunlop, P. L. Nara, et al. 1994. Efficient neutralization of primary isolates of HIV-1 by a recombinant human monoclonal antibody. *Science* **266:**1024–1027.

Cano, P., B. Fan, and S. Stass. 1998. A geometric study of the amino acid sequence of class I HLA molecules. *Immunogenetics* **48:**324–334.

Cecilia, D., V. N. KewalRamani, J. O'Leary, B. Volsky, P. Nyambi, et al. 1998. Neutralization profiles of primary human immunodeficiency virus type 1 isolates in the context of coreceptor usage. *J. Virol.* **72:**6988–6996.

Chang, J., R. Joswiak, B. Wang, T. Ng, Y. C. Ge, W. Bolton, et al. 1998. Unique HIV type 1 V3 region sequences derived from 6 different regions of brain: region-specific evolution within host-determined quasispecies. *AIDS Res. Hum. Retrovir.* **14:**25–30.

Chelvanayagam, G. 1997. A roadmap for HLA-DR peptide binding specificities. *Hum. Immunol.* **58:**61–69.

Chelvanayagam, G., I. B. Jakobsen, X. Gao, and S. Easteal. 1996. Structural comparison of major histocompatibility complex class I molecules and homology modelling of five distinct human leukocyte antigen-A alleles. *Protein Eng.* **9:**1151–1164.

Chelvanayagam, G. 1996. A roadmap for HLA-A, HLA-B, and HLA-C peptide binding specificities. *Immunogenetics* **45:**15–26.

Chiappelli, F. 2007. Immunity, p. 485–492. *In* G. Fink, B. McEwen, E. R. de Kloet, R. Rubin, G. Chrousos, A. Steptoe, N. Rose, I. Craig, and G. Feuerstein (ed.), *Encyclopaedia of Stress.* Elsevier, The Netherlands.

Clements, J. E., M. Li, L. Gama, B. Bullock, L. M. Carruth, J. L. Mankowski, and M. C. Zink. 2005. The CNS is a viral reservoir in SIV-infected macaques on combined antiretroviral therapy: a model for HIV patients on HAART. *J. Neurovirol.* **11:**180–189.

Cohen, J. 2003. AIDS vaccine still alive as booster after second failure in Thailand. *Science* **302:**1309–1310.

Cohen, J. 2005a. Hedged bet: an unusual AIDS vaccine trial. *Science* **309:**1003.

Cohen, J. 2005b. Prevention cocktails: combining tools to stop HIV's spread. *Science* **309:**1002–1005.

Dallasta, L. M., L. A. Pisarov, J. E. Esplen, J. V. Werley, A. V. Moses, J. A. Nelson, et al. 1999. Blood-brain barrier tight junction disruption in HIV encephalitis. *Am. J. Pathol.* **155:**1915–1927.

De Groot, A. S., H. Sbai, J. Frost, C. Saint-Aubin, et al. 2001. Designing HIV-1 vaccines to reflect viral diversity and the global context of HIV/AIDS. *AID Science* **1:**1–16.

De Groot, A. S., L. Marcon, E. A. Bishop, D. Rivera, M. Kutzler, D. B. Weiner, and W. Martin. 2005. HIV vaccine development by computer assisted design: the GAIA vaccine. *Vaccine* **23:**2136–2148.

Di Stefano, M., S. Wilt, F. Gray, M. Dubois-Dalq, and F. Chlodi. 1996. HIV type 1 V3 sequences and the development of dementia during AIDS. *AIDS Res. Hum. Retrovir.* **12:**471–476.

Doytchinova, I. A., P. Guan, and D. R. Flower. 2004. Identifying human MHC supertypes using bioinformatic methods. *J. Immunol.* **172:**4314–4323.

Doytchinova, I. A., and D. R. Flower. 2005. *In silico* identification of supertypes for class II MHCs. *J. Immunol.* **174:**7085–7095.

Elovaara, I., E. Nykyri, E. Poutiainen, L. Hokkanen, R. Raininko, and J. Suni. 1993. CSF follow-up in HIV-1 infection: intracathecal production of HIV-specific and unspecific IgG, and β-2 microglobulin increase with duration of HIV-1 infection. *Acta Neurol. Scand.* **87:**388–392.

Ensoli, B. 2005. Criteria for selection of HIV vaccine candidates—general principles. *Microbes Infect.* **7:**1433–1435.

Fu, S., A. C. Yopp, X. Mao, D. Chen, N. Zhang, C. Chen, M. Mao, Y. Ding, and J. S. Bromberg. 2004. CD4+ CD25+ CD62+ T-regulatory cell subset has optimal suppressive and proliferative potential. *Am. J. Transplant.* **4:**65–78.

Golding, H., G. M. Shearer, K. Hillman, P. Lucas, J. Manischewitz, R. A. Zajac, M. Clerici, R. E. Gress, R. N. Boswell, and B. Golding. 1989. Common epitope in human immunodeficiency virus (HIV) I-GP41 and HLA class II elicits immunosuppressive autoantibodies capable of contributing to immune dysfunction in HIV I-infected individuals. *J. Clin. Investig.* **83:**1430–1435.

Graham, B. S., M. J. McElrath, R. I. Connor, D. H. Schwartz, G. J. Gorse, M. C. Keefer, M. J. Mulligan, T. J. Matthews, S. M. Wolinsky, D. C. Montefiori, S. H. Vermund, J. S. Lambert, L. Corey, R. B. Belshe, R. Dolin, P. F. Wright, B. T. Korber, M. C. Wolff, P. E. Fast, et al. 1998. Analysis of intercurrent human immunodeficiency virus type 1 infections in phase I and II trials of candidate AIDS vaccines. *J. Infect. Dis.* **177:**310–319.

Gray, R. H., M. J. Wawer, R. Brookmeyer, N. K. Sewankambo, D. Serwadda, F. Wabwire-Mangen, T. Lutalo, X. Li, T. van Cott, T. C. Quinn, and the Rakai Project Team. 2001. Probability of HIV-1 transmission per coital act in monogamous, heterosexual, HIV-1-discordant couples in Rakai, Uganda. *Lancet* **357:**1149–1153.

Hasko, G., P. Pacher, E. S. Vizi, and P. Illes. 2005. Adenosine receptor signaling in the brain immune system. *Trends Pharmacol. Sci.* **26:**511–516.

Haynes, B. F., J. V. Torres, A. J. Langlois, D. P. Bolognesi, M. B. Gardner, T. J. Palker, R. M. Scearce, D. M. Jones, M. A. Moody, C. McDanal, et al. 1993. Induction of HIVMN neutralizing antibodies in primates using a prime-boost regimen of hybrid synthetic gp120 envelope peptides. *J. Immunol.* **151:**1646–1653.

Javaherian, K., A. J. Langlois, G. J. LaRosa, A. T. Profy, D. P. Bolognesi, W. C. Herlihy, S. D. Putney, and T. J. Matthews. 1990. Broadly neutralizing antibodies elicited by the hypervariable neutralizing determinant of HIV-1. *Science* **250:**1590–1593.

Johnston, M. I. 1997. HIV vaccines: problems and prospects. *Hosp. Pract.* **32:**125–128, 131–140.

Kangueane, P., M. K. Sakharkar, P. R. Kolatkar, and E. C. Ren. 2001. Towards the MHC-peptide combinatorics. *Hum. Immunol.* 62:539–556.

Kangueane, P., and M. K. Sakharkar. 2005. T-Epitope Designer: A HLA-peptide binding prediction server. *Bioinformation* 1:21–24.

Kangueane, P., M. K. Sakharkar, G. Rajaseger, S. Bolisetty, B. Sivasekari, B. Zhao, M. Ravichandran, P. Shapshak, and S. Subbiah. 2005. A framework to sub-type HLA supertypes. *Front. Biosci.* 10:879–886.

Kawashima, I., S. J. Hudson, V. Tsai, S. Southwood, K. Takesako, E. Appella, A. Sette, and E. Celis. 1998. The multiepitope approach for immunotherapy for cancer: identification of several CTL epitopes from various tumor-associated antigens expressed on solid epithelial tumors. *Hum. Immunol.* 59:1–14.

Klein, E., and R. J. Ho. 2000. Challenges in the development of an effective HIV vaccine: current approaches and future directions. *Clin. Ther.* 22:295–314.

Korber, B. M., K. J. Kunstman, B. K. Patterson, et al. 1994. Genetic differences between blood- and brain-derived viral sequences from human immunodeficiency virus type 1-infected patients: evidence of conserved elements in the V3 region of the envelope protein of brain-derived sequences. *J. Virol.* 68:7467–7481.

Koup, R. A., J. T. Safrit, Y. Cao, C. A. Andrews, G. McLeod, W. Borkowsky, C. Farthing, and D. D. Ho. 1994. Temporal association of cellular immune responses with the initial control of viremia in primary human immunodeficiency virus type 1 syndrome. *J. Virol.* 68:4650–4655.

Kozlowski, P. A., and M. R. Neutra. 2003. The role of mucosal immunity in prevention of HIV transmission. *Curr. Mol. Med.* 3:217–228.

Kwong, P. D., R. Wyatt, J. Robinson, R. W. Sweet, J. Sodroski, and W. A. Hendrickson. 1998. Structure of an HIV gp120 envelope glycoprotein in complex with the CD4 receptor and a neutralizing human antibody. *Nature* 393:648–659.

Kwong, P. D., M. L. Doyle, D. J. Casper, C. Cicala, S. A. Leavitt, S. Majeed, T. D. Steenbeke, M. Venturi, I. Chaiken, M. Fung, H. Katinger, P. W. Parren, J. Robinson, D. Van Ryk, L. Wang, D. R. Burton, E. Freire, R. Wyatt, J. Sodroski, W. A. Hendrickson, and J. Arthos. 2002. HIV-1 evades antibody-mediated neutralization through conformational masking of receptor-binding sites. *Nature* 420:678–682.

Lassmann, H., F. Zimprich, K. Rossler, and K. Vass. 1991. Inflammation in the nervous system. Basic mechanisms and immunological concepts. *Rev. Neurol.* 147:763–781.

Lee, M. R., D. D. Ho, and M. E. Gurney. 1987. Functional interaction and partial homology between human immunodeficiency virus and neuroleukin. *Science* 237:1047–1051.

Letvin, N. L. 1998. Progress in the development of an HIV-1 vaccine. *Science* 280:1875–1880.

Letvin, N. L., S. Robinson, D. Rohne, M. K. Axthelm, J. W. Fanton, M. Bilska, T. J. Palker, H. X. Liao, B. F. Haynes, and D. C. Montefiori. 2001. Vaccine-elicited V3 loop-specific antibodies in rhesus monkeys and control of a simian-human immunodeficiency virus expressing a primary patient human immunodeficiency virus type 1 isolate envelope. *J. Virol.* 75:4165–4175.

Liu, E., J. F. Cote, and K. Vuori. 2003. Negative regulation of FAK signaling by SOCS proteins. *EMBO J.* 22:5036–5046

Lorin, C., F. Delebecque, V. Labrousse, L. Da Silva, F. Lemonnier, M. Brahic, and F. Tangy. 2005. A recombinant live attenuated measles vaccine vector primes effective HLA-A0201-restricted cytotoxic T lymphocytes and broadly neutralizing antibodies against HIV-1 conserved epitopes. *Vaccine* 23:4463–4472.

Lund, O., M. Nielsen, C. Kesmir, A. G. Petersen, C. Lundegaard, P. Worning, C. Sylvester-Hvid, K. Lamberth,

G. Roder, S. Justesen, S. Buus, and S. Brunak. 2004. Definition of supertypes for HLA molecules using clustering of specificity matrices. *Immunogenetics* 55:797–810.

McKenzie, L. M., J. Pecon-Slattery, M. Carrington, and S. J. O'Brien. 1999 Taxonomic hierarchy of HLA class I allele sequences. *Genes Immun.* 1:120–129.

McMichael, A. J., and T. Hanke. 2003. HIV vaccines 1983–2003. *Nat. Med.* 9:874–880.

Minagar, A., P. Shapshak, E. M. Duran, A. S. Kablinger, J. S. Alexander, R. E. Kelley, R. Seth, and T. Kazic. 2004. Gene expression in HIV-associated dementia, Alzheimer's disease, multiple sclerosis, and schizophrenia. *J. Neurosci. Res.* 224:3–17.

Moore, J. P. 1997. Coreceptors: implications for HIV pathogenesis and therapy. *Science* 276:51–52.

Moore, J. P., A. Trkola, B. Korber, L. J. Boots, J. A. Kessler II, F. E. McCutchan, J. Mascola, D. D. Ho, J. Robinson, and A. J. Conley. 1995. A human monoclonal antibody to a complex epitope in the V3 region of gp120 of human immunodeficiency virus type 1 has broad reactivity within and outside clade B. *J. Virol.* 69:122–130.

Mortara, L., F. Letourneur, H. Gras-Masse, et al. 1998. Selection of virus variants and emergence of virus escape mutants after immunization with an epitope vaccine. *J. Virol.* 72:1403–1410

Nickle, D. C., M. A. Jensen, G. S. Gottlieb, D. Shriner, G. H. Learn, A. G. Rodrigo, and J. I. Mullins. 2003. Consensus and ancestral state HIV vaccines. *Science* 299:1515–1518.

Oldstone, M. B. A. 1987. Molecular mimicry and autoimmune disease. *Cell* 50:819–820.

Oldstone, M. B. A. 1989. Virus induced autoimmunity: molecular mimicry as a route to autoimmune disease. *J. Autoimmun.* 2:187–194.

Osborn, J. E. 1995. The rocky road to an AIDS vaccine. *J. Acquir. Immune Defic. Syndr. Hum. Retrovirol.* 9:26–29.

Pachter, J. S., H. E. de Vries, and Z. Fabry. 2003. The blood-brain barrier and its role in immune privilege in the central nervous system. *J. Neuropathol. Exp. Neurol.* 62:593–604.

Parren, P. W., and D. R. Burton. 2001. The antiviral activity of antibodies in vitro and in vivo. *Adv. Immunol.* 77:195–262.

Parren, P. W., P. A. Marx, A. J. Hessell, A. Luckay, J. Harouse, C. Cheng-Mayer, J. P. Moore, and D. R. Burton. 2001. Antibody protects macaques against vaginal challenge with a pathogenic R5 simian/human immunodeficiency virus at serum levels giving complete neutralization in vitro. *J. Virol.* 75:8340–8347.

Patterson, L. J., F. Robey, A. Muck, K. Van Remoortere, K. Aldrich, E. Richardson, W. G. Alvord, P. D. Markham, M. Cranage, and M. Robert-Guroff. 2001. A conformational C4 peptide polymer vaccine coupled with live recombinant vector priming is immunogenic but does not protect against rectal SIV challenge. *AIDS Res. Hum. Retrovir.* 17:837–849.

Pellequer, J. L., and E. Westhof. 1993. PREDITOP: a program for antigenicity prediction. *J. Mol. Graph.* 11:204–210.

Perrella, O., A. Perrella, M. Perrella, C. Sbreglia, and G. Borgia. 2003. Cytokines and AIDS dementia complex. *AIDS* 17:134–136.

Perry, V. H. 2004. The influence of systemic inflammation on inflammation in the brain: implications for chronic neurodegenerative disease. *Brain Behav. Immun.* 18:407–413.

Pert, C. B., J. M. Hill, M. R. Ruff, R. M. Berman, W. G. Robey, L. O. Arthur, F. W. Ruscetti, and W. L. Farrar. 1986. Octapeptides deduced from the neuropeptide receptor-like pattern of antigen T4 in brain potently inhibit human immunodeficiency virus receptor binding and T-cell infectivity. *Proc. Natl. Acad. Sci. USA* 83:9254–9258.

Poignard, P., E. O. Saphire, P. W. Parren, and D. R. Burton. 2001. gp120: biologic aspects of structural features. *Annu. Rev. Immunol.* 19:253–274.

Power, C., J. C. McArthur, R. T. Johnson, D. E. Griffin, J. D. Glass, S. Perryman, and B. Chesebro. 1994. Demented and non-demented patients with AIDS differ in brain derived human immunodeficiency virus type 1 envelope sequences. *J. Virol.* **68:**4643–4649.

Reitter, J. N., R. E. Means, and R. C. Desrosiers. 1998. A role for carbohydrates in immune evasion in AIDS. *Nat. Med.* **4:**679–684.

Resnick, L., J. R. Berger, P. Shapshak, and W. W. Tourtellotte. 1988. Early penetration of the blood-brain-barrier by HTLV-III/LAV. *Neurology* **38:**9–15.

Richman, D. D., T. Wrin, S. J. Little, and C. J. Petropoulos. 2003. Rapid evolution of the neutralizing antibody response to HIV type 1 infection. *Proc. Natl. Acad. Sci. USA* **100:**4144–4149.

Robey, F. A., and M. Robert-Guroff. 2001. A defined conformational epitope from the C4 domain of HIV type 1 glycoprotein 120: anti-cyclic C4 antibodies from HIV-positive donors magnify glycoprotein 120 suppression of interleukin 2 produced by T cells. *AIDS Res. Hum. Retrovir.* **17:**533–541.

Romagnani, S. 1992. Human TH1 and TH2 subsets: regulation of differentiation and role in protection and immunopathology. *Int. Arch. Allergy Immunol.* **98:**279–285.

Salemi, M., S. L. Lamers, S. Yu, T. de Oliveira, W. M. Fitch, and M. S. McGrath. 2005. Phylodynamic analysis of HIV-1 in distinct brain compartments provides a model for the neuropathogenesis of AIDS. *J. Virol.* **79:**11343–11352.

Sattentau, Q. J., and J. P. Moore. 1995. Human immunodeficiency virus type 1 neutralization is determined by epitope exposure on the gp120 oligomer. *J. Exp. Med.* **182:**185–196.

Sbai, H., A. Mehta, and A. S. De Groot. 2001. Use of T cell epitopes for vaccine development. *Curr. Drug Targets Infect. Disord.* **1:**283–293.

Schonning, K., A. Bolmstedt, J. Novotny, O. S. Lund, S. Olofsson, and J. E. Hansen. 1998. Induction of antibodies against epitopes inaccessible on the HIV type 1 envelope oligomer by immunization with recombinant monomeric glycoprotein 120. *AIDS Res. Hum. Retrovir.* **14:**1451–1456.

Scognamiglio, P., D. Accapezzato, M. A. Casciaro, A. Cacciani, M. Artini, G. Bruno, M. L. Chircu, J. Sidney, S. Southwood, S. Abrignani, A. Sette, and V. Barnaba. 1999. Presence of effector CD8⁺ T cells in hepatitis C virus-exposed healthy seronegative donors. *J. Immunol.* **162:**6681–6689.

Sette, A., and J. Sidney. 1998. HLA supertypes and supermotifs: a functional perspective on HLA polymorphism. *Curr. Opin. Immunol.* **10:**478–482.

Sette, A., and J. Sidney. 1999. Nine major HLA class I supertypes account for the vast preponderance of HLA-A and -B polymorphism. *Immunogenetics* **50:**201–212.

Shapshak, P., I. Nagano, K. Q. Xin, W. Bradley, et al. 1995. HIV-1 heterogeneity and cytokines: neuropathogenesis in the brain immune axis and substance abuse, p. 225–236. *In* B. Sharp, T. Eisenstein, J. Madden, and H. Friedman (ed.), *The Brain Immune Axis and Substance Abuse.* Plenum Press, New York, NY.

Shapshak, P., K. A. Crandall, K. Goodkin, et al. 1996. HIV-1 Neuropathogenesis and abused drugs: current views: problems and solutions. *Adv. Exp. Med. Biol.* **402:**171–186.

Shapshak, P., D. M. Segal, K. A. Crandall, R. K. Fujimura, B. T. Zhang, K. Q. Xin, K. Okuda, C. Petito, C. Eisdorfer, and K. Goodkin. 1999. Independent evolution of HIV-1 in different brain regions. *AIDS Res. Hum. Retrovir.* **15:**811–820.

Shapshak, P., R. Duncan, A. Nath, J. Turchan, P. Kangueane, S. A. M. Shapshak, H. Rodriguez, E. M. Duran, F. Ziegler, E. Amaro, A. Lewis, A. Rodriguez, A. Minagar, W. Davis, R. Seth, F. Chiappelli, and T. Kazic. 2006. Gene chromosomal organization and expression in cultured human neurons exposed to cocaine and HIV-1 proteins gp120 and tat: drug abuse and neuroAIDS. *Front. Biosci.* **11:**1774–1793.

Shapshak, P., R. Duncan, J. E. Torres-Munoz, E. M. Duran, A. Minagar, and C. K. Petito. 2004. Analytic approaches to differential gene expression in AIDS vs. control brains. *Front. Biosci.* **9:**2935–2946.

Sidney, J., H. M. Grey, S. Southwood, E. Celis, P. A. Wentworth, M. F. del Guercio, R. T. Kubo, R. W. Chesnut, and A. Sette. 1996. Definition of an HLA-A3-like supermotif demonstrates the overlapping peptide-binding repertoires of common HLA molecules. *Hum. Immunol.* **45:**79–93.

Singer, E. J., K. Syndulko, P. Shapshak, L. Resnick, and W. W. Tourtellotte. 1994. Cerebrospinal fluid p24 antigen levels and intrathecal immunoglobulin G synthesis are associated with cognitive disease severity in HIV-1. *AIDS* **8:**197–204.

Speth, C., M. P. Dierich, and S. Sopper. 2005. HIV-infection of the central nervous system: the tight rope walk of innate immunity. *Mol. Immunol.* **42:**213–228.

Stanhope, P. E., M. L. Clements, and R. F. Siliciano. 1993. Human CD4⁺ cytolytic T lymphocyte responses to a human immunodeficiency virus type 1 gp160 subunit vaccine. *J. Infect. Dis.* **168:**92–100.

Thomson, S. A., A. B. Jaramillo, M. Shoobridge, K. J. Dunstan, B. Everett, C. Ranasinghe, S. J. Kent, K. Gao, J. Medveckzy, R. A. Ffrench, and I. A. Ramshaw. 2005. Development of a synthetic consensus sequence scrambled antigen HIV-1 vaccine designed for global use. *Vaccine* **23:**4647–4657.

Toda, M. 2003. Immuno-viral therapy as a new approach for the treatment of brain tumors. *Drug News Perspect.* **16:**223–229.

Van Cott, T. C., J. R. Mascola, L. D. Loomis-Price, F. Sinangil, N. Zitomersky, J. McNeil, M. L. Robb, D. L. Birx, and S. Barnett. 1999. Cross-subtype neutralizing antibodies induced in baboons by a subtype E gp120 immunogen based on an R5 primary human immunodeficiency virus type 1 envelope. *J. Virol.* **73:**4640–4650.

van Marle, G., and C. Power. 2005. Human immunodeficiency virus type 1 genetic diversity in the nervous system: evolutionary epiphenomenon or disease determinant. *J. Neurovirol.* **11:**107–128.

Walker, C. M., D. J. Moody, D. P. Stites, and J. A. Levy. 1986. CD8⁺ lymphocytes can control HIV infection in vitro by suppressing virus replication. *Science* **234:**1563–1566.

Wei, X., J. M. Decker, S. Wang, H. Hui, J. C. Kappes, X. Wu, J. F. Salazar-Gonzalez, M. G. Salazar, J. M. Kilby, M. S. Saag, N. L. Komarova, M. A. Nowak, B. H. Hahn, P. D. Kwong, and G. M. Shaw. 2003. Antibody neutralization and escape by HIV-1. *Nature* **422:**307–312.

Weller, R. O., B. Engelhardt, and M. J. Phillips. 1996. Lymphocyte targeting of the central nervous system: a review of afferent and efferent CNS-immune pathways. *Brain Pathol.* **6:**275–288.

Wesselingh, S. L., C. Power, J. D. Glass, W. R. Tyor, J. C. McArthur, J. M. Farber, J. W. Griffin, and D. E. Griffin. 1993. Intracerebral cytokine messenger RNA expression in acquired immunodeficiency syndrome dementia. *Ann. Neurol.* **33:**6576–6582.

Whatmore, A. M., N. Cook, G. A. Hall, S. Sharpe, E. W. Rud, and M. P. Cranage. 1995. Repair and evolution of nef in vivo modulates simian immunodeficiency virus virulence. *J. Virol.* **69:**5117–5123.

Wyatt, R., and J. Sodroski. 1998. The HIV-1 envelope glycoproteins: fusogens, antigens and immunogens. *Science* **280:**1884–1888.

Xin, K. Q., K. Hamajima, S. Sasaki, A. Honsho, T. Tsuji, N. Ishii, X. R. Cao, Y. Lu, P. Shapshak, and K. Okuda. 1998. Intranasal administration of HIV-1 DNA vaccine with IL-2 expression plasmid enhances cell-mediated immunity against HIV. Immunology **94:**438–444.

Yagi, H., T. Nomura, K. Nakamura, S. Yamazaki, T. Kitawaki, S. Hori, M. Maeda, M. Onodera, T. Uchiyama, S. Fujii, and S. Sakaguchi. 2004. Crucial role of FOXP3 in the development and function of human CD25+ CD4+ regulatory T cells. *Int. Immunol.* **16:**1643–1656.

Young, J. A. 1988. HIV and HLA similarity. *Nature* **333:**215.

Zeng, W., D. C. Jackson, J. Murray, K. Rose, and L.E. Brown. 2000. Totally synthetic lipid-containing polyoxime peptide constructs are potent immunogens. *Vaccine* **18:**1031–1039.

Zhao, B., V. S. Mathura, G. Rajaseger, S. Moochhala, M. K. Sakharkar, and P. Kangueane. 2003. A novel MHCp binding prediction model. *Hum. Immunol.* **64:**1123–1143.

Zinckgraf, J. W., J. M. Winchell, and L. K. Silbart. 1999. Antibody responses to a mucosally delivered HIV-1 gp120-derived C4/V3 peptide. *J. Reprod. Immunol.* **45:**99–112.

Zou, L., B. Barnett, H. Safah, V. F. Larussa, M. Evdemon-Hogan, P. Mottram, S. Wei, O. David, T. J. Curiel, and W. Zou. 2004. Bone marrow is a reservoir for CD4+CD25+ regulatory T cells that traffic through CXCL12/CXCR4 signals. *Cancer Res.* **64:**8451–8455.

PATHOPHYSIOLOGICAL ISSUES

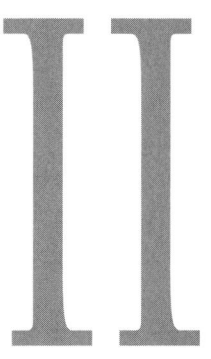

10

Neurovirological Aspects of HIV Infection in the HAART Era

ZAHIDA PARVEEN, EDWARD ACHEAMPONG, ROGER J. POMERANTZ,
AND MUHAMMAD MUKHTAR

HIV-1 targets mainly the immune system by depleting circulatory lymphocytes as well as ravaging the central nervous system (CNS) due to its neurotropic nature (Freed, 2004). A series of devastating clinical conditions, manifested in the CNS of certain HIV-1-infected individuals, are attributed to infection of cells in the brain parenchyma (Diesing et al., 2002; Lawrence and Major, 2002; Kaul et al., 2005; Kaul and Lipton, 2006). HIV-1-associated dementia (HAD) (also known as AIDS dementia complex), characterized by cognitive dysfunction, motor difficulties, coordination abnormalities, and other neurological signs and symptoms, develops to variable degrees in children and adults. The molecular mechanisms involved in these HIV-1-induced dysfunctions of the CNS remain incompletely explained (Kramer-Hammerle et al., 2005; Toborek et al., 2005). Besides direct invasion of the brain by the virus, other paradigms associated with HAD pathophysiology are (i) neurotoxicities (apoptosis) associated with specific HIV-1 proteins like gp41, gp120, Tat, Nef, and Vpr (Rappaport et al., 1999; Pomerantz, 2004; Acheampong et al., 2005); (ii) proinflammatory cytokines, chemokines, and oxidative stress responses (Bautista, 2001); and (iii) excitotoxicity, altered neurotransmitter release, and autoimmune disorders associated with the presence of anti-CNS antibodies in HAD patients (Mukhtar et al., 2005). Studies have demonstrated that the major reservoirs for productive infection in cells within the CNS of HIV-1-infected individuals are microglia and monocyte/macrophages, although infection of other CNS-based cell types (including microvascular endothelial cells [MVECs], astrocytes, and neuronal elements) also appears to occur at low levels (Bagasra et al., 1996; Mukhtar et al., 2000; Kramer-Hammerle et al., 2005).

Several studies have also proposed that both viral proteins and potentially proinflammatory cytokines may be involved in the manifestations of the deleterious effects of HIV-1 on the CNS.

The advent of HAART in the mid-1990s has significantly reduced the morbidity and mortality associated with HIV-1 infection, and the AIDS pandemic is now considered a chronic disorder (Nath and Sacktor, 2006). However, people having no access to HAART are still at the mercy of the viral infection and associated disorders. As far as neurological disorders are concerned, even in the era of HAART, we are still burdened with the AIDS-associated neurodegeneration either at lesser frequency or in different forms (Gonzalez-Scarano and Martin-Garcia, 2005; Nunn, 2006). Improved survival in elderly populations as a result of HAART has completely changed the dynamics of the HIV-1-associated neurological complications. The number of individuals living with HIV into their fifties and beyond is expected to grow. According to one estimate, in the United States alone, more than 60,000 HIV-1-infected individuals are expected to live to age 50 or older in the coming years. The National Institute of Mental Health (NIMH) of the U.S. National Institutes of Health (NIH), in anticipation of the urgency of this issue, organized a meeting to discuss clinical and basic research priorities on CNS-related comorbidities and complications in HIV-1-infected older populations (Mental Health Research Issues in HIV Infection and Aging, National Institute of Mental Health Workshop; NIMH, Washington, DC, 2002).

The major objectives of this meeting were to determine ways to differentiate between AIDS-related and aging-specific health challenges, as the aging process is associated with a plethora of health problems such as Alzheimer's disease, osteoporosis, prostate cancer, and diabetes. How the HIV-1-infected individuals on HAART respond to the aging phenomena still needs to be resolved. Besides extensive discussion on several issues, the overall recommendations of this meeting were to set forth aging research priorities among HIV-1-infected individuals, particularly in

Zahida Parveen and Edward Acheampong, Department of Medicine, Thomas Jefferson University, Philadelphia, PA 19107. **Roger J. Pomerantz,** Tibotec Inc., Yardley, PA 19067. **Muhammad Mukhtar,** Department of Biochemistry, Pir Mehr Ali Shah Arid Agriculture University Rawalpindi, Rawalpindi 46300, Pakistan.

the area of neurocognition and neuropsychiatric disorders in addition to neurodegeneration.

Several studies in the past have described neurotropic features of HIV-1 to better understand the mechanism of neuropathogenesis; however, no conclusive determinants involved in this aspect of viral pathogenesis have been elucidated. As described in other chapters of this volume, HIV-1 entry into permissive cells is mediated by the CD4 receptor acting in concert with a number of chemokine receptors. Of these chemokine receptors, CXCR4 and CCR5 are critical in determining whether the tropism of each individual viral strain is T cells (X4 strains), macrophages (R5 strains), or dual-tropic (X4R5). The roles of other chemokine receptors and CD4-independent infection of various cell types have also been described (Harouse et al., 1989). The chemokine receptors CXCR4 and CCR5 have been reported to play important roles in CD4-independent entry of HIV and determine the viral tropism (Edinger et al., 1997). The mechanisms of infection of CNS cells may be quite different. Surprisingly, CNS tissues are devoid of CD4, implying the existence of CD4-independent mechanisms for entry/infection (Li et al., 1990; Mukhtar et al., 2002). Moreover, we have previously reported that various chemokine receptor ligands are unable to inhibit viral attachment to cells of the blood-brain barrier (BBB), particularly brain MVECs, suggesting that there are chemokine receptor-independent pathways as well (Mukhtar et al., 2002). Infection of various cell types in the brain has been a controversial issue. A leading theory based on the "Trojan horse" hypothesis suggests that HIV present in the brain is derived from monocytes. This theory is also supported by several other studies suggesting that most of the brain-derived HIV-1 isolates are macrophage tropic (R5) in nature.

Besides chemokine receptors, several studies in the past have focused on the role of cholesterol-rich microdomains (rafts) in the plasma membrane of susceptible cells (Liao et al., 2003; Nguyen and Taub, 2004). The observation of HIV-1 entry into human primary macrophage as formation of macropinosomes in the intracellular vesicles further supported the idea that the virus entry route might involve alternative mechanisms besides viral envelope-receptor interactions (Marechal et al., 2001). This concept has been further elaborated in a study on brain MVECs that suggests interrelationships between macropinocytosis, lipid rafts, and the mitogen-activated protein kinase signaling pathway for viral entry into these cells (Liu et al., 2002), although actual infection was not examined. Using HIV-1 binding and internalization assays performed with primary human brain MVECs treated, or left untreated, with various cholesterol-depleting agents that disrupt lipid rafts, we found a cholesterol- and lipid-raft-independent mechanism in the infectious entry of HIV-1 into primary human brain MVECs (Argyris et al., 2003). As a positive control, we found that cholesterol-depleting agents disrupted HIV-1 binding and entry into T lymphocytes. The lack of CD4 and the inability of chemokine receptors' ligands and lipid raft disrupting agents to block HIV-1 infectivity/entry into neuronal cells will be the major challenges for understanding HIV-1 neuropathogenesis, particularly among populations having access to HAART.

EFFECTS OF HAART ON HIV-1 NEUROPATHOGENESIS

HIV-1 frequently infects the CNS of individuals soon after seroconversion (Resnick et al., 1988; Spector et al., 1993). Studies have demonstrated that microglia and monocyte/

macrophages are major cellular reservoirs for highly productive HIV-1 infection in the CNS (Bell et al., 1993; Gosztonyi et al., 1994). As well, several studies have demonstrated HIV-1 provirus and low-level replication, in vivo, within MVECs, astrocytes, and neuronal elements. These studies utilized immunocytochemistry and in situ PCR (Nuovo et al., 1994; Bagasra et al., 1996; Mukhtar et al., 2002). In addition, other studies have also demonstrated limited replication of HIV-1, in vitro as well as in vivo, in brain MVECs (Moses and Nelson, 1994; Bagasra et al., 1996). HIV-1 replication has been evaluated in some detail in human fetal and adult astrocytes, both in vitro and in vivo (Saito et al., 1994; Ranki et al., 1995). These studies suggest a restricted form of HIV-1 replication in astrocytic cells, characterized mainly by the expression of multiply spliced HIV-1 mRNA, which encode certain viral regulatory gene products (e.g., Rev, Tat, and especially Nef) (Saito et al., 1994; Ranki et al., 1995). Furthermore, a study demonstrating HIV-1 long-terminal-repeat-directed transcriptional alterations in the neuronal elements of transgenic mice is of potential interest, when viewed alongside other in vivo data from humans (Corboy et al., 1992). Of note, certain populations of neurons are infectible by HIV-1 and simian immunodeficiency virus (SIV) both in vitro and in vivo (Lane et al., 1996; Canto-Nogues et al., 2005).

Although clinical trials utilizing combinations of reverse transcriptase (RT) inhibitors and viral protease inhibitors in HAART have shown important efficiency in altering HIV-1 replication in vivo, these approaches may have several weaknesses in targeting HIV-1 reservoirs within the CNS (Pomerantz, 2002; von Giesen et al., 2002). First, the ability of some of these compounds to cross the BBB is not always efficient, leading to concentrations of some of these antiretroviral drugs that are lower in the CNS than in the peripheral blood (Aweeka et al., 1999; Tashima et al., 1999). This is due to the effects of the P-glycoprotein of the BBB on protease inhibitors and to active efflux pumps altering the levels of nucleoside analog RT inhibitors in the CNS (van der Sandt et al., 2001; Thomas, 2004). In addition, intracerebral concentrations of these agents, and in some cases active metabolites, are poorly described for various CNS-based cells (Pomerantz, 2001).

Of importance, viral kinetic studies have demonstrated a rapid turnover for HIV-1 virions in vivo (Perelson et al., 1996, 1997). These studies have also shown relatively rapid destruction of acutely infected CD4$^+$ T lymphocytes in vivo. Nevertheless, a small percentage of cells have been demonstrated, in these kinetic studies, to be either restrictively infected and/or long-lasting cells, which do not demonstrate rapid destruction after infection with HIV-1. These small but important fractions of cells in the human body, which may be infected and do not rapidly turn over, have been hypothesized to some extent to be in potential sanctuary sites (such as the CNS or testes) or to be nonproliferating and/or postmitotic cells (such as various cell types within the adult CNS) (Chun et al., 1997a, 1997b; Finzi et al., 1997). Regions in the body which are protected by MVEC tight layers (i.e., CNS, retina, and testes) are critical sites for possible HIV-1 reservoirs for patients on HAART (Pialoux et al., 1997; Pomerantz, 1999). Low but detectable levels of such cell infections have been shown in lymphoid tissue and peripheral blood of HIV-1-infected individuals on virally suppressive HAART (Cavert et al., 1997; Chun et al., 1997a, 1997b). Of note, in a few cases it has been demonstrated that there is worsening of HAD symptoms in the CNS of patients on triple anti-HIV-1 therapy, although the levels of virus in the peripheral blood are dramatically reduced (Dougherty and McArthur,

2002). Nevertheless, most patients with HAD on suppressive HAART have gained stability of HAD signs and symptoms, and some patients have cognitive improvement (Tozzi et al., 1999; Sacktor et al., 2000). Of interest is a study in which it was demonstrated that HIV-1 RNA in cerebrospinal fluid (CSF) is produced both from the peripheral blood and from the brain parenchyma in infected individuals (Ellis et al., 2000). This study supports the notion that the remission of HAART-associated neurological disorders might be relevant to the decrease in peripheral viral load. Conversely the brain and retina are difficult tissues to obtain from healthy HIV-1-infected individuals on virally suppressive HAART, and analysis of HIV-1 persistence and HIV-1 residual disease in a tissue obtained from a true blood-retinal barrier is almost impossible.

HAART-ASSOCIATED CHANGES IN THE BRAIN

The efficacy of HAART in controlling HIV-1 and associated infections is manifested as decreased plasma viral load and restoration of circulating T-lymphocyte populations (Daniel et al., 1999; Langford et al., 2003). However, the potential of HAART to eradicate virus as envisioned by several investigators has faded (Siliciano, 2005). It is prudent to mention here that levels of HIV-1 RNA in the CSF of HIV-1-infected individuals are considered to be a better predictor of neurocognitive impairments than levels in plasma (Brew et al., 1997; Ellis et al., 1997). Moreover, HAART-related control of CNS infections is due to viral control in plasma and not in the CNS-based cells. Some studies have suggested that the penetration of the antiretrovirals through the BBB is an issue (Solas et al., 2003); however, there are very limited data to substantiate these claims (Eggers et al., 2003; Evers et al., 2004).

The effects of HAART on cellular elements involved in the pathogenesis of HAD are still an active area of investigation (Table 1). Macrophages/microglia are considered to play a major role in the pathogenesis of HAD as well as in neuroinflammatory responses. Formation of multinucleated giant cells (MNGC) is a hallmark of HAD and is considered

to be a reliable marker of HIV-1 encephalopathy in brain autopsy of virally infected individuals (Davies et al., 1997). In earlier studies the levels of influx/activation of macrophages/microglia in autopsied brain tissues of HAD patients were considered to be a correlate of HAD severity (Glass et al., 1995; Fischer-Smith et al., 2001). Recently in a study to determine HIV-1-associated neuropathologies, Anthony et al. compared the microglial populations in the brains of patients from the pre- and post-HAART eras in Edinburgh, United Kingdom. The basal ganglia and the hippocampus, the two areas involved in cognitive function, revealed that HAART-treated cases have a significantly higher number of microglia/macrophages in basal ganglia (Anthony et al., 2005). Conversely, a recent update on neuropathology of HIV in the HAART era suggests that combination therapy has been very helpful in improving HIV-related immunological abnormalities and reducing AIDS-related opportunistic infections (Bell, 2004). This has led to improved survival rate of infected individuals; however, the higher prevalence of HIV-associated cognitive impairment and HIV encephalitis is very troubling. Such findings need further investigation in solving the mystery of persistent viral reservoirs as well as providing important information about development of strategies that could lead to the control of HIV-1-induced activation of microglial cells. On the other hand, persistent inflammatory responses (increased influx of microglia) could predispose individuals on HAART to neurodegeneration. In a recent report elevated levels of β-amyloid precursor protein were observed in the HAART era brain tissues compared with age- and gender-matched historical controls (Green et al., 2005). It is possible that prolonged HAART in conjunction with the aging process could elevate the levels of amyloid precursor protein, which has been reported in high amounts in several other dementias. Efforts have also been directed toward understanding overall pathogenesis of HAD and its correlates. A recent study has shown that HAD precedes an upregulation of antioxidant machinery (HAD onset) of the brain, followed by an accumulation of sphingomyelin (moderate cognitive disorder) and finally by production of ceramides, and

TABLE 1 Effects of HAART on HAD and associated neurological disorders

HAD manifestation	Description	Relative incidence	Reference(s)
HIV encephalitis	A pathological correlate of HAD, manifested as formation of MNGC from brain resident microglia/macrophage fusion	Decreased with HAART	Gray et al., 2003
HAD-associated opportunistic infections	AIDS patients are prone to several opportunistic infections (OI) of brain. Frequent OI are fungal (*Cryptococcus neoformans*, *Candida albicans*), protozoan (*Toxoplasma gondii*), and viral (herpes, polyomavirus).	Decreased with HAART	Gray et al., 2003; Pozio, 2004
AIDS-associated CNS lymphoma	Mainly non-Hodgkin's B-cell tumors develop in the brain of people infected with HIV-1	No significant change	Clayton and Mughal, 2004; Baeuerle et al., 2005
Peripheral neuropathy	HAD is associated with several types of peripheral neuropathies; however, DSPN and ATN are most prevalent.	Increased with HAART	Blanchard, 2004
Minor cognitive motor disorder	Major manifestations are loss of memory and decreases in computational and other higher cortical functions.	Increased with HAART	McArthur et al., 2003; Gonzalez-Scarano and Martin-Garcia, 2005

reactive aldehydes are indicators of severe cognitive decline (Bandaru et al., 2007).

HAART AND PERIPHERAL NEUROPATHY

HIV-1-associated neurological symptoms extend from CNS to the peripheral and visual nervous system disorders. HIV-1-associated peripheral neuropathies include chronic inflammatory demyelinating polyneuropathy, mononeuropathy multiplex, progressive lumbosacral polyradiculopathy, and distal symmetric polyneuropathy (DSPN). The most prevalent and clinically important is DSPN (Casanova-Sotolongo et al., 2003). Another disorder, antiretroviral drug toxic neuropathy (ATN), associated with the dideoxynucleoside (ddC, D4T, and ddI), is identical to DSPN. Both of these neuropathies result in painful conditions in feet and legs in addition to numbness.

HIV-1-associated immunological responses and viral replication vary in neuropathic etiology, and previous studies have failed to establish a link between peripheral neuropathies and immunological parameters (Brinley et al., 2001). This is also the case for infiltration of immune cells into the brain. It is believed that the toxic microenvironment from HIV-1-infected microglia is the root cause of DSPN. This is due to the fact that previous methodologies have failed to isolate virus or its transcript from the peripheral nerves. Pathologically, DSPN is associated with damage to distal regions of nerve fibers. Autopsy studies reveal peripheral nerve abnormalities in almost every patient who died from AIDS, suggesting gradual nerve damage before apparent clinical symptoms of DSPN.

The exact etiology of AIDS-associated peripheral neuropathies is still an active area of investigation. It has been reported that viral load prior to HAART is a risk factor for DSPN in later stages (Childs et al., 1999). It has also been observed that neurocognitive impairments at the initiation of HAART predict lifelong neuropsychological severity and persistence (Tozzi et al., 2007). Besides several other unknown factors, the genetic makeup of an individual may determine the predisposition of the individual to drug responses. ATN, a form of sensory neuropathy with associated dideoxynucleoside antiretrovirals, has recently been linked to a person's genotype. It has been found that an inherited mutation in human mitochondria determines the predisposition of individuals to risks of peripheral neuropathy. A good example is the prevalence of the association of haplotype T with peripheral neuropathies in the Caucasian population (Hulgan et al., 2005). In the future the notion of personalized medicine based on individual genotype will be very helpful in determining the drug toxicities in an individual or cases in which personal genotype determines the predisposition of an individual toward a certain disorder (Mukhtar, 2005).

According to the Johns Hopkins HIV Clinical Cohort, usage of HAART has elevated the incidence of DSPN among the HIV-infected population from 17.3/1,000 in 1994 to 31.1/1,000 by the year 2000 (Blanchard, 2004). The diagnostic criteria have also been an issue, as the procedures for the identification of peripheral neuropathies are still evolving. It is possible that in the near future a more reliable diagnostic procedure will help in resolving the issue of HIV-1-associated peripheral neuropathies in the HAART era. A recently described global screening tool, "Neuroscreen," has shown promise for assessing neuropsychological function and DSPN (Ellis et al., 2004).

HAART AND HAD-ASSOCIATED APOPTOSIS

HAART dramatically reduces the levels of HIV-1 in systemic circulation and also controls virally associated opportunistic infections. Similarly, HAD has also been lessened in patients on HAART. However, the cytopathic effects of HAART, particularly neurotoxicities, still persist in patients undergoing the therapy (Sperber and Shao, 2003). Such toxic stimuli could be precursors for the programmed cell death (apoptosis) usually observed in HIV-1 pathogenesis. Of importance, apoptosis has been considered to be one of the mechanisms for CD4$^+$ T-lymphocyte depletion during AIDS progression (Yue et al., 2005). Initially, the Fas/Fas ligand (also known as CD95 and APO-1) apoptotic pathway was recognized as one of the pathways of T-cell death during HIV-1 infection (Alderson et al., 1995), but a recent study has proposed that type I interferon-regulated interactions with tumor necrosis factor (TNF)-related apoptosis-induced ligand and its death receptor 5 (DR5) induce apoptosis of HIV-1-exposed CD4$^+$ T cells (Herbeuval et al., 2005). Particularly, this study showed that a decreased viral load and increased CD4$^+$ counts of HAART-responsive patients correlate with a proportionate decrease in the levels of CD4$^+$ T-cell mRNA. Whether similar apoptotic mechanisms operate in HAD is yet to be explored, although studies have suggested that apoptosis of neuronal elements leads to a neuronal loss noted in patients with HAD (Adle-Biassette et al., 1995; Gray et al., 2001; Ozdener, 2005). Increased apoptosis has been described in neurons, astrocytes, and MVECs in the CNS of macaques infected with a neurovirulent strain of SIV (Adamson et al., 1996). These findings have been confirmed in animal models and extended the data on increased apoptosis of neurons, astrocytes, and MVECs in patients with HAD, compared to nondemented HIV-1-infected individuals (Shi et al., 1996). Numerous hypotheses regarding neuronal cell injury or death within HIV-1-infected individuals have been provided. During HIV-1 infection, macrophages and microglia can be activated by HIV-1, resulting in the release of specific viral products (Persidsky et al., 1996; Zheng et al., 1999; Garden, 2002), which may induce apoptosis in bystander cells (Andreau et al., 2004). In CNS-based cells, it has been shown that HIV-1 infection can lead to the production and release of neurotoxic proinflammatory cytokines (Barak et al., 2002). These proinflammatory cytokines including TNF-α and interleukin-1β (IL-1β) have been shown to mediate both neurotoxic reactions and parallel neurocognitive dysfunction in individuals with HAD (Shi et al., 1998). In addition, other studies have shown that the production by the virus of neurotoxic viral proteins can be directly deleterious to neurons. The CXCR4 and CCR5 chemokine receptors expressed on neurons may induce cell death by facilitating HIV-1 gp120 binding (Weissman et al., 1997). The expression of the natural ligand for CXCR4, SDF-1-α, has been reported to be up-regulated in individuals with HAD-stimulating neurotoxicity (Hesselgesser and Horuk, 1999). SDF-1-α production is up-regulated in astrocytes by factors secreted by activated macrophages (Zheng et al., 1999). This reported increase in SDF-1-α levels in the CNS of HAD patients may contribute to neuronal apoptosis. It has been shown that blocking access of virus to the chemokine receptors seems to prevent the occurrence of apoptosis (Zheng et al., 1999). Of importance, neurons do not express the CD4 protein, the primary receptor for efficient HIV-1 entry into cells. However, HIV-1 gp120 released from infected cells can bind to CXCR4 expressed on neurons in a CD4-independent mechanism and initiate neuronal apoptosis (Hesselgesser and Horuk, 1999; Zheng et al., 1999). It has been shown that addition of gp120 to pure neuronal or neuroblastoma cell lines in nanomolar amounts is toxic to these cells in vitro (Kaul et al., 2001). In vivo, gp120 (Zhang et al., 2003) has been shown to cause neuronal dysfunction and death in rodents (Bagetta et al., 1996). In addition to the factors indicated above, oxidative stress has also been implicated in neuronal death. Oxidative stress, which occurs as a consequence of macrophage activation, is manifested as depletion of endogenous antioxidant moieties and increased production of reactive oxygen species like oxygen and nitric oxide (NO) free radicals. Elevated expression of NO synthase, an enzyme responsible for generation of NO free radicals in AIDS dementia, further supports the potential of oxidative stress in BBB breakdown and neuronal damage (Rafalowska, 1998). Furthermore, peroxynitrite, the major effector of oxidative stress, has been reported to damage neurons by targeting neurofilament, a critical neuronal structural protein (Coyle and Puttfarcken, 1993). Thus, the interactions of soluble inflammatory products and viral proteins and other pathologic processes that work through neuronal receptors in the HIV-1-infected nervous system result in neuronal death in HAD (Zheng et al., 1999).

The mechanisms involved in the induction of CNS-based apoptosis during HIV-1 infection may be the cumulative effects induced by various HIV-1 proteins, such as gp120 (Jana and Pahan, 2004; Nosheny et al., 2004); Tat (Kruman et al., 1998; Singh et al., 2004); Vpr (Patel et al., 2000, 2002); and possibly Nef (Acheampong et al., 2005). At mechanistic levels an interesting study has also suggested that CNS apoptosis may be secondary to the expression of c-kit proto-oncogene stimulated by HIV-1 Nef as reported in an in vitro analysis of an astrocytic cell line (He et al., 1997b). Certainly, specific proinflammatory cytokines (e.g., TNF-α) and/or N-methyl-D-aspartate (NMDA) excitatory receptor stimulation may also lead to apoptosis of select CNS cell types in HAD. The mechanisms of neuronal death either through direct inflammatory responses or induced by individual HIV-1 proteins suggest initiation of several avenues of the apoptotic cascade. Of note, HIV-1 protein Nef has been demonstrated to be overexpressed in pediatric and adult astrocytes (Tornatore et al., 1994; Ranki et al., 1995), to induce BBB disruption in rats (Sporer et al., 2000), and to lead to leukocyte recruitment to the CNS (Koedel et al., 1999). Other HIV-1 proteins have also been shown to exert diverse deleterious effects on CNS cellular elements both in vitro and in vivo.

The beneficial effects of HAART are increases in the number of CD4+ T cells and reductions in viremia. Whether this effect of HAART on elevation of T-cell levels is mediated by inhibition of T-cell apoptosis or some other mechanisms has not been extensively studied. A study by Roger et al. showed that HAART eliminates apoptosis among HIV-1-infected individuals without any relationship to plasma viremia (Roger et al., 1999). Similarly, control of apoptosis and HAD neurological symptoms is most probably due to the control of systemic viremia and not the beneficial effects of HAART on the CNS. It has been proposed that adjunctive therapies focusing on inhibition of proapoptotic machinery could be an excellent investigational step in controlling HAD in the era of HAART (Kolson, 2002).

DYNAMICS OF HIV-1 IN THE BRAIN IN HAART ERA

As indicated earlier, HIV-1 enters the brain during the early stages of viral infection. However, whether or not there is productive infection by the early penetrating virus is still unknown. A technical obstacle involved with the isolation of the virus from the brain is another issue, since most of the primary brain isolates have been obtained and sequenced from postmortem brain tissues. This situation increases the risk of sampling error. The SIV model has been quite helpful in resolving this issue. This model is a real mimic of AIDS and HAD in humans, and likewise HAART could ameliorate neurological symptoms in the SIV model. To resolve the issue of viral dynamics in the brain and systemic circulation, brain and tissue specimens from two animals with clear symptoms of SIV encephalitis were analyzed. Phylogenetic analyses of SIV envelope (env) sequences from MNGCs (a hallmark of encephalitis), brain, and spleen tissue revealed that genotypically MNGC sequences were closer to brain isolates, suggesting viral replication in the brain. Furthermore, a small percentage of sequences showed a phylogenetic relationship to the original inoculum, suggesting early penetration of virus into the brain (Ryzhova et al., 2002). The complex anatomical structure of the brain of humans and the presence of the BBB and blood-retinal barrier also warrant studies on HIV-1 dynamics among various compartments of the brain. A study to dissect the association between genetic differences and regional variability revealed minimal gene flow among various regions of the brain (Shapshak et al., 1999). This particular study took into consideration the four regions of the brain, i.e., frontal lobe, basal ganglia, medial temporal lobe, and nonmedial temporal lobe. Another recent study compared the phenotypic and genotypic features of the virus from autopsied brain, choroid plexus, and spleen tissue of patients with and without dementia. The study involved comparison of viral env and pol gene sequences from viral genomic DNA isolated either directly from tissues or coculturing methodology for retrieval of viral quasispecies.

Several studies in the past have compared viral evolution in the human brain with the systemic circulation (Ball et al., 1994; Bratanich et al., 1998; Ritola et al., 2005; Salemi et al., 2005). Most of these studies have focused on the HIV-1 surface env protein (Burkala et al., 2005; Ritola et al., 2005) isolated from brain tissues and the CSF. Due to limited HIV-1 replication in the CNS-based cells, the CSF is considered to be the most reliable surrogate for viral sampling and studying viral dynamics, although one has to consider the fact that the virus present in the CSF also originates both from the infected cells in the CNS and from peripheries. In the past several efforts have been made to determine the origin of the CSF viral pool. Several laboratories have used heteroduplex tracking assay, a technique that involves the amplification of the target exon through PCR followed by hybridization with PCR-amplifiable synthetic DNA (Wood et al., 1993). This method could reliably differentiate closely related genetic variants within a complex viral population as well as viral dynamics. The application of heteroduplex tracking assay methodologies to study HIV-1 dynamics in the CSF has suggested that short-lived CD4+ T cells trafficking between the CNS and peripheral compartments maintain HIV-1 in the CSF (Harrington et al., 2005). Other important findings of this study were that during antiretroviral therapy the virus present in the CSF declined rapidly, with an estimated half-life of 1 to 3 days. An issue with brain tissues/CSF isolates has been the nature of coreceptor usage. So far most of the brain isolates appear to be macrophage tropic in nature (He et al., 1997a). Very few studies have touched this important issue of viral dynamics in the brain, although a very elaborate study suggested that macrophage tropism, irrespective of coreceptor usage, defines HIV-1 neurotropism (Gorry et al., 2001). Viral dynamics and cellular trafficking into the brain of HIV-1-infected individuals are important issues that need to be dissected carefully in the future in order to understand the neuroprotective nature of currently available antiretrovirals as well as to facilitate future therapeutics design. The availability of complementary sophisticated technologies has made possible the isolation and study of viral dynamics at the level of individual cell type. The study of each cellular element has important implications in HAD, as limited HIV-1 infection/replication has been reported in various CNS cell types. Particularly, restricted replications in astrocytes are quite intriguing (Fang et al., 2005). Using laser capture microdissection, subtractive hybridization, and Affymetrix GeneChip analyses, the David Volsky group reported that HIV-1 infection modulates overall gene expression in astrocytes (Wang et al., 2004). Changes in the expression of various genes might provide an environment conducive to viral persistence in the brain. Technological strategies used in this study will provide a paradigm to isolate HIV-1 from individual cell types and its characterization. Along the same lines, phylodynamics (a statistical procedure that combines epidemiological and evolutionary behavior of viral pathogens with the immune system) analyses of HIV-1 env DNA sequences from different brain compartments showed significant interchange of env among different brain compartments, suggesting the potential of viral transfer and replication in various regions of this specialized area of the immune system (Salemi et al., 2005).

Viral genome dynamics also play an important role in immune evasion as well as emergence of drug-resistant quasispecies. There is a wealth of literature on the development of antiretroviral resistance mutations among people on HAART regimen. Clinical studies have extensively proven the relationship between viral genome mutations, particularly in HIV-1 protease and RT (Kiessling et al., 2005). Sophisticated genomic technologies have been a major tool in an attempt to overcome antiretroviral-drug resistance issues. Very few studies have addressed the issue of HAART and the development of drug resistance mutations in brain. It is essential to fully understand drug resistance mutation patterns in the brain for successful viral eradication protocols. In a study comparing HIV-1 protease and RT gene derived from different regions of the brain, sequence analyses revealed independent evolution of drug resistance mutations in various regions of the CNS (Smit et al., 2004). Since it is possible that brain resident virus could be involved in the emergence of drug-resistant viruses among people failing on HAART, a well-designed study for the determination of the viral genome dynamics in various regions of the brain will be essential for the development of effective therapeutics.

Although significant data are emerging regarding viral dynamics and evolution in the brain, this particular aspect of HIV-1 is still controversial and actively being pursued. The availability of well-characterized brain tissues from the National NeuroAIDS Tissue Consortium and the availability of animal models as described above (Ryzhova et al., 2002) will assist in resolving the controversies associated with viral evolution in the brain and its relationship to drug-resistant variants.

NEUROPROTECTIVE STRATEGIES FOR HAD

Although there have been considerable efforts on the development of an effective pharmacotherapy for HAD, a cure for this disease has eluded scientists so far. However, concerted efforts have been made to develop ways to augment antiretroviral therapy to provide neuroprotection against HAD. Among the approaches in use today are neuroprotection via caspase inhibitors, NMDA receptor blockers, poly(ADP-ribose) polymerase inhibitors, antioxidants, cytokines, chemokine receptor antagonists, and p38 mitogen-activated protein kinase inhibitors.

Recently, Corasaniti et al. reported that the caspase-1 inhibitor acetyl-Tyr-Val-Ala-Asp-2,6-dimethylbenzoyloxy-methylketone inhibits gp-120-induced cytosolic cytochrome c elevation in the neocortex of rat brain (Corasaniti et al., 2005). The same group had reported earlier that another caspase-1 inhibitor, Ac-Tyr-Val-Ala-Asp-chloromethyl-ketone minimized neuronal cell loss in the neocortex of rats (Corasaniti et al., 2003). This study also showed that the endogenous antagonist of IL-1 receptor type 1 (IL-1ra), an inhibitor of IL-1β, protected rat neuronal cells from apoptosis. Since caspases are involved in apoptotic cell death and have also been implicated in HIV-related neuronal damage (Deshpande et al., 2005), administration of therapeutic concentration to HIV-1-infected individuals may be helpful in minimizing neuronal loss in those individuals. However, the use of caspase inhibitors to control HAD may not be available for the foreseeable future, since formulations that can cross the BBB and can also be used in humans have not been developed.

Glycogen synthase kinase-3 beta (GSK-3β) is a serine-threonine kinase that participates in the regulation of many fundamental cellular processes including Wnt signaling during development and carbohydrate metabolism in the cell (Hoeflich et al., 2000). GSK-3β participates in apoptosis in several cell types, and increased GSK-3β activity promotes apoptosis via activation of the mitochondrial cell death pathway (Bijur et al., 2000). It has also been reported that the inhibition of GSK-3β is one of the mechanisms by which phosphatidylinositol 3-kinase activation protects neurons from apoptosis (Hetman et al., 2002). A report also suggests that HIV-1 Tat and platelet-activating factor induce the activity of GSK-3β to pathologic levels in neurons (Maggirwar et al., 1999). The same study also revealed that the end point of GSK-3β activation, after exposure to HIV-1 Tat and platelet-activating factor, was neuronal apoptosis (Maggirwar et al., 1999). Thus, the administration of GSK-3β inhibitors to individuals with HAD could be a valuable part of the therapeutic regimen for HAD. Drugs that can inhibit GSK-3β activity are attractive candidates for inhibiting neuronal apoptosis and could be proposed as adjunctive therapy with HAART. An anticonvulsant agent, sodium valporate, has been previously reported to protect neurons from HIV-1 envelope protein neurotoxicities by inhibiting GSK-3β enzymatic activity and tau protein phosphorylation (Dou et al., 2003). Of particular importance is a study suggesting the potential of valporate in eradicating HIV-1 reservoirs, particularly in resting CD4 T cells in vivo. In this eradication protocol, valproic acid was administered with HAART to four volunteers previously on HAART with undetectable viremia. After 4 months of treatment with this modality an average of 75% drop in infected resting CD4 cells was observed in three patients (Lehrman et al., 2005).

It has been shown that NMDA receptor antagonists can protect neurons against apoptosis induced by HIV/gp120 or infected macrophages (Kaul et al., 2001). The NMDA receptor is a Ca^{2+}-permeable, ligand-gated ion channel in neurons and a member of the ionotropic glutamate receptor family (Mukhtar et al., 2005). Overstimulation of NMDA receptor results in the influx of excessive intracellular Ca^{2+}, production of nitric oxide, and eventually the development of neurodegenerative disorders including HAD (Mukhtar et al., 2005). The open-channel blocker memantine inhibits NMDA receptor activity while preserving physiological activity (Lipton, 1992). It seems likely therefore that the inclusion of NMDA receptor activity inhibitors in future therapeutic strategies for HAD will impact the lives of individuals with this HIV-1 neurodegenerative disorder.

Furthermore, since the production of neurotoxic and proapoptotic mediators in HAD is also associated with increased influx of activated macrophages/microglia into the brain, drugs having inhibitory effects on enhanced transmigration of infected cells could have a great potential in controlling virus-mediated neurodegeneration. Certain anti-inflammatory and antimicrobial agents might be potentially beneficial for HAD. This proof of concept has been verified in an SIV model of HAD in which an antibiotic (minocycline) was shown to reduce encephalitis and neuroinflammatory markers associated with viral infection (Zink et al., 2005). There are several other antimicrobial agents that could be explored for their neuroprotective effects.

The beneficial effect of HAART is longevity of HIV-1-infected individuals; however, an increase in plasma lipids, the side effect of administration of protease inhibitor (a constituent of HAART therapy), still persists (Grover et al., 2005). In the past, lipid-lowering drugs, the statins, have been widely used to overcome protease inhibitor side effects among HIV-1-infected individuals (Grinspoon, 2005). Recent controversial reports have further expanded the potential usage of statins in controlling HIV-1 replication (del Real et al., 2004; Giguere and Tremblay, 2004; Gilbert et al., 2005; Moncunill et al., 2005; Waters et al., 2005) in addition to their lipid-lowering effects. According to one of these reports, lovastatin, a member of the statin family of 3-hydroxy-3-methyl-glutaryl-coenzyme A reductase inhibitors, potently inhibited viral replication in vitro and in vivo in a small group of chronically HIV-1-infected individuals (del Real et al., 2004). In addition, we have discovered that pretreatment of HIV-1-infected monocytes and T cells with another statin, atorvastatin, potently inhibited HIV-1-induced enhanced transmigration through an in vitro BBB model (Mukhtar et al., 2003), as well as infection-associated oxidative stress (Acheampong et al., 2003). Such effects may arise from inhibition of cholesterol biosynthesis or through cholesterol-independent actions (known as "pleiotropic" effects) (Calabro and Yeh, 2005). Because there are now a wide variety of clinically available statins with different physicochemical and pharmacokinetic characteristics, it will be prudent to compare HIV-1-associated beneficial effects of statins.

Statins are widely used to control coronary artery disorders; however, a growing body of evidence suggests additional clinical benefits of statins, particularly neuroprotective effects (Delanty et al., 2001). Several studies have shown the beneficial effects of statins in cerebral ischemia and stroke (Vaughan and Delanty, 1999; Yrjanheikki et al., 2005). The molecular mechanism involved in statin-associated neuroprotection in an ischemic model has been recently dissected and involves up-regulation in the expression of tissue plasminogen activator and endothelial nitric oxide synthase (Asahi et al., 2005). Of particular interest relevant to HAD are neuroprotective effects of statins against glutamate-induced excitotoxicity in vitro (Bosel et al., 2005) and increased Akt phosphorylation in vivo that may have inhibitory effects on apoptosis (Kretz et al., 2005). As neuronal demise in HAD individuals precedes apoptotic cascades and excitotoxicities (Mukhtar et al., 2005), the identification of drugs such as statins that have the potential of inhibiting cytotoxic cascades in brain compartments becomes very important. An advantage with these drugs is their safety profile, although a few studies have documented neurotoxicities associated with statins (Gazarin et al., 2002; Baker and Tarnopolsky, 2005). Currently, there are several statins on the market, and comparative clinical studies will help to identify a statin that could be used by HIV-1-infected individuals for controlling lipodystrophies as well as neurotoxicities.

FUTURE CHALLENGES

HAART has significantly controlled the incidence of HAD by reducing the levels of systemic viral replication; however, it has exposed people infected with HIV to a new form of neurological disorder described as milder cognitive and motor disorders (Gonzalez-Scarano and Martin-Garcia, 2005). It is also being feared that HAART-associated survival will increase the number of individuals with true symptoms of Alzheimer's disease, an important issue to be considered for future health care planners (Alisky, 2007). Along similar lines, the issue of immune reconstitution inflammatory syndrome, which further deteriorates neurological functions of HIV-1-infected individuals on HAART, is also of concern (Patel et al., 2006; Riedel et al., 2006).

Several other challenges encountered with the use of HAART in controlling neurological disorders are the side effects associated with the current therapeutic regimen, such as adverse drug reactions associated with normal aging (e.g., metabolic changes, kidney functions, and drug penetration) in elderly populations. HAART itself is associated with metabolic abnormalities and could initiate/accelerate other systemic dysfunctions.

The era of HAART now allows both clearer investigations of classical questions in human retrovirology and the generation of new clinical problems (Pomerantz and Horn, 2003). Mechanisms of (i) viral latency and (ii) hidden or "cryptic" viral replication can also now be addressed without the "noise" of active virally producing cells and high levels of cell-free virions, as virally suppressive HAART "unveils" viral persistence. Furthermore, approaches toward possible viral eradication or at least the long-term remission can be rationally studied. Nevertheless, it is critical to note that true viral eradication may be extremely difficult due to the presence of viral infections in sanctuary sites such as the brain (Canto-Nogues et al., 2005).

CONCLUSIONS

Several studies in the past and long-term experience with HAART suggest that the HIV-1-associated severe neurological disorder, HAD, has been significantly reduced in countries where the health care infrastructure could afford this costly treatment. Challenges associated with HAART treatment are the increase in HIV-1-infected aging populations, antiretroviral cytotoxicities, viral compartmentalization, and minor cognitive motor disorder encountered by people on HAART. These will be an active area of investigation dedicated to realizing the long-awaited dream of finding a cure for this viral pandemic. Modern technologies are providing us with a better understanding of HAD as well as its persistence in the era of HAART. In addition to several others, the efforts of the United Nations Programme on HIV/AIDS (UNAIDS) are highly commendable for providing resources to poor countries where viral infection is rampant.

We thank Rita Victor and Brenda Gordon for excellent secretarial assistance. This work was supported mainly by a Pfizer Atorvastatin Research Award (ARA) and in part by U.S. Public Health Service grants MH074375-01A1 to M.M. and MH074359 to Z.P. M.M. also acknowledges support from the Higher Education Commission of Pakistan.

REFERENCES

Acheampong, E., Z. Parveen, A. Mengistu, N. Ngoubilly, X. D. Cheng, R. J. Pomerantz, and M. Mukhtar. 2003. Statins control HIV-1 and ethanol-induced oxidative stress in human post-mitotic neurons. *Free Radic. Biol. Med.* **35**:499.

Acheampong, E. A., Z. Parveen, L. W. Muthoga, M. Kalayeh, M. Mukhtar, and R. J. Pomerantz. 2005. Human immunodeficiency virus type 1 Nef potently induces apoptosis in primary human brain microvascular endothelial cells via the activation of caspases. *J. Virol.* **79**:4257–4269.

Adamson, D. C., T. M. Dawson, M. C. Zink, J. E. Clements, and V. L. Dawson. 1996. Neurovirulent simian immunodeficiency virus infection induces neuronal, endothelial, and glial apoptosis. *Mol. Med.* **2**:417–428.

Adle-Biassette, H., Y. Levy, M. Colombel, F. Poron, S. Natchev, C. Keohane, and F. Gray. 1995. Neuronal apoptosis in HIV infection in adults. *Neuropathol. Appl. Neurobiol.* **21**:218–227.

Alderson, M. R., T. W. Tough, T. Davis-Smith, S. Braddy, B. Falk, K. A. Schooley, R. G. Goodwin, C. A. Smith, F. Ramsdell, and D. H. Lynch. 1995. Fas ligand mediates activation-induced cell death in human T lymphocytes. *J. Exp. Med.* **181**:71–77.

Alisky, J. M. 2007. The coming problem of HIV-associated Alzheimer's disease. *Med. Hypotheses* **69**:1140–1143.

Andreau, K., J. L. Perfettini, M. Castedo, D. Metivier, V. Scott, G. Pierron, and G. Kroemer. 2004. Contagious apoptosis facilitated by the HIV-1 envelope: fusion-induced cell-to-cell transmission of a lethal signal. *J. Cell Sci.* **117**:5643–5653.

Anthony, I. C., S. N. Ramage, F. W. Carnie, P. Simmonds, and J. E. Bell. 2005. Influence of HAART on HIV-related CNS disease and neuroinflammation. *J. Neuropathol. Exp. Neurol.* **64**:529–536.

Argyris, E. G., E. Acheampong, G. Nunnari, M. Mukhtar, K. J. Williams, and R. J. Pomerantz. 2003. Human immunodeficiency virus type 1 enters primary human brain microvascular endothelial cells by a mechanism involving cell surface proteoglycans independent of lipid rafts. *J. Virol.* **77**:12140–12151.

Asahi, M., Z. Huang, S. Thomas, S. Yoshimura, T. Sumii, T. Mori, J. Qiu, S. Amin-Hanjani, P. L. Huang, J. K. Lia, E. H. Lo, and M. A. Moskowitz. 2005. Protective effects of statins involving both eNOS and tPA in focal cerebral ischemia. *J. Cereb. Blood Flow Metab.* **25**:722–729.

Aweeka, F., A. Jayewardene, S. Staprans, S. E. Bellibas, B. Kearney, P. Lizak, T. Novakovic-Agopian, and R. W. Price. 1999. Failure to detect nelfinavir in the cerebrospinal fluid of HIV-1-infected patients with and without AIDS dementia complex. *J. Acquir. Immune Defic. Syndr. Hum. Retrovirol.* **20**:39–43.

Baeuerle, M., M. Schmitt-Haendle, A. Taubald, S. Mueller, H. Walter, C. Pfeiffer, B. Manger, and T. Harrer. 2005.

Severe HIV-1 encephalitis and development of cerebral non-Hodgkin lymphoma in a patient with persistent strong HIV-1 replication in the brain despite potent HAART-case report and review of the literature. *Eur. J. Med. Res.* **10**:309–316.

Bagasra, O., E. Lavi, L. Bobroski, K. Khalili, J. P. Pestaner, and R. J. Pomerantz. 1996. Cellular reservoirs of HIV-1 in the central nervous system of infected individuals: identification by the combination of in situ polymerase chain reaction and immunohistochemistry. *AIDS* **10**:573–585.

Bagetta, G., M. T. Corasaniti, W. Malorni, G. Rainaldi, L. Berliocchi, A. Finazzi-Agro, and G. Nistico. 1996. The HIV-1 gp120 causes ultrastructural changes typical of apoptosis in the rat cerebral cortex. *Neuroreport* **7**:1722–1724.

Baker, S. K., and M. A. Tarnopolsky. 2005. Statin-associated neuromyotoxicity. *Drugs Today* **41**:267–293.

Ball, J. K., E. C. Holmes, H. Whitwell, and U. Desselberger. 1994. Genomic variation of human immunodeficiency virus type 1 (HIV-1): molecular analyses of HIV-1 in sequential blood samples and various organs obtained at autopsy. *J. Gen. Virol.* **75**(Pt. 4):67–79.

Bandaru, V. V., J. C. McArthur, N. Sacktor, R. G. Cutler, E. L. Knapp, M. P. Mattson, and N. J. Haughey. 2007. Associative and predictive biomarkers of dementia in HIV-1-infected patients. *Neurology* **68**:1481–1487.

Barak, O., I. Goshen, T. Ben-Hur, J. Weidenfeld, A. N. Taylor, and R. Yirmiya. 2002. Involvement of brain cytokines in the neurobehavioral disturbances induced by HIV-1 glycoprotein120. *Brain Res.* **933**:98–108.

Bautista, A. P. 2001. Free radicals, chemokines, and cell injury in HIV-1 and SIV infections and alcoholic hepatitis. *Free Radic. Biol. Med.* **31**:1527–1532.

Bell, J. E. 2004. An update on the neuropathology of HIV in the HAART era. *Histopathology* **45**:549–559.

Bell, J. E., A. Busuttil, J. W. Ironside, S. Rebus, Y. K. Donaldson, P. Simmonds, and J. F. Peutherer. 1993. Human immunodeficiency virus and the brain: investigation of virus load and neuropathologic changes in pre-AIDS subjects. *J. Infect. Dis.* **168**:818–824.

Bijur, G. N., P. De Sarno, and R. S. Jope. 2000. Glycogen synthase kinase-3beta facilitates staurosporine- and heat shock-induced apoptosis. Protection by lithium. *J. Biol. Chem.* **275**:7583–7590.

Blanchard, P. 2004. Update on peripheral neuropathy in HIV-infection. *HIV Treat. Bull.* **5**(3): http://www.i-base.info/pub/htb/v5/htb5-3/Update.html.

Bosel, J., F. Gandor, C. Harms, M. Synowitz, U. Harms, P. C. Djoufack, D. Megow, U. Dirnagl, H. Hortnagl, K. B. Fink, and M. Endres. 2005. Neuroprotective effects of atorvastatin against glutamate-induced excitotoxicity in primary cortical neurones. *J. Neurochem.* **92**:1386–1398.

Bratanich, A. C., C. Liu, J. C. McArthur, T. Fudyk, J. D. Glass, S. Mittoo, G. A. Klassen, and C. Power. 1998. Brain-derived HIV-1 tat sequences from AIDS patients with dementia show increased molecular heterogeneity. *J. Neurovirol.* **4**:387–393.

Brew, B. J., L. Pemberton, P. Cunningham, and M. G. Law. 1997. Levels of human immunodeficiency virus type 1 RNA in cerebrospinal fluid correlate with AIDS dementia stage. *J. Infect. Dis.* **175**:963–966.

Brinley, F. J., Jr., C. A. Pardo, and A. Verma. 2001. Human immunodeficiency virus and the peripheral nervous system workshop. *Arch. Neurol.* **58**:1561–1566.

Burkala, E. J., J. He, J. T. West, C. Wood, and C. K. Petito. 2005. Compartmentalization of HIV-1 in the central nervous system: role of the choroid plexus. *AIDS* **19**:675–684.

Calabro, P., and E. T. Yeh. 2005. The pleiotropic effects of statins. *Curr. Opin. Cardiol.* **20**:541–546.

Canto-Nogues, C., S. Sanchez-Ramon, S. Alvarez, C. Lacruz, and M. A. Munoz-Fernandez. 2005. HIV-1 infection of neurons might account for progressive HIV-1-associated encephalopathy in children. *J. Mol. Neurosci.* **27:**79–89.

Casanova-Sotolongo, P., P. Casanova-Carrillo, and C. Casanova-Carrillo. 2003. Diseases of the peripheral and visual nervous system during infection with human immunodeficiency virus. *Rev. Neurol.* **37:**481–485. (In French.)

Cavert, W., D. W. Notermans, K. Staskus, S. W. Wietgrefe, M. Zupancic, K. Gebhard, K. Henry, Z. Q. Zhang, R. Mills, H. McDade, C. M. Schuwirth, J. Goudsmit, S. A. Danner, and A. T. Haase. 1997. Kinetics of response in lymphoid tissues to antiretroviral therapy of HIV-1 infection. *Science* **276:**960–964.

Childs, E. A., R. H. Lyles, O. A. Selnes, B. Chen, E. N. Miller, B. A. Cohen, J. T. Becker, J. Mellors, and J. C. McArthur. 1999. Plasma viral load and CD4 lymphocytes predict HIV-associated dementia and sensory neuropathy. *Neurology* **52:**607–613.

Chun, T. W., L. Carruth, D. Finzi, X. Shen, J. A. DiGiuseppe, H. Taylor, M. Hermankova, K. Chadwick, J. Margolick, T. C. Quinn, Y. H. Kuo, R. Brookmeyer, M. A. Zeiger, P. Barditch-Crovo, and R. F. Siliciano. 1997a. Quantification of latent tissue reservoirs and total body viral load in HIV-1 infection. *Nature* **387:**183–188.

Chun, T. W., L. Stuyver, S. B. Mizell, L. A. Ehler, J. A. Mican, M. Baseler, A. L. Lloyd, M. A. Nowak, and A. S. Fauci. 1997b. Presence of an inducible HIV-1 latent reservoir during highly active antiretroviral therapy. *Proc. Natl. Acad. Sci. USA* **94:**13193–13197.

Clayton, A., and T. Mughal. 2004. The changing face of HIV-associated lymphoma: what can we learn about optimal therapy inl the post highly active antiretroviral therapy era? *Hematol. Oncol.* **22:**111–120.

Corasaniti, M. T., C. Bellizzi, R. Russo, C. Colica, D. Amantea, and G. Di Renzo. 2003. Caspase-1 inhibitors abolish deleterious enhancement of COX-2 expression induced by HIV-1 gp120 in human neuroblastoma cells. *Toxicol. Lett.* **139:**213–219.

Corasaniti, M. T., D. Amante, R. Russo, S. Piccirilli, A. Leta, M. Corazzari, G. Nappi, and G. Bagetta. 2005. 17beta-Estradiol reduces neuronal apoptosis induced by HIV-1 gp120 in the neocortex of rat. *Neurotoxicology* **26:**893–903.

Corboy, J. R., J. M. Buzy, M. C. Zink, and J. E. Clements. 1992. Expression directed from HIV long terminal repeats in the central nervous system of transgenic mice. *Science* **258:**1804–1808.

Coyle, J. T., and P. Puttfarcken. 1993. Oxidative stress, glutamate, and neurodegenerative disorders. *Science* **262:**689–695.

Daniel, V., C. Susal, A. Melk, R. Weimer, M. Kropelin, R. Zimmermann, A. Huth-Kuhne, C. Uhle, and G. Opelz. 1999. Reduction of viral load and immune complex load on CD4+ lymphocytes as a consequence of highly active antiretroviral treatment (HAART) in HIV-infected hemophilia patients. *Immunol. Lett.* **69:**283–289.

Davies, J., I. P. Everall, S. Weich, J. McLaughlin, F. Scaravilli, and P. L. Lantos. 1997. HIV-associated brain pathology in the United Kingdom: an epidemiological study. *AIDS* **11:**1145–1150.

Delanty, N., C. J. Vaughan, and N. Sheehy. 2001. Statins and neuroprotection. *Expert Opin. Investig. Drugs* **10:**1847–1853.

del Real, G., S. Jimenez-Baranda, E. Mira, R. A. Lacalle, P. Lucas, C. Gomez-Mouton, M. Alegret, J. M. Pena, M. Rodriguez-Zapata, M. Alvarez-Mon, A. C. Martinez, and S. Manes. 2004. Statins inhibit HIV-1 infection by down-regulating Rho activity. *J. Exp. Med.* **200:**541–547.

Del Valle, L., and S. Pina-Oviedo. 2006. HIV disorders of the brain; pathology and pathogenesis. *Front. Biosci.* **11:**718–732.

Deshpande, M., J. Zheng, K. Borgmann, R. Persidsky, L. Wu, C. Schellpeper, and A. Ghorpade. 2005. Role of

activated astrocytes in neuronal damage: potential links to HIV-1-associated dementia. *Neurotox. Res.* **7:**183–192.

Diesing, T. S., S. Swindells, H. Gelbard, and H. E. Gendelman. 2002. HIV-1-associated dementia: a basic science and clinical perspective. *AIDS Read.* **12:**358–368.

Dou, H., K. Birusingh, J. Faraci, S. Gorantla, L. Y. Poluektova, S. B. Maggirwar, S. Dewhurst, H. A. Gelbard, and H. E. Gendelman. 2003. Neuroprotective activities of sodium valproate in a murine model of human immunodeficiency virus-1 encephalitis. *J. Neurosci.* **23:**9162–9170.

Dougherty, R. H., and J. McArthur. 2002. Progression of HIV-associated dementia treated with highly active antiretroviral therapy, abstr. P06.035. *Neurology* **58:**A441.

Edinger, A. L., J. L. Mankowski, B. J. Doranz, B. J. Margulies, B. Lee, J. Rucker, M. Sharron, T. L. Hoffman, J. F. Berson, M. C. Zink, V. M. Hirsch, J. E. Clements, and R. W. Doms. 1997. CD4-independent, CCR5-dependent infection of brain capillary endothelial cells by a neurovirulent simian immunodeficiency virus strain. *Proc. Natl. Acad. Sci. USA* **94:**14742–14747.

Eggers, C., K. Hertogs, H. J. Sturenburg, J. van Lunzen, and H. J. Stellbrink. 2003. Delayed central nervous system virus suppression during highly active antiretroviral therapy is associated with HIV encephalopathy, but not with viral drug resistance or poor central nervous system drug penetration. *AIDS* **17:**1897–1906.

Ellis, R., K. Robertson, L. Moo, D. Clifford, Y. Yang, C. Yiannoutsos, and S. Evans. 2004. NARC007: clinical validation of the ACTG NeuroScreen, abstr. no. 493. *11th Conf. Retrovir. Opportun. Infect.*

Ellis, R. J., A. C. Gamst, E. Capparelli, S. A. Spector, K. Hsia, T. Wolfson, I. Abramson, I. Grant, and J. A. McCutchan. 2000. Cerebrospinal fluid HIV RNA originates from both local CNS and systemic sources. *Neurology* **54:**927–936.

Ellis, R. J., K. Hsia, S. A. Spector, J. A. Nelson, R. K. Heaton, M. R. Wallace, I. Abramson, J. H. Atkinson, I. Grant, J. A. McCutchan, et al. 1997. Cerebrospinal fluid human immunodeficiency virus type 1 RNA levels are elevated in neurocognitively impaired individuals with acquired immunodeficiency syndrome. *Ann. Neurol.* **42:**679–688.

Evers, S., A. Rahmann, S. Schwaag, A. Frese, D. Reichelt, and I. W. Husstedt. 2004. Prevention of AIDS dementia by HAART does not depend on cerebrospinal fluid drug penetrance. *AIDS Res. Hum. Retrovir.* **20:**483–491.

Fang, J., E. Acheampong, R. Dave, F. Wang, M. Mukhtar, and R. J. Pomerantz. 2005. The RNA helicase DDX1 is involved in restricted HIV-1 Rev function in human astrocytes. *Virology* **336:**299–307.

Finzi, D., M. Hermankova, T. Pierson, L. M. Carruth, C. Buck, R. E. Chaisson, T. C. Quinn, K. Chadwick, J. Margolick, R. Brookmeyer, J. Gallant, M. Markowitz, D. Ho, D. D. Richman, and R. F. Siliciano. 1997. Identification of a reservoir for HIV-1 in patients on highly active antiretroviral therapy. *Science* **278:**1295–1300.

Fischer-Smith, T., S. Croul, A. E. Sverstiuk, C. Capini, D. L'Heureux, E. G. Regulier, M. W. Richardson, S. Amini, S. Morgello, K. Khalili, and J. Rappaport. 2001. CNS invasion by CD14+/CD16+ peripheral blood-derived monocytes in HIV dementia: perivascular accumulation and reservoir of HIV infection. *J. Neurovirol.* **7:**528–541.

Freed, E. O. 2004. HIV-1 and the host cell: an intimate association. *Trends Microbiol.* **12:**170–177.

Garden, G. A. 2002. Microglia in human immunodeficiency virus-associated neurodegeneration. *Glia* **40:**240–251.

Gazarin, S., H. Abd-El-Hady, O. Gheith, M. Rasem, M. Saad, K. El-Sayed, M. Sobh, and G. Amer. 2002. Neuromuscular toxicity in nephrotic patients treated with fluvastatin. *J. Nephrol.* **15:**690–695.

Giguere, J. F., and M. J. Tremblay. 2004. Statin compounds reduce human immunodeficiency virus type 1 replication by preventing the interaction between virion-associated host intercellular adhesion molecule 1 and its natural cell surface ligand LFA-1. *J. Virol.* **78:**12062–12065.

Gilbert, C., M. Bergeron, S. Methot, J. F. Giguere, and M. J. Tremblay. 2005. Statins could be used to control replication of some viruses, including HIV-1. *Viral Immunol.* **18:**474–489.

Glass, J. D., H. Fedor, S. L. Wesselingh, and J. C. McArthur. 1995. Immunocytochemical quantitation of human immunodeficiency virus in the brain: correlations with dementia. *Ann. Neurol.* **38:**755–762.

Gonzalez-Scarano, F., and J. Martin-Garcia. 2005. The neuropathogenesis of AIDS. *Nat. Rev. Immunol.* **5:**69–81.

Gorry, P. R., G. Bristol, J. A. Zack, K. Ritola, R. Swanstrom, C. J. Birch, J. E. Bell, N. Bannert, K. Crawford, H. Wang, D. Schols, E. De Clercq, K. Kunstman, S. M. Wolinsky, and D. Gabuzda. 2001. Macrophage tropism of human immunodeficiency virus type 1 isolates from brain and lymphoid tissues predicts neurotropism independent of coreceptor specificity. *J. Virol.* **75:**10073–10089.

Gosztonyi, G., J. Artigas, L. Lamperth, and H. D. Webster. 1994. Human immunodeficiency virus (HIV) distribution in HIV encephalitis: study of 19 cases with combined use of in situ hybridization and immunocytochemistry. *J. Neuropathol. Exp. Neurol.* **53:**521–534.

Gray, F., H. Adle-Biassette, F. Chretien, G. Lorin de la Grandmaison, G. Force, and C. Keohane. 2001. Neuropathology and neurodegeneration in human immunodeficiency virus infection. Pathogenesis of HIV-induced lesions of the brain, correlations with HIV-associated disorders and modifications according to treatments. *Clin. Neuropathol.* **20:**146–155.

Gray, F., F. Chretien, A. V. Vallat-Decouvelaere, and F. Scaravilli. 2003. The changing pattern of HIV neuropathology in the HAART era. *J. Neuropathol. Exp. Neurol.* **62:**429–440.

Green, D. A., E. Masliah, H. V. Vinters, P. Beizai, D. J. Moore, and C. L. Achim. 2005. Brain deposition of beta-amyloid is a common pathologic feature in HIV positive patients. *AIDS* **19:**407–411.

Grinspoon, S. K. 2005. Metabolic syndrome and cardiovascular disease in patients with human immunodeficiency virus. *Am. J. Med.* **118**(Suppl. 2):S23–S28.

Grover, S. A., L. Coupal, N. Gilmore, and J. Mukherjee. 2005. Impact of dyslipidemia associated with Highly Active Antiretroviral Therapy (HAART) on cardiovascular risk and life expectancy. *Am. J. Cardiol.* **95:**586–591.

Harouse, J. M., C. Kunsch, H. T. Hartle, M. A. Laughlin, J. A. Hoxie, B. Wigdahl, and F. Gonzalez-Scarano. 1989. CD4-independent infection of human neural cells by human immunodeficiency virus type 1. *J. Virol.* **63:**2527–2533.

Harrington, P. R, D. W. Haas, K. Ritola, and R. Swanstrom. 2005. Compartmentalized human immunodeficiency virus type 1 present in cerebrospinal fluid is produced by short-lived cells. *J. Virol.* **79:**7959–7966.

He, J., Y. Chen, M. Farzan, H. Choe, A. Ohagen, S. Gartner, J. Busciglio, X. Yang, W. Hofmann, W. Newman, C. R. Mackay, J. Sodroski, and D. Gabuzda. 1997a. CCR3 and CCR5 are co-receptors for HIV-1 infection of microglia. *Nature* **385:**645–649.

He, J., C. M. deCastro, G. R. Vandenbark, J. Busciglio, and D. Gabuzda. 1997b. Astrocyte apoptosis induced by HIV-1 transactivation of the c-kit protooncogene. *Proc. Natl. Acad. Sci. USA* **94:**3954–3959.

Herbeuval, J. P., J. C. Grivel, A. Boasso, A. W. Hardy, C. Chougnet, M. J. Dolan, H. Yagita, J. D. Lifson, and G. M. Shearer. 2005. CD4+ T cell death induced by infectious and noninfectious HIV-1: role of type I interferon-dependent, TRAIL/DR5-mediated apoptosis. *Blood* **106:**3524–3531.

Hesselgesser, J., and R. Horuk. 1999. Chemokine and chemokine receptor expression in the central nervous system. *J. Neurovirol.* **5:**13–26.

Hetman, M., S. L. Hsuan, A. Habas, M. J. Higgins, and Z. Xia. 2002. ERK1/2 antagonizes glycogen synthase kinase-3beta-induced apoptosis in cortical neurons. *J. Biol. Chem.* **277:**49577–49584.

Hoeflich, K. P., J. Luo, E. A. Rubie, M. S. Tsao, O. Jin, and J. R. Woodgett. 2000. Requirement for glycogen synthase kinase-3beta in cell survival and NF-kappaB activation. *Nature* **406:**86–90.

Hulgan, T., D. W. Haas, J. L. Haines, M. D. Ritchie, G. K. Robbins, R. W. Shafer, D. B. Clifford, A. R. Kallianpur, M. Summar, and J. A. Canter. 2005. Mitochondrial haplogroups and peripheral neuropathy during antiretroviral therapy: an adult AIDS clinical trials group study. *AIDS* **19:**1341–1349.

Jana, A., and K. Pahan. 2004. Human immunodeficiency virus type 1 gp120 induces apoptosis in human primary neurons through redox-regulated activation of neutral sphingomyelinase. *J. Neurosci.* **24:**9531–9540.

Kaul, M., G. A. Garden, and S. A. Lipton. 2001. Pathways to neuronal injury and apoptosis in HIV-associated dementia. *Nature* **410:**988–994.

Kaul, M., and S. A. Lipton. 2006. Mechanisms of neuronal injury and death in HIV-1 associated dementia. *Curr. HIV Res.* **4:**307–318.

Kaul, M., J. Zheng, S. Okamoto, H. E. Gendelman, and S. A. Lipton. 2005. HIV-1 infection and AIDS: consequences for the central nervous system. *Cell Death Differ.* **12**(Suppl.1):878–892.

Kiessling, A. A., S. J. Eyre, and B. D. Desmarais. 2005. Detection of drug-resistant HIV-1 strains. *Methods Mol. Biol.* **304:**287–313.

Koedel, U., B. Kohleisen, B. Sporer, F. Lahrtz, V. Ovod, A. Fontana, V. Erfle, and H. W. Pfister. 1999. HIV type 1 Nef protein is a viral factor for leukocyte recruitment into the central nervous system. *J. Immunol.* **163:**1237–1245.

Kolson, D. L. 2002. Neuropathogenesis of central nervous system HIV-1 infection. *Clin. Lab. Med.* **22:**703–717.

Kramer-Hammerle, S., I. Rothenaigner, H. Wolff, J. E. Bell, and R. Brack-Werner. 2005. Cells of the central nervous system as targets and reservoirs of the human immunodeficiency virus. *Virus Res.* **111:**194–213.

Kretz, A., C. Schmeer, S. Tausch, and S. Isenmann. 2005. Simvastatin promotes heat shock protein 27 expression and Akt activation in the rat retina and protects axotomized retinal ganglion cells in vivo. *Neurobiol. Dis.* **21:**421–430.

Kruman, I. I., A. Nath, and M. P. Mattson. 1998. HIV-1 protein Tat induces apoptosis of hippocampal neurons by a mechanism involving caspase activation, calcium overload, and oxidative stress. *Exp. Neurol.* **154:**276–288.

Lane, J. H., A. F. Tarantal, D. Pauley, M. Marthas, C. J. Miller, and A. A. Lackner. 1996. Localization of simian immunodeficiency virus nucleic acid and antigen in brains of fetal macaques inoculated in utero. *Am. J. Pathol.* **149:**1097–1104.

Langford, T. D., S. L. Letendre, G. J. Larrea, and E. Masliah. 2003. Changing patterns in the neuropathogenesis of HIV during the HAART era. *Brain Pathol.* **13:**195–210.

Lawrence, D. M., and E. O. Major. 2002. HIV-1 and the brain: connections between HIV-1-associated dementia, neuropathology and neuroimmunology. *Microbes Infect.* **4:**301–308.

Lehrman, G., I. B. Hogue, S. Palmer, C. Jennings, C. A. Spina, A. Wiegand, A. L. Landay, R. W. Coombs, D. D. Richman, J. W. Mellors, J. M. Coffin, R. J. Bosch, and

D. M. Margolis. 2005. Depletion of latent HIV-1 infection in vivo: a proof-of-concept study. *Lancet* **366**:549–555.

Li, X. L., T. Moudgil, H. V. Vinters, and D. D. Ho. 1990. CD4-independent, productive infection of a neuronal cell line by human immunodeficiency virus type 1. *J. Virol.* **64**:1383–1387.

Liao, Z., D. R. Graham, and J. E. Hildreth. 2003. Lipid rafts and HIV pathogenesis: virion-associated cholesterol is required for fusion and infection of susceptible cells. *AIDS Res. Hum. Retrovir.* **19**:675–687.

Lipton, S. A. 1992. Memantine prevents HIV coat protein-induced neuronal injury in vitro. *Neurology* **42**:1403–1405.

Liu, N. Q., A. S. Lossinsky, W. Popik, X. Li, C. Gujuluva, B. Kriederman, J. Roberts, T. Pushkarsky, M. Bukrinsky, M. Witte, M. Weinand, and M. Fiala. 2002. Human immunodeficiency virus type 1 enters brain microvascular endothelia by macropinocytosis dependent on lipid rafts and the mitogen-activated protein kinase signaling pathway. *J. Virol.* **76**:6689–6700.

Maggirwar, S. B., N. Tong, S. Ramirez, H. A. Gelbard, and S. Dewhurst. 1999. HIV-1 Tat-mediated activation of glycogen synthase kinase-3beta contributes to Tat-mediated neurotoxicity. *J. Neurochem.* **73**:578–586.

Marechal, V., M. C. Prevost, C. Petit, E. Perret, J. M. Heard, and O. Schwartz. 2001. Human immunodeficiency virus type 1 entry into macrophages mediated by macropinocytosis. *J. Virol.* **75**:11166–11177.

McArthur, J. C., N. Haughey, S. Gartner, K. Conant, C. Pardo, A. Nath, and N. Sacktor. 2003. Human immunodeficiency virus-associated dementia: an evolving disease. *J. Neurovirol.* **9**:205–221.

Moncunill, G., E. Negredo, L. Bosh, J. Vilarrasa, M. Witvrouw, A. Llano, B. Clotet, and J. A. Este. 2005. Evaluation of the anti-HIV activity of statins. *AIDS* **19**:1697–1700.

Moses, A. V., and J. A. Nelson. 1994. HIV infection of human brain capillary endothelial cells-implications for AIDS dementia. *Adv. Neuroimmunol.* **4**:239–247.

Mukhtar, M. 2005. Evolution of biomarkers: drug discovery to personalized medicine. *Drug Discov. Today* **10**:121–128.

Mukhtar, M., E. Acheampong, Z. Parveen, and R. J. Pomerantz. 2005. T-cells and excitotoxicity—HIV-1 and other neurodegenerative disorders. *Neuromol. Med.* **7**:265–273.

Mukhtar, M., H. Duke, M. BouHamdan, and R. J. Pomerantz. 2000. Anti-human immunodeficiency virus type 1 gene therapy in human central nervous system-based cells: an initial approach against a potential viral reservoir. *Hum. Gene Ther.* **11**:347–359.

Mukhtar, M., S. Harley, P. Chen, M. BouHamdan, C. Patel, E. Acheampong, R. J. Pomerantz. 2002. Primary isolated human brain microvascular endothelial cells express diverse HIV/SIV-associated chemokine coreceptors and DC-SIGN and L-SIGN. *Virology* **297**:78–88.

Mukhtar, M., A. Mengistu, E. Acheampong, J. Sullivan, G. Nunnari, E. G. Argyris, M. Kalayeh, R. J. Pomerantz, and K. J. Williams. 2003. Statins block enhanced expression of matrix metalloproteinases (MMPs) by virally infected monocytes and T-cells and thereby normalize their transvascular transmigration. A novel therapeutic approach to HIV-1 neuroinvasion. *Circulation* **108**:487.

Nath, A., and N. Sacktor. 2006. Influence of highly active antiretroviral therapy on persistence of HIV in the central nervous system. *Curr. Opin. Neurol.* **19**:358–361.

Nguyen, D. H., and D. D. Taub. 2004. Targeting lipids to prevent HIV infection. *Mol. Interv.* **4**:318–320.

Nosheny, R. L., A. Bachis, E. Acquas, and I. Mocchetti. 2004. Human immunodeficiency virus type 1 glycoprotein gp120 reduces the levels of brain-derived neurotrophic factor in vivo: potential implication for neuronal cell death. *Eur. J. Neurosci.* **20**:2857–2864.

Nunn, M. F. 2006. NeuroAIDS: a neuroscience problem with global impact. *Curr. HIV Res.* **4**:245–247.

Nuovo, G. J., F. Gallery, P. MacConnell, and A. Braun. 1994. In situ detection of polymerase chain reaction-amplified HIV-1 nucleic acids and tumor necrosis factor-alpha RNA in the central nervous system. *Am. J. Pathol.* **144**:659–666.

Ozdener, H. 2005. Molecular mechanisms of HIV-1 associated neurodegeneration. *J. Biosci.* **30**:391–405.

Patel, A. K., K. K. Patel, S. D. Shah, and J. Desai. 2006. Immune reconstitution syndrome presenting with cerebral varicella zoster vasculitis in HIV-1-infected patient: a case report. *J. Int. Assoc. Physicians AIDS Care* (Chicago) **5**:157–160.

Patel, C. A., M. Mukhtar, and R. J. Pomerantz. 2000. Human immunodeficiency virus type 1 Vpr induces apoptosis in human neuronal cells. *J. Virol.* **74**:9717–9726.

Patel, C. A., M. Mukhtar, S. Harley, J. Kulkosky, and R. J. Pomerantz. 2002. Lentiviral expression of HIV-1 Vpr induces apoptosis in human neurons. *J. Neurovirol.* **8**:86–99.

Perelson, A. S., P. Essunger, Y. Cao, M. Vesanen, A. Hurley, K. Saksela, M. Markowitz, and D. D. Ho. 1997. Decay characteristics of HIV-1-infected compartments during combination therapy. *Nature* **387**:188–191.

Perelson, A. S., A. U. Neumann, M. Markowitz, J. M. Leonard, and D. D. Ho. 1996. HIV-1 dynamics in vivo: virion clearance rate, infected cell life-span, and viral generation time. *Science* **271**:1582–1586.

Persidsky, Y., J. Limoges, R. McComb, P. Bock, T. Baldwin, W. Tyor, A. Patil, H. S. Nottet, L. Epstein, H. Gelbard, E. Flanagan, J. Reinhard, S. J. Pirruccello, and H. E. Gendelman. 1996. Human immunodeficiency virus encephalitis in SCID mice. *Am. J. Pathol.* **149**:1027–1053.

Pialoux, G., S. Fournier, A. Moulignier, J. D. Poveda, F. Clavel, and B. Dupont. 1997. Central nervous system as a sanctuary for HIV-1 infection despite treatment with zidovudine, lamivudine and indinavir. *AIDS* **11**:1302–1303.

Pomerantz, R. J. 1999. Residual HIV-1 disease in the era of highly active antiretroviral therapy. *N. Engl. J. Med.* **340**:1672–1674.

Pomerantz, R. J. 2001. Residual HIV-1 infection during antiretroviral therapy: the challenge of viral persistence. *AIDS* **15**:1201–1211.

Pomerantz, R. J. 2002. Reservoirs of human immunodeficiency virus type 1: the main obstacles to viral eradication. *Clin. Infect. Dis.* **34**:91–97.

Pomerantz, R. J. 2004. Effects of HIV-1 Vpr on neuroinvasion and neuropathogenesis. *DNA Cell Biol.* **23**:227–238.

Pomerantz, R. J., and D. L. Horn. 2003. Twenty years of therapy for HIV-1 infection. *Nat. Med.* **9**:867–873.

Pozio, E. 2004. Highly Active AntiRetroviral Therapy and opportunistic protozoan infections. *Parassitologia* **46**:89–93. (In Italian.)

Rafalowska, J. 1998. HIV-1-infection in the CNS. A pathogenesis of some neurological syndromes in the light of recent investigations. *Folia Neuropathol.* **36**:211–216.

Ranki, A., M. Nyberg, V. Ovod, M. Haltia, I. Elovaara, R. Raininko, H. Haapasalo, and K. Krohn. 1995. Abundant expression of HIV Nef and Rev proteins in brain astrocytes in vivo is associated with dementia. *AIDS* **9**:1001–1008.

Rappaport, J., J. Joseph, S. Croul, G. Alexander, L. Del Valle, S. Amini, and K. Khalili. 1999. Molecular pathway involved in HIV-1-induced CNS pathology: role of viral regulatory protein, Tat. *J. Leukoc. Biol.* **65**:458–465.

Resnick, L., J. R. Berger, P. Shapshak, and W. W. Tourtellotte. 1988. Early penetration of the blood-brain-barrier by HIV. *Neurology* **38**:9–14.

Riedel, D. J., C. A. Pardo, J. McArthur, and A. Nath. 2006. Therapy insight: CNS manifestations of HIV-associated immune reconstitution inflammatory syndrome. *Nat. Clin. Pract. Neurol.* **2:**557–565.

Ritola, K., K. Robertson, S. A. Fiscus, C. Hall, and R. Swanstrom. 2005. Increased human immunodeficiency virus type 1 (HIV-1) env compartmentalization in the presence of HIV-1-associated dementia. *J. Virol.* **79:**10830–10834.

Roger, P. M., J. P. Breittmayer, C. Arlotto, P. Pugliese, C. Pradier, G. Bernard-Pomier, P. Dellamonica, and A. Bernard. 1999. Highly active anti-retroviral therapy (HAART) is associated with a lower level of CD4+ T cell apoptosis in HIV-infected patients. *Clin. Exp. Immunol.* **118:**412–416.

Ryzhova, E. V., P. Crino, L. Shawver, S. V. Westmoreland, A. A. Lackner, and F. Gonzalez-Scarano. 2002. Simian immunodeficiency virus encephalitis: analysis of envelope sequences from individual brain multinucleated giant cells and tissue samples. *Virology* **297:**57–67.

Sacktor, N. C., R. L. Skolasky, R. H. Lyles, D. Esposito, O. A. Selnes, and J. C. McArthur. 2000. Improvement in HIV-associated motor slowing after antiretroviral therapy including protease inhibitors. *J. Neurovirol.* **6:**84–88.

Saito, Y., L. R. Sharer, L. G. Epstein, J. Michaels, M. Mintz, M. Louder, K. Golding, T. A. Cvetkovich, and B. M. Blumberg. 1994. Overexpression of nef as a marker for restricted HIV-1 infection of astrocytes in postmortem pediatric central nervous tissues. *Neurology* **44:**474–481.

Salemi, M., S. L. Lamers, S. Yu, T. de Oliveira, W. M. Fitch, and M. S. McGrath. 2005. Phylodynamic analysis of human immunodeficiency virus type 1 in distinct brain compartments provides a model for the neuropathogenesis of AIDS. *J. Virol.* **79:**11343–11352.

Shapshak, P., D. M. Segal, K. A. Crandall, R. K. Fujimura, B. T. Zhang, K. Q. Xin, K. Okuda, C. K. Petito, C. Eisdorfer, and K. Goodkin. 1999. Independent evolution of HIV type 1 in different brain regions. *AIDS Res. Hum. Retrovir.* **15:**811–820.

Shi, B., U. De Girolami, J. He, S. Wang, A. Lorenzo, J. Busciglio, and D. Gabuzda. 1996. Apoptosis induced by HIV-1 infection of the central nervous system. *J. Clin. Investig.* **98:**1979–1990.

Shi, B., J. Raina, A. Lorenzo, J. Busciglio, and D. Gabuzda. 1998. Neuronal apoptosis induced by HIV-1 Tat protein and TNF-alpha: potentiation of neurotoxicity mediated by oxidative stress and implications for HIV-1 dementia. *J. Neurovirol.* **4:**281–290.

Siliciano, R. F. 2005. Scientific rationale for antiretroviral therapy in 2005: viral reservoirs and resistance evolution. *Top. HIV Med.* **13:**96–100.

Singh, I. N., R. J. Goody, C. Dean, N. M. Ahmad, S. E. Lutz, P. E. Knapp, A. Nath, and K. F. Hauser. 2004. Apoptotic death of striatal neurons induced by human immunodeficiency virus-1 Tat and gp120: Differential involvement of caspase-3 and endonuclease G. *J. Neurovirol.* **10:**141–151.

Smit, T. K., B. J. Brew, W. Tourtellotte, S. Morgello, B. B. Gelman, and N. K. Saksena. 2004. Independent evolution of human immunodeficiency virus (HIV) drug resistance mutations in diverse areas of the brain in HIV-infected patients, with and without dementia, on antiretroviral treatment. *J. Virol.* **78:**10133–10148.

Solas, C., A. Lafeuillade, P. Halfon, S. Chadapaud, G. Hittinger, and B. Lacarelle. 2003. Discrepancies between protease inhibitor concentrations and viral load in reservoirs and sanctuary sites in human immunodeficiency virus-infected patients. *Antimicrob. Agents Chemother.* **47:**238–243.

Spector, S. A., K. Hsia, D. Pratt, J. Lathey, J. A. McCutchan, J. E. Alcaraz, J. H. Atkinson, S. Gulevich, M. Wallace, I. Grant, et al. 1993. Virologic markers of human immunodeficiency virus type 1 in cerebrospinal fluid. *J. Infect. Dis.* **168:**68–74.

Sperber, K., and L. Shao. 2003. Neurologic consequences of HIV infection in the era of HAART. *AIDS Patient Care STDs* **17:**509–518.

Sporer, B., U. Koedel, R. Paul, B. Kohleisen, V. Erfle, A. Fontana, and H. W. Pfister. 2000. Human immunodeficiency virus type-1 Nef protein induces blood-brain barrier disruption in the rat: role of matrix metalloproteinase-9. *J. Neuroimmunol.* **102:**12–30.

Tashima, K. T., A. M. Caliendo, M. Ahmad, J. M. Gormley, W. D. Fiske, J. M. Brennan, and T. P. Flanigan. 1999. Cerebrospinal fluid human immunodeficiency virus type 1 (HIV-1) suppression and efavirenz drug concentrations in HIV-1-infected patients receiving combination therapy. *J. Infect. Dis.* **180:**862–864.

Thomas, S. A. 2004. Anti-HIV drug distribution to the central nervous system. *Curr. Pharm. Des.* **10:**1313–1324.

Toborek, M., Y. W. Lee, G. Flora, H. Pu, I. E. Andras, E. Wylegala, B. Hennig, and A. Nath. 2005. Mechanisms of the blood-brain barrier disruption in HIV-1 infection. *Cell. Mol. Neurobiol.* **25:**181–199.

Tornatore, C., R. Chandra, J. R. Berger, Jr., and E. O. Major. 1994. HIV-1 infection of subcortical astrocytes in the pediatric central nervous system. *Neurology* **44:**481–487.

Tozzi, V., P. Balestra, S. Galgani, P. Narciso, F. Ferri, G. Sebastiani, C. D'Amato, C. Affricano, F. Pigorini, F. M. Pau, A. De Felici, and A. Benedetto. 1999. Positive and sustained effects of highly active antiretroviral therapy on HIV-1-associated neurocognitive impairment. *AIDS* **13:** 1889–1897.

Tozzi, V., P. Balestra, R. Bellagamba, A. Corpolongo, M. F. Salvatori, U. Visco-Comandini, C. Vlassi, M. Giulianelli, S. Galgani, A. Antinori, and P. Narciso. 2007. Persistence of neuropsychologic deficits despite long-term highly active antiretroviral therapy in patients with HIV-related neurocognitive impairment: prevalence and risk factors. *J. Acquir. Immune Defic. Syndr.* **45:**174–182.

van der Sandt, I. C., C. M. Vos, L. Nabulsi, M. C. Blom-Roosemalen, H. H. Voorwinden, A. G. de Boer, and D. D. Breimer. 2001. Assessment of active transport of HIV protease inhibitors in various cell lines and the in vitro blood-brain barrier. *AIDS* **15:**483–491.

Vaughan, C. J., and N. Delanty. 1999. Neuroprotective properties of statins in cerebral ischemia and stroke. *Stroke* **30:**1969–1973.

von Giesen, H. J., H. Koller, A. Theisen, and G. Arendt. 2002. Therapeutic effects of nonnucleoside reverse transcriptase inhibitors on the central nervous system in HIV-1-infected patients. *J. Acquir. Immune Defic. Syndr.* **29:**363–367.

Wang, Z., G. Trillo-Pazos, S. Y. Kim, M. Canki, S. Morgello, L. R. Sharer, H. A. Gelbard, Z. Z. Su, D. C. Kang, A. I. Brooks, P. B. Fisher, and D. J. Volsky. 2004. Effects of human immunodeficiency virus type 1 on astrocyte gene expression and function: potential role in neuropathogenesis. *J. Neurovirol.* **10**(Suppl. 1)**:**S25–S32.

Waters, L., J. Stebbing, R. Jones, S. Mandalia, M. Bower, M. Stefanovic, M. Nelson, and B. Gazzard. 2005. The effect of statins on HIV rebound and blips. *J. Acquir. Immune Defic. Syndr.* **39:**637–638.

Weissman, D., R. L. Rabin, J. Arthos, A. Rubbert, M. Dybul, R. Swofford, S. Venkatesan, J. M. Farber, and A. S. Fauci. 1997. Macrophage-tropic HIV and SIV envelope proteins induce a signal through the CCR5 chemokine receptor. *Nature* **389:**981–985.

Wood, N., L. Tyfield, and J. Bidwell. 1993. Rapid classification of phenylketonuria genotypes by analysis of heteroduplexes generated by PCR-amplifiable synthetic DNA. *Hum. Mutat.* **2:**131–137.

Yrjanheikki, J., J. Koistinaho, M. Kettunen, R. A. Kauppinen, K. Appel, M. Hull, and B. L. Fiebich. 2005. Long-term protective effect of atorvastatin in permanent focal cerebral ischemia. *Brain Res.* **1052:**174–179.

Yue, F. Y., C. M. Kovacs, R. C. Dimayuga, X. X. Gu, P. Parks, R. Kaul, and M. A. Ostrowski. 2005. Preferential apoptosis of HIV-1-specific CD4+ T cells. *J. Immunol.* **174:**2196–2204.

Zhang, K., F. Rana, C. Silva, J. Ethier, K. Wehrly, B. Chesebro, and C. Power. 2003. Human immunodeficiency virus type 1 envelope-mediated neuronal death: uncoupling of viral replication and neurotoxicity. *J. Virol.* **77:**6899–6912.

Zheng, J., M. R. Thylin, A. Ghorpade, H. Xiong, Y. Persidsky, R. Cotter, D. Niemann, M. Che, Y. C. Zeng, H. A. Gelbard, R. B. Shepard, J. M. Swartz, and H. E. Gendelman. 1999. Intracellular CXCR4 signaling, neuronal apoptosis and neuropathogenic mechanisms of HIV-1-associated dementia. *J. Neuroimmunol.* **98:**185–200.

Zink, M. C., J. Uhrlaub, J. DeWitt, T. Voelker, B. Bullock, J. Mankowski, P. Tarwater, J. Clements, and S. Barber. 2005. Neuroprotective and anti-human immunodeficiency virus activity of minocycline. *JAMA* **293:**2003–2011.

The Spectrum of Neuro-AIDS Disorders:
Pathophysiology, Diagnosis, and Treatment
Edited by K. Goodkin et al.
©2008 ASM Press, Washington, DC

11

Neuroimmunology and the Pathogenesis of HIV-1 Encephalitis in the HAART Era: Implications for Neuroprotective Treatment

SETH W. PERRY AND HARRIS A. GELBARD

HIV DEMENTIA: PREVALENCE AND CHARACTERIZATION

Human immunodeficiency virus (HIV) infection of the central nervous system (CNS) was identified shortly after AIDS was defined as a disease (Epstein et al., 1984). At that time, the virus now known as HIV was called HTLV-III/LAV. The symptomology and pathophysiological correlates resulting from HIV infection of the CNS have been identified by several names, including, in rough chronological order, AIDS encephalopathy, AIDS dementia complex, subacute HIV encephalitis (or just HIV encephalitis), and HIV-associated dementia. In 1991, a revision of the terminology was made by the American Academy of Neurology AIDS Task Force, which developed the term HIV-1-associated cognitive motor complex (HIV-CMC), to encompass both the milder HIV-1-associated minor cognitive motor disorder (HIV-MCMD) and the more severe HIV-1-associated dementia complex (HIV-DC) (American Academy of Neurology AIDS Task Force, 1991). For simplicity, in this work, we refer to the general syndrome of HIV-CMC as simply HIV dementia, or HAD.

HAD is a slowly progressing subcortical dementia with cognitive, motor, and psychiatric symptoms currently affecting between 3 and 20% of AIDS patients (depending on the population and selection criteria used) (Lopez et al., 1999; Berger and Arendt, 2000). With over 39,000,000 AIDS cases worldwide (World Health Organization, 2004) and thousands more infected each day, this represents a significant number of individuals afflicted with HAD.

Although the advent of highly active antiretroviral therapies (HAART) has made great strides in extending life for AIDS patients, this longer life span may present increasing

opportunity for HAD to develop. HAART can reduce viral burden and thus delay the onset of HAD, but it does not prevent HAD. Accordingly, with the advent of HAART, the lifetime incidence of HAD had dropped from 25% (with some estimates up to 50%) to less than 10% (by most estimates) of infected persons (Sacktor et al., 2001), but it has been rising again since 2001 (McArthur, 2004). In addition, the incidence rate for developing HAD or MCMD, a milder form of HAD, has been and remains around 25 to 40%, despite HAART (McArthur, 2004). Moreover, the prevalence—that is, the total number of cases—of HAD may be increasing, due to HAART-extended life spans and the increasing resistance to HAART seen in current AIDS patient populations. Only small fractions of HIV-infected individuals worldwide have access to any drug treatment, let alone current HAART therapies, for their condition. By most accounts, HAD is the most common cause of dementia worldwide in persons aged under 40 years and is in itself a significant independent risk factor for death by AIDS (Ellis et al., 1997). Development of HAD is also increasingly being seen at higher CD4 counts, suggesting increased incidence in otherwise healthier individuals (Sacktor et al., 2001). This may be due to a protected reservoir of HIV in the brain, resulting from the relatively privileged immune status of the brain, and limited penetration of many retroviral drugs across the blood-brain barrier (BBB). Taken together, this evidence indicates that HAD will remain a significant complication of HIV infection with a high rate of morbidity, as well as a significant disease state in and of itself.

Diagnosis of HAD is made by exclusion of opportunistic infections, malignancies, and metabolic and psychiatric disorders, although any or all of these can and often do occur concurrently with HAD (Diesing et al., 2002), thus confounding the diagnosis, complicating the treatment, and usually negatively impacting the outcome. In such cases, definitive diagnosis of HAD is greatly aided by a neuropsychological profile demonstrating specific deficits seen with the syndrome. Clinically, HAD manifests itself with mild

Seth W. Perry and Harris A. Gelbard, Center for Aging and Developmental Biology, Kornberg Medical Research Institute, Departments of Neurology, Pediatrics, Microbiology and Immunology, University of Rochester Medical Center, Rochester, NY 14642.

concentration difficulties, cognitive slowing, and forgetfulness early in the disease. Motor deficits are somewhat less common but can include gait disturbance and impaired hand coordination. Social withdrawal, apathy, mania, and anhedonia are common behavioral changes. These milder initial symptoms progress at variable rates to include delirium (confusion, inability to recognize surroundings, and sometimes hallucinations), frank dementia, muteness, paraparesis, and ultimately, coma and death (Gelbard et al., 1995; Diesing et al., 2002).

HIV-1 encephalitis, the histo- and neuropathological correlate of CNS HIV infection and HAD, occurs in most but not all cases of HAD (Ryan et al., 2002). Pathologically, HAD is characterized by a number of features, including dendritic vacuolization and synaptic pruning, both with and without neuronal loss; reactive astrocytosis and microgliosis; disruption of the BBB with macrophage infiltration and fluid accumulation resulting in myelin pallor; and formation of microglial nodules and multinucleated giant cells, which result from the fusion of brain macrophages and microglia with uninfected cells (Lipton, 1998; Kaul et al., 2001; Diesing et al., 2002). The most common feature of HAD, formation of multinucleated giant cells, is found throughout the brain but predominantly in deep brain structures and subcortical white matter (Diesing et al., 2002).

HIV IN THE BRAIN: CAUSATIVE MECHANISMS OF HAD

HIV penetrates the brain early in the course of infection, but symptoms associated with HAD do not occur until much later. This may be due in part to relatively scarce infections of brain cells. Neurons themselves are rarely if ever directly infected with HIV; only one postmortem case has shown evidence for neuronal infection (Nuovo et al., 1994). Many dispute whether neuronal infection occurs at all (Lipton, 1998; Diesing et al., 2002). At best, it is a rare occurrence. Astrocytes and brain microvascular endothelial cells are infected more frequently than neurons but are only restrictively infected (Saito et al., 1994; Tornatore et al., 1994; Moses et al., 1996), meaning that they can be infected but do not propagate the virus to cause further infections. Brain macrophages and microglia, collectively termed mononuclear phagocytes (MP), represent by far the predominantly infected cell types in HAD. As a result, the number of productively infected cells in the CNS is relatively small, since MP constitute only 12% of the cells in the CNS (Minagar et al., 2002) and not all of these will be infected.

With such a small proportion of native CNS cells actually infected with HIV, and few if any of these being neurons, the central question of HAD research has been how to account for the variable and rapidly progressing neurological deficits seen with HAD in the absence of widespread CNS infection. More specifically, any plausible hypothesis for the cause of HAD must account for several perplexing features of HAD that separate it from most other viral infections of the CNS: (i) HAD does not develop until long after HIV infection, and even long after the virus enters the CNS; (ii) neuronal dysfunction and degeneration occur without significant infection of neurons; and (iii) disease occurs without widespread infection of CNS cells, and disease severity does not correlate with viral burden in the brain. Research over the last decade points to several key concepts that address these issues and serve as the basis for our understanding of the pathogenesis of HAD.

Infiltration from the Periphery

Infiltration of infected and/or activated immune cells from the periphery is increased with HIV infection and likely to be essential for development of HAD. It is uncertain whether HIV itself can cross either an intact or compromised BBB to directly infect brain cells, or whether it must be transported across the BBB in an infected cell. HIV is found in the brain early in infection, but the mechanism of transport is uncertain. However, the similar human T-cell leukemia virus type 1 (HTLV-1) virus can be actively transported across the BBB by transcytosis through endothelial cells (Romero et al., 2000). The probability of direct viral passage may also increase with the progressive BBB disruption that occurs as HIV disease progresses. Regardless, what is certain is that infected peripheral immune cells cross an increasingly compromised BBB as HIV disease advances. HIV-infected peripheral monocytes in particular, which differentiate into macrophages upon entering the brain parenchyma, are thought to be principal mediators of viral entry into the CNS and subsequent HAD initiation.

Increased trafficking of activated or infected immune cells into the brain results from at least several factors linked to the HIV disease state. Normally, the BBB restricts and regulates passage of polar organics, ions, proteins, and cells from the bloodstream to the CNS. Multiple changes occur as a result of the HIV-induced inflammatory responses that increase passage of many of these substances across the BBB.

First, peripheral (and CNS) immune responses result in the secretion of various chemoattractants by activated MPs and astrocytes, including the chemotactic cytokines (also known as chemokines) macrophage inflammatory protein-1 alpha and macrophage chemotactic protein-1 (MCP-1) and the proinflammatory cytokines tumor necrosis factor alpha (TNF-α) and interleukin-1 beta (IL-1β), all of which serve to increase recruitment and trafficking of leukocytes (Diesing et al., 2002; Ryan et al., 2002).

Second, adhesion molecules such as intercellular adhesion molecule-1, vascular cell adhesion molecule-1, platelet endothelial cell adhesion molecule-1, and E-selectin are expressed on brain microvascular endothelial cells of the BBB and serve to regulate leukocyte trafficking across the BBB. A number of proinflammatory mediators, including cytokines, reactive oxygen species (ROS), and eicosanoids, up-regulate these and other adhesion molecules on brain microvascular endothelial cells during inflammation, thus facilitating increased leukocyte migration into the brain (Bolton et al., 1998; Huber et al., 2001; Diesing et al., 2002).

Finally, increased leukocyte migration alters the physical integrity of the BBB's tight junctions by inducing the breakdown of occludin and ZO1 and the reorganization of the actin cytoskeleton (Huber et al., 2001). Similar changes and increases in BBB permeability are seen after exposure to numerous substances produced by activated MPs and astrocytes, including TNF-α, IL-1β, gamma interferon, histamine, vascular endothelial growth factor, and fibroblast growth factor (Huber et al., 2001). Taken together, all of these factors serve to enhance leukocyte trafficking and migration across the BBB as a result of the immune reaction initiated by HIV.

Once across the BBB, these infiltrating infected and/or activated immune cells set in motion a cascade of inflammatory products which trigger a self-perpetuating cycle of further infections, inflammatory responses, and immune activation of neuroglia in autocrine and paracrine fashions. Infiltrating infected cells can infect or activate native CNS macrophages, microglia, and astrocytes, which may further infect or activate neighboring cells. Infiltrating activated cells can further activate native CNS cells in a paracrine fashion without themselves being infected, or they can act in an autocrine fashion to perpetuate the inflammatory immune response. The CNS immune response may also be further perpetuated by inflammatory signals originating in the periphery, such as the cytokines TNF-α and IL-β, among others. Importantly, since antiretrovirals often exhibit poor CNS penetration, the CNS can serve as a latent reservoir of virus, which may "reseed" infections in the presence of a weakened immune system late in the disease process, thus beginning the cycle anew (Diesing et al., 2002).

This peripherally triggered, self-amplifying cycle of CNS infection, cell immunoactivation, and inflammation is thought to be critical to the development of HAD, largely due to neurotoxic effects of the intercellular signaling molecules that mediate and perpetuate this response. This is discussed in more detail below. The apparent reliance on infiltrating immune cells to initiate HAD, as well as the relative scarcity of infected native brain cells, may be reasons why, at least in adults, HAD rarely occurs before the onset of advanced HIV disease (Kaul et al., 2001). Children infected with HIV from birth, however, are more likely to have cognitive and learning impairments without evidence of advanced HIV disease (Gelbard et al., 1995), perhaps from the effects of HIV infection on the developing nervous system such as inhibition of neural progenitor cell proliferation (Krathwohl et al., 1997). Although HIV is thought to enter the brain and CNS early in the disease, perhaps even with seroconversion, HAD does not develop until much later for reasons that are not fully understood. One explanation for this delayed onset of HAD is that significant immune dysregulation and consequent BBB disruption must have occurred before there is "sufficient entry of infected or activated immune cells into the brain to cause neuronal injury" (Kaul et al., 2001).

Individual and Synergistic Effects

These activated immune cells and astrocytes in the CNS secrete a milieu of cytokines, viral gene products, and other molecules that are both individually and synergistically toxic to neurons under some conditions.

Passage of infected cells or virus across the BBB results in the presence of activated immune cells in the brain, primarily macrophages and microglia but also astrocytes, which are thought to be directly causal to developing HAD. In fact, disease severity is best correlated with the number of activated macrophages, rather than viral burden or level of HIV gene products (Glass et al., 1995), suggesting that activated immune cells are critical mediators of the disease. Activated immune cells including macrophages, microglia, and astrocytes up-regulate production and secretion of a multitude of substances that can be toxic to neurons, some of which include the proinflammatory cytokines TNF-α and IL-1β; HIV gene products Tat, Nef, and gp120; the phospholipid mediators (eicanasoids) arachidonic acid and its derivative, platelet-activating factor (PAF); the excitatory amino acids glutamate and quinolate; ROS; and nitric oxide (Lipton, 1998; Epstein and Gelbard, 1999; Diesing et al., 2002).

Although all of these molecules have been shown to have deleterious effects on neurons under some circumstances, it is important to note that (with the exception of the HIV viral proteins) all of these substances are endogenously produced in the brain and as such serve routine cell signaling and even neuroprotective functions under some conditions.

Thus, when considering the contribution of these molecules to the neuropathogenesis of HAD (or any neurodegenerative disease, for that matter), it will be imperative for future studies to consider additional factors such as onset, timing, duration, cellular and neuroanatomical "neighborhood," and synergies of nervous system exposures to these molecules. For more-detailed discussions of the paradoxical nature of these and other molecules in CNS disease, please see Stoll et al., 2000; Stoll, 2002; Biber et al., 2002; Perry et al., 2002; Rock et al., 2004; Cartier et al., 2005; and Marchetti and Abbracchio, 2005.

Aside from their individual neurotoxic effects, the contributions of these compounds to initiating HAD are further magnified by several factors. First, most of them can be produced by a number of separate pathways implicated in HAD. For example, the cytokines TNF-α and IL-1β can be produced by activated macrophages, microglia, or astrocytes. Second, all of these substances either are themselves ROS or result directly or indirectly in the production of ROS somewhere downstream (Mollace et al., 2001). Third, many of these compounds act through, or induce production of, each other. For example, Tat induces production of TNF-α (New et al., 1998), which in turn acts through PAF (Perry et al., 1998). Finally, several of these compounds, such as Tat and TNF-α (Shi et al., 1998) and TNF-α and IL-1β (Venters et al., 2000), have been shown to exert synergistic effects with one another, and it is probable that other members of the group are capable of synergy as well (Perry et al., 2002). These complex and interdependent relationships serve to amplify the effects that these neurotoxins may have together, relative to the effect that each might have alone.

As a group, these substances have been shown to induce neuronal cell death and dysfunction by three primary disruptive mechanisms: (i) excitotoxicity via glutamate or other excitatory amino acid receptors, (ii) oxidative stress via production of free radicals and ROS, and (iii) calcium dysregulation. These broad mechanisms may converge to a final common mechanism of cell death such as apoptosis or remain separate and simultaneous contributors to neuronal demise by distinct pathways. Other pathways of neuronal disruption may also be employed in similar convergent or divergent fashion. Moreover, in addition to acting directly on neurons themselves, many of these HIV neurotoxins exert effects on neurons by acting indirectly, through disruption of glial functions. For example, TNF-α decreases extracellular glutamate uptake by astrocytes (Fine et al., 1996), rendering neurons more susceptible to excitotoxic cell death.

Aside from the demonstrated neurotoxicity of these compounds, using in vivo and in vitro models of HAD, elevated levels of most of these compounds have been found in the cerebrospinal fluid (CSF) and brain of HAD patients, including, but not limited to, PAF (Gelbard et al., 1994); quinolinate (Heyes et al., 1991); TNF-α, IL-1β, and other cytokines; arachidonic acid; free radicals; and nitric oxide (Xiong et al., 2000). The level of PAF in CSF correlates with the severity of clinical dementia (Gelbard et al., 1994), as do levels of TNF-α mRNA in microglia and astrocytes (Wesselingh et al., 1993, 1997). The levels of quinolinate (Heyes et al., 1991) and other excitotoxins (Giulian et al., 1996) have been found to correlate with disease status as well, although it is unclear whether this effect is causal or secondary to the disease state. Brain levels of gp120 mRNA have been correlated with severity of damage in a gp120-overexpressing transgenic mouse model of HAD (Toggas et al., 1994). These findings provide further support for the roles of these compounds in the pathology of HAD.

Taken together, these data have resulted in a consensus that HIV-associated dementia results in large part from a barrage of neurotoxic molecules being produced and released from infected and/or activated brain macrophages, microglia, astrocytes, and perhaps the virus itself in some cases. The synergy of effects seen with many of these molecules is of great importance, in that it allows for a much greater magnitude and range of effect than those observed with individual concentrations of compounds. Even further magnifying the relative effect of these neurotoxic substances is the fact that they may have long-lasting effects after only brief exposures. This concept is discussed next.

Long-Lasting Effects of Brief Exposure to Neurotoxic Molecules

Continuous exposure to these noxious molecules is not necessary for progressive neuronal dysfunction and death. For many years, one mystery of HAD has been how the magnitude of neurological dysfunction seen could be achieved without a large number of infected cells or an excessive supply of neurotoxic molecules. Certainly, levels of identified neurotoxins are higher than those found in control populations, but not to a degree that would justify the extent of deficits seen. Therefore, the finding that transient exposure to these molecules was sufficient to set in motion an ongoing cascade of events leading to neuronal dysfunction or death was critical to better understanding the disease.

There are at least two ways this can occur. Most directly, it has been found that only brief exposures to HIV gene products such as Tat and gp120 can induce progressive neuronal dysfunction eventually leading to cell death. For example, a transient Tat exposure sufficiently dysregulates intracellular calcium signaling to result in cell death (Haughey et al., 1999). Secondly, and perhaps of greater importance, brief or temporary exposures of glial or other immune cells to HIV neurotoxins such as Tat, TNF-α, and PAF trigger a self-amplifying cascade of further immune activation and production of chemokines, cytokines, and other neurotoxic molecules. These mechanisms allow HIV neurotoxins to exert effects greater than the magnitude of their presence and allow neurotoxicity to be separated by time and space from the initial insult, thus enabling significant dysfunction despite a limited presence of infected cells and neurotoxic molecules. For example, it was recently found that Tat infused into rat brains could be antero- and retrogradely transported to cause neuronal damage and dysfunction in brain regions distal from the injection site (Bruce-Keller et al., 2003).

In summary, the current model suggests that HAD is initiated once there is sufficient immune dysfunction to allow infiltration of high numbers of activated immune cells across a compromised BBB, resulting in a self-amplifying feedback loop of CNS inflammatory and immune responses, with consequent production of a neurotoxic cocktail of inflammatory cell and viral products with individual, synergistic, and long-acting effects, even after transient exposure. As a whole, this three-part conceptual understanding of the elements leading to HAD helps reconcile how this virally induced neurodegenerative disease can occur with significant delay relative to HIV infection and CNS viral entry, while HIV infection in the brain may be relatively limited and infections of neurons themselves remain rare or nonexistent, and while disease severity does not correlate with the overall number of HIV-1-infected cells in the brain (Epstein and Gelbard, 1999).

Although this progress has significantly enhanced our understanding of HAD and provides a model that addresses many of the paradoxes that HAD presents, many questions regarding the precise mechanisms leading to neuronal destruction remain unanswered. Thus, it will be critical that future work further develop our understandings of the precise mechanisms of neuronal death and dysfunction and how these mechanisms may lead to the pathology seen with HAD.

OTHER KEY MOLECULES AND SIGNALING PATHWAYS

As a consequence of these generalized pathogenic mechanisms, numerous molecules and signaling pathways are secreted and activated that are thought to be involved in precipitating the pathophysiology of HAD, many of which share functions in both normal cellular signaling and other neurodegenerative diseases. These include, but are not limited to, (i) HIV-1 gene proteins such as gp120, Tat, Nef, and Rev; (ii) excitatory amino acids such as quinolinate, cysteine, and glutamate; (iii) cytokines, including TNF-α, IL-1β, and IL-6; (iv) lipid species including arachidonic acid, ceramide, and PAF; (v) free-radical species such as superoxide anion (O_2^-) and nitric oxide (NO$^{\cdot}$); (vi) chemokines such as fractalkine and SDF-1α; and (vii) other factors yet to be identified. We now briefly discuss a few of these areas that we have not yet covered, as they relate to HAD. For more comprehensive overviews of the many mechanisms thought to contribute to the pathogenesis of HAD, please see Gonzalez-Scarano and Martin-Garcia, 2005; Kramer-Hammerle et al., 2005; Saksena and Smit, 2005; Kaul and Lipton, 2004; and Lipton, 1998.

For thorough clinically oriented discussions of HIV dementia in the age of HAART, please see McArthur, 2004; Gray et al., 2003; Langford et al., 2003; and Sperber and Shao, 2003.

Chemokines and Their Receptors

Chemokines, or "chemoattractant cytokines," were originally identified as regulators of leukocyte trafficking during inflammatory responses but have since been ascribed physiological roles including cell adhesion, phagocytosis, cytokine secretion, and cell cycle control outside the nervous system (Cartier et al., 2005). Within the nervous system, there is increasing evidence that they serve similar functions, in addition to possibly participating in the control of neuronal migration and synaptic activity (Cartier et al., 2005). Moreover, altered regulation of chemokines and their receptors is increasingly thought to be a significant pathogenic factor in numerous peripheral and CNS diseases (Cartier et al., 2005), including HIV dementia.

The issue of whether BBB integrity is compromised during the course of HIV-1 infection remains unresolved. Since monocytes traffic across the BBB and target focal inflammatory infiltrates in HAD and the relative numbers of monocyte-differentiated brain-resident macrophages and microglia in these infiltrates correlate with the degree of neurologic deficit, molecules which promote monocyte chemotaxis across the BBB are of cardinal importance in determining the temporal course of neurologic disease after HIV-1 infection.

Several kinds of chemokine receptors that are endogenously expressed in the brain may function as coreceptors for HIV-1 in the CNS (e.g., CCR3, CCR5, and CXCR4) (Cartier et al., 2005) and have helped to identify populations of glia at risk for infection (Tong et al., 2000; Sanders et al., 1998; Vallat et al., 1998). Macrophages localized to areas exhibiting the histopathologic correlates of HIV encephalitis express β-chemokines, MCP-1, macrophage inflammatory protein-1α, and RANTES, suggesting roles for chemokines in the formation of inflammatory infiltrates and microglial nodules (Tong et al., 2000; Sanders et al., 1998). In addition, Tat can stimulate astrocytes to release MCP-1 in vitro, and MCP-1 levels are elevated in brain and CSF of patients with HAD (Conant et al., 1998), suggesting that HIV-1 gene products like Tat initiate a cycle of inflammation through chemokine production and downstream signaling events that may include abnormal trafficking of monocytes across the BBB. Finally, CXCR4 gene-deleted transgenic mice suffer from abnormal cerebellar neuronal migration (Zou et al., 1998). Together, these data strongly suggest that chemokines and their receptors modulate development of the CNS, mediate immunologic communications between neurons and glia, and participate in the pathogenic effects of viral infections and other immunologic or inflammatory insults of the CNS.

One of the more recently discovered chemokines, fractalkine, is a large (373-residue) protein containing the chemokine domain attached to a mucin-like stalk and is derived from nonhemopoietic cells (Bazan et al., 1997). Fractalkine is predominantly expressed in neurons of the CNS, and its receptor CX3CR1 is expressed by microglia (Harrison et al., 1998). In its soluble form, it shows strong chemoattractant activity for T cells and monocytes, whereas its membrane-bound form is induced on activated endothelial cells and promotes leukocyte adhesion (Bazan et al., 1997). However, membrane-anchored fractalkine may be cleaved into a soluble, secreted form in the neuropil, where it retains its chemotactic properties. These features may make fractalkine unique among the chemokines in that it may be anchored in neuronal membranes with a mucin stalk that will arrest invading monocytes regardless of whether they express integrin counterreceptors.

Importantly, fractalkine has been shown to substantially protect against gp120-induced neuronal apoptosis in cultured rat hippocampal neurons (Meucci et al., 1998), suggesting that this molecule may help protect against the neuropathogenic effects of HIV-1. Accordingly, our laboratory has demonstrated that fractalkine expression is localized to cytoplasmic structures having a vesicular appearance in glutamatergic neurons. Moreover, we showed that in brain tissue from pediatric patients with HIV encephalitis and progressive encephalopathy (HIVEPE-positive), fractalkine is up-regulated in neurons adjacent to macrophages and microglia when compared with HIV-positive/HIVEPE-negative or HIV-negative pediatric controls. We also demonstrated that fractalkine convincingly mediates monocyte trafficking across an endothelial cell/astrocyte bilayer and in another in vitro model is neuroprotective against the neurotoxic effects of Tat and PAF on primary rat cortical neurons (Tong et al., 2000).

These results suggest that fractalkine may play a dual role in the neuropathogenesis of HIV-1-associated neurologic disease. Specifically, fractalkine may induce chemotaxis of peripheral monocytes into brain parenchyma with focal inflammatory infiltrates, thus potentiating production of neurotoxins, as well as provide neuroprotection to glutamatergic neurons by as yet unknown mechanisms. Because fractalkine is unique in its molecular structure, understanding how membrane-bound and soluble fractalkine of neuronal origin promotes monocyte chemotaxis across the BBB may be of paramount importance in arresting the formation of focal inflammatory infiltrates that contribute to neurologic

disease. Furthermore, understanding how fractalkine affords neuroprotection to glutamatergic neurons may benefit the development of new neuroprotective strategies.

We refer the interested reader to two excellent, comprehensive reviews covering the roles of fractalkine (Cotter et al., 2002) and chemokines in general (Cartier et al., 2005) in HAD.

ROS

Intracellular oxidizing agents (i.e., any molecule with a tendency to remove electrons from another molecule in an oxidation-reduction reaction) participate in, and are produced by, endogenous intracellular functions, yet in some circumstances can also have deleterious effects on the cell. Many intracellular oxidizing agents and free radicals are derived from reactions involving molecular oxygen (O_2), hence the terms "reactive oxygen species" and "oxidative stress." A primary source of ROS is the mitochondria, which generate superoxide ($°O_2$) during the molecular conversion of O_2 to water (H_2O) (i.e., respiration), principally from complex III of the electron transport chain (Nicholls, 2002). Excess O_2 elsewhere in the cell can be reduced to $°O_2^-$ by other oxidizing agents as well. Extramitochondrial sources of ROS include plasma membrane oxidases, particularly, NADPH oxidase, peroxisomes, and the endoplasmic reticulum (Sauer et al., 2001).

Oxidative damage can occur primarily on two levels: (i) direct oxidative damage to tissue, proteins, and other cell molecules, thus rendering them functionally impaired or terminally damaged; or (ii) ROS-mediated activation of signal transduction cascades such as mitogen-activated protein kinase, extracellular regulated kinase 1/2, c-Jun-N-terminal kinase, or transcription factors such as nuclear factor kappa-B and activator protein 1. Many of these molecules and pathways may have either toxic or protective effects depending on the cell type and situation, and very little is known about the precise mechanisms by which ROS activate signal transduction pathways and transcription factors.

ROS-mediated damage is thought to have functional significance for a broad range of diseases affecting both the immune system and the nervous system, including HIV infection, cancer, Parkinson's disease, Alzheimer's disease, and others. In HIV infection, oxidative stress may be involved in viral replication, inflammatory response, loss of immune function, decreased immune cell proliferation, sensitivity to drug toxicity, and chronic weight loss (for a review, see Pace and Leaf, 1995).

There is considerable evidence to suggest that oxidative stress may participate significantly in the pathophysiology of HAD. Many inflammatory mediators involved in HAD, including TNF-α and IL-1β, have been shown to induce oxidative stress, perhaps in significant part through Ca^{2+} dysregulation and subsequent production of nitric oxide synthase (leading to $OONO^-$). Antioxidant therapies have demonstrated some efficacy in alleviating symptoms associated with HAD (Dana Consortium, 1997). In addition, ROS levels are higher in the brains of HAD patients than in controls, and levels of the key antioxidant glutathione are lower (reviewed by Mollace et al., 2001). ROS-related injury is also thought to contribute to increased BBB permeability in HAD, thus leading to greater influx of infected immune cells and virotoxins into the brain (Mollace et al., 2001). More specifically, ROS generation by both Tat (Kumar et al., 1998) and TNF-α has been shown to activate c-Jun-N-terminal kinase and activator protein 1, a pathway that is generally toxic to neurons (Spiegel et al., 1998; Casaccia-Bonnefil et al., 1999). Excitotoxicity involving excessive activation of glutamate receptors, Ca^{2+} influx, and ROS production may be a common final mediator of cell death for many HIV neurotoxins, including Tat, TNF-α, PAF, gp120, and IL-1β. ROS production, in turn, leads to increased glutamate release and decreased glutamate uptake (Lipton, 1998; Epstein and Gelbard, 1999). Other properties particular to neurons, including generation of action potentials and synaptic communication, place heavy energetic demands on the cell, and therefore, neurons may be particularly susceptible to the effects of oxidative stress. Some of our own recent data support that some key indicators of oxidative stress in a neuron may include increased levels of ROS (Perry et al., 2004, 2005), increased activity of the DNA repair enzyme poly-ADP-ribose synthetase (H. A. Gelbard and S. Perry, unpublished data), and changes in mitochondrial membrane potential (Perry et al., 2005). Many of these interactions are diagrammed in Fig. 1.

Thus, there is ample evidence implicating the generation of ROS, or oxidative stress, as a significant cause of neuronal dysfunction or death in a number of neurological diseases. As such, oxidative stress may be a final common mediator of both synaptic and somal neuronal cell stress in both HAD and other neurodegenerative disorders (Mattson and Liu, 2002).

HIV Gene Products

Several HIV viral transcription proteins have been implicated in the pathogenesis of HIV dementia, the best known of which are Tat, Nef, and gp120 (for reviews, see Lipton, 1998, and Nath, 2002). Of these molecules, the HIV transcriptional activator Tat has shown a plethora of effects, and in fact Tat's proclivity for achieving cell entry has made it an attractive candidate as reagent for gene and drug delivery as well (nicely reviewed by Nori and Kopecek, 2005). Importantly, TNF-α and PAF are relevant downstream mediators of Tat that show similar effects and act synergistically with Tat. Tat induces production of TNF-α (New et al., 1998; Sawaya et al., 1998), which in turn acts through PAF (Perry et al., 1998).

Tat, or transactivating protein, is formed from two exons and is an 86- to 101-amino-acid nonstructural transcription regulator essential for HIV transcriptional activity and replication. Tat protein is found in the brain of patients with HAD, as demonstrated by Western blot analysis and mRNA detection (Nath, 2002), as are antibodies to Tat, also found in HAD brain (Zauli and Gibellini, 1996). While all HIV gene products can be released to the extracellular space by a variety of passive release mechanisms including lysis of infected cells (Nath, 2002), Tat is unique in that it is the

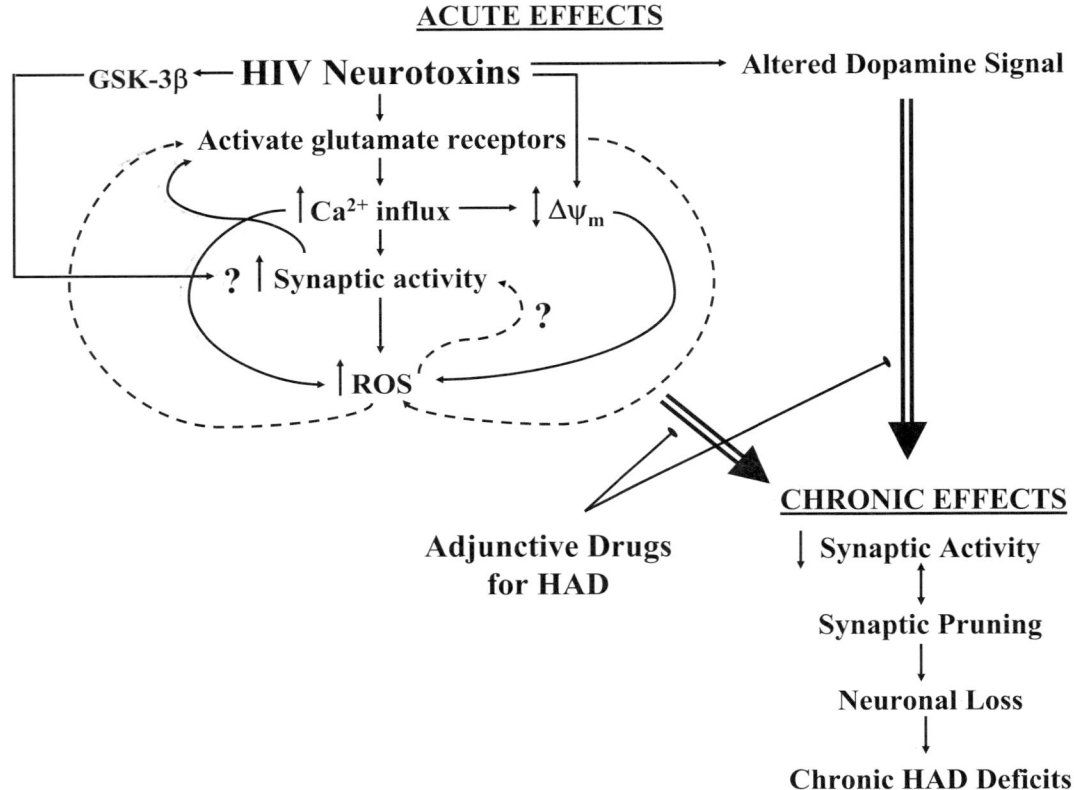

FIGURE 1 Schematic diagram of some purported HIV neurotoxin-induced neuronal dysfunctions in HIV dementia. Candidate HIV neurotoxins such as Tat, TNF-α, PAF, gp120, and others are thought to activate excitotoxic pathways involving glutamate receptor activation, calcium influx, increased excitotoxic synaptic activity, alterations in mitochondrial membrane potential ($\Delta\psi_m$), productions of ROS, and ultimately synapse loss and neuronal cell death if left unchecked. Alterations in the activity of GSK-3β or other signal transduction pathways (not diagrammed here) may lead to changes in synaptic activity and/or direct neuronal apoptosis. The goal of adjunctive therapeutics for HAD is to interrupt the cycle of cellular dysfunction before deficits become chronic and before significant synapse loss and/or neuronal cell death occurs.

only HIV viral protein actively secreted by infected glial cells (Tardieu et al., 1992), thus increasing the probability that it will be found in the extracellular space at higher concentrations than other HIV gene products.

Exactly how Tat interacts with the cell surface to mediate its effects is unclear, but in many cases this likely involves the two most adhesive regions of the protein: the highly basic heparin sulfate-binding region from the first exon, and the integrin-binding Arg-Gly-Asp (RGD) region of the carboxy-terminal portion from the second exon (ADD) (Nath, 2002). There are no known Tat receptors, although at least one HIV gene product, Vpr, is capable of pore (ion channel) formation in cell membranes (Nath, 2002). Whether this also occurs with Tat is uncertain. Moreover, whether Tat actually needs to gain entry into the cell to exert its effects is also uncertain, but this probably varies with the demonstrated effect. For example, Tat-induced alterations in transcriptional regulation may require cell entry, whereas Tat is thought to be capable of inducing neuronal depolarization by interfering with the zinc element of N-methyl-D-aspartate receptors exclusively on the extracellular membrane (Haughey et al., 2001; Song et al., 2003).

Tat is thought to affect neuronal functions in several ways: (i) by acting directly on neurons themselves; (ii) indirectly, by affecting glial functions, which in turn affect neurons; (iii) indirectly, by antigenically stimulating glial cells to produce molecules such as TNF-α and PAF, which in turn act either directly or indirectly on neurons; and (iv) by stimulating HIV replication and production of other HIV gene products detrimental to neurons. In addition, Tat is also an efficient regulator of the host genome (Nath, 2002), exerting transcriptional control over numerous cellular genes in a variety of cell types (Sawaya et al., 1998). For example, and of particular significance for HAD, Tat increases TNF-α levels in neuronal cells by increasing the transcriptional activity of its promoter (Sawaya et al., 1998). Tat also interacts with the transcription factor Pur-α in glial cells (Wortman et al., 2000). These mechanisms provide yet another avenue for Tat to exert effects in brain, i.e., by directly altering endogenous cellular gene expression of neurons or glia.

Finally, Tat has been shown to have a number of even more direct effects on neurons, including apoptosis (New et al., 1998), excessive depolarization and calcium influx leading to cell demise (Haughey et al., 1999), and downregulation of the tyrosine hydroxylase promoter in a neuronal cell line (Zauli et al., 2000).

GSK-3β

Tat has also been shown to act through glycogen synthase kinase-3β (GSK-3β), a constitutively active kinase member of the Wnt (wingless in *Drosophila* + proto-oncogene *int-1*) signaling pathway with a rapidly growing number of identified roles in the nervous system, including neuronal migration and neurodevelopment, cell death, and synaptic structure and function. Previous data from our and collaborators' laboratories indicate that Tat and its downstream mediator PAF induce apoptotic cell death via up-regulation of GSK-3β activity in cerebellar granule neurons (Maggirwar et al., 1999; Tong et al., 2001), and PAF also mediates neuronal migration in cerebellar granule neurons by GSK-3β activation (Tong et al., 2001).

In addition, there are several lines of evidence that make GSK-3β a compelling candidate for involvement in psychiatric and neurodegenerative disorders (reviewed by Martinez et al., 2002) and that link GSK-3β with control of redox status (reviewed by Chong et al., 2005). GSK-3β

has long been known as a critical mediator of animal development, playing key roles in cell fate determination and dorsoventral patterning (Klein and Melton, 1996), but its roles in the nervous system, including neuronal migration, axonal remodeling, synaptogenesis, and synaptic plasticity, have only recently been revealed (Packard et al., 2003). GSK-3β and downstream mediators like β-catenin induce changes in key structural and synaptic proteins that allow them to mediate these functional effects. These include destabilization of microtubule-associated proteins, thus allowing for axonal restructuring (Hall et al., 2002); recruitment of synaptic vesicle proteins such as synapsin I and increased presynaptic activity (Hall et al., 2002); and increased recruitment of postsynaptic proteins to the dendritic arbor, including S-SCAM and PSD-95, indicating increased postsynaptic size and density (Murase et al., 2002; Nishimura et al., 2002) (Fig. 1).

Lending further support for the possible role of GSK-3β in psychiatric disease, the GSK-3β inhibitor lithium chloride (LiCl) has been shown to act through GSK-3β to impart its effect on synaptic function. LiCl dramatically increases the probability of vesicle release at drosophila larval neuromuscular junctions (Acharya et al., 1998); and activation of the Wnt signaling pathway, the endogenous inhibitory pathway for GSK-3β, results in increased synapsin I levels and clustering, an effect that can be mimicked by LiCl (Hall et al., 2002). In the first report, an inositol-dependent mechanism is suggested, whereas the second report finds that LiCl is not acting through an inositol-dependent pathway, consistent with the growing body of evidence suggesting that the inositol and Wnt (GSK-3β) signaling pathways are two distinct mechanisms by which LiCl may regulate synaptic function (Klein and Melton, 1996; Salinas and Hall, 1999).

GSK-3β's primary substrate, β-catenin, may serve as an intermediary for many of GSK-3β's and LiCl's effects on synaptic function, as it has been shown that depolarization drives β-catenin into dendritic spines, where β-catenin directly increases the size and intensity of synapsin I clusters and the frequency of miniature excitatory postsynaptic currents (Murase et al., 2002). In other words, inhibition of GSK-3β (by LiCl or other mechanisms) and the resultant increased levels of β-catenin (phosphorylation of β-catenin by GSK-3β, its primary kinase, lead to increased degradation via the ubiquitin pathway), which may in turn lead to increased synaptic activity and plasticity. These or similar effects may at least in part explain the mood-stabilizing effects of lithium-based drugs. GSK-3β may also act to increase synaptic activity by direct interaction with several dynamin-like vesicular proteins shown to participate in exocytotic functions (Chen et al., 2000), but whether these interactions result in increased vesicular release is currently unknown. Any of all of these mechanisms may, at least in part, underlie the neuronal dysfunctions observed in HAD.

The Dopamine System

Motor deficits seen in HAD, notably tremor, dyskinesia, and impaired gait, often resemble those of Parkinson's disease, a disease caused by selective loss of dopaminergic neurons from the substantia nigra. In the HAD brain, neuronal loss is greatest in the basal ganglia and substantia nigra regions, areas which contain high populations of dopamine (DA) neurons (Gelbard et al., 1995). Finally, dopaminergic neurons may be particularly susceptible to oxidative stress, due to the chemical structure of dopamine, which renders it easily oxidized. This may result in a selective vulnerability of dopaminergic neurons in diseases such as Parkinson's disease and HAD.

There are a number of factors both related and unrelated to oxidative stress that might result in loss of DA neurons. One of those factors is alteration of the neuron's DA supply. Loss of dopaminergic neurons from the substantia nigra could occur due to either an excess intracellular dopamine supply or a deficient intracellular dopamine supply. Excess intracellular dopamine could lead to increased oxidative stress, as well as increased metabolic stress from increased synaptic activity, leading to a vicious cycle of further oxidative stress. Deficient intracellular dopamine might lead to decreased excitation of postsynaptic neurons and consequent withdrawal of trophic support leading to loss of the presynaptic DA neuron.

In findings specifically relevant to HAD, Tat treatment has been shown to down-regulate production of the dopamine precursor, tyrosine hydroxylase, in PC-12 cells (Zauli et al., 2000). In addition, in vivo positron emission tomography studies have shown the brains of HIV patients with dementia, but not those without dementia, to have significantly lower levels of dopamine transporters, but not D2 dopamine receptors, than seronegative controls (Wang et al., 2004). Finally, and significantly because of the high rate of drug abuse among HIV-infected populations, Tat and methamphetamine have been shown to act synergistically to reduce striatal dopamine availability in an in vivo animal model (Maragos et al., 2002). We refer the reader to reviews by Berger and Arendt (2000) and Nath et al. (2000) for a more detailed treatment of this topic.

NEURONAL CELL DEATH: NOT THE ONLY STORY

Early research on HAD, and many neurodegenerative diseases for that matter, tended to focus on frank loss of neurons as a critical mediator of the disease. While selective neuronal loss does occur and undoubtedly contributes to, and correlates with, HAD severity, it is not the best correlate for disease severity (Kaul et al., 2001). Instead, the best predictor of disease severity is the number of activated macrophages and microglia in the brain (Glass et al., 1995). Another significant and equally important correlate for HAD severity is decreased synaptic and dendritic density in the brains of HAD-afflicted individuals (Masliah et al., 1997; Everall et al., 1999). Other correlates have already been mentioned above.

Together, these data indicate that significant and clinically appreciable neuronal dysfunction can and does occur even in the absence of neuronal cell death. In other words, neurons do not have to die for HAD to occur. In fact, initiation of HAART after HAD onset can lead to an improvement of neurological symptoms in some individuals. Presumably, then, HAART may help ameliorate HAD symptoms in those individuals in whom significant neuronal loss has not already occurred. This strongly suggests that many of the symptoms of HAD result from an (at least partially) reversible metabolic encephalopathy. As such, intervention before significant cell death occurs is critical to controlling the outcome of this disease.

For most neurodegenerative diseases, cellular stress and aberrant neuronal function are likely to precede commitment to neuronal cell death (Fig. 1). Disruption of cellular energetics or synaptic transmission, function, or organization is arguably a first step in any neuronal demise. In fact, a growing body of evidence suggests that disruptions at the synapse may be principally determinative to whether a neuron undergoes cell death. This concept has been coined "synaptic apoptosis" (Gilman and Mattson, 2002; Mattson and Liu, 2002). Equally important, however, the same mechanisms that can trigger synaptic apoptosis (i) may simply result in degeneration of axons and dendrites or synaptic remodeling without cell death and (ii) may be reversibly activated once initiated, thus avoiding neuronal loss, and perhaps contributing to synaptic plasticity (Mattson and Liu, 2002).

HAD illustrates these concepts nicely, in that disease severity correlates with reduction in the neuronal arbor even in the absence of neuronal loss, and some neurologic deficits are reversible with timely HAART intervention. The precise mechanisms leading to neuronal loss, or neuronal dysfunction in the absence of neuronal demise, are not fully understood. However, in addition to the information already provided above, there is a great deal of literature indicating that candidate HIV neurotoxins participate in a number of effects on synaptic function including altered glutamatergic transmission and increased receptor sensitivity (Epstein and Gelbard, 1999), PAF-mediated synaptic facilitation in the striatum (H. A. Gelbard, unpublished data) and hippocampus (Bazan et al., 1993), and TNF-α-mediated up-regulation of AMPA receptors at the synapse (Beattie et al., 2002). TNF-α also induces changes in the actin/tubulin synaptic network and in expression levels of actin and tubulin proteins (Petrache et al., 2003), yet another effect which may lead to altered synaptic structure and function. Tat is highly excitatory to neurons and does not desensitize with repeated or prolonged exposure, leading to excessive depolarization and calcium influx and eventual cell demise (Cheng et al., 1998; Haughey et al., 1999, 2001). Tat also induces many effects on microtubule dynamics, interacting strongly with, and inhibiting, polymerization of several microtubule proteins, including actin-associated tubulin by binding with it at the microtubule-associated protein-binding domain to exert pathogenic effects (Battaglia et al., 2001). Finally, we have recently reported that the HIV neurotoxins Tat, TNF-α, and PAF contribute to increased synaptic activity, increased mitochondrial membrane potential, enhanced oxidative stress, and neuritic damage that may, at least in part, model the clinical symptomology of HAD (Perry et al., 2005). Furthering these data, we also find that Tat induces alterations in key synaptic proteins that may be corroborative with increased synaptic activity (Fig. 2).

NEUROPROTECTIVE STRATEGIES FOR HIV DEMENTIA

Although the advent of HAART steadily reduced the incidence of HAD until 2001, HAD incidence has been on the rise again since then, and the prevalence of HAD has also increased during the HAART era (McArthur, 2004). In fact, in an autopsy comparison of pre- and post-HAART cases, a very recent report found that in the hippocampus, microglial and macrophage activation (a key indicator of neuroinflammation and HAD neuropathology) was higher in post-HAART cases than in either pre-HAART or control cases. In the basal ganglia, activated, CD68-positive macrophages/microglia were more prevalent in post-HAART brains than in control (but not pre-HAART or presymptomatic) brains (Anthony et al., 2005). These results suggest that even with HAART, significant neuropathologic features of HAD continue to afflict brain areas critical for cognitive and other functions, underscoring the

Target Protein (Western Blot)	**Expression Level** (Tat treatment relative to Control)
p-Synapsin	+ 62% ± 22%
Synapsin 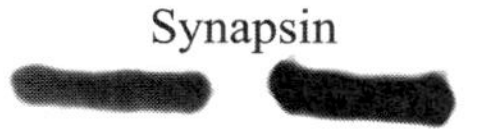 Control 2.5 ug/ml Tat	+ 44% ± 02%
CaM kinase II	+ 84% ± 35%

FIGURE 2 Tat upregulates synaptic proteins in rat cortical neurons. Treatment of rat cortical neurons for 24 h with 2.5 μg of Tat/ml up-regulated several key proteins involved in synaptic structure and function, including phosphorylated synapsin, total synapsin, and calcium calmodulin kinase II. Semiquantitative changes in protein expression were determined by densitometric analysis of mean band intensities from Western blots and were expressed as change with Tat treatment relative to control. A representative example of control and Tat synapsin bands (cut from blot film image after digital background subtraction) is shown. Percent values were generated from the average band intensity of duplicate samples (from separate treatment wells) per condition, run on the same gel. Treatment conditions were performed in duplicate or triplicate for at least two separate blots per target protein, and all changes were significant ($P < 0.05$, analysis of variance and Student's t test).

need for adjuvant neuroprotective therapies for HAD in the HAART era.

A number of phase 1 and phase 2 clinical trials for candidate HAD therapeutics have been performed, including the calcium channel antagonist nimodipine; the proprietary antioxidant OPC-14117; the monoamine oxidase-B inhibitor selegiline; the PAF antagonist lexipafant; the N-methyl-D-aspartate antagonist memantine; and the TNF antagonist CPI-1189 (for a review and summary, see Turchan et al., 2003). While most of the tested agents have been found to be safe, the trials have suffered from a lack of robust effects on HAD symptoms. Moreover, trials to date have relied on neuropsychological assessments of efficacy, yet the relationship of changes in neuropsychological performance to improvements in function has not been demonstrated (McArthur, 2004). Therefore, the need for effective therapeutic treatments for HAD continues.

Perhaps one of the more promising treatments in the pipeline for HIV infection both within and outside the CNS is the anticonvulsant valproic acid (also known as sodium valproate). Recent studies have been encouraging. For peripheral HIV infection, Lehrman and colleagues (2005) have recently demonstrated that a regimen of valproic acid and enfuvirtide-intensified HAART treatment significantly improved clearance of HIV from latently infected CD4$^+$ cells. However, in this study, the small sample size, lack of matched controls, and uncertainty regarding what happens to the pool of latently infected cells once the treatments are discontinued are all factors that must be judiciously addressed before the broader impacts of this study can be known (Smith, 2005). In rodent in vivo models of the CNS, valproic acid protects neurons against gp120-induced damage, induces neurite outgrowth, and protects severe combined immunodeficient (SCID) mice against the neurodegenerative effects of HIV-1-infected monocyte-derived

macrophages (Dou et al., 2003). See Dou et al. (2004) for further discussion of the therapeutic potential of valproate as an adjunctive therapy for HAD.

While these studies are encouraging, further questions remain. For example, based largely (although not exclusively) on a single early report (Chen et al., 1999), many of valproate's effects have been thought to be mediated by inhibition of GSK-3β. However, despite another encouraging report that lithium has similar protective effects against the neurotoxic effects of monocyte-derived macrophages in SCID mice (Dou et al., 2005), and despite associative evidence for decreased GSK-3β activity with valproate or lithium treatment in these CNS models of HAD (i.e., alterations in levels of nonexclusive GSK-3β substrate proteins such as β-catenin and *tau*) (Dou et al., 2003, 2005), GSK-3β inhibition has not been proven to be the causative mechanism behind valproate's (or lithium's) protective effects in either the Lehrman (2005) or HAD CNS models above (Dou et al., 2003, 2005). In fact, valproate may not even inhibit GSK-3β activity in significant portions of the brain (Ryves et al., 2005); in other words, GSK-3β inhibition by valproic acid may be a regionally dependent phenomenon. More-recent evidence suggests that inhibition of histone deacetylase may underlie some of the protective actions of valproate against HIV effects in the periphery (Ylisastigui et al., 2004) and in the CNS (reviewed by Chuang, 2005), although the extracellular signal-regulated kinase pathway may also mediate some of valproate's effects in the CNS (Hao et al., 2004). Sorting out these disparate effects will be critical to realizing whatever potential exists for valproate as an adjunctive therapy for HAD.

Even more novel, yet still largely unexplored, areas of adjunctive therapeutics for HIV dementia are the mitochondrial uncouplers. Several reports have indicated that mitochondrial hyperpolarization may represent an important feature of HIV infection both in the periphery (Matarrese et al., 2003) and the CNS (Perry et al., 2005; Norman et al., 2007), and mitochondrial uncouplers have already been shown to confer neuroprotection against some CNS insults (Korde et al., 2005; Jin et al., 2004). Moreover, the mitochondrial uncoupler 2,4-dinitrophenol protects against neuronal damage from the candidate HIV toxin quinolinate (Maragos et al., 2003). These studies infer significant potential for mitochondrial uncouplers as adjuvant therapies for HAD and other neurodegenerative diseases, pending the development of such compounds with clinically tolerable profiles. As a rule, the currently known uncoupling compounds such as 2,4-dinitrophenol are likely too toxic for safe human use (Korde et al., 2005; Maragos and Korde, 2004). For additional discussion of the import of mitochondrial uncouplers as neuroprotective agents for HAD and other neurodegenerative diseases, please see Perry and Gelbard (2005) and Maragos and Korde (2004), respectively.

Thus, we have several emerging possibilities for adjunctive neuroprotective therapies for HIV dementia in the age of HAART, yet further work remains. The mechanisms by which these putative agents maintain or restore CNS function must be further delineated, and such reagents must be brought to phase 3 clinical trials with real, functional assessments of their efficacy. With time, however, one or all of these putative therapeutics may represent successful adjunctive therapies for the debilitating effects of HIV in the CNS, with the hope of interrupting the cycle of neuronal dysfuction in HAD before more chronic deficits occur (Fig. 1).

CONCLUSIONS

Although our understanding of the causative mechanisms of HAD has progressed greatly over the last decade, the precise molecular mechanisms leading to neuronal dysfunction and death in the context of HAD have not been fully characterized. Fortunately, this situation is changing, and there is growing evidence to suggest that reversible (or irreversible) neuronal dysfunction from cellular and synaptic stress may be key components of this and other neurodegenerative diseases. Furthering our understanding of these mechanisms will allow continued development of therapeutics that interrupt the kinds of neuronal dysfunctions identified here that we believe, if left unchecked, lead to, or are concurrent with, neuronal cell death and represent the underlying pathophysiologic basis of HIV dementia.

Moreover, these ongoing investigations will have relevance to a variety of neurodegenerative diseases, since a (perhaps lengthy) period of neuronal dysfunction likely precedes neuronal cell death in many or even most diseases of the nervous system. Thus, it is our hope and expectation that future studies of HAD will not only aid HIV-infected patients but also further our understanding of relevant mechanisms of neuronal dysfunction that impact disease progression in other disorders of the nervous system as well. Towards that goal, we hope the information we have provided here serves as a useful starting point for those wishing to enhance their understanding of HIV dementia and its significant relationships to other CNS disorders, with the ultimate goal of designing more effective treatments for these devastating conditions.

This work was supported by NIH grants MH64570, MH56838, MH071176, NS31492, and T32 AI49815.

REFERENCES

Acharya, J., R. Delgado, K. Jalink, P. Labarca, and C. Zuker. 1998. Synaptic defects and compensatory regulation of inositol metabolism in inositol polyphosphate 1-phosphatase mutants. *Neuron* 20:1219–1229.

American Academy of Neurology AIDS Task Force. 1991. Nomenclature and research case definitions for neurologic manifestations of human immunodeficiency virus-type 1 (HIV-1) infection. Report of a Working Group of the American Academy of Neurology AIDS Task Force. *Neurology* 41:778–785.

Anthony, I., J. Bell, F. Carnie, and S. Ramage. 2005. Influence of HAART on HIV-related CNS disease and neuroinflammation. *J. Neuropathol. Exp. Neurol.* 64:529–536.

Battaglia, P., F. Gigliani, A. Macchini, and S. Zito. 2001. A *Drosophila* model of *HIV-Tat*-related pathogenicity. *J. Cell Sci.* 114:2787–2794.

Bazan, J. F., K. B. Bacon, G. Hardiman, W. Wang, K. Soo, D. Rossi, D. R. Greaves, A. Zlotkin, and T. J. Schall. 1997. A new class of membrane-bound chemokine with a CX3C motif. *Nature* 385:640–644.

Bazan, N., G. Clark, and C. Zorumski. 1993. The activation of phospholipase A2 and release of arachidonic acid and other lipid mediators at the synapse: the role of platelet-activating factor. *J. Lipid Mediat.* 6:421–427.

Beattie, E., M. Beattie, J. Bresnahan, B. Ha, R. Malenka, W. Morishita, D. Stellwagen, and M. Von Zastrow. 2002. Control of synaptic strength by glial TNF-alpha. *Science* 295:2282–2285.

Berger, J., and G. Arendt. 2000. HIV dementia: the role of the basal ganglia and dopaminergic systems. *J. Psychopharmacol.* 14:214–221.

Biber, K., H. Boddeke, I. Dijkstra, and M. Zuurman. 2002. Chemokines in the brain: neuroimmunology and beyond. *Curr. Opin. Pharmacol.* 2:63–68.

Bolton, S., D. Anthony, and V. Perry. 1998. Loss of the tight junction proteins occludin and zonula occludens-1 from cerebral vascular endothelium during neutrophil-induced blood-brain barrier breakdown in vivo. *Neuroscience* 86:1245–1257.

Bruce-Keller, A., A. Chauhan, F. Dimayuga, J. Gee, J. Keller, and A. Nath. 2003. Synaptic transport of human immunodeficiency virus-Tat protein causes neurotoxicity and *gliosis* in rat brain. *J. Neurosci.* 23:8417–8422.

Cartier, L., M. Dubois-Dauphin, O. Hartley, and K. Krause. 2005. Chemokine receptors in the central nervous system: role in brain inflammation and neurodegenerative diseases. *Brain Res. Brain Res. Rev.* 48:16–42.

Casaccia-Bonnefil, P., M. Chao, and C. Gu. 1999. Neurotrophins in cell survival/death decisions. *Adv. Exp. Med. Biol.* 468:275–282.

Chen, C. H., S. L. Hwang, S. L. Howng, C. K. Chou, and Y. R. Hong. 2000. Three rat brain alternative splicing dynamin-like protein variants: interaction with the glycogen synthase kinase *3beta* and action as a substrate. *Biochem. Biophys. Res. Commun.* 268:893–898.

Chen, G., L. Huang, Y. Jiang, and H. Manji. 1999. The mood-stabilizing agent valproate inhibits the activity of glycogen synthase kinase-3. *J. Neurochem.* 72:1327–1330.

Cheng, J., J. Geiger, S. Hochman, B. Knudsen, M. Ma, D. Magnuson, and A. Nath. 1998. Neuronal excitatory properties of human immunodeficiency virus type 1 Tat protein. *Neuroscience* 82:97–106.

Chong, Z. Z., F. Li, and K. Maiese. 2005. Oxidative stress in the brain: novel cellular targets that govern survival during neurodegenerative disease. *Prog. Neurobiol.* 75:207–246.

Chuang, D. 2005. The antiapoptotic actions of mood stabilizers: molecular mechanisms and therapeutic potentials. *Ann. N. Y. Acad. Sci.* 1053:195–204.

Conant, K., R. Gallo, A. Garzino-Demo, W. Halliday, E. Major, J. McArthur, A. Nath, and C. Power. 1998. Induction of monocyte chemoattractant protein-1 in HIV-1 Tat-stimulated astrocytes and elevation in AIDS dementia. *Proc. Natl. Acad. Sci. USA* 95:3117–3121.

Cotter, R., D. Erichsen, A. Lopez, H. Peng, L. Ryan, C. Williams, and J. Zheng. 2002. Fractalkine (*CX3CL1*) and brain inflammation: implications for HIV-1-associated dementia. *J. Neurovirol.* 8:585–598.

Dana Consortium on the Therapy of HIV Dementia and Related Cognitive Disorders. 1997. Safety and tolerability of the antioxidant OPC-14117 in HIV-associated cognitive impairment. *Neurology* 49:142–146.

Diesing, T., H. Gelbard, H. Gendelman, and S. Swindells. 2002. HIV-1-associated dementia: a basic science and clinical perspective. *AIDS Read.* 12:358–368.

Dou, H., K. Birusingh, S. Dewhurst, J. Faraci, H. Gelbard, H. Gendelman, S. Gorantla, S. B. Maggirwar, and L. Poluektova. 2003. Neuroprotective activities of sodium valproate in a murine model of human immunodeficiency virus-1 encephalitis. *J. Neurosci.* 23:9162–9170.

Dou, H., J. Bradley, S. Dewhurst, B. Ellison, H. Gendelman, A. Kasiyanov, S. Maggirwar, L. Poluektova, and H. Xiong. 2005. Neuroprotective mechanisms of lithium in murine human immunodeficiency virus-1 encephalitis. *J. Neurosci.* 25:8375–8385.

Dou, H., H. Gelbard, H. Gendelman, J. Kingsley, and R. Mosley. 2004. Neuroprotective strategies for HIV-1 associated dementia. *Neurotox. Res.* 6:503–521.

Ellis, R., I. Abramson, J. Atkinson, R. Deutsch, I. Grant, R. Heaton, T. Marcotte, J. McCutchan, J. Nelson, L. Thal, M. Wallace, et al. 1997. Neurocognitive impairment is an independent risk factor for death in HIV infection. *Arch. Neurol.* 54:416–424.

Epstein, L., E. Cho, M. Myenhofer, B. Navia, R. Price, and L. Sharer. 1984. HTLV-III/LAV-like retrovirus particles in the brains of patients with AIDS encephalopathy. *AIDS Res.* **1**:447–454.

Epstein, L., and H. Gelbard. 1999. HIV-1-induced neuronal injury in the developing brain. *J. Leukoc. Biol.* **65**:453–457.

Everall, I., J. Atkinson, R. Ellis, I. Grant, R. Heaton, M. Mallory, T. Marcotte, E. Masliah, J. McCutchan, et al. 1999. Cortical synaptic density is reduced in mild to moderate human immunodeficiency virus neurocognitive disorder. *Brain Pathol.* **9**:209–217.

Fine, S., R. Angel, S. Dewhurst, L. Epstein, H. Gelbard, S. Perry, and J. Rothstein. 1996. Tumor necrosis factor alpha inhibits glutamate uptake by primary human astrocytes. Implications for pathogenesis of HIV-1 dementia. *J. Biol. Chem.* **271**:15303–15306.

Gelbard, H., B. Blumberg, L. Epstein, H. James, A. Kazee, S. Perry, Y. Saito, and L. Sharer. 1995. Apoptotic neurons in brains from paediatric patients with HIV-1 encephalitis and progressive encephalopathy. *Neuropathol. Appl. Neurobiol.* **21**:208–217.

Gelbard, H., Y. Choi, K. Dzenko, P. Genis, H. Nottet, S. Swindells, M. Jett, R. White, L.Wang, D. Zhang, S. Lipton, W. Tourtellotte, L. Epstein, and H. Gendelman. 1994. Platelet-activating factor: a candidate human immunodeficiency virus type 1-induced neurotoxin. *J. Virol.* **68**:4628–4635.

Gilman, C. P., and M. P. Mattson. 2002. Do apoptotic mechanisms regulate synaptic plasticity and growth-cone motility? *Neuromol. Med.* **2**:197–214.

Giulian, D., J. Li, X. Li, S. N. Lin, C. Noonan, R. Schwarcz, D. Tom, E. Wendt, and J. Yu. 1996. Study of receptor-mediated neurotoxins released by HIV-1-infected mononuclear phagocytes found in human brain. *J. Neurosci.* **16**:3139–3153.

Glass, J., H. Fedor, J. McArthur, and S. Wesselingh. 1995. Immunocytochemical quantitation of human immunodeficiency virus in the brain: correlations with dementia. *Ann. Neurol.* **38**:755–762.

Gonzalez-Scarano, F., and J. Martin-Garcia. 2005. The neuropathogenesis of AIDS. *Nat. Rev. Immunol.* **5**:69–81.

Gray, F., F. Chretien, A. Vallat-Decouvelaere, and F. Scaravilli. 2003. The changing pattern of HIV neuropathology in the HAART era. *J. Neuropathol. Exp. Neurol.* **62**:429–440.

Hall, A., A. Brennan, K. Cleverley, R. Goold, F. Lucas, P. Salinas, and P. Gordon-Weeks. 2002. Valproate regulates GSK-3-mediated axonal remodeling and synapsin I clustering in developing neurons. *Mol. Cell. Neurosci.* **20**:257–270.

Hao, Y., G. Chen, T. Creson, F. Du, T. Gould, P. Li, H. Manji, P. Yuan, and L. Zhang. 2004. Mood stabilizer valproate promotes ERK pathway-dependent cortical neuronal growth and neurogenesis. *J. Neurosci.* **24**:6590–6599.

Harrison, J., S. Adhikari, K. Bacon, P. Botti, S. Chen, L. Feng, Y. Jiang, D. Maciejewski, R. K. McNamara, M. Salafranca, W. Streit, D. Thompson, and Y. Xia. 1998. Role for neuronally derived fractalkine in mediating interactions between neurons and CX3CR1-expressing microglia. *Proc. Natl. Acad. Sci. USA* **95**:10896.

Haughey, N., J. Geiger, C. Holden, and A. Nath. 1999. Involvement of inositol 1,4,5-trisphosphate-regulated stores of intracellular calcium in calcium dysregulation and neuron cell death caused by HIV-1 protein tat. *J. Neurochem.* **73**:1363–1374.

Haughey, N., J. Geiger, M. Mattson, A. Nath, and J. Slevin. 2001. HIV-1 Tat through phosphorylation of NMDA receptors potentiates glutamate excitotoxicity. *J. Neurochem.* **78**:457–467.

Heyes, P., B. Brew, J. Keilp, A. Martin, M. Mouradian, R. Price, A. Sadler, A. Salazar, J. Sidtis, and J. Yergey. 1991. Quinolinic acid in cerebrospinal fluid and serum in HIV-1 infection: relationship to clinical and neurological status. *Ann. Neurol.* **29**:202–209.

Huber, J., T. Davis, and R. Egleton. 2001. Molecular physiology and pathophysiology of tight junctions in the blood-brain barrier. *Trends Neurosci.* **24**:719–725.

Jin, Y., N. Dragicevic, W. Maragos, M. McEwen, S. Nottingham, J. Springer, and P. Sullivan. 2004. The mitochondrial uncoupling agent 2,4-dinitrophenol improves mitochondrial function, attenuates oxidative damage, and increases white matter sparing in the contused spinal cord. *J. Neurotrauma* **21**:1396–1404.

Kaul, M., G. Garden, and S. Lipton. 2001. Pathways to neuronal injury and apoptosis in HIV-associated dementia. *Nature* **410**:988–994.

Kaul, M., and S. Lipton. 2004. Signaling pathways to neuronal damage and apoptosis in human immunodeficiency virus type 1-associated dementia: chemokine receptors, excitotoxicity, and beyond. *J. Neurovirol.* **10**:97–101.

Klein, P., and D. Melton. 1996. A molecular mechanism for the effect of lithium on development. *Proc. Natl. Acad. Sci. USA* **93**:8455–8459.

Korde, A., L. Craddock, W. Maragos, and S. Pettigrew. 2005. The mitochondrial uncoupler 2,4-dinitrophenol attenuates tissue damage and improves mitochondrial homeostasis following transient focal cerebral ischemia. *J. Neurochem.* **94**:1676–1684.

Kramer-Hammerle, S., J. Bell, R. Brack-Werner, I. Rothenaigner, and H. Wolff. 2005. Cells of the central nervous system as targets and reservoirs of the human immunodeficiency virus. *Virus Res.* **111**:194–213.

Krathwohl, M. D., R. Hromas, D. R. Brown, H. E. Broxmeyer, and K. H. Fife. 1997. Functional characterization of the C—C chemokine-like molecules encoded by molluscum contagiosum virus types 1 and 2. *Proc. Natl. Acad. Sci. USA* **94**:9875–9880.

Kumar, A., B. Aggarwal, S. Dhawan, and S. Manna. 1998. HIV-Tat protein activates c-Jun N-terminal kinase and activator protein-1. *J. Immunol.* **161**:776–781.

Langford, T., S. Letendre, G. Larrea, and E. Masliah. 2003. Changing patterns in the neuropathogenesis of HIV during the HAART era. *Brain Pathol.* **13**:195–210.

Lehrman, G., R. Bosch, J. Coffin, R. Coombs, I. Hogue, C. Jennings, A. Landay, D. Margolis, J. Mellors, S. Palmer, D. Richman, C. Spina, and A. Wiegand. 2005. Depletion of latent HIV-1 infection in vivo: a proof-of-concept study. *Lancet* **366**:549–555.

Lipton, S. 1998. Neuronal injury associated with HIV-1: approaches to treatment. *Annu. Rev. Pharmacol. Toxicol.* **38**:159–177.

Lopez, O., J. Becker, M. Dew, J. Sanchez, and J. Wess. 1999. Neurological characteristics of HIV-infected men and women seeking primary medical care. *Eur. J. Neurol.* **6**:205–209.

Maggirwar, S., S. Dewhurst, H. Gelbard, S. Ramirez, and N. Tong. 1999. HIV-1 Tat-mediated activation of glycogen synthase kinase-3beta contributes to Tat-mediated neurotoxicity. *J. Neurochem.* **73**:578–586.

Maragos, W., W. Cass, M. Guseva, A. Nath, J. Pauly, J. Turchan, and K. Young. 2002. Human immunodeficiency virus-1 Tat protein and methamphetamine interact synergistically to impair striatal dopaminergic function. *J. Neurochem.* **83**:955–963.

Maragos, W., J. Dean, K. Rockich, and K. Young. 2003. Pre- or post-treatment with the mitochondrial uncoupler 2,4-dinitrophenol attenuates striatal quinolinate lesions. *Brain Res.* **966**:312-316.

Maragos, W., and A. Korde. 2004. Mitochondrial uncoupling as a potential therapeutic target in acute central nervous system injury. *J. Neurochem.* **91**:257–262.

Marchetti, B., and M. Abbracchio. 2005. To be or not to be (inflamed)-is that the question in anti-inflammatory drug therapy of neurodegenerative disorders? *Trends Pharmacol. Sci.* **26**:517–525.

Martinez, A., M. Alonso, A. Castro, and I. Dorronsoro. 2002. Glycogen synthase kinase 3 (GSK-3) inhibitors as new promising drugs for diabetes, neurodegeneration, cancer, and inflammation. *Med. Res. Rev.* **22**:373–384.

Masliah, E., C. Achim, J. Atkinson, R. Ellis, I. Grant, R. Heaton, M. Mallory, T. Marcotte, J. McCutchan, J. Nelson, C. Wiley, et al. 1997. Dendritic injury is a pathological substrate for human immunodeficiency virus-related cognitive disorders. *Ann. Neurol.* **42**:963–972.

Matarrese, P., A. Cassone, L. Gambardella, S. Vella, R. Cauda, and W. Malorni. 2003. Mitochondrial membrane hyperpolarization hijacks activated T lymphocytes toward the apoptotic-prone phenotype: homeostatic mechanisms of HIV protease inhibitors. *J. Immunol.* **170**:6006.

Mattson, M., and D. Liu. 2002. Energetics and oxidative stress in synaptic plasticity and neurodegenerative disorders. *Neuromol. Med.* **2**:215–231.

McArthur, J. 2004. HIV dementia: an evolving disease. *J. Neuroimmunol.* **157**:3–10.

Meucci, O., T. Bushell, A. Fatatis, P. Gray, R. Miller, and A. Simen. 1998. Chemokines regulate hippocampal neuronal signaling and gp120 neurotoxicity. *Proc. Natl. Acad. Sci. USA* **95**:14500.

Minagar, A., C. Eisdorfer, R. Fujimura, M. Heyes, R. Ownby, and P. Shapshak. 2002. The role of macrophage/microglia and astrocytes in the pathogenesis of three neurologic disorders: HIV-associated dementia, Alzheimer disease, and multiple sclerosis. *J. Neurol. Sci.* **202**:13–23.

Mollace, V., P. Clayette, C. Muscoli, H. S. Nottet, D. Salvemini, M. Perno, and C. Turco. 2001. Oxidative stress and neuroAIDS: triggers, modulators and novel antioxidants. *Trends Neurosci.* **24**:411–416.

Moses, A., S. Stenglein, J. Strussenberg, K. Wehrly, and J. Nelson. 1996. Sequences regulating tropism of human immunodeficiency virus type 1 for brain capillary endothelial cells map to a unique region on the viral genome. *J. Virol.* **70**:3401–3406.

Murase, S., E. Mosser, and E. Schuman. 2002. Depolarization drives beta-Catenin into neuronal spines promoting changes in synaptic structure and function. *Neuron* **35**:91–105.

Nath, A. 2002. Human immunodeficiency virus (HIV) proteins in neuropathogenesis of HIV dementia. *J. Infect. Dis.* **2**:S193–S198.

Nath, A., C. Anderson, J. Bell, R. Booze, K. Hauser, M. Jones, C. Mactutus, W. Maragos, and M. Mattson. 2000. Neurotoxicity and dysfunction of dopaminergic systems associated with AIDS dementia. *J. Psychopharmacol.* **14**:222–227.

New, D., S. Dewhurst, L. G. Epstein, H. Gelbard, and S. Maggirwar. 1998. HIV-1 Tat induces neuronal death via tumor necrosis factor-alpha and activation of non-N-methyl-D-aspartate receptors by a NFkappaB-independent mechanism. *J. Biol. Chem.* **273**:17852–17858.

Nicholls, D. G. 2002. Mitochondrial function and dysfunction in the cell: its relevance to aging and aging-related disease. *Int. J. Biochem. Cell Biol.* **34**:1372.

Nishimura, W., Y. Hata, J. Iida, N. Tanaka, and I. Yao. 2002. Interaction of synaptic scaffolding molecule and Beta-catenin. *J. Neurosci.* **22**:757–765.

Nori, A., and J. Kopecek. 2005. Intracellular targeting of polymer-bound drugs for cancer chemotherapy. *Adv. Drug Deliv. Rev.* **57**:609–636.

Norman, J. P., S. W. Perry, K. A. Kasischke, D. J Volsky, and H. A. Gelbard. 2007. HIV-1 trans activator of transcription protein elicits mitochondrial hyperpolarization and respiratory deficit, with dysregulation of complex IV and nicotinamide adenine dinucleotide homeostasis in cortical neurons. *J. Immunol.* **178**:869–876.

Nuovo, G., A. Braun, F. Gallery, and P. MacConnell. 1994. In situ detection of polymerase chain reaction-amplified HIV-1 nucleic acids and tumor necrosis factor-alpha RNA in the central nervous system. *Am. J. Pathol.* **144**:659–666.

Pace, G., and C. Leaf. 1995. The role of oxidative stress in HIV disease. *Free Radic. Biol. Med.* **19**:523–528.

Packard, M., V. Budnik, and D. Mathew. 2003. Wnts and TGF beta in synaptogenesis: old friends signalling at new places. *Nat. Rev. Neurosci.* **4**:113–120.

Perry, S., M. Bellizzi, S. Dewhurst, and H. Gelbard. 2002. Tumor necrosis factor-alpha in normal and diseased brain: conflicting effects via intraneuronal receptor crosstalk? *J. Neurovirol.* **8**:611–624.

Perry, S., G. Dbaibo, S. Dewhurst, K. Dzenko, L. Epstein, J. Hamilton, Y. Hannun, L. Tjoelker, and J. Whittaker. 1998. Platelet-activating factor receptor activation. An initiator step in HIV-1 neuropathogenesis. *J. Biol. Chem.* **273**:17660–17664.

Perry, S., S. Dewhurst, H. Gelbard, A. Litzburg, J. Norman, and D. Zhang. 2005. HIV-1 transactivator of transcription protein induces mitochondrial hyperpolarization and synaptic stress leading to apoptosis. *J. Immunol.* **174**:4333–4344.

Perry, S., and H. Gelbard. 2005. Adjunctive therapies for HIV-1 associated neurologic disease. *Neurotox. Res.* **8**:161–166.

Perry, S., H. Gelbard, A. Litzburg, and J. Norman. 2004. Antioxidants are required during the early critical period, but not later, for neuronal survival. *J. Neurosci. Res.* **78**:482.

Petrache, I., A. Birukova, J. Garcia, H. Gelbard, S. Ramirez, and A. Verin. 2003. The role of the microtubules in tumor necrosis factor-alpha-induced endothelial cell permeability. *Am. J. Respir. Cell Mol. Biol.* **28**:574–581.

Rock, R., M. Cheeran, G. Gekker, S. Hu, J. Lokensgard, P. Peterson, and W. Sheng. 2004. Role of microglia in central nervous system infections. *Clin. Microbiol. Rev.* **17**:942–964.

Romero, I., M. Prevost, E. Perret, P. Adamson, J. Greenwood, P. Couraud, and S. Ozden. 2000. Interactions between brain endothelial cells and human T-cell leukemia virus type 1-infected lymphocytes: mechanisms of viral entry into the central nervous system. *J. Virol.* **74**:6021–6030.

Ryan, L. A., R. L. Cotter, W. E. Zink II, H. E. Gendelman, and J. Zheng. 2002. Macrophages chemokines and neuronal injury in HIV-1-associated dementia. *Cell. Mol. Biol.* **48**:137–150.

Ryves, W., E. Dalton, A. Harwood, and R. Williams. 2005. GSK-3 activity in neocortical cells is inhibited by lithium but not carbamazepine or valproic acid. *Bipolar Disord.* **7**:260–265.

Sacktor, N., J. Becker, B. Cohen, C. Kleeberger, R. Lyles, E. Miller, O. Selnes, and R. Skolasky. 2001. HIV-associated neurologic disease incidence changes: Multicenter AIDS Cohort Study, 1990-1998. *Neurology* **56**:257–260.

Saito, Y., B. Blumberg, A. Cvetkovich, L. Epstein, K. Golding, M. Louder, J. Michaels, M. T. Mintz, and L. Sharer. 1994. Overexpression of nef as a marker for restricted HIV-1 infection of astrocytes in postmortem pediatric central nervous tissues. *Neurology* **44**:474–481.

Saksena, N., and T. Smit. 2005. HAART & the molecular biology of AIDS dementia complex. *Indian J. Med. Res.* **121**:256–269.

Salinas, P., and A. Hall. 1999. Lithium and synaptic plasticity. *Bipolar Disord.* **1**:87–90.

Sanders, V., C. Achim, C. Pittman, G. Wang, M. White, and C. Wiley. 1998. Chemokines and receptors in HIV encephalitis. *AIDS* **12**:1021.

Sauer, H., J. Hescheler, and M. Wartenberg. 2001. Reactive oxygen species as intracellular messengers during cell growth and differentiation. *Cell. Physiol. Biochem.* **11**:173–186.

Sawaya, B., S. Amini, J. Brady, L. Denisova, K. Khalili, and P. Thatikunta. 1998. Regulation of TNFalpha and TGFbeta-1 gene transcription by HIV-1 Tat in CNS cells. *J. Neuroimmunol.* **87**:33–42.

Shi, B., J. Busciglio, D. Gabuzda, A. Lorenzo, and J. Raina. 1998. Neuronal apoptosis induced by HIV-1 Tat protein and

TNF-alpha: potentiation of neurotoxicity mediated by oxidative stress and implications for HIV-1 dementia. *J. Neurovirol.* **4**:281–290.

Smith, S. M. 2005. Valproic acid and HIV-1 latency: beyond the sound bite. *Retrovirology* **2**:56.

Song, L., J. Geiger, S. Hochman, A. Moore, and A. Nath. 2003. Human immunodeficiency virus type 1 Tat protein directly activates neuronal N-methyl-D-aspartate receptors at an allosteric zinc-sensitive site. *J. Neurovirol.* **9**:399–403.

Sperber, K., and L. Shao. 2003. Neurologic consequences of HIV infection in the era of HAART. *AIDS Patient Care STDs* **17**:509–518.

Spiegel, S., O. Cuvillier, L. Edsall, T. Kohama, R. Menzeleev, Z. Olah, A. Olivera, G. Pirianov, D. Thomas, Z. Tu, J. Van Brocklyn, and F. Wang. 1998. Sphingosine-1-phosphate in cell growth and cell death. *Ann. N. Y. Acad. Sci.* **845**:11–18.

Stoll, G. 2002. Inflammatory cytokines in the nervous system: multifunctional mediators in autoimmunity and cerebral ischemia. *Rev. Neurol.* **158**:887–891.

Stoll, G., S. Jander, and M. Schroeter. 2000. Cytokines in CNS disorders: neurotoxicity versus neuroprotection. *J. Neural Transm.* **59**:81–89.

Tardieu, M., O. Boespflug, C. Hery, L. Montagnier, and S. Peudenier. 1992. Human immunodeficiency virus type 1-infected monocytic cells can destroy human neural cells after cell-to-cell adhesion. *Ann. Neurol.* **32**:11–17.

Toggas, S., C. Abraham, E. Masliah, L. Mucke, G. Rall, and E. Rockenstein. 1994. Central nervous system damage produced by expression of the HIV-1 coat protein gp120 in transgenic mice. *Nature* **367**:188–193.

Tong, N., A. Brooks, H. Bal, D. Dairaghi, S. Dewhurst, H. Gelbard, H. Gendelman, L. Epstein, S. Fine, H. Guo, H. James, S. Kinnear, T. Schall, L. Sharer, and Q. Zhang. 2000. Neuronal fractalkine expression in HIV-1 encephalitis: roles for macrophage recruitment and neuroprotection in the central nervous system. *J. Immunol.* **164**:1333–1339.

Tong, N., S. Dewhurst, H. Gelbard, H. Guo, S. Maggirwar, S. Ramirez, and J. Sanchez. 2001. Activation of glycogen synthase kinase 3 beta (GSK-3beta) by platelet activating factor mediates migration and cell death in cerebellar granule neurons. *Eur. J. Neurosci.* **13**:1913–1922.

Tornatore, C., J. Berger, R. Chandra, and E. Major. 1994. HIV-1 infection of subcortical astrocytes in the pediatric central nervous system. *Neurology* **44**:481–487.

Turchan, J., N. Sacktor, V. Wojna, K. Conant, and A. Nath. 2003. Neuroprotective therapy for HIV dementia. *Curr. HIV Res.* **1**:373–383.

Vallat, A., J. Bell, U. De Girolami, D. Gabuzda, F. Gray, J. He, W. Marasco, A. Mhashilkar, B. Shi, C. Keohane, and T. Smith. 1998. Localization of HIV-1 co-receptors CCR5 and CXCR4 in the brain of children with AIDS. *Am. J. Pathol.* **152**:167.

Venters, H., R. Dantzer, and K. Kelley. 2000. Tumor necrosis factor-alpha induces neuronal death by silencing survival signals generated by the type I insulin-like growth factor receptor. *Ann. N. Y. Acad. Sci.* **917**:210–220.

Wang, G., L. Chang, T. Ernst, J. Fowler, J. Logan, F. Telang, and N. Volkow. 2004. Decreased brain dopaminergic transporters in HIV-associated dementia patients. *Brain* **127**:2452–2458.

Wesselingh, S., J. Farber, J. Glass, D. Griffin, J. Griffin, and C. Power. 1993. Intracerebral cytokine messenger RNA expression in acquired immunodeficiency syndrome dementia. *Ann. Neurol.* **33**:576–582.

Wesselingh, S., J. Glass, D. Griffin, J. Griffin, J. McArthur, and K. Takahashi. 1997. Cellular localization of tumor necrosis factor mRNA in neurological tissue from HIV-infected patients by combined reverse transcriptase/polymerase chain reaction in situ hybridization and immunohistochemistry. *J. Neuroimmunol.* **74**:1–8.

World Health Organization. 2004. *AIDS Epidemic Update 2004.* Joint United Nations Program on HIV/AIDS and World Health Organization (UNAIDS/WHO), World Health Organization, Geneva, Switzerland.

Wortman, M., J. Brady, L. Chepenik, G. Gallia, R. Gordon, E. Johnson, J. Kim, K. Khalili, and C. Krachmarov. 2000. Interaction of HIV-1 Tat with Puralpha in nuclei of human glial cells: characterization of RNA-mediated protein-protein binding. *J. Cell. Biochem.* **77**:65–74.

Xiong, H., H. Gendelman, T. Lewis, Y. Persidsky, Y. Zeng, and J. Zheng. 2000. HIV-1 infected mononuclear phagocyte secretory products affect neuronal physiology leading to cellular demise: relevance for HIV-1-associated dementia. *J. Neurovirol.* **1**:S14–S23.

Ylisastigui, L., N. Archin, R. Bosch, G. Lehrman, and D. Margolis. 2004. Coaxing HIV-1 from resting CD4 T cells: histone deacetylase inhibition allows latent viral expression. *AIDS* **18**:1101–1108.

Zauli, G., S. Capitani, D. Dowd, D. Gibellini, M. Mazzoni, P. Mirandola, D. Milani, L. Rodella, P. Secchiero, and M. Vitale. 2000. HIV-1 Tat-mediated inhibition of the tyrosine hydroxylase gene expression in dopaminergic neuronal cells. *J. Biol. Chem.* **275**:4159–4165.

Zauli, G., and D. Gibellini. 1996. The human immunodeficiency virus type-1 (HIV-1) Tat protein and Bcl-2 gene expression. *Leuk. Lymphoma* **23**:551–560.

Zou, Y., A. Kottman, M. Kuroda, D. Littman, and I. Taniuchi. 1998. Function of the chemokine receptor CXCR4 in haematopoiesis and in cerebellar development. *Nature* **393**:595.

The Spectrum of Neuro-AIDS Disorders:
Pathophysiology, Diagnosis, and Treatment
Edited by K. Goodkin et al.
©2008 ASM Press, Washington, DC

12

Chemokines and the Neuropathogenesis of HIV-1 Infection

DAWN EGGERT, ERIC ANDERSON, JIALIN ZHENG, AND HOWARD E. GENDELMAN

Human immunodeficiency virus type 1 (HIV-1)-associated neurocognitive disorder (HAND) manifests during the later stages of viral infection and associated immunosuppression as a spectrum of neurological and psychiatric symptoms (Gendelman et al., 1994; Kieburtz and Schiffer, 1989; Marder et al., 1996; Navia et al., 1986b; Antinori et al., 2007). Behavioral, motor, and sensory impairments are present in varying degrees, but cognitive deficiency predominates. The clinical syndrome usually occurs late in the course of disease and rapidly evolves from subtle cognitive changes (forgetfulness and apathy) and physical slowing to florid mental and physical deterioration with memory loss, behavioral abnormalities, incontinence, hallucinations, seizures, coma, and in the very latest stages, death (Gelbard and Epstein, 1995; Janssen et al., 1991; Navia et al., 1986b; American Academy of Neurology AIDS Task Force, 1991). Although the incidence of HAND has dropped dramatically since the introduction of highly active antiretroviral therapy (HAART), from 20% of adults and 50% of children to <10% of all infected subjects (Sacktor et al., 2001), neurological dysfunction remains prevalent at or above previous levels. Clearly, resistance to antiretroviral therapy continues to grow with viral strain mutations that parallel the impaired ability of drugs to penetrate the blood-brain barrier (BBB). Indeed, recent evidence strongly suggests that viral mutations within cells that can ultimately cross the BBB may lead to HIV drug resistance (Chew et al., 2005). This suggests that HAND will continue to be a significant complication of advanced HIV-1 disease (Carpenter et al., 2000; Krebs et al., 2000; McArthur et al., 1999).

HAND is commonly associated with a multinucleated giant cell (MNGC) encephalitis termed HIV encephalitis

(HIVE) (Navia et al., 1986a). Importantly, it occurs in most, but not all, cases of dementia related to HIV-1 infection. Immune activation and productive viral replication of mono- and multinuclear phagocytes (MP) (perivascular and parenchymal brain macrophage and microglia), with the formation of microglial nodules, reactive astrocytosis, myelin pallor, and neuronal dropout, characterize the viral encephalitis. Moreover, brain inflammation, produced as a consequence of MP infection, produces a chemotactic gradient resulting in continuous monocyte transendothelial migration and BBB compromise during disease (Anderson et al., 2002; Boven et al., 2000; Cho and Miller, 2002; Williams and Hickey, 2002).

MPs are the principal cell type infected in the brain. Astrocytes are infected in a restricted manner and at low levels. Moreover, infections occur with a subset of viral strains (Thompson et al., 2004). To date, no conclusive evidence has shown that brain endothelial cells are infected by HIV. MP neurotoxic factors include cellular and viral proteins produced as a consequence of viral infection and immune activation (Aquaro et al., 2000; Conant et al., 1998; Gabuzda et al., 1998; Gendelman, 1997; Glass et al., 1995; Koenig et al., 1986; Nath and Geiger, 1998; Perno et al., 1994; Strizki et al., 1996; Wiley et al., 1986; Zheng and Gendelman, 1997). Significant astrogliosis is observed in brain areas with axonal and dendritic damage. The operative mechanisms by which MP become activated and affect neuronal damage are incompletely understood (Miller, 2005). This paper strives to describe what is known about MP activation and neuronal dysfunction with a focus on chemokines.

Mounting evidence suggests that chemokines affect the pathogenesis of HAND. First, there is a state of "immune privilege" within the central nervous system (CNS) that is, in part, an evolutionary adaptation (Streilein, 1995) for which increasing evidence suggests that functional immunity is quite operative in the brain. Support for CNS privilege comes from multiple sources, including the prolonged survival of allografts (Poltorak and Freed, 1991; Rao et al., 1989) in brain and the presence of the BBB (Annunziata, 2003).

Dawn Eggert, Eric Anderson, and Howard E. Gendelman, Laboratory of Neuroregeneration, Department of Pharmacology and Experimental Neuroscience, University of Nebraska Medical Center, Omaha, NE 68398-5880. Jialin Zheng, Laboratory of Neurotoxicology, Department of Pharmacology and Experimental Neuroscience, Center for Neurovirology and Neurodegenerative Disorders, University of Nebraska Medical Center, Omaha, NE 68398-5880.

However, each is affected by immune signals by which chemokines and their receptors are principal components (Speth et al., 2005). Second, the maintenance of nervous system function requires protection from a variety of environmental insults occurring during inflammatory activities, such as HIVE. Interplay between the peripheral and CNS immune systems is operative and leads to HIV penetration into the brain from blood and the eventual development of HIVE and HAND (Anderson et al., 2002; Garden, 2002). Third, chemokines (chemotactic cytokines) and chemokine receptors are an important part of the immune response that affects cell migration, activation, and tissue homeostasis (Richard et al., 2002; Shields and Adams, 2002). Fourth, following local production, chemokines induce leukocyte cytoskeletal changes, for example, actin polymerization, optimizing cell migration to areas of microbial infection or degeneration. Chemokines induce leukocyte differentiation from stem cells in bone marrow and thymic differentiation of T lymphocytes. They are also involved in angiogenesis, tumor development, and viral pathogenesis (Chen et al., 2005; Richard et al., 2002; Shields and Adams, 2002). Fifth, chemokines and chemokine receptors have been shown to play a critical role in the development of the nervous system and in disease (Cho and Miller, 2002; Kaul, 2008).

Within the past several years the links between chemokines, chemokine receptors, and HIV pathogenesis have become both clear and significant (Cartier et al., 2005; Cocchi et al., 1995; Deng et al., 1996; Dragic et al., 1996; Feng et al., 1996; Michael, 2002; O'Brien et al., 2002; Rizzardi and Pantaleo, 2002). Because of the role played by chemokines and their receptors in HIV entry and viral dissemination together with their role in a plethora of physiologic and inflammatory neurodegenerative events, chemokines represent a major focus for research into the neurology of AIDS (Miller, 2005). Indeed, chemokine receptors play a critical role in the early stages of HIV cell entry, including protection against HIV infection. Chemokine receptors CCR5 and CXCR4 are the major coreceptors for viral entry into CD4$^+$ T lymphocytes and macrophages (Cocchi et al., 1995; Deng et al., 1996; Feng et al., 1996; Joly and Pinto, 2005). As essential components of neural and glial physiology, chemokines and their receptors are also involved in the balance between neuroprotection and neurodegeneration, both of which affect the tempo of HAND in its human host (Gonzalez-Scarano and Martin-Garcia, 2005). These observations have elicited intensive research interest into chemokine biology of HIV CNS disease (Miller, 2005).

The importance of chemokines in the pathogenesis of HIV infection of the nervous system is underscored by inflammatory activities. Indeed, inflammatory responses manifested in the brain during HIV-1 infection of the nervous system lead to the development of a chemoattractant gradient that results in the formation of MNGC during HIVE (Williams and Hickey, 2002). These giant cells are a mixture of resident microglia and infiltrating blood-derived macrophages. Moreover, ongoing inflammatory responses in brain also change innate microglial function, manifest after prolonged exposures, leading to a level of microglial unresponsiveness to environmental cues (Ghorpade et al., 2005). This enables inflammatory monocyte-derived macrophages (MDM) to enter the brain, become infected, and expand the cellular sources of neurotoxic factors leading to the pathological and clinical aspects of disease (Gendelman et al., 2005; Wormser, 2004).

Chemokine receptors are critical for the infection of perivascular macrophages and microglia. It has also been shown that chemokines and their receptors play a more direct role in the neuropathogenesis of HIV-1 infection. This occurs through the expression of chemokine receptors by neurons and glia (Miller, 2005). Indeed, the interactions of HIV-1 gp120 with neuronal chemokine receptors can lead to dysfunction or apoptosis of neurons (Cho and Miller, 2002; Cotter et al., 2002; Ryan et al., 2002). It is interesting that opposing outcomes to the cell can occur after engagement of the identical receptor on neurons by specific proteins. For example, gp120 and stromal cell-derived factor 1 (SDF-1) both interact with CXCR4, initiating intracellular signaling pathways that lead to either neuronal or cell survival (Khan et al., 2004). The presence of chemokine receptors on neural cells also supports the notion that chemokines can regulate neuronal physiology.

HIV NEUROPATHOGENESIS

Infection of the CNS by HIV occurs early and remains persistent throughout the life of an infected person (Nottet and Gendelman, 1995). Disease is manifested as a consequence of ongoing viral infection and immune activation of MP. This results in autocrine and paracrine amplifications of immune neurotoxins, activation of the local complement systems, and engagement of a variety of neural receptors including chemokines (Kramer-Hammerle et al., 2005). The pathogenesis of HAND revolves around the numbers of virus-infected and immunocompetent brain MP (Glass et al., 1995) and the resultant secretion of neurotoxins. Immune activation of infected MP results in the secretion and amplification of factors that cause neuronal damage and subsequent cognitive dysfunction.

Although the importance of MP activation in HAND pathogenesis has been widely recognized, the process by which it occurs remains undefined (Kadiu et al., 2005). HIV-1 infection may predispose MPs to immune activation through intracellular events that lower the cytosolic signal transduction threshold necessary for macrophage activation and subsequent production of secretory factors (Cotter et al., 1999; Genis et al., 1992; Nottet and Gendelman, 1995; Persidsky et al., 1996; Kaul and Lipton, 2006). MP may be "primed" by HIV in this way to be active upon future immune stimulation. Tat and gp120, both HIV-1 proteins, can engage MP receptors and induce intracellular events (Chauhan and Nath, 2005). These may either alter the threshold for activation de novo or induce it (Conant et al., 1998; Jones et al., 1998; Lipton, 1994; Nath et al., 1999; New et al., 1998; Perry et al., 1998). Neurons express functional changes such as oxidative stress and perturbed cellular calcium homeostasis, thereby affecting excitotoxicity when exposed to HIV-1 gp120 and Tat (Mattson et al., 2005; Erdmann et al., 2006).

Peripheral immune challenge may also induce a response from infected MP, resulting in secretion of chemokines and cytokines, which impairs BBB function, and subsequently affecting widespread inflammation within the CNS (Fiala et al., 1998; Nottet et al., 1996; Persidsky et al., 1997, 1999). Leukocyte transendothelial migration into the CNS may be augmented by such events and, when combined with changes in cellular migratory capabilities and up-regulated adhesion molecules, cause amplification of the cellular sources of toxic molecules including virus and viral proteins in the nervous system (Ghorpade et al., 2001; McManus et al., 2000; Nottet et al., 1996; Weiss et al., 1999; Wu et al., 2000). BBB permeability can be changed with the interaction of brain microvascular endothelial cells (BMVEC) and cytokines (for example, tumor necrosis factor alpha [TNF-α] and interleukin-1 beta [IL-1β]), arachidonic acid and its metabolites, and nitric oxide (NO), as well as viral proteins such as Tat and HIV-1 gp120, and ultimately enhance cell trafficking into the brain (Persidsky et al., 2000). These observations clearly underline the importance of chemokines in their abilities to affect recruitment and activation of monocytes and macrophages during HAND.

Activated MP secretes an abundance of cellular and viral neurotoxins which include glutamate (Jiang et al., 2001), arachidonic acid (Nottet et al., 1995), platelet-activating factor (PAF) (Gelbard et al., 1994; Serradji et al., 2004), TNF-α (Gelbard et al., 1993; Pulliam et al., 2004; Talley et al., 1995), IL-1β (Pulliam et al., 2004), quinolinic acid (Guillemin et al., 2005; Heyes et al., 1991; Kerr et al., 1998), Ntox (Giulian et al., 1996), NO (Adamson et al., 1996; Anderson et al., 2002), HIV-1 gp120 (Brenneman et al., 1988; Conti et al., 2004), gp41 (Adamson et al., 1996), and Tat (Liou et al., 2004; Ma and Nath, 1997; Magnuson et al., 1995; Nath et al., 1996; New et al., 1997, 1998; Shi et al., 1998). Excessive calcium influx and overstimulation of glutamate receptors resulting from secreted excitatory amino acids can induce excitotoxicity in neurons, leading to formation of NO and superoxide anion (free radicals) and subsequent neuronal apoptosis (Rodriguez et al., 2000). Multiple effector mechanisms, from both microglia and astrocytes, are believed to be operative in disease and explain the diffuse compromise of neural function characteristic of HAND (Garden, 2002; Gendelman et al., 1997; Lipton and Gendelman, 1995; Williams and Hickey, 2002).

Neuropathological signatures of HAND include neuronal loss leading to alterations in dendritic arbor and decreased synaptic density (Gabuzda et al., 1998; Gelbard et al., 1994; Gendelman et al., 1997; Lipton and Gendelman, 1995; Nath and Geiger, 1998; New et al., 1998; Shi et al., 1996, 1998). Several questions remain as to how neuronal loss occurs during HIVE and HAND. First, how the major features of HAND neuronal injury of altered dendritic arbor and synaptic density (Everall et al., 1994; Wiley et al., 1991) are linked to specific MP secretory activities and are affected by antiretroviral and adjunctive therapies remains unclear (Aquaro et al., 1997, 1998, 2000; Fox et al., 2000; Gendelman et al., 1998; Limoges et al., 2000; Perno et al., 1988, 1994, 1998; Cook-Easterwood et al., 2007). Second, how the normal protective functions of MP are altered or reversed following immune activation remains unclear (Lazarov-Speigler et al., 1998a; Wiley et al., 2000; Zeev-Brann et al., 1998; Zheng et al., 2001a, 2001b; Sun et al., 2008). Third, the manner in which mutual receptor interactions between HIV gp120 and chemokines occur could be significant in the ultimate outcome of neuronal loss versus cellular protection. Fourth, determining how activation of chemokine receptors occurs in the brain inflammation is critical, as this process affects specific signaling events such as calcium mobilization and influx, both critical for neuronal homeostasis.

In order to address these questions and further define the relationship among HIV-1 infection, MP activation, chemokine production, and neuronal demise, laboratory assays were developed to mimic HIV-1-associated neuronal injury. The effects of virus-infected and/or immune-activated MP secretory products on aspects of neuronal morphology were quantitatively assessed. Assays were developed using rat cortical and hippocampal neurons and human cortical neurons exposed to secretory products from HIV-1-infected and activated human MDM. Assays for alterations in neuronal

dendritic arbor and cell loss include the quantification of neurofilament, neuron-specific enolase, and microtubule-associated protein 2 (MAP-2) by enzyme-linked immunosorbent assay and demonstrate that MP produce both neurotrophic and toxic factors (Lazarov-Speigler et al., 1998a; Wiley et al., 2000; Zeev-Brann et al., 1998; Zheng et al., 2001a). MDM conditioned media (MCM) enhance neuronal survival and differentiation, and several of the neurotrophic factors made by MDM are beginning to be defined (Shibata et al., 2003). In contrast, MCM obtained from MDM infected with HIV-1$_{ADA}$ and activated by lipopolysaccharide induces neuronal cell death, characterized by neuronal apoptosis (Zheng et al., 2001b), altered dendritic arbor, and decreased neuronal density (Zheng et al., 2001a). Utilizing a spectrum of HIV-1 strains to infect human MDM, productive viral replication was shown to be necessary, but not sufficient, for MP induction of neuronal injury. Virion-free HIV-1-infected and immune-activated MDM supernatants induced neuronal demise. Similar responses were observed with MCM from human fetal microglia, further supporting the role of HIV-1-infected and immune-activated brain MP in overall neurotoxic responses (Zheng et al., 2001a). Alterations in glutamate-mediated neuronal signaling were observed from neurons treated with secretory products from both HIV-1-infected and immune-activated MDM (Zheng et al., 2001b). Long-term potentiation inhibition was found in rat hippocampal slices (Xiong et al., 1999a, 199b) exposed to secretory products from both HIV-1-infected and immune-activated MDM. MK 801, an N-methyl D-aspartate receptor antagonist, partially blocked HIV-1-infected and immune-activated MDM-mediated neuronal injury (Jiang et al., 2001; Xiong et al., 2003; Zheng et al., 2001b). These data support a primary role for immune activation and HIV-1 infection in MP-mediated neuronal dysfunction.

Reseeding of the brain by HIV-1 late in the disease, with profound infiltration of MP into the CNS, likely heralds an expansion in viral load with subsequent immunologic activation. Nevertheless, there is no correlation between the quantity of HIV gene expression in the brain and the degree of neurological impairment. Inherent changes in both the secretory and migratory capabilities of macrophages in the periphery and the brain allow such processes to continue unabated as HIV disease progresses (Anderson et al., 2002; Boven et al., 2000).

In support of this theory, recent works demonstrate the emergence of specific monocyte subsets in patients with HAND. CD14/CD16- and CD14/CD69-positive monocytes may exhibit enhanced migratory and neurotoxic potential (Fischer-Smith et al., 2001; Pulliam et al., 1997; Williams et al., 2001), making these monocyte subsets crucial to disease pathogenesis. Evidence, supported by enhanced monocyte trafficking during late-stage HIV disease, underscores the potential importance of peripheral immune activity in HAND pathogenesis (Fischer-Smith et al., 2004). Chung and colleagues (Chung et al., 2002) have demonstrated that potassium channels, expressed in macrophages, are vital for MP movement through the BBB and that monocyte/macrophage migration could be inhibited by voltage- and calcium-activated potassium channel blockers. Thus, alterations in cell volume, differentiation, and shape represent pivotal factors in macrophage migration into and throughout the nervous system and may be affected by the immune environment occurring during progressive HIVE/HAND. Multiple ionic macrophage signaling responses are mediated by both CCR5 and CXCR4 upon activation by HIV-1 gp120 (Liu et al., 2000). Upregulation of soluble markers of MP activation within the plasma of infected patients with cognitive dysfunction and brain atrophy further supports the importance of peripheral monocyte activation in cell trafficking and for HAND pathogenesis (Ryan et al., 2001).

HIV TARGET CELLS WITHIN THE NERVOUS SYSTEM

Mononuclear Phagocytes

MP are the principal target cells for HIV infection in the brain and are a significant source of neurotoxins during disease (Gabuzda et al., 1986; Genis et al., 1992; Koenig et al., 1986). However, under steady-state conditions, MP function to eliminate microbial pathogens and other foreign material via phagocytosis and intracellular killing, as well as adaptive immune mechanisms. MP serve an important innate immune function through the secretion of their trophic factors, such as brain-derived neurotrophic factor, nerve growth factor, neurotrophin-3, glial-derived neurotrophic factor, and basic fibroblast growth factor (Batchelor et al., 1999; Caroleo et al., 2001; Elkabes et al., 1996; Heese et al., 1998; Kullander et al., 1997; Lazarov-Spiegler et al., 1998b, 1996; Rapalino et al., 1998; Zeev-Brann et al., 1998; Zheng et al., 2001a), required for tissue homeostasis. In the brain, macrophages nurture neural cells by secreting neurotrophins, thereby providing the necessary environment for neurons to function normally and thrive (Gendelman and Folks, 1999). The normal innate immune function of MP has been exploited to therapeutic advantage in neurodegenerative disorders (Rapalino et al., 1998); however, it remains unclear how the macrophage evolves from a neurotrophic cell to a neurotoxic cell.

Specific signaling pathways may arise following MP immune activation, which can regulate protective or destructive innate immune function of macrophages (Shibata et al., 2003). Viral infection and immune activation of MP could serve to change a protective cell into a destructive one, leading to neuronal injury and ultimately cell death. Perturbations in cell signaling pathways may underlie such molecular events. Neurotrophins engage Trk receptors, which are expressed on neural cells, thereby activating signaling pathways by phosphorylation of cytoplasmic tyrosine residues. Trk receptors convert Ras to an active conformation inducing the microtubule-associated protein kinase cascade (ERK1/2), which is involved in cellular transcription and growth (Segal and Greenberg, 1996; Shi et al., 1996; Soontornniyomkij et al., 1998; Zheng et al., 2001b). Interactions between neurotrophins and Trk receptors affect cell survival, differentiation, axon and dendrite patterning and growth, and expression of ion channels and neurotransmitters (Huang and Reichardt, 2003).

Microglia represent up to 10% of the parenchymal brain cell population in some regions. Three distinct MP are found in the brain parenchyma, ramified "resting" microglia, activated "amoeboid" microglia, and perivascular macrophages, all of which are targets for virus. Neighboring elliptical microglia contact each other in series and in parallel, forming a neural network. Unlike microglia, parenchymal and perivascular macrophages usually present an amoeboid appearance, and in morphology and function these cells more closely resemble tissue macrophages found in other organs. Recent studies by several groups support the idea that the perivascular macrophages are preferentially infected, thereby posing the greatest threat as vehicles of dissemination of virus and sources of neurotoxic activities (Pulliam et al., 1997; Rappaport et al., 2001; Williams et al., 2001; Williams and Hickey, 2002; Fisher-Smith et al., 2008).

T cells expressing the CD40 ligand (soluble and bound forms) can activate both infected and noninfected monocytes that express TNF-α CD40 receptors. The decline in CD4⁺ T lymphocytes allows macrophages to express a metabolically active, tissue-destructive phenotype. Another proposed mechanism relies on the fact that proinflammatory cytokines can trigger the activation of monocytes independent of lymphocytes. Indeed, late-stage HIV-1 patients with dementia show elevated serum TNF receptors (Ryan et al., 2001). The above examples illustrate the fact that multiple mechanisms have been proposed for the initiation of brain inflammatory responses during HAND (Anderson et al., 2002; Cotter et al., 2002; Zheng and Gendelman, 1997). Brain macrophages, when activated, secrete a variety of neurotoxic immune and viral factors. Changes in macrophage immunity lead to gp120-mediated cell fusion, MNGC formation, disruption of neuronal homeostasis, and ultimately to disease. It should be noted that the role of macrophages in disease pathogenesis and persistence is not limited to the CNS, as submucosal macrophages in the gut and cervix are thought to be the first cells infected by virus (Zhu et al., 1996). It is likely that memory CD4⁺ T lymphocytes sustain the viral population throughout the course of disease, as these cells become HIV-1 positive 6 h after viral exposure (Gupta et al., 2002) and may be a common link for viral dissemination in the lymph nodes and inevitably to the brain.

Astrocytes

In prior years, astrocytes were believed to lack functional excitability, having no role in signal integration, and to exist solely as supporters of nerve cell structure and function. Certainly, during steady-state conditions, astrocytes contribute to the structural scaffolding of both neurons and glia and participate in neuronal sustenance (Haydon, 2001). Astrocytes have been demonstrated to participate in synaptic integration by releasing glutamate through calcium-regulated exocytosis-like processes which may follow activation of CXCR4 by SDF-1 (Bezzi et al., 2001). Altered glutamate transport, such as the release of excessive glutamate resulting in inhibition of glutamate uptake coupled with enhanced glutamate secretion, results in neuronal injury. Such events may lead to neuronal excitotoxicity and apoptosis (Bezzi et al., 2001). By virtue of their status as the most abundant cell type in the CNS, their homeostatic functions, and their close juxtaposition to neurons, astrocytes may play a very prominent role in disease. After exposure of astrocytes to TNF-α, IL-1β, and/or phorbol esters, latent infection may become reactivated (Tornatore et al., 1994). HIV may gain sanctuary, protecting the virus against antiretroviral therapy in astrocytes, but this is only speculation.

Fas ligand (FasL) may play a role in neurotoxicity occurring as a consequence of HAND, as it is significantly up-regulated on astrocytes after exposure to TNF-α, IL-1β, and IL-6 (Ghorpade et al., 2003). However, the magnitude and relative role of FasL, compared to other neurotoxic pathways in human disease, are not yet known. Indeed, increased FasL expression has been observed in lymphocytes, monocytes, and cerebrospinal fluid (CSF) in HIV-1-infected patients, but it is not yet known whether FasL-mediated neurotoxicity is part of the pathogenic process of neural damage during HIVE/HAND (Ghorpade and Gendelman, 2003). Secretion of other soluble neurotoxic factors by astrocytes can lead to paracrine neuroimmune activation, an up-regulation of apoptotic factors such as Fas and FasL, and, ultimately, increased neuronal cell death by distinct mechanisms.

Astrocytes, while infected at a restricted level, may serve as a reservoir for HIV within the CNS and may be capable of transfer of infection to MP (Brack-Werner, 1999; Eugenin and Berman, 2007). Recently, studies using laser capture microdissection have shown astrocytes with HIV-1 DNA (Thompson et al., 2004; Trillo-Pazos et al., 2003). Astrocyte infection by HIV is CD4 and CXCR4 independent (Sabri et al., 1999). It is not known, however, whether alterations in astrocyte phenotype and function are beneficial or detrimental in regards to neuronal function. Cumulative excitotoxic effects perpetuated by activated astrocytes may substantially increase the amount of neuronal damage caused by HIV infection. Production of chemokines such as MCP-1 by endothelial cells and astrocytes affects the migration of leukocytes across the BBB, playing a critical role in HAND pathogenesis. MCP-1, a chemoattractant produced mainly by astrocytes, clearly accelerates monocyte entry into the brain and may be induced after glial exposure to cellular (TNF-α, gamma interferon, and IL-1β) and/ or viral (for example Tat) neurotoxins (Weiss et al., 1998). Astrocytes can affect the BBB by altering its permeability. In the normal brain, astrocytes produce tissue inhibitors of metalloproteinases and stabilize barrier integrity, thereby promoting normal function. In comparison, astrocytes in the diseased brain have down-regulated tissue inhibitor of matrix metalloproteinase 1, allowing an increased concentration of matrix metalloproteinases. Such processes provide clues on how BBB disruption can occur in the later stages of viral infection and disease (Suryadevara et al., 2003).

BBB

Under steady-state conditions, the BBB serves to regulate passage of immune cells and immune products. Brain microvasculature endothelial cells (BMVEC), connected to each other by a series of tight junctions, are involved in cell trafficking and molecule transport between the CNS and the bloodstream. HIV bypasses the regulatory functions of the BBB and enters the brain early after viral exposure (Kramer-Hammerle et al., 2005; Price, 1993). In experimental simian immunodeficiency virus infection, viral entry into the brain occurs a few days to a few weeks after viral inoculation (Chakrabarti et al., 1991; Davis et al., 1992; Lackner et al., 1994). Cell-mediated (NK and HIV-1-specific antiviral cytotoxic lymphocytes) and humoral immune responses, induced in the early stages of the disease, appear to curb HIV-1 infection. Only after years of progressive viral infection, often coupled with profound immunosuppression, does development of clinical neurological disease take place (Price, 2000), suggesting viral replication is necessary, but not sufficient, to induce clinical neurological injury. The mechanism by which the virus actually enters the brain is not exactly defined, and several possibilities exist, including the idea that free virus infects the brain endothelial cells or that virus gains entry to the CNS directly with infecting intermediate cells. Alternatively, the virus is carried into the brain through infected and immunoactivated leukocytes (Albright et al., 2003; Williams and Hickey, 2002). While most patients with HAND and advanced immunosuppression have high levels of virus in their brains (Achim et al., 1994; Wiley and Achim, 1994), there is no correlation between the presence or severity of neurologic disease and the absolute levels of virus in the brain or CSF (Kure et al.,

1990; Wiley and Achim, 1994). This suggests that viral and cellular factors amplify the production of one another, playing prominent roles in the disease onset and progression. Additionally, there remains still no clear explanation as to why only a subset of patients develop HAND and others remain unaffected. This may revolve around host or viral factors or a combination of both. Neuroimmune activation is likely precipitated by virus replication occurring in the face of a profound CD4+ T-cell depletion (Garden, 2002; Nishimura et al., 2005). Transendothelial migration of monocytes may be instigated by similar processes, and in some individuals, this migration may be affected by the secretory activities of activated brain macrophages.

Changes to the BBB can occur because of HIV-1 invasion and cytokines such as TNF-α and IL-1β, viral proteins including Tat and gp120, as well as contact with HIV-1-infected macrophages (Persidsky et al., 1999), and these changes can lead to activation of BMVEC. Activation can allow cells carrying virus to cross the BBB, infecting other cells such as microglia. During the disease, disruption of the BBB occurs through the up-regulation of adhesion molecules on the surface of BMVEC (Nottet et al., 1996), helping to allow macrophage infiltration into the brain, as well as altering the cell morphology of the BBB and permitting entry of normally excluded cells and immune factors. Increased expression of intercellular adhesion molecule 1 and vascular cell adhesion molecule, among others, as a consequence of brain inflammation instigates the passage of monocytes into the brain parenchyma (Nottet et al., 1996). BMVEC can be stimulated by the viral proteins such as Tat to produce MCP-1 (Toborek et al., 2003) and up-regulate IL-8, for attraction of lymphocytes into the brain (Hofman et al., 1999). Despite considerable immune activation occurring during advanced HIV-1 infection throughout most of the course of viral infection, disruption of the BBB remains minimal and it is only very late in the disease that the BBB integrity and function break down.

A prominent neuropathological finding with HIV infection is perivascular infiltration of monocytes across the BBB (Price et al., 1998). Postmortem studies of HIVE patients have revealed that the integrity of the BBB was damaged, as demonstrated by fibrinogen leakage (Petito and Cash, 1992). Other studies conclude that tight junction disruption, fibrinogen leakage, accumulation of HIV-1-infected brain macrophages, and astrocytosis also contribute to disrupting the integrity of the BBB (Dallasta et al., 1999; Maclean et al., 2005). A likely scenario involves the "priming" of macrophages by viral infection, thereby lowering the signaling threshold necessary for activation (Genis et al., 1992; Nottet et al., 1995) and facilitating BBB migration. Indeed, MP activation results in BBB impairment, not only in the secretion of cytokines and chemokines, but also in the up-regulation of adhesion molecules, which facilitate cell trafficking into the brain (Nottet et al., 1996). In one recent study, antibodies to intercellular adhesion molecule 1, integrin very late antigen-4 (VLA-4), and MCP-1 demonstrated significant monocyte migration across the BBB (Seguin et al., 2003).

Cells become targets for viral infection upon entry into tissue and differentiation into macrophages. Undifferentiated peripheral monocytes are infected at low frequency and are present in the circulation for limited time periods usually measured in hours for lentiviral infections (Gendelman and Gendelman, 1992; Gendelman et al., 1984, 1985, 1986). MDM or CD4+ T lymphocytes carry virus into the brain during disease. Free progeny virus can cross the BBB, infecting MDM in the perivascular space. Endothelial activation during progressive HIV-1 infection has been postulated to allow migration of MDM into the CNS, and this may be accomplished through the ability of HIV-1 gp120 to induce viral adsorptive endocytosis and transcytosis in brain endothelia. During disease, a principal component for how virus-infected monocytes and macrophages penetrate the BBB is the ability of these cells to change shape and volume. The ability of cells to swell and then restore their cell volume toward normal upon exposure to hyposmicity is achieved by the efflux of potassium and chloride channels with consequent loss of water. Such ion channels appear to be regulated by immune activation and viral infection, facilitating the movement of infected cells across the BBB in disease.

CHEMOKINES: AN OVERVIEW

"Chemotactic cytokines," or chemokines, are a large family of small (8- to 10-kDa), structurally related proteins that affect numerous biological functions and are produced by a variety of different cell types including blood leukocytes, endothelial cells, glia, and neurons. They help to regulate the migration, recruitment, accumulation, and activation of leukocytes (Wu et al., 2000) and are copiously produced in all tissues including the brain (Kutsch et al., 2000). The regulation of chemokines is affected by a plethora of environmental cues including bacterial lipopolysaccharide, proinflammatory cytokines, and viruses. Chemokines are classified into four families based on the number and relative positions of the N-terminal-conserved cysteine residues (Richard et al., 2002; Shields and Adams, 2002). They consist of 92 to 125 amino acids with four conserved cysteines linked by disulfide bonds. Four subfamilies are designated CC, CXC, C, and CX3C. The prefix CC designates the chemokines with two adjacent cysteines, while CXC designates chemokines containing two cysteines separated by one amino acid. The human chemokine genes are clustered on chromosomes 4 (CXC chemokines) and 17 (CC chemokines). The CXC chemokines include IL-8, melanoma growth stimulatory activity (MGSA), inducible protein 10 (IP-10), and SDF-1. The CC class includes RANTES, MCP-1, and macrophage inflammatory protein (MIP)-1α,β. Fractalkine (FKN) is part of the CX3C group. The group of C chemokines includes lymphotactin.

Since the initial identification of the first chemokine, IL-8, over 15 years ago, over 40 chemokines have now been identified (Shields and Adams, 2002). Chemokines are part of a large family of molecules with important physiologic functions ranging from cell development and growth to angiogenesis and neoplasia, cellular migration, inflammation, and interactions with microglial pathogens (Baggiolini et al., 1997). Each of the chemokines recognizes a particular subset of leukocytes. IL-8 and MGSA attract neutrophils (Rajagopalan and Rajarathnam, 2004), SDF-1 and IP-10 attract T lymphocytes (Poggi et al., 2004), eotaxin attracts eosinophils (Yamamoto et al., 2005), and RANTES and MCP-1 attract T cells and monocytes (Schall and Bacon, 1994). Many chemokines are found in the CNS (Table 1). Target cells are acted on by chemokines binding to cell surface chemokine receptors. Chemokine receptors are a family of seven transmembrane G-protein-coupled receptors and are also divided into four groups: α-chemokine receptors (such as CXCR2 and CXCR4); β-chemokine receptors (such as CCR5, CCR4, CCR3, and CCR2); γ-chemokine receptor (XCR1); and δ-chemokine receptors (CX3CR1) (Gabuzda et al., 1998; Hesselgesser and Horuk, 1999; Klein et al., 1999; Miller and Meucci, 1999; van der Meer et al., 2000). These receptors belong to the superfamily of receptors which signal through the GTP-binding, seven-transmembrane proteins (Baggiolini et al., 1997).

There are four classification groups of chemokine receptors: shared, specific, promiscuous, and viral (Premack and Schall, 1996); these receptors interact with a broad range of ligands belonging to a specific chemokine subfamily (shared

TABLE 1 Chemokines and their receptors in the brain

Cell type	Chemokines	Receptors	References
Monocytes/ macrophages	CCL2/MCP-1, CCL3/MIP-1α, CCL4/MIP-1β, CCL5/RANTES, CXCL8/IL-8, CXCL10/IP-10	CCR2, CCR3, CCR4, CCR5, CXCR4, CX3CR1, CXCR3	Bernasconi et al., 1996; Cinque et al., 1998; Kelder et al., 1998; Coleman and Flood, 1987; Gabuzda et al., 2002; Cartier et al., 2005; Rappert et al., 2004
Microglia	CCL15/HCC-2, CCL23/MPIF-1, CCL4/MIP-1β, CCL5/RANTES, CCL8/MCP-2, CXCL6/GCP-2, CXCL12/SDF-1, CX3CL1/FKN	CCR1, CCR2, CCR3, CCR5, CXCR1, CXCR4, CX3CR1	Kalehua et al., 2004; Bernasconi et al., 1996; Cinque et al., 1998; Kelder et al., 1998; Joly and Pinto, 2005; Chen et al., 2005; Cartier et al., 2005
Astrocytes	CCL5/RANTES, CCL2/MCP-1, CCL8/MCP-2, CCL15/HCC-2, CCL22/MDC, CCL20/MIP-3α, CCL28MEC, CXCL6/GCP-2, CXCL2/Gro-β, CXCL12/SDF-1, CX3CL1/FKN	CCR1, CCR2, CCR3, CCR4, CCR5, CCR6, CCR10, CXCR1, CXCR2, CXCR4, CX3CR1	Cartier et al., 2005; Conant et al., 1998; Dorf et al., 2000; Kalehua et al., 2004; El-Hage et al., 2005
Neurons	CCL3/MIP-1α, CCL15/HCC-2, CCL8/MCP-2, CXCL1/Gro-α, CXCL3/Gro-γ, CXCL12/SDF-1	CCR1, CCR2, CCR3, CCR5, CXCR1, CXCR2, CXCR4, CXCR5	Cartier et al., 2005; Coughlan et al., 2000; Bajetto et al., 2002
Endothelium	CCL23/MPIF-1, CCL15/HCC-2, CCL3/MIP-1α, CCL22/MDC, CCL5/RANTES, CCL8/MCP-2, CXCL12/SDF-1	CCR1, CCR2, CCR3, CCR4, CCR5, CXCR4	Cartier et al., 2005; Dzenko et al., 2005

group). Conversely, one chemokine can interact with several receptors. Cytomegalovirus US28 (Randolph-Habecker et al., 2002) and herpesvirus saimiri (ECRF3) (Rosenkilde et al., 2004) both encode chemokine receptors.

CHEMOKINES AND HIV CORECEPTORS

Fusion between certain amino acids of HIV-1 gp41 and the plasma membrane of $CD4^+$ T lymphocytes allows entry of HIV-1 after interactions with CD4 and a coreceptor (Miyauchi et al., 2005). Studies show that the β-chemokines, RANTES, MIP-1α, and MIP-1β can block viral infectivity mediated by macrophage-tropic (M-tropic) viruses in vitro (Cocchi et al., 1995). This observation prompted further research into identifying the viral coreceptor. CXCR4, originally named Fusin or Lestr, with the biological function to bind SDF-1 (Bleul et al., 1996a, 1996b; Chen et al., 2005; Oberlin et al., 1996), was demonstrated to block the entry of T-cell-tropic (T-tropic) strains (Feng et al., 1996; Gorry et al., 2005). To date, all HIV strains studied use chemokine receptors for viral entry (Berger and Major, 1999; Edinger et al., 1999). There is a genetic polymorphism in the V3 loop of the HIV envelope glycoprotein gp120 which determines whether the CCR5, CXCR4, or CXCR3 coreceptor is used and, thus, the type of host cell preferentially infected (Yamaguchi-Kabata et al., 2004).

The definition of HIV as a neurovirulent, neuroinvasive, or neurotropic virus has received much attention (Gendelman et al., 2005). One issue revolves around the ability to separate M-tropic from neurotropic signatures (Gabuzda and Wang, 1999; Lipton and Gendelman, 1995). This has received much attention in recent years. Indeed, M-tropic virus contributes to disease pathogenesis and can be isolated from brain tissue throughout HIV disease (Brew et al., 1990, 1996a, 1996b; Brew and Miller, 1996; Gray et al., 2005). M-tropic isolates replicate well in cultured human microglia from both adult and fetal tissue (Ghorpade et al., 1998a; Strizki et al., 1996), inducing neurotoxic responses and proinflammatory cytokine production (Genis et al., 1992; Kedzierska and Crowe, 2002). Nonetheless, HIV isolates that propagate in MDM also infect microglia. Molecular analysis of the HIV-1 envelope revealed that determinants for MDM and microglial tropism mapped to identical regions of the genome, consistent with the concept of dual tropism (Sharpless et al., 1992). This tropism is largely determined by the V3 hypervariable region of HIV-1 gp120. The V3 hypervariable region function is associated with the post-CD4 binding interactions including proteolytic cleavage and fusion and coreceptor usage and viral infection, rather than the HIV-1 gp120-CD4 requirement (Dong et al., 2005).

Using V3 loop sequences for determining tropism has been controversial. Residues thought to be critical for neurovirulence were also found in the majority of nondemented patients (Reddy et al., 1996). Neuroinvasiveness, associated with the proline determinant at position 305, was absent in brain-derived isolates (Di Stefano et al., 1996). Phylogenetic studies of the V3 envelope of strains derived from all brain regions indicate that there is independent regional evolution of HIV quasispecies after crossing into the brain, with some sequences more associated with regional neuropathology (Chang et al., 1998; Di Stefano et al., 1996). These quasispecies maintain replicative homeostasis that drives expansion and generates escape mutations. In addition to the V3 region, the V1/V2 regions may contribute to neuroinvasiveness either independently or in concert.

MDM and microglial pathways for viral infection are similar if not identical. CD4 is expressed by microglia, as well as a number of chemokine receptors including CCR5, CCR3, and CXCR4 (Cartier et al., 2005; Lavi et al., 1997; Vallat et al., 1998), but microglia are most susceptible to infection by R5 (M-tropic) viruses (Gorry et al., 2005; Lavi et al., 1997; Shieh et al., 1998). Qualitative differences between MDM and microglia for the use of chemokine receptors may exist, as evidenced by experiments showing lack of HIV inhibition by monoclonal antibodies to CCR5 and CCR3 and suggesting that additional coreceptors may also be used by microglia (Ghorpade et al., 1998b). A lack of strong up-regulation of CCR4 and CCR5 chemokine receptors on macrophages, in response to transforming growth factor alpha, also suggests that other coreceptors may be used (Flynn et al., 2003). Chemokine receptor expression by brain macrophages and microglia may influence viral evolution within the brain reservoir, leading to neurovirulence, but M-tropic strains alone may not be sufficient to cause clinical neurologic impairment. It is now generally accepted that HIV is neuroinvasive rather than neurotropic or neurovirulent, since the principal target cell in brain remains the MP.

However, M-tropic viruses are not the only strains that can be found in diseased brain tissue. The biology of HIV-1 T-cell interactions is thus relevant and important for both peripheral disease and ongoing disease in brain. T-tropic strains are associated with the α-chemokine receptor CXCR4, but T cells may be infected by either M- or T-tropic strains (Holm and Gabuzda, 2005). A proapoptotic response may be induced by interactions of ENV with CXCR4 on uninfected T cells and may lead to their destruction.

The importance of CCR5 for HIV-1 transmission was underscored by the observation that certain individuals who had been repeatedly exposed to HIV-1, but remained uninfected, have a defect for CCR5 expression (Liu et al., 1996a). $CD4^+$ T lymphocytes from these individuals were highly resistant to in vitro infection by primary macrophage-tropic HIV but were easily infected with viruses adapted to grow in transformed T-cell lines (Liu et al., 1996a). These noninfectable individuals were found to be homozygous for a defective CCR5 allele containing an internal 32-bp deletion (CCR5 Δ32) resulting in a truncated protein that is apparently not expressed on the cell surface. CCR5 Δ32 homozygous individuals comprise 1% of the Caucasian population, while heterozygous individuals comprise 20%. Heterozygous individuals for the deletion have been shown to progress more slowly to AIDS than wild-type homozygous individuals, suggesting that CCR5 expression may be altered in these individuals, thereby directly affecting HIV-1 replication in vivo. Recently, CCR5 Δ32 frequency was found to be higher in an exposed seronegative population (Liu et al., 2004). The effect of HIV resistance due to CCR5 Δ32 may be influenced more by gene dosage, homozygosity versus heterozygosity, than by receptor sequestration (Venkatesan et al., 2002). Additional mutations associated with HIV resistance include chemokine receptor CCR2b, the ligand SDF-1, and the copy number of the CCL3L1 gene (Smith, 1991; Smith and Hale, 1997; Winkler et al., 1998; Arenzana-Seisedos and Partmentier, 2006).

At least nine other chemokine receptors, or structurally related molecules, have been described as supporting HIV-1 envelope-mediated membrane fusion or viral entry in vitro. These include CCR2b (Doranz et al., 1996), CCR3 (Bazan et al., 1998), BOB/GPR15 (Farzan et al., 1997a, 1997b), BONZO/STRL33/TYMSTR (Farzan et al., 1997a, 1997b), GPR1 (Farzan et al., 1997a, 1997b), CCR8 (Horuk et al., 1998),

V28/CX3CR1 (Rucker et al., 1997), and APJ (Choe et al., 1998a, 1998b). Comparisons of coreceptor usage by primary HIV-1 isolates of several genetic subtypes reveal that most HIV strains use CCR5 or CXCR4 efficiently (Dooms et al., 2000).

CHEMOKINES AND CELL TRAFFICKING

Chemokines appear to be key regulators of monocyte recruitment during HAND. Endothelial cells, microglia, and astrocytes are major cellular sources of β-chemokines (for example, MCP-1) in the CNS during HIVE, setting up an inflammatory chemoattractant gradient. β-Chemokines bind to chemokine receptors on monocytes and regulate cell transendothelial migration into the brain. FKN, a brain chemokine expressed by neurons, astrocytes, and endothelial cells (Cotter et al., 2002; Tong et al., 2000), can promote adhesion and migration of leukocytes across the BBB (Imai et al., 1999; Tong et al., 2000). It is likely that endothelial membrane bound FKN also plays a role in the recruitment of monocytes into the brain (Ancuta et al., 2004).

Questions remain about how HIV-1-infected MDM enter the brain including the following: (i) the exact identification and relative abundance of chemokines produced by macrophages, astrocytes, and other inflammatory cells; (ii) the pathobiological conditions under which chemokines are produced; (iii) paracrine and autocrine regulation of chemokines and proinflammatory cytokines in microglia, astrocytes, endothelial cells, and neurons; and (iv) the role of chemokines in glial activation and HIVE.

Infected monocytes, macrophages, and perhaps CD4+ T lymphocytes act as vehicles through which virus enters the brain. Microglia and astrocytes produce chemokines and control monocyte migration across the BBB (Persidsky et al., 1999). Activated microglia, and to a lesser extent astrocytes, express major histocompatibility complex class I and II antigens and adhesion molecules and secrete cytokines and reactive oxygen intermediates. All are shown to be important factors contributing to HAND (Lipton and Gendelman, 1995). Although the event(s) triggering monocyte invasion into the nervous system remains unknown, it likely involves the secretion of macrophage-attractant chemokines and the up-regulation of adhesion molecules on activated endothelial and immune cells. Proinflammatory factors induce α and β chemokines (such as IL-8, interferon-γ [IFN-γ], IP-10, growth-related oncogene α, MIP-1α, MIP-1β, RANTES, and MCP-1) found in infected brain tissue and may also participate directly in the disease process. Virus and activated macrophage entry into the brain is likely precipitated by BBB damage heralded by activation of brain MP. Neuronal damages, as well as alterations in the integrity of tight junctions and/or regulation of macrophage immune function, occur as consequences of viral and cellular secretory products and are crucial to HIV-1 brain transport.

BMVEC secrete a variety of chemokines upon stimulation by the proinflammatory cytokines including MCP-1, MIP-1α, RANTES, MGSA, IP-10, monokine induced by IFN-γ (MIG), and FKN or neurotactin. These cells also express CXCR4 and CCR5, which may change dependent on the cytokine environment. For example, proinflammatory cytokines up-regulate chemokines and their receptors by endothelial cells, facilitating the entry of HIV into the brain. Leukocyte migration from the blood to the brain is a complex process involving rolling, tight adhesion and transendothelial migration. The stage of brain endothelial cell activation, as well as interactions with cellular factors produced as a consequence of leukocyte secretory activities, regulates how monocytes and some lymphocytes enter the brain parenchyma during disease.

CHEMOKINES AND NEUROGENESIS

Chemokines and their link to neurogenesis are a relatively new area of research. Direct migration, proliferation, and differentiation are steps suggested to be involved in neurogenesis (Fallon et al., 2000). SDF-1 has been suggested to play a role in neural progenitor cell (NPC) migration and has been found to be up-regulated in the cortex, thalamus, and hippocampus during a 2-week postnatal period (Tham et al., 2001). Studies of the neural migration and progenitor cell migration in the hippocampus, dentate gyrus, and cerebral cortex seem to implicate the interaction between SDF-1 and CXCR4 (Lu et al., 2002; Liapi et al., 2008). Deletion of genes for either CXCR4, the receptor for SDF-1, or SDF-1 is embryonically lethal in mice, and embryonic mouse brains from CXCR4 homozygous mutant mice were examined and found to have cerebellar morphology abnormalities (Lu et al., 2002). Other chemokines and chemokines thought to be involved in neurogenesis include the CCR3 receptor, implicated in inhibition of NPC proliferation, and FKN for survival promotion of NPCs. Evidence also suggests that inhibition of neurogenesis may be linked to inflammatory chemokine production (Krathwohl and Kaiser, 2004). Understanding how chemokines influence neurogenesis will lead to better understanding of how neural repair and neurogenesis are affected by inflammation in diseases such as HAND (Zheng et al., 2005).

CHEMOKINES AND NEURONAL AND GLIAL FUNCTION

A number of α-chemokine receptors are expressed on leukocytes, astrocytes, and neurons. For example, CXCR4 is found on neurons, microglia, and astrocytes (Albright et al., 1999; Banisadr et al., 2000; Broder and Collman, 1997; Coughlan et al., 2000; Endres et al., 1996; Ghorpade et al., 1998b; He et al., 1997; Horuk et al., 1997; Lavi et al., 1997; Luster, 1998; Mackay, 1996; Vallat et al., 1998; Flynn et al., 2003) and has been shown to play a substantive role in receptor-mediated apoptosis and cell function (Hesselgesser et al., 1998b; Khan et al., 2004; Zheng et al., 1999a, 1999b; Zou et al., 1998; Babcock et al., 2003). Neurons also express CXCR2 (Chen et al., 2005; Coughlan et al., 2000; Horuk et al., 1997) and CXCR5 (Kouba et al., 1993). CXCR2 and CXCR4 are expressed diffusely throughout the cell (Coughlan et al., 2000). Preliminary data, from others and our laboratory, suggest that CXCR5 is expressed predominantly on human neuronal dendrites and is also expressed at low levels of microglia and astrocytes (Flynn et al., 2003).

As HIV-1 gp120 can instigate signal transduction by binding to chemokine receptors (Davis et al., 1997; Guntermann et al., 1999; Weissman et al., 1997; Tran et al., 2005), the identification of neuronal chemokines is linked to tissue homeostasis and disease. Virion or endogenous ligand activation of neuron-expressed chemokine receptors may alter intracellular signaling events and cause apoptosis (Ohagen et al., 1999; Zheng et al., 1999b; Kaul et al., 2004). Ligands that stimulate neuron-expressed CXCR4, including HIV-1 gp120 and SDF-1α, can elicit both neuronal dysfunction and apoptosis (Hesselgesser et al., 1998a; Khan et al., 2004; Pandey and Bolsover, 2000; Sanders et al., 2000; Zheng et al., 1998, 1999b).

Activated MP secrete β-chemokines (Conant et al., 1998; Cotter et al., 2001; Cotter et al., 1999; Desbaillets et al., 1994; Kelder et al., 1998; Kornbluth et al., 1998; McManus et al., 2000; Persidsky, 1999), and receptors for β-chemokines include CCR2, CCR3, CCR4, CCR5, and CCR8. Macrophages and microglia express CCR3 and CCR5 (Albright et al., 1999; Ghorpade et al., 1998b; He et al., 1997; Lavi et al., 1997; Vallat et al., 1998; Brandimarti et al., 2004) and affect the regulation of HIV-1 infection (Cotter et al., 2001; Kitai et al., 2000). Unlike α-chemokine receptors, the major expression of β-chemokine receptors in the brain has been reported in macrophages, microglia, and astrocytes. Differential utilization of CCR5 and CXCR4 by brain X4, R5, and R5X4 viruses for macrophages and microglia infection has been suggested to underlie neurovirulence of HIV-1 and induce disease (Yi et al., 2005; Dunfee et al., 2006; Gorry et al., 2002).

Altogether, the importance of chemokine receptors in HIV neuropathogenesis was brought to the forefront when these receptors were found to be expressed on neurons. Most brain cells express chemokine receptors, and the interactions of virus with these receptors may initiate apoptotic death of neurons. The CXCR4 receptor, depending on the ligand bound to it, can respond in either an apoptotic or an antiapoptotic way (Khan et al., 2004), and this outcome may be modified by chemokines acting at the same receptors. Chemokine receptor expression on neurons suggests that these molecules affect neuronal homeostatic function (Miller and Meucci, 1999; Krathwohl and Kaiser, 2004). Cultured human fetal neurons express CXCR2, CXCR4, CCR1, and CCR5 (Hesselgesser et al., 1997), whereas human neural precursor cells show a high level of expression of CXCR4 (Ni et al., 2004). This receptor expression presents a scenario in which HIV-1 could damage neurons directly, although HIV-1 does not infect neurons. HIV-1 gp120 may bind CXCR4, initiating signal transduction pathway(s), leading to cellular dysfunction or apoptosis (Hesselgesser et al., 1998b; Zheng et al., 1999a, 1999b, 1999c; Mattson et al., 2005). HIV-1 gp120-induced damage can be inhibited by chemokine receptor agonists (Miller, 2005). Resultant neuronal damage may then elicit the secretion of brain-derived chemokines to recruit macrophages to the site of injury (Cartier et al., 2005; Cotter et al., 2002; Erichsen et al., 2003). In this way, the neurons themselves serve as a means to perpetuate the damage brought about by macrophage-produced neurotoxins.

SDF-1α and FKN are constitutively produced in the brain and are likely to play an important role in CNS homeostasis, whereas other chemokines, such as MIP-1α, MIP-1β, MCP-1, and RANTES, are induced by inflammatory stimuli. In neurodegenerative diseases with an inflammatory component, such as Alzheimer's disease, stroke, and HAND, these chemokines are likely to be involved in the pathogenesis (Letendre et al., 1999; Minami and Satoh, 2000; Sanders et al., 1998).

Astrocytes do express several receptors linked to HIV infection including CCR5, CCR3, and CXCR4 (Boutet et al., 2001; Schweighardt et al., 2001); however, expression of these receptors is not linked to viral infection. Astrocytes produce a number of chemokines including IL-8, MCP-1, RANTES, and IL-10 in response to the proinflammatory cytokines IFN-γ, IL-1β, and TNF-α (Croitoru-Lamoury et al., 2003; Hesselgesser and Horuk, 1999), which may affect disease pathogenesis. HIV-infected peripheral blood lymphocytes and monocytes can be attracted to the brain by these chemokines, and viral gene products, such as Tat, and astrocyte MCP-1 production may also facilitate monocyte transmigration across the BBB (Chauhan et al., 2003)

by increasing the permeability of the BBB (Stamatovic et al., 2005). During HAND, MP, astrocytes, and/or neurons produce high levels of chemokines that affect cell migration, neural signaling, and apoptosis and incite cascades of neuroinflammatory reactions regulating viral replication (Albright et al., 1999; Broder and Collman, 1997; Cotter et al., 2001; Endres et al., 1996; Ghorpade et al., 1998b; He et al., 1997; Kitai et al., 2000; Lavi et al., 1997; Luster, 1998; Mackay, 1996; Shieh et al., 1998; Vallat et al., 1998; Vicenzi et al., 2000; Zheng et al., 1999a; Liu et al., 1996b). Brain MP, astrocytes, and neurons may also directly participate as effector cells in disease pathogenesis independent of peripheral immune responses. Alpha- and β-chemokines, such as IL-8, IP-10, growth-related oncogene α, MIP-1α, MIP-1β, RANTES, and MCP-1, are produced in infected brain tissue by HIV-1-infected and immunoactivated MP and astrocytes (Conant et al., 1998; Cotter et al., 1999; Desbaillets et al., 1994; Kornbluth et al., 1998; Persidsky, 1999). Neuronal injury, induced by HIV-1 viral proteins or cytokines, may itself trigger chemokine secretion, which may serve as a damage signal to recruit macrophages and microglia to the site of injury, serving to stimulate brain inflammation independent of peripheral immune responses (Fig. 1) (Cotter et al., 2002; Erichsen et al., 2003; Jung et al., 2000; Tong et al., 2000; Zheng et al., 2001b; Zujovic et al., 2000).

CX3CR1, a recently discovered receptor, is highly expressed on neurons and MP (Boehme et al., 2000; Chapman et al., 2000a, 2000b; Dorf et al., 2000; Harrison et al., 1998; Imai et al., 1997; Meucci et al., 2000; Tong et al., 2000) and is up-regulated in astrocytes under inflammatory conditions (Hulshof et al., 2003). FKN, the ligand for CX3CR1, is expressed on the neuronal cell surface and astrocytes (Erichsen et al., 2003). Unlike other chemokine types, the polypeptide chain of the human CX3C motif is predicted to be part of a 373-amino-acid protein that carries the chemokine domain on top of an extended mucin-like stalk (Bazan et al., 1997). The only known ligand for the CX3CR1 is human FKN. FKN exists as a membrane-bound protein with adhesion properties, and when cleaved as a soluble protein, FKN is chemotactic for monocytes and lymphocytes (Chapman et al., 2000a, 2000b; Imai et al., 1997; Tong et al., 2000; Yoshikawa et al., 2004). Neuronal FKN RNA is not responsive to glutamate stimulation; however, FKN protein is detected in supernatants from cultured neurons treated with glutamate. This response is prevented by matrix metalloproteases inhibitors (Chapman et al., 2000a). These findings suggest that elevated FKN may be due to protein cleaved from injured neurons (Chapman et al., 2000a; Zheng et al., 2001a, 2001b). Thus, FKN induces chemotaxis by providing a chemotactic gradient to direct cell migration. However, it is not certain if this mechanism requires signal transduction or receptor-mediated G protein activation (Chapman et al., 2000b; Haskell et al., 1999, 2000; Shiraishi et al., 2000). FKN may also have neuroprotective abilities, as NO, IL-6, and TNF-α production were suppressed in microglia treated by fractalkine (Mizuno et al., 2003; Re and Przedborski, 2006).

Since MP activation is associated with neuronal injury in HAND, we proposed that FKN regulates MP effector function. It was reported that FKN is up-regulated in brain tissue and CSF of patients with HAND (Meucci et al., 2000; Tong et al., 2000; Kastenbauer et al., 2003). HIV-1 progeny virions (IIIB and ADA), gp120, and TNF-α-induced neuronal apoptosis in human neuronal cultures coincide with an increase in FKN production (Erichsen et al., 2003; Meucci et al., 2000). Moreover, FKN can effect chemotaxis of primary monocytes across an artificial BBB and is

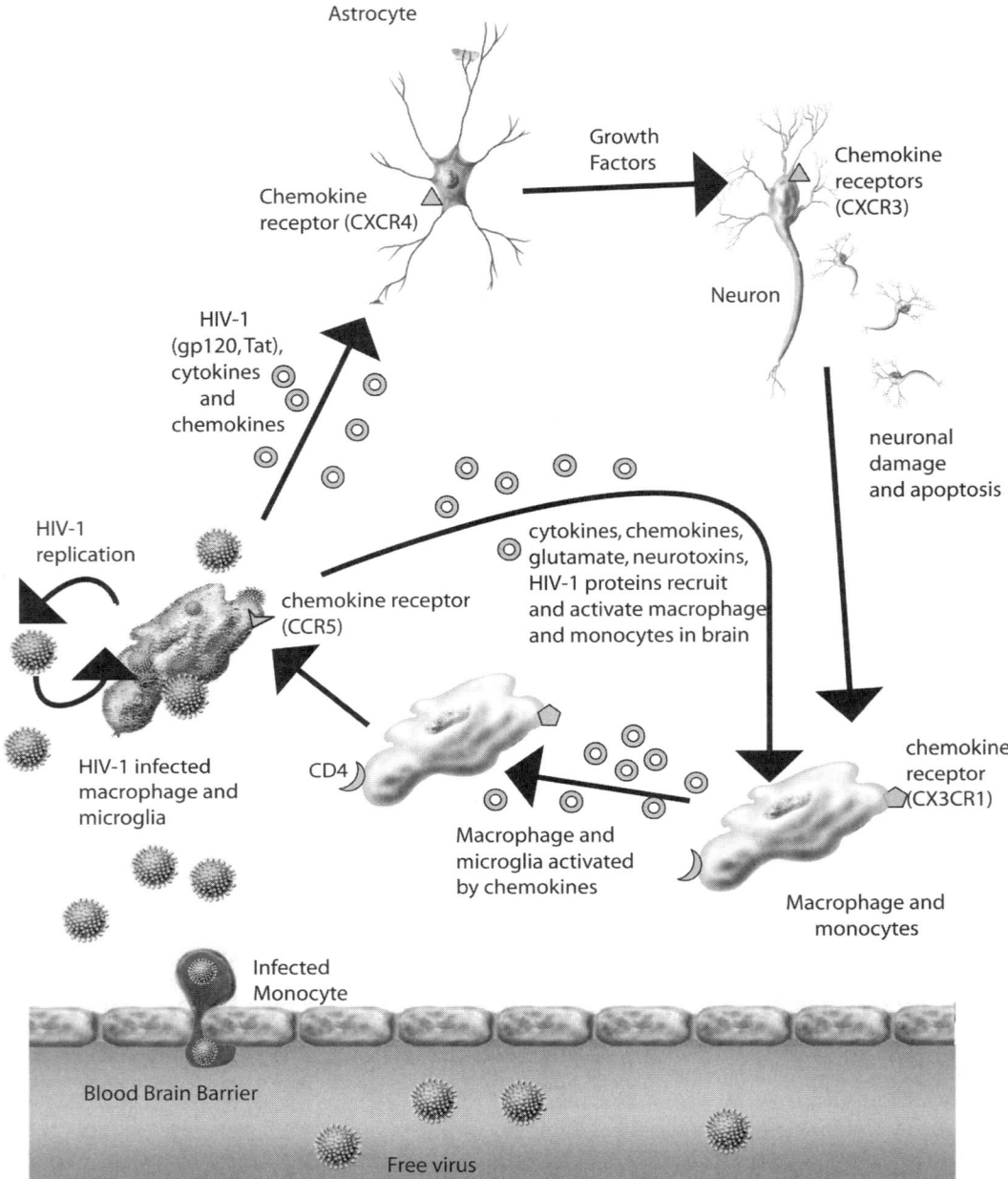

FIGURE 1 A proposed pathophysiological mechanism for how chemokines and their receptors influence the neuropathogenesis of HIV-1 infection. Transendothelial migration of monocytes into the nervous system is affected by chemokines produced by activated microglia and astrocytes. Productive HIV-1 infection is sustained in infected macrophages, although the process by which these macrophages become immunoactivated remains incompletely understood. Macrophages secrete a variety of factors, including cytokines and α and β chemokines, which affect CNS inflammation and neuronal function. Neural compromise is a consequence of intracellular signal transduction alterations induced by chemokines, HIV-1 gp120, Tat, and whole virions. Neural survival and apoptosis may be induced by chemokines.

neuroprotective to cultured neurons. Recent evidence suggests that FKN in its soluble form antagonizes MCP-1 and transendothelial migration of monocytes (Vitale et al., 2004). These results, taken together, demonstrate potential roles for FKN in MP migration and activation, both critical events in HAND pathogenesis.

CONCLUSIONS

The neuropathogenesis of HIV-1 infection revolves around inflammatory factors secreted from virus-infected and immunocompetent brain MP. One principal inflammatory factor is chemokines. Chemokines and their chemokine receptors are expressed in the nervous system, and their engagement affects neuronal and glial function. MP, astrocytes, and neuronal chemokines together with HIV-1 gp120 affect neuronal signaling pathways by binding to chemokine receptors, contributing to neuronal injury and repair. A chemokine gradient produced during HAND influences the transendothelial migration of monocytes into the brain during disease. This leads to an expanded reservoir for HIV and an increase in brain inflammation, both influencing neuronal destruction. Indeed, HIV-1 infection and immune activation work in synergy to stimulate chemokine secretion. Overall, it is likely that elucidation of the mechanisms whereby chemokines are regulated and affect neuronal injury in HAND will provide novel means for therapeutic interventions as well as having broad applicability in other neurodegenerative disorders.

We thank Nell Ingraham and Robin Taylor for outstanding administrative and graphic support. This work was supported, in part, by National Institutes of Health research grants 2 R37 NS36126, PO1 NS31492, 2RO1 NS134239, P20RR 15635, PO1A1050244, P30 A142845, 1RO1 NSA136127, 1 RO1 NS 41858, 1RO1 NS41862, and 1RO1 NS43113.

REFERENCES

Achim, C. L., R. Wang, D. K. Miners, and C. A. Wiley. 1994. Brain viral burden in HIV infection. *J. Neuropathol. Exp. Neurol.* 53:284–294.

Adamson, D. C., B. Wildemann, M. Sasaki, J. D. Glass, J. C. McArthur, V. I. Christov, T. M. Dawson, and V. L. Dawson. 1996. Immunologic NO synthase: elevation in severe AIDS dementia and induction by HIV-1 gp41. *Science* 274:1917–1926.

Albright, A. V., J. T. Shieh, T. Itoh, B. Lee, D. Pleasure, M. J. O'Connor, R. W. Doms, and F. Gonzalez-Scarano. 1999. Microglia express CCR5, CXCR4, and CCR3, but of these, CCR5 is the principal coreceptor for human immunodeficiency virus type 1 dementia isolates. *J. Virol.* 73:205–213.

Albright, A. V., S. A. Soldan, and F. Gonzalez-Scarano. 2003. Pathogenesis of human immunodeficiency virus-induced neurological disease. *J. Neurovirol.* 9:222–227.

American Academy of Neurology AIDS Task Force. 1991. Nomenclature and research case definitions for neurologic manifestations of human immunodeficiency virus-type 1 (HIV-1) infection. Report of a Working Group of the American Academy of Neurology AIDS Task Force. *Neurology* 41:778–785.

Ancuta, P., A. Moses, and D. Gabuzda. 2004. Transendothelial migration of CD16+ monocytes in response to fractalkine under constitutive and inflammatory conditions. *Immunobiology* 209:11–20.

Anderson, E., W. Zink, H. Xiong, and H. E. Gendelman. 2002. HIV-1-associated dementia: a metabolic encephalopathy perpetrated by virus-infected and immune-competent mononuclear phagocytes. *J. Acquir. Immune Defic. Syndr.* 31(Suppl. 2):S43–S54.

Annunziata, P. 2003. Blood-brain barrier changes during invasion of the central nervous system by HIV-1. Old and new insights into the mechanism. *J. Neurol.* 250:901–906.

Antinori, A., G. Arendt, J. T. Becker, B. J. Brew, D. A. Byrd, M. Cherner, D. B. Clifford, P. Cinque, L. G. Epstein, K. Goodkin, M. Gisslen, I. Grant, R. K. Heaton, J. Joseph, K. Marder, C. M. Marra, J. C. McArthur, M. Nunn, R. W. Price, L. Pulliam, K. R. Robertson, N. Sacktor, V. Valcour, and V. E. Wojna. 2007. Updated research nosology for HIV-associated neurocognitive disorders. *Neurology* 69:1789–1799.

Aquaro, S., E. Balestra, A. Cenci, M. Francesconi, R. Calio, and C. F. Perno. 1997. HIV infection in macrophage: role of long-lived cells and related therapeutical strategies. *J. Biol. Regul. Homeost. Agents* 11:69–73.

Aquaro, S., R. Calio, E. Balestra, P. Bagnarelli, A. Cenci, A. Bertoli, B. Tavazzi, D. Di Pierro, M. Francesconi, D. Abdelahad, and C. F. Perno. 1998. Clinical implications of HIV dynamics and drug resistance in macrophages. *J. Biol. Regul. Homeost. Agents* 12:23–27.

Aquaro, S., S. Panti, M. C. Caroleo, E. Balestra, A. Cenci, F. Forbici, G. Ippolito, A. Mastino, R. Testi, V. Mollace, R. Calio, and C. F. Perno. 2000. Primary macrophages infected by human immunodeficiency virus trigger CD95-mediated apoptosis of uninfected astrocytes. *J. Leukoc. Biol.* 68:429–435.

Arenzana-Seisdedos, F., and M. Partmentier. 2006. Genetics of resistance to HIV infection: role of co-receptors and co-receptor ligands. *Semin. Immunol.* 18:387–403.

Babcock, A. A., W. A. Kuziel, S. Rivest, and T. Owens. 2003. Chemokine expression by glial cells directs leukocytes to sites of axonal injury in the CNS. *J. Neurosci.* 23:7922–7930.

Baggiolini, M., B. Dewald, and B. Moser. 1997. Human chemokines: an update. *Annu. Rev. Immunol.* 15:675–705.

Bajetto, A., R. Bonavia, S. Barbero, and G. Schettini. 2002. Characterization of chemokines and their receptors in the central nervous system: physiopathological implications. *J. Neurochem.* 82:1311–1329.

Banisadr, G., E. Dicou, T. Berbar, W. Rostene, A. Lombet, and F. Haour. 2000. Characterization and visualization of (125I) stromal cell-derived factor-1alpha binding to CXCR4 receptors in rat brain and human neuroblastoma cells. *J. Neuroimmunol.* 110:151–160.

Batchelor, P. E., G. T. Liberatore, J. Y. Wong, M. J. Porritt, F. Frerichs, G. A. Donnan, and D. W. Howells. 1999. Activated macrophages and microglia induce dopaminergic sprouting in the injured striatum and express brain-derived neurotrophic factor and glial cell line-derived neurotrophic factor. *J. Neurosci.* 19:1708–1716.

Bazan, H. A., G. Alkhatib, C. C. Broder, and E. A. Berger. 1998. Patterns of CCR5, CXCR4, and CCR3 usage by envelope glycoproteins from human immunodeficiency virus type 1 primary isolates. *J. Virol.* 72:4485–4491.

Bazan, J., K. Bacon, G. Hardiman, W. Wang, K. Soo, D. Rossi, D. Greaves, A. Zlotnik, and T. Schall. 1997. A new class of membrane-bound chemokine with a CX3C motif. *Nature* 385:640–644.

Berger, J. R., and E. O. Major. 1999. Progressive multifocal leukoencephalopathy. *Semin. Neurol.* 19:193–200.

Bernasconi, S., P. Cinque, G. Peri, S. Sozzani, A. Crociati, W. Torri, E. Vicenzi, L. Vago, A. Lazzarin, G. Poli, and A. Mantovani. 1996. Selective elevation of monocyte chemotactic protein-1 in the cerebrospinal fluid of AIDS patients with cytomegalovirus encephalitis. *J. Infect. Dis.* 174:1098–1101.

Bezzi, P., M. Domercq, L. Brambilla, R. Galli, D. Schols, E. De Clercq, A. Vescovi, G. Bagetta, G. Kollias, J. Meldolesi, and A. Volterra. 2001. CXCR4-activated astrocyte glutamate release via TNFalpha: amplification by microglia triggers neurotoxicity. *Nat. Neurosci.* **4:**702–710.

Bleul, C. C., M. Farzan, H. Choe, C. Parolin, I. Clark-Lewis, J. Sodroski, and T. A. Springer. 1996a. The lymphocyte chemoattractant SDF-1 is a ligand for LESTR/fusin and blocks HIV-1 entry. *Nature* **382:**829–833.

Bleul, C. C., R. C. Fuhlbrigge, J. M. Casasnovas, A. Aiuti, and T. A. Springer. 1996b. A highly efficacious lymphocyte chemoattractant, stromal cell-derived factor 1 (SDF-1). *J. Exp. Med.* **184:**1101–1109.

Boehme, S. A., F. M. Lio, D. Maciejewski-Lenoir, K. B. Bacon, and P. J. Conlon. 2000. The chemokine fractalkine inhibits Fas-mediated cell death of brain microglia. *J. Immunol.* **165:**397–403.

Boutet, A., H. Salim, P. Leclerc, and M. Tardieu. 2001. Cellular expression of functional chemokine receptor CCR5 and CXCR4 in human embryonic neurons. *Neurosci. Lett.* **311:**105–108.

Boven, L. A., J. Middel, E. C. Breij, D. Schotte, J. Verhoef, C. Soderland, and H. S. Nottet. 2000. Interactions between HIV-infected monocyte-derived macrophages and human brain microvascular endothelial cells result in increased expression of CC chemokines. *J. Neurovirol.* **6:**382–389.

Brack-Werner, R. 1999. Astrocytes: HIV cellular reservoirs and important participants in neuropathogenesis. *AIDS* **13:**1–22.

Brandimarti, R., M. Z. Khan, A. Fatatis, and O. Meucci. 2004. Regulation of cell cycle proteins by chemokine receptors: a novel pathway in human immunodeficiency virus neuropathogenesis? *J. Neurovirol.* **10**(Suppl. 1):108–112.

Brenneman, D. E., G. L. Westbrook, S. P. Fitzgerald, D. L. Ennist, K. L. Elkins, M. R. Ruff, and C. B. Pert. 1988. Neuronal cell killing by the envelope protein of HIV and its prevention by vasoactive intestinal peptide. *Nature* **335:**639–642.

Brew, B., R. Bhalla, M. Paul, H. Gallardo, J. C. McArthur, M. K. Schwartz, and R. W. Price. 1990. Cerebrospinal fluid neopterin in human immunodeficiency virus type 1 infection. *Ann. Neurol.* **28:**556–560.

Brew, B. J., L. Evans, C. Byrne, L. Pemberton, and L. Hurren. 1996a. The relationship between AIDS dementia complex and the presence of macrophage tropic and non-syncytium inducing isolates of human immunodeficiency virus type 1 in the cerebrospinal fluid. *J. Neurovirol.* **2:**152–157.

Brew, B. J., and J. Miller. 1996. Human immunodeficiency virus type 1-related transient neurological deficits. *Am. J. Med.* **101:**257–261.

Brew, B. J., S. L. Wesselingh, M. Gonzales, M. P. Heyes, and R. W. Price. 1996b. How HIV leads to neurological disease. *Med. J. Aust.* **164:**233–234.

Broder, C. C., and R. G. Collman. 1997. Chemokine receptors and HIV. *J. Leukoc. Biol.* **62:**20–29.

Caroleo, M. C., N. Costa, L. Bracci-Laudiero, and L. Aloe. 2001. Human monocyte/macrophages activate by exposure to LPS overexpress NGF and NGF receptors. *J. Neuroimmunol.* **113:**193–201.

Carpenter, C. C., D. A. Cooper, M. A. Fischl, J. M. Gatell, B. G. Gazzard, S. M. Hammer, M. S. Hirsch, D. M. Jacobsen, D. A. Katzenstein, J. S. Montaner, D. D. Richman, M. S. Saag, M. Schechter, R. T. Schooley, M. A. Thompson, S. Vella, P. G. Yeni, and P. A. Volberding. 2000. Antiretroviral therapy in adults: updated recommendations of the International AIDS Society-USA Panel. *JAMA* **283:**381–390.

Cartier, L., O. Hartley, M. Dubois-Dauphin, and K. H. Krause. 2005. Chemokine receptors in the central nervous system: role in brain inflammation and neurodegenerative diseases. *Brain Res. Brain Res. Rev.* **48:**16–42.

Chakrabarti, L., M. Hurtrel, M. A. Maire, R. Vazeux, D. Dormont, L. Montagnier, and B. Hurtrel. 1991. Early viral replication in the brain of SIV-infected rhesus monkeys. *Am. J. Pathol.* **139:**1273–1280.

Chang, J., R. Jozwiak, B. Wang, T. Ng, Y. C. Ge, W. Bolton, D. E. Dwyer, C. Handle, R. Osborn, A. C. Cunningham, and N. D. Saksena. 1998. Unique HIV type 1 V3 region sequences derived from six different regions of brain: region-specific evolution within host-determined quasispecies. *AIDS Res. Hum. Retrovir.* **14:**25–30.

Chapman, G. A., K. Moores, D. Harrison, C. A. Campbell, B. R. Stewart, and P. J. Trijbos. 2000a. Fractalkine cleavage from neuronal membranes represents an acute event in the inflammatory response to excitotoxic brain damage. *J. Neurosci.* **20:**RC87.

Chapman, G. A., K. E. Moores, J. Gohil, T. A. Berkhout, L. Patel, P. Green, C. H. Macphee, and B. R. Stewart. 2000b. The role of fractalkine in the recruitment of monocytes to the endothelium. *Eur. J. Pharmacol.* **392:**189–195.

Chauhan, A., and A. Nath. 2005. Mechanisms of neuronal demise in HIV dementia: role of HIV-1 Tat, p. 193–199. *In* H. E. Gendelman, I. Grant, I. P. Everall, S. A. Lipton, and S. Swindells (ed.), *The Neurology of AIDS*, 2nd ed. Oxford University Press, New York, NY.

Chauhan, A., J. Turchan, C. Pocernich, A. Bruce-Keller, S. Roth, D. A. Butterfield, E. O. Major, and A. Nath. 2003. Intracellular human immunodeficiency virus Tat expression in astrocytes promotes astrocyte survival but induces potent neurotoxicity at distant sites via axonal transport. *J. Biol. Chem.* **278:**13512–13519.

Chen, S., D. L. Tuttle, J. T. Oshier, H. J. Knot, W. J. Streit, M. M. Goodenow, and J. K. Harrison. 2005. Transforming growth factor-beta 1 increases CXCR4 expression, stromal-derived factor-1alpha-stimulated signalling and human immunodeficiency virus-1 entry in human monocyte-derived macrophages. *Immunology* **114:**565–574.

Chew, C. B., S. J. Potter, B. Wang, Y. M. Wang, C. O. Shaw, D. E. Dwyer, and N. K. Saksena. 2005. Assessment of drug resistance mutations in plasma and peripheral blood mononuclear cells at different plasma viral loads in patients receiving HAART. *J. Clin. Virol.* **33:**206–216.

Cho, C., and R. J. Miller. 2002. Chemokine receptors and neural function. *J. Neurovirol.* **8:**573–584.

Choe, H., M. Farzan, M. Konkel, K. Martin, Y. Sun, L. Marcon, M. Cayabyab, M. Berman, M. E. Dorf, N. Gerard, C. Gerard, and J. Sodroski. 1998a. The orphan seven-transmembrane receptor apj supports the entry of primary T-cell-line-tropic and dualtropic human immunodeficiency virus type 1. *J. Virol.* **72:**6113–6118.

Choe, H., K. A. Martin, M. Farzan, J. Sodroski, N. P. Gerard, and C. Gerard. 1998b. Structural interactions between chemokine receptors, gp120 Env and CD4. *Semin. Immunol.* **10:**249–257.

Chung, I., M. Zelivyanskaya, and H. E. Gendelman. 2002. Mononuclear phagocyte biophysiology influences brain transendothelial and tissue migration: implication for HIV-1-associated dementia. *J. Neuroimmunol.* **122:**40–54.

Cinque, P., L. Vago, M. Mengozzi, V. Torri, D. Ceresa, E. Vicenzi, P. Transidico, A. Vagani, S. Sozzani, A. Mantovani, A. Lazzarinand, and G. Poli. 1998. Elevated cerebrospinal fluid levels of monocyte chemotactic protein-1 correlate with HIV-1 encephalitis and local viral replication. *AIDS* **12:**1327–1332.

Cocchi, F., A. L. DeVico, A. Garzino-Demo, S. K. Arya, R. C. Gallo, and P. Lusso. 1995. Identification of RANTES, MIP-1alpha, and MIP-1beta as the major HIV-suppressive factors produced by CD8+ T cells. *Science* **270:**1811–1815.

Coleman, P., and D. Flood. 1987. Neuron numbers and dendritic extent in normal aging and Alzheimer's disease. *Neurobiol. Aging* **8:**521–545.

Conant, K., A. Garzino-Demo, A. Nath, J. C. McArthur, W. Halliday, C. Power, R. C. Gallo, and E. O. Major. 1998. Induction of monocyte chemoattractant protein-1 in HIV-1 Tat-stimulated astrocytes and elevation in AIDS dementia. *Proc. Natl. Acad. Sci. USA* **95:**3117–3121.

Conti, L., L. Fantuzzi, M. Del Corno, F. Belardelli, and S. Gessani. 2004. Immunomodulatory effects of the HIV-1 gp120 protein on antigen presenting cells: implications for AIDS pathogenesis. *Immunobiology* **209:**99–115.

Cook-Easterwood, J., L. D. Middaugh, W. C. Griffen, 3rd, I. Khan, and W. R. Tyor. 2007. Highly active antiretroviral therapy of cognitive dysfunction and neuronal abnormalities in SCID mice with HIV encephalitis. *Exp. Neurol.* **205:**506–512.

Cotter, R., C. Williams, L. Ryan, D. Erichsen, A. Lopez, H. Peng, and J. Zheng. 2002. Fractalkine (CX3CL1) and brain inflammation: implications for HIV-1-associated dementia. *J. Neurovirol.* **8:**585–598.

Cotter, R., J. Zheng, M. Che, D. Niemann, Y. Liu, J. He, E. Thomas, and H. E. Gendelman. 2001. Regulation of HIV-1 infection, b-chemokine production, and CCR5 expression in CD40L-stimulated macrophages: immune control of viral entry. *J. Virol.* **75:**4308–4320.

Cotter, R. L., W. J. Burke, V. S. Thomas, J. F. Potter, J. Zheng, and H. E. Gendelman. 1999. Insights into the neurodegenerative process of Alzheimer's disease: a role for mononuclear phagocyte-associated inflammation and neurotoxicity. *J. Leukoc. Biol.* **65:**416–427.

Coughlan, C. M., C. M. McManus, M. Sharron, Z. Gao, D. Murphy, S. Jaffer, W. Choe, W. Chen, J. Hesselgesser, H. Gaylord, A. Kalyuzhny, V. M. Lee, B. Wolf, R. W. Doms, and D. L. Kolson. 2000. Expression of multiple functional chemokine receptors and monocyte chemoattractant protein-1 in human neurons. *Neuroscience* **97:**591–600.

Croitoru-Lamoury, J., G. J. Guillemin, F. D. Boussin, B. Mognetti, L. I. Gigout, A. Cheret, B. Vaslin, R. Le Grand, B. J. Brew, and D. Dormont. 2003. Expression of chemokines and their receptors in human and simian astrocytes: evidence for a central role of TNF alpha and IFN gamma in CXCR4 and CCR5 modulation. *Glia* **41:**354–370.

Dallasta, L. M., L. A. Pisarov, J. E. Esplen, J. V. Werley, A. V. Moses, J. A. Nelson, and C. L. Achim. 1999. Blood-brain barrier tight junction disruption in human immunodeficiency virus-1 encephalitis. *Am. J. Pathol.* **155:**1915–1927.

Davis, C. B., I. Dikic, D. Unutmaz, C. M. Hill, J. Arthos, M. A. Siani, D. A. Thompson, J. Schlessinger, and D. R. Littman. 1997. Signal transduction due to HIV-1 envelope interactions with chemokine receptors CXCR4 or CCR5. *J. Exp. Med.* **186:**1793–1798.

Davis, L. E., B. L. Hjelle, V. E. Miller, D. L. Palmer, A. L. Llewellyn, T. L. Merlin, S. A. Young, R. G. Mills, W. Wachsman, and C. A. Wiley. 1992. Early viral brain invasion in iatrogenic human immunodeficiency virus infection. *Neurology* **42:**1736–1739.

Deng, H., R. Liu, W. Ellmeier, S. Choe, D. Unutmaz, M. Burkhart, P. Di Marzio, S. Marmon, R. E. Sutton, C. M. Hill, C. B. Davis, S. C. Peiper, T. J. Schall, D. R. Littman, and N. R. Landau. 1996. Identification of a major co-receptor for primary isolates of HIV-1. *Nature* **381:**661–666.

Desbaillets, I., M. Tada, N. de Tribolet, A. C. Diserens, M. F. Hamou, and E. G. Van Meir. 1994. Human astrocytomas and glioblastomas express monocyte chemoattractant protein-1 (MCP-1) in vivo and in vitro. *Int. J. Cancer* **58:**240–247.

Di Stefano, M., S. Wilt, F. Gray, M. Dubois-Dalcq, and F. Chiodi. 1996. HIV type 1 V3 sequences and the development of dementia during AIDS. *AIDS Res. Hum. Retrovir.* **12:**471–482.

Dong, X. N., Y. Wu, J. Ying, and Y. H. Chen. 2005. The antigenic tip GPGRAFY of the V3 loop on HIV-1 gp120: genetic variability and subtypes. *Immunol. Lett.* **101:**112–114.

Dooms, H., T. Van Belle, M. Desmedt, P. Rottiers, and J. Grooten. 2000. Interleukin-15 redirects the outcome of a tolerizing T-cell stimulus from apoptosis to anergy. *Blood* **96:**1006–1012.

Doranz, B. J., J. Rucker, Y. Yi, R. J. Smyth, M. Samson, S. C. Peiper, M. Parmentier, R. G. Collman, and R. W. Dome. 1996. A dual-tropic primary HIV-1 isolate that uses fusin and the β chemokine receptor CKR5, CKR3, and CKR-2b as fusion cofactors. *Cell* **85:**1149–1158.

Dorf, M. E., M. A. Berman, S. Tanabe, M. Heesen, and Y. Luo. 2000. Astrocytes express functional chemokine receptors. *J. Neuroimmunol.* **111:**109–121.

Dragic, T., V. Litwin, G. P. Allaway, S. R. Martin, Y. Huang, K. A. Nagashima, C. Cayanan, P. J. Maddon, R. A. Koup, J. P. Moore, and W. A. Paxton. 1996. HIV-1 entry into CD4+ cells is mediated by the chemokines receptor CC-CKR-5. *Nature* **381:**667–673.

Dunfee, R., E. R. Thomas, P. R. Gorry, J. Wang, P. Ancuta, and D. Gabuzda. 2006. Mechanisms of HIV-1 neurotropism. *Curr. HIV Res.* **4:**267–278.

Dzenko, K. A., L. Song, S. Ge, W. A. Kuziel, and J. S. Pachter. 2005. CCR2 expression by brain microvascular endothelial cells is critical for macrophage transendothelial migration in response to CCL2. *Microvasc. Res.* **70:**53–64.

Edinger, A. L., C. Blanpain, K. J. Kunstman, S. M. Wolinsky, M. Parmentier, and R. W. Doms. 1999. Functional dissection of CCR5 coreceptor function through the use of CD4-independent simian immunodeficiency virus strains. *J. Virol.* **73:**4062–4073.

El-Hage, N., J. A. Gurwell, I. N. Singh, P. E. Knapp, A. Nath, and K. F. Hauser. 2005. Synergistic increases in intracellular Ca2+, and the release of MCP-1, RANTES, and IL-6 by astrocytes treated with opiates and HIV-1 Tat. *Glia* **50:**91–106.

Elkabes, S., E. M. DiCicco-Bloom, and I. B. Black. 1996. Brain microglia/macrophages express neurotrophins that selectively regulate microglial proliferation and function. *J. Neurosci.* **16:**2508–2521.

Endres, M. J., P. R. Clapham, M. Marsh, M. Ahuja, J. D. Turner, A. McKnight, J. F. Thomas, B. Stoebenau-Haggarty, S. Choe, P. J. Vance, T. N. C. Wells, C. A. Powers, S. S. Sutterwala, R. W. Doms, N. R. Landau, and J. A. Hoxie. 1996. CD4-independent infection by HIV-2 is mediated by fusin/CXCR4. *Cell* **87:**745–756.

Erdmann, N. B., N. P. Whitney, and J. Zheng. 2006. Potentiation of excitotoxicity in HIV-1 associated dementia and the significance of glutaminase. *Clin. Neurosci. Rex.* **6:**315–328.

Erichsen, D., A. L. Lopez, H. Peng, D. Niemann, C. Williams, M. Bauer, S. Morgello, R. L. Cotter, L. A. Ryan, A. Ghorpade, H. E. Gendelman, and J. Zheng. 2003. Neuronal injury regulates fractalkine: relevance for HIV-1 associated dementia. *J. Neuroimmunol.* **138:**144-155.

Eugenin, E. A., and J. W. Berman. 2007. Gap junctions mediate human immunodeficiency virus-bystander killing in astrocytes. *J. Neurosci.* **27:**12844–12850.

Everall, I. P., J. D. Glass, J. McArthur, E. Spargo, and P. Lantos. 1994. Neuronal density in the superior frontal and temporal gyri does not correlate with the degree of human immunodeficiency virus-associated dementia. *Acta Neuropathol.* **88:**538–544.

Fallon, J., S. Reid, R. Kinyamu, I. Opole, R. Opole, J. Baratta, M. Korc, T. L. Endo, A. Duong, G. Nguyen, M. Karkehabadhi, D. Twardzik, S. Patel, and S. Loughlin. 2000. In vivo induction of massive proliferation, directed migration, and differentiation of neural cells in the adult mammalian brain. *Proc. Natl. Acad. Sci. USA* **97:**14686–14691.

Farzan, M., H. Choe, K. Martin, L. Marcon, W. Hofmann, G. Karlsson, Y. Sun, P. Barrett, N. Marchand, N. Sullivan, N. Gerard, C. Gerard, and J. Sodroski. 1997a. Two orphan seven transmembrane segment receptors which are expressed in CD4-positive cells support simian immunodeficiency virus infection. *J. Exp. Med.* **186:**405–411.

Farzan, M., H. Choe, K. A. Martin, Y. Sun, M. Sidelko, C. R. Mackay, N. P. Gerard, J. Sodroski, and C. Gerard.

1997b. HIV-1 entry and macrophage inflammatory protein-1beta-mediated signaling are independent functions of the chemokine receptor CCR5. *J. Biol. Chem.* **272:**6854–6857.

Feng, Y., C. C. Broder, P. E. Kennedy, and E. A. Berger. 1996. HIV-1 entry cofactor: functional cDNA cloning of a seven-transmembrane, G protein-coupled receptor. *Science* **272:**872–877.

Fiala, M., X. H. Gan, L. Zhang, S. D. House, T. Newton, M. C. Graves, P. Shapshak, M. Stins, K. S. Kim, M. Witte, and S. L. Chang. 1998. Cocaine enhances monocyte migration across the blood-brain barrier. Cocaine's connection to AIDS dementia and vasculitis. *Adv. Exp. Med. Biol.* **437:**199–205.

Fischer-Smith, T., S. Croul, A. Adeniyi, K. Rybicka, S. Morgello, K. Khalili, and J. Rappaport. 2004. Macrophage/microglial accumulation and proliferating cell nuclear antigen expression in the central nervous system in human immunodeficiency virus encephalopathy. *Am. J. Pathol.* **164:**2089–2099.

Fischer-Smith, T., S. Croul, A. E. Sverstiuk, C. Capini, D. L'Heureux, E. G. Regulier, M. W. Richardson, S. Amini, S. Morgello, K. Khalili, and J. Rappaport. 2001. CNS invasion by CD14+/CD16+ peripheral blood-derived monocytes in HIV dementia: perivascular accumulation and reservoir of HIV infection. *J. Neurovirol.* **7:**528–541.

Fischer-Smith, T., E. M. Tedaldi, and J. Rappaport. 2008. CD163/CD16 coexpression by circulating monocytes/macrophages in HIV: potential biomarkers for HIV infection and AIDS progression. *AIDS Res. Hum. Retrovir.* **24:**417–421.

Flynn, G., S. Maru, J. Loughlin, I. A. Romero, and D. Male. 2003. Regulation of chemokine receptor expression in human microglia and astrocytes. *J. Neuroimmunol.* **136:**84–93.

Fox, H. S., M. R. Weed, S. Huitron-Resendiz, J. Baig, T. F. Horn, P. J. Dailey, N. Bischofberger, and S. J. Henriksen. 2000. Antiviral treatment normalizes neurophysiological but not movement abnormalities in simian immunodeficiency virus-infected monkeys. *J. Clin. Investig.* **106:**37–45.

Gabuzda, D., J. He, A. Ohagen, and A. Vallat. 1998. Chemokine receptors in HIV-1 infection of the central nervous system. *Immunology* **10:**203–213.

Gabuzda, D., and J. Wang. 1999. Chemokine receptors and virus entry in the central nervous system. *J. Neurovirol.* **5:**643–658.

Gabuzda, D., J. Wang, and P. Gorry. 2002. HIV-1-associated dementia, p. 345–360. *In* R. M. Ransohoff, K. Suzuki, A. E. I. Proudfoot, W. F. Hickey, and J. K. Harrison (ed.), *Chemokines and the Nervous System.* Elsevier Science, Amsterdam, The Netherlands.

Gabuzda, D. H., D. D. Ho, M. S. D. L. Monte, T. R. Rota, and R. A. Sobel. 1986. Immunohistochemical identification of HTLV-III antigen in brains of patients with AIDS. *Ann. Neurol.* **20:**289–295.

Garden, G. A. 2002. Microglia in human immunodeficiency virus-associated neurodegeneration. *Glia* **40:**240–251.

Gelbard, H., H. Nottet, K. Dzenko, M. Jett, P. Genis, R. White, L. Wang, Y. B. Choi, D. Zhang, S. Lipton, S. Swindells, L. Epstein, and H. Gendelman. 1994. Platelet-activating factor: a candidate human immunodeficiency virus type-1 infection neurotoxin. *J. Virol.* **68:**4628–4635.

Gelbard, H. A., K. Dzenko, D. Diloreto, C. D. Cerro, M. D. Cerro, and L. G. Epstein. 1993. Neurotoxic effects of tumor necrosis factor in primary human neuronal cultures are mediated by activation of the glutamate AMPA receptor subtypes implications for AIDS neuropathogenesis. *Dev. Neurosci.* **15:**417–422.

Gelbard, H. A., and L. G. Epstein. 1995. HIV-1 encephalopathy in children. *Curr. Opin. Pediatr.* **7:**655–662.

Gendelman, H., and S. Gendelman. 1992. Neurological aspects of human immunodeficiency virus infection, p. 229–254. *In*

S. Specter, M. Bendinelli, and H. Friedman (ed.), *Neuropathogenic Viruses and Immunity.* Plenum Press, New York, NY.

Gendelman, H. E., J. H. Atkinson, I. P. Everall, R. G. Gonzaliz, I. Grant, R. Heaton, D. L. Kolson, S. A. Lipton, J. McArthur, A. Nath, C. Power, S. Swindells, and B. Wigdahl. 2005. Overview: a panel discussion on current and future insights into the neurological, behavioral, and motor consequences of HIV-1 infection, p. 1–11. *In* H. E. Gendelman, I. Grant, I. P. Everall, S. A. Lipton, and S. Swindells (ed.), *The Neurology of AIDS*, 2nd ed. Oxford University Press, New York, NY.

Gendelman, H. E., and D. G. Folks. 1999. Innate and acquired immunity in neurodegenerative disorders. *J. Leukoc. Biol.* **65:**407–409.

Gendelman, H. E., P. Genis, M. Jett, Q. H. Zhai, and H. S. Nottet. 1994. An experimental model system for HIV-1-induced brain injury. *Adv. Neuroimmunol.* **4:**189–193.

Gendelman, H. E., O. Narayan, S. Kennedy-Stoskopf, J. E. Clements, and G. H. Pezeshkpour. 1984. Slow virus-macrophage interactions. Characterization of a transformed cell line of sheep alveolar macrophages that express a marker for susceptibility to ovine-caprine lentivirus infections. *Lab. Investig.* **51:**547–555.

Gendelman, H. E., O. Narayan, S. Kennedy-Stoskopf, P. G. Kennedy, Z. Ghotbi, J. E. Clements, J. Stanley, and G. Pezeshkpour. 1986. Tropism of sheep lentiviruses for monocytes: susceptibility to infection and virus gene expression increase during maturation of monocytes to macrophages. *J. Virol.* **58:**67–74.

Gendelman, H. E., O. Narayan, S. Molineaux, J. E. Clements, and Z. Ghotbi. 1985. Slow, persistent replication of lentiviruses: role of tissue macrophages and macrophage precursors in bone marrow. *Proc. Natl. Acad. Sci. USA* **82:**7086–7090.

Gendelman, H. E., Y. Persidsky, A. Ghorpade, J. Limoges, M. Stins, M. Fiala, and R. Morrisett. 1997. The neuropathogenesis of the AIDS dementia complex. *AIDS* **11:**S35–S45.

Gendelman, H. E., J. Zheng, C. L. Coulter, A. Ghorpade, M. Che, M. Thylin, R. Rubocki, Y. Persidsky, F. Hahn, J. Reinhard, and S. Swindells. 1998. Suppression of inflammatory neurotoxins by highly active antiretroviral therapy in human immunodeficiency virus-associated dementia. *J. Infect. Dis.* **178:**1000–1007.

Genis, P., M. Jett, E. Bernton, T. Boyle, H. Gelbard, K. Dzenko, R. Keane, L. Resnick, Y. Mizrachi, D. Volsky, L. Epstein, and H. Gendelman. 1992. Cytokines and arachidonic metabolites produced during human immunodeficiency virus (HIV)-infected macrophage-astroglia interactions: implications for the neuropathogenesis of HIV disease. *J. Exp. Med.* **176:**1703–1718.

Ghorpade, A., and H. E. Gendelman. 2003. Non-neuronal cells and their interactions in AIDS-associated dementia, p. 9901–9920. *In* L. Hertz (ed.), *Non-Neuronal Cells of the Nervous System: Function and Dysfunction.* Elsevier, New York, NY.

Ghorpade, A., S. Holter, K. Borgmann, R. Persidsky, and L. Wu. 2003. HIV-1 and IL-1 beta regulate Fas ligand expression in human astrocytes through the NF-kappa B pathway. *J. Neuroimmunol.* **141:**141–149.

Ghorpade, A., A. Nukuna, M. Che, S. Haggerty, Y. Persidsky, E. Carter, L. Carhart, L. Shafer, and H. E. Gendelman. 1998a. Human immunodeficiency virus neurotropism: an analysis of viral replication and cytopathicity for divergent strains in monocytes and microglia. *J. Virol.* **72:**3340–3350.

Ghorpade, A., R. Persidskaia, R. Suryadevara, M. Che, X. J. Liu, Y. Persidsky, and H. E. Gendelman. 2001. Mononuclear phagocyte differentiation, activation and viral infection regulate matrix metalloproteinase expression: implications for human immunodeficiency virus type 1-associated dementia. *J. Virol.* **75:**6572–6583.

Ghorpade, A., Y. Persidsky, S. Swindells, K. Borgmann, R. Persidsky, S. Holter, R. Cotter, and H. E. Gendelman. 2005. Neuroinflammatory responses from microglia recovered from HIV-1-infected and seronegative subjects. *J. Neuroimmunol.* **163:**145–156.

Ghorpade, A., M. Q. Xia, B. T. Hyman, Y. Persidsky, A. Nukuna, P. Bock, M. Che, J. Limoges, H. E. Gendelman, and C. R. Mackay. 1998b. Role of the β-chemokine receptors CCR3 and CCR5 in human immunodeficiency virus type 1 infection of monocytes and microglia. *J. Virol.* **72:**3351–3361.

Giulian, D., J. Yu, L. Xia, D. Tom, J. Li, S. N. Lin, R. Schwarz, and C. Noonan. 1996. Study of receptor-mediated neurotoxins released by HIV-1 infected mononuclear phagocytes found in human brain. *J. Neurosci.* **16:**3139–3153.

Glass, J. D., H. Fedor, S. L. Wesselingh, and J. C. McArthur. 1995. Immunocytochemical quantitation of human immunodeficiency virus in the brain: correlations with dementia. *Ann. Neurol.* **38:**755–762.

Gonzalez-Scarano, F., and J. Martin-Garcia. 2005. The neuropathogenesis of AIDS. *Nat. Rev. Immunol.* **5:**69–81.

Gorry, P. R., M. Churchill, S. M. Crowe, A. L. Cunningham, and D. Gabuzda. 2005. Pathogenesis of macrophage tropic HIV-1. *Curr. HIV Res.* **3:**53–60.

Gorry, P. R., J. Taylor, G. H. Holm, A. Mehle, T. Morgan, M. Cayabyab, M. Farzan, H. Wang, J. E. Bell, K. Kunstman, J. P. Moore, S. M. Wolinsky, and D. Gabuzda. 2002. Increased CCR5 affinity and reduced CCR5/CD4 dependence of a neurovirulent primary human immunodeficiency virus type 1 isolate. *J. Virol.* **76:**6277–6292.

Gray, L., J. Sterjovski, M. Churchill, P. Ellery, N. Nasr, S. R. Lewin, S. M. Crowe, S. L. Wesselingh, A. L. Cunningham, and P. R. Gorry. 2005. Uncoupling coreceptor usage of human immunodeficiency virus type 1 (HIV-1) from macrophage tropism reveals biological properties of CCR5-restricted HIV-1 isolates from patients with acquired immunodeficiency syndrome. *Virology* **337:**384–398.

Guillemin, G. J., S. J. Kerr, and B. J. Brew. 2005. Involvement of quinolinic acid in AIDS dementia complex. *Neurotox. Res.* **7:**103–123.

Guntermann, C., B. J. Murphy, R. Zheng, A. Qureshi, P. A. Eagles, and K. E. Nye. 1999. Human immunodeficiency virus-1 infection requires pertussis toxin sensitive G-protein-coupled signalling and mediates cAMP downregulation. *Biochem. Biophys. Res. Commun.* **256:**429–435.

Gupta, P., K. B. Collins, D. Ratner, S. Watkins, G. J. Naus, D. V. Landers, and B. K. Patterson. 2002. Memory CD4(+) T cells are the earliest detectable human immunodeficiency virus type 1 (HIV-1)-infected cells in the female genital mucosal tissue during HIV-1 transmission in an organ culture system. *J. Virol.* **76:**9868–9876.

Harrison, J. K., Y. Jiang, S. Chen, Y. Xia, D. Maciejewski, R. K. McNamara, W. J. Streit, M. N. Salafranca, S. Adhikari, D. A. Thompson, P. Botti, K. B. Bacon, and L. Feng. 1998. Role for neuronally derived fractalkine in mediating interactions between neurons and CX3CR1-expressing microglia. *Proc. Natl. Acad. Sci. USA* **95:**10896–10901.

Haskell, C. A., M. D. Cleary, and I. F. Charo. 1999. Molecular uncoupling of fractalkine-mediated cell adhesion and signal transduction. Rapid flow arrest of CX3CR1-expressing cells is independent of G-protein activation. *J. Biol. Chem.* **274:**10053–10058.

Haskell, C. A., M. D. Cleary, and I. F. Charo. 2000. Unique role of the chemokine domain of fractalkine in cell capture. Kinetics of receptor dissociation correlate with cell adhesion. *J. Biol. Chem.* **275:**34183–34189.

Haydon, P. G. 2001. GLIA: listening and talking to the synapse. *Nat. Rev. Neurosci.* **2:**185–193.

He, J., Y. Chen, M. Farzan, H. Choe, A. Ohagen, S. Gartner, J. Busciglio, X. Yang, W. Hofmann, W. Newman, C. R. Mackay, J. Sodroski, and D. Gabuzda. 1997. CCR3 and CCR5 are co-receptors for HIV-1 infection of microglia. *Nature* **385:**645–649.

Heese, K., C. Hock, and U. Otten. 1998. Inflammatory signals induce neurotrophin expression in human microglial cells. *J. Neurochem.* **70:**699–707.

Hesselgesser, J., M. Halks-Miller, V. DelVecchio, S. C. Peiper, J. Hoxie, D. L. Kolson, D. Taub, and R. Horuk. 1997. CD4-independent association between HIV-1 gp120 and CXCR4: functional chemokine receptors are expressed in human neurons. *Curr. Biol.* **7:**112-121.

Hesselgesser, J., and R. Horuk. 1999. Chemokine and chemokine receptor expression in the central nervous system. *J. Neurovirol.* **5:**13–26.

Hesselgesser, J., M. Liang, J. Hoxie, M. Greenberg, L. F. Brass, M. J. Orsini, D. Taub, and R. Horuk. 1998a. Identification and characterization of the CXCR4 chemokine receptor in human T cell lines: ligand binding, biological activity, and HIV-1 infectivity. *J. Immunol.* **160:**877–883.

Hesselgesser, J., D. Taub, P. Baskar, M. Greenberg, J. Hoxie, D. L. Kolson, and R. Horuk. 1998b. Neuronal apoptosis induced by HIV-1 gp120 and the chemokine SDF-1alpha mediated by the chemokine receptor CXCR4. *Curr. Biol.* **8:**595–598.

Heyes, M. P., B. B. Brew, A. Martin, R. W. Price, A. Salazar, J. J. Sidtis, J. A. Yergey, M. M. Mouradian, A. E. Sadler, J. Keilp, R. Rubinow, and S. P. Markey. 1991. Quinolinic acid in cerebrospinal fluid and serum in HIV-1 infection: relationship to clinical and neurological status. *Ann. Neurol.* **29:**202–209.

Hofman, F. M., P. Chen, F. Incardona, R. Zidovetzki, and D. R. Hinton. 1999. HIV-1 tat protein induces the production of interleukin-8 by human brain-derived endothelial cells. *J. Neuroimmunol.* **94:**28–39.

Holm, G. H., and D. Gabuzda. 2005. Distinct mechanisms of CD4+ and CD8+ T-cell activation and bystander apoptosis induced by human immunodeficiency virus type 1 virions. *J. Virol.* **79:**6299–6311.

Horuk, R., J. Hesselgesser, Y. Zhou, D. Faulds, M. Halks-Miller, S. Harvey, D. Taub, M. Samson, M. Parmentier, J. Rucker, B. J. Doranz, and R. W. Doms. 1998. The CC chemokine I-309 inhibits CCR8-dependent infection by diverse HIV-1 strains. *J. Biol. Chem.* **273:**386–391.

Horuk, R., A. W. Martin, Z. Wang, L. Schweitzer, A. Gerassimides, H. Guo, Z. Lu, J. Hesselgesser, H. D. Perez, J. Kim, J. Parker, T. J. Hadley, and S. C. Peiper. 1997. Expression of chemokine receptors by subsets of neurons in the central nervous system. *J. Immunol.* **158:**2882–2890.

Huang, E. J., and L. F. Reichardt. 2003. Trk receptors: roles in neuronal signal transduction. *Annu. Rev. Biochem.* **72:**609–642.

Hulshof, S., E. S. van Haastert, H. F. Kuipers, P. J. van den Elsen, C. J. De Groot, P. van der Valk, R. Ravid, and K. Biber. 2003. CX3CL1 and CX3CR1 expression in human brain tissue: noninflammatory control versus multiple sclerosis. *J. Neuropathol. Exp. Neurol.* **62:**899–907.

Imai, T., K. Hieshima, C. Haskell, M. Baba, M. Nagira, M. Nishimura, M. Kakizaki, S. Takagi, H. Nomiyama, T. J. Schall, and O. Yoshie. 1997. Identification and molecular characterization of fractalkine receptor CX3CR1, which mediates both leukocyte migration and adhesion. *Cell* **91:**521–530.

Imai, Y., T. Kimura, A. Murakami, N. Yajima, K. Sakamaki, and S. Yonehara. 1999. The CED-4-homologous protein FLASH is involved in Fas-mediated activation of caspase-8 during apoptosis. *Nature* **398:**777–785.

Janssen, R., D. Cornblath, L. Epstein, R. Foa, J. McArthur, R. Price, A. Asbury, A. Beckett, D. Benson, T. Bridge, C. Leventhal, P. Satz, A. Saykin, J. Sidtis, and S. Tross. 1991. Nomenclature and research case definitions for neurological manifestations of human immunodeficiency virus type 1 (HIV-1) infection. *Neurology* **41**:778–785.

Jiang, Z., C. Piggee, M. P. Heyes, C. Murphy, B. Quearry, M. Bauer, J. Zheng, H. E. Gendelman, and S. P. Markey. 2001. Glutamate is a mediator of neurotoxicity in secretions of activated HIV- 1-infected macrophages. *J. Neuroimmunol.* **117**:97–107.

Joly, M., and J. M. Pinto. 2005. CXCR4 and CCR5 regulation and expression patterns on T- and monocyte-macrophage cell lineages: implications for susceptibility to infection by HIV-1. *Math Biosci.* **195**:92–126.

Jones, M., K. Olafson, M. R. Del Bigio, J. Peeling, and A. Nath. 1998. Intraventricular injection of human immunodeficiency virus type 1 (HIV- 1) tat protein causes inflammation, gliosis, apoptosis, and ventricular enlargement. *J. Neuropathol. Exp. Neurol.* **57**:563–570.

Jung, S., J. Aliberti, P. Graemmel, M. J. Sunshine, G. W. Kreutzberg, A. Sher, and D. R. Littman. 2000. Analysis of fractalkine receptor CX(3)CR1 function by targeted deletion and green fluorescent protein reporter gene insertion. *Mol. Cell. Biol.* **20**:4106–4114

Kadiu, I., J. G. Glanzer, J. Kipnis, H. E. Gendelman, and M. P. Thomas. 2005. Mononuclear phagocytes in the pathogenesis of neurodegenerative diseases. *Neurotox. Res.* **8**:25–50.

Kalehua, A. N., J. E. Nagel, L. M. Whelchel, J. J. Gides, R. S. Pyle, R. J. Smith, J. W. Kusiak, and D. D. Taub. 2004. Monocyte chemoattractant protein-1 and macrophage inflammatory protein-2 are involved in both excitotoxin-induced neurodegeneration and regeneration. *Exp. Cell Res.* **297**:197–211.

Kastenbauer, S., U. Koedel, M. Wick, B. C. Kieseier, H. P. Hartung, and H. W. Pfister. 2003. CSF and serum levels of soluble fractalkine (CX3CL1) in inflammatory diseases of the nervous system. *J. Neuroimmunol.* **137**:210–217.

Kaul, M. 2008. HIV's double strike at the brain: neuronal toxicity and compromised neurogenesis. *Front Biosci.* **13**:2484–2494.

Kaul, M., and S. A. Lipton. 2006. Mechanisms of neuroimmunity and neurodegeneration associated with HIV-1 infection and AIDS. *J. Neuroimmune Pharmacol.* **1**:138–151.

Kaul, R., J. Rutherford, S. L. Rowland-Jones, J. Kimani, J. I. Onyango, K. Fowke, K. MacDonald, J. J. Bwayo, A. J. McMichael, and F. A. Plummer. 2004. HIV-1 Env-specific cytotoxic T-lymphocyte responses in exposed, uninfected Kenyan sex workers: a prospective analysis. *AIDS* **18**:2087–2089.

Kedzierska, K., and S. M. Crowe. 2002. The role of monocytes and macrophages in the pathogenesis of HIV-1 infection. *Curr. Med. Chem.* **9**:1893–1903.

Kelder, W., J. C. McArthur, T. Nance-Sproson, D. McClernon, and D. E. Griffin. 1998. β-Chemokines MCP-1 and RANTES are selectively increased in cerebrospinal fluid of patients with human immunodeficiency virus-associated dementia. *Ann. Neurol.* **44**:831–835.

Kerr, S. J., P. J. Armati, G. J. Guillemin, and B. J. Brew. 1998. Chronic exposure of human neurons to quinolinic acid results in neuronal changes consistent with AIDS dementia complex. *AIDS* **12**:355–363.

Khan, M. Z., R. Brandimarti, J. P. Patel, N. Huyn, J. Wang, Z. Huang, A. Fatatis, and O. Meucci. 2004. Apoptotic and antiapoptotic effects of CXCR4: is it a matter of intrinsic efficacy? Implications for HIV neuropathogenesis. *AIDS Res. Hum. Retrovir.* **20**:1063–1071.

Kieburtz, K., and R. Schiffer. 1989. Neurologic manifestations of human immunodeficiency virus infections. *Neurol. Clin.* **7**:447–468.

Kitai, R., M. L. Zhao, N. Zhang, L. L. Hua, and S. C. Lee. 2000. Role of MIP-1beta and RANTES in HIV-1 infection of microglia: inhibition of infection and induction by IFNbeta. *J. Neuroimmunol.* **110**:230–239.

Klein, R., K. Williams, X. Alvarez-Hernandez, S. Westmoreland, T. Force, A. Lackner, and A. Luster. 1999. Chemokine receptor expression and signaling in macaque and human fetal neurons and astrocytes: implications for the neuropathogenesis of AIDS. *J. Immunol.* **163**:1636–1646.

Koenig, S., H. E. Gendelman, J. M. Orenstein, M. C. D. Canto, G. H. Pezeshkpour, M. Yungbluth, F. Janotta, A. Aksamit, M. A. Martin, and A. S. Fauci. 1986. Detection of AIDS virus in macrophages in brain tissue from AIDS patients with encephalopathy. *Science* **233**:1089–1093.

Kornbluth, R. S., K. Kee, and D. D. Richman. 1998. CD40 ligand (CD154) stimulation of macrophages to produce HIV-1-suppressive beta-chemokines. *Proc. Natl. Acad. Sci. USA* **95**:5205–5210.

Kouba, M., M. V. Anetti, X. Wang, M. Schafer, and V. Hollt. 1993. Cloning of a novel putative G-protein-coupled receptor (NLR) which is expressed in neuronal and lymphatic tissue. *FEBS Lett.* **321**:173–178.

Kramer-Hammerle, S., I. Rothenaigner, H. Wolff, J. E. Bell, and R. Brack-Werner. 2005. Cells of the central nervous system as targets and reservoirs of the human immunodeficiency virus. *Virus Res.* **111**:194–213.

Krathwohl, M. D., and J. L. Kaiser. 2004. Chemokines promote quiescence and survival of human neural progenitor cells. *Stem Cells* **22**:109–118.

Krebs, F. C., H. Ross, J. McAllister, and B. Wigdahl. 2000. HIV-1-associated central nervous system dysfunction. *Adv. Pharmacol.* **49**:315–385.

Kullander, K., A. Kylberg, and T. Ebendal. 1997. Specificity of neurotrophin-3 determined by loss-of-function mutagenesis. *J. Neurosci. Res.* **50**:496–503.

Kure, K., K. M. Weidenheim, W. D. Lyman, and D. W. Dickson. 1990. Morphology and distribution of HIV-1 gp41-positive microglia in subacute AIDS encephalitis. Pattern of involvement resembling a multisystem degeneration. *Acta Neuropathol.* **80**:393–400.

Kutsch, O., J. Oh, A. Nath, and E. N. Benveniste. 2000. Induction of the chemokines interleukin-8 and IP-10 by human immunodeficiency virus type 1 tat in astrocytes. *J. Virol.* **74**:9214–9221.

Lackner, A. A., P. Vogel, R. A. Rames, D. Kluge, and M. Marthas. 1994. Early events in tissues during infection with pathogenic (SIVmac239) and nonpathogenic (SIVmac1A11) molecular clones of simian immunodeficiency virus. *Am. J. Pathol.* **145**:428–439.

Lavi, E., J. M. Strizki, A. M. Ulrich, W. Zhang, L. Fu, Q. Wang, M. O'Connor, J. A. Hoxie, and F. Gonzalez-Scarano. 1997. CXCR-4 (fusin), a co-receptor for the type 1 human immunodeficiency virus (HIV-1) is expressed in the human brain in a variety of cell types, including microglia and neurons. *Am. J. Pathol.* **151**:1035–1042.

Lazarov-Spiegler, O., O. Rapalino, G. Agranov, and M. Schwartz. 1998a. Restricted inflammatory reaction in the CNS: a key impediment to axonal regeneration? *Mol. Med. Today* **4**:337–442.

Lazarov-Spiegler, O., A. S. Solomon, and M. Schwartz. 1998b. Peripheral nerve-stimulated macrophages simulate a peripheral nerve-like regenerative response in rat transected optic nerve. *Glia* **24**:329–337.

Lazarov-Spiegler, O., A. S. Solomon, A. B. Zeev-Brann, D. L. Hirschberg, V. Lavie, and M. Schwartz. 1996. Transplantation of activated macrophages overcomes central nervous system regrowth failure. *FASEB J.* **10**:1296–1302.

Letendre, S. L., E. R. Lanier, and J. A. McCutchan. 1999. Cerebrospinal fluid beta chemokine concentrations in neurocognitively impaired individuals infected with human immunodeficiency virus type 1. *J. Infect. Dis.* **180**:310–319.

Liapi, A., J. Pritchett, O. Jones, N. Fujii, J. G. Parnavelas, and B. Nadarajah. 2008. Stromal-derived factor-1 signalling regulates radial and tangential migration in the developing cerebral cortex. *Dev. Neurosci.* **30:**117–131.

Limoges, J., Y. Persidsky, L. Poluektova, J. Rasmussen, W. Ratanasuwan, M. Zelivyanskaia, D. McClernon, E. Lanier, and H. Gendelman. 2000. Evaluation of antiretroviral drug efficacy for HIV-1 encephalitis in SCID mice. *Neurology* **54:**379–389.

Liou, L. Y., C. H. Herrmann, and A. P. Rice. 2004. HIV-1 infection and regulation of Tat function in macrophages. *Int. J. Biochem. Cell Biol.* **36:**1767–1775.

Lipton, S. 1994. HIV coat protein gp120 induces soluble neurotoxins in culture medium. *Neurosci. Res. Commun.* **15:**31–37.

Lipton, S. A., and H. E. Gendelman. 1995. Dementia associated with the acquired immunodeficiency syndrome. *N. Engl. J. Med.* **16:**934–940.

Liu, H., Y. Hwangbo, S. Holte, J. Lee, C. Wang, N. Kaupp, H. Zhu, C. Celum, L. Corey, M. J. McElrath, and T. Zhu. 2004. Analysis of genetic polymorphisms in CCR5, CCR2, stromal cell-derived factor-1, RANTES, and dendritic cell-specific intercellular adhesion molecule-3-grabbing noninte-grin in seronegative individuals repeatedly exposed to HIV-1. *J. Infect. Dis.* **190:**1055–1058.

Liu, R., W. A. Paxton, S. Choe, D. Ceradini, S. R. Martin, R. Horuk, M. E. MacDonald, H. Stuhlmann, R. A. Koup, and N. R. Landau. 1996a. Homozygous defect in HIV-1 core-ceptor accounts for resistance of some multiply-exposed individuals to HIV-1 infection. *Cell* **86:**367–377.

Liu, X., C. N. Kim, J. Yang, R. Jemmerson, and X. Wang. 1996b. Induction of apoptotic program in cell-free extracts: requirement for dATP and cytochrome c. *Cell* **86:**147–157.

Liu, Y., X. P. Tang, J. C. McArthur, J. Scott, and S. Gartner. 2000. Analysis of human immunodeficiency virus type 1 gp160 sequences from a patient with HIV dementia: evidence for monocyte trafficking into brain. *J. Neurovirol.* **6**(Suppl. 1): S70–S81.

Lu, M., E. A. Grove, and R. J. Miller. 2002. Abnormal development of the hippocampal dentate gyrus in mice lacking the CXCR4 chemokine receptor. *Proc. Natl. Acad. Sci. USA* **99:**7090–7095.

Luster, A. D. 1998. Chemokines-chemotactic cytokines that mediate inflammation. *N. Engl. J. Med.* **338:**436–445.

Ma, M., and A. Nath. 1997. Molecular determinants for cellular uptake of Tat protein of human immunodeficiency virus type 1 in brain cells. *J. Virol.* **71:**2495–2499.

Mackay, C. R. 1996. Chemokine receptors and T cell chemotaxis. *J. Exp. Med.* **184:**799–802.

Maclean, A. G., G. E. Belenchia, D. N. Bieniemy, T. A. Moroney-Rasmussen, and A. A. Lackner. 2005. Simian immunodeficiency virus disrupts extended lengths of the blood-brain barrier. *J. Med. Primatol.* **34:**237–242.

Magnuson, D. S., B. E. Knudsen, J. D. Geiger, R. M. Brownstone, and A. Nath. 1995. Human immunodeficiency virus type 1 tat activates non-N-methyl-D-aspartate excitatory amino acid receptors and causes neurotoxicity. *Ann. Neurol.* **37:**373–380.

Marder, K., S. Albert, G. Dooneief, Y. Stern, G. Ramachandran, and L. Epstein. 1996. Clinical confirmation of the American Academy of Neurology algorithm for HIV-1-associated cognitive/motor disorder. *Neurology* **47:**1247–1253.

Mattson, M. P., N. J. Haughey, and A. Nath. 2005. Cell death in HIV dementia. *Cell Death Differ.* **12**(Suppl. 1):893–904.

McArthur, J. C., N. Sacktor, and O. Selnes. 1999. Human immunodeficiency virus-associated dementia. *Semin. Neurol.* **19:**129–150.

McManus, C. M., K. Weidenheim, S. E. Woodman, J. Nunez, J. Hesselgesser, A. Nath, and J. W. Berman. 2000. Chemokine and chemokine-receptor expression in human glial elements: induction by the HIV protein, Tat, and chemokine autoregulation. *Am. J. Pathol.* **156:**1441–1453.

Meucci, O., A. Fatatis, A. A. Simen, and R. J. Miller. 2000. Expression of CX3CR1 chemokine receptors on neurons and their role in neuronal survival. *Proc. Natl. Acad. Sci. USA* **97:**8075–8080.

Michael, N. L. 2002. Chemokine receptors as HIV-1 coreceptors, p. 75–91. *In* T. R. O'Brien (ed.), *Chemokine Receptors and AIDS.* Marcel Dekker, Inc., New York, NY.

Miller, R. 2005. *Chemokines, HIV-1, and the central nervous system,* p. 181–191. *In* H. E. Gendelman, I. Grant, I. P. Everall, S. A. Lipton, and Susan Swindells (ed.), *The Neurology of AIDS,* 2nd ed. Oxford University Press, New York, NY.

Miller, R. J., and O. Meucci. 1999. AIDS and the brain: is there a chemokine connection? *Trends Neurosci.* **22:**471–479.

Minami, M., and M. Satoh. 2000. Chemokines as mediators for intercellular communication in the brain. *Nippon Yakurigaku Zasshi* **115:**193–200.

Miyauchi, K., J. Komano, Y. Yokomaku, W. Sugiura, N. Yamamot, and Z. Matsuda. 2005. Role of the specific amino acid sequence of the membrane-spanning domain of human immunodeficiency virus type 1 in membrane fusion. *J. Virol.* **79:**4720–4729.

Mizuno, T., J. Kawanokuchi, K. Numata, and A. Suzumura. 2003. Production and neuroprotective functions of fractalkine in the central nervous system. *Brain Res.* **979:**65–70.

Nath, A., K. Conant, P. Chen, C. Scott, and E. O. Major. 1999. Transient exposure to HIV-1 Tat protein results in cytokine production in macrophages and astrocytes. A hit and run phenomenon. *J. Biol. Chem.* **274:**17098–17102.

Nath, A., and J. Geiger. 1998. Neurobiological aspects of human immunodeficiency virus infection: neurotoxic mechanisms. *Prog. Neurobiol.* **54:**19–33.

Nath, A., K. Psooy, C. Martin, B. Knudsen, D. Magnuson, N. Haughey, and J. D. Geiger. 1996. Identification of a human immunodeficiency virus type 1 Tat epitope that is neuroexcitatory and neurotoxic. *J. Virol.* **70:**1475–1480.

Navia, B. A., E. S. Cho, C. K. Petito, and R. W. Price. 1986a. The AIDS dementia complex. II. Neuropathology. *Ann. Neurol.* **19:**525–535.

Navia, B. A., B. D. Jordan, and R. W. Price. 1986b. The AIDS dementia complex. I. Clinical features. *Ann. Neurol.* **19:**517–524.

New, D. R., M. Ma, L. G. Epstein, A. Nath, and H. A. Gelbard. 1997. Human immunodeficiency virus type-1 tat protein induces death by apoptosis in primary human neuron cultures. *J. Neurovirol.* **3:**168–173.

New, D. R., S. B. Maggirwar, L. G. Epstein, S. Dewhurst, and H. A. Gelbard. 1998. HIV-1 Tat induces neuronal death via tumor necrosis factor alpha and activation of non-NMDA receptors by a NFkB-independent mechanism. *J. Biol. Chem.* **273:**17852–17858.

Ni, H. T., S. Hu, W. S. Sheng, J. M. Olson, M. C. Cheeran, A. S. Chan, J. R. Lokensgard, and P. K. Peterson. 2004. High-level expression of functional chemokine receptor CXCR4 on human neural precursor cells. *Brain Res. Dev. Brain Res.* **152:**159–169.

Nishimura, Y., C. R. Brown, J. J. Mattapallil, T. Igarashi, A. Buckler-White, B. A. Lafont, V. M. Hirsch, M. Roederer, and M. A. Martin. 2005. Resting naive CD4+ T cells are massively infected and eliminated by X4-tropic simian-human immunodeficiency viruses in macaques. *Proc. Natl. Acad. Sci. USA* **102:**8000–8005.

Nottet, H. S., and H. E. Gendelman. 1995. Unraveling the neuroimmune mechanisms for the HIV-1-associated cognitive/motor complex. *Immunol. Today* **16:**441–448.

Nottet, H. S., M. Jett, C. R. Flanagan, Q. H. Zhai, Y. Persidsky, A. Rizzino, E. W. Bernton, P. Genis, T. Baldwin, J. H. Schwartz, C. J. LaBenz, and H. E. Gendelman. 1995. A regulatory role for astrocytes in HIV-1 encephalitis. An overexpression of eicosanoids, platelet-activating factor, and tumor necrosis factor-alpha by activated HIV-1-infected monocytes is attenuated by primary human astrocytes. *J. Immunol.* **154**:3567–3581.

Nottet, H. S., Y. Persidsky, V. G. Sasseville, A. N. Nukuna, P. Bock, Q. H. Zhai, L. R. Sharer, R. D. McComb, S. Swindells, C. Roderland, and H. E. Gendelman. 1996. Mechanisms for the transendothelial migration of HIV-1-infected monocytes into brain. *J. Immunol.* **156**:1284–1295.

Oberlin, E., A. Amara, F. Bachelerie, C. Bessia, J. L. Virelizier, F Arenzana-Seisdedos, O. Schwartz, J. M. Heard, I. Clark-Lewis, D. F. Legler, M. Loetscher, M. Baggiolini, and B. Moser. 1996. The CXC chemokine SDF-1 is the ligand for LESTR/fusin and prevents infection by T-cell-line-adapted HIV-1. *Nature* **382**:833–835.

O'Brien, T. R., N. L. Michael, H. W. Sheppard, and S. Buchbinder. 2002. HIV-1 infection in patients with the CCR5-Δ32 homozygous genotype, p. 215–225. *In* T. R. O'Brien (ed.), *Chemokine Receptors and AIDS.* Marcel Dekker, Inc., New York, NY.

Ohagen, A., S. Ghosh, J. He, K. Huang, Y. Chen, M. Yuan, R. Osathanondh, S. Gartner, B. Shi, G. Shaw, and D. Gabuzda. 1999. Apoptosis induced by infection of primary brain cultures with diverse human immunodeficiency virus type 1 isolates: evidence for a role of the envelope. *J. Virol.* **73**:897–906.

Pandey, V., and S. R. Bolsover. 2000. Immediate and neurotoxic effects of HIV protein gp120 act through CXCR4 receptor. *Biochem. Biophys. Res. Commun.* **274**:212–215.

Perno, C. F., S. Aquaro, B. Rosenwirth, E. Balestra, P. Peichl, A. Billich, N. Villani, and R. Calio. 1994. In vitro activity of inhibitors of late stages of the replication of HIV in chronically infected macrophages. *J. Leukoc. Biol.* **56**:381–386.

Perno, C. F., F. M. Newcomb, D. A. Davis, S. Aquaro, R. W. Humphrey, R. Calio, and R. Yarchoan. 1998. Relative potency of protease inhibitors in monocytes/macrophages acutely and chronically infected with human immunodeficiency virus. *J. Infect. Dis.* **178**:413–422.

Perno, C. F., R. Yarchoan, D. A. Cooney, N. R. Hartman, S. Gartner, M. Popovic, Z. Hao, T. L. Gerrard, Y. A. Wilson, D. G. Johns, et al. 1988. Inhibition of human immunodeficiency virus (HIV-1/HTLV-IIIBa-L) replication in fresh and cultured human peripheral blood monocytes/macrophages by azidothymidine and related 2′,3′- dideoxynucleosides. *J. Exp. Med.* **168**:1111–1125.

Perry, S. W., J. A. Hamilton, L. W. Tjoelker, G. Dbaibo, K. A. Dzenko, L. G. Epstein, Y. Hannun, J. S. Whittaker, S. Dewhurst, and H. A. Gelbard. 1998. Platelet-activating factor receptor activation. An initiator step in HIV-1 neuropathogenesis. *J. Biol. Chem.* **273**:17660–17664.

Persidsky, Y. 1999. Model systems for studies of leukocyte migration across the blood-brain barrier. *J. Neurovirol.* **5**:579–590.

Persidsky, Y., A. Ghorpade, J. Rasmussen, J. Limoges, X. J. Liu, M. Stins, M. Fiala, D. Way, K. S. Kim, M. H. Witte, M. Weinand, L. Carhart, and H. E. Gendelman. 1999. Microglial and astrocyte chemokines regulate monocyte migration through the blood-brain barrier in human immunodeficiency virus-1 encephalitis. *Am. J. Pathol.* **155**:1599–1611.

Persidsky, Y., J. Limoges, R. McComb, P. Bock, T. Baldwin, W. Tyor, A. Patil, H. S. Nottet, L. Epstein, H. Gelbard, E. Flanagan, J. Reinhard, S. J. Pirruccello, and H. E. Gendelman. 1996. Human immunodeficiency virus encephalitis in SCID mice. *Am. J. Pathol.* **149**:1027–1053.

Persidsky, Y., M. Stins, D. Way, M. W. Witte, M. Weinand, K. S. Kim, P. Bock, H. E. Gendelman, and M. Fiala. 1997. A model for monocyte migration through the blood-brain barrier during HIV-1 encephalitis. *J. Immunol.* **158**:499–510.

Persidsky, Y., J. Zheng, D. Miller, and H. E. Gendelman. 2000. Mononuclear phagocytes mediate blood-brain barrier

compromise and neuronal injury during HIV-1-associated dementia. *J. Leukoc. Biol.* **68**:413–422.

Petito, C. K., and K. S. Cash. 1992. Blood-brain barrier abnormalities in the acquired immunodeficiency syndrome: immunohistochemical localization of serum proteins in postmortem brain. *Ann. Neurol.* **32**:658–666.

Poggi, A., R. Carosio, D. Fenoglio, S. Brenci, G. Murdaca, M. Setti, F. Indiveri, S. Scabini, E. Ferrero, and M. R. Zocchi. 2004. Migration of V delta 1 and V delta 2 T cells in response to CXCR3 and CXCR4 ligands in healthy donors and HIV-1-infected patients: competition by HIV-1 Tat. *Blood* **103**:2205–2213.

Poltorak, M., and W. J. Freed. 1991. BN rats do not reject F344 brain allografts even after systemic sensitization. *Ann. Neurol.* **29**:377–388.

Premack, B. A., and T. J. Schall. 1996. Chemokine receptors: gateways to inflammation and infection. *Nat. Med.* **2**:1174–1178.

Price, D. L., S. S. Sisodia, and D. R. Borchelt. 1998. Genetic neurodegenerative diseases: the human illness and transgenic models. *Science* **282**:1079–1083.

Price, J. 1993. Organizing the cerebrum. *Nature* **362**:590–591.

Price, R. W. 2000. The two faces of HIV infection of cerebrospinal fluid. *Trends Microbiol.* **8**:387–391.

Pulliam, L., R. Gascon, M. Stubblebine, D. Mcguire, and M. S. McGrath. 1997. Unique monocyte subset in patients with AIDS dementia. *Lancet* **349**:692–695.

Pulliam, L., B. Sun, and H. Rempel. 2004. Invasive chronic inflammatory monocyte phenotype in subjects with high HIV-1 viral load. *J. Neuroimmunol.* **157**:93–98.

Rajagopalan, L., and K. Rajarathnam. 2004. Ligand selectivity and affinity of chemokine receptor CXCR1. Role of N-terminal domain. *J. Biol. Chem.* **279**:30000–30008.

Randolph-Habecker, J. R., B. Rahill, B. Torok-Storb, J. Vieira, P. E. Kolattukudy, B. H. Rovin, and D. D. Sedmak. 2002. The expression of the cytomegalovirus chemokine receptor homolog US28 sequesters biologically active CC chemokines and alters IL-8 production. *Cytokine* **19**:37–46.

Rao, K., R. D. Lund, H. W. Kunz, and T. J. Gill. 1989. The role of MHC and non-MHC antigens in the rejection of intracerebral allogeneic neural grafts. *Transplantation* **48**:1018–1021.

Rapalino, O., O. Lazarov-Spiegler, E. Agranov, G. J. Velan, E. Yoles, M. Fraidakis, A. Solomon, R. Gepstein, A. Katz, M. Belkin, M. Hadani, and M. Schwartz. 1998. Implantation of stimulated homologous macrophages results in partial recovery of paraplegic rats. *Nat. Med.* **4**:814–821.

Rappaport, A., M. Shaked, M. Landau, and E. Dolev. 2001. Sweet's syndrome in association with Crohn's disease: report of a case and review of the literature. *Dis. Colon Rectum* **44**:1526–1529.

Rappert, A., I. Bechmann, T. Pivneva, J. Mahlo, K. Biber, C. Nolte, A. D. Kovac, C. Gerard, H. W. Boddeke, R. Nitsch, and H. Kettenmann. 2004. CXCR3-dependent microglial recruitment is essential for dendrite loss after brain lesion. *J. Neurosci.* **24**:8500–8509.

Re, D. B., and S. Przedborski. 2006. Fractalkine: moving from chemotaxis to neuroprotection. *Nat. Neurosci.* **9**:859–861.

Reddy, R. T., C. L. Achim, D. A. Sirko, S. Tehranchi, and the HMR Group. 1996. Sequence analysis of the V3 loop in brain and spleen of patients with HIV encephalitis. *AIDS Res. Hum. Retrovir.* **12**:477–482.

Richard, R. M., S. E. Snyderman, and B. Haribabu. 2002. Chemokine receptor expression and regulatory mechanisms, p. 31–51. *In* T. R. O'Brien (ed.), *Chemokine Receptors and AIDS.* Marcel Dekker, Inc., New York, NY.

Rizzardi, G. P., and G. Pantaleo. 2002. Pathogenesis of HIV-1 infection, p. 51–75. *In* T. R. O'Brien (ed.), *Chemokine Receptors and AIDS.* Marcel Dekker, Inc., New York, NY.

Rodriguez, M. J., F. Bernal, N. Andres, Y. Malpesa, and N. Mahy. 2000. Excitatory amino acids and neurodegeneration: a hypothetical role of calcium precipitation. Int. J. Dev. Neurosci. 18:299–307.

Rosenkilde, M. M., K. A. McLean, P. J. Holst, and T. W. Schwartz. 2004. The CXC chemokine receptor encoded by herpesvirus saimiri, ECRF3, shows ligand-regulated signaling through Gi, Gq, and G12/13 proteins but constitutive signaling only through Gi and G12/13 proteins. J. Biol. Chem. 279:32524–32533.

Rucker, J., A. L. Edinger, M. Sharron, M. Samson, B. Lee, J. F. Berson, Y. Yi, B. Margulies, R. G. Collman, B. J. Doranz, M. Parmentier, and R. W. Doms. 1997. Utilization of chemokine receptors, orphan receptors, and herpesvirus-encoded receptors by diverse human and simian immunodeficiency viruses. J. Virol. 71:8999–9007.

Ryan, L. A., R. L. Cotter, W. E. Zink, H. E. Gendelman, and J. Zheng. 2002. Macrophages, chemokines and neuronal injury in HIV-1 associated dementia. Cell. Mol. Biol. 48:137–150.

Ryan, L. A., J. Zheng, M. Brester, D. Bohac, F. Hahn, J. Anderson, W. Ratanasuwan, H. E. Gendelman, and S. Swindells. 2001. Plasma levels of soluble cd14 and tumor necrosis factor-alpha type II receptor correlate with cognitive dysfunction during human immunodeficiency virus type 1 infection. J. Infect. Dis. 184:699–706.

Sabri, F., E. Tresoldi, M. Di Stefano, S. Polo, M. C. Monaco, A. Verani, J. R. Fiore, P. Lusso, E. Major, F. Chiodi, and G. Scarlatti. 1999. Nonproductive human immunodeficiency virus type 1 infection of human fetal astrocytes: independence from CD4 and major chemokine receptors. Virology 264:370–384.

Sacktor, N., R. H. Lyles, R. Skolasky, C. Kleeberger, O. A. Selnes, E. N. Miller, J. T. Becker, B. Cohen, and J. C. McArthur. 2001. HIV-associated neurologic disease incidence changes: Multicenter AIDS Cohort Study, 1990-1998. Neurology 56:257–560.

Sanders, V. J., I. P. Everall, R. W. Johnson, E. Masliah, et al. 2000. Fibroblast growth factor modulates HIV coreceptor CXCR4 expression by neural cells. J. Neurosci. Res. 59:671–679.

Sanders, V. J., C. A. Pittman, M. G. White, G. Wang, C. A. Wiley, and E. L. Achim. 1998. Chemokines and receptors in HIV encephalitis. AIDS 12:1021–1026.

Schall, T. J., and K. B. Bacon. 1994. Chemokines, leukocyte trafficking, and inflammation. Curr. Opin. Immunol. 6:865–873.

Schweighardt, B., J. T. Shieh, and W. J. Atwood. 2001. CD4/CXCR4-independent infection of human astrocytes by a T-tropic strain of HIV-1. J. Neurovirol. 7:155–162.

Segal, R. A., and M. E. Greenberg. 1996. Intracellular signaling pathways activated by neurotrophic factors. Annu. Rev. Neurosci. 19:463–489.

Seguin, R., K. Biernacki, R. L. Rotondo, A. Prat, and J. P. Antel. 2003. Regulation and functional effects of monocyte migration across human brain-derived endothelial cells. J. Neuropathol. Exp. Neurol. 62:412–419.

Serradji, N., M. Martin, O. Bensaid, S. Cisternino, C. Rousselle, N. Dereuddre-Bosquet, J. Huet, C. Redeuilh, A. Lamouri, C. Z. Dong, P. Clayette, J. M. Scherrmann, D. Dormont, and F. Heymans. 2004. Structure-activity relationships in platelet-activating factor. 12. Synthesis and biological evaluation of platelet-activating factor antagonists with anti-HIV-1 activity. J. Med. Chem. 47:6410–6419.

Sharpless, N. E., E. Verdin, C. V. Kufta, I. S. Y. Chen, and M. Dubois-Dalcq. 1992. Human immunodeficiency virus type 1 tropism for brain microglial cells is determined by a region of the env glycoprotein that controls macrophage tropism. J. Virol. 66:2588–2593.

Shi, B., U. D. Girolami, J. He, S. Wang, A. Lorenzo, J. Busciglio, and D. Gabuzda. 1996. Apoptosis induced by HIV-1 infection of the central nervous system. J. Clin. Investig. 98:1979–1990.

Shi, B., J. Rainha, A. Lorenzo, J. Busciglio, and D. Gabuzda. 1998. Neuronal apoptosis induced by HIV-1 Tat protein and TNF-α: potentiation of neurotoxicity mediated by oxidative stress and implications for HIV-1 dementia. J. Neurovirol. 4:281–290.

Shibata, A., M. Zelivyanskaya, J. Limoges, K. A. Carlson, S. Gorantla, C. Branecki, S. Bishu, H. Xiong, and H. E. Gendelman. 2003. Peripheral nerve induces macrophage neurotrophic activities: regulation of neuronal process outgrowth, intracellular signaling and synaptic function. J. Neuroimmunol. 142:112–129.

Shieh, J. T. C., A. V. Albright, M. Sharron, S. Gartner, J. Strizki, R. W. Doms, and F. Gonzalez-Scarano. 1998. Chemokine receptor utilization by human immunodeficiency virus type 1 isolates that replicate in microglia. J. Virol. 72:4243–4249.

Shields, P. L., and D. H. Adams. 2002. Chemokines and chemokine receptor interactions and functions, p. 1–31. In T. R. O'Brien (ed.), Chemokine Receptors and AIDS. Marcel Dekker, Inc., New York, NY.

Shiraishi, K., S. Fukuda, T. Mori, K. Matsuda, T. Yamaguchi, C. Tanikawa, M. Ogawa, Y. Nakamura, and H. Arakawa. 2000. Identification of fractalkine, a CX3C-type chemokine, as a direct target of p53. Cancer Res. 60:3722–3726.

Smith A. 1991. Symbol Modalities Test. Western Psychological Services, Los Angeles, CA.

Smith, G. M., and J. H. Hale. 1997. Macrophage/microglia regulation of astrocytic tenascin: synergistic action of transforming growth factor-beta and basic fibroblast growth factor. J. Neurosci. 17:9624–9633.

Soontornniyomkij, V., G. Wang, C. A. Pittman, C. A. Wiley, and C. L. Achim. 1998. Expression of brain-derived neurotrophic factor protein in activated microglia of human immunodeficiency virus type 1 encephalitis. Neuropathol. Appl. Neurobiol. 24:453–460.

Speth, C., M. P. Dierich, and S. Sopper. 2005. HIV-infection of the central nervous system: the tightrope walk of innate immunity. Mol. Immunol. 42:213–228.

Stamatovic, S. M., P. Shakui, R. F. Keep, B. B. Moore, S. L. Kunkel, N. Van Rooijen, and A. V. Andjelkovic. 2005. Monocyte chemoattractant protein-1 regulation of blood-brain barrier permeability. J. Cereb. Blood Flow Metab. 25:593–606.

Streilein, J. W. 1995. Unraveling immune privilege. Science 270:1158–1159.

Strizki, J. M., A. V. Albright, H. Sheng, M. O'Connor, L. Perrin, and F. Gonzalez-Scarano. 1996. Infection of primary human microglia and monocyte-derived macrophages with human immunodeficiency virus type 1 isolates: evidence of differential tropism. J. Virol. 70:7654–7662.

Sun, J., J. H. Zheng, M. Zhoa, S. Lee, and H. Goldstein. 2008. Increased in vivo activation of microglia and astrocytes in the brains of mice transgenic for an infectious R5 human immunodeficiency virus type 1 provirus and for CD4-specific expression of human cyclin T1 in response to stimulation by lipopolysaccharides. J. Virol. 82:5562–5572.

Suryadevara, R., S. Holter, K. Borgmann, R. Persidsky, C. Labenz-Zink, Y. Persidsky, H. E. Gendelman, L. Wu, and A. Ghorpade. 2003. Regulation of tissue inhibitor of metalloproteinase-1 by astrocytes: links to HIV-1 dementia. Glia 44:47–56.

Talley, A. K., S. Dewhurst, S. W. Perry, S. C. Dollard, S. Gummuluru, S. M. Fine, D. New, L. G. Epstein, H. E. Gendelman, and H. A. Gelbard. 1995. Tumor necrosis factor alpha-induced apoptosis in human neuronal cells: protection by the antioxidant N-acetylcysteine and the genes bcl-2 and crmA. *Mol. Cell. Biol.* **15:**2359–2366.

Tham, T. N., F. Lazarini, I. A. Franceschini, F. Lachapelle, A. Amara, and M. Dubois-Dalcq. 2001. Developmental pattern of expression of the alpha chemokine stromal cell-derived factor 1 in the rat central nervous system. *Eur. J. Neurosci.* **13:**845–856.

Thompson, K. A., M. J. Churchill, P. R. Gorry, J. Sterjovski, R. B. Oelrichs, S. L. Wesselingh, and C. A. McLean. 2004. Astrocyte specific viral strains in HIV dementia. *Ann. Neurol.* **56:**873–877.

Toborek, M., Y. W. Lee, H. Pu, A. Malecki, G. Flora, R. Garrido, B. Hennig, H. C. Bauer, and A. Nath. 2003. HIV-Tat protein induces oxidative and inflammatory pathways in brain endothelium. *J. Neurochem.* **84:**169–179.

Tong, N., S. W. Perry, Q. Zhang, H. J. James, H. Guo, A. Brooks, H. Bal, S. A. Kinnear, S. Fine, L. G. Epstein, D. Dairaghi, T. J. Schall, H. E. Gendelman, S. Dewhurst, L. R. Sharer, and H. A. Gelbard. 2000. Neuronal fractalkine expression in HIV-1 encephalitis: roles for macrophage recruitment and neuroprotection in the central nervous system. *J. Immunol.* **164:**1333–1339.

Tornatore, C., K. Meyers, W. Atwood, K. Conant, and E. Major. 1994. Temporal patterns of human immunodeficiency virus type 1 transcripts in human fetal astrocytes. *J. Virol.* **68:**93–102.

Tran, P. B., D. Ren, and R. J. Miller. 2005. The HIV-1 coat protein gp120 regulates CXCR4-mediated signaling in neural progenitor cells. *J. Neuroimmunol.* **160:**68–76.

Trillo-Pazos, G., A. Diamanturos, L. Rislove, T. Menza, W. Chao, P. Belem, S. Sadiq, S. Morgello, L. Sharer, and D. J. Volsky. 2003. Detection of HIV-1 DNA in microglia/macrophages, astrocytes and neurons isolated from brain tissue with HIV-1 encephalitis by laser capture microdissection. *Brain Pathol.* **13:**144–154.

Vallat, A. V., U. D. Girolami, J. He, A. Mhashikar, W. Marasco, B. Shi, F. Gray, J. Bell, C. Keohane, T. W. Smith, and D. Gabuzda. 1998. Localization of HIV-1 co-receptors CCR5 and CXCR4 in the brain of children with AIDS. *Am. J. Pathol.* **152:**167–178.

van der Meer, P., A. M. Ulrich, F. Gonzalez-Scarano, and E. Lavi. 2000. Immunohistochemical analysis of CCR2, CCR3, CCR5, and CXCR4 in the human brain: potential mechanisms for HIV dementia. *Exp. Mol. Pathol.* **69:**192–201.

Venkatesan, S., A. Petrovic, D. I. Van Ryk, M. Locati, D. Weissman, and P. M. Murphy. 2002. Reduced cell surface expression of CCR5 in CCR5Delta 32 heterozygotes is mediated by gene dosage, rather than by receptor sequestration. *J. Biol. Chem.* **277:**2287–2301.

Vicenzi, E., M. Alfano, S. Ghezzi, A. Gatti, F. Veglia, A. Lazzarin, S. Sozzani, A. Mantovani, and G. Poli. 2000. Divergent regulation of HIV-1 replication in PBMC of infected individuals by CC chemokines: suppression by RANTES, MIP-1alpha, and MCP-3, and enhancement by MCP-1. *J. Leukoc. Biol.* **68:**405–412.

Vitale, S., A. Schmid-Alliana, V. Breuil, M. Pomeranz, M. A. Millet, B. Rossi, and H. Schmid-Antomarchi. 2004. Soluble fractalkine prevents monocyte chemoattractant protein-1-induced monocyte migration via inhibition of stress-activated protein kinase 2/p38 and matrix metalloproteinase activities. *J. Immunol.* **172:**585–592.

Weiss, J., S. Downie, W. Lyman, and J. Berman. 1998. Astrocyte-derived monocyte-chemoattractant protein-1 directs the transmigration of leukocytes across a model of the human blood-brain barrier. *J. Immunol.* **161:**6896–6903.

Weiss, J. M., A. Nath, E. O. Major, and J. W. Berman. 1999. HIV-1 Tat induces monocyte chemoattractant protein-1-mediated monocyte transmigration across a model of the human blood-brain barrier and up-regulates CCR5 expression on human monocytes. *J. Immunol.* **163:**2953–2959.

Weissman, D., R. Rabin, J. Arthos, A. Rubbert, M. Dybul, R. Swofford, S. Venkatesan, J. Farber, and A. Fauci. 1997. Macrophage-tropic HIV and SIV envelope proteins induce a signal through the CCR5 chemokine receptor. *Nature* **389:**981–985.

Wiley, C. A., and C. Achim. 1994. Human immunodeficiency virus encephalitis is the pathological correlate of dementia in acquired immunodeficiency syndrome. *Ann. Neurol.* **36:**673–676.

Wiley, C. A., C. L. Achim, R. Hammond, S. Love, E. Masliah, L. Radhakrishnan, V. Sanders, and G. Wang. 2000. Damage and repair of DNA in HIV encephalitis. *J. Neuropathol. Exp. Neurol.* **59:**955–965.

Wiley, C. A., E. Masliah, M. Morey, C. Lemere, R. Teresa, M. Grafe, L. Hansen, and R. Terry. 1991. Neocortical damage during HIV infection. *Ann. Neurol.* **29:**651–657.

Wiley, C. A., R. D. Schrier, J. A. Nelson, P. W. Lampert, and M. B. A. Oldstone. 1986. Cellular localization of human immunodeficiency virus infection within the brains of acquired immune deficiency syndrome patients. *Proc. Natl. Acad. Sci. USA* **83:**7089–7093.

Williams, K. C., S. Corey, S. V. Westmoreland, D. Pauley, H. Knight, C. deBakker, X. Alvarez, and A. A. Lackner. 2001. Perivascular macrophages are the primary cell type productively infected by simian immunodeficiency virus in the brains of macaques: implications for the neuropathogenesis of AIDS. *J. Exp. Med.* **193:**905–915.

Williams, K. C., and W. F. Hickey. 2002. Central nervous system damage, monocytes and macrophages, and neurological disorders in AIDS. *Annu. Rev. Neurosci.* **25:**537–562.

Winkler, C., W. Modi, M. W. Smith, G. Nelson, X. Wu, M. Carrington, M. Dean, T. Honjo, K. Tashiro, D. Yabe, S. Buchbinder, E. Vittinghoff, J. J. Goedert, T. O'Brien, L. P. Jacobson, R. Detels, S. Donfield, A. Willoughby, E. G. D. Vlahov, and J. Phair. 1998. Genetic restriction of AIDS pathogenesis by an SDF-1 chemokine gene variant. *Science* **279:**389–393.

Wormser, G. P. 2004. *AIDS and Other Manifestations of HIV Infection*, 4th ed. Elsevier Academic Press, San Diego, CA.

Wu, D. T., S. E. Woodman, J. M. Weiss, C. M. McManus, T. G. D'Aversa, J. Hesselgesser, E. O. Major, A. Nath, and J. W. Berman. 2000. Mechanisms of leukocyte trafficking into the CNS. *J. Neurovirol.* **6**(Suppl. 1)**:**S82–S85.

Xiong, H., J. Boyle, M. Winkelbauer, S. Gorantla, J. Zheng, A. Ghorpade, Y. Persidsky, K. A. Carlson, and H. E. Gendelman. 2003. Inhibition of long-term potentiation by interleukin-8: implications for human immunodeficiency virus-1-associated dementia. *J. Neurosci. Res.* **71:**600–607.

Xiong, H., Y. C. Zeng, J. Zheng, M. Thylin, and H. E. Gendelman. 1999a. Soluble HIV-1 infected macrophage secretory products mediate blockade of long-term potentiation: a mechanism for cognitive dysfunction in HIV-1-associated dementia. *J. Neurovirol.* **5:**519–528.

Xiong, H., J. Zheng, M. Thylin, and H. E. Gendelman. 1999b. Unraveling the mechanisms for neurotoxicity in HIV-1-associated dementia: inhibition of neuronal synaptic transmission by macrophage secretory products. *AIDS Res. Hum. Retrovir.* **15:**57–63.

Yamaguchi-Kabata, Y., M. Yamashita, S. Ohkura, M. Hayami, and T. Miura. 2004. Linkage of amino acid variation and evolution of human immunodeficiency virus type 1 gp120 envelope glycoprotein (subtype B) with usage of the second receptor. *J. Mol. Evol.* **58:**333–340.

Yamamoto, H., M. Nagata, and Y. Sakamoto. 2005. CC chemokines and transmigration of eosinophils in the presence of vascular cell adhesion molecule 1. *Ann. Allergy Asthma Immunol.* **94:**292–300.

Yi, Y., F. Shaheen, and R. G. Collman. 2005. Preferential use of CXCR4 by R5X4 human immunodeficiency virus type 1 isolates for infection of primary lymphocytes. *J. Virol.* **79:**1480–1486.

Yoshikawa, M., T. Nakajima, K. Matsumoto, N. Okada, T. Tsukidate, M. Iida, N. Otori, S. Haruna, H. Moriyama, T. Imai, and H. Saito. 2004. TNF-alpha and IL-4 regulate expression of fractalkine (CX3CL1) as a membrane-anchored proadhesive protein and soluble chemotactic peptide on human fibroblasts. FEBS Lett. 561:105–110.

Zeev-Brann, A. B., O. Lazarov-Spiegler, T. Brenner, and M. Schwartz. 1998. Differential effects of central and peripheral nerves on macrophages and microglia. Glia 23:181–190.

Zheng, J., and H. E. Gendelman. 1997. The HIV-1 associated dementia complex: a metabolic encephalopathy fueled by viral replication in mononuclear phagocytes. Curr. Opin. Neurol. 10:319–325.

Zheng, J., A. Ghorpade, D. Niemann, R. L. Cotter, M. R. Thylin, L. Epstein, J. M. Swartz, R. B. Shepard, X. Liu, A. Nukuna, and H. E. Gendelman. 1999a. Lymphotropic virions affect chemokine receptor-mediated neural signaling and apoptosis: implications for human immunodeficiency virus type 1-associated dementia. J. Virol. 73:8256–8267.

Zheng, J., H. Peng, J. Rose, and S. Herek. 2005. Neurogenesis and its links to brain development, developmental therapeutics, and the pathogenesis of neurodegenerative disorders including HIV-1-associated dementia, p. 239–253. In H. E. Gendelman, I. Grant, I. P. Everall, S. A. Lipton, and S. Swindells (ed.), The Neurology of AIDS, 2nd ed. Oxford University Press, New York, NY.

Zheng, J., M. Thylin, A. Ghorpade, R. Cotter, Y. Persidsky, and H. E. Gendelman. 1998. CXCR4 mediates neuronal dysfunction by HIV-1 infected macrophage secretory product: importance for HIV-1 associated dementia. Abstr. Soc. Neurosci. 24:776.6.

Zheng, J., M. Thylin, A. Ghorpade, H. Xiong, Y. Persidsky, R. Cotter, D. Niemann, M. Che, Y. Zeng, H. Gelbard, R. Shepard, J. Swartz, and H. E. Gendelman. 1999b. Intracellular CXCR4 signaling, neuronal apoptosis and neuropathogenic mechanisms of HIV-1-associated dementia. J. Neuroimmunol. 98:185–200.

Zheng, J., M. R. Thylin, R. L. Cotter, A. L. Lopez, A. Ghorpade, Y. Persidsky, H. Xiong, G. B. Leisman, M. H. Che, and H. E. Gendelman. 2001a. HIV-1 infected and immune competent mononuclear phagocytes induce quantitative alterations in neuronal dendritic arbor: relevance for HIV-1-associated dementia. Neurotox. Res. 3:443–459.

Zheng, J., M. R. Thylin, A. Ghorpade, H. Xiong, Y. Persidsky, R. Cotter, D. Niemann, M. Che, Y. C. Zeng, H. A. Gelbard, R. B. Shepard, J. M. Swartz, and H. E. Gendelman. 1999c. Intracellular CXCR4 signaling, neuronal apoptosis and neuropathogenic mechanisms of HIV-1-associated dementia. J. Neuroimmunol. 98:185–200.

Zheng, J., M. R. Thylin, Y. Persidsky, C. E. Williams, R. L. Cotter, W. Zink, L. Ryan, A. Ghorpade, K. Lewis, and H. E. Gendelman. 2001b. HIV-1 infected immune competent mononuclear phagocytes influence the pathways to neuronal demise. Neurotox. Res. 3:461–484.

Zhu, S., D. Cerutis, J. Anderson, and M. Toews. 1996. Regulation of hamster alpha1B-adrenoceptors expressed in CHO cells. Eur. J. Pharm. 299:205–212.

Zou, Y. R., A. H. Kottmann, M. Kuroda, I. Taniuchi, and D. R. Littman. 1998. Function of the chemokine receptor CXCR4 in haematopoiesis and in cerebellar development. Nature 393:595–599.

Zujovic, V., J. Benavides, X. Vigé, C. Carter, and V. Taupin. 2000. Fractalkine modulates TNF-alpha secretion and neurotoxicity induced by microglial activation. Glia 29:305–315.

The Spectrum of Neuro-AIDS Disorders:
Pathophysiology, Diagnosis, and Treatment
Edited by K. Goodkin et al.
©2008 ASM Press, Washington, DC

13

Cerebrospinal Fluid Markers in the Management of Central Nervous System HIV Infection and the AIDS Dementia Complex

MAGNUS GISSLÉN, LARS HAGBERG, PAOLA CINQUE, BRUCE BREW,
AND RICHARD W. PRICE

"When *I* use a word," Humpty Dumpty said, in rather a scornful tone, "it means just what I choose it to mean—neither more nor less."

Through the Looking *Glass*, Lewis Carroll

THE NEED FOR LABORATORY DIAGNOSIS OF ADC AND ASSESSMENT OF DISEASE ACTIVITY

The major clinical and pathological features of the AIDS dementia complex (ADC), or synonymously, AIDS dementia, HIV-associated dementia, and minor cognitive motor disorder, were characterized almost 20 years ago (Navia et al., 1986a, 1986b). Despite major advances in diagnostic methods, identification of ADC relies on clinical recognition and often uncertain clinical or neuropsychological testing (Navia and Price, 2005; Price, 1995) (for a series of recent reviews from multiple viewpoints, see Gendelman et al., 2005). ADC remains a syndromic diagnosis without confirmatory objective laboratory measures. Indeed the role of the laboratory in ADC is to exclude alternatives rather than more directly establishing a positive diagnosis (Navia and Price, 2005). The problem of ADC diagnosis has confounded not only general physicians and patients at risk but also experts in the neurology of AIDS, despite accumulated individual and collective experience. As a consequence, there is a clear need for development of more objective, laboratory-based testing.

A second, related problem is the need for measures that can assess whether ADC is pathologically active or quiescent. This need stems particularly from the salutary effect of combination antiretroviral therapy (ART) on ADC. ART has reduced the incidence of ADC in regions of the world where it has achieved widespread use (d'Arminio Monforte et al., 2004; Sacktor, 2002). Moreover, it is clear from a number of reports that ART can arrest and at least partially reverse the clinical impairment of ADC (Eggers et al., 2003; Marra et al., 2003; Robertson et al., 2004; Spudich et al., 2005b). However, the degree of effectiveness of treatment is at times uncertain, and laboratory measures that more objectively assess treatment outcomes are needed.

The issue of disease activity is likewise important for patients with confounding neurological diseases or susceptibilities. Thus, HIV-infected patients with a history of head trauma, drug or alcohol abuse, nutritional vulnerability, or psychiatric disease present a considerable problem in diagnosis and management. Not only do these conditions confound the diagnosis of ADC when present in the background, but also they are associated with increased risk of HIV infection and with difficulty in gaining access to and adhering to ART. In our own experience, this background is particularly prominent in patients who now present with new onset ADC, so that those currently at highest risk also present the greatest problem in diagnosis. It would be particularly valuable to be able to discriminate the static encephalopathies associated with these conditions from active ADC. This problem is only likely to increase as the HIV-infected population ages, and dissecting the HIV-related component from an array of common disorders, including Alzheimer's disease, cerebrovascular diseases, or other pathologies, becomes a more common exercise. Newer, atypical central nervous system (CNS) diseases have also emerged during the treatment era that must be distinguished from ADC (Ammassari et al., 2000).

In the developed world with access to contemporary technologies, confident diagnosis of major opportunistic

Magnus Gisslén and Lars Hagberg, Departments of Infectious Diseases, Göteborg University, Sahlgrenska University Hospital, Sweden. **Paola Cinque,** Clinic of Infectious Diseases, San Raffaele Scientific Institute, Milan, Italy. **Bruce Brew,** Neurology, University of New South Wales and St. Vincent's Hospital, Sydney, Australia. **Richard W. Price,** Department of Neurology, University of California–San Francisco, San Francisco General Hospital, San Francisco, CA 94110.

infections (OIs) is usually possible and these diagnoses are readily distinguished from more severe ADC. Thus, neuroanatomical imaging, particularly using magnetic resonance imaging, combined with identification of organisms in cerebrospinal fluid (CSF) usually allows accurate diagnosis. With respect to CSF diagnosis, OIs are often confirmed by identification of the offending pathogen or its components by morphological stain of the organism, antigen detection (cryptococcal meningitis), culture (*Mycobacterium tuberculosis*), antibody profile (for example, serum antibody signifying susceptibility to recurrent toxoplasmosis), or nucleic acid amplification (notable examples are JC virus in progressive multifocal leukoencephalopathy, Epstein-Barr virus in primary CNS lymphoma, and cytomegalovirus causing encephalitis) (Cinque et al., 1997). Among the common OIs, only cytomegalovirus encephalitis commonly presents difficulty in distinguishing it from ADC on imaging and routine CSF examination (Cinque et al., 1998a, 1998b; Morgello et al., 1987).

Diagnosis of ADC in relation to CNS HIV infection differs from these OIs for which detection of the organism in the CSF implies disease etiology. The fundamental difficulty is that although ADC is caused by HIV itself (Cinque et al., 1998a, 1998b; Nath and Berger, 2004; Wiley and Achim, 1994), the presence of HIV in CSF has little diagnostic specificity. In fact, HIV reaches the CNS during primary infection and characteristically can be detected in the CSF throughout the course of systemic infection by nucleic acid hybridization methods irrespective of the presence of neurological disease (Bossi et al., 1998; Gisslen et al., 1998, 1999; Spudich et al., 2005b). Indeed, one of the cardinal pathogenetic questions in relation to CNS disease and HIV is how the virus can be present in the CNS for years without apparent neurological sequelae and subsequently lead to more invasive encephalitis and ADC at a later time in some patients. Whatever the answer, the diagnostic corollary of this question is that detection of HIV in CSF does not establish an ADC diagnosis. Furthermore, CSF HIV RNA may be elevated by the presence of CNS OIs or CSF pleocytosis (Brew et al., 1997b; Martin et al., 1998; Morris et al., 1998).

One of the major difficulties of interpreting CSF findings relates to the uncertain origin of its individual components (Ransohoff et al., 2003). Thus, while the fluid originates in the choroid plexus of the cerebral ventricles, it may be modified within the leptomeningeal compartment. With the exception of neural markers (see below) it is not always certain whether a particular marker originates in the brain, in the perivascular space, or within the leptomeninges. We have viewed the CSF as both a model of, and window into, the CSF. CSF may directly reflect brain infection, provide insight to the extent that CSF infection parallels that in brain, or mislead as the fluid diverges from the brain extracellular fluid (Price, 2000). Hence, its interpretation in relation to cerebral disease must always be tempered by this reservation.

In this brief commentary we consider an approach to more certain ADC diagnosis using CSF analysis. (An alternative approach to objective ADC diagnosis involves the use of newer neuroimaging techniques, including functional and anatomical imaging; however, this is not considered here.) We describe a pathogenetically based approach using a combination of CSF markers.

PATHOGENETIC SCHEMA OF ADC AS THE BASIS FOR CSF MARKER DIAGNOSIS

In simple terms, ADC pathogenesis can be considered to result from the evolving interactions of three factors: the

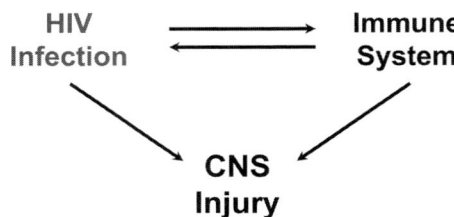

FIGURE 1   The three principal components of HIV-1-related neurodegeneration and ADC.

driving force, HIV; the modulating influence, immune dysregulation; and the target, CNS (Fig. 1).

The relationship among this trinity varies as systemic disease and immunosuppression progress. Systemic HIV infection is the ultimate driver and both perturbs the immune system and serves as the source for CNS HIV infection. The immune system sustains progressive damage that is measured by the blood CD4 count and underlies vulnerability to OIs. Importantly, alteration of the immune system is likely important in permitting progressive HIV infection of the CNS and in determining its pathogenic character (Price, 2000). Macrophages in the perivascular spaces and parenchyma and related microglia appear to play a pivotal role both in sustaining this late parenchymal infection (HIV encephalitis) and in producing neurotoxins that cause brain dysfunction and neural cell death (Gonzalez-Scarano and Baltuch, 1999; Williams et al., 2001, 2005; Williams and Hickey, 2002). However, the transformation of macrophages into virus and toxin producers within the CNS appears to require advanced immune dysregulation, though the specifics of this transformation are poorly understood.

The details of the current concepts of these pathogenic factors have been reviewed elsewhere (Gonzalez-Scarano and Martin-Garcia, 2005). As presented in Fig. 1 in its simplest terms, the interaction of these three factors helps to frame an approach to categorizing candidate diagnostics and to applying a combinatorial approach to define ADC using markers that apply to each: viral markers, immune-system-related markers, and brain markers.

Viral Markers

Initial reports of CSF HIV concentrations measured by nucleic acid amplification held the hope that measuring the viral load in CSF might serve as a diagnostic marker of ADC, and indeed when patient groups are examined, there is a general association of high CSF HIV RNA concentrations and ADC/HIV encephalitis (Brew et al., 1997a). However, it also soon became evident that CSF viral load alone was insufficiently specific to establish this diagnosis (Ellis et al., 1997; McArthur et al., 1997), particularly in an individual patient. Subsequent observations have suggested that high CSF HIV or concentrations substantially exceeding that of plasma HIV might increase the probability of ADC but likely apply to a minority of patients and also lack clear specificity (Cinque et al., 1998a, 1998b). For these reasons the CSF HIV RNA concentration as a diagnostic test of ADC has fallen from favor (see below).

Beyond the concentration of CSF HIV, investigators have also pursued whether more-detailed analysis of CSF virus might help in diagnosis. This has not yet borne practical fruit. While neurotropic or neuropathogenetic genotypes have been suggested to associate with ADC (Power et al., 1995, 2004), identification of sequences has not been secure enough to migrate to clinical practice. ADC has also been associated with preferential use of the CCR5 coreceptor by macrophage-tropic strains (R5 variants), and a commercial assay of receptor use is available (Coakley et al., 2005). However, most CSF HIV prefers this receptor even in the absence of ADC (Spudich et al., 2005a), so that this property is not diagnostically useful.

A number of studies have shown that CSF HIV exhibits compartmentalization with respect to blood virus, that is, virus populations in the CSF differ from those of blood (Strain et al., 2005; Wong et al., 1997). Moreover, the degree of compartmentalization of CSF and divergence of the CSF population from that of plasma may vary with the stage of infection. These differences between populations have been shown in a number of ways, including differences in viral characteristics, viral drug resistance, and, more directly, by sequence analysis of clonal populations (Chiodi et al., 1989; Cunningham et al., 2000; Di Stefano et al., 1995; Korber et al., 1994; Lanier et al., 2001; Reddy et al., 1996; Spudich et al., 2005a; Strain et al., 2005; Venturi et al., 2000). A convenient way of examining these differences is the heteroduplex tracking assay (HTA), and in a series of papers, Swanstrom and colleagues have shown that (i) primary infection shows minimal compartmentalization; (ii) chronic asymptomatic infection enhanced compartmentalization sustained by rapidly turning over cells, presumably T cells; and (iii) ADC exhibits the greatest degree of compartmentalization (Harrington et al., 2005; Ritola et al., 2004, 2005). These observations are consistent with concepts of early transitory, common amplified, and late autonomous CNS infections contributing variably to virus identified in CSF (Spudich et al., 2005b). It is possible that measuring the degree of compartmentalization or identifying macrophage-derived or brain-derived strains will eventually provide a more specific diagnostic measure of ADC, but this remains to be tested.

Immunological Markers

Elevations in CSF immunological markers were identified before the introduction of quantitative nucleic acid hybridization tests for HIV RNA, and several have been consistently shown to be elevated in ADC patients and to correlate with severity. Among those that have been characterized best are beta-2-microglobulin, neopterin, quinolinic acid, and monocyte chemotactic protein 1 (MCP-1) (Brew et al., 1990, 1992; Conant et al., 1998; Fuchs et al., 1989; Heyes et al., 1991; Kelder et al., 1998; Letendre et al., 2004; McArthur et al., 1992; Monteiro de Almeida et al., 2005), but other "footprints" of immunological or other host responses have been reported (Cinque et al., 2004; Conant et al., 1999; Griffin et al., 1990, 1991, 1994; Letendre et al., 1999; Sabri et al., 2001; Sporer et al., 2000, 2003). However, none of these measurements has entered mainstream clinical practice related to ADC diagnosis. Perhaps the principal reason is that none has been shown to be specific for ADC. They may be elevated in other inflammatory conditions, including HIV-related OIs (Lazzarin et al., 1992; Heyes et al., 1992; Hagberg et al., 1993; Bernasconi et al., 1996; Kolb et al., 1999; Abdulle et al., 2002, 2005; Cinque, 2005), and are sometimes elevated in neurologically asymptomatic subjects, particularly in the presence of a CSF pleocytosis (Abdulle et al., 2002; Gisslen et al., 1999). Thus, while there are group differences between ADC and neurologically normal individuals, the nonspecificity of elevated immune markers has discouraged clinical application to the individual patient. Also, the major impetus for study of these markers has been pathogenetic exploration, and work has not been extended to rigorously test their practical clinical application.

Brain Markers

The use of brain-specific markers to document neurodegeneration has been pursued in a variety of neurological diseases, but until more recently, not with the same enthusiasm in ADC. Candidate markers in this category include molecular products of neurons, astrocytes, oligodendrocytes, and microglia (Andersson et al., 1998; Berger et al., 1994; Brew et al., 2005; Gisslen et al., 1996; Green et al., 2000; Hagberg et al., 2000; Miller et al., 2000; Pemberton and Brew, 2001; Sporer et al., 2004). Although detection of several of these markers in the CSF of ADC patients has been reported, none have yet moved to clinical practice.

As an example, we have recently evaluated a neuron-specific marker, the light chain of neurofilament protein, which has proved to be a sensitive marker in other neurodegenerations (Norgren et al., 2003; Rosengren et al., 1996, 1999). We have found this protein to be elevated after ART interruption in 3 of 8 subjects studied (Gisslen et al., 2005) and in the great majority of ADC patients (Hagberg et al., 2000; our unpublished data). We view this as a prototype neural marker with an advantage over other classes of markers—it clearly originates in neural tissue and thus is not a simple product of inflammation. However, its elevation is unspecific with respect to the underlying neurodegenerative process and it is also found in some CNS OIs.

Other brain products have also been pursued and include markers of increased blood-brain barrier permeability such as CSF albumin (usually presented as a ratio to blood albumin) or products of brain injury pathways such as oxidative enzymes or metabolites (Andersson et al., 2001; Haughey et al., 2004).

An Approach Using a Combined Panel of CSF Markers

Given the nonspecificity of each of the types of markers briefly reviewed above, we suggest that an attractive avenue using current information is to develop a combinatorial approach assessing markers from each of the three factors highlighted earlier. In part, markers from each of the categories can make up for deficiencies of the others. Here is the approach that we are now testing.

HIV Marker: CSF HIV RNA

Unless compartmentalization measures migrate to the clinic or a specific neuropathic genotype can be identified that is readily assessed, measurement of total HIV RNA concentration is the major candidate in the HIV marker category. Although, as discussed earlier, detection of HIV RNA in CSF is not diagnostically specific, this measurement is still useful. Pathologically meaningful HIV encephalitis is unlikely in the absence of detectable CSF HIV when using sensitive methods (Havlir et al., 2001), though this needs to be established with certainty. Absence of CSF HIV also provides therapeutically practical information and suggests that further adjustments of ART are not likely to be helpful.

Immunological Marker

In the immunological marker category, the most promising measurements are those of CSF neopterin and MCP-1 (Abdulle et al., 2002, 2005; Brew et al., 1990; Hagberg et al., 1993; Letendre et al., 2004; Monteiro de Almeida et al.,

2005; Sevigny et al., 2004). Both are easily measured using commercial assays and are indicators of macrophage activation or taxis; thus, they detect an important pathogenic component of parenchymal brain HIV infection. Both have been well documented to be elevated in ADC, though they have not been rigorously tested for specificity. However, we suggest that one or the other of these measurements might be of ancillary value when measured along with the other two types. Interpreted pathogenically in concert with CSF HIV, their elevation suggests not only that HIV infection is present but also that macrophages are activated—processes necessary for, if not sufficient to cause, HIV encephalitis. Elevation of these markers may be particularly helpful in the case of HIV-infected patients presenting with neurological impairment due to another, less inflammatory cause (Alzheimer's disease, etc.) in which neural markers may be perturbed and HIV is detected but levels of macrophage activation are less marked.

Neural Marker

Neural markers are under exploration, with our own group pursuing the value of neurofilament protein (Gisslen et al., 2005; Norgren et al., 2003) as discussed above. A neural marker is most helpful in documenting that the CNS is currently sustaining injury. While unspecific as to the cause, spillover of neural markers in CSF separates active from static brain degeneration. It remains to be determined how sensitive individual candidate markers of this type are in this clinical setting.

We view the combination of these three classes of markers as a promising approach to more-specific ADC diagnosis, though clearly this needs direct empirical testing. However, even as one pursues the use of these markers alone or in combination, one needs to recognize that none will be entirely specific for ADC. All are frequently elevated in major OIs, and each can be raised alone or in combination with at least one of the other marker classes in other diseases. Hence, use of these markers must still be interpreted in a broader context, taking into account the clinical picture, and, in many cases, complemented by anatomical imaging using magnetic resonance imaging or computed tomography scanning. This does not vitiate their usefulness but only recognizes the commonality of brain injury pathways in a number of inflammatory disorders other than ADC in the context of HIV infection.

Since all these markers decrease during effective ART, they likely can also be used to evaluate treatment effects in patients with ADC.

CONCLUSIONS

The uncertainty of ADC diagnosis more than 20 years after its initial characterization remains a conspicuous shortcoming both in the clinic and in clinical trials. There is still a pressing need to develop objective, laboratory-based markers to aid in predicting development of ADC, establishing ADC diagnosis, and appraising disease activity, including treatment responses. While it is likely that the foundation has been laid with a number of exploratory studies already published, these have fallen short of practical clinical application. This deficiency warrants a renewed effort to further develop and analyze recognized markers and to explore novel markers.

Our own studies contributing to this essay were supported by grants from National Institutes of Health (R01 NS043103, R01 NS37660, R01 MH62701, and M01-RR00083), from the Medical Faculty of Göteborg University (ALFGBG-2874), from Västra Götalandsregionens FoU-anslag (VGFOUREG-3283), and from the Research Foundation of Swedish Physicians against AIDS.

REFERENCES

Abdulle, S., L. Hagberg, B. Svennerholm, D. Fuchs, and M. Gisslen. 2002. Continuing intrathecal immunoactivation despite two years of effective antiretroviral therapy against HIV-1 infection. *AIDS* **16**:2145–2149.

Abdulle, S., L. Hagberg, and M. Gisslen. 2005. Effects of antiretroviral treatment on blood-brain barrier integrity and intrathecal immunoglobulin production in neuroasymptomatic HIV-1-infected patients. *HIV Med.* **6**:164–169.

Ammassari, A., A. Cingolani, P. Pezzotti, D. De Luca, R. Murri, M. Giancola, L. Larocca, and A. Antinori. 2000. AIDS-related focal brain lesions in the era of highly active antiretroviral therapy. *Neurology* **55**:1194–1200.

Andersson, L., P. Fredman, A. Lekman, L. Rosengren, and M. Gisslen. 1998. Increased cerebrospinal fluid ganglioside GD3 concentrations as a marker of microglial activation in HIV type 1 infection. *AIDS Res. Hum. Retrovir.* **14**:1065–1069.

Andersson, L., L. Hagberg, D. Fuchs, B. Svennerholm, and M. Gisslen. 2001. Increased blood-brain barrier permeability in neuro-asymptomatic HIV-1-infected individuals-correlation with cerebrospinal fluid HIV-1 RNA and neopterin levels. *J. Neurovirol.* **7**:542–547.

Berger, J., M. Kumar, A. Kumar, J. Fernandez, and B. Levin. 1994. Cerebrospinal fluid dopamine in HIV-1 infection. *AIDS* **8**:67–71.

Bernasconi, S., P. Cinque, G. Peri, S. Sozzani, A. Crociati, W. Torri, E. Vicenzi, L. Vago, A. Lazzarin, G. Poli, and A. Mantovani. 1996. Selective elevation of monocyte chemotactic protein-1 in the cerebrospinal fluid of AIDS patients with cytomegalovirus encephalitis. *J. Infect. Dis.* **174**:1098–1101.

Bossi, P., N. Dupin, A. Coutellier, F. Bricaire, C. Lubetzki, C. Katlama, and V. Calvez. 1998. The level of human immunodeficiency virus (HIV) type 1 RNA in cerebrospinal fluid as a marker of HIV encephalitis. *Clin. Infect. Dis.* **26**:1072–1073.

Brew, B., R. Bhalla, M. Paul, H. Gallardo, J. McArthur, M. Schwartz, and R. Price. 1990. Cerebrospinal fluid neopterin in human immunodeficiency virus type 1 infection. *Ann. Neurol.* **28**:556–560.

Brew, B., R. Bhalla, M. Paul, J. Sidtis, J. Keilp, A. Sadler, H. Gallardo, J. McArthur, M. Schwartz, and R. Price. 1992. Cerebrospinal fluid beta 2-microglobulin in patients with AIDS dementia complex: an expanded series including response to zidovudine treatment. *AIDS* **6**:461–465.

Brew, B., L. Pemberton, P. Cunningham, and M. Law. 1997a. Levels of human immunodeficiency virus type 1 RNA in cerebrospinal fluid correlate with AIDS dementia stage. *J. Infect. Dis.* **175**:963–966.

Brew, B., L. Pemberton, P. Cunningham, and M. Law. 1997b. Levels of human immunodeficiency virus type 1 RNA in cerebrospinal fluid correlate with AIDS dementia stage. *J. Infect. Dis.* **175**:963–966.

Brew, B., L. Pemberton, K. Blennow, A. Wallin, and L. Hagberg. 2005. CSF amyloid beta42 and tau levels correlate with AIDS dementia complex. *Neurology* **65**:1490–1492.

Chiodi, F., A. Valentin, B. Keys, S. Schwartz, B. Asjo, S. Gartner, M. Popovic, J. Albert, V. Sundqvist, and E. Fenyo. 1989. Biological characterization of paired human immunodeficiency virus type 1 isolates from blood and cerebrospinal fluid. *Virology* **173**:178–187.

Cinque, P., B. J. Brew, M. Gisslén, L. Hagberg, and R. W. Price. 2007. Cerebrospinal fluid markers in central nervous system HIV infection and AIDS dementia complex,

p. 261–300. *In* P. Portegies and J. Berger (ed.), *Handbook of Clinical Neurology: AIDS and HIV Dementias*, 3rd series, vol. 85. Elsevier.

Cinque, P., G. Cleator, T. Weber, P. Monteyne, C. Sindic, G. Gerna, A. van Loon, and P. Klapper. 1998a. Diagnosis and clinical management of neurological disorders caused by cytomegalovirus in AIDS patients. European Union Concerted Action on Virus Meningitis and Encephalitis. *J. Neurovirol.* **4:**120–132.

Cinque, P., M. Nebuloni, M. Santovito, R. Price, M. Gisslen, L. Hagberg, A. Bestetti, G. Vago, A. Lazzarin, F. Blasi, and N. Sidenius. 2004. The urokinase receptor is overexpressed in the AIDS dementia complex and other neurological manifestations. *Ann. Neurol.* **55:**687–694.

Cinque, P., P. Scarpellini, L. Vago, A. Linde, and A. Lazzarin. 1997. Diagnosis of central nervous system complications in HIV-infected patients: cerebrospinal fluid analysis by the polymerase chain reaction. *AIDS* **11:**1–17.

Cinque, P., L. Vago, D. Ceresa, F. Mainini, M. Terreni, A. Vagani, W. Torri, S. Bossolasco, and A. Lazzarin. 1998b. Cerebrospinal fluid HIV-1 RNA levels: correlation with HIV encephalitis. *AIDS* **12:**389–394.

Coakley, E., C. Petropoulos, and J. Whitcomb. 2005. Assessing chemokine co-receptor usage in HIV. *Curr. Opin. Infect. Dis.* **18:**9–15.

Conant, K., A. Garzino-Demo, A. Nath, J. McArthur, W. Halliday, C. Power, R. Gallo, and E. Major. 1998. Induction of monocyte chemoattractant protein-1 in HIV-1 Tat-stimulated astrocytes and elevation in AIDS dementia. *Proc. Natl. Acad. Sci. USA* **95:**3117–3121.

Conant, K., J. McArthur, D. Griffin, L. Sjulson, L. Wahl, and D. Irani. 1999. Cerebrospinal fluid levels of MMP-2, 7, and 9 are elevated in association with human immunodeficiency virus dementia. *Ann. Neurol.* **46:**391–398.

Cunningham, P., D. Smith, C. Satchell, D. Cooper, and B. Brew. 2000. Evidence for independent development of resistance to HIV-1 reverse transcriptase inhibitors in the cerebrospinal fluid. *AIDS* **14:**1949–1954.

d'Arminio Monforte, A., P. Cinque, A. Mocroft, F. Goebel, F. Antunes, C. Katlama, U. Justesen, S. Vella, O. Kirk, and J. Lundgren. 2004. Changing incidence of central nervous system diseases in the EuroSIDA cohort. *Ann. Neurol.* **55:**320–328.

Di Stefano, M., F. Sabri, T. Leitner, B. Svennerholm, L. Hagberg, G. Norkrans, and F. Chiodi. 1995. Reverse transcriptase sequence of paired isolates of cerebrospinal fluid and blood from patients infected with human immunodeficiency virus type 1 during zidovudine treatment. *J. Clin. Microbiol.* **33:**352–355.

Eggers, C., K. Hertogs, H. Sturenburg, J. van Lunzen, and H. Stellbrink. 2003. Delayed central nervous system virus suppression during highly active antiretroviral therapy is associated with HIV encephalopathy, but not with viral drug resistance or poor central nervous system drug penetration. *AIDS* **17:**1897–1906.

Ellis, R., K. Hsia, S. Spector, J. Nelson, R. Heaton, M. Wallace, I. Abramson, J. Atkinson, I. Grant, J. McCutchan, et al. 1997. Cerebrospinal fluid human immunodeficiency virus type 1 RNA levels are elevated in neurocognitively impaired individuals with acquired immunodeficiency syndrome. *Ann. Neurol.* **42:**679–688.

Fuchs, D., F. Chiodi, J. Albert, B. Asjo, L. Hagberg, A. Hausen, G. Norkrans, G. Reibnegger, E. Werner, and H. Wachter. 1989. Neopterin concentrations in cerebrospinal fluid and serum of individuals infected with HIV-1. *AIDS* **3:**285–288.

Gendelman, H., I. Grant, I. Everall, S. Lipton, and S. Swindells. 2005. *The Neurology of AIDS.* Oxford University Press, Oxford, United Kingdom.

Gisslen, M., P. Fredman, G. Norkrans, and L. Hagberg. 1996. Elevated cerebrospinal fluid sulfatide concentrations as a sign of increased metabolic turnover of myelin in HIV type I infection. *AIDS Res. Hum. Retrovir.* **12:**149–155.

Gisslen, M., D. Fuchs, B. Svennerholm, and L. Hagberg. 1999. Cerebrospinal fluid viral load, intrathecal immunoactivation, and cerebrospinal fluid monocytic cell count in HIV-1 infection. *J. Acquir. Immune Defic. Syndr.* **21:**271–276.

Gisslen, M., L. Hagberg, D. Fuchs, G. Norkrans, and B. Svennerholm. 1998. Cerebrospinal fluid viral load in HIV-1-infected patients without antiretroviral treatment: a longitudinal study. *J. Acquir. Immune Defic. Syndr. Hum. Retrovirol.* **17:**291–295.

Gisslen, M., L. Rosengren, L. Hagberg, S. Deeks, and R. Price. 2005. Cerebrospinal fluid signs of neuronal damage after antiretroviral treatment interruption in HIV-1 infection. *AIDS Res. Ther.* **2:**6.

Gonzalez-Scarano, F., and G. Baltuch. 1999. Microglia as mediators of inflammatory and degenerative diseases. *Annu. Rev. Neurosci.* **22:**219–240.

Gonzalez-Scarano, F., and J. Martin-Garcia. 2005. The neuropathogenesis of AIDS. *Nat. Rev. Immunol.* **5:**69–81.

Green, A., G. Giovannoni, M. Hall-Craggs, E. Thompson, and R. Miller. 2000. Cerebrospinal fluid tau concentrations in HIV infected patients with suspected neurological disease. *Sex. Transm. Infect.* **76:**443–446.

Griffin, D., J. McArthur, and D. Cornblath. 1990. Soluble interleukin-2 receptor and soluble CD8 in serum and cerebrospinal fluid during human immunodeficiency virus-associated neurologic disease. *J. Neuroimmunol.* **28:**97–109.

Griffin, D., J. McArthur, and D. Cornblath. 1991. Neopterin and interferon-gamma in serum and cerebrospinal fluid of patients with HIV-associated neurologic disease. *Neurology* **41:**69–74.

Griffin, D., S. Wesselingh, and J. McArthur. 1994. Elevated central nervous system prostaglandins in human immunodeficiency virus-associated dementia. *Ann. Neurol.* **35:**592–597.

Hagberg, L., L. Dotevall, G. Norkrans, M. Larsson, H. Wachter, and D. Fuchs. 1993. Cerebrospinal fluid neopterin concentrations in central nervous system infection. *J. Infect. Dis.* **168:**1285-1288.

Hagberg, L., D. Fuchs, L. Rosengren, and M. Gisslen. 2000. Intrathecal immune activation is associated with cerebrospinal fluid markers of neuronal destruction in AIDS patients. *J. Neuroimmunol.* **102:**51–55.

Harrington, P., D. Haas, K. Ritola, and R. Swanstrom. 2005. Compartmentalized human immunodeficiency virus type 1 present in cerebrospinal fluid is produced by short-lived cells. *J. Virol.* **79:**7959–7966.

Haughey, N., R. Cutler, A. Tamara, J. McArthur, D. Vargas, C. Pardo, J. Turchan, A. Nath, and M. Mattson. 2004. Perturbation of sphingolipid metabolism and ceramide production in HIV-dementia. *Ann. Neurol.* **55:**257–267.

Havlir, D., R. Bassett, D. Levitan, P. Gilbert, P. Tebas, A. Collier, M. Hirsch, C. Ignacio, J. Condra, H. Gunthard, D. Richman, and J. Wong. 2001. Prevalence and predictive value of intermittent viremia with combination HIV therapy. *JAMA* **286:**171–179.

Heyes, M., B. Brew, A. Martin, R. Price, A. Salazar, J. Sidtis, J. Yergey, A. Mouradian, A. Sadler, J. Keilp, D. Rubinow, and S. Markey. 1991. Quinolinic acid in cerebrospinal fluid and serum in HIV-1 infection: relationship to clinical and neurological status. *Ann. Neurol.* **29:**202–209.

Heyes, M. P., K. Saito, J. S. Crowley, L. E. Davis, M. A. Demitrack, M. Der, L. A. Dilling, J. Elia, M. J. Kruesi, A. Lackner, et al. 1992. Quinolinic acid and kynurenine pathway metabolism in inflammatory and non-inflammatory neurological disease. *Brain* **115**(Pt. 5):1249–1273.

Kelder, W., J. McArthur, T. Nance-Sproson, D. McClernon, and D. Griffin. 1998. Beta-chemokines MCP-1 and RANTES are selectively increased in cerebrospinal fluid of patients with human immunodeficiency virus-associated dementia. *Ann. Neurol.* **44:**831–835.

Kolb, S. A., B. Sporer, F. Lahrtz, U. Koedel, H. W. Pfister, and A. Fontana. 1999. Identification of a T cell chemotactic factor in the cerebrospinal fluid of HIV-1-infected individuals as interferon-gamma inducible protein 10. *J. Neuroimmunol.* **93:**172–181.

Korber, B., K. Kunstman, B. Patterson, M. Furtado, M. McEvilly, R. Levy, and S. Wolinsky. 1994. Genetic differences between blood- and brain-derived viral sequences from human immunodeficiency virus type 1-infected patients: evidence of conserved elements in the V3 region of the envelope protein of brain-derived sequences. *J. Virol.* **68:**7467–7481.

Lanier, E., G. Sturge, D. McClernon, S. Brown, M. Halman, N. Sacktor, J. McArthur, J. Atkinson, D. Clifford, R. Price, D. Simpson, G. Torres, J. Catalan, K. Marder, C. Power, C. Hall, C. Romero, and B. Brew. 2001. HIV-1 reverse transcriptase sequence in plasma and cerebrospinal fluid of patients with AIDS dementia complex treated with Abacavir. *AIDS* **15:**747–751.

Lazzarin, A., A. Castagna, G. Cavalli, M. Amprimo, M. Vaj, C. Parravicini, G. Costanzi, P. Ronchi, C. Foppa, M. Moroni, and R. Turconi. 1992. Cerebrospinal fluid beta 2-microglobulin in AIDS related central nervous system involvement. *J. Clin. Lab. Immunol.* **38:**175–186.

Letendre, S., E. Lanier, and J. McCutchan. 1999. Cerebrospinal fluid beta chemokine concentrations in neurocognitively impaired individuals infected with human immunodeficiency virus type 1. *J. Infect. Dis.* **180:**310–319.

Letendre, S., J. Marquie-Beck, K. Singh, S. de Almeida, J. Zimmerman, S. Spector, I. Grant, and R. Ellis. 2004. The monocyte chemotactic protein-1-2578G allele is associated with elevated MCP-1 concentrations in cerebrospinal fluid. *J. Neuroimmunol.* **157:**193–196.

Marra, C., D. Lockhart, J. Zunt, M. Perrin, R. Coombs, and A. Collier. 2003. Changes in CSF and plasma HIV-1 RNA and cognition after starting potent antiretroviral therapy. *Neurology* **60:**1388–1390.

Martin, C., J. Albert, P. Hansson, P. Pehrsson, H. Link, and A. Sonnerborg. 1998. Cerebrospinal fluid mononuclear cell counts influence CSF HIV-1 RNA levels. *J. Acquir. Immun. Defic. Syndr. Hum. Retrovirol.* **17:**214–219.

McArthur, J., D. McClernon, M. Cronin, T. Nance-Sproson, A. Saah, M. St Clair, and E. Lanier. 1997. Relationship between human immunodeficiency virus-associated dementia and viral load in cerebrospinal fluid and brain. *Ann. Neurol.* **42:**689-698.

McArthur, J., T. Nance-Sproson, D. Griffin, D. Hoover, O. Selnes, E. Miller, J. Margolick, B. Cohen, H. Farzadegan, and A. Saah. 1992. The diagnostic utility of elevation in cerebrospinal fluid beta 2-microglobulin in HIV-1 dementia. Multicenter AIDS Cohort Study. *Neurology* **42:**1707–1712.

Miller, R., A. Green, G. Giovannoni, and E. Thompson. 2000. Detection of 14-3-3 brain protein in cerebrospinal fluid of HIV infected patients. *Sex. Transm. Infect.* **76:**408.

Monteiro de Almeida, S., S. Letendre, J. Zimmerman, D. Lazzaretto, A. McCutchan, and R. Ellis. 2005. Dynamics of monocyte chemoattractant protein type one (MCP-1) and HIV viral load in human cerebrospinal fluid and plasma. *J. Neuroimmunol.* **169:**144–152.

Morgello, S., E. Cho, S. Nielsen, O. Devinsky, and C. Petito. 1987. Cytomegalovirus encephalitis in patients with acquired immunodeficiency syndrome: an autopsy study of 30 cases and a review of the literature. *Hum. Pathol.* **18:**289–297.

Morris, L., E. Silber, P. Sonnenberg, S. Eintracht, S. Nyoka, S. Lyons, D. Saffer, H. Koornhof, and D. Martin. 1998. High human immunodeficiency virus type 1 RNA load in the cerebrospinal fluid from patients with lymphocytic meningitis. *J. Infect. Dis.* **177:**473–476.

Nath, A., and J. Berger. 2004. HIV dementia. *Curr. Treat. Options Neurol.* **6:**139–151.

Navia, B., E. Cho, C. Petito, and R. Price. 1986a. The AIDS dementia complex. II. Neuropathology. *Ann. Neurol.* **19:**525–535.

Navia, B., B. Jordan, and R. Price. 1986b. The AIDS dementia complex. I. Clinical features. *Ann. Neurol.* **19:**517–524.

Navia, B., and R. Price. 2005. An overview of the clinical and biological features of the AIDS dementia complex, p. 339–356. *In* H. Gendelman, I. Grant, I. Everall, S. Lipton, and S. Swindells (ed.), *The Neurology of AIDS.* Oxford University Press, Oxford, United Kingdom.

Norgren, N., L. Rosengren, and T. Stigbrand. 2003. Elevated neurofilament levels in neurological diseases. *Brain Res.* **987:**25–31.

Pemberton, L., and B. Brew. 2001. Cerebrospinal fluid S-100beta and its relationship with AIDS dementia complex. *J. Clin. Virol.* **22:**249–253.

Power, C., K. Zhang, and G. van Marle. 2004. Comparative neurovirulence in lentiviral infections: the roles of viral molecular diversity and select proteases. *J. Neurovirol.* **10:**113–117.

Power, C., J. McArthur, R. Johnson, D. Griffin, J. Glass, R. Dewey, and B. Chesebro. 1995. Distinct HIV-1 env sequences are associated with neurotropism and neurovirulence. *Curr. Top. Microbiol. Immunol.* **202:**89–104.

Price, R. 1995. Management of AIDS dementia complex and HIV-1 infection of the nervous system. *AIDS* **9(A):**S221–S236.

Price, R. 2000. The two faces of HIV infection of cerebrospinal fluid. *Trends Microbiol.* **8:**387–391.

Ransohoff, R., P. Kivisakk, and G. Kidd. 2003. Three or more routes for leukocyte migration into the central nervous system. *Nat. Rev. Immunol.* **3:**569–581.

Reddy, R., C. Achim, D. Sirko, S. Tehranchi, F. Kraus, F. Wong-Staal, and C. Wiley. 1996. Sequence analysis of the V3 loop in brain and spleen of patients with HIV encephalitis. *AIDS Res. Hum. Retrovir.* **12:**477–482.

Ritola, K., C. Pilcher, S. Fiscus, N. Hoffman, J. Nelson, K. Kitrinos, C. Hicks, J. Eron, and R. Swanstrom. 2004. Multiple V1/V2 env variants are frequently present during primary infection with human immunodeficiency virus type 1. *J. Virol.* **78:**11208–11218.

Ritola, K., K. Robertson, S. Fiscus, C. Hall, and R. Swanstrom. 2005. Increased human immunodeficiency virus type 1 (HIV-1) env compartmentalization in the presence of HIV-1-associated dementia. *J. Virol.* **79:**10830–10834.

Robertson, K., W. Robertson, S. Ford, D. Watson, S. Fiscus, A. Harp, and C. Hall. 2004. Highly active antiretroviral therapy improves neurocognitive functioning. *J. Acquir. Immune Defic. Syndr.* **36:**562–566.

Rosengren, L., J. Karlsson, J. Karlsson, L. Persson, and C. Wikkelso. 1996. Patients with amyotrophic lateral sclerosis and other neurodegenerative diseases have increased levels of neurofilament protein in CSF. *J. Neurochem.* **67:**2013–2018.

Rosengren, L., J. Karlsson, M. Sjogren, K. Blennow, and A. Wallin. 1999. Neurofilament protein levels in CSF are increased in dementia. *Neurology* **52:**1090–1093.

Sabri, F., A. De Milito, R. Pirskanen, I. Elovaara, L. Hagberg, P. Cinque, R. Price, and F. Chiodi. 2001. Elevated levels of soluble Fas and Fas ligand in cerebrospinal fluid of patients with AIDS dementia complex. *J. Neuroimmunol.* **114:**197–206.

Sacktor, N. 2002. The epidemiology of human immunodeficiency virus-associated neurological disease in the era of highly active antiretroviral therapy. *J. Neurovirol.* **8:** 115–121.

Sevigny, J., S. Albert, M. McDermott, J. McArthur, N. Sacktor, K. Conant, G. Schifitto, O. Selnes, Y. Stern, D. McClernon, D. Palumbo, K. Kieburtz, G. Riggs, B. Cohen, L. Epstein, and K. Marder. 2004. Evaluation of HIV RNA and markers of immune activation as predictors of HIV-associated dementia. *Neurology* **63:**2084–2090.

Sporer, B., S. Kastenbauer, U. Koedel, G. Arendt, and H. Pfister. 2003. Increased intrathecal release of soluble fractalkine in HIV-infected patients. *AIDS Res. Hum. Retrovir.* **19:**111–116.

Sporer, B., U. Koedel, F. Goebel, and H. Pfister. 2000. Increased levels of soluble Fas receptor and Fas ligand in the cerebrospinal fluid of HIV-infected patients. *AIDS Res. Hum. Retrovir.* **16:**221–226.

Sporer, B., U. Missler, O. Magerkurth, U. Koedel, M. Wiesmann, and H. Pfister. 2004. Evaluation of CSF glial fibrillary acidic protein (GFAP) as a putative marker for HIV-associated dementia. *Infection* **32:**20–23.

Spudich, S., W. Huang, A. Nilsson, C. Petropoulos, T. Liegler, J. Whitcomb, and R. Price. 2005a. HIV-1 chemokine coreceptor utilization in paired cerebrospinal fluid and plasma samples: a survey of subjects with viremia. *J. Infect. Dis.* **191:**890–898.

Spudich, S., A. Nilsson, N. Lollo, T. Liegler, C. Petropoulos, S. Deeks, E. Paxinos, and R. Price. 2005b. Cerebrospinal fluid HIV infection and pleocytosis: relation to systemic infection and antiretroviral treatment. *BMC Infect. Dis.* **5:**98.

Strain, M., S. Letendre, S. Pillai, T. Russell, C. Ignacio, H. Gunthard, B. Good, D. Smith, S. Wolinsky, M. Furtado, J. Marquie-Beck, J. Durelle, I. Grant, D. Richman, T. Marcotte, J. McCutchan, R. Ellis, and J. Wong. 2005. Genetic composition of human immunodeficiency virus type 1 in cerebrospinal fluid and blood without treatment and during failing antiretroviral therapy. *J. Virol.* **79:**1772–1788.

Venturi, G., M. Catucci, L. Romano, P. Corsi, F. Leoncini, P. Valensin, and M. Zazzi. 2000. Antiretroviral resistance mutations in human immunodeficiency virus type 1 reverse transcriptase and protease from paired cerebrospinal fluid and plasma samples. *J. Infect. Dis.* **181:**740–745.

Wiley, C., and C. Achim. 1994. Human immunodeficiency virus encephalitis is the pathological correlate of dementia in acquired immunodeficiency syndrome. *Ann. Neurol.* **36:**673–676.

Williams, K., S. Corey, S. Westmoreland, D. Pauley, H. Knight, C. deBakker, X. Alvarez, and A. Lackner. 2001. Perivascular macrophages are the primary cell type productively infected by simian immunodeficiency virus in the brains of macaques: implications for the neuropathogenesis of AIDS. *J. Exp. Med.* **193:**905–915.

Williams, K., and W. Hickey. 2002. Central nervous system damage, monocytes and macrophages, and neurological disorders in AIDS. *Annu. Rev. Neurosci.* **25:**537–562.

Williams, K., S. Westmoreland, J. Greco, E. Ratai, M. Lentz, W. Kim, R. Fuller, J. Kim, P. Autissier, P. Sehgal, R. Schinazi, N. Bischofberger, M. Piatak, J. Lifson, E. Masliah, and R. Gonzalez. 2005. Magnetic resonance spectroscopy reveals that activated monocytes contribute to neuronal injury in SIV neuroAIDS. *J. Clin. Investig.* **115:**2534–2545.

Wong, J., C. Ignacio, F. Torriani, D. Havlir, N. Fitch, and D. Richman. 1997. In vivo compartmentalization of human immunodeficiency virus: evidence from the examination of pol sequences from autopsy tissues. *J. Virol.* **71:**2059–2071.

The Spectrum of Neuro-AIDS Disorders:
Pathophysiology, Diagnosis, and Treatment
Edited by K. Goodkin et al.
©2008 ASM Press, Washington, DC

14

The Neuropathology of
HIV Pre- and Post-HAART

JUTTA K. NEUENBURG

Before the introduction of highly active antiretroviral therapy (HAART) in 1995–1996, clinical HIV-associated dementia was a common complication of HIV disease, especially in late-stage patients. Signs of HIV encephalopathy, the neuropathological correlate of clinical HIV dementia, were seen in brain tissue as early as 1984 (Moskowitz et al., 1984) and were described consistently throughout the early epidemic (Sharer et al., 1985; Navia et al., 1986; Petito et al., 1986; Lang et al., 1989; Levy et al., 1989; Budka, 1991b).

HIV encephalopathy is characterized mainly by infected and uninfected monocytes (which in tissue are called macrophages) and monocyte-derived HIV giant cells in brain tissue. HIV infection causes activation of monocytes and macrophages. Among other effects, activated monocytes and macrophages secrete chemokines and other neurotoxic substances that attract more infected and uninfected monocytes to the brain. Continued trafficking of monocytes from bone marrow via blood to the brain during HIV infection can lead to a "burn-out" of the bone marrow. Thus, anemia is one of the best predictors of clinical HIV dementia.

Not all HIV-infected persons with abundant monocytes and macrophages in brain tissue are clinically demented. Signs of HIV encephalopathy can also be found in brain tissue of nondemented HIV-infected patients at autopsy. Host factors appear to play a role in the detrimental effects of activated monocytes and macrophages: certain host/genetic factors increase the risk of developing HIV-associated brain disease (Gonzalez et al., 2002), suggesting that other factors might be protective in nondemented persons with HIV encephalopathy. However, clinical HIV dementia is more closely correlated with the abundance of monocytes and macrophages in brain tissue than with the extent of HIV infection in the brain (Glass et al., 1995). Therefore, activated monocytes and macrophages in brain tissue are important in the pathogenesis of HIV brain disease. For example, macrophages produce the neurotoxin quinolinic acid and may increase nitric oxide production. HIV increases the levels of inducible nitric oxide synthetase in cell cultures containing macrophages and astrocytes (Hori et al., 1999; Klatt, 2005). Although neurons and glial cells are not directly infected by HIV, the release of cytokines and viral factors from monocytes and macrophages and microglial cells, which are brain-resident macrophages, can lead to neuronal damage and neuronal apoptosis (Clifford, 2002).

The wide variability in viral production by HIV-infected macrophages, HIV genotype, and production of different toxins in brains (Cunningham et al., 1997; Klatt, 2005) may explain the variability in neuropathologic findings among different patients and even between different areas of the brain in the same person. Because of these variations, autopsy reports before the introduction of HAART showed that the number of HIV-infected patients with neuropathological signs of HIV encephalopathy was greater than the number of clinically demented patients. In one study, 205 patients had HIV encephalopathy at autopsy, but only 55% of them had been diagnosed with clinical dementia (Vago et al., 1990). Thus, central nervous system (CNS) lesions can be detected postmortem in patients who were not known to suffer from cognitive decline or HIV dementia, and CNS involvement is more widespread than assumed (Neuen-Jacob et al., 1993). Other studies emphasize that none of the neuropathological features of HIV infection correlate precisely with the clinical expression of HIV dementia (Budka, 1991a, 1991b; Bell, 1998; Gray et al., 2001).

After the introduction of ART, the frequency of AIDS-related deaths in countries with access to antiretroviral drugs decreased dramatically (Brodt et al., 1997). Accordingly, the number of autopsies dropped, and patients rarely presented with clinical HIV dementia in the clinics. Therefore, patients treated with HAART are less likely to develop HIV dementia and are expected to have fewer CNS lesions at autopsy. However, because of the rarity of HIV autopsies of persons who died while on HAART, it has been difficult

Jutta Neuenburg, Department of Neurology, University of California, San Francisco, Gladstone Institute of Virology and Immunology, San Francisco, CA 94158.

to determine if HIV encephalopathy has decreased as rapidly as clinical dementia.

This chapter presents (i) unifying neuropathological criteria for diagnosing HIV encephalopathy to decrease variability in diagnostic terms and criteria, (ii) an overview of the neuropathology of HIV infection, and (iii) data to show that HAART can reduce the severity of HIV encephalopathy but does not prevent monocyte trafficking to the brain.

FRANKFURT NEUROPATHOLOGY STUDY (1985–1990)

To determine the prevalence of HIV encephalopathy in autopsies before and after the introduction of HAART in 1995–1996, a group of physicians in Frankfurt, Germany, reevaluated neuropathology reports of autopsies performed on 436 HIV-infected patients between 1985 and 1999 at the Edinger Institute. All reports were classified according to strictly defined criteria (Neuenburg et al., 2002). Clinical data were available for 371 of these patients, who had been closely monitored at the Infectious Disease Clinic at Frankfurt University Hospital. Because clinical neurological evaluations were incomplete and could not be matched with the neuropathologic findings, a neuropathological definition of HIV dementia/HIV encephalopathy was used. The term "dementia" usually requires a clinical evaluation and, as mentioned above, is not always consistent with the neuropathologic findings, especially in HIV disease.

Neuropathological Classification of HIV Encephalopathy

To determine the extent of directly HIV-associated brain pathology, referred to as HIV encephalopathy, two Frankfurt physicians (W. Schlote and J. Neuenburg) evaluated the histopathological records of the 436 cases based on the criteria from the Consensus Report (Budka et al., 1991a, 1991b). Patients were divided into four groups according to defined criteria (Tables 1 and 2): no HIV encephalopathy, mild HIV encephalopathy, moderate HIV encephalopathy, or severe HIV encephalopathy. Required signs of HIV encephalopathy were multiple disseminated foci composed of monocytes, macrophages, microglia, and multinucleated HIV giant cells; the presence of HIV antigen or HIV leukoencephalopathy with diffuse white matter changes; and in cases of severe HIV encephalopathy, cerebral atrophy (Tables 1 and 2; Color Plates 3 and 4).

Neuropathological Classifications of Other Neuro-AIDS Complications

CMV

The diagnosis of cytomegalovirus (CMV) infection of the brain required the identification of cells with the characteristic cytoplasmic and intranuclear inclusions of CMV. The microglial nodular encephalitis that is often present in CMV-infected brains (Lang et al., 1989) was insufficient for the diagnosis. Immunohistochemistry and in situ hybridization were used in all cases.

TABLE 1 Frankfurt criteria for diagnosing HIV encephalopathy, related to Consensus Report[a] (also see Table 2)

Criterion no.	Clinical finding(s)	Comments
1	Nodular encephalitis Nodular microglia Microglial nodules Granular encephalitis	These inflammatory lesions are nonspecific and can be caused by HIV or any opportunistic disease (Kato et al., 1987; Budka, 1989); not diagnostic alone for any HIV encephalopathy.
2	HIV encephalitis HIV meningitis	Multiple disseminated foci composed of microglia, macrophages, and multinucleated giant cells Without multinucleated giant cells, HIV antigen or nucleic acids determined by immunohistochemistry or in situ hybridization required. Multinucleated giant cells are diagnostic (Sharer et al., 1985; Budka, 1986) when other histopathological findings are consistent with HIV encephalitis (Budka, 1991a, 1991b).
3	HIV leukoencephalopathy	Diffuse damage to white matter, including myelin loss, reactive astrogliosis, macrophages, and multinucleated giant cells but little or no inflammatory infiltrates (Lang et al., 1989). Without multinucleated giant cells, HIV antigen or nucleic acids as determined by immunohistochemistry or in situ hybridization required. Affects cerebral and cerebellar white matter mostly symmetric. Myelin loss evident as diffuse pallor in myelin stains and mono- or multinucleated macrophages with incorporated myelin debris (usually located perivascular) is a sign of myelin breakdown. White matter pallor without multinucleated giant cells or the local demonstration of HIV cannot lead to the diagnosis of HIV leukoencephalopathy (Navia et al., 1986).
4	HIV giant cells Multinucleated giant cells HIV macrophages Macrophage encephalitis	PAS-positive mono- or multinuclear macrophages, also called multinucleated giant cells or HIV giant cells, unequivocally prove HIV encephalopathy.
5	Cerebral atrophy	Required for severe HIV encephalopathy.

[a]Budka et al., 1991.

TABLE 2 Criteria for diagnosing mild, moderate, severe, any HIV encephalopathy[a]

Diagnosis	Criteria
Mild HIV encephalopathy	2 without multinuclear giant cells
Moderate HIV encephalopathy	3 or 4 or 2 with multinuclear giant cells
Severe HIV encephalopathy . . .	5 with 2 or 3
Any HIV encephalopathy	2; 3 or 4; 5 with 2 or 3
Not diagnostic	1

[a]Numbers refer to criteria in Table 1; data are from Neuenburg et al., 2002.

Toxoplasmosis

To diagnose cerebral toxoplasmosis, pseudocysts had to be present. Immunohistochemistry was used in all cases.

Fungi

To diagnose aspergillosis, Grocott stain in combination with morphology was used. To diagnose cryptococcosis, Grocott stain in combination with the typical mucinous capsules surrounding the fungi was used.

PML

The diagnosis of progressive multifocal leukencephalopathy (PML) required multiple sharply demarcated areas of demyelination and enlarged nuclei of oligodendrocytes. In situ hybridization with probes for JC virus was used.

Herpes

To diagnose herpes encephalitis, intranuclear inclusions and areas of necrosis had to be present.

Lymphoma

Malignant lymphomas were diagnosed by standard surgical pathology criteria. The size, number, distribution, and morphology of the lymphomatous lymphocytes allowed for ready distinction from inflammatory or reactive lymphoid infiltrates. Immunohistochemistry with B- and T-cell antibodies was used.

Demographics

Patients were divided into four groups according to the date of death and the type of ART available in Germany: 32 patients died before 1987 (before zidovudine was available), 170 died between 1987 and 1992 (monotherapy with nucleoside analogue reverse transcriptase inhibitors), 127 died between 1993 and 1995 (dual nucleoside analogue reverse transcriptase inhibitor combinations), and 42 died between 1996 and 1999 (HAART including a protease inhibitor [PI]). Access to the latest ART in Germany was widespread. In the population who died in the era of HAART, 57% received that therapy, 21% followed a PI-containing regimen, and 36% followed a non-PI-containing regimen. The overall mean age was 40.5 years; the mean ages of the four groups were very similar (39.9, 40.1, 41.7, and 40.1 years for the eras, respectively). Most (90.6%) autopsy cases were male and had homosexuality as a risk factor (83.6%). The remaining subjects had one or more of the following histories: intravenous drug use, commercial sex work, transfused blood products, or nosocomial infections. The number of autopsies peaked in 1987–1992, reflecting the decreasing mortality after the introduction of HAART.

Main Results

HIV Encephalopathy

Overall, HIV encephalopathy was found in 38% of all autopsy cases (34, 34, 37, and 60% in the eras, respectively) (Table 3 and Fig. 1). Throughout the study period, HIV encephalopathy was the most common histological finding and the only neuro-AIDS complication that increased over time; the prevalence of CMV, toxoplasmosis, cryptococcosis, and CNS lymphoma (related to Epstein-Barr virus) decreased (Fig. 1 and Table 3). The second most common complication was CMV (25.3%), followed by CNS lymphoma (9.4%), toxoplasmosis (7.0%), PML (3.5%), and cryptococcosis (1.1%). CNS tuberculosis and CNS herpes were rare (0.2 and 0.8%, respectively). Luetic encephalitis (neurosyphilis) was not found (see "Neuropathology" below for definition).

Further, the prevalence of HIV encephalopathy peaked in the era of HAART (1996–1999) and then declined. The incidence of brain CMV, toxoplasmosis, cryptococcosis, and lymphoma declined after peaking in 1987–1992. PML peaked before ART in 1993–1995. The incidence of cerebral tuberculosis and herpes remained low throughout. CNS aspergillosis was seen only in the first two periods, before 1987 (0.7%) and from 1988 to 1992 (1.4%). Thereafter, aspergillosis was still diagnosed clinically (lung) but was not seen in our neuropathology series.

TABLE 3 HIV-related brain pathology at autopsy[a]

Group (n = 371)	% of cases				P value
	1987 (n = 32)	1987–1992 (n = 170)	1993–1995 (n = 127)	1996–1999 (n = 42)	
HIV encephalopathy					
Any	34.4	33.5	37.0	59.5	0.014
Severe HIV	6.3	3.5	3.2	0	0.17
CMV	21.9	35.9	15.7	9.5	0.0005
Lymphoma	15.6	11.2	7.9	2.4	0.029
Toxoplasmosis	10.8	9	5.7	5.1	0.14
Aspergillosis	9.4	3.5	0	0	0.0021
PML	6.3	1.2	7.1	0	0.80
Cryptococcosis	3.1	1.2	0.8	0	0.23
Herpes	6.3	0	0	2.4	0.30
Tuberculosis	0	0	0.7	0	0.52

[a]Data are from Neuenburg et al., 2002.

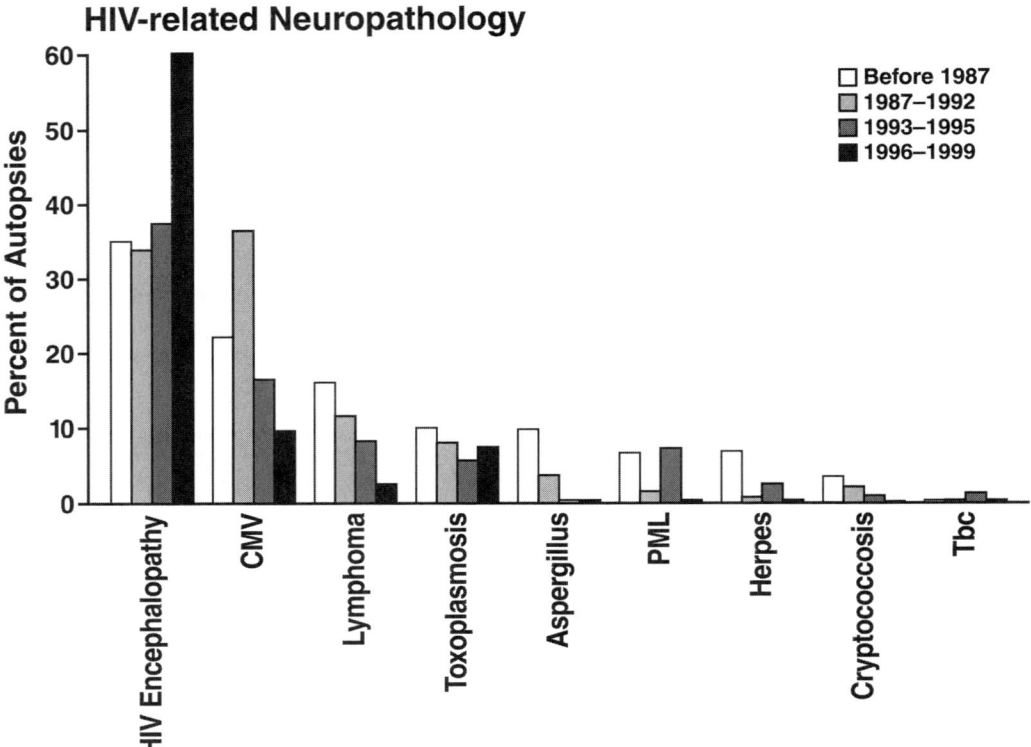

FIGURE 1 In the era of HAART (1996 to 1999), the prevalence of AIDS-related opportunistic infections of the brain is decreasing, but the prevalence of HIV encephalopathy is increasing. Data are from Neuenburg et al., 2002.

Overall, 85% of cases had CNS alterations related to HIV disease either directly (HIV encephalopathy) or secondarily (opportunistic infections), consistent with reports of other studies throughout the epidemic (Table 4). In 16.5% of cases, both direct and secondary HIV-related neuropathologies were found simultaneously, mostly HIV encephalopathy and CMV. Only 1.4% showed three different CNS diseases related to HIV disease; 38% of patients had opportunistic brain lesions without HIV encephalopathy.

Non-HIV-related CNS pathology

Other CNS pathologies included leptomeningeal fibroses (21% of cases) and hydrocephalus (20%). Both findings are expected. HIV-infected persons have a higher incidence of meningitis/encephalitis and cerebral atrophy. Intracranial hemorrhage was found in 12% of cases and included subarachnoid and subdural bleeding (4 and 2%, respectively) as well as mass and focal hemorrhages; 12% seems high but might reflect preselection of hospitalized patients. Increased intracranial pressure was found in 10% of the patients, and signs of ischemia or stroke were found in 9%. Although 9% seems low in view of recent findings that show increased incidence of cardiovascular and cerebrovascular events in HIV patients treated with HAART, only 9 of 436 patients were on PI therapy, so the incidence is comparable to that in other studies (Klatt, 2005). Brain edema was found in 3% of patients. Rare diagnoses were vacuolar myelopathy (0.9%; cord samples were not routinely available), central pontine myelinolyses (0.5%), and carcinoma metastases (0.2%). No neuropathology was found in 3% of cases.

Opportunistic Infections

The incidence of opportunistic infections of the CNS has declined with advances in ART (Brodt et al., 1997; Brew and Dore, 2000; Gray et al., 2001). Cerebral CMV and CNS lymphoma decreased after the introduction of HAART, even after controlling for CD4 count. In contrast, the frequency of direct HIV-related neuropathology at autopsy increased, especially after HAART became widely available (1996 to 1999). This finding is consistent with previous reports of increasing HIV encephalopathy from 1982 to 1993 (Maehlen et al., 1995; Sacktor et al., 2001) and persistence of mild HIV encephalitis through 1998 (Masliah et al., 2000). Mild clinical dementia also appears to be on the rise (Ives et al., 2001; Sacktor et al., 2002).

Why Has HIV Encephalopathy Increased in the Era of HAART?

To gain insight into the forces driving HIV encephalopathy and to understand the increase in its prevalence, a multivariate statistical analysis was performed. ART was the best predictor of signs of HIV encephalopathy ($P = 0.0073$), followed by last CD4 count ($P = 0.017$), nadir CD4 count ($P = 0.025$), and time since first clinical visit, reflecting disease duration ($P = 0.063$). Although the last CD4 count was an independent predictor of HIV encephalopathy, the independent effects of ART could not be accurately assessed. Most treated patients died in the last era. Thus, HIV therapy was confounded with the last era (Neuenburg et al., 2002). Nevertheless, the fact that ART was the best predictor of signs

TABLE 4 CNS involvement and prevalence of opportunistic and HIV-related diseases in autopsy series[a]

Pathology	% of all autopsies							
	Moskowitz et al., 1984	Anders et al., 1986	Petito et al., 1986	Nielsen and Davis, 1988	Levy et al., 1989	Lang et al., 1989	Neuen-Jacob et al., 1993	Neuenburg et al., 2000
CNS involvement	73.0	74.0	>80.0	70–80.0	75.0	88.0		85.0
Toxoplasmosis	30.8	9.1	10.0			26.0	21.4	7.6
Cryptococcosis	1.9	16.7	<3.0			4.0	4.3	0.9
CMV	3.8	21.2	26.0			10.0	8.6	23.4
PML	3.8	9.1	<3.0			7.0	2.9	3.4
HIV encephalopathy	9.6		28.0			16.0	20.0	36.5
Tuberculosis	1.9							0.2
Herpes			<3.0			1.0		0.7
Lymphoma	1.9	4.5	6.0			7.0	10.0	8.5

[a]Data are from Neuenburg et al., 2002.

of HIV encephalopathy prompted further research (see "San Francisco Study," below).

Decreasing Prevalence of Severe HIV Encephalopathy during HAART

In contrast to the increasing prevalence of mild and moderate encephalopathy, severe HIV encephalopathy was uncommon overall (3.2% of all cases) and was not detected in the era of HAART. Although there were too few cases for statistical analysis, the trends suggest that HAART may prevent severe direct HIV pathology of the CNS but has a limited effect in preventing CNS damage.

A reported autopsy series similarly found no evidence of severe encephalitis in the ART era, except for one case of persistent dementia on ART with evidence of "burnt out" HIV-induced pathological changes (Gray et al., 2001). ART may not prevent HIV encephalopathy, but the Frankfurt study suggests that the severity seen before 1996 no longer occurs. HIV encephalopathy may take a long time, maybe decades, to develop. If some contributing factors are eliminated, the time may be even longer. For instance, decreased viral burden and decreased overall inflammation might slow the rate of encephalopathic changes. Systemic therapy decreases the viral burden in plasma and in tissue compartments (Gupta et al., 1997; Price et al., 2001), thereby decreasing the severity of pathological changes. However, the entry of HIV in compartments over time cannot be prevented, and pathological changes in the mild and moderate categories are seen.

Also, systemic therapy might not decrease immune cell activation to the level of uninfected persons (Neuenburg et al., 2005a). Activated immune cells might still reach the brain tissue compartment and contribute to the encephalopathic changes that accumulate over time. The severe cases of HIV dementia and HIV encephalopathy seen before the introduction of HAART were probably due to massive systemic inflammation, with high viral loads in cerebrospinal fluid (CSF) and blood and massive trafficking of HIV-infected and uninfected monocytes/macrophages from bone marrow via blood to the brain.

Systemic inflammation also makes the blood-brain barrier more permeable. At circumventricular organs—specialized brain regions that lack a tight blood-brain barrier—adhesion molecules might function differently in inflammation (Roth et al., 2004). In cells within the circumventricular organs, receptors for inflammatory cytokines and bacterial fragments are constitutively expressed; their expression is upregulated in systemic inflammation (Roth et al., 2004). In HIV-infected patients with high viral loads, these differences might further enhance monocyte trafficking. Conversely, patients on systemic ART who have low systemic viral load may have reduced, but nevertheless continuous, monocyte trafficking into tissues.

Long-Term Survival Appears To Increase the Risk for HIV Encephalopathy

The length of HIV infection is an important factor for HIV encephalopathy (Neuenburg et al., 2002). In the Frankfurt study, HIV encephalopathy and HAART were associated with increased time since the first clinical visit, reflecting a longer duration of HIV infection. HAART might also be associated with a survival benefit, because patients seeking ART are more likely to be in proper medical care for other conditions. HIV encephalopathy was also associated with lower CD4 counts (current and nadir), which also indicate longer disease duration. However, the independent effects of duration of infection, time period, and ART could not be evaluated, because these variables were strongly correlated.

The rising prevalence of HIV encephalopathy at time of death may reflect a longer survival time after initial HIV infection in the era of HAART. Importantly, however, the mean ages in all periods did not differ substantially (mean age, ~40 years in all four groups). In the last era, the mean ages of persons with and without any HIV encephalopathy are similar as well: 39.9 and 40.3 years, respectively. Therefore, the increased prevalence of HIV encephalopathy in the era of HAART cannot be attributed to older age at death; rather, the length of HIV infection is important.

HIV infection may be more pathogenic for CNS tissue later in the course of disease. Lentiviruses such as HIV have CNS tropism (Gardner et al., 1995), and lentiviral diseases take decades to develop. HIV may be neurotropic as well, and human autopsy series from 1984 through 1999 demonstrated high proportions of subjects dying with CNS pathology, including evidence of pathology directly related to HIV infection of the brain (Table 4).

Further emphasizing the role of disease duration in HIV brain disease, subjects in later stages of disease (as judged by CD4 cell count) were more likely to have increases in CSF viral load during HAART (Staprans et al., 1999), indicating localized HIV replication in the CNS. Viral genetic analysis also suggests that HIV replicates in the brain only during the late stages of HIV infection. The increases in HIV encephalopathy might suggest that, once HIV acquires neurotropic properties, the effects of neurotropism are not fully reversed by HAART. Alternatively, despite HAART, monocytes might continue trafficking to the brain, perhaps because of incomplete suppression of viral replication, especially in tissues such as the brain, where penetration of drugs may be impaired by the blood-brain barrier.

Summary

The findings from the Frankfurt study show that HAART prolongs life, decreases opportunistic CNS infections, and leads to reduced severity of HIV encephalopathy. However, HAART does not prevent monocyte trafficking to the brain.

NEUROPATHOLOGY: DIAGNOSIS OF NEURO-AIDS COMPLICATIONS

HIV Encephalopathy

Gross examination of the brain and spinal cord at autopsy may reveal no lesions specific for HIV encephalopathy. Brain atrophy is present in severe cases and can be mild to marked, with hydrocephalus ex vacuo. Subcortical lesions are most prominent in hemispheric white matter and deep gray nuclei such as the basal ganglia. Multiple areas should be sampled for histologic examination. Microscopic findings with HIV encephalopathy usually demonstrate increased numbers of macrophages and multinucleated giant cells and diffuse myelin pallor. Areas of active HIV encephalitis contain abundant HIV RNA and DNA localized to macrophages and microglia, but also uninfected macrophages. Neurons and astrocytes usually are uninfected.

Microscopic examination of the brain at autopsy in HIV infection usually reveals subacute encephalitis in varying degrees consisting of multiple disseminated foci composed of monocytes, macrophages, microglia, and multinucleated HIV giant cells. These manifestations are often located near small blood vessels ("perivascular cuffing"), especially in the basal ganglia, deep cerebral white matter, and brainstem. They can also appear scattered in the gray matter or leptomeninges. Multinucleated giant cells are the hallmark of HIV infection of the brain. HIV can be demonstrated in their cytoplasm. Even with aggressive ART, the CNS remains an important reservoir for HIV infection (Schrager and D'Souza, 1998). In some cases of HIV encephalopathy, multinucleated giant cells are not present, but large amounts of HIV antigen may be found in macrophages and microglia (Clifford, 2002).

HIV can be detected in tissues by immunohistochemical methods using antibodies to p24, gp41, or gp120. HIV encephalopathy can occur in all stages of HIV infection. Perivascular or leptomeningeal lymphocytic infiltration can occur even in persons with asymptomatic HIV infection. In CSF samples, an increasing level of HIV RNA can correlate with the presence of HIV encephalopathy and usually correlates with the number of white cells (Neuenburg et al., 2004).

Microglial nodules can be found in both gray and white matter throughout the brain, including the brainstem, at any stage of HIV infection. They are not HIV specific and may be present with viral, protozoal, or bacterial infection, neoplasia, or traumatic focal necrosis. Microglial nodules are small, focal collections of cells, thought to arise from brain-resident glial cells that are mixed with invading systemic inflammatory cells, including reactive astrocytes, lymphocytes, and monocytes. They are often located near small capillaries that may have plump endothelial cells with nearby hemosiderin-laden macrophages that sometimes can give rise to large multinucleated cells (up to 25 μm in diameter) with irregular nuclei and scant cytoplasm. Most of the astroglial cells in microglial nodules have round or oblong nuclei with scant cytoplasm. Small foci of necrosis may be seen in or close to the nodules. As mentioned earlier, HIV and other infectious agents, such as CMV and Toxoplasma gondii, may be found. In cases of CMV infection, microglial nodules are often periventricular. In some microglial nodules, HIV-infected cells may be seen with immunohistochemical staining. In those cases, HIV encephalopathy is likely the cause. Sometimes, no infectious agent can be demonstrated. Therefore, in the Frankfurt study, the presence of HIV antigen was required for the diagnosis of HIV encephalopathy.

HIV leukoencephalopathy produces diffuse bilateral damage to cerebral white matter that can be seen on magnetic resonance imaging (MRI) scans and may involve the cerebellum (Ekholm and Simon, 1988; Budka, 1989; Budka, 1991a, 1991b). Myelin loss is found mainly in the deep white matter, with a tendency to spare the subcortical U fibers and the more compact myelin bundles of corpus callosum, internal capsules, optic radiations, and descending tracts in the brainstem. In HIV-infected patients, especially those with HIV encephalopathy, motor-evoked potentials, which measure pyramid tract conduction time, can be delayed (Neuenburg, 1997). Grossly, the lesions may resemble multiple sclerosis plaques.

Examination of the mostly perivascular lesions by light microscopy shows myelin debris in macrophages, reactive astrocytosis, hemosiderin in macrophages, multinucleated giant cells, and little or no inflammation. If multinucleated giant cells are absent, the presence of HIV antigen in macrophages is required for the diagnosis. Vacuolar myelin swellings can occur, as well as axonal damage. Oligodendroglial cells usually appear normal. A multifocal pontine leukoencephalopathy can be seen in HIV-infected patients but is rare.

Is there a "new" leukoencephalopathy in the era of HAART? Although HIV-infected patients have shown improvement of white matter disease after going on HAART (Thurnher et al., 2000), not all patients improve consistently (Filippi et al., 1998). Some patients who are responding well, both virologically and immunologically, to HAART can actually have progressive white matter lesions on MRI (Filippi et al., 1998; Joerg Madlener, personal communication). Between 1991 and 1999, focal mass lesions declined significantly, but focal white matter lesions without mass effect or contrast enhancement became the most frequently seen focal brain lesions (Ammassari et al., 2000). The etiology of these lesions is not clear. Host factors most certainly play a role.

CMV

The prevalence of CMV in AIDS patients at autopsy has been declining because of prophylaxis and therapy for ocular

CMV lesions and HAART. CMV encephalitis does not cause a specific clinical syndrome. Headache, disorientation, confusion, cognitive dysfunction, focal neurologic deficits, and impaired memory can be present, or neurological symptoms can be absent. The abrupt onset of mental status changes, along with radiologic findings of periventricular or meningeal contrast enhancement and hydrocephalus, can suggest CMV meningoencephalitis. Although isolated CMV infection of the CNS is possible, CMV is usually disseminated throughout the brain; CMV retinitis can be concomitant. Analysis of CSF may reveal increased protein and a mild lymphocytic pleocytosis. The cells with inclusions typically seen in CMV infections in tissue are generally not seen in the CSF. The pathologic findings of CMV infection of the brain correlate poorly with the degree of neurologic problems. The most common pattern of involvement is an encephalitis, which tends to progress as HIV disease advances; therefore, the incidence and prevalence of CMV brain involvement have decreased since the introduction of HAART. Grossly, no specific lesions are seen.

Microscopically, CMV can cause meningoencephalomyelitis, most often periventricular, in the brainstem (most often pons or medulla), basal ganglia, cerebrum (with gray and white matter equally involved), and cerebellum; CMV lesions may also be found in the meninges or beneath the pia mater on gyral surfaces. Histologic patterns include ventriculitis, necrotizing vasculitis, and microglial nodules. Large violaceous intranuclear and small basophilic intracytoplasmic inclusions can be present in microglial nodules, ependymal cells, astrocytes, or even neurons, but CMV inclusions can be difficult to find, even in microglial nodules, the most common feature.

Toxoplasmosis

Toxoplasmosis is the most common focal brain lesion in AIDS. It occurs most often in the advanced stages of HIV infection with a CD4 count of <100 cells/μl. If treated early, it has a good prognosis. The prevalence of toxoplasmosis at autopsy has been decreasing because of drug prophylaxis, and it now appears in <10% of cases (Jellinger et al., 2000). In most cases, toxoplasmosis is thought to result from reactivation of a latent infection. The immunoglobulin G antibody is useful only if absent; a large percentage of the population usually is positive without any symptoms.

The most common presenting symptoms are fever, headache, focal neurological signs, confusion, or altered consciousness. The most common focal neurologic signs include hemiparesis, ataxia, and cranial nerve palsies. Seizures are less frequent, depending on how close the lesions are to the cortex.

On computed tomography (CT) scans, toxoplasmosis lesions can resemble lymphomas, malignant tumor metastases, or abscesses. The CT findings include focal or multiple lesions (usually two or three) that appear as hypodense masses with ring or nodular contrast enhancement and surrounding edema and mass effect. In rare cases, lesions do not display contrast enhancement. If the mass effect is substantial, cortisone therapy is indicated and can have a positive effect on the concomitant vasculitis (Husstedt, 1998).

By MRI, toxoplasmosis lesions appear as hypointense on T1-weighted images and as discrete foci of high signal intensity with moderate edema on T2-weighted images. Typically, there is moderate to intense ring enhancement after administration of contrast media (Chang et al., 1995).

In HIV infection, serum antitoxoplasma antibodies are usually but not always present. However, if serologic tests are positive and the CD4 lymphocyte count is <200/μl, prophylaxis with trimethoprim-sulfamethoxazole may be useful (Gallant et al., 1994).

T. gondii encephalitis leads to necrotizing abscesses with acute and chronic inflammation, macrophage infiltration, and vascular proliferation. These lesions can be large or small, single or widespread. Usually, they are found in subcortical white matter and deep gray nuclei, and less often they are found in cerebral cortex. The numerous free tachyzoites at the periphery of necrotizing lesions are very destructive, and there is a significant inflammatory response with a variety of inflammatory cells. True cysts or pseudocysts containing *T. gondii* bradyzoites may not be surrounded by an inflammatory response until the wall of the cyst ruptures. Accompanying vasculitis can be present, possibly an allergic response. Endothelial proliferation in some blood vessels has been observed.

T. gondii lesions may organize and contain numerous lipid-laden macrophages. They have a fibrous capsule with collagen, typical for brain abscesses that can be identified in surgical biopsies. A lymphoplasmacytic infiltrate is typically present. Healing may lead to cystic lesions with macrophages and surrounding gliosis. Organizing and cystic lesions contain few detectable organisms; therefore, immunohistochemical staining with antibody to *T. gondii* helps to identify the tachyzoites and make a proper diagnosis.

Treatment with oral pyrimethamine and sulfadiazine results in a good clinical response and recovery within 4 to 6 weeks in most cases. Small residual neurologic deficits can persist. Toxicity of pyrimethamine to bone marrow can be reduced by concomitant folinic acid therapy. An alternative therapy consists of clindamycin with pyrimethamine. Treatment with leucovorin is also effective, and clindamycin and clarithromycin have been used. Relapses are common and usually due to lack of maintenance therapy (Husstedt, 1998). Lifelong maintenance of pyrimethamine therapy (with or without sulfadiazine) is necessary to prevent relapses. The lack of a response to antitoxoplasma therapy in 1 to 2 weeks suggests that the lesion might not be due to toxoplasmosis.

Lymphoma

Most HIV-related non-Hodgkin's lymphomas of the CNS are primary neoplasms. Metastases of systemic lymphomas are more often meningeal but can be inside the CNS as well. CNS lymphomas are of the diffuse, high-grade, large-cell tumors of B-lymphocyte origin and are thought to be a mass of B lymphocytes infected with Epstein-Barr virus. On CT scans, single or multiple lesions are hyperdense with solid or ring-like contrast enhancement. They can appear as multiple discrete ring-enhancing lesions and be very similar to toxoplasmosis lesions. The lesions often are near a ventricle, in the basal ganglia, or near subarachnoid space and frequently have edema and mass effect. By MRI, the lesions are hyperintense on T1-weight images and isointense to hyperintense masses with moderate edema and mass effect on T2-weight images, and they show homogenous or ring enhancement after administration of contrast media. A periventricular location (particularly in deep white matter), a solitary lesion, homogenous enhancement of a lesion greater than 2 cm in diameter, and limited edema or mass effect suggest lymphoma rather than toxoplasmosis.

The treatment is radiotherapy, which leads to a decrease in lesion size, hypodensity of lesions, and loss of contrast enhancement. Gallium-67 scintigraphy has a high sensitivity for detecting lymphoma; thallium-201 scintigraphy can help distinguish tumor from edema, posttherapy effect, and infections. Widespread CNS lymphomas sometimes shed cells into CSF (meningeosis) that can be detected cytologically. Meningeosis should be treated with chemotherapy (methotrexate) to prevent relapse.

Grossly, the most common pattern for CNS lymphomas is widespread infiltration, either unifocal or multifocal, without a discrete mass. Most are located above the tentorium.

Microscopically, lymphomas usually are high grade and most are of an immunoblastic or large-cell type; almost all express bcl-2. They can be difficult to classify, particularly in small biopsy samples with necrotic areas. Whether a prominent mass is seen or not, generally there is extensive perivascular spread in the brain or spinal cord, and necrosis may also be extensive. The prognosis is poor, with survival of 1 to 2 months without treatment and 6 to 8 months with treatment (Husstedt, 1998).

Cryptococcosis

Cryptococcus neoformans is a fungus found in bird excrement and in soil. Inhalation of fungus-containing dust leads to a pneumonia in immunocompromised hosts, and organisms spread to the CNS through the systemic circulation (Husstedt, 1998), causing meningitis. Cryptococcal leptomeningitis and encephalitis do not result in extensive inflammatory cell reactions to *C. neoformans* in patients with AIDS, possibly because of their immunocompromised status. The most common presenting features are headache, fever, nausea, vomiting, and malaise. Some patients have a clinical benefit from lumbar puncture to release intracranial pressure.

CT scans can be without pathological findings or show discrete lesions that are hypodense with or without contrast enhancement. By MRI, lesions are discrete and hypointense on T1-weighted images but appear as nonenhancing, hyperintense "soap bubbles" that are well circumscribed without edema on T2-weighted images (Chang et al., 1995).

Cryptococcal meningitis is diagnosed by latex agglutination antigen testing of the CSF; the serum should be examined as well. The India ink preparation is used to detect fungi directly in CSF. Other CSF findings include a mildly elevated protein, normal or low glucose, and lymphocytic pleocytosis. White blood cells may not be numerous in the CSF in HIV-infected patients because of the poor inflammatory response to cryptococci.

Histologically, the fungi can be poorly encapsulated and accompanied by a sparse inflammatory reaction with few lymphocytes or macrophages. Thus, a grossly apparent gelatinous exudate may not be present, though the patient may have clinical symptoms of meningitis. A methenamine silver stain can identify the organisms in tissues.

Acute infections are treated with intravenous amphotericin B followed by oral fluconazole for 2 to 6 weeks (Husstedt, 1998). Prophylaxis is necessary for patients with CD4 lymphocyte counts of <100/μl. Many patients with treated cryptococcosis will have a recurrence without prophylaxis. Amphotericin B, flucytosine, and triazoles (fluconazole and itraconazole) can be used. In some cases, HAART has resulted in an immune reconstitution syndrome with extensive inflammation around established foci of infection and onset of more severe symptoms.

Aspergillosis

CNS aspergillosis is due to a fungal infection. There are at least 40 different *Aspergillus* species of medical significance. CNS aspergillosis is rare in HIV-infected patients (Zelman and Mossakowski, 1998; Neuenburg et al., 2002). Usually, *Aspergillus* causes a sinus infection and pulmonary complication in immunocompromised patients. Sinusitis is frequently seen among HIV-infected patients. Invasive aspergillus sinusitis can lead to brain or orbital involvement and mastoid or other bony disease. Invasive pulmonary aspergillosis can precede or occur concomitantly with CNS aspergillosis. Aspergillosis is more frequent in advanced HIV disease, and the prognosis is poor (Teh et al., 1995). Surgical intervention and systemic antifungal therapy are indicated.

PML

PML results from human papovavirus (subgroup polyoma virus) infection that primarily affects the white matter of the brain. The virus is named JC virus after the initials of the first patient from whom it was isolated. PML is seen most frequently in patients with late-stage HIV disease, though it also occurs in other immunocompromised patients. Depending on the brain location of the lesions, neurological clinical findings include hemianopsia, dysarthria, gait imbalance, limb dystaxia, hemiparesis, cognitive impairment, and cortical blindness. The CSF is typically normal, though some patients may have mild protein elevations and mild pleocytosis. Oligoclonal bands may be present as well. The diagnosis can be established by brain biopsy, but less invasive techniques are preferred, including PCR to detect JC virus DNA in CSF, blood leukocytes, and urine.

CT imaging studies show asymmetric multifocal isodense to hypodense lesions in the white matter with minimal to no enhancement and rarely with hemorrhage or mass effect. Without ART, the lesions tend to become larger and more numerous and decrease in density over weeks to months. MRI scans (T2-weighted spin-echo) are more sensitive for detecting small lesions in the white matter, particularly in the posterior fossa. By MRI, there are white matter hypointense areas on T2-weighted images and hyperintense lesions on T1-weighted images, with minimal or no enhancement after intravenous injection of contrast media. Involvement of the "U" fibers creates a sharp border with the cortex. Parietal and occipital lobe involvement is common. Lesions can be unilateral, bilateral, single, or multiple and usually are not symmetric. HIV leukoencephalopathy is distinguished from PML by diffuse, less intense lesions on T2-weighted images that are not visible on T1-weighted images and by noninvolvement of "U" fibers; moreover, bilateral lesions in HIV leukoencephalopathy tend to be symmetrical.

JC virus targets oligodendrocytes, causing focal areas of white matter damage a few millimeters in diameter that may coalesce. Abnormalities of white matter range from myelin pallor to demyelination to necrosis. The gray-white matter junction is typically involved, and adjacent cortical gray matter and white matter tracts in cerebellum, brainstem, and cervical spinal cord may also be involved. Usually, the lesions are centered around capillaries.

Microscopically, PML involves mainly the myelin-producing oligodendrocytes, which are lysed by the infection. The resulting PML lesions are characterized by demyelination with perivascular monocytes, astrocytosis with bizarre or enlarged astrocytes (with occasional mitotic figures), and central lipid-laden macrophages. At the lesion periphery, large "ballooned" oligodendrocytes infected with JC virus may be found that have enlarged "ground glass" nuclei containing viral antigen. JC virus in brain tissue can be identified with immunohistochemical staining or in situ hybridization. HIV-containing multinucleated giant cells and a perivascular mononuclear infiltrate composed predominantly of T cells may be present.

In some patients beginning HAART, "inflammatory" lesions may be found. By MRI, these lesions show contrast enhancement due to mononuclear infiltrates. This variant of PML may be related to immune reconstitution after ART.

PML has a poor prognosis, with a mortality rate of 30 to 50% within 3 months for most AIDS patients. However, the survival time after diagnosis has improved dramatically after the introduction of HAART. A higher CD4 lymphocyte count is a favorable prognostic factor, and about 10% of patients may have a more prolonged course with remission and improvement of neurological symptoms. Intravenous cytarabine (Ara-C) has been utilized for therapy before HAART; it may be beneficial but is very toxic. Post-HAART, other agents have been evaluated, including, most notably cidofovir, which unfortunately has been found not to be effective (Marra et al., 2002). The impact of HAART itself (particularly with high-dose zidovudine) (Wyen et al., 2005), delta-ala-peptide T amide, topotecan (Royal et al., 2003), and alpha interferon has also been evaluated, with the data supporting efficacy predominantly for HAART treatment (see chapter 26, this volume). However, it should be noted that PML may occur as an immune reconstitution inflammatory syndrome event (Martinez et al., 2006)—a toxicity of HAART—as well.

BK Virus

BK virus is a polyoma virus that resembles JC virus and simian virus 40. Named after the initials of the first patient from whom it was isolated, BK virus can cause tubulointerstitial nephropathy, interstitial desquamative pneumonitis, and subacute meningoencephalitis. Polyomavirus antigen and BK virus DNA have been found postmortem in various cell types of the kidney, lung, and CNS (Vallbracht et al., 1993). Generally, BK virus is associated with renal disease in transplant patients (Hammarin et al., 1996), but it can cause encephalitis in immunocompetent and immunocompromised patients. In HIV-infected patients, BK virus infection is very rare (Vallbracht et al., 1993; Lesprit et al., 2001; Garavelli and Boldorini, 2002; Behzad-Behbahani et al., 2003; Gray et al., 2003). Besides various cytopathic effects including increased nuclear size, basophilic intranuclear inclusions are a prominent histopathological feature (Vallbracht et al., 1993).

Herpes

Herpes simplex virus type 1 (HSV-1) occasionally leads to a meningoencephalitis in HIV-infected patients. Varicellazoster virus (VZV) and even HSV-2 have been identified in brain lesions of HIV-infected patients who have had a clinical and radiologic picture similar to that of PML. These cases can mimic PML; however, CT or MRI scans may show evidence of hemorrhage, a mass effect, or gray matter involvement. Grossly, areas of necrosis can appear most commonly in temporal lobe, inferior frontal lobe, insula, or cingulate gyrus. Microscopically, the lesions can have petechiae with fibrinoid necrosis, perivascular mononuclear inflammatory cell infiltrates, and Cowdry type A inclusions in neurons or glial cells. The diagnosis can be confirmed by immunohistochemical staining for HSV.

HSV infection of the CNS can have a varied clinical presentation, including confusion, fever, headache, epilepsy, anxiety, depression, memory loss, and focal neurological signs. CSF PCR confirms the diagnosis. If treated early, most patients respond to therapy with acyclovir or valacyclovir.

Patients with VZV skin rash or peripheral nervous system involvement (e.g., Bell's paralysis) can have concomitant meningitis with a mildly elevated CSF white blood cell count. In patients with HIV infection, VZV involvement of the CNS can vary in pattern and severity. Multifocal leukoencephalitis involves mainly the deep white matter and gray-white junction. Ventriculitis and periventriculitis can be accompanied by vasculitis and necrosis of the ventricular wall. The large amount of virus present leads to intranuclear Cowdry type A inclusions. In severe cases, acute hemorrhagic meningo-myeloradiculitis with necrotizing vasculitis, focal necrotizing myelitis, and leptomeningeal arterial vasculopathy with cerebral infarction develop. Patients with characteristic VZV skin eruptions are less likely to develop CNS symptoms. Conversely, cases with brain involvement may not have skin lesions. However, VZV infections can involve skin, viscera, spinal cord, and brain and clinically lead to headache, confusion, and focal signs. The clinical course can be protracted. Patients, especially those who are elderly, can develop postherpetic neuralgia lasting more than 4 to 6 weeks after resolution of the skin lesions of VZV.

Tuberculosis

Mycobacterial infections of the CNS in patients with HIV infection are uncommon. The diagnosis can be made by CSF culture or by acid-fast staining of biopsy or autopsy tissue. Possible lesions are small tuberculomas, abscesses, communicating hydrocephalus, and infarction. Concomitant pulmonary tuberculosis is expected.

Typical radiographic findings include meningeal enhancement, enhancing parenchymal lesions, multiloculated abscesses, basal ganglia infarction, and cisternal enhancement. The prognosis is poor (Husstedt, 1998). *Mycobacterium avium* complex in the CNS is also uncommon but can be an incidental finding at autopsy in patients who had disseminated *Mycobacterium avium* complex infection. No gross pathologic findings are typically present; histologically, there can be small foci containing perivascular lymphocytes and macrophages. The clinical findings usually suggest a meningitis or encephalitis.

Neurosyphilis

Syphilis infection usually involves three stages. Primary syphilis is usually limited to skin. Secondary neurosyphilis is asymptomatic in most cases. In secondary syphilis, VDRL can be positive or falsely negative in CSF, the CSF white blood cell count can be slightly elevated, and CSF protein can be elevated (Husstedt, 1998). If secondary neurosyphilis is symptomatic, it can lead to fever, headaches, and cranial nerve abnormalities. Tertiary neurosyphilis is very rare; it can manifest in a brain vasculitis affecting larger vessels and lead to multiple infarcts and syndromes (Husstedt, 1998).

HIV-infected persons have an increased incidence of neurosyphilis. Often, this is reactivated syphilis because of the acquired immunosuppression, or the disease may be accelerated when CD4 counts drop (unless treated). The involvement is more often meningovascular than encephalitic.

Clinical findings can include acute or chronic meningitis, cranial and peripheral neuropathies, dementia, cerebrovascular disease, and myelopathy. High-dose penicillin therapy should readily be initiated based upon clinical suspicion (Husstedt, 1998). However, serologic or clinical relapse may occur, even repeatedly, especially in patients with a positive

CSF VDRL or a rash of secondary syphilis. Relapses can occur over a year after initial therapy (Malone et al., 1995).

Spinal Cord

Vacuolar myelopathy of the spinal cord is a consequence of HIV infection but is not usually associated with myelitis. (Myelitis in HIV infection is very rare.) Vacuolar myelopathy presents with slowly progressive spastic paraparesis, loss of vibratory and position sense, and increased urinary frequency/urgency or incontinence. In males, erectile dysfunction can be present.

Vacuolar myelopathy is characterized by vacuolar intramyelinic swellings of white matter and macrophage infiltration. Vacuoles may appear in macrophages and axons. The vacuoles are 10 to 50 μm in diameter and appear in the posterior and lateral columns in a pattern similar to that of subacute combined degeneration. For unknown reasons, the disease usually begins in the mid to low thoracic cord (producing a clinical thoracic cord syndrome) and extends rostrally as it becomes more severe. Severe lesions can also have clearing of macrophages from the centers of foci of involvement. Vacuolar myelopathy does not lead to Wallerian degeneration. MRI findings for vacuolar myelopathy might be increased signal symmetrically from affected white matter tracts on T2-weighted scans on contiguous slices. Opportunistic infections of the spinal cord are rare and include tuberculosis and lymphoma.

Others

Fungal Infections

Nocardiosis is a fungal infection caused by Nocardia asteroides that usually affects the lung and other organs in immunocompromised patients but can also disseminate and lead to CNS involvement, sometimes forming cerebral nocardia abscesses (Adair et al., 1987; Ogg et al., 1997; Marcus et al., 1999; Lee et al., 2000; Pintado et al., 2003).

Histoplasmosis is a fungal infection caused by Histoplasma capsulatum that can lead to meningitis and focal brain lesions when disseminated (Knapp et al., 1999; Nicolas et al., 2003; Wheat et al., 2005).

Blastomycosis is a fungal infection caused by Blastomyces dermatitidis. CNS involvement can occur with dissemination, which is more likely in advanced HIV disease and has a high mortality rate (Harding, 1991).

Bacterial Infections

Bacterial infections in HIV-infected patients can lead to purulent leptomeningitis, cerebritis, and abscesses, especially in persons with a history of intravenous drug use. Bacterial infection is typically due to septicemia resulting from a local infection, usually pneumonia. Staphylococcus aureus, Streptococcus pneumoniae, Pseudomonas aeruginosa, and Haemophilus influenzae should be considered in such a setting. Listeria monocytogenes should also be included as a possible pathogen, especially if gastrointestinal disease is present. Microscopically, a septic infarct as a result of an embolism or vasculitis with surrounding hemorrhage can be found.

Ischemic lesions in HIV disease may be accompanied by a vasculopathy consisting of hyaline thickening of small vessels, perivascular space dilation, rarefaction, and pigment deposition, with vessel wall mineralization and possibly perivascular inflammatory cell infiltrates. Rarely, intravascular thrombi are seen. Subarachnoid, intraventricular, or intracerebral hemorrhage without a demonstrable opportunistic infection or evidence of trauma can also be found in some HIV-infected patients. The cause can be a vasculitis from systemic bacterial infection, when neutrophilic infiltrates in and around small cerebral vessels are seen. CNS hemorrhages may also be due to direct endothelial damage resulting from the chronic HIV infection.

Bartonella henselae infection can lead to bacteremia and can cause bacillary angiomatosis with skin, bone, and liver involvement (Santos et al., 2000) and lead to encephalitis, myelitis, cerebral arteritis, and retinitis (Dougherty et al., 1996; George et al., 1998; Koehler et al., 2003).

Mycoplasmata are bacteria with an intracellular localization in the host. Mycoplasma fermentans (strain incognitus) has been identified in brain tissue of some AIDS patients with acute or subacute encephalitis when no other opportunistic agent was found (Lo et al., 1989; Miller-Catchpole et al., 1991). Inflammation and necrosis may or may not be present with M. fermentans. Strain incognitus has also been identified in HIV-infected patients in thymus, liver, spleen, lymph node, and placenta (Lo et al., 1989).

Protozoan Infections

Trypanosoma cruzi is a protozoan that causes Chagas' disease. In immunocompromised hosts, T. cruzi can cause mass lesions and an acute necrotizing encephalitis (Gluckstein et al., 1992; Cohen et al., 1998; Lazo et al., 1998; Silva et al., 1999). Trypanosomes can be found in CSF and have to be considered when patients do not respond to antitoxoplasmosis therapy. Histologically, T. cruzi can be distinguished from T. gondii by the presence of amastigote-filled macrophages.

Microsporidia are obligate intracellular protozoa that cause chronic diarrhea in HIV-infected patients (Pol et al., 1993). Cerebral microsporidiosis can occur with dissemination (Tosoni et al., 2002), resulting in the appearance of spores in CSF and multiple small ring-enhancing lesions by MRI.

Neurocysticercosis is the most frequent helminthic infection of the CNS and has been reported in HIV-infected patients. Cysticercosis is caused by Taenia solium larvae.

Giant cysts and racemose forms of neurocysticercosis seem to be more frequent in HIV-infected patients and may be secondary to an uncontrolled parasitic growth because of an impaired cell-mediated immune response (Delobel et al., 2004).

CLINICAL DEMENTIA AFTER THE INTRODUCTION OF HAART

HIV dementia seemed to decrease after the introduction of HAART (Brew and Dore, 2000; Gray et al., 2003). Some authors found that HAART led to a 95% reduction in events defining CNS AIDS, including HIV dementia, compared with untreated patients (d'Arminio Monforte et al., 2000). The EuroSIDA cohort found a drastically reduced incidence of HIV dementia after the introduction of HAART (d'Arminio Monforte et al., 2004). HAART also appears to delay the development of AIDS-associated mild neurocognitive impairment (Deutsch et al., 2001). New neuropsychological impairment was twice as common in the pre-HAART group as in the post-HAART group and occurred sooner in the course of HIV infection (Deutsch et al., 2001). These studies suggest that the course of HIV dementia may be prolonged and milder, but not nonexistent, when HAART is available.

In contrast, a survey of HIV-related neurological complications in AIDS patients in Japan showed that the frequency of the main neurological complications of AIDS did not change after the introduction of HAART (Kishida, 2004). Such therapy would be expected to alter the clinical pattern of HIV dementia from severe subacute progressive dementia in the terminal stage of HIV infection to slowly progressive neurological deficits occurring without immune deficiency (Kishida, 2004). The reason for the unchanged frequency might be that the severity of HIV dementia was not considered in incidence reports, and in fact, dementia cases might have been less severe after HAART was introduced.

HAART is clearly recommended for the treatment of HIV dementia (Kandaneatratchi et al., 2003). Although the incidence of HIV dementia has been reduced, the prevalence is increasing as people with HIV survive longer (Kandaneatratchi et al., 2003). Studies show that HIV dementia symptoms improve when HAART is administered (A. McCutchan, presented at the 11th Conference on Retroviruses and Opportunistic Infections [CROI], San Francisco, CA, 2004); however, it is possible that minimal alterations of cognitive functions persist. For instance, forgetfulness, overall slowness, problems concentrating or reading, and difficulty in problem solving could persist even though the patient is overall better. In summary, most studies show that HAART is beneficial in treating and preventing HIV dementia, but beneficial effects have not been reported consistently. Whether drugs are penetrating CSF or not does not seem to make a difference (A. Antinori, presented at the 11th CROI, San Francisco, CA, 2004).

Moreover, in different countries and continents, clinical dementia in HIV disease is still being diagnosed after the introduction of HAART in 1996. From 1990 to 1998, clinical dementia remained stable, whereas most HIV-related opportunistic infections decreased in incidence after the introduction of ART in 1996 (Ives et al., 2001). The prevalence of minor HIV-associated cognitive impairment appears to be rising among treated patients with increased survival times, and this may be a particular risk for older individuals (Bell, 2004).

In the Multicenter AIDS Cohort Study, even though the incidence of HIV dementia decreased after the introduction of HAART, the proportion of new cases of HIV dementia with a CD4 count in a higher range (i.e., 201 to 350/μl) since 1996 appeared to be increasing (Sacktor et al., 2001). Further, neuropsychological testing of patients before and after the introduction of HAART revealed that even though fewer patients presented with HIV dementia, there was no significant difference between groups (Sacktor et al., 2002). Thus, even though HAART has reduced the incidence of HIV dementia, HIV-associated cognitive impairment continues to be a major clinical problem among patients with advanced infection. This conclusion was confirmed by a study which also showed that HIV-related neurocognitive deficits can be related to cardiovascular risk factors like diabetes mellitus (Valcour et al., 2005).

Similarly, since the introduction of HAART, a proportional increase in HIV dementia, compared with other AIDS-defining diseases, and an increase in the median CD4 cell count at diagnosis have been found in Australia (Dore et al., 1999). These changes further suggest that HAART is less effective for HIV dementia than for other HIV-related complications.

In addition, the proportion of HIV dementia among AIDS-defining diseases increased from the pre-HAART to the HAART period (Dore et al., 2002). Interestingly,

median survival increased from 19.6 months for AIDS cases diagnosed pre-HAART to 39.6 months for those diagnosed during HAART (Dore et al., 2002). In another analysis, the median survival after diagnosis of HIV dementia increased to a greater extent than that for all other AIDS illnesses, from 11.9 months pre-HAART to 48.2 during HAART (Dore et al., 2003). The increase in survival among those with HIV dementia and a low CD4 cell count (<100 cells/μl) at diagnosis was most striking. The authors conclude that although there has been a proportional increase in HIV dementia at AIDS diagnosis, survival after diagnosis of HIV dementia has improved markedly in the era of HAART.

Summary

HAART prolongs life, decreases opportunistic CNS infections, and leads to reduced severity of HIV dementia. However, it cannot prevent the development of clinical dementia entirely. The findings from the Frankfurt study raise the question of whether HIV-infected living persons on ART have increased numbers of activated monocytes in their brain tissue, which might be reflected in the CSF.

SAN FRANCISCO STUDY (2002–2004)

HAART slows, but does not prevent, the development of clinical dementia in HIV-infected patients. Radiological methods cannot show microscopic changes, such as enrichment of monocytes in brain tissue. Even with contrast enhancement, CT and MRI cannot detect these subtle changes. Is there a way to measure brain monocyte content in patients receiving HAART without performing a brain biopsy?

CSF can be sampled repeatedly with a minimally invasive technique. Interstitial fluid drains from the perivascular space of the brain, which contains an abundance of HIV-infected and uninfected activated monocytes in HIV brain disease (Fischer-Smith et al., 2001), into the CSF. Thus, the monocyte content in CSF reflects the monocyte content of the perivascular space. Activated monocytes stain positive for CD16, and many of them stain positive for p24 HIV capsid protein, a sign of HIV infection (Fischer-Smith et al., 2001). CD16 can be measured by flow cytometry on blood and CSF monocytes.

Does ART Increase the Number of Activated Monocytes in CSF?

To assess the effects of HAART on activated monocytes in CSF, a group of physicians in San Francisco examined monocytes in the blood and CSF of HIV patients (Neuenburg et al., 2005a, 2005b). Three groups were recruited: 22 "treatment successes" with low plasma viral loads (<500 copies/ml), 16 "treatment failures" with higher plasma viral loads (>500 copies/ml) during therapy, and 38 subjects off ART. Of the patients on ART, 27 were on a PI-containing regimen and 11 were on a non-PI-containing regimen. Activated monocytes in the CSF were analyzed with six-color flow cytometry. Clinical characteristics that can affect monocyte activation, including plasma lipids, were also assessed.

The mean percentage of activated CD16$^+$ monocytes in CSF was highest in the treatment successes (Fig. 2A). These patients also had much lower plasma and CSF viral loads than those who were off therapy or for whom treatment was failing. The absolute cell counts mirrored the results for percentages of CD14$^+$/CD16$^+$ monocytes in CSF (Fig. 2C).

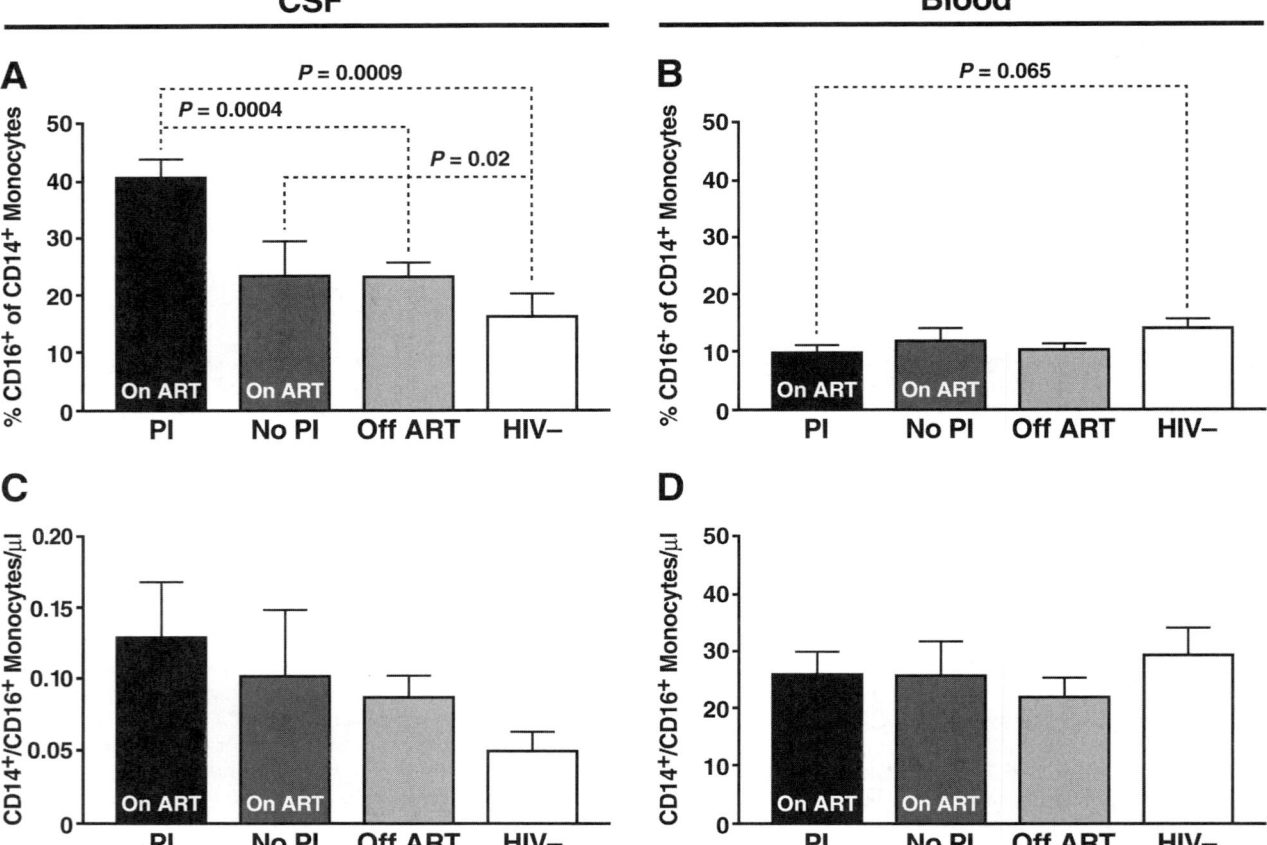

FIGURE 2 Percentages and absolute counts of activated monocytes (CD14+/CD16+) in the CSF and blood. Patients on PI-containing regimens had a higher percentage of activated monocytes in CSF than uninfected controls (HIV–), patients off treatment (Off ART), or patients on a non-PI-containing regimen (No PI) (A). Absolute counts of activated monocytes in CSF show a similar profile (C). In blood, the highest percentage of activated monocytes was found in the uninfected controls (B). Absolute counts of activated monocytes in blood did not differ significantly but were highest in uninfected controls (D). Data are from Neuenburg et al., 2005a, 2005b.

Those who were on a PI-containing regimen had a higher percentage of activated monocytes in CSF than uninfected controls ($P = 0.0009$), patients off treatment, and patients on non-PI-containing regimens (Fig. 2A). Multivariate analysis demonstrated that there was no effect of the recruitment group membership (virological success versus failure) after the use of PIs was considered in the model. Further, CSF viral load was an independent predictor for activated monocytes in CSF.

These findings suggest that both PI treatment and CSF viral load increase the percentage (and number) of activated monocytes in CSF. How PIs increase monocyte trafficking to the CSF is unknown. An understanding of this mechanism might lead to insights into how HIV encephalopathy, which involves activated monocytes, might be prevented.

Activated Monocytes: the Link between HIV Encephalopathy and Atherosclerosis

HAART, especially regimens that include a PI, can increase atherosclerosis, which can lead to coronary artery disease (Neumann et al., 2002; Cotter, 2003; Mooser, 2003;

Vittecoq et al., 2003; Hsue et al., 2004a), transient ischemic attacks (Hsue et al., 2004b), and strokes (Zunker et al., 1996; Menge et al., 2000; Evers et al., 2003).

The pathogenesis of both atherosclerosis and HIV encephalopathy involves activated monocytes. Monocyte activation has been associated with high levels of plasma lipids (Panasenko et al., 1991; Aviram, 1996), which are elevated during HAART (Periard et al., 1999).

Among HIV-infected patients in the San Francisco study, most plasma lipids (total cholesterol, calculated low-density lipoprotein cholesterol [LDL-C], and oxidized LDL-C levels) were highest in the treatment successes and patients on PIs and lowest in patients off therapy. High-density lipoprotein cholesterol (HDL-C) levels were similar in the various groups. Triglyceride and oxidized LDL-C levels were higher in all HIV-infected groups than in uninfected controls. Total plasma cholesterol and calculated LDL-C were higher in HIV-infected groups on ART than in HIV-infected patients off treatment and uninfected controls, which showed comparable results.

A particular modified lipid, oxidized LDL-C (Harrison and Ohara, 1995; Steinberg, 1997; Landmesser and Harrison,

2001), can bind to scavenger receptor CD36 on monocytes (Palinski et al., 1996; Steinberg, 1997; Martens et al., 1998). CD36, a component of the innate immune system, helps remove damaged or apoptotic cells displaying damaged outer lipid membranes; CD36 is also involved in the pathogenesis of atherosclerosis (Han et al., 1997; Febbraio et al., 2000).

HAART may lead to an atherogenic lipid profile with increased LDL-C and total cholesterol (Berthold et al., 1999; Periard et al., 1999; Bonnet et al., 2001; Fantoni et al., 2002; Badiou et al., 2003) and reduced scavenger receptor CD36 expression on monocytes while increasing CD36 mRNA. Altered expression of CD36 facilitates the development of cholesterol-ester-accumulating activated monocytes, which are essential in the pathogenesis of atherosclerosis (Serghides et al., 2002; Dressman et al., 2003).

Interestingly, one of the ligands of CD36, thrombospondin type 1, binds to a domain in CD36 that spans amino acids 93 to 110, the so-called CLESH domain (CD36-LIMP-2-Emp-structural-homology domain). This domain appears in HIV gp120 domains C2 and C3 (Leonard et al., 1990; Crombie et al., 1998; Silverstein and Febbraio, 2000). Therefore, anti-HIV-gp120-antibodies could theoretically contribute to monocyte trafficking by binding to and activating CD36 on monocytes. (CD36 is also expressed on thrombocytes. Before the introduction of HAART, anti-HIV-gp120 antibodies, which are abundant in plasma of patients with high plasma viral loads, frequently caused idiopathic thrombocytopenia purpura by binding to thrombocytes.) Whether CD36 on monocytes also plays a role in monocyte trafficking to the brain and CSF is unknown.

Monocytes expressing chemokine receptor 2 (CCR2), the predominant chemotaxis receptor on monocytes, are involved in monocyte trafficking to the CNS in monkeys infected with simian immunodeficiency virus (Zink et al., 2001). The ligand for CCR2, monocyte chemoattractant protein 1 (MCP-1), also known as CCL2, plays a key role in monocyte trafficking to the CSF (Bernasconi et al., 1996; Zink et al., 2001) and into vessel walls in atherosclerosis (Charo and Peters, 2003; Charo and Taubman, 2004). Increased CCR2 expression increases chemotaxis: a 70% increase in CCR2 expression on monocytes can lead to a doubling of chemotaxis (Han et al., 2004).

High levels of LDL-C, a well-established risk factor for cardiovascular and cerebrovascular disease, also increase CCR2 expression on monocytes (Han et al., 1998, 1999) and therefore facilitate monocyte trafficking. C-reactive protein (CRP), another risk factor for vascular diseases, also increases CCR2 expression on monocytes (Han et al., 2004). Coincubation of monocytes with CRP and cholesterol synergistically enhances MCP-1-mediated chemotaxis (Han et al., 2004).

In the San Francisco study, subjects who were on ART had higher levels of plasma lipids and activated monocytes than those who were not on ART. However, the percentage and number of activated monocytes in CSF did not directly correlate with any particular plasma lipid. Therefore, it is currently unknown whether monocyte activation by lipids is important in treated HIV disease.

However, although ART treatment improves HIV-related brain disorders in the short term, it may increase the numbers of activated monocytes in tissues, such as the brain and vessel walls, and may cause long-term complications. Preventive measures for arteriosclerosis, which might decrease monocyte activation and trafficking, taken by persons on ART might also prevent the development of HIV-related brain disease.

Enrichment of activated monocytes in CSF might reflect enrichment of activated monocytes in the perivascular area of the brain. Thus, understanding the mechanisms leading to an abundance of activated monocytes in CSF might help elucidate the pathogenesis of HIV encephalopathy. Enrichment of activated monocytes in CSF might be driven by multiple factors that could have additive effects and could also be cardiovascular risk factors. HIV infection, HAART, elevated plasma lipids, and activated monocytes in plasma and bone marrow can contribute to monocyte trafficking (Fig. 3). Studies are under way to identify the determinants of monocyte activation in CSF.

Summary

HAART, especially regimens that include a PI, is associated with an increase in the percentage and number of activated monocytes in CSF. CSF viral load is associated with an increase in the percentage and number of activated monocytes in CSF. HAART reduces the severity of HIV-associated dementia and encephalopathy. However, HAART does not seem to prevent monocyte trafficking to the brain in HIV infection.

SUMMARY

HAART is the treatment of choice for HIV dementia. Although ART was the best predictor for signs of HIV encephalopathy in the Frankfurt study, ART is without doubt beneficial for HIV brain disease.

However, the research presented in this chapter and other studies suggests that HIV dementia and HIV encephalopathy are diseases that are ongoing in patients on HAART (Clifford, 2002), even though the onset of disease is delayed, its course is prolonged, and its symptoms are milder. After the introduction of HAART, severe clinical HIV dementia/HIV encephalopathy decreased in prevalence, and mild and moderate clinical HIV dementia/HIV encephalopathy increased. Patients on ART, especially PI-containing ART, have higher percentages and numbers of activated monocytes in CSF. It is unknown whether patients with beginning HIV encephalopathy should be on ART without PIs. Although HAART can prevent opportunistic infections of the CNS and reduces the risk for HIV dementia/HIV encephalopathy, it cannot eliminate the risk for HIV dementia/HIV encephalopathy.

CALL FOR RESEARCH

In the San Francisco study, an increased CSF viral load was associated with increased activation of CSF monocytes. Expression of foreign antigen inside the brain could cause monocytes to invade brain tissue. Brain tissue is exposed to virus early in HIV infection, and some cells become infected (Miyake et al., 2004). This foreign antigen might lead to activation of resident macrophages, which can secrete chemokines that attract more monocytes from the circulation. When the HIV-infected patient starts ART and immune function is partially restored, trafficking of monocytes to the CSF may be further augmented. This process of monocyte trafficking from bone marrow via blood to brain tissue might represent immune restoration during treatment that fails to eliminate viral antigens entirely. Research is needed to clarify whether monocyte trafficking to the brain is a phenomenon associated with immune restoration.

In addition, there is some evidence that HIV-infected persons on HAART can have increased atherosclerosis. It

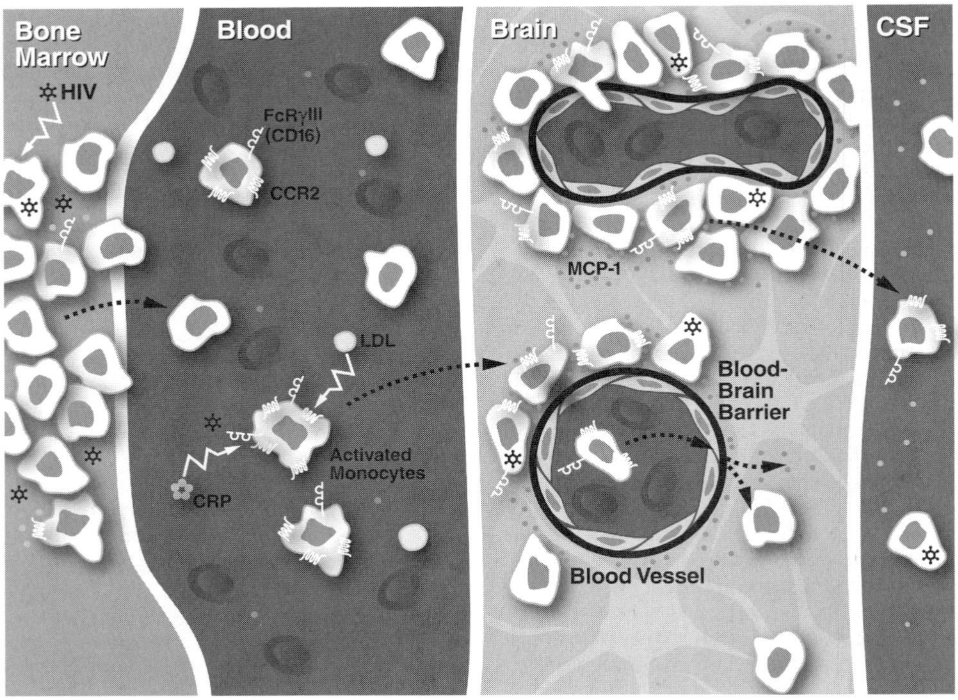

FIGURE 3 Proposed model of increased monocyte trafficking to the central nervous system in HIV infection and during ART. HIV infection leads to increased monocyte trafficking from bone marrow via blood into the perivascular area of the brain, which drains into the CSF. HIV can activate monocytes, and the activated monocytes are usually CD16$^+$. ART can lead to increased levels of LDL cholesterol in plasma; HIV and maybe ART lead to increased levels of CRP (which binds to Fcγ receptors [Stein et al., 2000], such as CD16). Increases in LDL and CRP can upregulate the expression of CCR2, a chemokine receptor that is important in monocyte trafficking through its ligand monocyte chemoattractant protein 1 (MCP-1). Increased expression of CCR2 increases chemotaxis.

is currently unknown how different pathogenetic factors in atherosclerosis and HIV infection influence each other. Important pathogenetic factors are the innate and adaptive immune system, antiretroviral and drug therapy, lipid metabolism, chronic HIV infection, overall inflammatory status, and immune activation. Furthermore, the pathogenesis of both atherosclerosis and HIV dementia/HIV encephalopathy involves trafficking of activated monocytes. Therefore,

reducing monocyte activation and trafficking might slow the development of atherosclerosis and HIV dementia/HIV encephalopathy as well. Similarly, since HIV encephalopathy and vascular encephalopathy may share pathogenetic mechanisms (Jellinger, 2004), preventive measures for vascular disease that decrease monocyte trafficking might delay the onset of brain disease in HIV-infected patients receiving ART. Research is needed to test the hypothesis that

TABLE 5 Hypothesized strategies for augmenting the beneficial effect of HAART on HIV dementia

Drug	Current indication	Rationale
Statins	Hyperlipidemia and high-normal plasma lipid levels	Might influence monocyte trafficking, decreases vascular risk factors; decreases lipids and CRP in plasma (Ridker et al., 2005); additional anti-inflammatory benefit (Mulhaupt et al., 2003; Galle, 2004; Paragh et al., 2004).
Nonsteroidal anti-inflammatory drugs including ASS	Various inflammatory conditions and arteriosclerosis	Might influence monocyte trafficking, might decrease vascular risk factors and inflammatory processes.
Folic acid	(Vitamin)	Decreases homocysteine levels in blood and vessels; this might decrease vascular risk factors (Paramonov et al., 2004) and might inhibit inflammatory processes that lead to demyelination (Glowinska et al., 2001; Cicconetti et al., 2004).
Thiazolidinediones	Diabetes mellitus	In addition to regulating blood glucose and therefore decreasing vascular risk, may decrease monocyte recruitment to vessel walls and inflammatory sites (Tanaka et al., 2005).
Antihypertensiva	Arterial hypertension	Decreases vascular risk factors.
Other antidiabetica	Diabetes mellitus	Decreases vascular risk factors.

interventions that reduce atherosclerosis may also reduce inflammatory processes in the CNS and CSF.

Recent studies are expanding the area of knowledge regarding the pathogenesis of immune activation in HIV disease (Brenchley et al., 2006a, 2006b; Grossmann et al., 2006; Ancuta et al., 2008). In particular, microbial translocation from the gastrointestinal tract is a likely cause of systemic immune activation in chronic HIV infection. Elevated plasma lipopolysaccharide level, an indicator of microbial translocation, induces monocyte activation and trafficking into brain tissue. This may prove to be a key mechanism in the pathogenesis of HAD.

TREATMENT IMPLICATIONS

The treatment of choice for HIV dementia and HIV-associated neurocognitive decline is HAART. It is currently unknown whether a PI-containing or a non-PI-containing regimen should be preferred. Further research is necessary to determine the effect of PIs on monocyte trafficking. Whether drugs are penetrating CSF or not does not seem to make a difference (Antinori, presented).

Additionally, careful monitoring of vascular risk factors is highly recommended for all HIV-infected persons on HAART. Vascular risk factors such as elevated plasma lipid and CRP levels could influence monocyte trafficking by altering CCR2 expression on monocytes (Han et al., 1998, 2004). Therefore, plasma lipids and plasma CRP should be lowered if they are found to be elevated. Further, other vascular risk factors such as elevated blood pressure, increased body weight, and cigarette smoking should be minimized, exercise should be recommended, and glucose tolerance/insulin resistance should be monitored. Hypothesized strategies for augmenting the beneficial effect of HAART on HIV dementia are shown in Table 5.

HAART has changed the course of HIV infection dramatically for most patients. However, the long-term effects of chronic antiretroviral medication may introduce new problems with brain and heart disease and perhaps other side effects. More study is necessary to monitor, prevent, and treat these problems.

I thank Wolfgang Schlote, Reinhardt Brodt, Eilke Helm, and Markus Bickel for their help with the Frankfurt study; all patients who participated in the San Francisco study; Robert M. Grant for critical reviewing of the manuscript; Gary Howard and Stephen Ordway from the Gladstone Editorial Department and Ron Gascon for editing the manuscript; John Carroll and Chris Goodfellow from the Gladstone Graphics Department for assistance with all figures as well as Mark Weinstein, Mike McGrath, Ron Gascon, Richard Reyes, and Jim Yampolsky for help with the micrographs.

REFERENCES

Adair, J. C., A. C. Beck, R. I. Apfelbaum, and J. R. Baringer. 1987. Nocardial cerebral abscess in the acquired immunodeficiency syndrome. *Arch. Neurol.* **44:**548–550.

Ammassari, A., A. Cingolani, P. Pezzotti, D. A. De Luca, R. Murri, M. L. Giancola, L. M. Larocca, and A. Antinori. 2000. AIDS-related focal brain lesions in the era of highly active antiretroviral therapy. *Neurology* **55:**1194–1200.

Ancuta, P., A. Kamat, K. J. Kunstman, E. Y. Kim, P. Autissier, A. Wurcel, T. Zaman, D. Stone, M. Mefford, S. Morgello, E. J. Singer, S. M. Wolinsky, and D. Gabuzda. 2008. Microbial translocation is associated with increased monocyte activation and dementia in AIDS patients. *PLoS ONE* **3:**e2516.

Anders, K. H., W. F. Guerra, U. Tomiyasu, M. A. Verity, and H. V. Vinters. 1986. The neuropathology of AIDS. UCLA experience and review. *Am. J. Pathol.* **124:**537–558.

Aviram, M. 1996. Interaction of oxidized low density lipoprotein with macrophages in atherosclerosis, and the antiatherogenicity of antioxidants. *Eur. J. Clin. Chem. Clin. Biochem.* **34:**599–608.

Badiou, S., C. M. De Boever, A. M. Dupuy, V. Baillat, J. P. Cristol, and J. Reynes. 2003. Small dense LDL and atherogenic lipid profile in HIV-positive adults: influence of lopinavir/ritonavir-containing regimen. *AIDS* **17:**772–774.

Behzad-Behbahani, A., P. E. Klapper, P. J. Vallely, G. M. Cleator, and A. Bonington. 2003. BKV-DNA and JCV-DNA in CSF of patients with suspected meningitis or encephalitis. *Infection* **31:**374–378.

Bell, J. E. 1998. The neuropathology of adult HIV infection. *Rev. Neurol.* **154:**816–829.

Bell, J. E. 2004. An update on the neuropathology of HIV in the HAART era. *Histopathology* **45:**549–559.

Bernasconi, S., P. Cinque, G. Peri, S. Sozzani, A. Crociati, W. Torri, E. Vicenzi, L. Vago, A. Lazzarin, G. Poli, and A. Mantovani. 1996. Selective elevation of monocyte chemotactic protein-1 in the cerebrospinal fluid of AIDS patients with cytomegalovirus encephalitis. *J. Infect. Dis.* **174:**1098–1101.

Berthold, H. K., K. G. Parhofer, M. M. Ritter, M. Addo, J. C. Wasmuth, K. Schliefer, U. Spengler, and J. K. Rockstroh. 1999. Influence of protease inhibitor therapy on lipoprotein metabolism. *J. Intern. Med.* **246:**567–575.

Bonnet, E., J. B. Ruidavets, J. Tuech, J. Ferrieres, X. Collet, J. Fauvel, P. Massip, and B. Perret. 2001. Apoprotein c-III and E-containing lipoparticles are markedly increased in HIV-infected patients treated with protease inhibitors: association with the development of lipodystrophy. *J. Clin. Endocrinol. Metab.* **86:**296–302.

Brenchley, J. M., D. A. Price, and D. C. Douek. 2006a. HIV disease: fallout from a mucosal catastrophe? *Nat. Immunol.* **7:**235–239.

Brenchley, J. M., D. A. Price, T. W. Schacker, T. E. Asher, G. Silvestri, S. Rao, Z. Kazzaz, E. Bornstein, O. Lambotte, D. Altmann, B. R. Blazar, B. Rodriguez, L. Teixeira-Johnson, A. Landay, J. N. Martin, F. M. Hecht, L. J. Picker, M. M. Lederman, S. G. Deeks, and D. C. Douek. 2006b. Microbial translocation is a cause of systemic immune activation in chronic HIV infection. *Nat. Med.* **12:**1365–1371.

Brew, B. J., and G. Dore. 2000. Decreasing incidence of CNS AIDS defining events associated with antiretroviral therapy. *Neurology* **55:**1424.

Brodt, H. R., B. S. Kamps, P. Gute, B. Knupp, S. Staszewski, and E. B. Helm. 1997. Changing incidence of AIDS-defining illnesses in the era of antiretroviral combination therapy. *AIDS* **11:**1731–1738.

Budka, H. 1986. Multinucleated giant cells in brain: a hallmark of the acquired immune deficiency syndrome (AIDS). *Acta Neuropathol.* **69:**253–258.

Budka, H. 1989. Human immunodeficiency virus (HIV)-induced disease of the central nervous system: pathology and implications for pathogenesis. *Acta Neuropathol.* **77:**225–236.

Budka, H. 1991a. The definition of HIV-specific neuropathology. *Acta Pathol. Jpn.* **41:**182–191.

Budka, H. 1991b. Neuropathology of human immunodeficiency virus infection. *Brain Pathol.* **1:**163–175.

Budka, H., C. A. Wiley, P. Kleihues, J. Artigas, A. K. Asbury, E. S. Cho, D. R. Cornblath, M. C. Dal Canto, U. DeGirolami, D. Dickson, L. G. Epstein, M. M. Esiri, F. Giangaspero, G. Gosztonyi, F. Gray, J. W. Griffin, D. Henin, Y. Iwasaki, R. S. Janssen, R. T. Johnson, P. Lantos, W. D. Lyman, J. C. McArthur, K. Nagashima, N. Peress, C. Petito, R. W. Price, R. H. Rhodes, M. L. Rosenblum, G. Said, F. Scaravilli, L. R. Sharer, and

H. V. Vinters. 1991. Consensus report HIV-associated disease of the nervous system: review of nomenclature and proposal for neuropathology-based terminology. *Brain Pathol.* **1**:143–152.

Chang, L., M. E. Cornford, F. L. Chiang, T. M. Ernst, N. C. Sun, and B. L. Miller. 1995. Radiologic-pathologic correlation. Cerebral toxoplasmosis and lymphoma in AIDS. *AJNR Am. J. Neuroradiol.* **16**:1653–1663.

Charo, I. F., and W. Peters. 2003. Chemokine receptor 2 (CCR2) in atherosclerosis, infectious diseases, and regulation of T-cell polarization. *Microcirculation* **10**:259–264.

Charo, I. F., and M. B. Taubman. 2004. Chemokines in the pathogenesis of vascular disease. *Circ. Res.* **95**:858–866.

Cicconetti, P., N. Riolo, C. Priami, L. Tafaro, and E. Ettore. 2004. Risk factors for cognitive impairment. *Recenti Prog. Med.* **95**:535–545. (In Italian.)

Clifford, D. B. 2002. AIDS dementia. *Med. Clin. N. Am.* **86**:537–550.

Cohen, J. E., E. C. Tsai, H. J. Ginsberg, and J. Godes. 1998. Pseudotumoral chagasic meningoencephalitis as the first manifestation of acquired immunodeficiency syndrome. *Surg. Neurol.* **49**:324–327.

Cotter, B. R. 2003. Epidemiology of HIV cardiac disease. *Prog. Cardiovasc. Dis.* **45**:319–326.

Crombie, R., R. L. Silverstein, C. MacLow, S. F. Pearce, R. L. Nachman, and J. Laurence. 1998. Identification of a CD36-related thrombospondin 1-binding domain in HIV-1 envelope glycoprotein gp120: relationship to HIV-1-specific inhibitory factors in human saliva. *J. Exp. Med.* **187**: 25–35.

Cunningham, A. L., H. Naif, N. Saksena, G. Lynch, J. Chang, S. Li, R. Jozwiak, M. Alali, B. Wang, W. Fear, A. Sloane, L. Pemberton, and B. Brew. 1997. HIV infection of macrophages and pathogenesis of AIDS dementia complex: interaction of the host cell and viral genotype. *J. Leukoc. Biol.* **62**:117–125.

d'Arminio Monforte, A., P. Cinque, A. Mocroft, F. D. Goebel, F. Antunes, C. Katlama, U. S. Justesen, S. Vella, O. Kirk, and J. Lundgren. 2004. Changing incidence of central nervous system diseases in the EuroSIDA cohort. *Ann. Neurol.* **55**:320–328.

d'Arminio Monforte, A., P. G. Duca, L. Vago, M. P. Grassi, and M. Moroni. 2000. Decreasing incidence of CNS AIDS-defining events associated with antiretroviral therapy. *Neurology* **54**:1856–1859.

Delobel, P., A. Signate, M. El Guedj, P. Couppie, M. Gueye, D. Smadja, and R. Pradinaud. 2004. Unusual form of neurocysticercosis associated with HIV infection. *Eur. J. Neurol.* **11**:55–58.

Deutsch, R., R. J. Ellis, J. A. McCutchan, T. D. Marcotte, S. Letendre, and I. Grant. 2001. AIDS-associated mild neurocognitive impairment is delayed in the era of highly active antiretroviral therapy. *AIDS* **15**:1898–1899.

Dore, G. J., P. K. Correll, Y. Li, J. M. Kaldor, D. A. Cooper, and B. J. Brew. 1999. Changes to AIDS dementia complex in the era of highly active antiretroviral therapy. *AIDS* **13**:1249–1253.

Dore, G. J., Y. Li, A. McDonald, H. Ree, and J. M. Kaldor. 2002. Impact of highly active antiretroviral therapy on individual AIDS-defining illness incidence and survival in Australia. *J. Acquir. Immune Defic. Syndr.* **29**:388–395.

Dore, G. J., A. McDonald, Y. Li, J. M. Kaldor, and B. J. Brew. 2003. Marked improvement in survival following AIDS dementia complex in the era of highly active antiretroviral therapy. *AIDS* **17**:1539–1545.

Dougherty, M. J., D. H. Spach, A. M. Larson, T. M. Hooton, and M. B. Coyle. 1996. Evaluation of an extended blood culture protocol to isolate fastidious organisms from patients with AIDS. *J. Clin. Microbiol.* **34**:2444–2447.

Dressman, J., J. Kincer, S. V. Matveev, L. Guo, R. N. Greenberg, T. Guerin, D. Meade, X. A. Li, W. Zhu, A. Uittenbogaard, M. E. Wilson, and E. J. Smart. 2003. HIV protease inhibitors promote atherosclerotic lesion formation independent of dyslipidemia by increasing CD36-dependent cholesteryl ester accumulation in macrophages. *J. Clin. Investig.* **111**:389–397.

Ekholm, S., and J. H. Simon. 1988. Magnetic resonance imaging and the acquired immunodeficiency syndrome dementia complex. *Acta Radiol.* **29**:227–230.

Evers, S., D. Nabavi, A. Rahmann, C. Heese, D. Reichelt, and I. W. Husstedt. 2003. Ischaemic cerebrovascular events in HIV infection: a cohort study. *Cerebrovasc. Dis.* **15**:199–205.

Fantoni, M., C. Del Borgo, C. Autore, and G. Barbaro. 2002. Metabolic disorders and cardiovascular risk in HIV-infected patients treated with antiretroviral agents. *Ital. Heart J.* **3**:294–299.

Febbraio, M., E. A. Podrez, J. D. Smith, D. P. Hajjar, S. L. Hazen, H. F. Hoff, K. Sharma, and R. L. Silverstein. 2000. Targeted disruption of the class B scavenger receptor CD36 protects against atherosclerotic lesion development in mice. *J. Clin. Investig.* **105**:1049–1056.

Filippi, C. G., G. Sze, S. J. Farber, M. Shahmanesh, and P. A. Selwyn. 1998. Regression of HIV encephalopathy and basal ganglia signal intensity abnormality at MR imaging in patients with AIDS after the initiation of protease inhibitor therapy. *Radiology* **206**:491–498.

Fischer-Smith, T., S. Croul, A. E. Sverstiuk, C. Capini, D. L'Heureux, E. G. Regulier, M. W. Richardson, S. Amini, S. Morgello, K. Khalili, and J. Rappaport. 2001. CNS invasion by CD14+/CD16+ peripheral blood-derived monocytes in HIV dementia: perivascular accumulation and reservoir of HIV infection. *J. Neurovirol.* **7**:528–541.

Gallant, J. E., R. D. Moore, and R. E. Chaisson. 1994. Prophylaxis for opportunistic infections in patients with HIV infection. *Ann. Intern. Med.* **120**:932–944.

Galle, J. 2004. Atherosclerosis and arteriitis: implications for therapy of cardiovascular disease. *Herz* **29**:4–11. (In German.)

Garavelli, P. L., and R. Boldorini. 2002. BK virus encephalitis in an HIV-seropositive patient. Preliminary data. *Recenti Prog. Med.* **93**:247. (In Italian.)

Gardner, M. B., and S. Dandekar. 1995. Neurobiology of simian and feline immunodeficiency virus infections. *Curr. Top. Microbiol. Immunol.* **202**:135–150.

George, T. I., G. Manley, J. E. Koehler, V. S. Hung, M. McDermott, and A. Bollen. 1998. Detection of *Bartonella henselae* by polymerase chain reaction in brain tissue of an immunocompromised patient with multiple enhancing lesions. Case report and review of the literature. *J. Neurosurg.* **89**:640–644.

Glass, J. D., H. Fedor, S. L. Wesselingh, and J. C. McArthur. 1995. Immunocytochemical quantitation of human immunodeficiency virus in the brain: correlations with dementia. *Ann. Neurol.* **38**:755–762.

Glowinska, B., M. Urban, J. Peczynska, B. Florys, and E. Szydlowska. 2001. Elevated concentrations of homocysteine in children and adolescents with arterial hypertension accompanying Type 1 diabetes. *Med. Sci. Monit.* **7**:1242–1249.

Gluckstein, D., F. Ciferri, and J. Ruskin. 1992. Chagas' disease: another cause of cerebral mass in the acquired immunodeficiency syndrome. *Am. J. Med.* **92**:429–432.

Gonzalez, E., B. H. Rovin, L. Sen, G. Cooke, R. Dhanda, S. Mummidi, H. Kulkarni, M. J. Bamshad, V. Telles, S. A. Anderson, E. A. Walter, K. T. Stephan, M. Deucher, A. Mangano, R. Bologna, S. S. Ahuja, M. J. Dolan, and S. K. Ahuja. 2002. HIV-1 infection and AIDS dementia are influenced by a mutant MCP-1 allele linked to increased monocyte infiltration of tissues and MCP-1 levels. *Proc. Natl. Acad. Sci. USA* **99:**13795–13800.

Gray, F., H. Adle-Biassette, F. Chretien, G. Lorin de la Grandmaison, G. Force, and C. Keohane. 2001. Neuropathology and neurodegeneration in human immunodeficiency virus infection. Pathogenesis of HIV-induced lesions of the brain, correlations with HIV-associated disorders and modifications according to treatments. *Clin. Neuropathol.* **20:**146–155.

Gray, F., F. Chretien, A. V. Vallat-Decouvelaere, and F. Scaravilli. 2003. The changing pattern of HIV neuropathology in the HAART era. *J. Neuropathol. Exp. Neurol.* **62:**429–440.

Grossmann, Z., M. Meier-Schellersheim, W. E. Paul, and L. J. Picker. 2006. Pathogenesis of HIV infection: what the virus spares is as important as what it destroys. *Nat. Med.* **12:**289–295.

Gupta, P., J. Mellors, L. Kingsley, S. Riddler, M. K. Singh, S. Schreiber, M. Cronin, and C. R. Rinaldo. 1997. High viral load in semen of human immunodeficiency virus type 1-infected men at all stages of disease and its reduction by therapy with protease and nonnucleoside reverse transcriptase inhibitors. *J. Virol.* **71:**6271–6275.

Hammarin, A. L., G. Bogdanovic, V. Svedhem, R. Pirskanen, L. Morfeldt, and M. Grandien. 1996. Analysis of PCR as a tool for detection of JC virus DNA in cerebrospinal fluid for diagnosis of progressive multifocal leukoencephalopathy. *J. Clin. Microbiol.* **34:**2929–2932.

Han, J., D. P. Hajjar, M. Febbraio, and A. C. Nicholson. 1997. Native and modified low density lipoproteins increase the functional expression of the macrophage class B scavenger receptor, CD36. *J. Biol. Chem.* **272:**21654–21659.

Han, K. H., K. O. Han, S. R. Green, and O. Quehenberger. 1999. Expression of the monocyte chemoattractant protein-1 receptor CCR2 is increased in hypercholesterolemia. Differential effects of plasma lipoproteins on monocyte function. *J. Lipid Res.* **40:**1053–1063.

Han, K. H., K. H. Hong, J. H. Park, J. Ko, D. H. Kang, K. J. Choi, M. K. Hong, S. W. Park, and S. J. Park. 2004. C-reactive protein promotes monocyte chemoattractant protein-1-mediated chemotaxis through upregulating CC chemokine receptor 2 expression in human monocytes. *Circulation* **109:**2566–2571.

Han, K. H., R. K. Tangirala, S. R. Green, and O. Quehenberger. 1998. Chemokine receptor CCR2 expression and monocyte chemoattractant protein-1-mediated chemotaxis in human monocytes. A regulatory role for plasma LDL. *Arterioscler. Thromb. Vasc. Biol.* **18:**1983–1991.

Harding, C. V. 1991. Blastomycosis and opportunistic infections in patients with acquired immunodeficiency syndrome. An autopsy study. *Arch. Pathol. Lab. Med.* **115:**1133–1136.

Harrison, D. G., and Y. Ohara. 1995. Physiologic consequences of increased vascular oxidant stresses in hypercholesterolemia and atherosclerosis: implications for impaired vasomotion. *Am. J. Cardiol.* **75:**75B–81B.

Hori, K., P. R. Burd, K. Furuke, J. Kutza, K. A. Weih, and K. A. Clouse. 1999. Human immunodeficiency virus-1-infected macrophages induce inducible nitric oxide synthase and nitric oxide (NO) production in astrocytes: astrocytic NO as a possible mediator of neural damage in acquired immunodeficiency syndrome. *Blood* **93:**1843–1850.

Hsue, P. Y., K. Giri, S. Erickson, J. S. MacGregor, N. Younes, A. Shergill, and D. D. Waters. 2004a. Clinical features of acute coronary syndromes in patients with human immunodeficiency virus infection. *Circulation* **109:**316-319.

Hsue, P. Y., J. C. Lo, A. Franklin, A. F. Bolger, J. N. Martin, S. G. Deeks, and D. D. Waters. 2004b. Progression of atherosclerosis as assessed by carotid intima-media thickness in patients with HIV infection. *Circulation* **109:**1603–1608.

Husstedt, I. W. 1998. *HIV und AIDS.* Springer-Verlag, Berlin, Germany.

Ives, N. J., B. G. Gazzard, and P. J. Easterbrook. 2001. The changing pattern of AIDS-defining illnesses with the introduction of highly active antiretroviral therapy (HAART) in a London clinic. *J. Infect.* **42:**134–139.

Jellinger, K. A. 2004. Pathology and pathophysiology of vascular cognitive impairment. A critical update. *Panminerva Med.* **46:**217–226.

Jellinger, K. A., U. Setinek, M. Drlicek, G. Bohm, A. Steurer, and F. Lintner. 2000. Neuropathology and general autopsy findings in AIDS during the last 15 years. *Acta Neuropathol.* **100:**213–220.

Kandanearatchi, A., B. Williams, and I. P. Everall. 2003. Assessing the efficacy of highly active antiretroviral therapy in the brain. *Brain Pathol.* **13:**104–110.

Kato, T., A. Hirano, J. F. Llena, and H. M. Dembitzer. 1987. Neuropathology of acquired immune deficiency syndrome (AIDS) in 53 autopsy cases with particular emphasis on microglial nodules and multinucleated giant cells. *Acta Neuropathol.* **73:**287–294.

Kishida, S. 2004. The neurology of HIV infection: clinical features of HIV encephalopathy and future problems in the HAART era. *Rinsho Shinkeigaku* **44:**852–854. (In Japanese.)

Klatt, E. C. 2005. Pathology of AIDS, version 15. Spencer S. Eccles Health Sciences Library, Salt Lake City, UT. http://www.medlib.med.utah.edu.

Knapp, S., M. Turnherr, G. Dekan, B. Willinger, G. Stingl, and A. Rieger. 1999. A case of HIV-associated cerebral histoplasmosis successfully treated with fluconazole. *Eur. J. Clin. Microbiol. Infect. Dis.* **18:**658–661.

Koehler, J. E., M. A. Sanchez, S. Tye, C. S. Garrido-Rowland, F. M. Chen, T. Maurer, J. L. Cooper, J. G. Olson, A. L. Reingold, W. K. Hadley, R. R. Regnery, and J. W. Tappero. 2003. Prevalence of *Bartonella* infection among human immunodeficiency virus-infected patients with fever. *Clin. Infect. Dis.* **37:**559–566.

Landmesser, U., and D. G. Harrison. 2001. Oxidant stress as a marker for cardiovascular events: Ox marks the spot. *Circulation* **104:**2638–2640.

Lang, W., J. Miklossy, J. P. Deruaz, G. P. Pizzolato, A. Probst, T. Schaffner, E. Gessaga, and P. Kleihues. 1989. Neuropathology of the acquired immune deficiency syndrome (AIDS): a report of 135 consecutive autopsy cases from Switzerland. *Acta Neuropathol.* **77:**379–390.

Lazo, J., A. C. Meneses, A. Rocha, M. S. Ferreira, J. O. Marquez, E. Chapadeiro, and E. R. Lopes. 1998. Chagasic meningoencephalitis in the immunodeficient. *Arq. Neuropsiquiatr.* **56:**93–97.

Lee, C. C., L. W. Loo, and M. S. Lam. 2000. Case reports of nocardiosis in patients with human immunodeficiency virus (HIV) infection. *Ann. Acad. Med. Singapore* **29:**119–126.

Leonard, C. K., M. W. Spellman, L. Riddle, R. J. Harris, J. N. Thomas, and T. J. Gregory. 1990. Assignment of intrachain disulfide bonds and characterization of potential glycosylation sites of the type 1 recombinant human immunodeficiency virus envelope glycoprotein (gp120) expressed in Chinese hamster ovary cells. *J. Biol. Chem.* **265:**10373–10382.

Lesprit, P., D. Chaline-Lehmann, F. J. Authier, T. Ponnelle, F. Gray, and Y. Levy. 2001. BK virus encephalitis in a patient with AIDS and lymphoma. *AIDS* **15:**1196–1199.

Levy, R. M., D. E. Bredesen, M. L. Rosenblum, and R. L. Davis. 1989. Central nervous system disorders in AIDS. *Immunol. Ser.* **44:**371–401.

Lo, S. C., M. S. Dawson, D. M. Wong, P. B. Newton III, M. A. Sonoda, W. F. Engler, R. Y. Wang, J. W. Shih, H. J. Alter, and D. J. Wear. 1989. Identification of *Mycoplasma incognitus* infection in patients with AIDS: an immunohistochemical, in situ hybridization and ultrastructural study. *Am. J. Trop. Med. Hyg.* **41:**601–616.

Maehlen, J., O. Dunlop, K. Liestol, J. H. Dobloug, A. K. Goplen, and A. Torvik. 1995. Changing incidence of

HIV-induced brain lesions in Oslo, 1983-1994: effects of zidovudine treatment. *AIDS* **9**:1165–1169.

Malone, J. L., M. R. Wallace, B. B. Hendrick, A. LaRocco, Jr., E. Tonon, S. K. Brodine, W. A. Bowler, B. S. Lavin, R. E. Hawkins, and E. C. Oldfield III. 1995. Syphilis and neurosyphilis in a human immunodeficiency virus type-1 seropositive population: evidence for frequent serologic relapse after therapy. *Am. J. Med.* **99**:55–63.

Marcus, C. D., S. D. Taylor-Robinson, I. J. Cox, J. Sargentoni, and S. Shaunak. 1999. Reversible alterations in brain metabolites during therapy for disseminated nocardiosis using proton magnetic resonance spectroscopy. *Metab. Brain Dis.* **14**:231–237.

Marra, C. M., N. Rajicic, D. E. Barker, B. A. Cohen, D. Clifford, M. J. D. Post, A. Ruiz, B. C. Bowen, M. L Huang, J. Queen-Baker, J. Andersen, S. Kelly, S. Shriver, and the Adult AIDS Clinical Trials Group 363 Team. 2002. A pilot study of cidofovir for progressive multifocal leukoencephalopathy in AIDS. *AIDS* **16**:1791–1797.

Martens, J. S., N. E. Reiner, P. Herrera-Velit, and U. P. Steinbrecher. 1998. Phosphatidylinositol 3-kinase is involved in the induction of macrophage growth by oxidized low density lipoprotein. *J. Biol. Chem.* **273**:4915–4920.

Martinez, J. V., J. V. Mazziotti, E. D. Efron, P. Bonardo, R. Jordan, G. Sevlever, M. Martinez, S. C. Verbanaz, Z. S. Salazar, M. F. Pardal, and R. Reisin. 2006. Immune reconstitution inflammatory syndrome associated with PML in AIDS: a treatable disorder. *Neurology* **67**:1692–1694.

Masliah, E., R. M. DeTeresa, M. E. Mallory, and L. A. Hansen. 2000. Changes in pathological findings at autopsy in AIDS cases for the last 15 years. *AIDS* **14**:69–74.

Menge, T., T. Neumann-Haefelin, H. J. von Giesen, and G. Arendt. 2000. Progressive stroke in an HIV-1-positive patient under protease inhibitors. *Eur. Neurol.* **44**:252–254.

Miller-Catchpole, R., M. Shattuck, P. Kandalaft, D. Variakojis, J. Anastasi, C. Abrahams, et al. 1991. The incidence and distribution of *Mycoplasma fermentans* (incognitus strain) in the Chicago AIDS autopsy series: an immunohistochemical study. *Mod. Pathol.* **4**:481–486.

Miyake, A., Y. Enose, S. Ohkura, H. Suzuki, T. Kuwata, T. Shimada, S. Kato, O. Narayan, and M. Hayami. 2004. The quantity and diversity of infectious viruses in various tissues of SHIV-infected monkeys at the early and AIDS stages. *Arch. Virol.* **149**:943–955.

Mooser, V. 2003. Atherosclerosis and HIV in the highly active antiretroviral therapy era: towards an epidemic of cardiovascular disease? *AIDS* **17**(Suppl. 1):S65–S69.

Moskowitz, L. B., G. T. Hensley, J. C. Chan, J. Gregorios, and F. K. Conley. 1984. The neuropathology of acquired immune deficiency syndrome. *Arch.Pathol. Lab. Med.* **108**:867–872.

Mulhaupt, F., C. M. Matter, B. R. Kwak, P. Pelli, N. R. Veillard, F. Burger, P. Graber, T. F. Luscher, and F. Mach. 2003. Statins (HMG-CoA reductase inhibitors) reduce CD40 expression in human vascular cells. *Cardiovasc. Res.* **59**:755–766.

Navia, B. A., E. S. Cho, C. K. Petito, and R. W. Price. 1986. The AIDS dementia complex. II. Neuropathology. *Ann. Neurol.* **19**:525–535.

Neuenburg, J. K. 1997. Motor evoked potentials in HIV-infection, p. 86. *In Medicine*. Johann Wolfgang Goethe-University, Frankfurt/Main, Germany.

Neuenburg, J. K., H. R. Brodt, B. G. Herndier, M. Bickel, P. Bacchetti, R. W. Price, R. M. Grant, and W. Schlote. 2002. HIV-related neuropathology, 1985 to 1999: rising prevalence of HIV encephalopathy in the era of highly active antiretroviral therapy. *J. Acquir. Immune Defic. Syndr.* **31**:171–177.

Neuenburg, J. K., H. R. Brodt, B. G. Herndier, and W. Schlote. 2000. Is there really a correlation between AIDS dementia and Kaposi's sarcoma? *AIDS* **14**:94–95 (Letter.)

Neuenburg, J. K., T. A. Cho, A. Nilsson, B. M. Bredt, S. J. Hebert, R. M. Grant, and R. W. Price. 2005a. T-cell activation and memory phenotypes in cerebrospinal fluid during HIV infection. *J. Acquir. Immune Defic. Syndr.* **39**:16–22.

Neuenburg, J. K., S. N. Furlan, P. Bacchetti, R. W. Price, and R. M. Grant. 2005b. Enrichment of activated monocytes in cerebrospinal fluid during antiretroviral therapy. *AIDS* **19**:1351–1359.

Neuenburg, J. K., E. Sinclair, A. Nilsson, C. Kreis, P. Bacchetti, R. W. Price, and R. M. Grant. 2004. HIV-producing T cells in cerebrospinal fluid. *J. Acquir. Immune Defic. Syndr.* **37**:1237–1244.

Neuen-Jacob, E., C. Figge, G. Arendt, B. Wendtland, B. Jacob, and W. Wechsler. 1993. Neuropathological studies in the brains of AIDS patients with opportunistic diseases. *Int. J. Legal Med.* **105**:339–350.

Neumann, T., M. Miller, S. Esser, G. Gerken, and R. Erbel. 2002. Atherosclerosis in HIV-positive patients. *Z. Kardiol.* **91**:879–888. (In German.)

Nicolas, X., H. Granier, J. P. Laborde, F. Talarmin, F. Zagnoli, A. Garin, A. M. Le Flohic, E. Moalic, D. Quinio, and F. Klotz. 2003. Disseminated and central nervous system *Histoplasma capsulatum* infection mimicking neoplasm: difficulties in diagnosis, failure in management. *Rev. Med. Interne* **24**:389–393. (In French.)

Nielsen, S. L., and R. L. Davis. 1988. Neuropathology of acquired immunodeficiency syndrome, p. 155–181. *In M. L. Rosenblum, R. M. Levy, and D. E. Bredesen (ed.), AIDS and the Nervous System*. Raven Press, New York, NY.

Ogg, G., W. A. Lynn, M. Peters, W. Curati, J. E. McLaughlin, and S. Shaunak. 1997. Cerebral nocardia abscesses in a patient with AIDS: correlation of magnetic resonance and white cell scanning images with neuropathological findings. *J. Infect.* **35**:311–313.

Palinski, W., S. Horkko, E. Miller, U. P. Steinbrecher, H. C. Powell, L. K. Curtiss, and J. L. Witztum. 1996. Cloning of monoclonal autoantibodies to epitopes of oxidized lipoproteins from apolipoprotein E-deficient mice. Demonstration of epitopes of oxidized low density lipoprotein in human plasma. *J. Clin. Investig.* **98**:800–814.

Panasenko, O. M., T. V. Vol'nova, A. N. Osipov, O. A. Azizova, and A. Vladimirov Yu. 1991. Free-radical generation by monocytes and neutrophils: a possible cause of plasma lipoprotein modification. *Biomed. Sci.* **2**:581–589.

Paragh, G., L. Mark, and E. Katona. 2004. The non-lipid effects of statins. *Orv. Hetil.* **145**:1903–1910. (In Hungarian.)

Paramonov, A. D., S. V. Moiseev, V. V. Fomin, M. V. Kopeleva, L. I. Stankevich, A. I. Martynov, and N. A. Mukhin. 2004. Hyperhomocysteinemia and acute phase proteins in various forms of ischemic heart disease. *Ter. Arkh.* **76**:67–70. (In Russian.)

Periard, D., A. Telenti, P. Sudre, J. J. Cheseaux, P. Halfon, M. J. Reymond, S. M. Marcovina, M. P. Glauser, P. Nicod, R. Darioli, V. Mooser, et al. 1999. Atherogenic dyslipidemia in HIV-infected individuals treated with protease inhibitors. *Circulation* **100**:700–705.

Petito, C. K., E. S. Cho, W. Lemann, B. A. Navia, and R. W. Price. 1986. Neuropathology of acquired immunodeficiency syndrome (AIDS): an autopsy review. *J. Neuropathol. Exp. Neurol.* **45**:635–646.

Pintado, V., E. Gomez-Mampaso, J. Cobo, C. Quereda, M. A. Meseguer, J. Fortun, E. Navas, and S. Moreno. 2003. Nocardial infection in patients infected with the human immunodeficiency virus. *Clin. Microbiol. Infect.* **9**:716–720.

Pol, S., C. A. Romana, S. Richard, P. Amouyal, I. Desportes-Livage, F. Carnot, J. F. Pays, and P. Berthelot. 1993. Microsporidia infection in patients with the human immunodeficiency virus and unexplained cholangitis. *N. Engl. J. Med.* **328**:95–99.

Price, R. W., E. E. Paxinos, R. M. Grant, B. Drews, A. Nilsson, R. Hoh, N. S. Hellmann, C. J. Petropoulos, and S. G. Deeks. 2001. Cerebrospinal fluid response to structured treatment interruption after virological failure. *AIDS* **15:**1251–1259.

Ridker, P. M., C. P. Cannon, D. Morrow, N. Rifai, L. M. Rose, C. H. McCabe, M. A. Pfeffer, and E. Braunwald. 2005. C-reactive protein levels and outcomes after statin therapy. *N. Engl. J. Med.* **352:**20–28.

Roth, J., E. M. Harre, C. Rummel, R. Gerstberger, and T. Hubschle. 2004. Signaling the brain in systemic inflammation: role of sensory circumventricular organs. *Front. Biosci.* **9:**290–300.

Royal, W., B. Dupont, D. McGuire, L. Chang, K. Goodkin, T. Ernst, M. J. Post, D. Fish, G. Pailloux, H. Poncelet, M. Concha, L. Apuzzo, and E. Singer. 2003. Topotecan in the treatment of acquired immunodeficiency syndrome-related progressive multifocal leukoencephalopathy. *J. Neurovirol.* **9:**411–419.

Sacktor, N., R. H. Lyles, R. Skolasky, C. Kleeberger, O. A. Selnes, E. N. Miller, J. T. Becker, B. Cohen, J. C. McArthur, and The Multicenter AIDS Cohort Study. 2001. HIV-associated neurologic disease incidence changes: Multicenter AIDS Cohort Study, 1990-1998. *Neurology* **56:**257–260.

Sacktor, N., M. P. McDermott, K. Marder, G. Schifitto, O. A. Selnes, J. C. McArthur, Y. Stern, S. Albert, D. Palumbo, K. Kieburtz, J. A. De Marcaida, B. Cohen, and L. Epstein. 2002. HIV-associated cognitive impairment before and after the advent of combination therapy. *J. Neurovirol.* **8:**136–142.

Santos, R., O. Cardoso, P. Rodrigues, J. Cardoso, J. Machado, A. Afonso, F. Bacellar, E. Marston, and R. Proenca. 2000. Bacillary angiomatosis by *Bartonella quintana* in an HIV-infected patient. *J. Am. Acad. Dermatol.* **42:**299–301.

Schrager, L. K., and M. P. D'Souza. 1998. Cellular and anatomical reservoirs of HIV-1 in patients receiving potent antiretroviral combination therapy. *JAMA* **280:**67–71.

Serghides, L., S. Nathoo, S. Walmsley, and K. C. Kain. 2002. CD36 deficiency induced by antiretroviral therapy. *AIDS* **16:**353–358.

Sharer, L. R., E. S. Cho, and L. G. Epstein. 1985. Multinucleated giant cells and HTLV-III in AIDS encephalopathy. *Hum. Pathol.* **16:**760.

Silva, N., L. O'Bryan, E. Medeiros, H. Holand, J. Suleiman, J. S. de Mendonca, N. Patronas, S. G. Reed, H. G. Klein, H. Masur, and R. Badaro. 1999. *Trypanosoma cruzi* meningoencephalitis in HIV-infected patients. *J. Acquir. Immune Defic. Syndr. Hum. Retrovirol.* **20:**342–349.

Silverstein, R. L., and M. Febbraio. 2000. CD36 and atherosclerosis. *Curr. Opin. Lipidol.* **11:**483–491.

Staprans, S., N. Marlowe, D. Glidden, T. Novakovic-Agopian, R. M. Grant, M. Heyes, F. Aweeka, S. Deeks, and R. W. Price. 1999. Time course of cerebrospinal fluid responses to antiretroviral therapy: evidence for variable compartmentalization of infection. *AIDS* **13:**1051–1061.

Stein, M. P., J. C. Edberg, R. P. Kimberly, E. K. Mangan, D. Bharadwaj, C. Mold, and T. W. Du Clos. 2000. C-reactive protein binding to FcgammaRIIa on human monocytes and neutrophils is allele-specific. *J. Clin. Investig.* **105:**369–376.

Steinberg, D. 1997. Low density lipoprotein oxidation and its pathobiological significance. *J. Biol. Chem.* **272:**20963–20966.

Tanaka, T., Y. Fukunaga, H. Itoh, K. Doi, J. Yamashita, T. H. Chun, M. Inoue, K. Masatsugu, T. Saito, N. Sawada, S. Sakaguchi, H. Arai, and K. Nakao. 2005. Therapeutic potential of thiazolidinediones in activation of peroxisome proliferator-activated receptor gamma for monocyte recruitment and endothelial regeneration. *Eur. J. Pharmacol.* **508:**255–265.

Teh, W., B. S. Matti, H. Marisiddaiah, and G. Y. Minamoto. 1995. Aspergillus sinusitis in patients with AIDS: report of three cases and review. *Clin. Infect. Dis.* **21:**529–535.

Thurnher, M. M., E. G. Schindler, S. A. Thurnher, H. Pernerstorfer-Schon, C. Kleibl-Popov, and A. Rieger. 2000. Highly active antiretroviral therapy for patients with AIDS dementia complex: effect on MR imaging findings and clinical course. *AJNR Am. J. Neuroradiol.* **21:**670–678.

Tosoni, A., M. Nebuloni, A. Ferri, S. Bonetto, S. Antinori, M. Scaglia, L. Xiao, H. Moura, G. S. Visvesvara, L. Vago, and G. Costanzi. 2002. Disseminated microsporidiosis caused by *Encephalitozoon cuniculi* III (dog type) in an Italian AIDS patient: a retrospective study. *Mod. Pathol.* **15:**577–583.

Vago, L., G. Trabattoni, A. Lechi, S. Cristina, and H. Budka. 1990. Neuropathology of AIDS dementia. A review after 205 post mortem examinations. *Acta Neurol.* **12:**32–35.

Valcour, V. G., C. M. Shikuma, B. T. Shiramizu, A. E. Williams, M. R. Watters, P. W. Poff, J. S. Grove, O. A. Selnes, and N. C. Sacktor. 2005. Diabetes, insulin resistance, and dementia among HIV-1-infected patients. *J. Acquir. Immune Defic. Syndr.* **38:**31–36.

Vallbracht, A., J. Lohler, J. Gossmann, T. Gluck, D. Petersen, H. J. Gerth, M. Gencic, and K. Dorries. 1993. Disseminated BK type polyomavirus infection in an AIDS patient associated with central nervous system disease. *Am. J. Pathol.* **143:**29–39.

Vittecoq, D., L. Escaut, G. Chironi, E. Teicher, J. J. Monsuez, M. Andrejak, and A. Simon. 2003. Coronary heart disease in HIV-infected patients in the highly active antiretroviral treatment era. *AIDS* **17**(Suppl. 1):S70–S76.

Wheat, L. J., C. E. Musial, and E. Jenny-Avital. 2005. Diagnosis and management of central nervous system histoplasmosis. *Clin. Infect. Dis.* **40:**844–852.

Wyen, C., C. Lehmann, G. Fatkenheuer, and C. Hoffmann. 2005. AIDS-related progressive multifocal leukoencephalopathy in the era of HAART: report of two cases and review of the literature. *AIDS Patient Care STDs* **19:**486–494.

Zelman, I. B., and M. J. Mossakowski. 1998. Opportunistic infections of the central nervous system in the course of acquired immune deficiency syndrome (AIDS). Morphological analysis of 172 cases. *Folia Neuropathol* **36:**129–144.

Zink, M. C., G. D. Coleman, J. L. Mankowski, R. J. Adams, P. M. Tarwater, K. Fox, and J. E. Clements. 2001. Increased macrophage chemoattractant protein-1 in cerebrospinal fluid precedes and predicts simian immunodeficiency virus encephalitis. *J. Infect. Dis.* **184:**1015–1021.

Zunker, P., D. G. Nabavi, A. Allardt, I. W. Husstedt, and G. Schuierer. 1996. HIV-associated stroke: report of two unusual cases. *Stroke* **27:**1694–1696.

The Spectrum of Neuro-AIDS Disorders:
Pathophysiology, Diagnosis, and Treatment
Edited by K. Goodkin et al.
©2008 ASM Press, Washington, DC

15

The Role of Viral Genetic Variability in HIV-Associated Neurocognitive Disorder

PAUL SHAPSHAK, ALIREZA MINAGAR, PANDJASSARAME KANGUEANE,
SIMON FROST, SERGEI L. KOSAKOVSKY POND, SELENE ZARATE, ELYSE SINGER,
DEBORAH COMMINS, ANNE DE GROOT, MIGUEL QUINONES-MATEU,
AND ERNEST TERWILLIGER

There have been great strides in our understanding of the neuro-AIDS component of the AIDS epidemic, and profound changes are currently occurring. This chapter is presented to assist the reader in understanding how we arrived at our current position in the neuro-AIDS epidemic.

We discuss the origins of HIV-1 and HIV-2, summarizing information pointing to multiple cross species of viruses in Africa from chimpanzees to humans to produce HIV-1 and from the sooty mangabey to produce HIV-2. Next, we review several findings that describe molecular epidemiologic issues of blood strains of HIV-1 and HIV-2. Point sources of these viruses are discussed, showing that their spread can be traced to specific founder viruses by using phylogenetic analysis. Risk factors are then touched upon, including drug abuse, sex, poverty, and social inequality of women. These remain the primary risks that the world grapples with to alleviate HIV spread.

In the highly active antiretroviral therapy (HAART) era, the existence of long-term HIV reservoirs appears to be a source of discontinuous evolution of HIV (appearance of strains that are out of a strict chronological progression of ancestor to progeny, where the temporal sampling of the tissue or fluid sources of virus is actually documented). Several paradigms for HIV molecular studies are discussed. Next, extensive changes in the neuropathological manifestations of HIV in the HAART era are described, both from the point of view of neuropathology and from psychiatric assessments. We describe the natural history and key features of HIV-associated dementia that have been altered by HAART. A description and analysis of HIV isolates and strains with different sequences that appear to be important for the pathogenesis of brain disease in neuro-AIDS are discussed.

Recent decreases in the heterogeneity of HIV sequences for many strains that have occurred in several places in the world including Southeast Asia are described, and their possible association with human behaviors such as drug abuse is considered. Reverse transcriptase (RT) fidelity and recombination, which impact on the heterogeneity of HIV, are discussed.

Finally, the following topics are examined because of their overall importance in understanding HIV infection and vaccine problems: (i) cellular immunity, CD8$^+$ cytotoxic T lymphocytes, and HIV infection; (ii) periphery, CD8$^+$ cytotoxic T lymphocytes, and HIV-1 infection; (iii) brain, CD8$^+$ cytotoxic T lymphocytes and vaccine against HIV-1 infection, and CD4$^+$ helper/inducer T lymphocytes and HIV-1 infection; (iv) receptors (coreceptors); and (v) humoral immunity. HIV strains from brain isolates show strain "speciation" with respect to brain regions as well as geographical locations of the infected patients. An understanding of these phenomena in conjunction with immunity and neuro-AIDS in future studies in greater detail should

Paul Shapshak, Division of Infectious Diseases and International Medicine, Tampa General Hospital, Departments of Internal Medicine and Psychiatry-Behavioral Medicine, USF Health, Tampa, FL 33606. **Alireza Minagar,** Departments of Neurology and Anesthesiology, Louisiana State University Health Sciences Center, Shreveport, LA 71301. **Pandjassarame Kangueane,** Biomedical Informatics, 17A Irulan Sundai Annex, Pondicherry 607402, India. **Simon Frost and Sergei L. Kosakovsky Pond,** Antiviral Research Center, Department of Pathology, University of California San Diego, San Diego, CA 92103. **Selene Zarate,** Department of Genetics, Independent University of Mexico City, San Lorenzo 290 Col. Del Valle, 03100 México, D.F, México. **Elyse Singer,** Department of Neurology, UCLA David Geffen School of Medicine, Los Angeles, CA 90024. **Deborah Commins,** Department of Pathology (Neuropathology), University of Southern California Keck School of Medicine, Los Angeles, CA 90089. **Anne De Groot,** EpiVax, Inc. and Biomedical Center, Brown University School of Medicine, Providence, RI 02912. **Miguel Quinones-Mateu,** Life Sciences Division, Diagnostic Hybrids, Athens, OH 45701. **Ernest Terwilliger,** Harvard Institute of Medicine, Boston, MA 02115.

provide road maps for vaccine development as well as other treatments (see chapter 6, this volume).

Since the start of the AIDS pandemic, the hallmark of HIV sequence analysis has been the extreme sequence heterogeneity of this virus due to its high mutation and recombination rates, leading to the evolution of new HIV strains. This increases the difficulty of developing an effective vaccine and increases the propensity for developing resistance to antiretroviral drugs.

HIV's genetic hypervariability and ability to recombine and escape from immune suppression are well known. However, simultaneously with the known expansion of its genetic variation, there are indications during the last several years that there also has been an increase in some homogeneous strains (less than 2% variability) of HIV associated with networks of drug abuse. Intrasubtype diversity in HIV-1 in variable proteins such as the envelope protein can reach 20%, and between-subtype distances can reach 35%. These changes appear to be associated with the accelerated spread of drug abuse worldwide (particularly injection drug abuse). New strains of HIV evolve through inter/intrasubtype recombination. As a result, the host-virus relationships are changing and influence HIV infection at the levels of strain, receptor, cytokine, and chemokine interactions; replication; and spread. A question that we do not address here is whether the strains that have appeared with limited sequence heterogeneity indicate bottlenecks in HIV-1 gene flow and evolution.

Another question is raised as to the existence of mechanisms by which strains coalesce to produce additional strains with the disappearance of some parental strains. Since the numbers of strains have increased and overlapping infections have been occurring (due to human mobile sexual and drug abuse high-risk behaviors), individuals increasingly become infected and reinfected with similar strains that they may transmit back and forth. Therefore, the number of individuals with infections of multiple HIV strains is increasing.

ORIGINS OF HIV-1 AND HIV-2

Genetic variability and sequence heterogeneity are key features of HIV. Its enzyme, RT, exhibits the ability to jump between nucleic acid strands during replication, resulting in recombination of different types of HIV that infect the same cell. This enzyme also incorporates mismatched (non-Watson-Crick) base pairs. There is thus a central lack of fidelity of HIV to propagate any particular sequence from one cell to the next, unlike what is observed with many other viruses.

Simian immunodeficiency virus (chimpanzee) (SIV-CPZ) is most likely the source of HIV-1, and SIV (sooty mangabey) (SIV-SMM) is the source of the distantly related HIV-2 (Peeters and Sharp, 2000). HIV-1 and HIV-2 infection of humans originated most likely in Africa and occurred several times (Essex, 1997). There are three main subgroups of HIV-1: (i) M, "main," consisting of the assortment of known subgroups (also known as clades) including A, B, C, D, E, F, G, etc.; (ii) N, "new," or non-M, non-O; and (iii) O, "outlier." The third group is found mainly in Cameroon and West Africa in a few thousand patients (Peeters and Sharp, 2000). HIV-2 was detected originally in Senegal in 1985 and also has subtypes or groups (including A through F) (McCutchan, 1999; Sarr et al., 2000). In addition to the fact that HIV-1 and HIV-2 most likely invaded humans each from separate subhuman primates, it appears that

HIV-1 infected humans separately at least three times from chimpanzees whereas HIV-2 apparently crossed from sooty mangabeys to humans at least seven times (McCutchan, 1999; Sarr et al., 2000). HIV-1 and HIV-2 later spread from Africa to other countries, and the strains that developed in all these locations (e.g., Senegal, Europe, Brazil, and India) show phylogenetic similarities (Kulkarni et al., 1999). Going further back in time beyond the last few hundred years, perhaps to a million years, phylogenetic analysis indicates that human T-cell leukemia virus type 1-like retroviruses crossed the species barriers back and forth among human and subhuman primates several times (Crandall, 1996). It is unclear yet whether anything similar occurred for HIV-1 and HIV-2 pandemics.

The original "authentic," i.e., historically accurate, first isolate of HIV is unknown. Several have been proposed including, for example, ZR.59, obtained from a blood sample collected in 1959 in the Democratic Republic of the Congo (Chang et al., 1993; Korber et al., 2000). For the United States, the HIV epidemic appears to stem from Haitian rather than Puerto Rican isolates (Gilbert et al., 2007).

BLOOD STRAINS OF HIV-1 AND HIV-2

Early and Recent Blood Strains

Several issues relating to the early events and spread of the HIV epidemic have not been resolved. These include concrete parameters involved in timing and differentiation of subtypes and the possible point sources involved in the spread of HIV strains. Thus, for example, studies in Ethiopia pinpoint the introduction of a subcluster, C', of the HIV-1 subtype C in 1982. Ethiopian isolates from 1988 to 1999 showed a correlation between chronological sampling of sequences and their synonymous distances from the reconstructed HIV-1 subtype C' subcluster common ancestor, using phylogenetic clustering algorithms (Abebe et al., 2001). Given the existence of a subtype C strain in Africa in 1982, the hypothesis was advanced that by the time HIV-1 B was detected in the United States in 1981 HIV must have already differentiated into at least several of the various subtypes. Both epidemiology and current molecular models for the evolution of HIV indicate that subtype differentiation events must have occurred prior to 1981.

HIV-1 and HIV-2 differ by 30 to 60% at the nucleic acid sequence level. Much effort has been expended to produce technology for HIV-2 testing, detection, surveillance, and epidemiology. There are more than 36 different enzyme-linked immunosorbent assays and Western blot immunological tests for HIV-2, many of which overlap with HIV-1 tests (Constantine et al., 1992). Furthermore, there are PCR-based tests that are specific for each HIV-1 and HIV-2 subtype. Assays include the Roche Amplicor 1 and 1.5, Chiron bDNA, and NASBA NucliSens. Roche Amplicor 1 detects B, C, and D equally, and Amplicor 1.5 detects A, B, C, D, CRF01_AE, and F equally (Alaeus et al., 1999; Clarke et al., 2000; Nkengasong et al., 1999; Pasquier et al., 1999; Triques et al., 1999). This laboratory has produced HIV-1- and HIV-2-specific PCR assays as well (Shapshak et al., 2002, 2005a, 2005b). Development of molecular techniques has always been important because, e.g., there are HIV-2-seronegative carriers of HIV-2 (in India), and the same occurs for HIV-1 (Kageyama et al., 2000).

Both HIV-1 A and HIV-2 A circulate in Senegal. The HIV-1 C2-V3 region was sequenced from commercial sex workers (CSWs). Twenty-three of 29 dually infected individuals had HIV-1 subtype A with subtypes C, D, or J. There were two separate subclusters of these viruses, one with, and one without, the CRF02_AG recombinant form IbNG. The non-IbNG-associated HIV-1 subtype A predominated in single infections (Sarr et al., 2000).

In vitro studies in cell culture showed that HIV-1 replication is inhibited by HIV-2 in dually infected cell cultures (Dern et al., 2001). Coinfections of individuals with HIV-1 and HIV-2 strains occur as well, and initial epidemiological investigations seemed to indicate that there may be differences in virulence of HIV-1 and HIV-2 that translate into a relative cross-clade suppression of HIV-1 by HIV-2 infection (Essex, 1997). These observations in fact have not translated into long-term reduction in the spread of HIV-1 or of HIV-2 anywhere. It is puzzling as to what the significance of these in vitro and in vivo observations may be in terms of HIV-1 and HIV-2 replicative fitness and pathogenicity, since overall, HIV-2 is considered to be less pathogenic than HIV-1 (Essex, 1997; Sarr et al., 2000). In India, the HIV-1 and HIV-2 epidemics seem to have occurred from point source spread without any interactive effects (Grez et al., 1994). There are HIV-1 and HIV-2 dually infected individuals in India, Thailand, Guinea-Bissau, Ivory Coast, and Portugal (Andersson et al., 1999; Dern et al., 2001; Grez et al., 1994; Kannangai et al., 1999; Xin et al., 1998). And there has been a resurgence of HIV-1 spread in Guinea-Bissau, quite to the contrary of prior speculations in spite of the prevalence of HIV-2 and the existence of dually infected individuals.

Recombinant forms of HIV-1 are spreading in the human population (Andersson et al., 1999). In Guinea-Bissau there is a single recombinant form, CRF02_AG, that is recombinant between HIV-1 strains A and G (identified as, e.g., IbNG, DJ263, and DJ264). This increased incidence of the new CRF02_AG recombinant form is analogous to the pandemic spread of HIV-1 CRF01_AE recombinants throughout Southeast Asia. Also, there was no special sub-grouping or clusters of HIV-1 or HIV-2 among the dually infected individuals compared to the individuals infected singly with HIV-1 or HIV-2. This indicates that there may be several mechanisms of spread occurring simultaneously: bottlenecks (strain narrowing), watersheds (strain expansion), and weaving (strain recombination). Thus, the complexity of HIV spread is greater than originally thought.

Kong et al. (1988) observed that a cloned isolate of HIV-2 derived from a patient in Senegal had decreased cytopathicity (cell killing) in vitro in cell culture compared to the laboratory-cultured strain HIV-2ROD. However, first, it should be noted that the HIV-2ROD laboratory strain may have become more virulent in cell culture and this may not be in direct correlation with the disease-producing effects of the virus that is spreading in the world. Second, although the virus entered cells via a CD4-dependent mechanism, Kong and colleagues (Kong et al., 1988) note that there appeared to be a slow entry step and speculated that alternative non-envelope proteins may be involved in infection. Another interpretation is that alternative secondary receptor utilization (analogous to chemokine receptors for HIV-1 strains) may be involved in the infection.

HIV-2 strains in India are being characterized. HIV-2 subtype A has six conserved amino acids in gp120. In the C2V3 region, of 153 amino acids (at positions 119, 142, 173, 174, 189, and 270), 6 amino acids were shared by HIV-2 Indian strains, respectively, as follows: Y (tyrosine), A (alanine), S (serine), K (lysine), S, and K (Sankale et al., 1995). Many of these strains have macrophage-tropic signatures that may be indicative of strains related to neuro-AIDS as

for HIV-1, for which there is an association of macrophage tropism with neuro-AIDS.

Risk Factors (Drug Abuse, Sex, Poverty, and Social Inequality of Women)

The basic risks for HIV infection are no mystery. Sexual activity, drug abuse (injection), transfusion, needle-sticks, and transplacental transmission are primary risks (Eisen et al., 1991; McCoy and Khoury, 1990). Secondary risks include poverty and noninjecting-drug abuse (McCoy and Khoury, 1990) because these are conditions that lead to the further breakdown of social behaviors that are normally barriers to the spread of HIV infection. There is an additional secondary risk for HIV infection that injection drug abusers are subject to specifically. When drug abusers share their needle/syringes (n/s), they are subject to a direct and primary transmission of HIV, since there is a high percentage of n/s used for drug abuse that contain HIV-1 (Shapshak et al., 2000). However, many injection drug abusers also share their paraphernalia (cottons and cookers) and wash-waters (that are infected with HIV). Therefore, even in the presence of needle exchange programs, the risks of spread of HIV exist when the paraphernalia and wash-waters are still shared (McCoy et al., 1994; Shah et al., 1996; Shapshak et al., 1994, 2000). In addition, the lack of empowerment of women, i.e., gender inequality, also contributes to infection of monogamous women from their risk-taking spouses (Solomon et al., 1998) (see chapter 13, this volume).

There is evidence that in other countries, just as in the United States, sexual and drug abuse activities increase the risk for the spread of both non-HIV infections (termed comorbid infections and including hepatitis viruses, herpesviruses, and bacterial and parasitic infections) and HIV infections. Measurements of the baseline immunological values for subjects (including HIV-negative ones) in various risk groups support this notion. For example, studies of female CSWs in the Vellore region in Tamil Nadu in Southern India showed that both HIV-positive and HIV-negative CSWs had hyperglobulinemia and elevated CD4 cells (Babu et al., 1997), indicating an inflammatory response to infection. (Immune activation increases risk for HIV replication.) In another example, the parasitic disease kala-azar indirectly increases the risk for the spread of HIV, hepatitis C virus (HCV), and hepatitis B virus in Northeastern India, because local physicians reuse n/s in their treatments of patients infected with kala-azar (Singh et al., 2000). The n/s then becomes the vector for the spread of these viruses (Shapshak et al., 2001).

Discontinuous Evolution for HIV-1 and HIV-2

It has been hypothesized that there are long-term viral reservoirs of HIV-1. These can exist in the context of T-cell latency as well as HAART (Finzi et al., 1999; Gunthard et al., 1999). The existence of these long-term HIV reservoirs may be a source of discontinuous evolution of HIV. We define discontinuous evolution of HIV as the appearance of strains that are out of a strict chronological progression of ancestor to progeny where the temporal sampling of the tissue or fluid sources of virus is actually documented. Thus, the C2-V3 region of HIV-2 was analyzed for two individuals by using peripheral blood mononuclear cells as sources of proviral DNA obtained in 1992, 1995, and 1997. The 1995 strains were antecedent phylogenetically to the 1992 and 1997 strains for one individual. This phenomenon is explained as the recrudescence of a clone in 1995 that had been quiescent in 1992 and thus undetected in the individual (Esteves et al., 2001).

Two other studies further address the issue of directionality versus stochasticity in HIV evolution and the problem of strain similarities among individuals who were not epidemiologically linked. Herbeck and colleagues (Herbeck et al., 2006) recently concluded that their data supported a model of convergent evolution of HIV upon transmission. Thus, they state that HIV evolves back to ancestral sequences when infecting a new host (Herbeck et al., 2006). This is counter to the paradigm of a stochastic factor generally accepted in HIV evolutionary studies. Liu and colleagues (Liu et al., 2005) demonstrated in molecular epidemiological studies that there is a remarkable homogeneity of sequences among injection drug users at distances of hundreds of miles. This is also unexpected based on prior stochastic models in the field. All these results cast serious doubt on the internal logic and assumptions of temporal and epidemiological paradigms made in highly critical prior publications, a lesson for the practitioner in the field as well as the serendipitous reader, and a matter of continued concern (Korber et al., 1995, 2000; Learn et al., 1996). It is important then to utilize a purely scientific approach in which the door is left open for paradigm shifts to occur and for constructive explanations of seemingly anomalous results with the passage of time.

CHANGES IN THE NEUROPATHOLOGICAL MANIFESTATIONS OF HIV IN THE HAART ERA

Prior to the advent of HAART, at least 50% of AIDS patients were reported to have had significant symptomatic central nervous system (CNS) involvement during life (Snider et al., 1983). An even higher percentage of AIDS patients were reported to have CNS abnormalities at autopsy, up to 80% in some analyses (Petito et al., 1986). These CNS abnormalities commonly included one or more opportunistic infections such as toxoplasmosis encephalitis, cytomegalovirus, encephalitis, *Cryptococcus neoformans* meningitis, atypical mycobacterial infections, disseminated tuberculosis, or progressive multifocal leukoencephalopathy (PML) (Ferrando and Lyketsos, 2006; Petito et al., 1986). In addition, unusual CNS neoplasms, in particular Epstein-Barr virus-associated primary CNS lymphoma (PCNSL), were also relatively common (Bell, 1998) (see chapters 26, 29, and 31, this volume). Such opportunistic complications were similar to those described in HIV-seronegative individuals with cancer, transplants, or other immunosuppressive conditions.

In addition to the opportunistic conditions associated with immunosuppression, approximately 30% of AIDS cases were found to have a "subacute encephalitis" (also known as HIV encephalitis [HIVE]) at autopsy (Petito et al., 1986). This HIVE, which was a new neuropathological entity unique to the AIDS epidemic, could be found alone or in addition to a CNS opportunistic condition. The key histopathological feature of HIVE was deemed to be HIV-infected multinucleated giant cells (MNGCs) (Budka, 1986; Petito et al., 1986) (see chapter 24, this volume). These MNGCs usually were found in deep cortical white matter and in the basal ganglia, typically in a perivascular location. They were accompanied by other signs of inflammation such as microglial nodules and often by varying degrees of white matter damage (HIV-associated leukoencephalopathy). In addition, the presence of HIV antigens such as p24 and gp41 in the brain (as determined by immunohistochemistry) or the presence of HIV nucleic acids (as determined by in situ hybridization or PCR) has also been accepted as being diagnostic of HIVE (Glass et al., 1995).

Navia and colleagues (Navia et al., 1986a) suggested that HIVE was the pathological correlate of a progressive dementia, frequently accompanied by degenerative changes in CNS motor systems and/or changes in behavior (such as apathy and irritability), that was observed in late-stage AIDS patients (Navia et al., 1986b). This clinical entity was initially called "AIDS dementia complex" (ADC). The hallmarks of this condition included memory loss, slowing of mental processing, psychomotor slowing, and declining cognition. The notion that ADC was a predominantly subcortical process was supported by the presence of other characteristics of subcortical pathology, e.g., central motor disorders (including corticospinal tract signs and Parkinsonian features such as bradykinesia, cogwheeling, and rigidity) in some patients (Glass et al., 1995). ADC was also frequently accompanied by behavioral changes and with an HIV-associated vacuolar myelopathy (see chapter 3, this volume). However, it has become apparent that these features do not invariably accompany ADC.

Subsequently, the American Academy of Neurology (AAN) refined the nomenclature for HIV-associated neurological disorders. Their terminology is the one that is still the most frequently used by researchers who study HIV neurology. The diagnosis of ADC was refined to include moderate to severe cognitive disorders, termed HIV-associated dementia (HAD); and a milder form of cognitive impairment, termed HIV-associated minor cognitive-motor disorder (American Academy of Neurology AIDS Task Force, 1991). The American Academy of Neurology criteria for HAD required both "an acquired abnormality in at least two cognitive (nonmotor) areas causing impairment in work or activities of daily living (ADLs), and either an abnormality of motor function or specified neuropsychiatric or psychosocial functions (e.g., motivation, emotional control, social behavior)." In short, this led to further subclassification of HAD according to the presence or absence of motor or behavioral features. In 2007, yet another refinement in the research nomenclature was published (Antinori et al., 2007), which introduced the overarching term "HIV-associated neurocognitive disorders" (HAND) (see chapter 1, this volume). It recognized a spectrum of neurocognitive impairments ranging from asymptomatic neurocognitive impairment to HIV-1-associated mild neurocognitive disorder to full-blown HAD. The new criteria elaborated the neuropsychological criteria necessary for the various diagnoses and the degree of severity of impact on activities of daily living. Finally, the new classification recognized the importance of comorbid conditions in the development of HAND. It remains to be seen whether these new criteria will be widely adopted. Additional work supports this view and the complexity imposed by comorbid findings due to drug abuse (Kopnisky et al., 2007). It is important not to lose sight of the interaction of drug abuse and the spread of HIV infection, both due to risky behaviors that drive each other epidemiologically and require analysis and treatment in tandem, a paradigm that has stood the test of time (Edlin et al., 1994; Nath et al., 2006) (see chapter 32, this volume).

The introduction of effective HAART has led to some impressive changes in the natural history of AIDS, slowing its progression and possibly turning AIDS into a chronic disease. The neuropathology of HIV in the post-HAART era, however, can be characterized by the phrase, "some things change, some things stay the same." The number of autopsy cases reporting a CNS opportunistic infection or PCNSL has decreased dramatically for HAART-treated patients (Bell, 2004; Gray et al., 2003; Langford et al., 2003; Masliah et al., 2000). Some HIV-associated conditions such as PML and PCNSL are no longer invariably rapidly fatal thanks to the immune reconstitution that can be achieved by instituting HAART (Lima et al., 2007). In the case of PML, successful control of the disease appears to require JC virus-specific cytotoxic T lymphocytes, although CD4$^+$ T cells play a contributory role (Du Pasquier et al., 2004). Despite the obvious improvements engendered by HAART, all the pre-HAART CNS diseases are still seen, albeit at a lower rate except for cirrhosis and arteriosclerosis, which show increased prevalence (Morgello et al., 2002). This is due to a number of factors, including late diagnosis, poor patient compliance with HAART, and the emergence of multidrug-resistant strains of HIV. In addition, new entities have emerged such as CNS immune reconstitution inflammatory syndrome (Torre et al., 2005; Vallat-Decouvelaere et al., 2003; Vendrely et al., 2005). This syndrome refers to the sudden clinical deterioration of an AIDS patient shortly after the initiation of HAART, which is typically associated with an improvement in CD4$^+$ subsets and a decline in viral load (immune reconstitution inflammatory syndrome appears to be due to a brisk inflammatory response by the newly reconstituted immune system to a previously silent infection such as PML [Nuttall et al., 2004]). The brain is deluged with an influx of CD8$^+$ cytotoxic lymphocytes, causing a leukoencephalitis. In some cases, a clinical response to corticosteroids has been reported (Venkataramana et al., 2006). In addition AIDS patients on HAART may show evidence at autopsy of "burned-out" opportunistic infections such as chronic PML (Gray et al., 2003). They also may have CNS lesions related to the long-term adverse effects of HAART itself, such as ischemic strokes (Boccara and Cohen, 2003) (see chapter 7, this volume).

The status of HIVE/HAD in the post-HAART era is interesting and controversial. Cognitive impairment associated with HIV infection remains a relatively common problem, estimated at approximately 20% (Sacktor et al., 2002), despite the widespread use of HAART (Cysique et al., 2004). In fact, although the incidence of new cases of HAD has reportedly decreased with the use of HAART, the actual prevalence of HAD has been reported to be stable or increased due to the longer survival of HIV-infected individuals (Sacktor et al., 2002; Cysique et al., 2004; McArthur, 2004; Dilley et al., 2005; Tozzi et al., 2005a). In addition to the longer retention of HAD-affected individuals in the population, the risk of developing HAD increases with time from seroconversion, even in the era of HAART (Bhaskaran et al., 2007).

It has been argued by some investigators that the natural history and key features of HAD have in fact been altered by HAART. In addition to the increased longevity of HAD patients (Dore et al., 2003; Tozzi et al., 2005b), changes in the neuropsychological features of the disease (Cysique et al., 2004), higher mean CD4$^+$ counts in afflicted individuals (Dore et al., 1999), and reduced levels of cerebrospinal fluid (CSF) HIV RNA in HAD-affected patients have been reported (McArthur et al., 2004; Cysique et al., 2005). It has also been observed that fewer HAART-treated individuals manifest the most severe and disabling forms of HAD in favor of milder disease (McArthur, 2004). Moreover, slowed neurodegenerative processes may be associated

with reductions in increased CSF neurofilament proteins in the CSF of treated patients (Mellgran et al., 2007). However, the prolonged survival of HIV-infected individuals has resulted in an increased incidence of comorbid conditions such as HCV-associated cirrhosis, cerebrovascular disease, drug abuse, and Alzheimer's disease, all of which can affect cognition (Alisky, 2007; Bell et al., 2006; Brew, 2004; Letendre et al., 2007). Several psychiatric conditions have also been recognized as comorbid with AIDS including psychological reactions, stress-distress spectrum and adjustment disorder, anxiety disorders, mood disorders, personality disorders, cognitive disorders, psychotic disorders, substance use disorders, and sleep disorders. These are all discussed extensively in the context of HIV infection in a recent set of review articles (Fernandez and Ruiz, 2006). In some cases, the comorbid condition may increase the likelihood of developing HAD and vice versa. For instance, there is extensive research supporting the view that drug abuse increases the risk of developing HIV-associated neurocognitive deficits (Bell et al., 2006; Kopnisky et al., 2007). Similarly it is possible that HIV infection may increase the risk of development of Alzheimer's disease (Alisky, 2007). Even in the absence of specific interactions between HIV and comorbid conditions, the simple presence of comorbid disorders complicates the neuromedical, neuropsychological, and neuropathological assessment of these patients. In addition, they add potentially confounding variables to any studies of HIVE/HAD that utilize data and/or tissue from these patients.

If HAART reduces the viral load in plasma and CSF, why do we continue to find cases of HAD and HIVE? Some of the remaining severe cases of HAD are seen in patients with low CD4$^+$ cell counts and a high HIV load and represent treatment failure due to either refusal of therapy, poor adherence, multidrug resistance, late diagnosis, or some additional mechanism that requires further study to decipher. More common are patients with lesser but nonetheless significant degrees of cognitive impairment that have been treated with HAART but did not return to baseline. This may represent a failure of current regimens to completely eradicate HIV in the brain, or it may represent stable cognitive dysfunction in patients who received late or inadequate treatment and sustained irreversible damage. In a prospective observational study of 1,160 HIV-positive adults who had received HAART from the AIDS Clinical Trials Group (Robertson et al., 2007), it was observed that a history of a low CD4$^+$ count (under 200 cells/µl) and increasing age were associated with an increased prevalence of cognitive dysfunction. The study was somewhat limited in that it did not employ either neuroimaging or CSF parameters. However, the study could not identify an immunological, demographic, or virological risk factor for the development of new incident cognitive impairment. This supports the notion that there may be irreparable damage to the CNS that does not resolve fully with treatment. It also indicates that there may be subtle factors, perhaps limited to the CNS (such as persistent infection in the CNS or sustained CNS inflammation), that promote the development of impairment in a HAART-treated individual. This study did not examine the subjects with neuroimaging or CSF tests. However, elevated CNS CSF neopterin levels (measure of activated macrophages) and CSF immunoglobulin G index (marker of B-cell activation) persist even after long-term, effective HAART (Yilmaz et al., 2007; Abdulle et al., 2005) (see chapter 17, this volume). This buttresses the idea that persistent immune activation may contribute to a neurocognitive disorder even in the face of HAART (Goodkin, 2006) (see chapter 1, this volume).

Some patients continue to experience slow cognitive decline despite apparently adequate treatment and despite undetectable CSF and plasma viral loads (Brew, 2004; McArthur et al., 2004). This is a new variation in the course of HAD, which in the pre-HAART era was typically characterized by a rapid decline leading to death (Navia et al., 1986b). This observation has led some investigators to propose that HAART has created subtypes of HAD (Brew, 2004). It has also led investigators to consider whether inflammatory damage to the CNS can persist despite low or absent antigenic stimulus (Anthony et al., 2005) or whether a persistent virus has evolved to adapt to the neural environment and/or HAART (Pillai et al., 2006; Strain et al., 2005).

The situation becomes even more complex when one considers the neuropathology of HIVE in the post-HAART era. There is considerable disagreement in the literature as to the prevalence of HIVE post-HAART, with reports ranging from approximately 7 to 25% of HIV autopsies (Anthony et al., 2005; Masliah et al., 2000). There are numerous reasons for this discrepancy. Possibly, patients who fail to take their HAART may be at increased risk of death; patients with a history of severe neurological symptoms are more likely to be autopsied; certainly, there may be differences between cohorts in the strains of virus they harbor; and some authors have presented data indicating that HIVE is more commonly associated with certain demographic factors including drug use (Bell et al., 1998, 2006).

A more mundane reason for the differences in the prevalence of HIVE, however, and one that is rarely addressed, is the differences in how the diagnosis is made. The diagnosis of HIVE may be based on examination of routine hematoxylin and eosin sections for the presence of MNGCs or may be based on detection of HIV antigens by immunohistochemistry or nucleic acids by PCR. This is not a minor issue; Glass and colleagues (Glass et al., 1995) found that MNGCs were present in only 25% of HIV-infected subjects with a premortem history of dementia who came to autopsy. Conversely, HIV antigens, detected immunohistochemically, were found in the brains of the majority of subjects, demented or not, at autopsy. In this pre-HAART autopsy study, the best correlate of dementia was the number of macrophages and microglia in the brain. Synaptic pruning and dendritic simplification have also been proposed as a key feature of HIVE (Masliah et al., 1997). Some HAART era studies (Brew, 2004) suggest that the presence of virus in the brain, as determined by CSF markers, no longer correlates with cognitive functioning. There are good reasons why this may hold true, and it may extend to immunohistochemical or PCR detection of virus. There are, of course, other factors that may affect the correlation between premortem cognition and postmortem pathology. The adequacy of the premortem diagnosis is one. Others include the number of areas sampled and the number and types of diagnostic tests applied to the brain tissue postmortem. For example, diagnostic tests for HCV were not available in the early days of the epidemic. Recent studies indicate that HCV may penetrate the CNS and infect astrocytes and macrophages/microglia, possibly affecting cognition (Forton et al., 2003; Letendre et al., 2007; Tozzi et al., 2005a). Further, the history of patient adherence to use of antiretrovirals is rarely available to the pathologist. The use of HAART, especially in some patient populations, can be irregular. It seems reasonable that a subject may have suffered irreversible virus-induced damage at some course in their illness, but subsequent HAART may then clear the virus and diminish the more overt signs of inflammation, such as MNGCs. Another possibility is that the entry of HIV into the brain early in the infection triggers a cascade of neurotoxic and inflammatory events that is self-sustaining, even in the absence of the virus, leading to progressive cognitive decline (Anthony et al., 2005). Finally, brain macrophages and microglia act as a reservoir for HIV in subjects on HAART (Dunfee et al., 2006b). The levels of virus may be too low to initiate MNGC formation and overt white matter damage but may be sufficient to maintain a low level of inflammation that results in cumulative damage over time. One of the practical consequences of this matter is that subjects with HIV-associated cognitive deficits may receive no specific neuropathologic diagnosis at autopsy. A second consequence is that without the diagnosis of HIVE, as based on the presence of MNGCs, the tissue of some subjects with a premortem history of HAD will be excluded from research studies. This group of subjects may actually be very interesting and important.

Anthony and colleagues (Anthony et al., 2005) have presented evidence that there is considerable ongoing inflammation in the brains of nondemented subjects who had been on HAART and died of causes unrelated to HIV such as HCV. In this study, they used image analysis techniques to quantify the number of microglia/macrophages present. It seems likely that such techniques may allow the detection of more subtle, yet functionally highly significant HIV-induced damage in the brain than routine examination of hematoxylin and eosin stained sections. Just as the disease itself has changed in the era of HAART, so changes may be required in the approach to neuropathological diagnosis. It should also be noted that these changes impact on the use of putative laboratory markers to assist in the diagnosis of HIV-related cognitive changes (Minagar et al., 2008).

Studies from different areas around the world may ultimately contribute to our understanding of the potential influence of viral genetics on the relationship between neuropathological findings and HAD. The neurological complications of HIV in areas of the world (Africa and Asia) where HIV clade C predominates have received relatively little attention. A recent report from India describes the neuropathology seen in 15 clade C-infected, antiretroviral-naïve individuals who died of CNS opportunistic infection (Mahadevan et al., 2007). Macrophages/microglia positive for p24 were seen in 14 of 15 brains. Despite the presence of numerous HIV-positive cells in most of the brains, no MNGCs were identified. The authors postulate that in their patient population, death from opportunistic infection supervenes before MNGCs (and HAD) develop. Alternatively, the clade C and B viruses may differ in their propensity for inducing formation of MNGCs.

It remains to be determined whether or not MNGCs would serve as a marker for HAD in patients infected with clade C HIV. In fact, it is unknown what the incidence of HAD would be in these individuals if opportunistic infections were better controlled. As the use of HAART spreads, more attention must be given to neuro-AIDS in populations outside North America and Europe.

BRAIN STRAINS OF HIV

HIV viral isolates and strains with different sequences appear to be important for the pathogenesis of brain disease in neuro-AIDS, and early studies identified HIV-1 isolates related to neuro-AIDS (Cheng-Mayer et al., 1991a, 1991b; Gilizia et al., 1996; Liu et al., 1990; Shioda et al., 1992). (We do not address non-B clades and the issues of their involvement in neuro-AIDS.) As with generalized AIDS, deciphering HIV-1-associated brain disease involves studying interactions between host and virus to increase our understanding of the biology of each. The toxicity of HIV-1B proteins (with emphasis on env and tat) and their involvement with activation of immune and brain cells including macrophage/microglia and astrocytes have been under extensive study (Gendelman, 2002; King et al., 2006; van Marle and Power, 2005; Nath et al., 2000; Ranga et al., 2004; Shapshak et al., 2006). An additional mechanism of pathogenesis in the brain involves the ability of the virus to enter cells in the brain mediated by the HIV-1 envelope protein. It is also of great concern whether envelope-mediated death is due to viral replication or toxicity. Zhang and colleagues (Zhang et al., 2003) dissected the two mechanisms. Possibly, on the one hand, the heterogeneity of sequences of HIV-1 gp120 in the brain is associated with neuronal death; most of these sequences are not associated with replicating virus. On the other hand, the smaller quantity of replicating virus is not associated with neurotoxicity. Furthermore, HIV env sequences from HIV-infected individuals with neuro-AIDS differ from those of individuals without neuro-AIDS (Power et al., 1998). This needs to be dealt with by both researcher and clinician alike.

HIV-1 shows one of the highest mutation rates known for any organism and thus has a high degree of heterogeneity. This heterogeneity further shows grouped molecular behavior, i.e., clades. It was early acknowledged that HIV-1 evolved into different quasispecies in brain, blood, and CSF (Korber et al., 1994; Shapshak et al., 1995, 1996). In time, it was accepted by researchers in the field that there was compartmentalization of HIV evolution in different regions of the body (Nickle et al., 2003b, 2003c; Strain et al., 2005; Wong et al., 1997). The question became primarily focused on what occurs in the brain. There have been many analyses of HIV load in different brain regions, such as those of Fujimura et al. (1997a, 1997b, 2005) and Kumar et al. (2007), to state a few; such analyses have also been well reviewed by Fujimura (2006) and Kumar et al. (2007). Of these studies, some indicated no preference by the virus for brain regions and some supported more-elevated virus loads in hippocampus and frontal cortex. It was further hypothesized that sequence heterogeneity would be detected in different regions of brain in AIDS patients. This was the case in several studies, and in addition, resistance to HAART was implicated in brain virus-associated pathogenesis (Cunningham et al., 1997; Shapshak et al., 1999; Smit et al., 2004; Chang et al., 1998). In some studies (Cunningham et al., 1997) quinolinic acid toxicity and association with neurovirulent strains of HIV were further supported. Additional phylogenetic analysis using recently developed methods further supported the model of neurovirulence of some HIV strains. The envelope gene of HIV-1 was sequenced directly from several regions of brain from three AIDS cases (Shapshak et al., 1999). Samples were screened for within-patient recombination by using a newly developed genetic algorithm maximum likelihood method (Kosakovsky Pond et al., 2006). Phylogenetic analysis (Fig. 1) revealed that sequences were compartmentalized and that there was little gene flow among regions (Slatkin-Maddison test; $p < 0.01$), supporting prior findings (Shapshak et al., 1999). Within-brain region genetic distances were smaller than genetic distances between brain regions, and standard tests of population subdivision were

significant (Table 1). Amino acid signature analysis in these envelope sequences showed that 15 majority amino acid signatures associated with known biological characteristics of the virus codon-based likelihood analyses (Frost el al., 2005) did not reveal a pattern of elevated selective pressure along branches involved in inferred migration events (Table 2). Salemi et al. (2005) analyzed clonal env V1-V2 and, separately, V3 sequences from multiple brain regions of a single AIDS case and argued that whereas sequences from different brain regions cluster nonrandomly in a phylogeny—an obvious pattern of compartmentalization—substantial gene flow was found between brain regions. However, the power of inference from a single sample of relatively short sequence fragments may be low, and complicating factors (recombination and differential selective pressure) need to be addressed more carefully. As more high-resolution sequence samples become available, further studies of molecular sequence data could further elucidate evolutionary patterns and dynamics of HIV-1 in different regions of the brain (Zárate et al., 2007).

There is increasing support for the notion that specific strains of HIV-1 infect the brain and contribute to neuro-AIDS in various forms including neuropathology, cognitive distress, and psychiatric disease (Chang et al., 1998; Gartner, 2000; Jurado et al., 1999; Power et al., 1994; Salemi et al., 2005; Shapshak et al., 1999). The involvement of brain regional evolution of HIV-1 in neuro-AIDS was supported by extensive and detailed studies (Salemi et al., 2005), supporting earlier findings of neurovirulent HIV-1 regional brain strains mentioned above. Furthermore, even in the era of HAART, when therapy has been able to reduce peripheral virus load, the brain remains a reservoir of HIV infection and source of reactivation (Clements et al., 2005; Minagar and Shapshak, 2006; Wang et al., 2005) as was originally anticipated earlier in the epidemic (Resnick et al., 1988; Singer et al., 1994). An integrative model combining several hypotheses is that HIV penetrates the brain early to late throughout disease (Gartner, 2006) and that superimposed on this is the regional evolution of HIV in the brain; the virus has a low likelihood of transmission within the brain (Cunningham et al., 1987; Chang et al., 1998; Shapshak et al., 1999; Zárate et al., 2007).

van Marle and Power (2005) extensively reviewed several issues related to HIV-1 and the human nervous system. They discussed issues including host genetics, HIV-1 evolution, viral diversity, turnover, neuroinvasion, and host response in the context of HAART and their impact on cognition in neuro-AIDS. They pointed out on the one hand that viral antigenic and genetic heterogeneity are lower in brain than in blood and CSF and on the other hand that viral diversity is greater in patients with HAD than in nondemented patients. These findings vary per viral gene analyzed. Furthermore, van Marle and Power (2005) summarized the involvement of the HIV genes with neuropathogenesis as follows: long terminal repeat with viral transcription, replication, and neurotropism; gag-pol with viral replication, neurotropism, and variability; Vpr with cell death; tat with viral transcription, replication, neurotropism, host transcription, neuroinflammation, apoptosis, and neurotoxin induction; env with neuroinvasion, neurotropism, apoptosis, neuroinflammation, and neurotoxin induction; and nef with apoptosis and neuroinflammation. In addition, host genetics including polymorphisms are discussed as well. They thus built a model based on mounting toxicity to characterize the pathogenesis of neuro-AIDS. The continued concern that requires clarification is that viral heterogeneity, expansion, and fitness

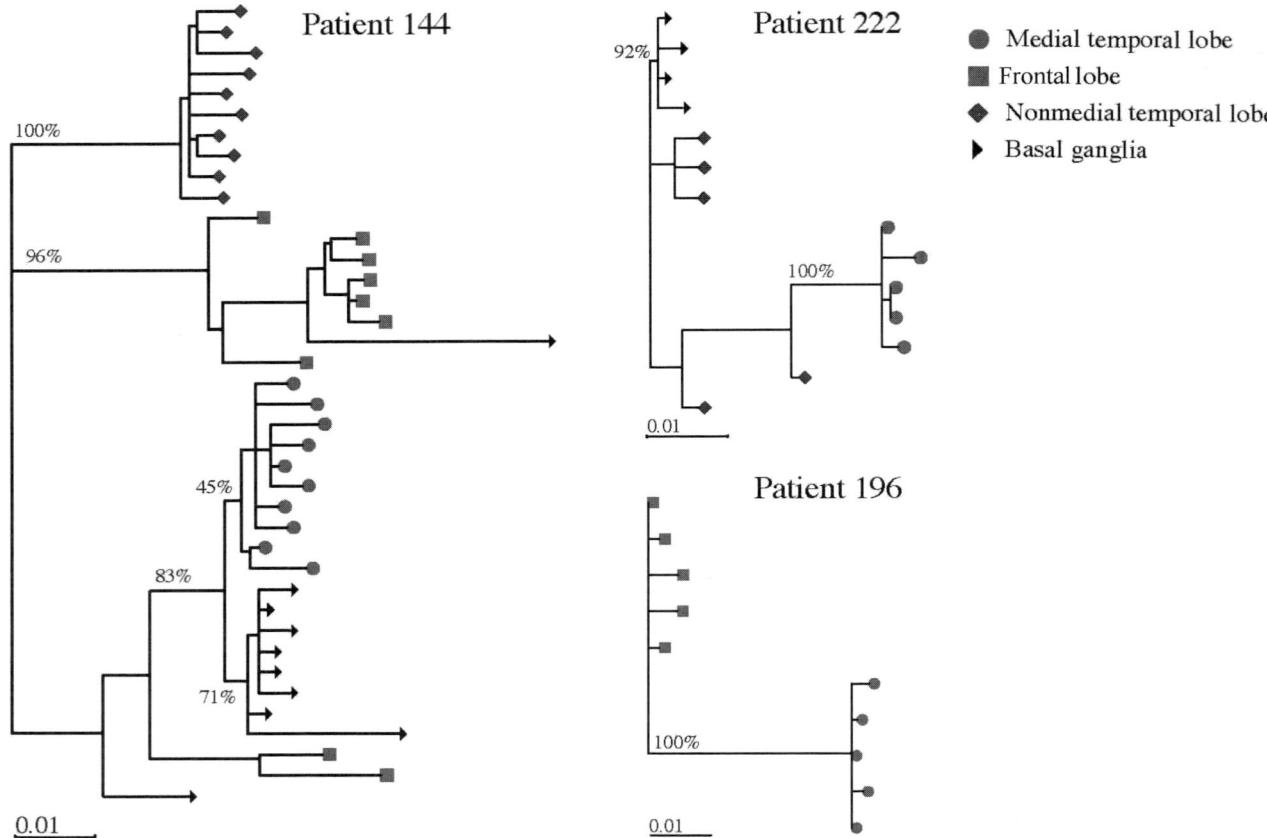

FIGURE 1 Maximum likelihood phylogenetic trees for env sequences from different brain regions. MG94 x TrN93 codon model was used to infer the trees, scaled on the expected number of nucleotide substitutions per site per unit time. Bootstrap support values for clade-separating branches were obtained via 1,000 neighbor-joining bootstrap trees.

are associated with neurological disease. Others have come to similar conclusions supporting the importance of macrophage tropism and CCR5 coreceptor use in neuro-AIDS (Dunfee et al., 2006a; Ohagen et al., 2003), supporting the earlier work reviewed by van Marle and Power (2005).

Host gene expression response is also a crucial aspect of the pathogenesis of AIDS and HAD, and many host genes are known to be involved in the pathogenesis of this disease. However, our understanding will be greatly accelerated with the advent of the new large-scale laboratory and information-processing (bioinformatics) methodologies for analysis of gene expression in human brain as well as in animal models. This is a burgeoning component of neuro-AIDS research and has been described and is reviewed extensively elsewhere. Suffice it to indicate a few examples of genes implicated in neuro-AIDS pathogenesis in these global analyses; such gene classes include those governing inflammation, signaling, transcription, synaptic plasticity, cytoskeleton, and axonal function, to name a few (Fellay et al., 2007; Levine et al., 2008; Masliah et al., 2004; Minagar et al., 2004; Roberts et al., 2003; Shapshak and Stengel, 2002; Shapshak et al., 2001, 2002, 2004, 2005a, 2006; Vahey et al., 2003). In concert with host gene expression is the study of host genetics itself and the susceptibility to neuro-AIDS. This important area is also extensively reviewed elsewhere (Gonzalez et al., 2005; Levine et al., 2008).

HETEROGENEITY/HOMOGENEITY

There is a recent decrease in the heterogeneity of HIV sequences for several strains, which has been found in several places in the world. This is possibly associated with human behaviors such as drug abuse. There are several examples of the recombination events associated with strain variation narrowing in the C2-V3 region of the envelope gene (Andersson et al., 1999; McCutchan, 1999; Peeters and Sharp, 2000; Sankalé et al., 1995). In addition, CRF01_ AE strains isolated and sequenced from 11 of 13 infected individuals in Thailand in 1998 and 1999 were less heterogeneous than CRF01_AE strains previously reported (from 1992 to 1995) from the same region (Kurosu et al., 2001). These changes occurred in the 5′ long terminal repeats and downstream sequences. In addition, changes occurred in the T-cell-specific factor 1alpha motif (which is located behind the 3′ terminus of nef) and the gag leader region of these isolates. Chang and colleagues (Chang et al., 1999) found a 24-nucleotide insertion in the primer-binding site common to the CRF01_AE and subtype G strains but not in HIV-1 subtypes B, C, and D. This insertion is not present in all A subtypes. The recombinant described by Kurosu and colleagues (Kurosu et al., 2001) had the insert. Analysis by Yu and colleagues (Yu et al., 2002) in Guangxi province in China demonstrated rapid spread of homogeneous

TABLE 1 Distance-based tests for viral population division[a]

Patient	Pairwise region comparisons					
	F-M	F-T	F-G	M-T	M-G	G-T
144	$d = 1.99\%$	$d = 1.97\%$	$d = 2.59\%$	$d = 0.96\%$	$d = 1.5\%$	$d = 1.50\%$
	$D = 5.32\%$	$D = 6.51\%$	$D = 5.05\%$	$D = 4.77\%$	$D = 2.0\%$	$D = 5.39\%$
	$F_{st} = 0.63^*$	$F_{st} = 0.70^*$	$F_{st} = 0.49^*$	$F_{st} = 0.80^*$	$F_{st} = 0.24^*$	$F_{st} = 0.72^*$
196	$d = 0.37\%$					
	$D = 3.7\%$					
	$F_{st} = 0.9^*$					
212				$d = 0.86\%$	$d = 0.34\%$	$d = 1.02\%$
				$D = 2.75\%$	$D = 3.12\%$	$D = 1.11\%$
				$F_{st} = 0.69^*$	$F_{st} = 0.89^*$	$F_{st} = 0.11^*$

[a]For sequences from every pair of brain regions (F, frontal lobe; T, nontemporal medial lobe; M, medial temporal lobe; G, basal ganglia), Tamura-Nei genetic distance measures were computed (d, mean within region; D, mean between regions distances). To assess the degree of subdivision, a standard F_{st} measure (Hudson et al., 1992) was evaluated. F_{st} takes values between 0 (completely mixed population) and 1 (completely subdivided population). Values significantly different from 0 ($P < 0.001$, permutation test) are marked with an asterisk.

CRF01_AE and also AG recombinant strains HIV-1. BC recombinants that span a 4-year time frame showed intersubject env V3 diversity of less than 0.2%. Similarly, over a 3-year duration CRF01_AE from injection drug users had an intersubject env V3 diversity of <1.6%. Different patterns of sequence variations occurred comparing the V3 and V4 regions for these recombinants.

RT Infidelity

Genomic hypervariability of HIV-1 is a major defense mechanism by which the invading virus eludes selective pressure that is imposed by the host immune system or therapeutic approaches. This genomic hypervariability occurs through three major mechanisms involving HIV replication. First, mutations can be generated by the virally encoded DNA polymerase, HIV-1 RT (Coffin, 1995), which is error prone and has a very low fidelity. HIV RT is involved in conversions of retroviruses' single-stranded genomic RNA to linear duplex DNA. Second, HIV RT also mediates strand transfer reactions that lead to recombination (Luo and Taylor, 1990; DeStefano et al., 1992), and this can amplify the mutations. Third, continuous replication increases the complexity of the viral population (Perelson et al., 1996).

The molecular mechanisms of HIV-1 RT infidelity have not been fully unraveled. Absence of a 3' to 5' proofreading activity is a presumptive factor (Williams and Loeb, 1992), but not the only one, since other retroviral RTs with no proofreading exonuclease possess a 10- to 18-fold-higher fidelity (Roberts et al., 1989) and recently the role of p53 as

an enhancer of the fidelity of DNA synthesis by HIV-1 RT was demonstrated (Bakhanashvili, 2001). Another potential mechanism for such high infidelity may be that the incorporation of mutagenic nucleotides by HIV-1 RT increases the rate of mutagenesis of HIV by the use of nucleotides that form noncomplementary base pairs at high frequency (Hizi et al., 1997).

RT Recombination

Recombination is a major means for genetic variability in retroviruses, particularly HIV-1. This high degree of genetic recombination plays a significant role in the dynamics of HIV-1 populations and can generate new pathogenic strains. Like all retroviruses, HIV-1 is a single-stranded plus-sense RNA virus and contains two copies of genomic RNA in each virion. Reverse transcription is a crucial step in viral replication. During this process the virally encoded enzyme RT uses the packaged RNA as a template to synthesize viral DNA. Since each virion contains two copies of RNA, it is possible for RT to switch from one copy of the viral RNA to the other copy during DNA formation and generate a recombinant containing some genetic data from each of the RNAs (switch-in-template phenomenon) (Hu et al., 2003; Luo and Taylor, 1990; Negroni and Buc, 2001). Recombination occurs at high frequency in HIV-1. The two major processes responsible for recombination consist of homologous and nonhomologous recombination. Homologous recombination is the most frequent source of genetic rearrangement in retroviruses, while nonhomologous recombination that

TABLE 2 Selective pressure on sequences by brain region[a]

Patient	dN/dS for indicated branch class				
	Frontal lobe	Nonmedial temporal lobe	Medial temporal lobe	Basal ganglia	Between-region migration events
144	0.84	0.53	0.41	0.50	0.50
196	1.44		1.05		0.63
212		0.33	0.46	7.94*	1.84

[a]We measured the average strength of selection on HIV-1 sequences from different brain regions. All branches in the phylogenetic tree were partitioned into those that involve sequences from a single region and those that were involved in inferred migration events. For each class of branch, a separate dN/dS was fitted using the MG94 x TRN93 model of codon evolution (Frost et al., 2005). A value of dN/dS significantly greater than one (as assessed by profile likelihood) indicates that positive selection had operated on a given class of branches. In only one case (marked by an asterisk) the test for selection was significant ($P = 0.05$).

involves regions of homology as short as a few nucleotides is much less effective in generating recombinant strains. The high rate of recombination has a significant influence on the pandemic and potential future treatments of HIV-1.

IMMUNITY

Cellular Immunity

CD8⁺ Cytotoxic T Lymphocytes and HIV Infection: Periphery

The cellular immune response plays a crucial role in the pathogenesis of HIV infection. HIV infection elicits cellular immune responses by both HIV-specific CD4⁺ helper/ inducer and CD8⁺ cytotoxic T lymphocytes. Progressive quantitative and qualitative depletion of CD4⁺ helper/ inducer T lymphocytes and consequent increased risk for development of opportunistic diseases are hallmarks of HIV disease.

The initial response of the immune system to HIV infection is similar in many ways to the immune response to other viruses and effectively removes most of the virus present in the circulation and T lymphocytes. The early response to HIV infection is colossal expansion of CD8⁺ cytotoxic T lymphocytes specific for peptides derived from HIV proteins. As many as 10% or more of circulating CD8⁺ cytotoxic T lymphocytes may be specific against HIV-derived proteins including core proteins, RT, envelope proteins, and regulatory proteins (Wilson et al., 2000; Kuroda et al., 1999). Such expansion of HIV-specific CD8⁺ cytotoxic T lymphocytes precedes the generation of neutralizing antibodies and is mainly responsible for reduction in viremia and transition to the clinically latent phase.

With progression of HIV infection, CD8⁺ T lymphocytes acquire an abnormal phenotype characterized by the expression of certain activation markers and the lack of CD25 interleukin-2 (IL-2) receptor. Development of such abnormal HIV-specific CD8⁺ T lymphocytes carries prognostic significance. Quantitative studies have demonstrated an inverse correlation between the frequency of HIV-specific CD8⁺ cytotoxic T-lymphocyte activity and plasma viral load at all stages of HIV infection (Ogg et al., 1998; Greenough et al., 1997) and between the frequency of these CD8⁺ cytotoxic T lymphocytes and the pace of CD4⁺ T-lymphocyte loss (Musey et al., 1997). Apart from this, patients whose CD8⁺ T lymphocytes express only HLA-DR and not CD38 following seroconversion develop a stabilization of their CD8⁺ T-lymphocyte count with a less aggressive course of disease. On the other hand, coexpression of HLA-DR and CD38 by CD8⁺ T lymphocytes is associated with a more accelerated course of HIV-1 infection, worse prognosis, and a faster drop of the CD8⁺ cytotoxic T-lymphocyte count.

Oligoclonal expansions of the CD8⁺ cytotoxic T lymphocytes, which are mainly composed of HIV-specific CD8⁺ cytotoxic T lymphocytes, are typical of HIV-1 infection. The disappearance of specific CD8⁺ cytotoxic T lymphocytes can be due to various factors, such as mutation of virus within the CD8⁺ cytotoxic T-lymphocyte recognition epitope and clonal exhaustion.

CD8⁺ Cytotoxic T Lymphocytes and HIV-1 Infection: Brain

HAD is one of the most common causes of dementia in HIV-infected individuals between 20 and 59 years of age. The spectrum of HIV-1 infection of brain includes HAD,

HIV-1-associated cognitive/motor disorder, subsyndromic neurocognitive impairment, and other neuropsychiatric and neurological disorders. The intriguing point is that despite the early brain invasion by HIV-1, the infection remains restricted for several years. The mechanisms of such restriction of infection are only partially understood and most probably involve both innate and acquired immunological responses which are pointed against the principal target of HIV-1 in brain, macrophages/microglia. CD8⁺ cytotoxic T lymphocytes play a major role in control of HIV-1 infection in brain (Sewell et al., 2000). Interactions of CNS macrophage/microglia, which function as antigen-presenting cells (Minagar et al., 2002), with CD8⁺ cytotoxic T lymphocytes can either restrict or eliminate HIV-1 in brain, while continuous viral proliferation occurs in the periphery (Poluektova et al., 2002) (see chapter 18, this volume).

CD8⁺ Cytotoxic T Lymphocytes and Vaccine against HIV-1 Infection

Accumulating evidence indicates that cellular and humoral immunity and other immunological responses have certain protective roles against HIV-1 infection. Among these, CD8⁺ cytotoxic T lymphocytes probably constitute the most crucial and robust component of protective immunity, which plays a significant role in the clearing of primary HIV-1 infection and control of chronic HIV-1 infection. These cells appear early in the course of HIV-1 infection and are temporally associated with the clearance of culturable virus from blood (Koup et al., 1994). These CD8⁺ cytotoxic T lymphocytes are often detected in high numbers during the asymptomatic phase of HIV-1 infection and decrease with progression to AIDS (Goulder et al., 1997). However, the pressure of these activated T lymphocytes may also be a significant factor for development of new mutants of HIV-1, which in turn can lead to epitope deletion, failure of antigen processing, and loss of major histocompatibility complex class I binding, impaired recognition by the T-cell receptor, and more resistance to pressure exerted by the immune system. Indeed, such HIV-1 escape from these effector cells is a determinant of disease progression in infected patients (De Groot et al., 2001; Sewell et al., 2000). Therefore, development of any prophylactic measure against HIV-1, such as a vaccine, is an empiric endeavor in which stimulation of both humoral and cellular immune responses appears to be a logical goal. Apart from the defective role of these immune responses in restraining the HIV-1 infection and preventing the generation of a potent vaccine, hypervariability of the HIV-1 strains is the other major obstacle in designing effective HIV-1 vaccines. A more optimistic finding is that individuals expressing HLA-A11 had cytotoxic T lymphocytes directed to a $G_{357}S$ escape variant of the $Gag_{349-359}$ epitope, thus supporting the notion of developing vaccines against both variant and wild-type forms of the CD8 epitopes. This may simultaneously counter the emergence of HIV escape cytotoxic T lymphocyte variants from primary epitopes (Allen et al., 2005).

There is a caveat related to statistics that should be stated in this type of immunology and virology research. Some publications are based on very small numbers of cases. This is often due to the limitations of available tissues and cases for analysis. Often increased numbers and types of specimens are analyzed so that analysis-of-variance-type statistics become more readily applicable rather than relying only on the Student t tests, as is done in many studies. Accepting results based on phylogenetics, microarray, and proteomics analyses is similarly replete with questions. But here again, multiple findings by the same and additional laboratories as well as various types of analyses of the data sets provide greater insight into the conclusions until additional, possibly confirmatory analyses are conducted.

Several approaches to contend with HIV variation are being considered. These include using isolates of a particular subtype, appropriate for the pandemic in a targeted geographic region, or using multivalent protein cocktails that include a spectrum of regional subtypes, in the hope that the immune responses elicited by one circulating strain will be sufficiently cross-reactive to protect from the other variants from the same subtype (Graham, 2002; Schultz and Bradac, 2001). Given the extraordinary variability of HIV strains, however, even within-clade diversity is an obstacle to protective immunity. For example, a recent case study of an HIV-1-positive patient showed that despite a robust immune response to an initial HIV infection, he acquired a second virus of the same subtype, only 12% different from the first (Altfeld et al., 2002). Alternative approaches include enhancing cross-reactivity of the population through the use of artificially generated sequences. These can be "central" sequences, either a consensus or reconstructed ancestor (Gaschen et al., 2002; Nickle et al., 2003a), which by design are more similar to prevalent strains than the strains are to each other and reduce the average number of amino acid differences between a vaccine candidate strain and circulating viruses by one-half. Another approach is to design polyepitope vaccines that consist of epitopes of the HIV-1 genome that are highly conserved across the various strains of HIV-1. The bioinformatics tools for attempting to manufacture wide-spectrum vaccines that can cross-react with a large number of these epitopes are available (De Groot et al., 2001). Although results are not too encouraging at this point, vaccines are under continued study (Smith, 2005).

CD4+ Helper/Inducer T Lymphocytes and HIV-1 Infection

Dysfunction and progressive reduction of CD4+ helper/inducer T lymphocytes are other significant features of HIV infection. During development of HIV infection, the percentage of CD4+ helper/inducer lymphocytes expressing CD28 and IL-2 production and IL-2 receptor expression by these cells are decreased. These defective CD28⁻ CD4+ T lymphocytes fail to respond to activation signals and express markers of terminal activation, such as HLA-DR, CD38, and CD45RO (Borthwick et al., 1994). The CD4+ helper/inducer T lymphocytes of HIV-infected patients also demonstrate abnormally low levels of CD40 ligand, which in turn may partially be responsible for B-lymphocyte dysfunction during pathogenesis of HIV-1 infection (Wolthers et al., 1997).

Various mechanisms that may be responsible for T-lymphocyte dysfunction during HIV infection include interference with CD4 expression by HIV gp120 (Hoxie et al., 1986), Nef (Garcia and Miller, 1991), and Vpu (Wiley et al., 1992), which in turn may impair the ability of the infected T lymphocytes to interact with appropriate major histocompatibility complex class II molecules. Preferential infection of CD4+ T lymphocyte memory cells by HIV, alone or in concert with the preferential susceptibility of these cells to the cytopathic effects of HIV infection, is another possible mechanism for loss of the function and number of these cells. HIV envelope glycoproteins, through mechanisms that are distinct from infection of CD4+ T lymphocytes, can contribute to dysfunction of these cells.

Receptors (Coreceptors)

HIV-1 particles interact with several receptors located on cell surfaces (Erdmann et al., 2006). T lymphocytes, macrophages, and probably dendritic cells are the principal host cells that are infected by HIV-1. However, a selective depletion of CD4+ helper/inducer lymphocytes is the prominent feature of HIV-1 infection, which appears to originate from selective tropism of HIV-1 for this subpopulation of inflammatory cells. The viral gp120 envelope protein exhibits high affinity for the CD4 molecule. Two different receptors, CD4 and a coreceptor, are usually needed for HIV-1 to infect cells. The chemokine receptor CCR5 is the coreceptor mainly used in vivo; however, HIV-1 variants that bind to another coreceptor, CXCR4 (fusin receptor), evolve during disease progression in some AIDS patients (see chapter 19, this volume).

Other receptors that can also interact with gp120 on viral particles are mannose-binding proteins on macrophages and DC-SIGN on dendritic cells; however, these interactions do not actively facilitate fusion and viral entry to cells (Clapham and McKnight, 2001).

Humoral Immunity

The role of the humoral immune response in preventing HIV-1 infection or deterring disease progression is not fully understood. However, the available data indicate that this arm of the immune system does not play a major role in protecting the organism and rather the cellular immunity or a combination of both is more crucial.

Soon after HIV-1 infection, potent anti-HIV-1 responses can be detected, which only down regulate and incompletely clear the circulating virus (Pantaleo et al., 1994; Daar et al., 1991; Moore et al., 1994; Koup et al., 1994). Antibodies against the viral core protein p24 appear within weeks of acute HIV-1 infection and may be involved in the decline of plasma viremia associated with primary infection (Sei et al., 1989; Clark et al., 1991). Loss of these anti-p24 antibodies is associated with progression of HIV infection (Weber et al., 1987; Sei et al., 1989; Clark et al., 1991).

B lymphocytes induced by HIV-1 infection generate neutralizing antibodies. These antibodies are capable of neutralizing the virus and can be detected 1 to 3 months following the initial infection. Antibodies can neutralize free virus before their entry into cells and may be responsible for at least some degree of control of viral replication in vivo (Sei et al., 1989; Weber et al., 1987). These neutralizing antibodies may be type specific or group specific. The variable loop 3 (V3) of the HIV-1 envelope gp120 protein is the principal target of most type-specific neutralizing antibodies (Goudsmit et al., 1988; Palker et al., 1988). The targets of group-specific neutralizing antibodies include epitopes within the HIV envelope gp41 protein, discontinuous conformational epitopes around the CD4 binding site of gp120, or carbohydrate determinants. However, more recently not much optimism has been expressed in the value of humoral immunity in the control against HIV infection (Lopalco, 2004).

CONCLUSIONS

HIV-1 continually changes genetically and employs various mechanisms to evade host immune pressure. Genetic recombination is a highly significant and effective mechanism associated with this genetic hypervariability that protects HIV-1 from immunity and eventually leads to profound immunosuppression and demise of AIDS patients. Any future efforts for development of more effective therapeutic and preventive measures should be based on the approach to overcome the mechanisms that HIV-1 utilizes to escape host defenses, particularly its genetic hypervariability.

We thank Karina Yusim (Los Alamos, NM) and Rebecca Geffin (Miami, FL) for discussions. This work was supported in part by NIH Grants DA 04787, DA 07909, DA12580, DA 14533, AG19952, and GM056529 (to P.S.) and NS 38841 (to E.S. and D.C.).

REFERENCES

Abdulle, S., L. Hagberg, and M. Gisslén. 2005. Effects of antiretroviral treatment on blood-brain barrier integrity and intrathecal immunoglobulin production in neuroasymptomatic HIV-1-infected patients. *HIV Med.* **6:**164–169.

Abebe, A., V. V. Lukashov, T. F. Rinke de Wit, B. Fisseha, B. Tegbaru, and A. Kliphuis. 2001. Timing of the introduction into Ethiopia of subcluster C9 of HIV-1 subtype C. *AIDS Res. Hum. Retrovir.* **17:**657–661.

Alaeus, A., E. Lilja, S. Herman, J. Spadoro, J. Wang, and J. Albert. 1999. Assay of plasma samples representing different HIV-1 genetic subtypes: an evaluation of new versions of the Amplicor HIV-1 Monitor assay. *AIDS Res. Hum. Retrovir.* **15:**889–894.

Alisky, J. 2007. The coming problem of HIV-associated Alzheimer's disease. *Med. Hypotheses* **69:**1140–1143.

Allen, T. M., X. G. Yu, E. T. Kalife, L. L. Reyor, M. Licherfeld, M. John, and M. Cheng. 2005. De novo generation of escape variant-specific CD81 T-cell responses following CTL escape in chronic HIV-1 infection. *J. Virol.* **79:**12952–12960.

Altfeld, M., T. M. Allen, X. G. Yu, M. N. Johnston, D. Agrawal, B. T. Korber, D. C. Montefiori, D. H. O'Connor, B. T. Davis, P. K. Lee, E. L. Maier, J. Harlow, P. J. Goulder, C. Brander, E. S. Rosenberg, and B. D. Walker. 2002. HIV-1 superinfection despite broad CD81 T-cell responses containing replication of the primary virus. *Nature* **420:**434–439.

American Academy of Neurology AIDS Task Force. 1991. Nomenclature and research case definitions for neurologic manifestations of human immunodeficiency virus-type 1 (HIV-1) infection. Report of a Working Group of the American Academy of Neurology AIDS Task Force. *Neurology* **41:**778–785.

Andersson, S., H. Norrgren, F. Dias, G. Biberfeld, and J. Albert. 1999. Molecular characterization of HIV-1 and HIV-2 in individuals from Guinea-Bissau with single or dual infections: predominance of a distinct HIV-1 subtype A/G recombinant in West Africa. *Virology* **262:**312–320.

Anthony, I. C., S. N. Ramage, F. W. Carnie, P. Simmonds, and J. E. Bell. 2005. Influence of HAART on HIV-related CNS disease and neuroinflammation. *J. Neuropathol. Exp. Neurol.* **64:**529–536.

Antinori, A., G. Arendt, J. T. Becker, B. J. Brew, D. A. Byrd, M. Cherner, D. B. Clifford, P. Cinque, L. G. Epstein, K. Goodkin, M. Gisslen, I. Grant, R. K. Heaton, J. Joseph, K. Marder, C. M. Marra, J. C. McArthur, M. Nunn, R. W. Price, L. Pulliam, K. R. Robertson, N. Sacktor, V. Valcour, and V. E. Wojna. 2007. Updated research nosology for HIV-associated neurocognitive disorders. *Neurology* **69:**1789–1799.

Babu, P. G., A. Pramilabai, G. Sripriya, S. Damodharan, and J. T. Jacob. 1997. Immunologic profiles of HIV-infected and uninfected commercial sex workers in the Vellore region of Southern India. *J. AIDS Hum. Retrovir.* **16:**357–361.

Bakhanashvili, T. 2001. P53 enhances the fidelity of DNA synthesis by human immunodeficiency virus type 1 reverse transcriptase. *Oncogene* **20:**7635–7644.

Bell, J., J. C. Arango, and I. Anthony. 2006. Neurobiology of multiple insults: HIV-1-associated brain disorders in those who use illicit drugs. *J. Neuroimmune Pharmacol.* **1:**182–191.

Bell, J. E. 1998. The neuropathology of adult HIV infection. *Rev. Neurol.* (Paris) **154:**816–829.

Bell, J. E. 2004. An update on the neuropathology of HIV in the HAART era. *Histopathology* **45:**549–559.

Bell, J. E., R. P. Brettle, A. Chiswick, and P. Simmonds. 1998. HIV encephalitis, proviral load and dementia in drug users and homosexuals with AIDS. Effect of neocortical involvement. *Brain* **121:**2043–2052.

Bhaskaran, K., C. Mussini, A. Antinori, A. S. Walker, M. Dorrucci, C. Sabin, A. Phillips, K. Porter, et al. 2008. Changes in the incidence and predictors of human immunodeficiency virus-associated dementia in the era of highly active antiretroviral therapy. *Ann. Neurol.* **63:**213–221.

Boccara, F., and A. Cohen. 2003. Coronary artery disease and stroke in HIV-infected patients: prevention and pharmacological therapy. *Adv. Cardiol.* **40:**163–184.

Borthwick, N. J., M. Bofill, W. M. Gombert, A. N. Akbar, E. Medina, K. Sagawa, M. C. Lipman, M. A. Johnson, and G. Janossy. 1994. Lymphocyte activation in HIV-1 infection. II. Functional defects of CD28- T cells. *AIDS* **8:**431–441.

Brew, B. J. 2004. Evidence for a change in AIDS dementia complex in the era of highly active antiretroviral therapy and the possibility of new forms of AIDS dementia complex. *AIDS* **1:**75–78.

Budka, H. 1986. Multinucleated giant cells in brain: a hallmark of the acquired immune deficiency syndrome (AIDS). *Acta Neuropathol.* (Berlin) **69:**253–258.

Chang, J., R. Joswiak, B. Wang, T. Ng, Y. C. Ge, and W. Bolton. 1998. Unique HIV type 1 V3 region sequences derived from 6 different regions of brain: region-specific evolution within host-determined quasispecies. *AIDS Res. Hum. Retrovir.* **14:**25–30.

Chang, S. Y., C. Apichartpiyakul, C. L. Kuiken, M. Essex, and T. H. Lee. 1999. Sequence features downstream of the primer binding site of HIV–1 subtype E shared by subtype G and a subset of subtype A. *AIDS Res. Hum. Retrovir.* **15:**1703–1706.

Chang, S. Y., B. H. Bowman, J. B. Weiss, R. E. Garcia, and T. White. 1993. The origin of HIV-1 isolate HTLV-IIIB. *Nature* **363:**466–469.

Cheng-Mayer, C., D. Seto, and J. A. Levy. 1991a. Altered host range of HIV-1 after passage through various human cell types. *Virology* **181:**288–294.

Cheng-Mayer, C., T. Shioda, and J. A. Levy. 1991b. Host range, replicative, and cytopathic properties of human immunodeficiency virus type 1 are determined by very few amino acid changes in *tat* and gp120. *J. Virol.* **65:**6931–6941.

Clapham, P. R., and A. McKnight. 2001. HIV-1 receptors and cell tropism. *Br. Med. Bull.* **58:**43–59.

Clark, S. J., M. S. Saag, W. D. Decker, S. Campbell-Hill, J. L. Roberson, P. J. Veldkamp, J. C. Kappes, B. H. Hahn, and G. M. Shaw. 1991. High titers of cytopathic virus in plasma of patients with symptomatic primary HIV-1 infection. *N. Engl. J. Med.* **32:**954–960.

Clarke, J. R., S. Galpin, R. Braganza, A. Ashraf, R. Russell, D. R. Churchill, J. N. Weber, and M. O. McClure. 2000. Comparative quantification of diverse serotypes of HIV-1 in plasma from a diverse population of patients. *J. Med. Virol.* **62:**445–449.

Clements, J. E., M. Li, L. Gama, B. Bullock, L. M. Carruth, J. L. Mankowski, and M. C. Zink. 2005. The CNS is a viral reservoir in SIV-infected macaques on combined antiretroviral therapy: a model for HIV patients on HAART. *J. Neurovirol.* **11:**180–189.

Coffin, J. M. 1995. HIV population dynamics in vivo: implications for genetic variation, pathogenesis, and therapy. *Science* **267:**483–489.

Constantine, N. T., J. D. Callahan, and D. M. Watts. 1992. *Retroviral Testing, Essentials for Quality Control and Laboratory Diagnosis,* p. 89–102. CRC Press, Ann Arbor, MI.

Crandall, K. 1996. Multiple interspecies transmissions of human and simian T-cell leukemia/lymphoma virus type 1 sequences. *Mol. Biol. Evol.* **13:**115–131.

Cunningham, A. L., H. Naif, N. Saksena, G. Lynch, J. Chang, S. Li, R. Jozwiak, M. Alali, B. Wang, W. Fear, A. Sloane, L. Pemberton, and B. J. Brew. 1997. HIV infection of macrophages and pathogenesis of AIDS dementia complex: interaction of the host cell and viral genotypes. *J. Leukoc. Biol.* **62:**117–125.

Cysique, L. A., B. J. Brew, M. Halman, J. Catalan, N. Sacktor, R. W. Price, S. Brown, J. H. Atkinson, D. B. Clifford, D. Simpson, G. Torres, C. Hall, C. Power, K. Marder, J. C. McArthur, W. Symonds, and C. Romero. 2005. Undetectable cerebrospinal fluid HIV RNA and beta-2 microglobulin do not indicate inactive AIDS dementia complex in highly active antiretroviral therapy-treated patients. *J. Acquir. Immune Defic. Syndr.* **39:**426–429.

Cysique, L. A., P. Maruff, and B. J. Brew. 2004. Prevalence and pattern of neuropsychological impairment in human immunodeficiency virus-infected/acquired immunodeficiency syndrome (HIV/AIDS) patients across pre- and post-highly active antiretroviral therapy eras: a combined study of two cohorts. *J. Neurovirol.* **10:**350–357.

Daar, E. S., T. Moudgil, R. D. Meyer, and D. D. Ho. 1991. Transient high levels of viremia in patients with primary human immunodeficiency virus type 1 infection. *N. Engl. J. Med.* **324:**961–964.

De Groot, A. S., H. Sbai, J. Frost, and C. Saint-Aubin. 2001. Designing HIV-1 vaccines to reflect viral diversity and the global context of HIV/AIDS. *Science* **1:**1–16.

Dern, K., H. Rubsamen-Waigmann, and R. E. Unger. 2001. Inhibition of HIV-1 replication by simultaneous infection of PBLs with HIV-1 and HIV-2. *AIDS Res. Hum. Retrovir.* **17:**295–309.

DeStefano, J. J., L. M. Mallaber, L. Rodriguez, P. J. Fay, and R. A. Bambara. 1992. Requirements for strand transfer between internal regions of heteropolymer templates by human immunodeficiency virus reverse transcriptase. *J. Virol.* **66:**6370–6380.

Dilley, J. W., S. Schwarcz, L. Loeb, L. Hsu, K. Nelson, and S. Scheer. 2005. The decline of incident cases of HIV-associated neurological disorders in San Francisco, 1991-2003. *AIDS* **19:**634–635.

Dore, G. J., P. K. Correll, Y. Li, J. M. Kaldor, D. A. Cooper, and B. J. Brew. 1999. Changes to AIDS dementia complex in the era of highly active antiretroviral therapy. *AIDS* **13:**1249–1253.

Dore, G. J., A. McDonald, Y. Li, J. M. Kaldor, and B. J. Brew. 2003. Marked improvement in survival following AIDS dementia complex in the era of highly active antiretroviral therapy. *AIDS* **17:**1539–1545.

Dunfee, R., E. R. Thomas, P. R. Gorry, J. Wang, J. Taylor, K. Kunstman, S. M. Wolinsky, and D. Gabuzda. 2006a. The HIV env variant N283 enhances macrophage tropism and is associated with brain infection and dementia. *Proc. Natl. Acad. Sci. USA* **103:**15160–15165.

Dunfee, R., E. R. Thomas, P. R. Gorry, J. Wang, P. Ancuta, and D. Gabuzda. 2006b. Mechanisms of HIV-1 neurotropism. *Curr. HIV Res.* **4:**267–278.

Du Pasquier, R., M. Kuroda, Y. Zheng, J. Jean-Jacques, N. Letvin, and I. Koralnik. 2004. A prospective study demonstrates an association between JC virus-specific cytotoxic T lymphocytes and the early control of progressive multifocal leukoencephalopathy. *Brain* **127:**1970–1978.

Edlin, B. R., K. L. Irwin, S. Faruque, C. B. McCoy, C. Word, Y. Serrano, J. A. Inciardi, B. P. Bowser, R. F. Schilling, and S. D. Holmberg. 1994. Intersecting epidemics--crack cocaine use and HIV infection among inner-city young adults. *N. Engl. J. Med.* **331:**1422–1427.

Eisen, L. N., T. M. Field, E. S. Bandstra, J. P. Roberts, C. Morrow, S. K. Larson, and B. M. Steele. 1991. Perinatal cocaine effects on neonatal stress behavior and performance on the Brazelton Scale. *Pediatrics* **88:**477–480.

Erdmann, N., Y. Huang, and J. Zheng. 2006. The relevance of chemokines and cytokines to the pathogenesis of HIV-1 associated dementia, p. 41–80. *In* A. Minagar and P. Shapshak (ed.), *Neuro-AIDS.* Nova Biomedical Books, New York, NY.

Essex, M. E. 1997. Origin of AIDS, p. 3–14. *In* V. T. de Vita, Jr., S. Hellman, and S. A. Rosenberg (ed.), *AIDS: Biology, Diagnosis, Treatment, and Prevention,* 4th ed. Lippincott-Raven Publishers, Philadelphia, PA.

Esteves, A., J. Piedade, C. Santos, T. Venenno, W. F. Canas-Ferreira, and R. Parreira. 2001. Follow-up study of intra-host HIV-2 variability reveals discontinuous evolution of C2V3 sequences. *AIDS Res. Hum. Retrovir.* **17:**253–256.

Fellay, J., K. V. Shianna, D. Ge, S. Colombo, B. Ledergerber, M. Weale, K. Zhang, C. Gumbs, et al. 19 July 2007, posting date. Identification of major determinants of the host control of HIV-1 through a whole-genome association study. *Science Express* doi:10.1126/science.1143767.

Fernandez, F., and P. Ruiz (ed.). 2006. *Psychiatric Aspects of HIV/AIDS,* p. 69–146. Lippincott Williams & Wilkins, Philadelphia, PA.

Ferrando, S. J., and C. G. Lyketsos. 2006. Psychiatric comorbidities in medically ill patients with HIV/AIDS, p. 198–211. *In* F. Fernandez and P. Ruiz (ed.), *Psychiatric Aspects of HIV/AIDS.* Lippincott Williams & Wilkins, Philadelphia, PA.

Finzi, D., J. Bankson, J. D. Siliciano, J. B. Margolick, K. Chadwisk, and T. Pierson. 1999. Latent infection of CD41 T cells provides a mechanism for lifelong persistence of HIV-1, even in patients on effective combination therapy. *Nat. Med.* **5:**512–517.

Forton, D. M., S. D. Taylor-Robinson, and H. C. Thomas. 2003. Cerebral dysfunction in chronic hepatitis C infection. *J. Viral Hepatol.* **10:**81–86.

Frost, S. D., S. J. Little, S. L. Pond, C. Chappey, Y. Liu, T. Wrin, C. J. Petropoulos, and D. D. Richman. 2005. Characterization of HIV-1 envelope variation and neutralizing antibody responses during transmission of HIV-1 subtype B. *J. Virol.* **79:**6523–6527.

Fujimura, R. K. 2006. Viral load on HIV-1 associated dementia: neuropathology and drug efficacy, p. 101–119. *In* A. Minagar and P. Shapshak (ed.), *Neuro-AIDS.* Nova Biomedical Books, New York, NY.

Fujimura, R. K., K. Goodkin, C. Petito, R. Douyon, D. Feaster, M. Concha, and P. Shapshak. 1997a. HIV-1 proviral DNA load across neuroanatomic regions of individuals with evidence for HIV-1-associated dementia. *J. Acquir. Immune Defic. Syndr. Hum. Retrovirol.* **16:**146–152.

Fujimura, R. K., I. Khamis, P. Shapshak, and K. Goodkin. 2005. Regional quantitative comparison of multispliced to unspliced ratios of HIV-1 RNA copy number in infected human brain. *J. Neuro-AIDS* **2:**45–60.

Fujimura, R. K., P. Shapshak, D. Feaster, M. Epler, and K. Goodkin. 1997b. A rapid method for comparative quantitative PCR of HIV-1 proviral DNA extracted from cryopreserved brain tissues. *J. Virol. Methods* **67:**177–187.

Garcia, J. V., and A. D. Miller. 1991. Serine phosphorylation-independent downregulation of cell-surface CD4 by nef. *Nature* **350:**508–511.

Gartner, S. 2000. HIV infection and dementia. *Science* **287:**602–604.

Gartner, S. 2006. Mechanism of HIV entry into the CNS, p. 15–40. *In* A. Minagar and P. Shapshak (ed.), *Neuro-AIDS.* Nova Biomedical Books, New York, NY.

Gaschen, B., J. Taylor, K. Yusim, B. Foley, F. Gao, D. Lang, V. Novitsky, B. Haynes, B. H. Hahn, T. Bhattacharya, and B. Korber. 2002. Diversity considerations in HIV-1 vaccine selection. *Science* **296:**2354–2360.

Gendelman, H. E. 2002. Neural immunity: friend or foe? *J. Neurovirol.* **8:**474–479.

Gilbert, M. T. P., A. Rambaut, G. Wlasiuk, T. J. Spira, A. E. Pitchenik, and M. Worobey. 2007. The emergence of HIV/AIDS in the Americas and beyond. *Proc. Natl. Acad. Sci. USA.* http://www.pnas.org/cgi/reprint/0705329104v2.

Gilizia, R. J., J. A. Levy, and D. E. Mosier. 1996. The envelope gp120 gene of human immunodeficiency virus type 1 determines the rate of cd4-positive t-cell depletion in scid mice engrafted with human peripheral blood leukocytes. *J. Virol.* **70:**4184–4187.

Glass, J. D., H. Fedor, S. L. Wesselingh, and J. C. McArthur. 1995. Immunocytochemical quantitation of human immunodeficiency virus in the brain: correlations with dementia. *Ann. Neurol.* **38:**755–762.

Gonzalez, E., H. Kulkarni, H. Bolivar, A. Mangano, R. Sanchez, G. Catano, et al. 2005. The influence of CCL3L1 gene-containing segmental duplications on HIV-1/AIDS susceptibility. *Science* **307:**1434–1439.

Goodkin, K. 2006. Virology, immunology, transmission, and disease stage, p. 11–22. *In* F. Fernandez and P. Ruiz (ed.), *Psychiatric Aspects of HIV/AIDS.* Lippincott Williams & Wilkins, Philadelphia, PA.

Goudsmit, J., C. Debouck, and R. H. Moloen. 1988. Human immunodeficiency virus type 1 neutralization epitope with conserved architecture elicits early type-specific antibodies in experimentally infected chimpanzees. *Proc. Natl. Acad. Sci. USA* **85:**4478–4482.

Goulder, P. J., R. E. Phillips, and R. A. Colbert. 1997. Late escape from an immunodominant cytotoxic T-lymphocyte response associated with progression to AIDS. *Nat. Med.* **3:**212–217.

Graham, B. S. 2002. Clinical trials of HIV vaccines. *Annu. Rev. Med.* **53:**207–221.

Gray, F., F. Chretien, A. V. Vallat-Decouvelaere, and F. Scaravilli. 2003. The changing pattern of HIV neuropathology in the HAART era. *J. Neuropathol. Exp. Neurol.* **62:**429–440.

Greenough, T. C., D. B. Brettler, M. Somasundaran, D. L. Panicali, and J. L. Sullivan. 1997. Human immunodeficiency virus type 1-specific cytotoxic T lymphocytes (CTL), virus load, and CD4 T cell loss: evidence supporting a protective role for CTIL in vivo. *J. Infect. Dis.* **176:**118–125.

Grez, N., U. Dietrich, P. Balfe, H. von Briesen, J. K. Maniar, G. Mhambre, E. L. Delwar, J. I. Mullins, and H. Rubsamen-Waigmann. 1994. Genetic analysis of HIV1 and HIV-2 mixed infections in India reveals a recent spread of HIV-1 and HIV-2 from a single ancestor for each of these viruses. *J. Virol.* **68:**2161–2168.

Gunthard, H., S. Frost, A. Leigh-Brown, C. Ignacio, K. Kee, A. Perelson, C. Spina, D. Havlir, M. Hezareh, D. Looney, D. Richman, and J. Wong. 1999. Evolution of envelope sequences of human immunodeficiency virus type 1 in cellular reservoirs in the setting of potent antiviral therapy. *J. Virol.* **73:**9404–9412.

Herbeck, J. T., D. C. Nickle, G. H. Learn, G. S. Gottlieb, M. E. Curlin, L. Heath, and J. I. Mullins. 2006. HIV-1 env evolves towards ancestral states upon transmission to a new host. *J. Virol.* **80:**1637–1644.

Hizi, A., A. S. Kamath-Loeb, K. D. Rose, and L. A. Loeb. 1997. Mutagenesis by human immunodeficiency virus reverse transcriptase: incorporation of O6-methyldeoxyguanosine triphosphate. *Mutat. Res.* **374:**41–50.

Hoxie, J. A., J. D. Alpers, and J. L. Rackowski. 1986. Alterations in T4 (CD4) protein and mRNA synthesis in cells infected with HIV. *Science* **234:**1123–1127.

Hu, W. S., T. Rhodes, T. Q. Dang, and V. Pathak. 2003. Retroviral recombination: review of genetic analyses. *Front. Biosci.* **8:**D143–D155.

Hudson, R. R., M. Slatkin, and W. P. Maddison. 1992. Estimation of levels of gene flow from DNA sequence data. *Genetics* **132:**583–589.

Jurado, A., P. Rahimi-Moghaddam, S. Bar-Jurado, J. S. Richardson, M. Jurado, and A. Shuaib. 1999. Genetic markers on HIV-1 gp120 C2-V3 region associated with the expression or absence of cognitive motor complex in HIV/AIDS. *J. NeuroAIDS* **2:**15–28.

Kageyama, S., J. K. Maniar, M. Iwasaki, J. Zhang, D. G. Saple, H. Tsuchie, A. Tanabe-Tochikura, K. Taniguchi, K. Shiraki, and T. Kurimura. 2000. Seronegative HIV-2 carriers in India. *Int. J. STD AIDS* **11:**31–37.

Kannangai, R., S. Ramalingam, R. C. Castillo, P. G. Babu, T. J. John, G. Sridharan, and D. H. Schwartz. 1999. HIV-2 status in Southern India. *Trans. R. Soc. Trop. Med. Hyg.* **93:**30–31.

King, J. E., E. A. Eugenin, C. M. Buckner, and J. W. Berman. 2006. HIV tat and neurotoxicity. *Microbes Infect.* **8:**1347–1357.

Kong, L. I., S. W. Lee, J. C. Kappes, J. S. Parkin, D. Decker, J. A. Hoxie, B. H. Hahn, and G. M. Shaw. 1988. West African HIV-2-related human retrovirus with attenuated cytopathicity. *Science* **240:**1525–1529.

Kopnisky, K. L., J. Bao, and Y. W. Lin. 2007. Neurobiology of HIV, psychiatric and substance abuse comorbidity research: workshop report. *Brain Behav. Immun.* **21:**428–441.

Korber, B., M. Muldoon, J. Theiler, F. Gao, R. Gupta, A. Lapedes, B. H. Hahn, S. Wolinsky, and T. Bhattacharya. 2000. Timing the ancestor of the HIV-1 pandemic strains. *Science* **288:**1789–1796.

Korber, B. T. M., K. J. Kunstman, B. K. Patterson, M. Furtado, M. M. McEvilly, R. Levy, and S. M. Wolinsky. 1994. Genetic differences between blood- and brain-derived viral sequences from HIV-1 infected patients: evidence of conserved elements in the V3 region of the env protein of brain-derived sequences. *J. Virol.* **68:**7467–7481.

Korber, B. T. M., G. Learn, J. I. Mullins, B. H. Hahn, and S. Wolinsky. 1995. Protecting HIV sequence databases. *Nature* (London) **378:**242–243.

Kosakovsky Pond, S. L., D. Posada, M. B. Gravenor, C. H. Woelk, and S. D. W. Frost. 2006. Automated phylogenetic detection of recombination using a genetic algorithm. *Mol. Biol. Evol.* **23:**1891–1901.

Koup, R., J. Safrit, and Y. Cao. 1994. Temporal association of cellular immune responses with the initial control of viremia in primary human immunodeficiency virus type 1 syndrome. *J. Virol.* **68:**4650–4655.

Kulkarni, S. S., S. Tripathy, R. S. Paranjape, N. S. Mani, D. R. Joshi, U. Patil, and D. A. Gadkari. 1999. Isolation and preliminary characterization of two HIV-2 strains from Pune, India. *Indian J. Med. Res.* **109:**123–130.

Kumar, A. M., I. Borodowsky, B. J. Fernandez, L. Gonzalez, and M. Kumar. 2007. Human immunodeficiency virus type 1 RNA levels in different regions of human brain: quantification using real-time reverse transcriptase–polymerase chain reaction. *J. Neurovirol.* **13:**210–224.

Kuroda, M. J., J. E. Schmitz, W. A. Charini, C. E. Nickerson, M. A. Lifton, C. I. Lord, M. A. Forman, and N. L. Letvin. 1999. Emergence of CTL coincides with clearance of virus during primary simian immunodeficiency virus infection in rhesus monkeys. *J. Immunol.* **162:**5127–5133.

Kurosu, T., T. Mukai, W. Auwanit, P. I. N. Ayuthaya, S. Saeng-Aroon, and K. Ikuta. 2001. Variable sequences in the LTR and its downstream region of some of HIV-1 CRF01_AE recently distributing among Thai carriers. *AIDS Res. Hum. Retrovir.* **17:**863–866.

Langford, T. D., A. Adame, A. Grigorian, I. Grant, J. A. McCutchan, R. J. Ellis, T. D. Marcotte, and E. Masliah. 2003. Changing patterns in the neuropathogenesis of HIV during the HAART era. *Brain Pathol.* **13:**195–210.

Learn, G. H., Jr., B. T. M. Korber, B. Foley, B. H. Hahn, S. M. Wolinsky, and J. I. Mullins. 1996. Maintaining the integrity of human immunodeficiency virus sequence databases. *J. Virol.* **70:**5720–5730.

Letendre, S., A. D. Paulino, E. Rockenstein, A. Adame, L. Crews, M. Cherner, R. Heaton, R. Ellis, I. P. Everall, I. Grant, and E. Masliah. 2007. Pathogenesis of hepatitis C virus coinfection in the brains of patients infected with HIV. *J. Infect. Dis.* **196:**361–370.

Levine, A. J., E. J. Singer, and P. Shapshak. 9 February 2008. The role of host genetics in the susceptibility for HIV-1-associated neurocognitive disorders. *AIDS Behav.* [Epub ahead of print.] doi: 10.1007/s 10461-008-3254.

Lima, M., R. Katz-Brull, R. Lenkinski, R. Nunez, D. Feinrider, and I. Koralnik. 2007. Remission of progressive multifocal leukoencephalopathy and primary central nervous system lymphoma in an HIV-infected patient. *Eur. J. Neurol.* **14:**598–602.

Liu, L., B. Su, and K. Zhuang. 2005. Genetic characterization of full-length HIV-1 genomes from 3 infected paid blood donors in Henan, China. *J. Acquir. Immune Defic. Syndr.* **40:**501–502.

Liu, Z. Q., C. Wood, J. A. Levy, and C. Cheng-Mayer. 1990. The viral envelope gene is involved in macrophage tropism of a human immunodeficiency virus type 1 strain isolated from brain tissue. *J. Virol.* **64:**6148–6153.

Lopalco, L. 2004. Humoral immunity in HIV-1 exposure: cause or effect of HIV resistance? *Curr. HIV Res.* **2:**127–139.

Luo, G., and J. Taylor. 1990. Template switching by reverse transcriptase during DNA synthesis. *J. Virol.* **64:**4321–4328.

Mahadevan, A., S. Shankar, P. Satishchandra, U. Ranga, Y. Chickabasaviah, V. Santosh, R. Vasanthapuram, C. Pardo, A. Nath, and M. Zink. 2007. Characterization of human immunodeficiency virus (HIV)-infected cells in infiltrates associated with CNS opportunistic infections in patients with HIV clade C infection. *J. Neuropathol. Exp. Neurol.* **66:**799–808.

Masliah, E., R. M. DeTeresa, M. E. Mallory, and L. A. Hansen. 2000. Changes in pathological findings at autopsy in AIDS cases for the last 15 years. *AIDS* **14:**69–74.

Masliah, E., R. K. Heaton, T. D. Marcotte, R. J. Ellis, C. A. Wiley, M. Mallory, C. L. Achim, J. A. McCutchan, J. A. Nelson, J. H. Atkinson, and I. Grant. 1997. Dendritic injury is a pathological substrate for human immunodeficiency virus-related cognitive disorders. *Ann. Neurol.* **42:**963–972.

Masliah, E., E. S. Roberts, D. Langford, I. Everall, L. Crews, A. Adame, E. Rockenstein, and H. S. Fox. 2004. Patterns of gene dysregulation in the frontal cortex of patients with HIV encephalitis. *J. Neuroimmunol.* **157:**163–175.

McArthur, J. C. 2004. HIV dementia: an evolving disease. *J. Neuroimmunol.* **157:**3–10.

McArthur, J. C., M. P. McDermott, D. McClernon, C. St Hillaire, K. Conant, K. Marder, G. Schifitto, O. A. Selnes, N. Sacktor, Y. Stern, S. M. Albert, K. Kieburtz, J. A. deMarcaida, B. Cohen, and L. G. Epstein. 2004. Attenuated central nervous system infection in advanced HIV/AIDS with combination antiretroviral therapy. *Arch. Neurol.* **61:**1687–1696.

McCoy, C. B., and E. L. Khoury. 1990. Drug use and the risk of AIDS. *Am. Behav. Sci.* **33:**419–431.

McCoy, C. B., P. Shapshak, J. E. Rivers, H. V. McCoy, N. L. Weatherby, D. D. Chitwood, S. M. Shah, J. A. Inciardi, D. C. McBride, and J. K. Watters. 1994. The risks of injection practices and compliance to risk reduction protocols in the prevention of HIV-1 among injecting drug users. *J. Acquir. Immune Defic. Syndr.* **7:**773–776.

McCutchan, F. E. 1999. Global diversity in human immunodeficiency viruses, p. 41–101. *In* K. A. Crandall (ed.), *The Evolution of HIV.* Johns Hopkins University Press, Baltimore, MD.

Mellgran, A., R. W. Price, L. Hagberg, L. Rosengren, B. J. Brew, and M. Gisslen. 2007. Antiretroviral treatment reduces increased CSF neurofilament protein (NFL) in HIV-1 infection. *Neurology* **69:**1536–1541.

Minagar, A., D. Commins, J. S. Alexander, R. Hoque, F. Chiappelli, E. J. Singer, B. Nikbin, and P. Shapshak. 2008. NeuroAIDS: characteristics and diagnosis of the neurological complications of AIDS. **12:**25–43.

Minagar, A., and P. Shapshak. 2006. HIV-associated dementia: clinical features and pathogenesis, p. 1–14. *In* A. Minagar and P. Shapshak (ed.), *Neuro-AIDS.* Nova Biomedical Books, New York, NY.

Minagar, A., P. Shapshak, E. M. Duran, A. S. Kablinger, J. A. Alexander, R. E. Kelley, R. Seth, and T. Kazic. 2004. Gene expression in HIV-associated dementia, Alzheimer's disease, multiple sclerosis, and schizophrenia. *J. Neurosci. Res.* **224:**3–17.

Minagar, A., P. Shapshak, R. Fujimura, R. Ownby, M. Heyes, and C. Eisdorfer. 2002. The role of macrophage/microglia and astrocytes in the pathogenesis of three neurologic disorders: HIV-associated dementia, Alzheimer disease, and multiple sclerosis. *J. Neurol. Sci.* **202:**13–23.

Moore, J. P., Y. Cao, D. D. Ho, and R. A. Koup. 1994. Development of the anti-gp120 antibody response during seroconversion to human immunodeficiency virus type 1. *J. Virol.* **68:**5142–5155.

Morgello, S., R. Mahboob, T. Yakoushina, S. Khan, and K. Hague. 2002. Autopsy finding in a HIV-infected population over 2 decades. *Arch. Pathol. Lab. Med.* **126:**182–190.

Musey, L., J. Hughes, and T. Schacker. 1997. Cytotoxic-T-cell responses, viral load, and disease progression in early human immunodeficiency virus type 1 infection. *N. Engl. J. Med.* **337:**1267–1274.

Nath, A., N. J. Haughey, M. Jones, J. E. Anderson, C. Bell, and J. D. Geiger. 2000. Synergistic neurotoxicity by HIV proteins tat and gp120: protection by memantine. *Ann. Neurol.* **7:**186–194.

Nath, A., K. F. Hauser, M. Prendergast, and J. Berger. 2006. Drug abuse and neuro-AIDS, p. 81–100. *In* A. Minagar and P. Shapshak (ed.), *Neuro-AIDS.* Nova Biomedical Books, New York, NY.

Navia, B. A., E. S. Cho, C. K. Petito, and R. W. Price. 1986a. The AIDS dementia complex. II. Neuropathology. *Ann. Neurol.* **19:**525–535.

Navia, B. A., B. D. Jordan, and R. W. Price. 1986b. The AIDS dementia complex. I. Clinical features. *Ann. Neurol.* **19:**517–524.

Negroni, M., and H. Buc. 2001. Mechanisms of retroviral recombination. *Annu. Rev. Genet.* **35:**275–302.

Nickle, D. C., M. A. Jensen, G. S. Gottlieb, D. Shriner, G. H. Learn, A. G. Rodrigo, and J. I. Mullins. 2003a. Consensus and ancestral state HIV vaccines. *Science* **299:**1515–1518.

Nickle, D. C., M. A. Jensen, D. Shriner, et al. 2003b. Evolutionary indicators of human immunodeficiency virus type 1 reservoirs and compartments. *J. Virol.* **77:**5540–5546.

Nickle, D. C., D. Shriner, J. E. Mittler, L. M. Frenkel, and J. I. Mullins. 2003c. Importance and detection of virus reservoirs and compartments of HIV infection 1. *Curr. Opin. Microbiol.* **6:**410–416.

Nkengasong, J. N., C. Bile, M. Kalou, C. Maurice, E. Boateng, M. Sassan-Morokro, M. Rayfield, D. Coulibaly, A. E. Greenberg, and S. Z. Wiktor. 1999. Quantification of RNA in HIV type 1 subtypes D and G by NucliSens and Amplicor assays in Abidjan, Ivory Coast. *AIDS Res. Hum. Retrovir.* **15:**495–498.

Nuttall, J. J., J. M. Wilmshurst, A. P. Ndondo, J. Yeats, C. Corcoran, G. D. Hussey, and B. S. Eley. 2004. Progressive multifocal leukoencephalopathy after initiation of highly active antiretroviral therapy in a child with advanced human immunodeficiency virus infection: a case of immune reconstitution inflammatory syndrome. *Pediatr. Infect. Dis. J.* **23**:683–685.

Ogg, G. S., X. Jin, S. Bonhoeffer, P. R. Dunbar, M. A. Nowak, and S. Monard. 1998. Quantitation of HIV-1-specific cytotoxic T lymphocytes and plasma load of viral RNA. *Science* **279**:2103–2106.

Ohagen, A., A. Devitt, K. J. Kunstman, P. R. Gorry, P. P. Rose, B. Korber, J. Taylor, R. Levy, R. L. Murphy, S. M. Wolinsky, and D. Gabuzda. 2003. Genetic and functional analysis of full-length HIV-1 env genes derived from brain and blood of patients with AIDS. *J. Virol.* **77**:12336–12345.

Palker, T. J., M. E. Clark, A. J. Langlois, T. J. Matthews, K. J. Weinhold, R. R. Randall, D. P. Bolognesi, and B. F. Haynes. 1988. Type-specific neutralization of the human immunodeficiency virus with antibodies to env-encoded synthetic peptides. *Proc. Natl. Acad. Sci. USA* **85**:1932–1936.

Pantaleo, G., J. F. Demarest, H. Soudeyns, C. Graziosi, F. Denis, J. W. Adelsberger, P. Borrow, M. S. Saag, G. M. Shaw, and R. P. Sekaly. 1994. Major expansion of CD81 T cells with a predominant V beta usage during the primary immune response to HIV. *Nature* **370**:463–467.

Pasquier, C., K. Sandres, G. Salama, J. Puel, and J. Izopet. 1999. Using RT-PCR and bDNA assays to measure non-clade B HIV-1 subtype RNA. *J. Virol. Methods* **81**:123–129.

Peeters, M., and P. M. Sharp. 2000. Genetic diversity of HIV-1: the moving target. *AIDS* **14**:129–140.

Perelson, A. S., A. U. Neumann, M. Markowitz, J. M. Leonard, and D. D. Ho. 1996. HIV-1 dynamics in vivo: virion clearance rate, infected cell life-span, and viral generation time. *Science* **271**:1582–1586.

Petito, C. K., E. S. Cho, W. Lemann, B. A. Navia, and R. W. Price. 1986. Neuropathology of acquired immunodeficiency syndrome (AIDS): an autopsy review. *J. Neuropathol. Exp. Neurol.* **45**:635–646.

Pillai, S. K., S. L. Pond, Y. Liu, B. M. Good, M. C. Strain, R. J. Ellis, S. Letendre, D. M. Smith, H. F. Günthard, I. Grant, T. D. Marcotte, J. A. McCutchan, D. D. Richman, and J. K. Wong. 2006. Genetic attributes of cerebrospinal fluid-derived HIV-1 env. *Brain* **129**(Pt. 7):1872–1883.

Poluektova, L. Y., D. H. Munn, Y. Persidsky, and H. E. Gendelman. 2002. Generation of CTL against virus-infected human brain macrophages in a murine model for HIV-1 encephalitis. *J. Immunol.* **168**:3941–3949.

Power, C., J. C. McArthur, A. Nath, K. Wehrly, M. Mayne, J. Nishio, T. Langelier, R. T. Johnson, and B. Chesebro. 1998. Neuronal death induced by brain-derived HIV-1 env genes differs between demented and nondemented AIDS patients. *J. Virol.* **72**:9045–9053.

Power, C., J. C. McArthur, R. T. Johnson, D. E. Griffin, J. D. Glass, S. Perryman, and B. Chesebro. 1994. Demented and non-demented patients with aids differ in brain-derived human immunodeficiency virus type 1 envelope sequences. *J. Virol.* **68**:4643–4649.

Ranga, U., R. Shankarappa, N. B. Siddappa, L. Ramakrishna, R. Nagendran, et al. 2004. Tat protein of HIV-1 subtype C strains is a defective chemokine. *J. Virol.* **78**:2586–2590.

Resnick, L., J. R. Berger, P. Shapshak, and W. W. Tourtellotte. 1988. Early penetration of the blood-brain-barrier by HTLV-III/LAV. *Neurology* **38**:9–15.

Roberts, E. S., M. A. Zandonatti, D. D. Watry, L. J. Madden, S. J. Henriksen, M. A. Taffe, and H. S. Fox. 2003. Induction of pathogenic sets of genes in macrophages and neurons in NeuroAIDS. *Am. J. Pathol.* **162**:2041–2057.

Roberts, J. D., B. D. Preston, L. A. Johnston, A. Soni, L. A. Loeb, and T. A. Kunkel. 1989. Fidelity of two retroviral reverse transcriptases during DNA-dependent DNA synthesis in vitro. *Mol. Cell. Biol.* **9**:469–476.

Robertson, K. R., M. Smurzynski, T. D. Parsons, K. Wu, R. J. Bosch, J. Wu, J. C. McArthur, A. C. Collier, S. R.

Evans, and R. J. Ellis. 2007. The prevalence and incidence of neurocognitive impairment in the HAART era. *AIDS* **21**:1915–1921.

Sacktor, N., M. P. McDermott, K. Marder, G. Schifitto, O. A. Selnes, J. C. McArthur, Y. Stern, S. Albert, D. Palumbo, K. Kieburtz, J. A. De Marcaida, B. Cohen, and L. Epstein. 2002. HIV-associated cognitive impairment before and after the advent of combination therapy. *J. Neurovirol.* **8**:136–142.

Salemi, M., S. L. Lamers, S. Yu, T. de Oliveira, W. M. Fitch, and M. S. McGrath. 2005. Phylodynamic analysis of human immunodeficiency virus type 1 in distinct brain compartments provides a model for the neuropathogenesis of AIDS. *J. Virol.* **79**:11343–11352.

Sankale, J. L., R. S. de la Tour, and B. Renjifo. 1995. Intrapatient variability of HIV-2 envelope V3 loop. *AIDS Res. Hum. Retrovir.* **11**:617–623.

Sarr, A. D., J. L. Sankale, D. L. Hamel, K. U. Travers, A. Gueye-Ndiaye, M. Essex, S. Mboup, and P. J. Kanki. 2000. Interaction with HIV-2 predicts HIV-1 genotypes. *Virology* **268**:402–410.

Schultz, A. M., and J. A. Bradac. 2001. The HIV vaccine pipeline, from preclinical to phase III. *AIDS* **5**:147–158.

Sei, Y., P. H. Tsang, F. N. Chu, I. Wallace, J. P. Roboz, P. S. Sarin, and J. G. Bekesi. 1989. Inverse relationship between HIV-1 p24 antigenemia, anti-p24 antibody and neutralizing antibody response in all stages of HIV-1 infection. *Immunol. Lett.* **20**:223–230.

Sewell, A. K., D. A. Price, A. Oxenius, A. D. Kelleher, and R. E. Phillips. 2000. Cytotoxic T lymphocyte responses to human immunodeficiency virus: control and escape. *Stem Cells* **18**:230–244.

Shah, S. M., P. Shapshak, J. E. Rivers, N. L. Weatherby, K. Q. Xin, R. V. Stewart, D. D. Chitwood, B. Page, D. C. Mash, D. Vlahov, and C. B. McCoy. 1996. Detection of HIV-1 DNA in needle/syringes, paraphernalia, and washes from shooting galleries in Miami: preliminary laboratory results. *J. Acquir. Immune Defic. Syndr.* **11**:301–306.

Shapshak, P., M. Alireza, M. Duran, F. Ziegler, W. Davis, R. Seth, and T. Kazic. 2005a. Gene expression in HIV associated dementia, p. 305–318. *In* A. Minagar and J. S. Alexander (ed.), *Inflammatory Disorders of the Nervous System, Clinical Aspects, Pathogenesis, and Management.* Humana Press, Totowa, NJ.

Shapshak, P., K. A. Crandall, K. Goodkin, et al. 1996. HIV-1. Neuropathogenesis and abused drugs. Current views: problems and solutions. *Adv. Exp. Med. Biol.* **23**:171–186.

Shapshak, P., R. Duncan, C. B. McCoy, and J. B. Page. 2005b. Real time reverse transcriptase PCR method for quantification of HIV gag RNA. *Front. Biosci.* **10**:135–142.

Shapshak, P., R. Duncan, A. Nath, J. Turchan, P. Kangueane, S. Shapshak, H. Rodriguez, E. M. Duran, F. Ziegler, E. Amaro, A. Lewis, A. Rodriguez, A. Minagar, W. Davis, R. Seth, F. Chiappelli, and T. Kazic. 2006. Gene chromosomal organization and expression in cultured human neurons exposed to cocaine and HIV-1 proteins gp120 and tat: drug abuse and NeuroAIDS. *Front. Biosci.* **11**:1774–1793.

Shapshak, P., R. Duncan, J. Torres-Munoz, M. Duran, A. Minagar, and C. Petito. 2004. Analytic approaches to differential gene expression in AIDS vs. control brains. *Front. Biosci.* **9**:2935–2946.

Shapshak, P., R. Duncan, J. E. Torres-Munoz, A. Minagar, and C. K. Petito. 2002. Preliminary gene expression studies in AIDS: problems and solutions. *Proceedings of the 2nd Virtual Conference on Genomics and Bioinformatics.* North Dakota State University, Fargo. http://www.ndsu.edu/virtual-genomics.

Shapshak, P., R. Fujimura, B. Page, D. Segal, J. Yang, S. Shah, G. Graham, J. Rivers, D. Chitwood, and C. McCoy. 2000. HIV-1 RNA load in needle/syringes from shooting galleries in Miami: a preliminary laboratory report. *Drug Alcohol Depend.* **58**:153–157.

Shapshak, P., C. McCoy, S. Shah, B. Page, J. Rivers, N. Weatherby, D. Chitwood, and D. Mash. 1994. Preliminary laboratory studies on inactivation of HIV-1 in needles and syringes containing infected blood using undiluted household bleach. *J. Acquir. Immune Defic. Syndr.* **7:**754–759.

Shapshak, P., I. Nagano, K. Q. Xin, W. Bradley, et al. 1995. HIV-1 heterogeneity and cytokines: neuropathogenesis. *Adv. Exp. Med. Biol.* **373:**225–238.

Shapshak, P., D. Segal, K. Crandall, R. Fujimura, B. Zhang, K. Xin, K. Okuda, C. Petito, C. Eisdorfer, and K. Goodkin. 1999. Independent evolution of HIV-1 in different brain regions. *AIDS Res. Hum. Retrovir.* **15:**811–820.

Shapshak, P., and R. Stengel. 2002. Discovering brain mechanisms and the rules of molecular biology. *6th World Multiconference on Systemics, Cybernetics and Informatics,* Orlando, FL, July 14–18. http://www.iiis.org/sci2002/.

Shapshak, P., J. Torres-Munos, and C. Petito. 2001. Bioinformatics in neurodegenerative diseases. *Proceedings of Virtual Conference on Genomics and Bioinformatics.* North Dakota State University, Fargo. http://www.ndsu/virtual-genomics.

Shioda, T., J. A. Levy, and C. Cheng-Mayer. 1992. Small amino acid changes in the V3 hypervariable region of gp120 can affect the T-cell-line and macrophage tropism of human immunodeficiency virus type 1. *Proc. Natl. Acad. Sci. USA* **89:**9434–9438.

Singer, E. J., K. Syndulko, P. Shapshak, L. Resnick, and W. W. Tourtellotte. 1994. Cerebrospinal fluid p24 antigen levels and intrathecal immunoglobulin G synthesis are associated with cognitive disease severity in HIV-1. *AIDS* **8:**197–204.

Singh, S., S. N. Dwivedi, R. Sood, and J. P. Wali. 2000. Hepatitis B, C, and HIV infections in multiply-injected Kala-azar patients in Delhi. *Scand. J. Infect. Dis.* **32:**3–6.

Smit, T. K., B. J. Brew, W. W. Tourtellotte, S. Morgello, B. B. Gelman, and N. K. Saksena. 2004. Independent evolution of HIV drug resistance mutations in diverse areas of the brain in HIV-infected patients, with and without dementia, on antiretroviral treatment. *J. Virol.* **78:**100133–100148.

Smith, K. A. 2005. The continuing HIV vaccine saga: naked emperors alongside fairy godmothers. *Med. Immun.* **4:**1–5.

Snider, W. D., D. M. Simpson, S. Nielsen, J. Gold, C. Metroka, and J. Posner. 1983. Neurological complications of acquired immune deficiency syndrome: analysis of 50 patients. *Ann. Neurol.* **14:**403–418.

Solomon, S., N. Kumarasamy, A. K. Ganesh, and R. E. Amalraj. 1998. Prevalence and risk factors of HIV-1 and HIV-2 infection in urban and rural areas in Tamil Nadu, India. *Int. J. STD AIDS* **9:**98–103.

Strain, M. C., S. Letendre, S. K. Pillai, T. Russell, C. C. Ignacio, H. F. Günthard, B. Good, D. M. Smith, S. M. Wolinsky, M. Furtado, J. Marquie-Beck, J. Durelle, I. Grant, D. D. Richman, T. Marcotte, J. A. McCutchan, R. J. Ellis, and J. K. Wong. 2005. Genetic composition of human immunodeficiency virus type 1 in cerebrospinal fluid and blood without treatment and during failing antiretroviral therapy. *J. Virol.* **79:**1772–1788.

Torre, D., F. Speranza, and R. Martegani. 2005. Impact of highly active antiretroviral therapy on organ-specific manifestations of HIV-1 infection. *HIV Med.* **6:**66–78.

Tozzi, V., P. Balestra, P. Lorenzini, R. Bellagamba, S. Galgani, A. Corpolongo, C. Vlassi, D. Larussa, M. Zaccarelli, P. Noto, U. Visco-Comandini, M. Giulianelli, G. Ippolito, A. Antinori, and P. Narciso. 2005a. Prevalence and risk factors for human immunodeficiency virus-associated neurocognitive impairment, 1996 to 2002: results from an urban observational cohort. *J. Neurovirol.* **11:**265–273.

Tozzi, V., P. Balestra, D. Serraino, R. Bellagamba, A. Corpolongo, P. Piselli, P. Lorenzini, U. Visco-Comandini, C. Vlassi, M. E. Quartuccio, M. Giulianelli, P. Noto, S. Galgani, G. Ippolito, A. Antinori, and P. Narciso. 2005b. Neurocognitive impairment and survival in a cohort of HIV-infected patients treated with HAART. *AIDS Res. Hum. Retrovir.* **21:**706–713.

Triques, K., J. Coste, J. L. Perret, T. Segarra, E. Mpoudi, J. Reynes, E. Delaporte, A. Butcher, K. Dreyer, S. Herman, J. Spadoro, and M. Peeters. 1999. Efficiencies of four versions of the amplicor HIV-1 monitor test for quantification of different subtypes of human immunodeficiency virus type 1. *J. Clin. Microbiol.* **37:**110–116.

Vahey, M. T., M. E. Nau, M. Taubman, J. Yalley-Ogunro, P. Silvera, and M. G. Lewis. 2003. Patterns of gene expression in PBMNCs of Rhesus macaques infected with SIVmac251 and exhibiting differential rates of disease progression. *AIDS Res. Hum. Retrovir.* **19:**369–387.

Vallat-Decouvelaere, A. V., F. Chretien, G. Lorin de la Grandmaison, R. Carlier, G. Force, and F. Gray. 2003. The neuropathology of HIV infection in the era of highly active antiretroviral therapy. *Ann. Pathol.* **23:**408–423.

van Marle, G., and C. Power. 2005. HIV-1 genetic diversity in the nervous system: evolutionary epiphenomenon or disease determinant. *J. Neurovirol.* **11:**107–128.

Vendrely, A., B. Bienvenu, J. Gasnault, J. B. Thiebault, D. Salmon, and F. Gray. 2005. Fulminant inflammatory leukoencephalopathy associated with HAART-induced immune restoration in AIDS-related progressive multifocal leukoencephalopathy. *Acta Neuropathol.* (Berlin) **109:**449–455.

Venkataramana, A., C. A. Pardo, J. C. McArthur, D. A. Kerr, D. N. Irani, J. W. Griffin, P. Burger, D. S. Reich, P. A. Calabresi, and A. Nath. 2006. Immune reconstitution inflammatory syndrome in the CNS of HIV-infected patients. *Neurology* **67:**383–388.

Wang, F. X., Y. Xu, J. Sullivan, E. Souder, E. G. Argyris, E. A. Acheampong, et al. 2005. IL-7 is a potent and proviral strain-specific inducer of latent HIV-1 cellular reservoirs of infected individuals on virally suppressive HAART. *J. Clin. Investig.* **115:**128–137.

Weber, J. N., P. R. Clapham, and R. A. Weiss. 1987. Human immunodeficiency virus infection in two cohorts of homosexual men: neutralizing sera and association of anti-gag antibody with prognosis. *Lancet* **i:**119–122.

Wiley, R. L., F. Maldarelli, M. A. Martin, and K. Strebel. 1992. Human immunodeficiency virus type 1 Vpu protein regulates the formation of intracellular gp160-CD4 complexes. *J. Virol.* **66:**226–234.

Williams, K. J., and L. A. Loeb. 1992. Retroviral reverse transcriptases: error frequencies and mutagenesis. *Curr. Top. Microbiol. Immunol.* **176:**165–180.

Wilson, J. D., G. S. Ogg, R. L. Allen, C. Davis, S. Shaunak, J. Downie, W. Dyer, C. Workman, S. Sullivan, A. J. McMichael, and S. L. Rowland-Jones. 2000. Direct visualization of HIV-1-specific cytotoxic T lymphocytes during primary infection. *AIDS* **14:**225–233.

Wolthers, K. C., S. A. Otto, S. M. Lens, R. A. Van Lier, F. Miedema, and L. Meyaard. 1997. Functional B cell abnormalities in HIV type 1 infection: role of CD40L and CD70. *AIDS Res. Hum. Retrovir.* **13:**1023–1029.

Wong, J. K., C. C. Ignacio, F. Torriani, D. Havlir, N. J. Fitch, and D. D. Richman. 1997. In vivo compartmentalization of human immunodeficiency virus: evidence from the examination of pol sequences from autopsy tissues. *J. Virol.* **71:**2059–2071.

Xin, K. Q., K. Hamajima, S. Sasaki, A. Honsho, T. Tsuji, N. Ishii, X. R. Cao, Y. Lu, P. Shapshak, and K. Okuda. 1998. Intranasal administration of HIV-1 DNA vaccine with IL-2 expression plasmid enhances cell-mediated immunity against HIV. *Immunology* **94:**438–444.

Yilmaz, A., R. W. Price, S. Spudich, D. Fuchs, L. Hagberg, and M. Gisslén. 2008. Persistent intrathecal immune activation in

HIV-1-infected individuals on antiretroviral therapy. *J. Acquir. Immune Defic. Syndr.* **47:**168–173.

Yu, X. F., W. Liu, J. Chen, W. Kong, B. Liu, Q. Zhu, F. Liang, F. McCutchan, S. Piyasirisilp, and S. Lai. 2002. Maintaining low HIV type 1 env genetic diversity among injection drug users infected with a B/C recombinant and CRF01_AE HIV type 1 in southern China. *AIDS Res. Hum. Retrovir.* **18:**167–170.

Zárate, S., S. L. Kosakovsky-Pond, P. Shapshak, and S. D. W. Frost. 2007. A comparative study of methods for detecting sequence compartmentalization in HIV-1. *J. Virol.* **81:**6643–6651.

Zhang, K., F. Rana, C. Silva, J. Ethier, K. Ehrly, B. Chesebro, and C. Power. 2003. HIV-1 envelope-mediated neuronal death: uncoupling of viral replication and neurotoxicity. *J. Virol.* **77:**6899–2003.

The Spectrum of Neuro-AIDS Disorders:
Pathophysiology, Diagnosis, and Treatment
Edited by K. Goodkin et al.
©2008 ASM Press, Washington, DC

16

Antioxidants and Brain Function in HIV/AIDS

GAIL SHOR-POSNER, ADRIANA CAMPA, MARIA-JOSE MIGUEZ-BURBANO,
GLORIA CASTILLO, AND GERALDINE MORENO-BLACK

Impaired neuroprotection, due to increased oxidative stress, has been implicated as a factor affecting neuronal degeneration in HIV/AIDS. The nervous system is protected from radical-mediated oxidative damage by a number of antioxidant defense systems. Deficiencies in micronutrients required for antioxidant defense, however, are prominent in HIV-1-seropositive individuals and likely to contribute to the impaired neuroprotection and subsequent neuronal degeneration resulting from increased oxidative stress in HIV disease. Thus, antioxidant therapies that protect the brain against toxic oxygen species may offer the potential to slow down or prevent progressive nerve cell death in HIV/AIDS. In addition to its critical role in detoxification, antioxidants may decrease HIV neuropathogenesis through regulation of specific cytokines, suppression of neuronal apoptosis, and protection against blood-brain barrier (BBB) damage. The role of biological antioxidants in maintaining adequate brain function in HIV-1 disease is reviewed in this chapter.

HIV NEUROCOGNITIVE FUNCTION IN THE ERA OF HAART

Cognitive impairment is the major neurological complication of HIV-1 infection, ranging in severity from a mild subclinical cognitive deficit to a dementing illness (HIV-1-associated dementia [HAD]). The presence of HAD has been associated with losses in the range of 20 to 50% of neurons in the frontal cortex (Ketzler et al., 1990) and characterized by deficits in attention, memory, and abstraction and severe slowing of cognitive and motor function. Higher risks have

been associated with increasing age, viral load, decreased CD4 cell count, and in some studies, intravenous drug use (Bell et al., 1996; Chiesi et al., 1996). In its less severe and more prevalent form, the effect has been described as minor cognitive motor disorder (American Academy of Neurology Task Force, 1991). Even in its mild form, cognitive impairment can affect compliance with treatment and functional ability (Heaton et al.,1994) and is associated with decreased survival (Mayeux et al., 1991; Wilkie et al., 1998).

The advent of protease inhibitors has raised the possibility of HIV-1 suppression and potential eradication, as well as potential neuropsychological benefit. Treatment with highly active antiretroviral therapy (HAART) appears to produce a beneficial effect on neurocognitive functioning (Cohen et al., 2001). Even with the introduction of HAART, however, HIV-associated cognitive impairment continues to be a major clinical problem (Sacktor et al., 2002). Studies have demonstrated that while performance in psychomotor tests (e.g., Purdue Pegboard dominant hand) improved continuously during HAART administration, memory test performance (e.g., Grober and Buschke free recall) tended to reach a plateau. A retrospective study in Australia (Dore et al., 1999) reported that with HAART the proportion of cases with AIDS dementia complex has increased, despite a reduction of infectious diseases compromising the central nervous system (CNS). A marked increase in the median CD4 cell count at AIDS dementia complex diagnosis has also been observed since the introduction of HAART (Dore et al., 1999; Price et al., 2007). These changes suggest that HAART may have a lesser impact on AIDS dementia complex than on other infectious diseases compromising the CNS. Moreover, viral persistence may occur in the CNS, and with longer survival time, it is reasonable to predict that the destructive effects of HIV-1 within the brain will include cognitive impairment (Boos, 2000).

HIV NEUROPATHOGENESIS

While etiologically and cognitively different, HIV-related subcortical dementia and cortical type dementia in Alzheimer's disease have strikingly similar pathogenic mechanisms

Gail Shor-Posner and Gloria Castillo, Department of Epidemiology and Public Health, Division of Disease Prevention, University of Miami Miller School of Medicine, Miami, FL 33136. Adriana Campa, Department of Dietetics and Nutrition, Florida International University, Stempel School of Public Health, Miami, FL 33199. Maria-Jose Miguez-Burbano, Department of Psychiatry & Behavioral Sciences, University of Miami Miller School of Medicine, Miami, FL 33136. Geraldine Moreno-Black, Department of Anthropology, University of Oregon, Eugene, OR 97403.

leading to neurotoxicity. In both dementia of aging and HIV-related dementia, chronically activated members of the microglia/macrophage groups, abnormal cytokine production, and increased oxidative stress have been implicated (Kusdra et al., 2002; Minagar et al., 2002; Pulliam et al., 1997; Rausch and Davis, 2001; Ryan et al., 2002; Smits et al., 2001).

Moreover, chronic oxidative stress has been reported during the early and advanced stages of HIV-1 infection (Favier et al., 1994), and evidence for oxidative stress has been demonstrated both in brain and in cerebrospinal fluid (Turchan et al., 2003a, 2003b). The pathological phenomenon of oxidative stress results from an imbalance between the production of reactive oxygen species and the defense systems which function to protect or destroy them (Favier et al., 1994). Reactive oxygen species, which include both radical and nonradical species, are essential for life and are formed constantly as a consequence of physiological metabolic reactions and nervous system function. While some free radicals are important for normal functioning, uncontrolled production is potentially harmful to life. The accumulation of radicals of oxygen, carbon, nitrogen, sulfur, and reactive nonradical oxygen species (hydrogen peroxide and singlet oxygen) leads to excessive lipid peroxidation, causing damage to lipids, proteins, carbohydrates, and nucleic acids. Excessive radical oxidative production can lead to abnormal production of certain cytokines that activate the immune system, which in turn induces free-radical generation and, consequently, reinitiation of the cycle. Increased microglial activation and cytokine expression, through the mediation of oxidative stress, may subsequently result in neuronal and cellular dysfunction (Gray et al., 2000; Shi et al., 1998).

Microglial activation, through the mediation of oxidative stress, appears to play a major role in neuronal apoptosis and consequent neuronal loss in HIV-1-infected individuals (Gray et al., 2000). Although all organs and proteins can potentially be modified by oxidative stress, the brain is particularly vulnerable, with the accumulation of free radicals leading to excessive lipid peroxidation and neuronal degeneration (Harman, 1982; Porta, 1988; Smith et al., 1991, 1996). Apoptotic stimuli (tumor necrosis factor alpha [TNF-α] and HIV-1 Tat protein) evidently potentiate the induction of neuronal apoptosis in the brains of AIDS patients by increasing oxidative stress (Shi et al., 1998; Eugenin et al., 2007). It has been recently demonstrated that Tat protein induces neurotoxicity and oxidative stress directly and indirectly (Chauhan et al., 2003; Pocernich et al., 2005; Pu et al., 2005). In HIV-positive drug users, the brain seems especially susceptible to the interaction of HIV and drugs (Shor-Posner et al., 2002). In support of this concept, the interaction of Tat protein with methamphetamine has been confirmed in an animal model (Maragos et al., 2002).

Elevated levels of interleukin-1β (IL-1β), IL-10, inducible nitric oxide synthase, and the antioxidant Cu-Zn superoxide dismutase (SOD) have also been demonstrated in brain tissue from demented AIDS patients (Boven et al., 1999). The proinflammatory cytokine IL-1β induces nitric oxide by up-regulating enzymatic inducible nitric oxide synthase in astrocytes, whereas IL-10 is a potent inhibitor of cytokine secretion by microphage and microglia. Production of the cytosolic antioxidant enzyme Cu-Zn SOD is increased in infected brain macrophages to prevent this neurotoxic effect (Coyle and Puttfarcken, 1993). Cultures of HIV-1-infected macrophages and astrocytes suggest that interactions between HIV-infected macrophages, microglial cells,

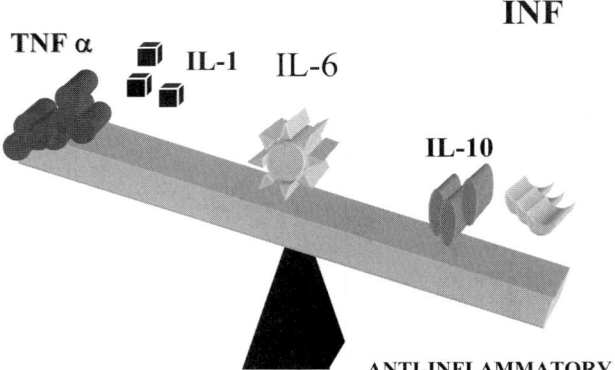

FIGURE 1 Cytokines in HIV neuropathogenesis. Imbalanced cytokines (proinflammatory versus anti-inflammatory) in the brain tissue of HIV-infected individuals.

and astrocytes are critical factors in the induction of events that lead to neuronal injury (Boven et al., 1999; Fine et al., 1996).

In addition, the cytokine TNF-α and the phospholipid mediator platelet-activating factor have been identified as potential neurotoxins secreted by HIV-infected monocytes. The pathway for neuronal damage appears to involve glutamate-mediated excitotoxicity. The toxicity attributed to TNF-α is mediated by the α-amino-3-hydroxy-5-methyl-4-isoxazole propionate receptor, whereas that related to platelet-activating factor is mediated by the N-methyl-D-aspartate receptor. Combined with oxidative stress, excitotoxicity may lead to HIV-1-induced neuronal apoptosis (Epstein and Gerbard, 1999) (Fig. 1).

Increased generation of both oxygen radicals and proinflammatory products including cytokines occurs early after HIV infection (Dobmeyer et al., 1997; Greenspan and Aruoma, 1994; Jariwalla, 1995; Jarstrand et al., 1990), affecting not only neuronal function but also the immune response as well as viral replication (Halliwell and Gutterbridge, 1985). Elevated levels of proinflammatory cytokines and oxygen radicals stimulate HIV replication (Roederer et al., 1990), through activation of nuclear factor κB (NF-κB), which is essential for the expression of HIV-controlled genes (Matsuyama et al., 1991; Staal et al., 1990; Schreck et al., 1991). Oxidative stress due to infection itself has been shown to facilitate NF-κB-dependent HIV transcription in ex vivo experiments, and in vitro studies suggest that this oxidative environment may facilitate HIV activation (Israel and Gougerot-Pocidalo, 1997). Consequently, the accumulation of oxygen radicals and proinflammatory cytokines can lead to a steady increase of viral load in HIV-infected cells.

ANTIOXIDANT DEFENSE IN BRAIN FUNCTION

Oxidative Stress

The potential importance of antioxidant nutrients in preventing and delaying the onset of neurodegenerative diseases has awakened a profound interest in this field. The brain, which exhibits intense metabolic activity, is protected from radical-mediated oxidative damage by a number of antioxidant defense systems. Large molecule "enzyme" antioxidants include SOD, which detoxifies catalase, and glutathione peroxidase (GPx), which acts to detoxify cellular peroxides. These enzymes must be synthesized by cells and are subject to regulatory mechanisms. Antioxidant nutrients, along with riboflavin (vitamin B$_2$), niacin (vitamin B$_3$), cyanocobalamin (vitamin B$_{12}$), folate, I-arginine, and omega-3 fatty acids, play key roles in modulating the function and activity of nitric oxide synthase that regulates nitric oxide production (Larrick, 1994).

Three essential nutrients (alpha-tocopherol, ascorbic acid, and beta-carotene) can directly interfere with free-radical generation and scavenge free radicals. Vitamin E (α-tocopherol) is the primary defense against potentially harmful lipid peroxidation in body fluids and cell membranes. Through its ability to trap free radicals and interrupt the chain reaction that damages brain cells, it may slow or prevent neurodegenerative changes associated with cognitive impairment (Abrams et al., 1993). Sulforaphane, glutathione, pantothenic acid, vitamin C, and molybdenum influence the activity and proper gene expression of the xenobiotic detoxification pathways that prevent the accumulation of endo- and exotoxins associated with neuronal destruction. Selenium and vitamin E seem to protect against the oxidative stress caused by magnesium-calcium imbalances in the mitochondrial membrane, which have been associated with many degenerative diseases including HIV/AIDS (Perlmutter, 1999) (Fig. 2).

Cytokine Regulation

Antioxidants may also decrease neuropathogenesis through regulation of specific proinflammatory cytokines that contribute to neurodegenerative changes and are evident in HIV-1 disease. Glutathione supplementation in vitro increases T-cell proliferation and suppresses the spontaneous release of TNF-α from peripheral blood mononuclear cells in HAART-treated HIV patients (Aukrust et al., 2003).

Selenium and zinc are two mineral trace elements linked to cytokine signaling in the immune system. Selenium has been shown to down-regulate the production of TNF-α (Haslett, 1998) and levels of TNF type II receptors in HIV-infected patients (Look et al., 1997). Selenium enhances IL-2 production in a dose-dependent manner, apparently through the increased expansion of high-affinity receptors (Roy et al., 1993). In addition, selenium seems to affect the production of TNF-α, which is prominent in the pathogenesis of anorexia and cachexia in chronic diseases (Haslett, 1998). Evidence for a selenium-cytokine mechanism of action has also been described in studies indicating the potential of selenium to decrease neuropathogenesis through suppression of IL-induced HIV-1 replication, neuronal apoptosis, and BBB damage (Hori et al., 1997; Look et al., 1997; Moutet et al., 1998).

The micronutrient zinc stimulates the secretion of IL-2 as well as the activity of thymulin and appears to prevent apoptosis. In in vitro models, zinc regulates levels of IL-2, the cytokine responsible for the earliest and most rapid expansion of T lymphocytes (Prasad, 2007). While the concentration of IL-1 in brain tissue is generally low, its expression is increased in response to injury or insult and elevated in the brain of patients with AIDS dementia complex. In studies of age-related neuronal changes, compromise in antioxidant defenses (increased lipid peroxidation and IL-1β) has been shown to be reversed in the cortex of the rat by dietary supplementation with antioxidant vitamins (O'Donnell and Lynch, 1998). Of interest, Hirano and colleagues (1998) have demonstrated that EPC-K1, a phosphodiester compound of vitamin E and vitamin C, has the ability to inhibit both DNA-binding activity and transactivation of NF-κB in a dose-dependent manner in astrocytoma cells. Moreover, treatment with this compound had a suppressive effect on HIV-1 promoter activation, supporting a potential role for antioxidants as inhibitory agents of HIV-1-related disorders.

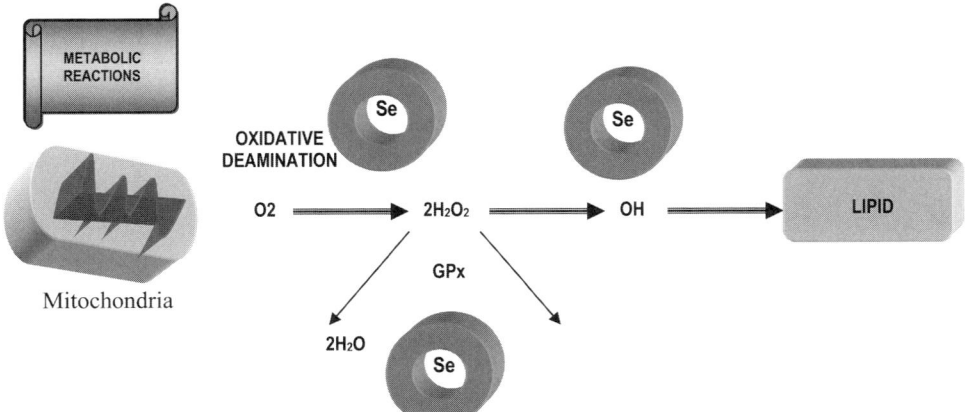

FIGURE 2   Potential action of selenium in reducing oxidative stress through its role in glutathione peroxidase activity, which protects the brain against lipoperoxidation. Cells are susceptible to the damaging actions of the small amounts of O_2^-, OH, and H_2O_2 that inevitably form during metabolism, especially in the reduction of oxygen by the electron transfer system of mitochondria. Free reactive oxygen species react with lipids, particularly polyunsaturated fatty acids, initiating a process known as lipid peroxidation, and subsequent production of new reactive species. Both O_2^- and H_2O_2 need to be quickly removed from the system and, in general, are reduced by enzyme detoxification, involving catalase and selenium-dependent glutathione peroxidase (Se-GPx), the major protective enzyme against excessive oxidative stress in the brain.

It should be noted that some nutrients are recognized pro-oxidants, involved in oxidative, free-radical-generating reactions. The proposed mechanisms of free-radical generation and neuron injury by nutrients vary with the condition. Iron in hemoglobin, for example, appears to facilitate the formation of more-reactive forms of activated oxygen in hemorrhagic trauma such as stroke (Sayed and Eaton, 1992). Wefers and Sies (1988) indicate that vitamin C can act as an antioxidant or as a pro-oxidant and have demonstrated that vitamin E is involved in switching vitamin C from a potentially damaging to a protective agent. Pharmacological doses of zinc have been implicated in neuronal apoptosis, and under pathological conditions, such as seizure, zinc release from the hippocampus may reach neurotoxic levels in extracellular concentrations. In Alzheimer's disease, zinc has been shown to bind to beta-amyloid, forming a potentially neurotoxic complex. Overstimulation of N-methyl-D-aspartate receptors by excitatory neurotransmitter amino acids in the mitochrondrial membrane has been proposed as a potential mechanism of oxidative stress in neurodegenerative diseases including Alzheimer's disease, and possibly AIDS neurodegeneration (Epstein and Gelbard, 1999; Yost and Kligman, 2001).

ANTIOXIDANTS AND THE BBB

Structural neuroimaging abnormalities, including opening of the BBB and moderate brain atrophy, appear to be common in HIV-1-infected patients, with and without cognitive impairment, and have been described as occurring even in the asymptomatic stage (Gray, 1997; Hassine et al., 1995). Although the opening of the BBB may facilitate viral entry, it is likely that specific immune responses inhibit viral replication during the early stage of HIV disease (Gray, 1997). The hallmark of AIDS dementia complex is productive viral replication by monocytes and macrophages, which appears to occur through breaches in the BBB (Persidsky, 1999), as documented by magnetic resonance imaging and single proton emission. The pioneering studies of Berger et al. (2000) have demonstrated increased basal ganglia enhancement in HIV-positive patients with moderate to severe dementia, immediately and 30 min after gadolinium contrast administration. Consistent with increased permeability of the BBB, decline of basal ganglia enhancement was slower in the demented than the nondemented patients. In other HIV studies, levels of nitric oxide metabolites have been correlated with BBB dysfunction (Giovannoni et al., 1998) and elevated in severe AIDS dementia (Adamson et al., 1996). Together, these findings support an important link between BBB disruption and cognitive impairment in HIV/AIDS.

There is some evidence to suggest that alterations in the BBB can be mediated, to some extent, by oxidative stress and host-derived factors such as cytokines, produced in response to the viral infection (Conant et al., 1998; Kruman et al., 1998). How blood barrier dysfunction occurs is not well understood, but the loss of BBB integrity may involve the destruction of capillary endothelial cell membranes by free radicals (Ikeda et al., 1997; Noseworthy and Bray, 1998). Synthetic antioxidants have been demonstrated to produce modulatory effects on the induction of cell adhesion molecule expression by IL-1α (Moynagh et al., 1994), and to prevent TNF-α-induced apoptosis (Bjugstad et al., 1998). In addition, altered glutathione oxidation/reduction ratios have been described in animals with diminished BBB integrity (Noseworthy and Bray, 2000). In patients with head trauma, significantly lower levels of vitamin C in plasma have been reported, and they were inversely correlated with the severity of neurological impairment as well as the major diameter of the lesion (Polidori et al., 2001).

As a component of various selenoproteins, selenium has important enzymatic actions that help to maintain membrane integrity (Diplock, 1994; Neve, 1996) and reduce the likelihood of further oxidative damage to biomolecules. Although natural antioxidants do not readily enter the brain, appreciable amounts of ascorbic acid, alpha tocopherol, and antioxidant enzymes (glutathione peroxidase and SOD) have been demonstrated in the BBB of the monkey and rat (Shukla et al., 1995). Moreover, altered antioxidant levels have been associated with a reduced BBB breakdown during pentylenetetrazol-induced seizures in animal studies (Oztas et al., 2001). Of interest, the magnitude of disruption of the BBB during epileptic seizures was reported to be significantly lower in rats treated with vitamin E and selenium. Since the presence of HIV in the brain involves migration of infected monocytes and lymphocytes across the vascular boundary, the development of novel therapies aimed at protecting the integrity of the BBB upon systemic HIV infection could be critical for controlling CNS infection.

ANTIOXIDANT STATUS IN HIV/AIDS

Alterations in nutritional status have long been acknowledged in various HIV-1-infected cohorts, including men who have sex with men, drug users, heterosexual adults, and children (Beach et al., 1992; Campa et al., 1999; Shor-Posner and Baum, 1996; Skurnick et al., 1996). The interaction between nutrition and HIV-1 infection is reciprocally disturbing, creating a fatal vicious cycle. Beyond the devastating effects of the disease on nutritional status, nutritional factors have the potential for influencing the rate of HIV-1 disease progression and mortality (Baum et al., 1997; Semba et al., 1993, Tang et al., 1997).

Coupled with the increased oxidative damage, and potentially aggravating it, perturbations in the antioxidant defense system, including changes in levels of ascorbic acid, tocopherols, carotenoids, zinc, selenium, and glutathione, have been observed in plasma as well as in various tissues (Beach et al., 1992; Favier et al., 1994; Pace and Leaf, 1995). In AIDS, diarrhea and destruction of the gastrointestinal lining by secondary infections or the virus itself are major contributors to micronutrient malabsorption. In addition, the hypermetabolic state produced by chronic HIV and other opportunistic infections may increase the need for the very antioxidant nutrients already compromised by poor intake and malabsorption (Grunfeld and Kotler, 1992). Deficiencies of antioxidant nutrients have been documented to influence the immunological responses of HIV-infected individuals. Decreased plasma levels of selenium, zinc, and vitamins A, E, and C have been described and associated with impaired antioxidant defense, as well as an increased risk for HIV-1 mortality (Baum et al., 1997; Lai et al., 2001; Sappey et al., 1994; Semba et al., 1993; Tang et al., 1997).

Additional studies indicate that enzymes involved in antioxidant defense are altered in HIV/AIDS. Specifically, levels of selenium and glutathione peroxidase decrease as HIV disease progresses (Cirelli et al., 1991). Moreover, clinically demented AIDS patients exhibit significantly increased expression of enzymes involved in oxidative stress, compared to nondemented patients (Boven et al., 1998). In patients with dementia of the Alzheimer's type, activities of enzymatic antioxidants are also higher, particularly where lipid peroxidation is most pronounced (Lovell et al., 1995).

Even with the introduction of HAART, initial studies do not overwhelmingly show improvements in serum micronutrient levels (Tang et al., 2005). In a small study of 20 HIV-infected patients, HAART was accompanied by both an improvement of glutathione-redox status and an increase in levels of antioxidant vitamins, without full normalization (Aukrust et al., 2003). Other studies suggest that antiretroviral therapy may reduce selenium and zinc deficiencies (Rousseau et al., 2000) as well as oxidative stress (Tang and Smit, 2000). In fact, in one recent cross-sectional study including 224 HIV-seropositive adolescents and young adults, there were none with selenium deficiency and there was no significant difference in plasma level from HIV-seronegative subjects (Stephenson et al., 2007). Conflicting findings have been reported in studies of cobalamin (vitamin B_{12}) status and HAART. Though Remacha et al. (2003) indicate a decrease in prevalence of low vitamin B_{12} in patients receiving HAART compared to previously studied non-HAART-treated patients, Woods et al. (2003) report that low levels of vitamin B_{12} can occur, even with supplementation, in patients using protease inhibitors. Considering the disparity in research findings and evidence that weight loss and wasting remain common complications for patients treated with HAART, as well as for those for whom HAART has failed or cannot be tolerated (Wanke et al., 2000), assessment of micronutrient status remains of critical importance.

ANTIOXIDANT NEUROPROTECTION

As oxidative damage has been implicated as one of the neuropathogenic factors in the development of HIV-related dementia, neuroprotective therapy that includes inhibitors of oxidative damage and/or cytokines could be promising therapeutic agents for preventing progressive nerve cell death and slowing the advance of dementia (McFadden, 1996; Shor-Posner et al., 2002; Turchan et al., 2003a, 2003b). Antioxidative treatment (daily intake of selenium, vitamin E, and vitamin C) has been reported to inhibit progression of mental deterioration in patients with multiple sclerosis (Clausen et al., 1988). Moreover, antioxidant therapies have been reported to slow the progression of Alzheimer's disease (Sano et al., 1997) and improve cognitive function in late life for those without dementia (Masaki et al., 2000). In several studies (Engelhart et al., 2002; Masaki et al., 1995, 2000; Morris et al., 1998), but not all (Luchsinger et al., 2003), antioxidant intake has been reported to reduce the risk of dementia.

In HIV subjects, daily antioxidant supplementation appears to reduce oxidative stress levels (Tang et al., 2005). There is additional evidence to suggest that antioxidant therapy may provide neuroprotection in HIV/AIDS. A randomized, double-blind, placebo-controlled trial in patients with mild HIV-associated cognitive impairment evaluated the effect of selegiline (deprenyl) and thioctic acid on cognitive function. The effectiveness of deprenyl, a monoamine oxidase-B inhibitor, in promoting cognitive improvement appears to involve its scavenger action and impact on antioxidant enzymes (Dana Consortium, 1998). In accord with these findings, chronic treatment with a synthetic antioxidant has been demonstrated to prevent TNF-α action in an animal model of AIDS dementia (Bjugstad et al., 1998). In addition, other novel protecting antioxidants have been screened for protective effects on the brain. L-deprenil, didox, imidate, diosgenin, and ebselen were found to block toxicity of cerebrospinal fluid in brain tissue from patients with HIV encephalitis and macaques with simian immunodeficiency

virus encephalitis (Turchan et al., 2003b). Nonpectic macrocyclic MN(II)s have also shown potential for future treatment. In particular, M40401, which mimics SOD enzymatic activity, has been shown in vitro to reduce oxidative stress and protect against apoptotic cell death (Mollace et al., 2001).

Antioxidant micronutrients may also have a protective role in preventing the development of neurodegenerative disease. In support of this suggestion, selenium depletion has been reported to constitute an important triggering factor for seizures and subsequent neuronal damage in patients with epilepsy (Raemaekers et al., 1994). Early studies with selenium therapy revealed symptomatic improvements and increased serum selenium concentrations in HIV patients (Cirelli et al., 1991). Moreover, an increase in enzymatic antioxidant defense systems, following supplementation with selenium, has been demonstrated in latently infected T lymphocytes (Sappey et al., 1994) and in HIV/AIDS patients receiving selenium daily for 1 year (Delmas-Beauvieux et al., 1996).

Selenium-Cytokine Mechanism in Neuroprotection

Radical-oxidative-induced production of certain cytokines can activate the immune system, which in turn stimulates free-radical generation, resulting in reinitiation of the cycle. The potential for selenium to decrease neuropathogenesis through suppression of IL-induced HIV-1 replication and neuronal apoptosis has been described in a number of investigations (Hori et al., 1997; Look et al., 1997; Moutet et al., 1998; Sappey et al., 1994). In vitro studies suggest that selenium, in the glutathione peroxidase system, inhibits IL-8 release by endothelial cells (Look et al., 1997). Selenium supplementation has been shown to suppress TNF-α-induced HIV-1 replication (Hori et al., 1997) and significantly reduce NF-κB-activation by IL-1 (Brigelius-Flohe et al., 1997). Thus, selenium may protect the neural cells from IL-1-induced superoxide production, thereby preventing neuronal apoptosis.

Look and colleagues (1997) have demonstrated that selenium levels are inversely correlated with levels of soluble TNF type II receptors in HIV-infected patients. Selenium's effect on TNF-α would also be expected to decrease IL-15 production (Lee et al., 1996; Stoeck et al., 1998), providing an important protective effect against cytotoxic effects and cell activation (Fig. 3).

Zinc

As an essential micronutrient for the growth and function of the brain, zinc appears to influence the concentration of neurotransmitters in the synaptic cleft and may be an inhibitory neuromodulator of glutamate release in the hippocampus (Takeda, 2004). Three decades ago, Henkin et al. (1975) described impaired neuromotor and cognitive performance in adults with severe zinc deficiency. More recently, pilot studies have suggested that even mild zinc deficiency may decrease cognitive function (Tucker and Sandstead, 1984), and low zinc nutrition appears to increase the risk of dementia in the elderly (Burnet, 1981; Tully et al., 1995). A number of reports have noted improved neuropsychological function with zinc repletion, in the context of repletion of other potentially limiting micronutrients (Ronaghy et al., 1974; Penland et al., 1997, 1999).

The importance of zinc in preserving the integrity of biological membranes has long been recognized, along with its role in the synthesis of coenzymes that mediate biogenic-amine synthesis and metabolism (Prasad et al., 1978). In HIV/AIDS studies, conflicting results on the role of zinc

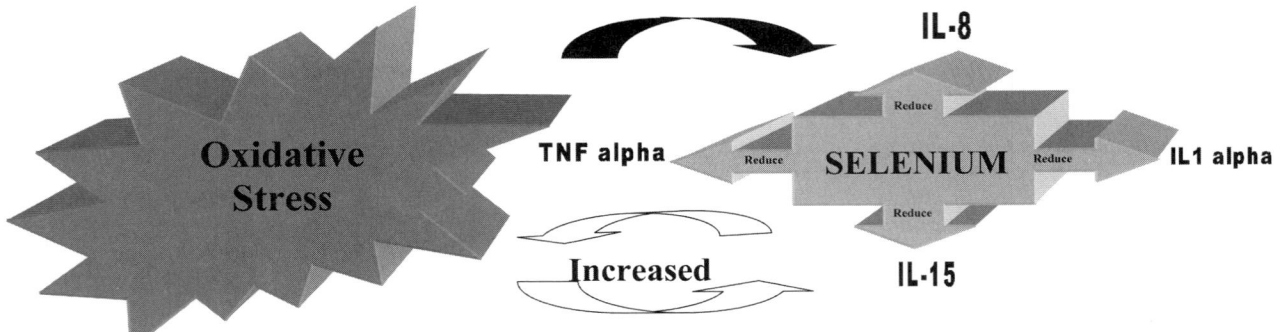

FIGURE 3   Selenium and cytokine regulation. The rationale for a selenium-cytokine mechanism of action in neuroprotection has been demonstrated in studies indicating the potential for selenium to decrease neuropathogenesis through suppression of IL-induced HIV-1 replication and neuronal apoptosis (Hori et al., 1997; Look et al., 1997; Moutet et al., 1998; Sappey et al., 1994).

status in disease progression have been described (Lai et al., 2001; Kupka and Fawzi, 2002). Nevertheless, important zinc-cytokine interactions have been revealed in in vitro experiments. Zinc has been shown to stimulate expression of the IL-2 gene by allowing regulatory proteins to bind to DNA (Schwabe and Rhodes, 1991). In other investigations, zinc has been demonstrated to increase the proliferation of T lymphocytes and the synthesis of IL-2 (Tanala et al., 1990). Zinc enables thymulin activity, and in turn, active cycling thymulin allows zinc to be recognized by T-lymphocyte receptors that promote T-cell differentiation (Prasad, 2007). Zinc also inhibits the endogenous endonuclease activated by calcium ions that is responsible for the apoptosis of CD4 cells induced by TNF (Tanala et al., 1990; Zhang et al., 1998).

Alpha-Tocopherol: Vitamin E

Vitamin E comprises a family of eight antioxidants, four tocopherols (alpha, beta, gamma, and delta) and four tocotrienols (also alpha, beta, gamma, and delta). The form of vitamin E found in the largest quantities in the blood and tissues is alpha-tocopherol, which functions to maintain cell membrane integrity and protect the fats in low-density lipoproteins from oxidation. In a multicenter clinical trial in individuals with moderately severe Alzheimer's disease, patients were administered selegiline (a monoamine oxidase β inhibitor), or alpha-tocopherol (vitamin E), or both, or a placebo. Treatment with vitamin E or selegiline was found to slow disease progression, as measured by the time required for institutionalization, loss of activity abilities, progression to severe dementia, or death (Sano et al., 1997). An earlier investigation (Parkinson Study Group, 1993) of patients showing clinical Parkinson's symptoms, the DATATOP (Deprenyl and Tocopherol Antioxidant Therapy of Parkinsonism) study, also administered selegiline and alpha-tocopherol. The results of this study, however, did not reveal a benefit from vitamin E therapy, possibly due to the substantial loss of neurons prior to treatment initiation.

In HIV-seropositive patients, short-term (3-month) daily supplementation with both vitamin E and vitamin C has been reported to reduce oxidative stress and produce a trend towards a reduction in viral load (Allard et al., 1998). Vitamin E supplementation has also been associated with a lower risk for cognitive impairment in an epidemiological study of Japanese-American men (Masaki et al., 1995, 2000) and with higher plasma levels of alpha-tocopherol in a rela-

tively healthy cohort of middle-aged and older individuals (Morris et al., 1998). Schmidt et al. (1998) report a reduced occurrence of incident Alzheimer's disease in association with vitamin C, which is capable of regenerating the antioxidant capacity of alpha-tocopherol, or vitamin E supplementation. However, vitamin E supplementation should not be used in the setting of the patient with vascular disease or diabetes mellitus, as this has been associated with an increased risk for heart failure (Lonn et al., 2005). This is particularly relevant for HIV-seropositive patients, who may develop vascular disease and diabetes mellitus as a toxocity of HIV medication therapies.

MICRONUTRIENTS AND PSYCHOLOGICAL WELL-BEING

It is important to note that, even in the era of HAART, HIV remains a serious psychological burden (Kilbourne et al., 2001; Zinkernagel et al., 2001). More symptoms of anxiety and stress have been described among HIV-seropositive subjects than among the general population, and a positive relationship between anxiety and HIV symptoms, fatigue, and physical limitations has been reported (Sewell et al., 2000). With the availability of antiretroviral therapies, there is some evidence that depressive symptoms may decrease (Brechtl et al., 2001; Judd et al., 2000) and that treatment may be protective for new-onset psychosis (di Ronchi et al., 2000). Alciati et al. (2001) suggest that new combination therapies may explain, at least in part, a decreased prevalence of current mood disorders in their study. Overall psychological improvement with antiretroviral therapy has also been reported by Rabkin and colleagues (2000). No significant effect was observed, nevertheless, on an individual basis. Those whose disease status reflected successful treatment were no more likely than others to be relieved of the psychological burdens of illness, underscoring the importance of alternative therapeutic strategies to enhance well-being.

Antioxidants

A role for antioxidants in reducing anxiety and stress is suggested by studies demonstrating psychological mediation of increased lipid peroxidation (Matsumoto et al., 1993) and is supported by the report of reactive oxygen species action in some neuropsychiatric disorders (Bilici et al., 2001). In accord with this proposal, lower plasma levels of alpha-tocopherol have been documented in people diagnosed with major depression (Owen et al., 2005), and a variety of mental and behavioral changes have been associated with zinc deficiency, including depression and paranoia (Prasad et al., 1978).

A number of investigations have demonstrated a beneficial effect of selenium therapy on mood status in healthy individuals. Utilizing the Profile of Mood States, Benton and Cook (1991) found a significant association between selenium intake and elevation in mood, specifically a decrease in anxiety. Furthermore, they found that this mood change during selenium supplementation was inversely correlated with the level of selenium in the diet. Similarly, Hawkes and Hornbostel (1996) reported that people with low levels of selenium might be susceptible to depressed moods. Penland and Finley (1995) also examined the effect of high/low dietary selenium in healthy men and showed a significant positive correlation between selenium-dependent enzyme activity in platelets and measures of mood.

In our studies of HIV-positive drug users, participants in a randomized, double-blind, placebo-controlled nutritional chemoprevention clinical trial were administered selenium therapy (200 µg/day) and monitored over a 12-month period (Shor-Posner et al., 2003). Psychosocial measures (State and Trait anxiety, BDI-depression, and POMS-mood state), clinical status (CD4 cell count and viral load), and plasma selenium levels were determined at baseline and compared with measurements obtained at the 12-month evaluation. At baseline, the majority of the study participants (32 men and 31 women) reported elevated levels of anxiety; 25% reported overall mood distress and moderate depression. Psychological burden was not influenced by current drug use, antiretroviral treatment, or viral load.

At the 12-month evaluation, selenium-treated HIV-positive individuals reported increased vigor and had less anxiety than placebo-treated subjects (Shor-Posner et al., 2003). The risk for state anxiety was almost four times higher and the risk for trait anxiety was nearly nine times greater in the placebo-treated group, controlling for antiretroviral therapy, CD4 cell decline, and years of education, suggesting that selenium therapy may be a beneficial treatment to decrease anxiety in persons who exhibit a high prevalence of psychological burden.

Group B Vitamins

Although the focus of this chapter has been on antioxidant action in neuroprotection, the B vitamins have long been recognized to have an important role in brain function and may also provide a protective action against excitotoxicity to the brain (Lin et al., 2004). Many neurological symptoms, ranging from peripheral neuropathies to global cognitive impairment, observed in HIV-infected individuals have also been demonstrated to be a consequence of B vitamin deficiency (Dreyfuss, 1988). Adequate status of cobalamin (vitamin B_{12}), pyridoxine (vitamin B_6), and folate protects the CNS against methylation defects and accumulation of homocysteine (Yost and Kligman, 2001).

Deficiencies of the B vitamins, on the other hand, are associated with poor development of the nervous system and dementia (Whitney and Rolfes, 1999). Pyridoxine deficiency has been hypothesized to be related to various mood states including depression and irritability, as well as to affective disorders. The mediating mechanism for the relationship between pyridoxine status and psychological distress has been postulated to involve change in central serotonin levels, as pyridoxine is a cofactor for 5-HTP decarboxylase, an enzyme in the biosynthesis pathway of serotonin. Assessment of pyridoxine status in HIV-infected individuals has revealed that normalizing pyridoxine status is related to a significant decline in overall psychological distress, controlling for life stressor burden, social support availability, and coping style (Shor-Posner et al., 1994). In a study of recently bereaved HIV-infected men, we have also demonstrated increased psychological distress in relationship to plasma pyridoxine deficiency (Baldewicz et al., 1998), highlighting the importance of maintaining adequate pyridoxine status in HIV disease.

Low cobalamin levels may potentiate neuropsychological impairment and have been associated with overall psychological distress (Healton et al., 1991; Newbold, 1989), as well as depressed mood (Carethers, 1988). Several investigations have indicated that depression (Geagea and Ananth, 1975; Verbanck and Oliver, 1991) and psychotic symptoms (Evans et al., 1983; Phillips and Kahaner, 1988; Zucker et al., 1981) are reversible with cobalamin supplementation. Our studies of nutritional status and neuropsychological function indicate that plasma cobalamin levels, which are frequently low among HIV/AIDS patients, may be related to some of the neuropsychological impairment noted in HIV disease. Specifically, our longitudinal investigations reveal that normalization of vitamin B_{12} status is associated with significant improvement, whereas becoming cobalamin deficient (<200 pg/ml) is related to a significant decline in the speed of accessing information from semantic memory (Shor-Posner et al., 1995). Moreover, our research group has demonstrated that cobalamin level may be physiologically related to depressed and anxious mood level, as well as to syndromal depression (Baldewicz et al., 2000). Further support for maintaining adequate vitamin B_{12} status in preventing neuropsychological symptoms in HIV-1 infection is provided from cobalamin therapy studies demonstrating a therapeutic response in HIV-1-seropositive subjects referred for neurological evaluation (Kieburtz et al., 1991) and resolution of HIV-associated dementia symptoms in a patient with low vitamin B_{12} levels (Herzlich and Schiano, 1993).

SUMMARY

HIV-associated dementia continues to be a major cause of morbidity and mortality, even in the era of HAART. Accordingly, much attention has focused on adjunctive therapies targeted at preserving, restoring, or enhancing systemic and brain immune responses that may prevent or slow the development of HIV-associated cognitive disorders. Antioxidant therapies that protect the brain may provide a safe and affordable strategy to inhibit processes associated with brain deterioration. This appears to be especially warranted in HIV-infected men and women who exhibit widespread deficiencies of micronutrients required for immune function and antioxidant defense that are likely to contribute to diminished neuroprotection.

This work was supported by NIH Fogarty (5D43TW00017-gsp).

REFERENCES

Abrams, B., D. Duncan, and I. Hertz-Picciotto. 1993. A prospective study of dietary intake and acquired immune deficiency syndrome in HIV-seropositive homosexual men. *J. Acquir. Immune Defic. Syndr.* **6**:949.

Adamson, D., B. Wildemann, M. Sasaki, J. Glass, J. McArthur, V. Christov, T. Dawson, and V. Dawson. 1996. Immunologic NO synthase: elevation in severe AIDS dementia and induction by HIV-1gp41. *Science* **274**:1917–1921.

Alciati, A., F. Starace, B. Scaramelli, M. Campaniello, B. Adriani, C. Mellado, and A. Cargnel. 2001. Has there been a decrease in the prevalence of mood disorders in HIV-seropositive individuals since the introduction of combination therapy? *Eur. Psychiatry* **16:**491–496.

Allard, J., E. Aghdassi, J. Chau, C. Tam C. Kovacs, I. Salit, and S. Walmsley. 1998. Effects of vitamin E and C supplementation on oxidative stress and viral load in HIV-infected subjects. *AIDS* **12:**1653–1659.

American Academy of Neurology Task Force. 1991. Nomenclature and research case definitions for neurologic manifestations of human immunodeficiency virus-type 1 (HIV-1) infection. *Neurology* **41:**778–785.

Aukrust, P., F. Muller, A. Svardal, T. Ueland, R. Berge, and S. Froland. 2003. Disturbed glutathione metabolism and decreased antioxidant levels in human immunodeficiency virus-infected patients during highly active antiretroviral therapy-potential immunomodulatory effects of antioxidants. *J. Infect. Dis.* **188:**232–238.

Baldewicz, T., K. Goodkin, N. Blaney, G. Shor-Posner, M. Kumar, F. Wilkie, M. Baum, and C. Eisdorfer. 2000. Cobalamin level is related to self-reported and clinically related mood and to syndromal depression in bereaved HIV-1+ and HIV-1 homosexual men. *J. Psychosom. Res.* **48:**177–185.

Baldewicz, T., K. Goodkin, D. Feaster, N. Blaney, M. Kumar, A. Kumar, G. Shor-Posner, and M. Baum. 1998. Plasma pyridoxine deficiency is related to increased psychological distress in recently bereaved homosexual men. *Psychosom. Med.* **60:**297–308.

Baum, M., G. Shor-Posner, S. Lai, G. Zhang, H. Lai, M. Fletcher, H. Sauberlich, and J. Page. 1997. High risk of HIV-related mortality is associated with selenium deficiency. *J. Acquir. Immune Defic. Syndr.* **15:**370–374.

Beach, R., E. Mantero-Atienza, G. Shor-Posner, J. Javier, J. Szapocznik, R. Morgan, H. Sauberlich, P. Cornwell, C. Eisdorfer, and M. Baum. 1992. Specific nutrient abnormalities in asymptomatic HIV-1 infection. *AIDS* **6:**701–708.

Bell, J., Y. Donaldson, S. Lowrie, C. McKenzie, R. Elton, A. Chiswick, R. Brettle, J. Ironside, and P. Simmonds. 1996. Influence of risk group and zidovudine therapy on the development of HIV encephalitis and cognitive impairment in AIDS patients. *AIDS* **10:**493–499.

Benton, D., and R. Cook. 1991. The impact of selenium supplementation on mood. *Biol. Psychiatry* **29:**1092–1098.

Berger, J., A. Nath, R. Greenberg, A. Andersen, R. Greene, R. Bognar, and M. Avison. 2000. Cerebrovascular changes in the basal ganglia with HIV dementia. *Neurology* **54:**921–926.

Bilici, M., H. Efe, M. Koroglu, H. Uyda, M. Bekaroglu, and O. Deger. 2001. Antioxidative enzyme activities and lipid peroxidation in major depression: alterations by antidepressant treatments. *J. Affect. Disord.* **64:**43–51.

Bjugstad, K., W. Flitter, W. Garland, G. Su, and G. Arendash. 1998. Preventive actions of a synthetic antioxidant in a novel animal model of AIDS dementia. *Brain Res.* **795:**349–357.

Boos, J. 2000. Chronic-treated HIV: a neurologic disease. *J. Urban Health* **7:**204–212.

Boven, L., L. Gomez, C. Hery, F. Gray, J. Verhoef, P. Portegies, M. Tardieu, and H. Nottet. 1999. Increased peroxynitrite activity in AIDS dementia complex: implications for the neuropathogenesis of HIV-1 infection. *Immunology* **162:**4319–4327.

Boven, L., J. Middel, C. Hery, F. Gray, P. Verhoef P. Portegies, M. Tardieu, and H. Nottet. 1998. Increased peroxynitrite activity and elevated neurotrophin levels in brains of patients with AIDS dementia complex. Neuroscience of HIV infection. *J. Neurovirol.* **4:**343.

Brechtl, J., W. Breitbart, M. Galietta, S. Krivo, and B. Rosenfeld. 2001. The use of highly active antiretroviral therapy (HAART) in patients with advanced HIV infection: impact on medical, palliative care, and quality of life outcomes. *J. Pain Symptom Manage.* **21:**41–51.

Brigelius-Flohe, R., B. Friedrichs, S. Maurer, M. Schultz, and R. Streicher. 1997. Interleukin 1-induced nuclear factor kappa B activation is inhibited by overexpression of phospholipid hydroperoxide glutathione peroxidase in a human endothelial cell line. *Biochem. J.* **328:**199–203.

Burnet, F. 1981. A possible role of zinc in the pathology of dementia. *Lancet* **1:**186–188.

Campa, A., G. Shor-Posner, F. Indacochea, G. Zhang, H. Lai, D. Asthana, G. Scott, and M. Baum. 1999. Mortality risk in selenium-deficient HIV-positive children. *J. Acquir. Immun. Defic. Syndr.* **20:**508–513.

Carethers, M. 1988. Diagnosing vitamin B12 deficiency: a common geriatric disorder. *Geriatrics* **43:**89–112.

Chauhan, A., J. Turchan, C. Pocernich, A. Bruce-Keller, S. Roth, D. Butterfield, E. Major, and A. Nath. 2003. Intracellular human immunodeficiency virus Tat expression in astrocytes promotes astrocyte survival but induces potent neurotoxicity at distant sites via axonal transport. *J. Biol. Chem.* **278:**13512–13519.

Chiesi, A., S. Vella, L. Dally, C. Pedersen, S. Danner, A. Johnson, S. Schwander, F. Goebel, H. Glauser, and F. Antunes. 1996. Epidemiology of AIDS dementia complex in Europe. *J. Acquir. Immune Defic. Syndr.* **11:**39–44.

Cirelli, A., M. Ciard, C. DeSimone, F. Sonce, R. Giordano, L. Ciaralli, and S. Constantini. 1991. Serum selenium concentration and disease progress in patients with HIV infection. *Clin. Biochem.* **24:**211–214.

Clausen, J., G. Jensen, and S. Nielsen. 1988. Selenium in chronic neurologic diseases. Multiple sclerosis and Batten's disease. *Biol. Trace Elem. Res.* **15:**179–203.

Cohen, R., R. Boland, R. Paul, K. Tashima, E. Schoenbaum, D. Celentano, P. Schuman, D. Smith, and C. Carpenter. 2001. Neurocognitive performance enhanced by highly active antiretrovial therapy in HIV-infected women. *AIDS* **15:**341–345.

Conant, K., A. Garzino-Demo A. Nath, J. McArthur, W. Halliday, C. Power, R. Gallo, and E. Major. 1998. Induction of monocyte chemoattractant protein-1 in HIV-1 Tat stimulated astrocytes and elevation in AIDS dementia. *Proc. Natl. Acad. Sci. USA* **95:**3117–3121.

Coyle, J., and P. Puttfarcken. 1993. Oxidative stress, glutamate, and neurodegenerative disorders. *Science* **262:**689.

Dana Consortium on the Therapy of HIV Dementia and Related Cognitive Disorders. 1998. A randomized, double-blind, placebo-controlled trial of deprenyl and thioctic acid in human immunodeficiency virus-associated cognitive impairment. *Neurology* **50:**645–651.

Delmas-Beauvieux, M., E. Peuchant, A. Couchoron, J. Constans, C. Sergeant, M. Simonoff, J. Pellegrin, B. Leng, C. Conri, and M. Clerc. 1996. The enzymatic antioxidant system in blood and glutathione status in human immunodeficiency virus (HIV)-infected patients: effects of supplementation with selenium or B-carotene. *Am. J. Clin. Nutr.* **64:**101–107.

Diplock, A. 1994. Antioxidants and disease prevention. *Mol. Aspects Med.* **15:**293–376.

di Ronchi, D., I. Faranca, P. Forti, G. Ravaghia, M. Borderi, R. Manfredi, and V. Volterra. 2000. Development of acute psychotic disorders and the HIV-1 infection. *Int. J. Psychiatry Med.* **30:**173–183.

Dobmeyer, T., S. Findhammer, J. Dobmeyer, S. Klein, B. Raffel, D. Hoelzer, E. Helm, D. Kabelitz, and R. Rossol. 1997. Ex vivo induction of apoptosis in lymphocytes is mediated by oxidative stress: role for lymphocyte loss in HIV infection. *Free Radic. Biol. Med.* **22:**775–785.

Dore, G., P. Correll, Y. Li, J. Kaldor, D. Cooper, and B. Brew. 1999. Changes to AIDS dementia complex in the era of highly active antiretroviral therapy. *AIDS* **9:**1249–1253.

Dreyfuss, P. 1988. Diet and nutrition in neurologic disorder, p. 1458–1470. *In* M. Shils and Y. Young (ed.), *Modern Nutrition in Health and Disease*. Lea & Febiger, Philadelphia, PA.

Engelhart, M., M. Geerlings, A. Ruitenberg, J. van Swieten, A. Hofman, J. Witteman, and M. Breteler. 2002. Dietary intake of antioxidants and risk of Alzheimer disease. *JAMA* 287:3223–3229.

Epstein, L., and H. Gerbard. 1999. HIV-1-induced neuronal injury in the developing brain. *J. Leukoc. Biol.* 65:453–457.

Eugenin, E. A., J. E. King, A. Nath, T. M. Calderon, R. S. Zukin, M. V. Bennett, and J. W. Berman. 2007. HIV-tat induces formation of an LRP-PSD-95-NMDAR-nNOS complex that promotes apoptosis in neurons and astrocytes. *Proc. Natl. Acad. Sci. USA* 104:3438–3443.

Evans, D., G. Edelsohn, and R. Golden. 1983. Organic psychosis without anemia or spinal cord symptoms in patients with vitamin B12 deficiency. *Am. J. Psychiatry* 140:218–221.

Favier, A., C. Sappey, P. Leclerc, P. Faure, and M. Micoud. 1994. Antioxidant status and lipid peroxidation in patients infected with HIV. *Chem. Biol. Interact.* 91:165.

Fine, S., R. Angel, S. Perry, L. Epstein, J. Rothstein, S. Dewhurst, and H. Gerbard. 1996. Tumor necrosis factor α inhibits glutamate uptake by primary human astrocytes: implications for pathogenesis of HIV-1 dementia. *J. Biol. Chem.* 27:15303.

Geagea, K., and J. Ananth. 1975. Response of a psychiatric patient to vitamin B12 therapy. *Dis. Nerv. Syst.* 36:343–344.

Giovannoni, G., R. Miller, S. Heales, J. Land, M. Harrison, and E. Thompson. 1998. Elevated cerebrospinal fluid and serum nitrate and nitrite levels in patients with central nervous system complications of HIV-1 infection: a correlation with blood-brain-barrier dysfunction. *J. Neurol. Sci.* 156:53–58.

Gray, F. 1997. Lesions of the central nervous system in the early stages of human immunodeficiency virus. *Rev. Neurol.* 153:629–640.

Gray, F., H. Adle-Biassette, F. Brion, T. Ereau, I. le Maner, V. Levy, and G. Crocket. 2000. Neuronal apoptosis in human immunodeficiency virus infection. *J. Neurovirol.* 6(Suppl. 1):S38–S43.

Greenspan, H., and O. Aruoma. 1994. Oxidative stress and apoptosis in HIV infection: a role for plant-derived metabolites with synergistic antioxidant activity. *Immunol. Today* 15:209.

Grunfeld, C., and D. Kotler. 1992. Wasting in the acquired immunodeficiency syndrome. *Semin. Liver Dis.* 12:175–187.

Halliwell, B., and J. Gutteridge. 1985. Oxygen radicals in the nervous system. *Trends Neurosci.* 8:22–26.

Harman, D. 1982. The free radical theory of aging, p. 255–275. *In* W. Pryor (ed.), *Free Radicals in Biology*. Academic Press, New York, NY.

Haslett, P. 1998. Anticytokine approaches to the treatment of anorexia and cachexia. *Semin. Oncol.* 25:53–57.

Hassine, D., F. Gray, R. Chekroun, F. Chretien, B. Marc, M. Durigon, and E. Schouman-Claeys. 1995. Early cerebral lesions in HIV infection. Postmortem radio-pathologic correlations in non-AIDS asymptomatic seropositive patients. *J. Neuroradiol.* 22:148–160.

Hawkes, W., and L. Hornbostel. 1996. Effects of dietary selenium on mood in healthy men living in a metabolic research unit. *Biol. Psychiatry* 39:121–128.

Healton, E., D. Savage, J. Brust, T. Garrett, and J. Lindenbaum. 1991. Neurologic aspects of cobalamin deficiency. *Medicine* 70:229–245.

Heaton, R., R. Velin, J. McCutchan, S. Gulevich, H. Atkinson, M. Wallace, H. Godfrey, D. Kirson, I. Grant, and the HNRC. 1994. Neuropsychological impairment in human immunodeficiency virus-infection: implications for employment. *Psychosom. Med.* 56:8–17.

Henkin, R., B. Patten, P. Re, and D. Bronzert. 1975. A syndrome of acute zinc loss. Cerebellar dysfunction, mental changes, anorexia, and taste and smell dysfunction. *Arch. Neurol.* 32:745–751.

Herzlich, B., and T. Schiano. 1993. Reversal of apparent AIDS dementia complex following treatment with vitamin B12. *J. Intern. Med.* 233:495–497.

Hirano, F., H. Tanaka, T. Miura, Y. Hirano, K. Okamoto, Y. Makino, and I. Makino. 1998. Inhibition of NH-kB-dependent transcription of human immunodeficiency virus 1 promoter by a phosphodiester compound of vitamin C and vitamin E, EPC-K1. *Immunopharmacology* 39:31–38.

Hori, K., D. Hatfield, F. Maldarelli, B. Lee, and K. Close. 1997. Selenium supplementation suppresses tumor necrosis factor alpha-induced human immunodeficiency virus replication in vitro. *AIDS* 13:1325–1332.

Ikeda, K., T. Nagashima, S. Wu, M. Yamaguchi, and N. Tamaki. 1997. The role of calcium ion in anoxide/regoxygenation damage of cultured brain capillary endothelial cells. *Acta Neurochir. Suppl.* 70:4–7.

Israel, N., and M. Gougerot-Pocidalo. 1997. Oxidative stress in human immunodeficiency virus infection. *Cell. Mol. Life Sci.* 53:864–870.

Jariwalla, R. 1995. Micronutrient imbalance in HIV infection and AIDS: relevance to pathogenesis and therapy. *J. Nutr. Environ. Med.* 5:297.

Jarstrand, C., B. Akerlund, and B. Lindeke. 1990. Glutathione and HIV infection. *Lancet* i:235.

Judd, F., A. Cockram, A. Komiti, A. Mijch, J. Hoy, and R. Bell. 2000. Depressive symptoms reduced in individuals with HIV/AIDS treated with highly active antiretroviral therapy: a longitudinal study. *Aust. N. Z. J. Psychiatry* 34:1015–1021.

Ketzler, S., S. Weiss, H. Hung, and H. Budka. 1990. Loss of neurons in the frontal cortex in AIDS brains. *Acta Kieb. Neuropathol.* 80:92–94.

Kieburtz, K., D. Giang, R. Schiffer, and N. Vakil. 1991. Abnormal vitamin B$_{12}$ metabolism in human immunodeficiency virus infection. Association with neurological dysfunction. *Arch. Neurol.* 48:312–314.

Kilbourne, A., A. Justice, L. Rabeneck, M. Rodriguez-Barrdas, S. Weissman, and The VACS 3 Project Team. 2001. General medical and psychiatric comorbidity among HIV-infected veterans in the post-HAART era. *J. Clin. Epidemiol.* 54:S22–S28.

Kruman, I., A. Nath, and M. Mattson. 1998. HIV-1 protein Tat induces apoptosis of hippocampal neurons by a mechanism involving caspase activation, calcium overload, and oxidative stress. *Exp. Neurol.* 154:276–288.

Kupka, R., and W. Fawzi. 2002. Zinc nutrition and HIV infection. *Nutr. Rev.* 60:69–79.

Kusdra, L., D. McGuire, and L. Pulliam. 2002. Changes in monocyte/macrophage neurotoxicity in the era of HAART. Implications for HIV-associated dementia. *AIDS* 16:31–38.

Lai, H., S. Lai, G. Shor-Posner, M. Fangcho, E. Trapido, and M. Baum. 2001. Plasma zinc, copper, copper:zinc ratio and survival in a cohort of HIV-1 infected homosexual men. *J. Acquir. Immune Defic. Syndr.* 27:56–62.

Larrick, J. 1994. Metabolism of arginine to nitric oxide: an area for nutritional manipulation of human disease? *J. Optimal Nutr.* 3:22–31.

Lee, Y., J. Satoh, D. Walker, and S. Kim. 1996. Interleukin-15 gene expression in human astrocytes and microglia in culture. *Neuroreport* 7:1062–1066.

Lin, Y., A. Desbois, S. Jiang, and S. Hou. 2004. Group B vitamins protect murine cerebellar granule cells from glutamate/NMDA toxicity. *Neuroreport* 15:2241–2244.

Lonn, E., J. Busch, S. Yusuf, P. Sheridan, J. Pogue, J. M. O. Arnold, C. Ross, A. Arnold, P. Sleight, J. Probstfield, and G. R. Dagenais. 2005. Effects of long term vitamin E supplementation on cardiovascular events and cancer in a randomized controlled trial. *New Engl. J. Med.* 293:1338–1347.

Look, M., J. Rockstroh, G. Rao, K. Kreuzer, S. Barton, H. Lemoch, T. Sudhop, J. Hoch, K. Stockings, U. Spengler, and T. Sauerbruch. 1997. Serum selenium, plasma glutathione (GSH) and erythrocyte glutathione peroxidase (GSH-PS) levels in asymptomatic versus symptomatic human immunodeficiency virus-1 (HIV-1) infection. *Eur. J. Clin. Nutr.* **51**:266–272.

Lovell, M., W. Ehmann, S. Butler, and W. Markesbery. 1995. Elevated thiobarbituric acid-reactive substances and antioxidant enzyme activity in the brain in Alzheimer's disease. *Neurology* **45**:1594–1601.

Luchsinger, J., M. Tang, S. Shea, and R. Mayeux. 2003. Antioxidant vitamin intake and risk of Alzheimer disease. *Arch. Neurol.* **60**:203–208.

Maragos, W., K. Young, J. Turchan, M. Guseva, J. Pauly, A. Nath, and W. Cass. 2002. Human immunodeficiency virus-1 Tat protein and methamphetamine interact synergistically to impair striatal dopaminergic function. *J. Neurochem.* **83**:955–963.

Masaki, K., K. Losonczy, G. Izmirlian, D. Foley, G. Ross, H. Petrovitch, R. Halik, and L. White. 2000. Association of vitamin E and C supplement use with cognitive function and dementia in elderly men. *Neurology* **54**:1265–1272.

Masaki, K., L. White, H. Petrovic, et al. 1995. Superior cognitive functioning in later life. *Neurology* **45**:A271–A272.

Matsumoto, T., T. Miike, R. Nelson, W. Trudeau, R. Lockey, and J. Yoddoi. 1993. Elevated serum levels of IL-8 in patients with HIV infection. *Clin. Exp. Immunol.* **93**:149.

Matsuyama, T., N. Kobayashi, and N. Yamamoto. 1991. Cytokines and HIV infection–is AIDS a tumor necrosis factor disease. *AIDS* **5**:1405.

Mayeux, R., Y. Stern, M. Tang, G. Todak, K. Masarder, M. Sano, M. Richard, Z. Stein, A. Ehrhardt, and J. Gorman. 1991. Mortality risks in gay men with human immunodeficiency virus infection and cognitive impairment. *Neurology* **43**:176–182.

McFadden, S. 1996. Phenotypic variation in xenobiotic metabolism and adverse environmental response: focus on sulfur-dependent detoxification pathways. *Toxicology* **111**:43–65.

Minagar, A., P. Shapshak, R. Fujimura, R. Ownby, M. Heyes, and C. Eisdorfer. 2002. The role of macrophage/microglia and astrocytes in the pathogenesis of three neurologic disorders: HIV-associated dementia, Alzheimer disease, and multiple sclerosis. *J. Neurol. Sci.* **202**:13.

Mollace, V., H. Nottet, P. Clayette, M. Turco, C. Muscoli, D. Salvemini, and C. Perno. 2001. Oxidative stress and neuroAIDS: triggers, modulators and novel antioxidants. *Trends Neurosci.* **24**:411–416.

Morris, M., L. Beckett, P. Scherr, L. Hebert, D. Bennett, T. Field, and D. Evans. 1998. Vitamin E and vitamin C supplement use and risk of incident Alzheimer disease. *Alzheimer Dis. Assoc. Disord.* **12**:121–126.

Moutet, M., P. d'Alessio, P. Malette, V. Devaux, and J. Chaudiere. 1998. Glutathione peroxidase mimics prevent TNF and neutrophil induced endothelial alterations. *Free Radic. Biol. Med.* **25**:270–281.

Moynagh, P., D. Williams, and L. O'Neill. 1994. Activation of NF-kappa B and induction of vascular cell adhesion molecule-1 and intracellular adhesion molecule-1 expression in human glial cells by IL-1. Modulation by antioxidants. *J. Immunol.* **153**:2681–2690.

Neve, J. 1996. Selenium as a risk factor for cardiovascular diseases. *J. Cardiovasc. Risk* **3**:42–47.

Newbold, H. 1989. Vitamin B-12: placebo or neglected therapeutic tool? *Med. Hypotheses* **28**:155–164.

Noseworthy, M., and T. Bray. 1998. Effect of oxidative stress on brain damage detected by MRI and in vivo 31P-NMR. *Free Radic. Biol. Med.* **24**:942–951.

Noseworthy, M., and T. Bray. 2000. Zinc deficiency exacerbates loss in blood-brain barrier integrity induced by hyperoxide measured by dynamic MRI. *Proc. Soc. Exp. Biol. Med.* **223**:175–182.

O'Donnell, E., and M. Lynch. 1998. Dietary antioxidant supplementation reverses age-related neuronal changes. *Neurobiol. Aging* **19**:461–467.

Owen, A., M. Batterham, Y. Probst, B. Grenyer, and L. Tapsell. 2005. Low plasma vitamin E in major depression: diet or disease? *Eur. J. Clin. Nutr.* **59**:304–306.

Oztas, B., S. Kilac, E. Dural, and T. Ispir. 2001. Influence of antioxidants on the blood-brain barrier permeability during epileptic seizures. *J. Neurosci. Res.* **66**:674–678.

Pace, G., and C. Leaf. 1995. The raise of oxidative stress in HIV disease. *Free Radic. Biol. Med.* **19**:523–528.

Parkinson Study Group. 1993. Effects of tocopherol and deprenyl on the progression of disability in early Parkinson's disease. *N. Engl. J. Med.* **328**:176–183.

Penland, J., and J. Finley. 1995. Dietary selenium and mood states in healthy young men. *N. Dakota Acad. Sci. Proc.* **49**:26.

Penland, J., H. Sandstead, N. Alcock, H. Dayal, X. Chen, J. Li, F. Zhao, and J. Yang. 1997. A preliminary report: effects of zinc and micronutrient repletion on growth and neuropsychological function of urban Chinese children. *J. Am. Coll. Nutr.* **16**:268–272.

Penland, J., H. Sandstead, N. Egger, H. Dayal, N. Alcock, R. Plotkin, C. Rocco, and A. Zavaleta. 1999. Zinc, iron and micronutrient supplementation effectis on cognitive and psychomotor function of Mexican-American school children. *FASEB J.* **13**:A921.

Perlmutter, D. 1999. Functional therapeutics in neurodegenerative disease. *J. Applied Nutr.* **51**:3–13.

Persidsky, Y. 1999. Model systems for studies of leukocyte migration across the blood-brain barrier. *J. Neurovirol.* **5**:579–590.

Phillips, S., and K. Kahaner. 1988. An unusual presentation of vitamin B12 deficiency. *Am. J. Psychiatry* **145**:529.

Pocernich, C., R. Sultana, H. Mohmmad-Abdul, A. Nath, and D. Butterfield. 2005. HIV-dementia, Tat-induced oxidative stress, and antioxidant therapeutic considerations. *Brain Res. Brain Res. Rev.* **50**:14–26.

Polidori, M., P. Mecocci, and B. Frei. 2001. Plasma vitamin C levels are decreased and correlated with brain damage in patients with intracranial hemorrhage or head trauma. *Stroke* **32**:898–902.

Porta, E. 1998. Role of oxidative damage in the aging process, p. 1–52. *In* C. Chow (ed.), *Cellular Antioxidant Defense Mechanisms.* CRC Press, Boca Raton, FL.

Prasad, A. D. 2007. Zinc: mechanisms of host defense. *J. Nutrition* **137**:1345–1349.

Prasad, A., P. Rabbani, and A. Abbash. 1978. Experimental zinc deficiency in humans. *Ann. Intern. Med.* **89**:483.

Price, R. W., L. G. Epstein, J. T. Becker, P. Cinque, M. Gisslen, L. Pulliam, and J. C. McArthur. 2007. Biomarkers of HIV-1 CNS infection and injury. *Neurology* **69**:1781–1788.

Pu, H., J. Tian, I. Andras, K. Hayashi, G. Flora, B. Hennig, and M. Toborek. 2005. HIV Tat protein-induced alterations of ZO-1 expression are mediated by redox-regulated ERK1/2 activation. *J. Cereb. Blood Flow Metab.* **25**:1325–1335.

Pulliam, L., R. Gascon, M. Stubblebine, D. McGuire, and M. McGrath. 1997. Unique monocyte subset in patients with AIDS dementia. *Lancet* **349**:692–695.

Rabkin, J., S. Ferrando, S. Lin, M. Sewell, and M. McElhiney. 2000. Psychological effects of HAART: a 2-year study. *Psychosom. Med.* **62**:413–422.

Raemaekers, V., M. Calomme, D. Vanden Berghe, et al. 1994. Selenium deficiency triggering intractable seizures. *Neuropediatrics* **25**:217–223.

Rausch, D., and M. Davis. 2001. HIV in the CNS: pathogenic relationships to systemic HIV disease and other CNS diseases. *J. Neurovirol.* **7**:85–96.

Remacha, A., J. Cadafalch, P. Sarda, M. Barcelo, and M. Fuster. 2003. Vitamin B-12 metabolism in HIV-infected patients in the age of highly active antiretroviral therapy: role of homocysteine in assessing vitamin B-12 status. Am. J. Clin. Nutr. 77:420–424.

Roederer, M., F. Stall, P. Raju, S. Ela, and L. Herzenberg. 1990. Cytokine-stimulated human immunodeficiency virus replication is inhibited by N-acetyl-l-cysteine. Proc. Natl. Acad. Sci. USA 87:4884.

Ronaghy, H., J. Reinhold, M. Mahloudji, P. Ghavami, M. Fox, and J. Halsted. 1974. Zinc supplementation of malnourished schoolboys in Iran: increased growth and other effects. Am. J. Clin. Nutr. 27:112–121.

Rousseau, M., C. Molines, J. Moreau, and J. Delmont. 2000. Influence of highly active antiretroviral therapy on micronutrient profiles in HIV-infected patients. Ann. Nutr. Metab. 44:212–216.

Roy, M., L. Kiremidjian-Schumacher, H. Wishe, M. Cohen, and G. Stotzky. 1993. Selenium supplementation enhances the expression of interleukin 2 receptor subunits and internalization of interleukin 2. Proc. Soc. Exp. Biol. Med. 202:231–295.

Ryan, L., R. Cotter, W. Zink, H. Gendelman, and J. Zheng. 2002. Macrophages, chemokines and neuronal injury in HIV-1 associated dementia. Cell. Mol. Biol. 48:137–150.

Sacktor, N., M. McDermott, K. Marder, G. Schifitto, O. Selnes, J. McArthur, Y. Stern, S. Albert, D. Palumbo, K. Kieburtz, J. De Marcaida, B. Cohen, and L. Epstein. 2002. HIV-associated cognitive impairment before and after the advent of combination therapy. J. Neurovirol. 8:136–142.

Sano, M., C. Ernesto, R. Thomas, M. Klauber, K. Schafer, M. Grundman, P. Woodbury, J. Growdon, C. Cotman, E. Pfeiffer, L. Schneider, and L. Thal. 1997. A controlled trial of selegiline, alpha-tocopherol, or both as treatment for Alzheimer's disease. N. Engl. J. Med. 336:1216–1222.

Sappey, C., S. Legrand-Poels, M. Best-Belpomme, A. Favier, B. Rentier, and J. Piette. 1994. Stimulation of glutathione peroxidase activity decreases HIV type 1 activation after oxidative stress. AIDS 10:1451–1461.

Sayed, M., and J. Eaton. 1992. Hemoglobin-induced oxidant damage to the central nervous system, p. 23–32. In M. Moslen and C. Smith (ed.), Free Radical Mechanisms of Tissue Injury. CRC Press, Boca Raton, FL.

Schmidt, R., M. Hayn, B. Reinhart, G. Roob, H. Schmidt, M. Schumacher, N. Watzinger, and L. Launer. 1998. Plasma antioxidants and cognitive performance in middle-aged and older adults: results of the Austrian Stroke Prevention Study. J. Am. Geriatr. Soc. 46:1407–1410.

Schreck, R., P. Rieber, and P. Baeuerle. 1991. Reactive oxygen intermediates as apparently widely used messengers in the activation of the NF-kB transcription factor and HIV-1. EMBO J. 10:2247.

Schwabe, J., and D. Rhodes. 1991. Beyond zinc fingers: steroid hormone receptors have a novel structural motif for DNA recognition. Trends Biochem. Sci. 16:291.

Semba, R., N. Graham, W. Caiaffa, J. Margolick, L. Clement, and D. Vlahov. 1993. Increased mortality associated with vitamin A deficiency during human immunodeficiency virus type I infection. Arch. Intern. Med. 153:2149–2154.

Sewell, M., K. Goggin, J. Rabkin, S. Ferrando, M. McElhiney, and S. Evans. 2000. Anxiety syndromes and symptoms among men with AIDS: a longitudinal controlled study. Psychosomatics 41:294–300.

Shi, B., J. Raina, A. Lorenzo, J. Busciglio, and D. Gabuzda. 1998. Neuronal apoptosis induced by HIV-1 at protein and TNF-alpha: potentiation of neurotoxicity mediated by oxidative stress and implications for HIV-1 dementia. J. Neurovirol. 4:281–290.

Shor-Posner, G., and M. Baum. 1996. Nutritional alterations in HIV-1 seronegative drug users. Nutrition 12:555–556.

Shor-Posner, G., D. Feaster, N. Blaney, H. Rocca, E. Mantero-Atienza, J. Szapocznik, C. Eisdorfer, K. Goodkin, and M. Baum. 1994. Impact of vitamin B6 status on psychological distress in a longitudinal study of HIV-1 infection. Int. J. Psychiatry Med. 24:209–222.

Shor-Posner, G., R. Lecusay, M. Miguez, G. Moreno-Black, G. Zhang, N. Rodriguez, X. Burbano, M. Baum, and F. Wilkie. 2003. Psychological burden in the era of HAART: impact of selenium therapy. Int. J. Psychiatry Med. 33:555–569.

Shor-Posner, G., R. Lecusay, G. Morales, A. Campa, and M. Miguez-Burbano. 2002. Neuroprotection in HIV-positive drug users: implications for antioxidant therapy. J. Acquir. Immune Defic. Syndr. 31:S84–S88.

Shor-Posner, G., R. Morgan, F. Wilkie, C. Eisdorfer, and M. Baum. 1995. Plasma cobalamin levels affect information processing speed in a longitudinal study of HIV-1 disease. Arch. Neurol. 52:195–198.

Shukla, A., M. Dikshit, and R. Srimal. 1995. Status of antioxidants in brain microvessels of monkey and rat. Free Radic. Res. 22:303–308.

Skurnick, J., J. Bogden, H. Baker, F. Kemp, A. Sheffet, G. Qualtrone, and D. Louria. 1996. Micronutrient profiles in HIV-1-infected heterosexual adults. J. Acquir. Immune Defic. Syndr. 12:75–83.

Smith, C., J. Carney, P. Starke-Reed, C. Oliver, E. Stadtman, R. Floyd, and W. Markesbery. 1991. Excess brain protein oxidation and enzyme dysfunction in normal aging and in Alzheimer disease. Proc. Natl. Acad. Sci. USA 88:1540–1543.

Smith, M., G. Perry, P. Richey, L. Sayre, V. Anderson, M. Beal, and N. Jowall. 1996. Oxidative damage in Alzheimer's. Nature 382:120–121.

Smits, H., L. Boven, C. Pereira, J. Verhoef, and H. Nottet. 2001. Role of macrophage activation in the pathogenesis of Alzheimer's disease and human immunodeficiency virus type 1-associated dementia. Eur. J. Clin. Investig. 30:526–535.

Staal, F., M. Roederer, L. Herzenberg, and L. Herzenberg. 1990. Intracellular thiols regulate activation of nuclear factor kappa B and transcription of human immunodeficiency virus. Proc. Natl. Acad. Sci. USA 87:9943.

Stephenson, C. B., G. S. Marquis, S. D. Douglas, L. A. Kruzich, and C. M. Wilson. 2007. Glutathione, glutathione peroxidase, and selenium status in HIV-positive and HIV-negative adolescents and young adults. Am. J. Clin. Nutr. 85:173–181.

Stoeck, M., W. Kromer, and V. Gekeler. 1998. Induction of IL-15 mRNA and protein in A549 cells by pro-inflammatory cytokines. Immunobiology 199:14–22.

Takeda, A. 2004. Essential trace metals and brain function. Yakugaku Zasshi 124:577–585.

Tanala, Y., S. Shiozawa, I. Morito, and T. Fujita. 1990. Role of zinc in interleukin 2 mediated T-cell activation. Scand. J. Immunol. 31:547.

Tang, A., N. Graham, R. Semba, and A. Saah. 1997. Association between serum vitamin A and E levels and HIV-1 disease progression. AIDS 11:613–620.

Tang, A., J. Lanzillotti, K. Hendricks, J. Gerrior, M. Ghosh, M. Woods, and C. Wanke. 2005. Micronutrients: current issues for HIV care providers. AIDS 19:847–861.

Tang, A., and E. Smit. 2000. Oxidative stress in HIV-1-infected injection drug users. J. Acquir. Immune Defic. Syndr. 25:S12–S18.

Tucker, D., and H. Sandstead. 1984. Neuropsychological function in experimental zinc deficiency in humans, p. 139–152. In C. Frederickson, G. Howell, and E. Kasarskis (ed.), The Neurobiology of Zinc. Part B. Deficiency, Toxicity and Pathology. Alan R. Liss, New York, NY.

Tully, C., D. Snowdon, and W. Markesbery. 1995. Serum zinc, senile plaques and neurofibrillary tangles: findings from the Nun Study. Neuroreport 6:2105–2108.

Turchan, J., C. Pocernich, C. Gairola, A. Chauhan, G. Schifitto, D. Butterfield, S. Buch, O. Narayan, A. Sinai, J. Geiger J. Berger, H. Elford, and A. Nath. 2003a. Oxidative stress in HIV demented patients and protection ex vivo with novel antioxidants. *Neurology* **60:**307–314.

Turchan, J., N. Sacktor, V. Wojna, K. Conant, and A. Nath. 2003b. Neuroprotective therapy for HIV dementia. *Curr. HIV Res.* **1:**373–383.

Verbanck, P., and L. Oliver. 1991. Changing psychiatric symptoms in a patient with vitamin B12 deficiency. *J. Clin. Psychiatry* **52:**182–183.

Wanke, C., M. Silva, T. Knox, J. Forrester, D. Spiegelman, and S. Gorbach. 2000. Weight loss and wasting remain common complications in individuals infected with human immunodeficiency virus in the era of highly active antiretroviral therapy. *Clin. Infect. Dis.* **31:**803–805.

Wefers, H., and H. Seis. 1988. The protection by ascorbate and glutathione against lipid peroxidation is dependent on vitamin E. *Eur. J. Biochem.* **174:**353–357.

Whitney, E., and S. Rolfes. 1999. *Understanding Nutrition*, 8th ed., p. 290–435. West/Wadsworth, Belmont, CA.

Wilkie, F., R. Goodkin, R. Morgan, D. Feaster, M. Fletcher, N. Blaney, M. Baum, J. Szapocznik, and C. Eisdorfer. 1998. Mild cognitive impairment and risk of mortality in HIV-1 infection. *J. Neuropsychiatry Clin. Neurosci.* **10:**125–132.

Woods, M. N., A. M. Tang, J. Forrester, C. Jones, K. Hendricks, B. Ding, and T. A. Knox. 2003. Effect of dietary intake and protease inhibitors on serum vitamin B12 levels in a cohort of human immunodeficiency virus-positive patients. *Clin. Infect. Dis.* **37:**124–131.

Yost, H., and E. Kligman. 2001. Nutritional modulation of neurodegenerative disorders, p. 333–341. *In* R. Watson (ed.), *Handbook of Nutrition in the Aged*, 3rd ed. CRC Press, Boca Raton, FL.

Zhang, Z., P. Inserra, B. Liang, and R. Watson. 1998. Antioxidants and AIDS, p. 179–192. *In* R. Watson (ed.), *Nutrients and Foods in AIDS*. CRC Press, Boca Raton, FL.

Zinkernagel, C., P. Taffe, M. Rickenbach, R. Amiet, B. Ledergerber, A. Volkart, U. Rauchfleisch, A. Kiss, V. Werder, P. Vernazza, M. Battegay, and Swiss HIV Cohort Study. 2001. Importance of mental health assessment in HIV-infected outpatients. *J. Acquir. Immune Defic. Syndr.* **28:**240–249.

Zucker, D., R. Livingston, R. Nakra, and P. Clayton. 1981. B12 deficiency and psychiatric disorders: case report and literature review. *Biol. Psychiatry* **16:**197–205.

The Spectrum of Neuro-AIDS Disorders:
Pathophysiology, Diagnosis, and Treatment
Edited by K. Goodkin et al.
©2008 ASM Press, Washington, DC

17

Cell Cycle Proteins and the Pathogenesis of HIV-1 Encephalitis in the HAART Era

KELLY L. JORDAN-SCIUTTO AND CAGLA AKAY

The clinical syndrome HIV-associated dementia complex (HAD) is notable for cognitive, motor, and behavioral abnormalities that suggest a preponderance of subcortical damage (Grant et al., 1987; Navia et al., 1986; Pierce et al., 1998; Portegies et al., 1993). Early neurologic symptoms appear to be reversible (DeCarli et al., 1991; Portegies et al., 1993); however, later a progressive neurologic deficit becomes fixed. The neuropathology associated with HAD consists of perivascular chronic inflammatory cells, microglial nodules, and multinucleated giant cells (Navia et al., 1986). These features are the hallmarks of HIV encephalitis (HIVE), which was defined by histopathologic measurement of activated and/or infected macrophages and viral burden (Budka, 1991). Though most cases of HIVE exhibit a high central nervous system (CNS) viral burden (Wiley and Achim, 1994; Wiley et al., 1998), there are cases with high CNS viral burdens without documented evidence of HAD. This suggests that HIV needs to be present in the brain for a finite period of time to mediate neurological damage. These findings suggest that HAD occurs after a prolonged exposure of the brain to HIV-infected and/or -activated cells, which initially disrupts neuronal function in a reversible manner but ultimately results in neuronal loss.

HIVE: PROPOSED ETIOLOGIES

Although the etiology of HIVE is covered in greater detail in previous chapters, it is necessary to place the discussion of the role of cell cycle proteins within the context of what is known about HIV infection and progression to HIVE. It is now widely accepted that HIV enters the brain via infection of macrophages that cross the blood-brain barrier and differentiate into microglia (Kaul et al., 2001). Although a small percentage of neurons and glia may become infected (Nuovo et al., 1994; Saito et al., 1994; Tornatore et al., 1994), such infection is not productive. Instead, neuronal

damage correlates best with the presence of HIV-infected, activated macrophages (Gelbard et al., 1994). Currently two major theories have been proposed for the pathogenesis of neuronal damage in HIVE: (i) neurotoxicity of HIV proteins such as the HIV envelope and HIV tat transactivator proteins (Benos et al., 1994; Bernardo et al., 1994; Kaiser et al., 1990; Levi et al., 1993; Lipton, 1993; Savio and Levi, 1993; Toggas et al., 1994); and (ii) neurotoxicity of factors secreted by activated macrophages regardless of their infection status (Achim et al., 1994; Achim and Wiley, 1992, 1996; Brouwers et al., 1993; Crowe, 1995; Gelbard et al., 1994; Giulian et al., 1996; Heyes et al., 1998; Lipton et al., 1991; Lo et al., 1992; Masliah et al., 1992; Power et al., 1993, 1998; Price et al., 1988; Pulliam et al., 1994, 1996; Wiley and Achim, 1994; Wiley et al., 1998). HAD is likely caused by a combination of these two toxic events in vivo. Macrophage-secreted factors associated with HIV and neurologic damage in the CNS of AIDS patients include monokines, chemokines, neurotrophic factors (NTF), reactive oxygen species (ROS), excitotoxic molecules, and quinolinic acid. Macrophage-secreted factors act in a paracrine fashion to stimulate reactive CNS cells (i.e., astrocytes, microglia, etc.) to further increase the level and variety of signaling molecules in the neuronal extracellular milieu (Giulian et al., 1996). Factors such as cytokines, chemokines, NTF, excitotoxic molecules, and ROS activate distinct responses in neurons. Since both neurotrophic and neurotoxic factors are present, the neuronal response cannot be predicted simply by knowing the identity of all the stimuli.

DETERMINANTS OF NEURONAL VIABILITY

The neuronal interpretation of the conflicting signaling environment in HIVE ultimately determines viability. In neurons, factors such as NTF and chemokines have been reported to activate survival pathways as part of their signaling cascades, whereas ROS and cytokines can induce death via apoptosis or necrosis (Annunziato et al., 2003; Barzilai et al., 2003; Bibel and Barde, 2000; Boldyrev et al., 2000; D'Mello, 1998; Holmin and Mathiesen,

Kelly L. Jordan-Sciutto and Cagla Akay, Department of Pathology, University of Pennsylvania, Philadelphia, PA 19104-6030.

2000; Nicotera et al., 1997; Pulliam et al., 1998; Takikita et al., 2001). Further, in in vitro neuronal cultures, NTF have been shown to protect against death by ROS and HIV viral coat protein gp120 (Bachis et al., 2003). These experiments hint at the complexity of determining the mechanism of neuronal loss in HIVE. Common downstream targets of both the neuroprotective and neurotoxic factors implicated in HIVE are the regulators of cell cycle progression. As the key regulators of cell differentiation, division, senescence, and death, cell cycle proteins have been ascribed numerous roles in diseases as varied as cancer and neurodegeneration. This chapter discusses the known mechanisms by which cell cycle proteins regulate viability, which of these mechanisms are at play in regulating neuronal viability, evidence that cell cycle regulators are stimulated in HIV encephalitis, the implications of these findings in the post-HAART era, and their potential for additional therapy.

HOW CELL CYCLE PROTEINS REGULATE CELLULAR VIABILITY

The three cell cycle proteins implicated in regulating cell viability are retinoblastoma (pRb), E2F1, and p53 (Harbour and Dean, 2000). pRb and p53 are the two key targets of signaling pathways that regulate cellular decisions to divide, differentiate, or die. These tumor suppressor proteins are targeted for inactivation in virtually all cancers by direct or indirect mechanisms, suggesting that they are the master determinants of cell cycle progression. Understanding their activities and regulation in nonneuronal populations will provide the groundwork for appreciating their salient roles in neuronal response to neurodegenerative stimuli in HIV encephalitis.

Functions of pRb and E2F1

The pRb protein was the first member of the pocket protein family to be identified. Along with its family members, p107 and p130, pRb coordinates orderly progression through the cell cycle. Deletion of p107 and p130 can compensate for each other, but not for loss of pRb. Despite functional overlap, each of the three pocket protein family members has its own unique contribution to progression through the cell cycle. All three proteins contain a "pocket domain," which is the protein interaction motif known to bind and regulate members of the E2F family (E2F1 through E2F6) as well as interact with viral oncoproteins such as adenovirus E1A or simian virus 40 T antigen. A major difference between p107, p130, and pRb is the E2F family members that they bind. Whereas pRb binds to E2F1-3, p107 and p130 prefer E2F4 and 5. Much research has specifically defined the contribution of the pocket protein-E2F complexes to each phase of the cell cycle. Most important for this discussion are p130 and pRb. The p130-E2F4 complex binds E2F-containing promoters and represses their expression, which maintains the cells in G_0. In differentiated cells like neurons, E2F sites are largely occupied by p130-E2F4 complexes. In nonneuronal cells stimulated to proliferate, pRb assumes regulation of E2F sites by direct interaction with E2F1, 2, or 3 in G_1 phase (Fig. 1) (Adams and Kaelin, 1995; Kouzarides, 1995). While in complex with pRb, E2F1 represses transcription of genes necessary for S-phase progression, cell cycle control, and apoptosis (Cress et al., 1993; Flemington et al., 1993; Hagemeier et al., 1993; Helin et al., 1993a). Phosphorylation of pRb inactivates pRb by disrupting its interaction with E2F1

or E2F family members E2F2 and E2F3. Free of pRb, E2F1 activates expression of target genes which include DNA polymerase alpha, proliferating cell nuclear antigen, cyclin A, cyclin E, cyclin-dependent kinase 1 (CDK1) and CDK2, etc. (Farnham et al., 1993; LaThangue, 1994; Nevins, 1998; Scherr, 1998). Expression of these genes leads to progression through S phase. At the end of S phase, E2F1 activity is downregulated through phosphorylation by its own target gene products, cyclin A and CDK2, allowing progression to the G_2 phase of the cell cycle (Farnham et al., 1993; LaThangue, 1994).

In mitogenesis, phosphorylation of pRb usually occurs in response to signaling via growth factor binding to tyrosine kinase receptors such as platelet-derived growth factor (PDGF) binding to PDGF receptor. PDGF receptor and its family members signal an intracellular cascade of phosphorylation events resulting in production of D-type cyclins which bind CDK4 or CDK6, forming an active kinase that targets phosphorylation of pRb. Further phosphorylation of pRb occurs by newly synthesized cyclin E-CDK2, which leads to release of E2F1 and production of genes necessary for entry into S phase.

E2F1 regulates not only the genes necessary for DNA synthesis and cell cycle control but also those that induce cell death including APAF, BAX, and p14^{ARF} (DeGregori et al., 1997; Hallstrom and Nevins, 2003). When E2F1 is not inhibited by pRb as in the pRb$^{-/-}$ mice, massive neuronal loss occurs during neurogenesis at E14.5 (Clarke et al., 1992; Jacks et al., 1992; Lee et al., 1992). In pRb$^{-/-}$ E2F1$^{-/-}$ double-knockout mice, neurogenesis occurs normally (Tsai et al., 1998), suggesting that E2F1 activity is regulated by pRb in developing neurons and that deregulation of E2F1 results in apoptosis in these cells.

Although E2F1 is part of a family of proteins that contains seven known members, E2F1 appears to play a predominant role in regulating apoptosis via a p53-dependent mechanism by increasing transcription of p14^{ARF}, the p53-stabilizing protein (Fig. 1) (Bates et al., 1998). The newly synthesized p14^{ARF} protein interacts with MDM2, preventing MDM2-p53 interaction. MDM2 shuttles p53 into the cytoplasm and targets p53 for degradation by the proteosome. By blocking MDM2-p53 interaction, p14^{ARF} stabilizes p53, which can now induce apoptosis by activating expression of apoptotic genes. Thus, p14^{ARF} mediates E2F1-induced death in a p5-dependent manner. However, increased expression of E2F1 induces apoptosis in p53-deficient cells as well (Hsieh et al., 1997; Phillips et al., 1999; Pierce et al., 1998), indicating the existence of an alternate pathway. One mechanism for p53-independent apoptosis has been suggested to involve the death receptor cascade (Phillips et al., 1999). In this model, increased E2F1 expression results in a decrease in TRAF2 protein levels. TRAF2 is an inhibitor of death receptor-mediated apoptosis (Duckett and Thompson, 1997). Alternatively, promoters containing E2F-binding elements include BAX and APAF, two regulators of apoptotic activation, suggesting that E2F1 can induce apoptosis by increasing expression of proapoptotic gene products. These data suggest that E2F1 can induce apoptosis by several mechanisms, which can be p53 dependent and p53 independent.

Functions of p53

Although originally identified as a regulator of cell cycle progression, the tumor suppressor gene p53 plays a major role in adaptation of the cell to a multitude of stimuli (hypoxia, ionizing radiation, heat shock, genotoxicity, viral infection,

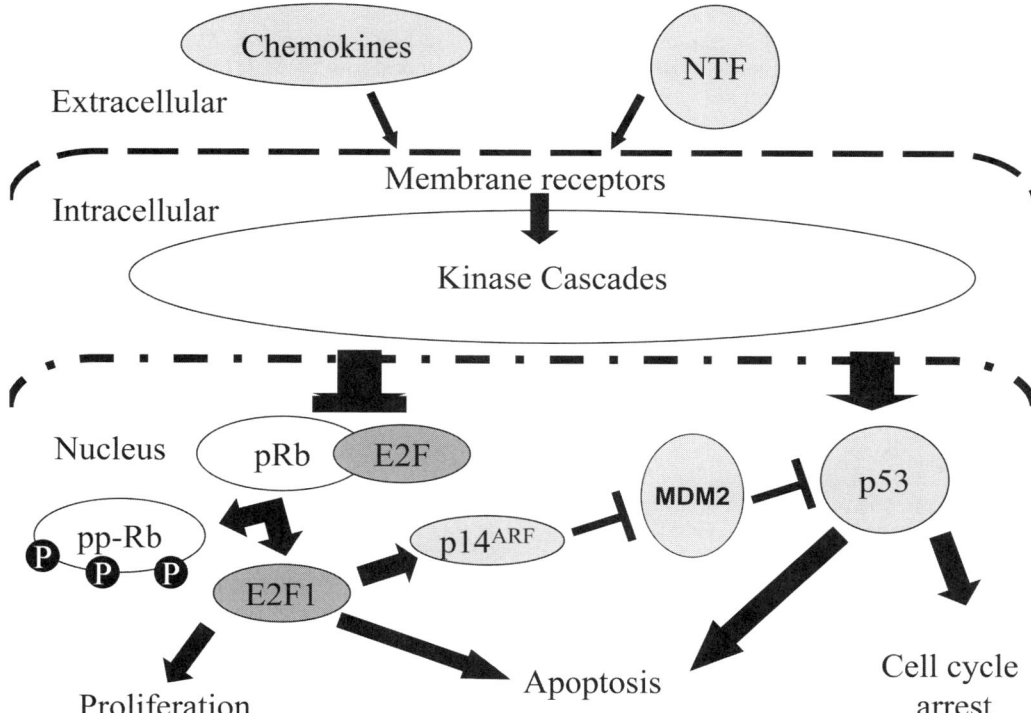

FIGURE 1 Potential cell cycle protein response to extracellular signaling of chemokines and NTF. NTF and chemokines bind membrane receptors and activate various intracellular kinase cascades. These cascades can result in activation of p53 and inactivation of pRb by phosphorylation. ppRb releases E2F1, allowing it to induce expression from promoters that can promote proliferation or apoptosis. E2F1 can also induce expression of p14^ARF, which will activate p53 by inhibiting MDM2-mediated degradation of p53. p53 activated by p14^ARF can lead to apoptosis or cell cycle arrest.

etc.) that are potentially lethal. Thus, it is not surprising that p53 stands at the crossroads of signaling pathways dictating whether a cell should exit the cell cycle, undergo apoptosis, contribute to differentiation, or become senescent. As such, p53 function has been intensely investigated from several perspectives. In dividing cells p53 is expressed at low levels and is targeted for proteosomal degradation through its association with the MDM2 protein. Following cellular stress, p53 levels are stabilized by posttranslational modifications (i.e., phosphorylation) or disruption of its interactions with MDM2 (as described earlier). When stabilized, p53 transactivates expression of genes whose products trigger cell cycle arrest, cell survival, or cell death. Cell cycle arrest results when p53 increases the mRNA levels of the CDK inhibitor p21cdki (Vogelstein et al., 2000). p21cdki is sufficient to cause G1 arrest by blocking activity of CDK phosphorylation of pRb (Poluha et al., 1997) but may not be the only p53 target capable of doing so, since p21cdki-deficient cells can still arrest in G1 by a p53-dependent mechanism (el-Deiry, 1998; el-Deiry et al., 1994). How p53 causes apoptosis is still not completely understood. It has been shown that p53 transcriptionally induces expression of the BCL-2 antagonist, BAX, which can induce apoptosis (el-Deiry, 1998; el-Deiry et al., 1994), as well as other apoptotic regulators including APAF1, PUMA, and NOXA. However, p53 can also cause apoptosis in the presence of protein and mRNA synthesis antagonists (Caelles et al., 1994). Therefore, p53 causes apoptosis by several mechanisms, some as yet undefined.

CELL CYCLE PROTEINS ALSO PARTICIPATE IN REGULATION OF NEURONAL DEATH

E2F1 and Phosphorylation of pRb in Neuronal Death

Using in vitro neuronal culture models, E2F1 and phosphorylation of pRb have been shown to be necessary and sufficient for neuronal cell death (Giovanni et al., 1999, 2000; Park et al., 1997b, 2000b). Increasing pRb phosphorylation by forced expression of cyclin D1 induces neuronal apoptosis, demonstrating that pRb phosphorylation is sufficient for neuronal death (Freeman et al., 1994; Kranenburg et al., 1996). Phosphorylation of pRb has been observed in several in vitro models of neuronal apoptosis including trophic factor withdrawal, DNA damage, low potassium levels, beta-amyloid treatment, and oxidative stress (Boutillier et al., 2000; Giovanni et al., 1999, 2000; Liu and Greene, 2001; Mirjany et al., 2002; Morris et al., 2001; Padmanabhan et al., 1999; Park et al., 1997a, 2000a, 2000b; Rideout et al., 2003; Trinh et al., 2001). Blocking pRb phosphorylation in many of these models prevents apoptosis as effectively as does blocking caspase activation, demonstrating that pRb phosphorylation is necessary for neuronal death. Once pRb is phosphorylated, it should release E2F1, which can induce apoptosis through p53-dependent or p53-independent pathways. Increased E2F1 expression in cerebellar granule neurons was sufficient to induce apoptosis (O'Hare et al., 2000). While no report has indicated a role for E2F1 in neuronal death due to DNA damage, neuronal cultures from E2F1$^{-/-}$ embryos were resistant to death by trophic factor withdrawal, low potassium levels, beta-amyloid treatment, and oxidative stress via dopamine treatment (Coulier et al., 1990; Giovanni et al., 2000; Hou et al., 2001; Trinh et al., 2001). Interestingly, p53 was not required for death in response to a subset of these toxins. The requirement for E2F1 and pRb phosphorylation to induce neuronal loss indicates that these proteins are part of the cascade leading to neuronal loss. Further investigation is necessary to determine if they are the ultimate targets for deciding between life and death in neurons for the subset of toxins associated with neurodegeneration in response to HIVE.

Role for p53 in Neuronal Death

As in cell cycle progression, pRb and E2F1 are only half the story for regulation of neuronal death. p53 has been implicated in neuronal loss in response to numerous and varied insults in vitro and in human neurodegenerative diseases. Roles for p53 have been ascertained in two ways: (i) by demonstrating an increase in p53 proteins levels, indicating stabilization of p53; or (ii) by inhibiting or genetically deleting p53 in neuronal cells and assessing protection from insult or disease progression. Table 1 summarizes the data supporting

a role for p53 in various models of neuronal loss (Morrison et al., 2003). As shown in this table, p53 is both upregulated in response to, and necessary for death due to, stimuli including excitotoxicity (e.g., glutamate), oxidative damage (e.g., dopamine and 6-hydroxydopamine), mitochondrial dysfunction (MPTP [1-methyl-4-phenyl-1,2,3,6-tetrahydropyridine]), DNA damage (e.g., ionizing radiation and hereditary DNA damage disorders), and neurodegenerative stimuli (e.g., Alzheimer's disease [AD], amyotrophic lateral sclerosis [ALS], Huntington's disease, HIVE, etc.). Although there appear to be some insults in which p53 is either not induced or not required for protection, p53 plays an undeniable role in a plethora of neuronal responses to toxicity.

While regulation of p53 is still a subject of intense investigation, there is already abundant evidence that p53 stability is regulated by phosphorylation. Exactly how phosphorylation of p53 leads to stability of the protein is not completely understood, but it has been suggested that phosphorylation disrupts and/or changes the interaction with MDM2, leading to increased p53 stability. At least two phosphorylation sites have been identified as important for increased p53 stability and/or DNA binding activity, serine 392 and serine 18. Kinases known to phosphorylate p53 in response

TABLE 1 Summary of neuronal insults in which p53 levels are induced and/or required for cell death[a]

Condition/treatment	Increased p53 levels	p53 loss is protective[b]	Type of study	Reference(s)
Adrenalectomy	Yes	Yes	In vivo	Sakhi et al., 1996
AD	Yes	ND	In vivo	de la Monte et al., 1997; Kitamura et al., 1997; Kohji et al., 1998
AB peptide		Yes/no	In vitro	Culmsee et al., 2001; Zhang et al., 2002/ Giovanni et al., 2000
AB transgenic mouse	Yes	ND	In vivo	LaFerla et al., 1996
ALS	Yes	No	In vivo	Kuntz et al., 2000; Prudlo et al., 2000
Angelman syndrome	Yes	ND	In vivo	Jiang et al., 1998
Developmental death		Yes	In vivo	Aloyz et al., 1998
Dopamine	Yes	No	In vitro	Daily et al., 1999
Excitotoxicity	Yes	Yes/no	In vivo/in vitro	Sakhi et al., 1994; Tan et al., 2002/Schauwecker and Steward, 1997
Genotoxic injury (bleomycin, camptothecin, cytosine arabinoside)	Yes	Yes	In vitro	Araki et al., 1998; Chen et al., 1999; Culmsee et al., 2001; Enokido et al., 1996a; Morris et al., 2001; Xiang et al., 1998
Glutamate	Yes	Yes	In vitro	Chen and Chuang, 1999; Culmsee et al., 2001; Uberti et al., 1998; Xiang et al., 1996
Hereditary DNA repair disorders	Yes	ND	In vivo	Kohji et al., 1998
HIVE	Yes	ND	In vivo	Garden et al., 2004
Huntington's disease	Yes	ND	In vitro	Steffan et al., 2000
6-Hydroxydopamine	Yes	No	In vitro	Blum et al., 1997; Hou et al., 2001
Hypoxia	Yes	Yes	In vitro	Banasiak and Haddad, 1998; Halterman et al., 1999
Ionizing radiation	Yes	Yes	In vitro	Enokido et al., 1996b; Johnson et al., 1998
Ischemia	Yes	Yes	In vivo	Chopp et al., 1992; Crumrine et al., 1994; Watanabe et al., 1999
Methamphetamine	Yes	Yes	In vivo	Hirata and Cadet, 1997
MPTP		Yes	In vivo	Trimmer et al., 1996
NGF withdrawal	Yes	Yes/no	In vivo	Aloyz et al., 1998; Vogel and Parada, 1998/ Sadoul et al., 1996
Rb deficiency	Yes	Yes	In vivo	Macleod et al., 1996
Spinal cerebellar ataxia		Yes	In vivo	Zhang et al., 2002
Traumatic brain injury	Yes	ND	In vivo	Muir et al., 1999; Napieralski et al., 1999

[a]Reprinted from *Experimental Neurology* (Strachan et al., 2005) with permission from the publisher.
[b]Yes/no, independent reports gave conflicting interpretations; ND, not determined.

to various stresses include DNA protein kinase, mutated in ataxia telangectasia, ataxia telangectasia-Rad3-related, jun-N-terminal kinase, and p38 kinase. Finally, increased p53 levels may also be attributed to activation of nuclear factor κB (NF-kB). NF-κB is a transcriptional regulator that is sequestered in the cytoplasm and released to the nucleus in response to a number of cellular stresses, both physiologic and pathologic. One can speculate that at least part of NF-κB-induced survival is mediated by increasing p53 levels. Whatever the mechanism, p53 needs to be stabilized to regulate survival or death.

As with p53 regulation, the mechanism of p53-mediated death in nonneuronal and neuronal cells is a subject of intense investigation. As a transcriptional regulator, at least one mechanism by which p53 exerts its effects on cell viability is via activation of p53 target gene promoters. Among p53-regulated genes are both cell survival and cell death proteins. Activation of p21^{cdki} expression leads to cell cycle arrest; however, the effects of expression of a CDK inhibitor in neuronal cells which are permanently postmitotic are not clear. To induce death in nonneuronal cells, p53 increases expression of the proapoptotic proteins BAX, APAF1, FAS, FAS ligand, PERP, NOXA, and PUMA, among others. While much work remains to be done to determine the specific role of these proteins in neuronal death, BAX has been shown to be capable of mediating p53-induced neuronal death. BAX is a BCL-2 antagonist. In response to stress, BAX translocates from the cytoplasm to the mitochondria, where it is believed to form pores in the mitochondrial membrane, leading to loss of the mitochondrial membrane potential and release of cytochrome c and mitochondrial Ca^{2+}. Cytochrome c and Ca^{2+} are key components for apoptosome formation (caspase 9, APAF1, cytochrome c, and Ca^{2+}), which leads to activation of the caspase cascade, a defining feature of apoptosis.

Understanding the role of p53 in neuronal death is further confounded by the discovery of p53 family members p63 and p73. While p63 and p73 appear to play more prominent roles in development, at least p73 has also been demonstrated to have the ability to induce apoptosis. Interestingly, p73 has also been found to be mutated in glioblastoma (Watanabe et al., 2002; Yu et al., 2004), implicating it in CNS cell type maintenance. Finally, p73 is a transcriptional target of E2F1, suggesting that it may mediate neuronal loss in models of death determined to be p53 independent. There is much work to be done to determine the specific roles of p53 and its family members in neuronal loss, but clearly these proteins are integral mediators of neuronal viability.

Cell Cycle Proteins in Response to NTF and Chemokines

While neuronal loss is a devastating and irreversible consequence of diseases like HIV encephalitis, it is not the complete story. Inflammatory infiltrates secrete molecules that are neuroprotective as well as neurotoxic. Therefore, we need to consider the role of cell cycle proteins in response to protective agents as well. As neurons are inherently postmitotic, minimal emphasis has been placed on investigating the impact of neuroprotective factors on cell cycle protein regulation; however, both NTF and chemokines bind receptors that are members of larger receptor families whose downstream targets include activation of cell cycle machinery. Therefore, it is important to understand the result of NTF and chemokine signaling on pRb phosphorylation, p53, and E2F1 activity in neurons. Investigations into NTF impact on cell cycle were initiated by Yan and colleagues

(Yan and Ziff, 1995), who demonstrated that nerve growth factor (NGF) did not stimulate pRb phosphorylation in the PC12 model of neuronal differentiation despite the increase in cyclin D1 levels and increased cyclin D1-pRb interaction. The lack of pRb phosphorylation was attributed to the concomitant increase in CDK inhibitor p21^{cdki}, which would inhibit cyclin D-CDK4 activity (Yan and Ziff, 1997). While these results indicate that NGF treatment stimulates part of the cell cycle cascade, the proliferation is inhibited by increase in inhibitors of CDKs. Interestingly, the inhibitor of cyclin D activity stimulated by NGF, p21^{cdki}, is a p53 target. Indeed treatment of PC12 cells with NGF induces p53 stability and nuclear translocation (Hughes et al., 2000). Further, NGF-induced growth arrest in PC12 cells is dependent on p53 and its induction of p21^{cdki}. Thus, NGF treatment does have the potential to stimulate phosphorylation of pRb, but this is kept in check by p53 activation of p21^{cdki}. However, these experiments have two caveats that suggest that the initial interpretations may not be relevant for differentiated neurons. First, PC12 cells are a transformed cell line, suggesting that they have aberrations in their cell cycle regulatory machinery. Therefore, studies using these cells may give a misleading picture of the players involved in the response of a differentiated neuron (like those present in brains of patients with HAD) to NGF. Second, the comparisons for cyclin D1 were made between NGF-treated cells and proliferating cells instead of unstimulated and NGF-treated cells. In a system more reflective of neurons in mature CNS, primary human and murine cortical neuronal cultures, which are neither transformed nor proliferating, were used to investigate pRb phosphorylation and p53 levels in response to NTF and chemokines. In contrast to the PC12 studies, neuronal response to NTF and chemokines increased cytoplasmic levels of E2F1 (Color Plate 5) and pRb phosphorylation (Jordan-Sciutto et al., 2001) (Color Plate 6). Both of these changes were blocked by inhibitors of CDKs. Substantiating these observations, Khan and colleagues (Khan et al., 2003) demonstrated that stimulation of the chemokine receptor CXCR4 by different ligands alters phosphorylation state and subcellular localization of pRb and E2F1 in cerebellar granule neurons and rat hippocampal neurons. Increased cytoplasmic E2F1 staining and phosphorylation of pRb has also been demonstrated in murine cortical neuron cultures responding to brain-derived neurotrophic factor (BDNF), NGF, RANTES, and monocyte chemotactic protein 1 (MCP1) (Strachan et al., 2005) (Color Plates 5 and 6). Interestingly, the increase in E2F1 staining appears to be a change in immunogenicity instead of an overall increase in protein levels (Strachan et al., 2005) (Color Plate 5), suggesting a change in E2F1 function and/or activity in response to neuroprotection. These findings suggest that pRb and E2F1 are downstream targets of chemokine and NTF signaling. However, evidence from these studies indicates that regulation of pRb and E2F1 by NTF and chemokine signaling is different in neurons (Table 2). Phosphorylation of pRb in response to NTF is dependent on translation and nuclear export, while the increase in available E2F1 is not, suggesting that the change in E2F1 is independent of pRb phosphorylation (Table 2). Further, the changes in E2F1 are dependent on cytoskeletal movement, whereas pRb phosphorylation is not. Thus, although pRb and E2F1 are downstream of NTF and chemokine signaling, their regulation and activities may be distinct from those observed in nonneuronal cells (Table 2). This is further supported by the localization of E2F1 in neuronal cells. As a transcriptional regulator, E2F1 is normally nuclear in

TABLE 2 Summary of cellular processes required for changes in ppRb and E2F1 localization and/or levels[a]

Process inhibited	E2F1	ppRb
Translation	−	+
Nuclear export	−	+
CDK	+	+
Microtubule depolymerization	+	−
Microfilament depolymerization	+	−

[a]+, process is required for change; −, process did not block altered localization or increased protein levels.

nonneuronal cells. However, E2F1 is predominantly cytoplasmic in neurons. Cytoplasmic E2F1 has also been observed in differentiated myocytes (Kiess et al., 1995), suggesting either that E2F1 is being sequestered in differentiated cells to prevent activation of cell cycle or apoptosis or that E2F1 has a novel role in the cytoplasm. In either scenario, further investigation of E2F1 regulation and activity in neurons is warranted.

Even less work has been done investigating the response of p53 to NTF or chemokine signaling in primary neurons. In addition to the observed increase in p53 in PC12 cells, p53 has been shown to be altered in primary human fetal neuroglial cultures responding to NTF and chemokines. Interestingly, there is not an increase in the overall levels of p53; instead there is a change in p53 localization. In response to NTF and chemokines, p53 immunostaining is predominantly nuclear in neuronal and astrocytic cells but predominantly cytoplasmic in untreated cells (Jordan-Sciutto et al., 2001). Nuclear localization of p53 without large increases in p53 levels is consistent with potential activation of differentiation, survival targets like p21[cdki], and not apoptotic targets as seen with large increases in p53. Consistent with these findings, Manes and colleagues have demonstrated that p53 is induced in response to CCR5 in breast cancer cells (Manes et al., 2003). Therefore, p53 is a potential target of chemokine and NTF signaling, but still much work needs to be done to understand the role of p53 in dictating neuronal survival, differentiation, and death.

CELL CYCLE PROTEINS IN OTHER NEURODEGENERATIVE DISEASES

Not only is there considerable evidence in vitro supporting a role for p53, E2F1, and pRb in regulation of neuronal death, but there is also in vivo evidence from several neurodegenerative diseases including AD, Parkinson's disease (PD), and ALS, as well as HIVE. Initial work implicating cell cycle proteins in neurodegenerative conditions came from studies in AD, the most common form of dementia among the elderly. Using an antibody to mitotic cells, Vincent and colleagues demonstrated increased staining for mitotic proteins in AD (Vincent et al., 1996). As the cell cycle is highly regulated by kinases and one of the pathologic hallmarks of AD, the neurofibrillary tangle, consists of a hyperphosphorylated protein called tau, it was reasoned that the cell cycle kinases were a likely candidate for aberrant activity in AD. This led to the identification of several cyclins, CDKs, and CDK inhibitors as having altered expression in AD including cyclin A, cyclin B, cyclin D, CDK4, CDK5, CDK inhibitors p16[ink4a] and p21[cdki], PCNA, and Ki67 (Arendt et al., 1996, 1998; Baumann et al., 1993; Busser et al., 1998; Hoozemans et al., 2002; Lew and Wang,

1995; McShea et al., 1997; Nagy et al., 1997; Vincent et al., 1996, 1997; Yang et al., 2001, 2003). Expression of many of these gene products is regulated by either p53 or E2F1-pRb complexes. Investigation into the expression of these proteins in AD revealed that indeed p53, E2F1, pRb, and the inactive phosphoisoform of pRb, phospho-pRb (ppRb), all exhibited increased staining and/or levels over age-matched controls in the hippocampus and mid-frontal cortex (de la Monte et al., 1997; Jordan-Sciutto et al., 2002a; Kitamura et al., 1997). Staining for p53 was observed to be predominantly nuclear in neurons of mid-frontal cortex. Staining for E2F1 was observed in the cytoplasm of cells with morphology of neurons and astrocytes of the mid-frontal cortex of AD patients. ppRb immunostaining was increased predominantly in the nuclei of neurons and astrocytes (Jordan-Sciutto et al., 2002a). Further, cells containing nuclear ppRb had cytoplasmic E2F1, indicating that these changes were occurring in the same cell. These findings are consistent with findings in vitro demonstrating that E2F1, ppRb, and p53 are similarly affected in primary cultured neurons responding to beta-amyloid treatment, one of the toxins associated with AD. Together, these findings indicate a role for these cell cycle proteins in neurodegenerative disease.

Consistent with the observations in AD, p53, E2F1, and pRb have been observed to exhibit altered expression patterns in several neurodegenerative diseases or their in vitro models. In the substantia nigra of patients with PD, increased ppRb staining was observed specifically in the neuromelanin-positive neurons that are targeted for destruction in disease (Jordan-Sciutto et al., 2003). Similarly, increased nuclear ppRb and cytoplasmic E2F1 have been observed in both the ventral horn motor neurons and neurons of the motor cortex of patients with ALS (Ranganathan and Bowser, 2003). Further, proteins that make up one of the pRb kinase complexes, cyclin D1 and CDK4, were also increased in the same neuronal populations in ALS. Increased p53 has been observed in ALS patient CNS; however, knocking out p53 in ALS transgenic mouse models does not confer protection from disease progression, suggesting that p53 may not be necessary for disease progression (Gonzalez de Aguilar et al., 2000; Kuntz et al., 2000; Martin, 2000). Despite the negative findings in the animal model, it is clear that these pathways are activated in disease, which suggests that these proteins are part of the neuronal response to neurodegenerative stimuli, though they may not be the sole mediators of death.

Taken together, these findings suggest that activation of cell cycle proteins may be a common neuronal response to toxic stimuli and/or the stimuli in neurodegenerative diseases. As we discuss in the next section, cell cycle protein activation is also a feature of HIVE, suggesting a common mechanism of neuronal response to toxic stimuli among these diseases, which can serve as potential targets for therapy in patients with neurodegenerative diseases. As proteomic approaches, cerebrospinal fluid analysis, and CD4[+] T-cell levels combined are more likely to presymptomatically determine those at risk for progression to HAD before diagnostics for AD and PD are available, patients with HIVE are likely to benefit first from therapies aimed at preventing neuronal loss by targeting cell cycle protein in combination with other therapeutics.

CELL CYCLE PROTEINS IN HIVE

Investigation into cell cycle proteins in HIVE is still in its early days; however, research thus far indicates that mechanisms of neuronal response to the degenerative stimuli in HIVE are similar to those seen in other neurodegenerative diseases. As observed in AD, cytoplasmic E2F1 and ppRb staining was increased in neurons of patients with HIVE compared to infected, nonencephalitic controls in hippocampus, mid-frontal cortex, and basal ganglia (Jordan-Sciutto et al., 2000, 2002b) (Color Plate 7), similar to findings in the simian model of disease, SIVE. In both HIVE and SIVE, quantification of staining revealed significantly more ppRb and E2F1 in mid-frontal cortex, hippocampus, and basal ganglia from cases diagnosed with encephalitis than in nonencephalitic, infected controls. Further, increased ppRb and E2F1 correlated with increased macrophage staining in mid-frontal cortex and putamen of SIVE (Jordan-Sciutto et al., 2002b), suggesting that the expression of these proteins correlates with disease processes. Finally, E2F DNA-binding complexes were altered in protein extracts from mid-frontal cortex and basal ganglia from SIVE compared to nonencephalitic controls, suggesting an alteration in E2F transcriptional activity during disease progression. As an in vitro model of HIVE, we treated primary rat cortical neurons with HIV-infected macrophage supernatants and observed increased E2F1 staining in neuronal cytoplasm and nucleus compared to mock-infected control supernatants (K. L. Jordan-Sciutto and D. L. Kolson, unpublished observations). E2F1 levels were also increased by Western blot analysis, indicating that E2F1 regulation is altered in response to HIV-infected macrophage-secreted factors that are implicated in HIVE (Jordan-Sciutto and Kolson, unpublished). Taken together, these findings indicate that neurons as well as other CNS cells exhibit altered pRb and E2F1 regulation, which is likely contributing to neuronal dysfunction and loss in HIVE and the simian model of disease.

At least one pathway of E2F1-induced apoptosis involves activation of p53. Consistent with activation of this pathway, two independent groups have shown that p53 expression is increased in neurons, astrocytes, and microglia of cortex from patients with HIVE compared to nonencephalitic controls (Garden et al., 2004; Silva et al., 2003). p53 levels are also increased in autopsy tissue as determined by Western blot analysis (Silva et al., 2003). Using another in vitro model of HIVE, Garden and colleagues treated primary murine cortical neurons directly with gp120 or with gp120-treated microglia, which should induce secretion of factors similar to those observed in encephalitis (Garden et al., 2004). In these studies, p53$^{-/-}$ neurons were not susceptible to HIV gp120- or gp120-stimulated microglial secreted factors. Further, stimulation of p53$^{-/-}$ microglia with gp120 did not alter viability of p53$^{+/+}$ neurons. These findings suggest that p53 is required by microglia to produce the toxins associated with neuronal loss in HIVE as well as for neuronal loss in response to these HIVE-associated toxins (Garden et al., 2004). Taken together, these findings indicate that p53 is a downstream target for neuronal response to HIVE-associated toxins.

Beyond E2F1, pRb, and p53, few, if any, other, cell cycle proteins have been implicated in disease progression. E2F1 family member E2F4 has been found to be predominantly nuclear in neurons in SIV and SIVE mid-frontal cortex and basal ganglia but does not change localization (Morgan et al., 2005). Studies need to be done to determine DNA-binding activity of E2F4 in SIVE and its interaction with p130. If p130-E2F4 complexes are unaltered, it suggests that only a subset of E2F targets are subject to changes in HIVE, as p130-E2F4 has been shown to regulate different subsets of E2F target promoters (Helin et al., 1993b; Ren et al., 2002; Takahashi et al., 2000). Further, E2F2, 3, 5, and 6 have yet

to be investigated; however, as these proteins are not highly expressed in CNS, they are not likely to be altered in the CNS pathogenesis of AIDS. Investigation of pRb family members p107 and p130 did not reveal apparent changes in either of these molecules in neurons, although there was a dramatic increase in both proteins in the macrophage/microglial population (Chalovich et al., 2005). Currently, there are no reports regarding p53 family members p63 and p73 in HIVE. Further investigation into p73 is warranted given its described role in regulating neuronal viability, its alternative expression in AD, and its transcriptional activation by E2F1 (Helin et al., 1993b; Pozniak et al., 2000; Ren et al., 2002; Takahashi et al., 2000).

With strong evidence supporting a role for E2F1, pRb, and p53 in HIVE, further investigation needs to be made into the mechanisms regulating their activity in neurons and disease. All three proteins are responsive to both neuroprotective molecules and neurotoxic molecules. Understanding the differences in E2F1, pRb, and p53 regulation under these distinct stimuli is necessary to understand how neurons interpret and respond to the conflicting signaling factors secreted by HIV-infected and/or -activated macrophages. In order to understand how these proteins are being regulated in HIVE, we need to know at least three key things: (i) how these proteins are regulated in neurons in HIVE, (ii) whether they have novel or distinct functions when they are mislocalized in neurons, and (iii) how HAART changes the neuronal response to these stimuli.

FUTURE IMPLICATIONS FOR NEURO-AIDS

Justification for investigating p53, pRb, and E2F1 in HIVE to this point has hinged upon their known roles in regulating death in both nonneuronal and neuronal cells. While neuronal loss is a key feature of end stages of HIVE, there is evidence to suggest that initially HAD occurs due to neuronal dysfunction, not neuronal loss. This was most clearly demonstrated by the observed cognitive improvement in HAD patients after antiretroviral interventions were introduced (DeCarli et al., 1991; Portegies et al., 1993). Therefore, the initial stages of cognitive decline are likely associated with neuronal dysfunction prior to neuronal loss. Consistent with this supposition, synaptic loss is also a key finding in HIVE as well as other neurodegenerative diseases. This has led to the conclusion that neurodegeneration in HIVE as well as other neurodegenerative diseases including AD is due to synaptic loss and dysfunction that culminate in neuronal loss (Selkoe and Schenk, 2003). This raises the question of whether cell cycle proteins contribute to neuronal dysfunction.

Roles for Cell Cycle Proteins in Neuronal Dysfunction

Roles for cell cycle proteins in synapse formation and synaptic transmission have not been demonstrated; however, there are several observations supporting a potential role for these proteins in this process. Synaptic dysfunction can be due to either disruption of signaling at the synapse or collapse of the neurite supporting the synapse. While roles in regulation of synaptic function are pure speculation at this point, there is some evidence that E2F1 and p53 may contribute to changes in neurite morphology. Both E2F1 and p53 have been shown to activate the family of proteases associated with apoptosis, the caspases. Many caspase target proteins are cytoskeletal components including spectrin, MAP2, actin, and tau (Siman et al., 2004). While mass activation of caspases does trigger apoptosis, there has been speculation that localized activation of caspases results in cleavage of cell cycle proteins leading to rearrangement of neuritis (Morrison et al., 2003). Another protease family associated with regulating cell death, calpains, shares many of the same targets as caspases. By activating caspases and/or calpains locally, neurite structure can be rapidly rearranged in response to prevailing signals (Morrison et al., 2003). Calpains have already been implicated in neurite outgrowth in response to trophic factors. These findings suggest a mechanism by which cell cycle proteins may regulate neurite stability in the cytoplasm. Further evidence for E2F1 in regulation of cytoskeleton comes from early observations that expression of a mutant E2F1 lacking the nuclear localization signal in fibroblasts disrupts actin and microtubule polymerization (Logan et al., 1994). Future investigations are needed to determine what effects this mutant may have in neuronal cells.

In addition to E2F1 and p53, a non-cell-cycle-associated CDK, CDK5, has been observed to regulate cytoskeletal rearrangement, nuclear movement, axonal migration, axonal transport, synaptic endocytosis, and neurite elongation (Jorda et al., 2005; O'Hare et al., 2005; Rashid et al., 2001; Shea et al., 2004; Smith et al., 2004; Xie et al., 2003). With such processes, disregulation of CDK5 could potentially impact both synaptic activity and neurite stability. Activation of CDK5 occurs by association with a noncyclin subunit, p35. Cleavage of p35 by calpain results in increased kinase activity. It is this more stable and active complex of CDK5-p25 that has been implicated in neuronal death. Increased expression of p25 can induce death, while inhibition of CDK5 activity blocks neuronal death. Further, increased CDK5 has been observed in AD, ALS, Pick's disease, and HAD (Baumann et al., 1993; Bu et al., 2002; Giovanni et al., 1999; Mapelli et al., 2005; O'Hare et al., 2005; Wang et al., 2007). The exact mechanism by which it may induce death is not clear; however, recent studies provide more insight to the possible pathways involved. In an in vitro model of PD, dopaminergic neuronal death was mediated by CDK5 phosphorylation of the transcription factor, myocyte enhancing factor 2 (MEF2) in the nucleus, resulting in suppression of its prosurvival functions (Smith et al., 2006). However, MEF2 phosphorylation by CDK5 was not observed in HAD tissue or an in vitro model of HAD (Wang et al., 2007). On the other hand, two studies conducted with the neuroblastoma cell line SH-SY5Y suggest a more conventional, CDK family-like function for CDK5. A recent work by Lee and colleagues showed CDK5-induced stabilization and activation of p53 by its phosphorylation at specific epitopes and inhibition of MDM2-mediated proteasomal degradation, resulting in genotoxic and oxidative stress-mediated death (Lee et al., 2007). In a second study, pRb phosphorylation by CDK5 was detected as an early event in neuronal death, suggesting an alternative link between CDK5 and neuronal death (Hamdane et al., 2005). Taken together, modulation of CDK5 has potential to exert effects on both neuronal function and neuronal viability.

Potential Therapies for HAD in the post-HAART Era

HAART was introduced in 1995 as an aggressive approach to take HIV viral load under control and increase CD4[+] cell counts by using two or more antiretroviral drugs. This strategy based on the concept of blocking viral replication at multiple points provided improved outcome for patients. With the advent of HAART, compliant patients experience a decrease in the incidence of opportunistic infections and dramatically reduced mortality rates. However, in the post-HAART era the prevalence of HAD, characterized by the loss of neurocognitive functions, seems to be increasing compared to that observed in the pre-HAART era. The reasons for this unexpected outcome of HAART are elusive; however, the longer life expectancy has been proposed to play a role (Valcour et al., 2004). Although little to no investigating has been made into the effects of HAART on cell cycle proteins in HIVE, it is unlikely that HAART will alter or prevent cell cycle protein activities in neurons of patients with HAD, as many of the HAART therapeutics do not cross the blood-brain barrier or prevent initial entry of virally infected macrophages into the CNS. However, studies to confirm this supposition are warranted. With the continued progression of HIV-infected, HAART-compliant patients to HAD, there is a greater need for a treatment for this disease. Currently, two therapies under consideration for other neurodegenerative disease, inhibition of caspases or inhibition of CDKs, may have potential impact on rescuing neuronal dysfunction and loss in HAD. As caspases and cdk5 both are hypothesized to regulate neurite outgrowth and potentially synaptic activity, inhibition of these activities has the potential for treatment. As cdk5 is neuron specific, it is an ideal target, which will likely have little effect on peripheral cells, which lack cdk5, so long as the therapeutic is highly specific for this cdk family member. As caspases have more global expression and are necessary for normal immune function and cancer surveillance, a caspase inhibitor is a riskier therapeutic unless it can be targeted to neurons. As E2F1, p53, and pRb are also ubiquitously expressed proteins, targeting them for therapy has similar issues. However, the localization of E2F1 and pRb in neurodegenerative diseases suggests that their neuronal activity is not analogous to their normal roles in nonneuronal cells. If alternative functions for these proteins in neurons are uncovered, it may be possible to target the neuron-specific activities in HIVE or other neurodegenerative conditions.

SUMMARY

The pathogenesis of HIVE is not completely understood; however, most available evidence supports a pathogenic role for macrophage-secreted factors of endogenous and/or viral origin. While it is likely that neuronal loss can be attributed to both groups of proteins, the endogenous macrophage-secreted factors can also participate in neuronal loss in the absence of viral infection in other neurodegenerative diseases. Increased macrophage infiltration and secretion of cytokines, chemokines, and NTF have been observed in several neurodegenerative diseases of the CNS including HIVE, AD, and PD (Beal, 2003; Hirsch et al., 2003; Ishizuka et al., 1997; McGeer and McGeer, 2003; Roberts et al., 2003; Streit et al., 2001; Wullner and Klockgether, 2003). Further, p53, E2F1, and hyperphosphorylated pRb exhibit increased immunoreactivity and altered subcellular distribution in HIVE, SIVE, AD, and PD (Garden et al., 2004; Jordan-Sciutto et al., 2000, 2002a, 2002b, 2003; Silva et al., 2003). These findings indicate that the neuronal response in chronic neurodegenerative conditions is comparable to that of lentiviral encephalitis and involves changes in the cell cycle machinery, including p53, pRb, and E2F1. By understanding the impact of macrophage-secreted factors such as cytokines, chemokines, NTF, and ROS on modulation of cell cycle regulatory proteins in neurons, we will gain a greater insight into neurodegenerative processes in HIVE and neurodegeneration as a whole and hopefully identify potential therapeutic targets for treatment of these devastating diseases.

REFERENCES

Achim, C. L., R. Wang, D. K. Miners, and C. A. Wiley. 1994. Brain viral burden in HIV-infection. *J. Neuropathol. Exp. Neurol.* **53:**284–294.

Achim, C. L., and C. A. Wiley. 1992. Expression of major histocompatibility complex antigens in the brains of patients with progressive multifocal leukoencephalopathy. *J. Neuropathol. Exp. Neurol.* **51:**257–263.

Achim, C. L., and C. A. Wiley. 1996. Inflammation in AIDS and the role of the macrophage in brain pathology. *Curr. Opin. Neurol.* **9:**221–225.

Adams, P., and W. J. Kaelin. 1995. Transcriptional control by E2F. *Semin. Cancer Biol.* **6:**99–108.

Aloyz, R., S. Bamji, C. Pozniak, J. Toma, J. Atwal, D. Kaplan, and F. Miller. 1998. p53 is essential for developmental neuron death as regulated by the TrkA and p75 neurotrophin receptors. *J. Cell Biol.* **143:**1691–1703.

Annunziato, L., S. Amoroso, A. Pannaccione, M. Cataldi, G. Pignataro, A. D'Alessio, R. Sirabella, A. Secondo, L. Sibaud, and G. F. Di Renzo. 2003. Apoptosis induced in neuronal cells by oxidative stress: role played by caspases and intracellular calcium ions. *Toxicol. Lett.* **139:**125–133.

Araki, T., Y. Enokido, N. Inamura, S. Aizawa, J. C. Reed, and H. Hatanaka. 1998. Changes in c-Jun but not Bcl-2 family proteins in p53-dependent apoptosis of mouse cerebellar granule neurons induced by DNA damaging agent bleomycin. *Brain Res.* **794:**239–247.

Arendt, T., M. Holzer, and U. Gartner. 1998. Neuronal expression of cycline dependent kinase inhibitors of the INK4 family in Alzheimer's disease. *J. Neural Transm.* **105:**949–960.

Arendt, T., L. Rodel, U. Gartner, and M. Holzer. 1996. Expression of the cyclin-dependent kinase inhibitor p16 in Alzheimer's disease. *Neuroreport* **7:**3047–3049.

Bachis, A., E. O. Major, and I. Mocchetti. 2003. Brain-derived neurotrophic factor inhibits human immunodeficiency virus-1/gp120-mediated cerebellar granule cell death by preventing gp120 internalization. *J. Neurosci.* **23:**5715–5722.

Banasiak, K. J., and G. G. Haddad. 1998. Hypoxia-induced apoptosis: effect of hypoxic severity and role of p53 in neuronal cell death. *Brain Res.* **797:**295–304.

Barzilai, A., D. Daily, R. Zilkha-Falb, I. Ziv, D. Offen, E. Melamed, and A. Shirvan. 2003. The molecular mechanisms of dopamine toxicity. *Adv. Neurol.* **91:**73–82.

Bates, S., A. C. Phillips, P. A. Clark, F. Stott, G. Peters, R. L. Ludwig, and K. H. Vousden. 1998. p14ARF links the tumour suppressors RB and p53. *Nature* **395:**124–125.

Baumann, K., E. M. Mandelkow, J. Biernat, H. Piwnica-Worms, and E. Mandelkow. 1993. Abnormal Alzheimer-like phosphorylation of tau-protein by cyclin-dependent kinases cdk2 and cdk5. *FEBS Lett.* **336:**417–424.

Beal, M. F. 2003. Mitochondria, oxidative damage, and inflammation in Parkinson's disease. *Ann. N. Y. Acad. Sci.* **991:**120–131.

Benos, D., B. Hahn, J. Bubien, S. Ghosh, N. Mashburn, M. Chaikin, G. Shaw, and E. Benveniste. 1994. Envelope glycoprotein gp120 of human immunodeficiency virus type1 alters ion-transport in astrocytes-implications for AIDS dementia Complex. *Proc. Natl. Acad. Sci. USA* **91:**494–498.

Bernardo, A., M. Patrizio, G. Levi, and T. Petrucci. 1994. Human immunodeficiency virus protein gp120 interferes with b-adrenergic receptor-mediated protein phosphorylation in cultured rat cortical astrocytes. *Cell. Mol. Neurobiol.* **14:**1367–1378.

Bibel, M., and Y. A. Barde. 2000. Neurotrophins: key regulators of cell fate and cell shape in the vertebrate nervous system. *Genes Dev.* **14:**2919–2937.

Blum, D., Y. Wu, M. F. Nissou, S. Arnaud, B. Alim Louis, and J. M. Verna. 1997. p53 and Bax activation in 6-hydroxydopamine-induced apoptosis in PC12 cells. *Brain Res.* **751:**139–142.

Boldyrev, A., R. Song, V. A. Dyatlov, D. A. Lawrence, and D. O. Carpenter. 2000. Neuronal cell death and reactive oxygen species. *Cell. Mol. Neurobiol.* **20:**433–450.

Boutillier, A. L., E. Trinh, and J. P. Loeffler. 2000. Caspase-dependent cleavage of the retinoblastoma protein is an early step in neuronal apoptosis. *Oncogene* **19:**2171–2178.

Brouwers, P., M. P. Heyes, H. A. Moss, P. L. Wolters, D. G. Poplack, S. P. Markey, and P. A. Pizzo. 1993. Quinolinic acid in the cerebrospinal fluid of children with symptomatic human immunodeficiency virus type 1 disease: relationships to clinical status and therapeutic response. *J. Infect. Dis.* **168:**1380–1386.

Bu, B., J. Li, P. Davies, and I. Vincent. 2002. Deregulation of cdk5, hyperphosphorylation, and cytoskeletal pathology in the Niemann-Pick type C murine model. *J. Neurosci.* **22:**6515–6525.

Budka, H. 1991. Neuropathology of human immunodeficiency virus infection. *Brain Pathol.* **1:**163–175.

Busser, J., D. S. Geldmacher, and K. Herrup. 1998. Ectopic cell cycle proteins predict the sites of neuronal cell death in Alzheimer's disease brain. *J. Neurosci.* **18:**2801–2807.

Caelles, C., A. Helmberg, and M. Karin. 1994. p53-dependent apoptosis in the absence of transcriptional activation of p53-target genes. *Nature* **370:**220–223.

Chalovich, E. M., M. A. Koike, M. A. Aras, M. Murphey-Corb, C. A. Wiley, and K. L. Jordan-Sciutto. 2005. Pocket proteins p107 and p130 exhibit increased expression in macrophages during SIV encephalitis. *Neuropathology* **25:**315–325.

Chen, R. W., and D. M. Chuang. 1999. Long term lithium treatment suppresses p53 and Bax expression but increases Bcl-2 expression. A prominent role in neuroprotection against excitotoxicity. *J. Biol. Chem.* **274:**6039–6042.

Chen, R. W., P. A. Saunders, H. Wei, Z. Li, P. Seth, and D. M. Chuang. 1999. Involvement of glyceraldehyde-3-phosphate dehydrogenase (GAPDH) and p53 in neuronal apoptosis: evidence that GAPDH is upregulated by p53. *J. Neurosci.* **19:**9654–9662.

Chopp, M., Y. Li, Z. G. Zhang, and S. O. Freytag. 1992. p53 expression in brain after middle cerebral artery occlusion in the rat. *Biochem. Biophys. Res. Commun.* **182:**1201–1207.

Clarke, A., E. Maandag, M. van Roon, N. M. van der Lugt, M. van der Balk, M. Hooper, A. Berns, and H. Riele. 1992. Requirement for a functional Rb-2 gene in murine development. *Nature* **359:**328–330.

Coulier, F., R. Kumar, M. Ernst, R. Klein, D. Martin-Zanca, and M. Barbacid. 1990. Human trk oncogenes activated by point mutation, in-frame deletion, and duplication of the tyrosine kinase domain. *Mol. Cell. Biol.* **10:**4202–4210.

Cress, W., D. Johnson, and J. Nevins. 1993. A genetic analysis of the E2F1 gene distinguishes regulation by RB, p107, and adenovirus E4. *Mol. Cell. Biol.* **13:**6314–6325.

Crowe, S. M. 1995. Role of macrophages in the pathogenesis of human immunodeficiency virus (HIV) infection. *Aust. N. Z. J. Med.* **25:**777–783.

Crumrine, R. C., A. L. Thomas, and P. F. Morgan. 1994. Attenuation of p53 expression protects against focal ischemic damage in transgenic mice. *J. Cereb. Blood Flow Metab.* **14:**887–891.

Culmsee, C., X. Zhu, Q. S. Yu, S. L. Chan, S. Camandola, Z. Guo, N. H. Greig, and M. P. Mattson. 2001. A synthetic inhibitor of p53 protects neurons against death induced by ischemic and excitotoxic insults, and amyloid beta-peptide. *J. Neurochem.* **77:**220–228.

Daily, D., A. Barzilai, D. Offen, A. Kamsler, E. Melamed, and I. Ziv. 1999. The involvement of p53 in dopamine induced apoptosis of cerebellar granule neurons and leukemic cells overexpressing p53. *Cell. Mol. Neurobiol.* **19:**261–276.

DeCarli, C., L. Fugate, J. Falloon, J. Eddy, D. Katz, R. Friedland, S. Rapoport, P. Brouwers, and P. Pizzo. 1991.

Brain growth and cognitive improvement in children with human immunodeficiency virus-induced encephalopathy after 6 months of continuous infusion zidovudine therapy. *J. Acquir. Immune Defic. Syndr.* **4:**585–592.

DeGregori, J., G. Leone, A. Miron, L. Jakoi, and J. Nevins. 1997. Distinct roles for E2F proteins in cell growth control and apoptosis. *Proc. Natl. Acad. Sci. USA* **94:**7245–7250.

de la Monte, S. M., Y. K. Sohn, and J. R. Wands. 1997. Correlates of p53- and Fas (CD95)-mediated apoptosis in Alzheimer's disease. *J. Neurol.Sci.* **152:**73–83.

D'Mello, S. R. 1998. Molecular regulation of neuronal apoptosis. *Curr. Top. Dev. Biol.* **39:**187–213.

Duckett, C., and C. Thompson. 1997. CD-30-dependent degradation of TRAF-2: implications for negative regulation of TRAF signaling and the control of cell survival. *Genes Dev.* **11:**2810–2821.

el-Deiry, W. S. 1998. Regulation of p53 downstream genes. *Semin. Cancer Biol.* **8:**345–357.

el-Deiry, W. S., J. W. Harper, P. M. O'Connor, V. E. Velculescu, C. E. Canman, J. Jackman, J. A. Pietenpol, M. Burrell, D. E. Hill, Y. Wang, et al. 1994. WAF1/CIP1 is induced in p53-mediated G1 arrest and apoptosis. *Cancer Res.* **54:**1169–1174.

Enokido, Y., T. Araki, S. Aizawa, and H. Hatanaka. 1996a. p53 involves cytosine arabinoside-induced apoptosis in cultured cerebellar granule neurons. *Neurosci. Lett.* **203:**1–4.

Enokido, Y., T. Araki, K. Tanaka, S. Aizawa, and H. Hatanaka. 1996b. Involvement of p53 in DNA strand break-induced apoptosis in postmitotic CNS neurons. *Eur. J. Neurosci.* **8:**1812–1821.

Farnham, R., J. Slansky, and R. Kollmar. 1993. The role of E2F in the mammalian cell cycle. *Biochim. Biophys. Acta* **1155:**125–131.

Flemington, E., S. Speck, and W. Kaelin. 1993. E2F1-mediated transactivation is inhibited by complex formation with the retinoblastoma susceptibility gene product. *Proc. Natl. Acad. Sci. USA* **90:**6914–6918.

Freeman, R., S. Estus, and E. Johnson, Jr. 1994. Analysis of cell cycle-related gene expression in postmitotic neurons: selective induction of cyclin D1 during programmed cell death. *Neuron* **12:**343–355.

Garden, G. A., W. Guo, S. Jayadev, C. Tun, S. Balcaitis, J. Choi, T. J. Montine, T. Moller, and R. S. Morrison. 2004. HIV associated neurodegeneration requires p53 in neurons and microglia. *FASEB J.* **18:**1141–1143.

Gelbard, H. A., H. S. L. M. Nottet, S. Swindells, M. Jett, K. A. Dzenko, P. Genis, R. White, L. Wang, Y. B. Choi, D. Zhang, S. A. Lipton, W. W. Tourtellotte, L. G. Epstein, and H. E. Gendelman. 1994. Platelet activating factor: a candidate HIV-1-induced neurotoxin. *J. Virol.* **68:**4628–4635.

Giovanni, A., E. Keramaris, E. Morris, S. Hou, M. O'Hare, N. Dyson, G. Robertson, R. Slack, and D. Park. 2000. E2F1 mediates death of B-amyloid-treated cortical neurons in a manner independent of p53 and dependent on Bax and Caspase 3. *J. Biol. Chem.* **275:**11553–11560.

Giovanni, A., F. Wirtz-Bruger, E. Keramaris, R. Slack, and D. Park. 1999. Involvement of cell cycle elements, cyclin-dependent kinases, pRb, and E2F-DP, in B-amyloid-induced neuronal death. *J. Biol. Chem.* **274:**19011–19016.

Giulian, D., J. H. Yu, X. Li, D. Tom, J. Li, E. Wendt, S. N. Lin, R. Schwarcz, and C. Noonan. 1996. Study of receptor-mediated neurotoxins released by HIV-1-infected mononuclear phagocytes found in human brain. *J. Neurosci.* **16:**3139–3153.

Gonzalez de Aguilar, J. L., J. W. Gordon, F. Rene, M. de Tapia, B. Lutz-Bucher, C. Gaiddon, and J. P. Loeffler. 2000. Alteration of the Bcl-x/Bax ratio in a transgenic mouse model of amyotrophic lateral sclerosis: evidence for the implication of the p53 signaling pathway. *Neurobiol. Dis.* **7:**406–415.

Grant, R., J. Wiley, and W. Winkelstein. 1987. Infectivity of the human immunodeficiency virus: estimates from a prospective study of homosexual men. *J. Infect. Dis.* **156:**189–193.

Hagemeier, C., A. Cook, and T. Kouzarides. 1993. The retinoblastoma protein binds E2F residues required for activation in vivo and TBP binding in vitro. *Nucleic Acids Res.* **21:**4998–5004.

Hallstrom, T. C., and J. R. Nevins. 2003. Specificity in the activation and control of transcription factor E2F-dependent apoptosis. *Proc. Natl. Acad. Sci. USA* **100:**10848–10853.

Halterman, M. W., C. C. Miller, and H. J. Federoff. 1999. Hypoxia-inducible factor-1alpha mediates hypoxia-induced delayed neuronal death that involves p53. *J. Neurosci.* **19:**6818–6824.

Hamdane, M., A. Bretteville, A. V. Sambo, K. Schindowski, S. Begard, A. Delacourte, P. Bertrand, and L. Buee. 2005. p25/Cdk5-mediated retinoblastoma phosphorylation is an early event in neuronal cell death. *J. Cell Sci.* **118:**1291–1298.

Harbour, J. W., and D. C. Dean. 2000. The Rb/E2F pathway: expanding roles and emerging paradigms. *Genes Dev.* **14:**2393–2409.

Helin, K., E. Harlow, and A. Fattaey. 1993a. Inhibition of E2F1 transactivation by direct binding of the retinoblastoma protein. *Mol. Cell. Biol.* **13:**6501–6508.

Helin, K., C. Wu, A. Fattaey, J. Lees, B. Dynlacht, C. Ngwu, and E. Harlow. 1993b. Heterodimerization of the transcription factors E2F-1 and DP-1 leads to cooperative trans-activation. *Genes Dev.* **7:**1850–1861.

Heyes, M. P., K. Saito, A. Lackner, C. A. Wiley, C. L. Achim, and S. P. Markey. 1998. Sources of the neurotoxin quinolinic acid in the brain of HIV-1 infected patients and retrovirus-infected macaques. *FASEB J.* **12:**881–896.

Hirata, H., and J. L. Cadet. 1997. p53-knockout mice are protected against the long-term effects of methamphetamine on dopaminergic terminals and cell bodies. *J. Neurochem.* **69:**780–790.

Hirsch, E. C., T. Breidert, E. Rousselet, S. Hunot, A. Hartmann, and P. P. Michel. 2003. The role of glial reaction and inflammation in Parkinson's disease. *Ann. N. Y. Acad. Sci.* **991:**214–228.

Holmin, S., and T. Mathiesen. 2000. Intracerebral administration of interleukin-1beta and induction of inflammation, apoptosis, and vasogenic edema. *J. Neurosurg.* **92:**108–120.

Hoozemans, J. J., M. K. Bruckner, A. J. Rozemuller, R. Veerhuis, P. Eikelenboom, and T. Arendt. 2002. Cyclin D1 and cyclin E are co-localized with cyclo-oxygenase 2 (COX-2) in pyramidal neurons in Alzheimer disease temporal cortex. *J. Neuropathol. Exp. Neurol.* **61:**678–688.

Hou, S. T., E. Cowan, T. Walker, N. Ohan, M. Dove, I. Rasqinha, and J. P. MacManus. 2001. The transcription factor E2F1 promotes dopamine-evoked neuronal apoptosis by a mechanism independent of transcriptional activation. *J. Neurochem.* **78:**287–297.

Hsieh, J.-K., S. Fredersdorf, T. Kouzarides, K. Martin, and X. Lu. 1997. E2F-1 induced apoptosis requires DNA binding but no transactivation and is inhibited by the Retinoblastoma protein through direct interaction. *Genes Dev.* **11:**1840–1852.

Hughes, A. L., L. Gollapudi, T. L. Sladek, and K. E. Neet. 2000. Mediation of nerve growth factor-driven cell cycle arrest in PC12 cells by p53. Simultaneous differentiation and proliferation subsequent to p53 functional inactivation. *J. Biol. Chem.* **275:**37829–37837.

Ishizuka, K., T. Kimura, R. Igata-yi, S. Katsuragi, J. Takamatsu, and T. Miyakawa. 1997. Identification of monocyte chemoattractant protein-1 in senile plaques and reactive microglia of Alzheimer's disease. *Psychiatry Clin. Neurosci.* **51:**135–138.

Jacks, T., A. Fazeli, E. Schmitt, R. Bronson, M. Goodell, and R. Weinerg. 1992. Effects of an Rb mutation in the mouse. *Nature* **359**:295–300.

Jiang, Y. H., D. Armstrong, U. Albrecht, C. M. Atkins, J. L. Noebels, G. Eichele, J. D. Sweatt, and A. L. Beaudet. 1998. Mutation of the Angelman ubiquitin ligase in mice causes increased cytoplasmic p53 and deficits of contextual learning and long-term potentiation. *Neuron* **21**:799–811.

Johnson, M. D., H. Xiang, S. London, Y. Kinoshita, M. Knudson, M. Mayberg, S. J. Korsmeyer, and R. S. Morrison. 1998. Evidence for involvement of Bax and p53, but not caspases, in radiation-induced cell death of cultured postnatal hippocampal neurons. *J. Neurosci. Res.* **54**:721–733.

Jorda, E. G., E. Verdaguer, A. Jimenez, S. G. Arriba, C. Allgaier, M. Pallas, and A. Camins. 2005. Evaluation of the neuronal apoptotic pathways involved in cytoskeletal disruption-induced apoptosis. *Biochem. Pharmacol.* **70**:470–480.

Jordan-Sciutto, K., L. Malaiyandi, and R. Bowser. 2002a. Altered distribution of cell cycle transcriptional regulators during Alzheimer's disease. *J. Neuropathol. Exp. Neurol.* **61**:358–367.

Jordan-Sciutto, K., B. Murray, C. Wiley, and C. Achim. 2001. Response of cell cycle proteins to neurotrophic factor and chemokine stimulation in human neuroglia. *Exp. Neurol.* **167**:205–214.

Jordan-Sciutto, K., G. Wang, M. Murphey-Corb, and C. Wiley. 2002b. Cell cycle proteins exhibit altered expression patterns in lentiviral-associated encephalitis. *J. Neurosci.* **22**:2185–2195.

Jordan-Sciutto, K., G. Wang, M. Murphy-Corb, and C. Wiley. 2000. Induction of cell cycle regulators in simian immunodeficiency virus encephalitis. *Am. J. Pathol.* **157**:497–507.

Jordan-Sciutto, K. L., R. Dorsey, E. M. Chalovich, R. R. Hammond, and C. L. Achim. 2003. Expression patterns of retinoblastoma protein in Parkinson disease. *J. Neuropathol. Exp. Neurol.* **62**:68–74.

Kaiser, P., J. Offermann, and S. Lipton. 1990. Neuronal injury due to HIV-1 envelope protein is blocked by anti-gp120 antibodies but not by anti-CD4 antibodies. *Neurology* **40**:1757–1761.

Kaul, M., G. A. Garden, and S. A. Lipton. 2001. Pathways to neuronal injury and apoptosis in HIV-associated dementia. *Nature* **410**:988–994.

Khan, M. Z., R. Brandimarti, B. J. Musser, D. M. Resue, A. Fatatis, and O. Meucci. 2003. The chemokine receptor CXCR4 regulates cell-cycle proteins in neurons. *J. Neurovirol.* **9**:300–314.

Kiess, M., R. M. Gill, and P. A. Hamel. 1995. Expression and activity of the retinoblastoma protein (pRB)-family proteins, p107 and p130, during L6 myoblast differentiation. *Cell Growth Differ.* **6**:1287–1298.

Kitamura, Y., S. Shimohama, W. Kamoshima, Y. Matsuoka, Y. Nomura, and T. Taniguchi. 1997. Changes in p53 in the brains of patients with Alzheimer's disease. *Biochem. Biophys. Res. Commun.* **232**:418–421.

Kohji, T., M. Hayashi, K. Shioda, M. Minagawa, Y. Morimatsu, K. Tamagawa, and M. Oda. 1998. Cerebellar neurodegeneration in human hereditary DNA repair disorders. *Neurosci. Lett.* **243**:133–136.

Kouzarides, T. 1995. Transcriptional control by the retinoblastoma protein. *Semin. Cancer Biol.* **6**:91–98.

Kranenburg, O., A. van der Eb, and A. Zantema. 1996. Cyclin D1 is an essential mediator of apoptotic neuronal cell death. *EMBO J.* **15**:46–54.

Kuntz, C., IV, Y. Kinoshita, M. F. Beal, L. A. Donehower, and R. S. Morrison. 2000. Absence of p53: no effect in a transgenic mouse model of familial amyotrophic lateral sclerosis. *Exp. Neurol.* **165**:184–190.

LaFerla, F. M., C. K. Hall, L. Ngo, and G. Jay. 1996. Extracellular deposition of beta-amyloid upon p53-dependent neuronal cell death in transgenic mice. *J. Clin. Investig.* **98**:1626–1632.

LaThangue, N. 1994. DRTF1/E2F: an expanding family of heterodimeric transcription factors implicated in cell-cycle control. *Trends Biochem. Sci.* **19**:108–114.

Lee, E.-H., C. Chang, N. Hu, Y.-C. Wang, C.-C. Lai, K. Herrup, and W.-H. Lee. 1992. Mice deficient for Rb are nonviable and show defects in neurogenesis and haematopoiesis. *Nature* **359**:288–294.

Lee, J. H., H. S. Kim, S. J. Lee, and K. T. Kim. 2007. Stabilization and activation of p53 induced by Cdk5 contributes to neuronal cell death. *J. Cell Sci.* **120**:2259–2271.

Levi, G., M. Patrizio, A. Bernardo, T. Petrucci, and C. Agresti. 1993. Human immunodeficiency virus coat protein gp120 inhibits the beta-adrenergic regulation of astroglial and microglial functions. *Proc. Natl. Acad. Sci. USA* **90**:1541–1545.

Lew, J., and J. H. Wang. 1995. Neuronal cdc2-like kinase. *Trends Biochem. Sci.* **20**:33–37.

Lipton, S. 1993. Human immunodeficiency virus-infected macrophages, gp120, and N-methyl-D-aspartate receptor-mediated neurotoxicity. *Ann. Neurol.* **33**:227–228.

Lipton, S. A., N. J. Sucher, P. K. Kaiser, and E. B. Dreyer. 1991. Synergistic effects of HIV coat protein and NMDA receptor-mediated neurotoxicity. *Neuron* **7**:111–118.

Liu, D. X., and L. A. Greene. 2001. Neuronal apoptosis at the G1/S cell cycle checkpoint. *Cell Tissue Res.* **305**:217–228.

Lo, T. M., C. J. Fallert, T. M. Piser, and S. A. Thayer. 1992. HIV-1 envelope protein evokes intracellular calcium oscillations in rat hippocampal neurons. *Brain Res.* **594**:189–196.

Logan, T., K. Jordan, and D. Hall. 1994. Altered shape and cell cycle characteristics of fibroblasts expressing the E2F1 transcription factor. *Mol. Biol. Cell* **5**:667–678.

Macleod, K. F., Y. Hu, and T. Jacks. 1996. Loss of Rb activates both p53-dependent and independent cell death pathways in the developing mouse nervous system. *EMBO J.* **15**:6178–6188.

Manes, S., E. Mira, R. Colomer, S. Montero, L. M. Real, C. Gomez-Mouton, S. Jimenez-Baranda, A. Garzon, R. A. Lacalle, K. Harshman, A. Ruiz, and A. C. Martinez. 2003. CCR5 expression influences the progression of human breast cancer in a p53-dependent manner. *J. Exp. Med.* **198**:1381–1389.

Mapelli, M., L. Massimiliano, C. Crovace, M. A. Seeliger, L. H. Tsai, L. Meijer, and A. Musacchio. 2005. Mechanism of CDK5/p25 binding by CDK inhibitors. *J. Med. Chem.* **48**:671–679.

Martin, L. J. 2000. p53 is abnormally elevated and active in the CNS of patients with amyotrophic lateral sclerosis. *Neurobiol. Dis.* **7**:613–622.

Masliah, E., C. L. Achim, N. Ge, R. DeTeresa, R. D. Terry, and C. A. Wiley. 1992. Spectrum of human immunodeficiency virus-associated neocortical damage. *Ann. Neurol.* **32**:321–329.

McGeer, E. G., and P. L. McGeer. 2003. Inflammatory processes in Alzheimer's disease. *Prog. Neuropsychopharmacol. Biol. Psychiatry* **27**:741–749.

McShea, A., P. Harris, K. Webster, A. Wahl, and M. Smith. 1997. Abnormal expression of the cell cycle regulators p16 and cdk4 in Alzheimer's disease. *Am. J. Pathol.* **150**:1933–1939.

Mirjany, M., L. Ho, and G. M. Pasinetti. 2002. Role of cyclooxygenase-2 in neuronal cell cycle activity and glutamate-mediated excitotoxicity. *J. Pharmacol. Exp. Ther.* **301**:494–500.

Morgan, K. L., E. M. Chalovich, G. D. Strachan, L. L. Otis, and K. L. Jordan-Sciutto. 2005. E2F4 expression patterns in SIV encephalitis. *Neurosci. Lett.* **382**:259–264.

Morris, E. J., E. Keramaris, H. J. Rideout, R. S. Slack, N. J. Dyson, L. Stefanis, and D. S. Park. 2001. Cyclin-dependent kinases and P53 pathways are activated independently and mediate Bax activation in neurons after DNA damage. *J. Neurosci.* **21**:5017–5026.

Morrison, R. S., Y. Kinoshita, M. D. Johnson, W. Guo, and G. A. Garden. 2003. p53-dependent cell death signaling in neurons. *Neurochem. Res.* **28**:15–27.

Muir, J. K., R. Raghupathi, D. L. Emery, F. M. Bareyre, and T. K. McIntosh. 1999. Postinjury magnesium treatment attenuates traumatic brain injury-induced cortical induction of p53 mRNA in rats. *Exp. Neurol.* **159**:584–593.

Nagy, Z., M. Esiri, A.-M. Cato, and A. D. Smith. 1997. Cell cycle markers in the hippocampus in Alzheimer's disease. *Acta Neuropathol.* **94**:6–15.

Napieralski, J. A., R. Raghupathi, and T. K. McIntosh. 1999. The tumor-suppressor gene, p53, is induced in injured brain regions following experimental traumatic brain injury. *Brain Res. Mol. Brain Res.* **71**:78–86.

Navia, B. A., E. S. Cho, C. K. Petito, and R. W. Price. 1986. The AIDS dementia complex. II. Neuropathology. *Ann. Neurol.* **19**:525–535.

Nevins, J. 1998. Towards an understanding of the functional complexity of the E2F and retinoblastoma families. *Cell Growth Differ.* **9**:585–593.

Nicotera, P., M. Ankarcrona, E. Bonfoco, S. Orrenius, and S. A. Lipton. 1997. Neuronal necrosis and apoptosis: two distinct events induced by exposure to glutamate or oxidative stress. *Adv. Neurol.* **72**:95–101.

Nuovo, G. J., F. Gallery, P. MacConnell, and A. Braun. 1994. In situ detection of polymerase chain reaction-amplified HIV-1 nucleic acids and tumor necrosis factor-alpha RNA in the central nervous system. *Am. J. Pathol.* **144**:659–666.

O'Hare, M. J., S. T. Hou, E. J. Morris, S. P. Cregan, Q. Xu, R. S. Slack, and D. S. Park. 2000. Induction and modulation of cerebellar granule neuron death by E2F-1. *J. Biol. Chem.* **275**:25358–25364.

O'Hare, M. J., N. Kushwaha, Y. Zhang, H. Aleyasin, S. M. Callaghan, R. S. Slack, P. R. Albert, I. Vincent, and D. S. Park. 2005. Differential roles of nuclear and cytoplasmic cyclin-dependent kinase 5 in apoptotic and excitotoxic neuronal death. *J. Neurosci.* **25**:8954–8966.

Padmanabhan, J., D. S. Park, L. A. Greene, and M. L. Shelanski. 1999. Role of cell cycle regulatory proteins in cerebellar granule neuron apoptosis. *J. Neurosci.* **19**:8747–8756.

Park, D., E. Morris, R. Bremmer, E. Keramaris, J. Padmanabhan, M. Rosenbaum, M. Shelanski, H. Geller, and L. Greene. 2000a. Involvement of Retinoblastoma family members and E2F/DP complexes in the death of neurons by DNA damage. *J. Neurosci.* **20**:3104–3114.

Park, D., E. Morris, L. Greene, and H. Geller. 1997a. G1/S cell cycle blockers and Inhibitors of cyclin-dependent kinases supression camptothecin-induced neuronal apoptosis. *J. Neurosci.* **17**:1256–1270.

Park, D. S., B. Levine, G. Ferrari, and L. A. Greene. 1997b. Cyclin dependent kinase inhibitors and dominant negative cyclin dependent kinase 4 and 6 promote survival of NGF-deprived sympathetic neurons. *J. Neurosci.* **17**:8975–8983.

Phillips, A., M. Ernst, S. Bates, N. Rice, and K. Vousden. 1999. E2F-1 potentiates cell death by blocking antiapoptotic signaling pathways. *Mol. Cell* **4**:771–781.

Pierce, A., I. Gimenez-Conti, R. Schneider-Broussard, L. Martinez, C. Conti, and D. Johnson. 1998. Increased E2F1 activity induces skin tumors in mice heterozygous and nullizygous for p53. *Proc. Natl. Acad. Sci. USA* **95**:8858–8863.

Poluha, W., C. M. Schonhoff, K. S. Harrington, M. B. Lachyankar, N. E. Crosbie, D. A. Bulseco, and A. H. Ross. 1997. A novel, nerve growth factor-activated pathway involving nitric oxide, p53, and p21WAF1 regulates neuronal differentiation of PC12 cells. *J. Biol. Chem.* **272**:24002–24007.

Portegies, P., R. H. Enting, J. deGans, P. R. Algra, M. M. Derix, J. M. Lange, and J. Goudsmit. 1993. Presentation and course of AIDS dementia complex: 10 years of follow-up in Amsterdam, The Netherlands. *AIDS* **7**:669–675.

Power, C., P. A. Kong, T. O. Crawford, S. Wesselingh, J. D. Glass, J. C. McArthur, and B. D. Trapp. 1993. Cerebral white matter changes in acquired immunodeficiency syndrome dementia: alterations of the blood-brain barrier. *Ann. Neurol.* **34**:339–350.

Power, C., J. C. McArthur, A. Nath, K. Wehrly, M. Mayne, J. Nishio, T. Langelier, R. T. Johnson, and B. Chesebro. 1998. Neuronal death induced by brain-derived human immunodeficiency virus type 1 envelope genes differs between demented and nondemented AIDS patients. *J. Virol.* **72**:9045–9053.

Pozniak, C. D., S. Radinovic, A. Yang, F. McKeon, D. R. Kaplan, and F. D. Miller. 2000. An anti-apoptotic role for the p53 family member, p73, during developmental neuron death. *Science* **289**:304–306.

Price, R. W., B. Brew, J. Sidtis, M. Rosenblum, A. C. Scheck, and P. Cleary. 1988. The brain in AIDS: central nervous system HIV-1 infection and AIDS dementia complex. *Science* **239**:586–592.

Prudlo, J., J. Koenig, J. Graser, E. Burckhardt, P. Mestres, M. Menger, and K. Roemer. 2000. Motor neuron cell death in a mouse model of FALS is not mediated by the p53 cell survival regulator. *Brain Res.* **879**:183–187.

Pulliam, L., J. A. Clarke, M. S. McGrath, D. Moore, and D. McGuire. 1996. Monokine products as predictors of AIDS dementia. *AIDS* **10**:1495–1500.

Pulliam, L., J. A. Clarke, D. McGuire, and M. S. McGrath. 1994. Investigation of HIV-infected macrophage neurotoxin production from patients with AIDS dementia. *Adv. Neuroimmunol.* **4**:195–198.

Pulliam, L., M. Zhou, M. Stubblebine, and C. M. Bitler. 1998. Differential modulation of cell death proteins in human brain cells by tumor necrosis factor alpha and platelet activating factor. *J. Neurosci. Res.* **54**:530–538.

Ranganathan, S., and R. Bowser. 2003. Alterations in G(1) to S phase cell-cycle regulators during amyotrophic lateral sclerosis. *Am. J. Pathol.* **162**:823–835.

Rashid, T., M. Banerjee, and M. Nikolic. 2001. Phosphorylation of Pak1 by the p35/Cdk5 kinase affects neuronal morphology. *J. Biol. Chem.* **276**:49043–49052.

Ren, B., H. Cam, Y. Takahashi, T. Volkert, J. Terragni, R. A. Young, and B. D. Dynlacht. 2002. E2F integrates cell cycle progression with DNA repair, replication, and G(2)/M checkpoints. *Genes Dev.* **16**:245–256.

Rideout, H. J., Q. Wang, D. S. Park, and L. Stefanis. 2003. Cyclin-dependent kinase activity is required for apoptotic death but not inclusion formation in cortical neurons after proteasomal inhibition. *J. Neurosci.* **23**:1237–1245.

Roberts, E. S., M. A. Zandonatti, D. D. Watry, L. J. Madden, S. J. Henriksen, M. A. Taffe, and H. S. Fox. 2003. Induction of pathogenic sets of genes in macrophages and neurons in NeuroAIDS. *Am. J. Pathol.* **162**:2041–2057.

Sadoul, R., A. L. Quiquerez, I. Martinou, P. A. Fernandez, and J. C. Martinou. 1996. p53 protein in sympathetic neurons: cytoplasmic localization and no apparent function in apoptosis. *J. Neurosci. Res.* **43**:594–601.

Saito, T., L. Sharer, L. Epstein, J. Michaels, M. Mintz, M. Lounder, K. Golding, T. Cvetkovich, and B. Blumberg. 1994. Overexpression of nef as a marker for restricted HIV-1 infection of astrocytes in postmortem pediatric central nervous tissues. *Neurology* **44**:474–481.

Sakhi, S., A. Bruce, N. Sun, G. Tocco, M. Baudry, and S. Schreiber. 1994. p53 induction is associated with neuronal damage in the central nervous system. *Proc. Natl. Acad. Sci. USA* **90:**7525–7529.

Sakhi, S., W. Gilmore, N. D. Tran, and S. S. Schreiber. 1996. p53-deficient mice are protected against adrenalectomy-induced apoptosis. *Neuroreport* **8:**233–235.

Savio, T., and G. Levi. 1993. Neurotoxicity of HIV coat protein gp120, NMDA receptors, and protein kinase C: a study with rat cerebellar granule cell cultures. *J. Neurosci. Res.* **34:**265–272.

Schauwecker, P. E., and O. Steward. 1997. Genetic determinants of susceptibility to excitotoxic cell death: implications for gene targeting approaches. *Proc. Natl. Acad. Sci. USA* **94:**4103–4108.

Scherr, C. 1998. Tumor surveillance via the ARF-p53 pathway. *Genes Dev.* **12:**2984–2991.

Selkoe, D. J., and D. Schenk. 2003. Alzheimer's disease: molecular understanding predicts amyloid-based therapeutics. *Annu. Rev. Pharmacol. Toxicol.* **43:**545–584.

Shea, T. B., J. T. Yabe, D. Ortiz, A. Pimenta, P. Loomis, R. D. Goldman, N. Amin, and H. C. Pant. 2004. Cdk5 regulates axonal transport and phosphorylation of neurofilaments in cultured neurons. *J. Cell Sci.* **117:**933–941.

Silva, C., K. Zhang, S. Tsutsui, J. K. Holden, M. J. Gill, and C. Power. 2003. Growth hormone prevents human immunodeficiency virus-induced neuronal p53 expression. *Ann. Neurol.* **54:**605–614.

Siman, R., T. K. McIntosh, K. M. Soltesz, Z. Chen, R. W. Neumar, and V. L. Roberts. 2004. Proteins released from degenerating neurons are surrogate markers for acute brain damage. *Neurobiol. Dis.* **16:**311–320.

Smith, P. D., M. P. Mount, R. Shree, S. Callaghan, R. S. Slack, H. Anisman, I. Vincent, X. Wang, Z. Mao, and D. S. Park. 2006. Calpain-regulated p35/cdk5 plays a central role in dopaminergic neuron death through modulation of the transcription factor myocyte enhancer factor 2. *J. Neurosci.* **26:**440–447.

Smith, P. D., M. J. O'Hare, and D. S. Park. 2004. Emerging pathogenic role for cyclin dependent kinases in neurodegeneration. *Cell Cycle* **3:**289–291.

Steffan, J. S., A. Kazantsev, O. Spasic-Boskovic, M. Greenwald, Y. Z. Zhu, H. Gohler, E. E. Wanker, G. P. Bates, D. E. Housman, and L. M. Thompson. 2000. The Huntington's disease protein interacts with p53 and CREB-binding protein and represses transcription. *Proc. Natl. Acad. Sci. USA* **97:**6763–6768.

Strachan, G. D., A. S. Kopp, M. A. Koike, K. L. Morgan, and K. L. Jordan-Sciutto. 2005. Chemokine- and neurotrophic factor-induced changes in E2F1 localization and phosphorylation of the retinoblastoma susceptibility gene product (pRb) occur by distinct mechanisms in murine cortical cultures. *Exp. Neurol.* **193:**455–468.

Streit, W. J., J. R. Conde, and J. K. Harrison. 2001. Chemokines and Alzheimer's disease. *Neurobiol. Aging* **22:**909–913.

Takahashi, Y., J. B. Rayman, and B. D. Dynlacht. 2000. Analysis of promoter binding by the E2F and pRB families in vivo: distinct E2F proteins mediate activation and repression. *Genes Dev.* **14:**804–816.

Takikita, S., T. Takano, T. Narita, M. Takikita, M. Ohno, and M. Shimada. 2001. Neuronal apoptosis mediated by IL-1 beta expression in viral encephalitis caused by a neuroadapted strain of the mumps virus (Kilham Strain) in hamsters. *Exp. Neurol.* **172:**47–59.

Tan, Z., R. Sankar, D. Shin, N. Sun, H. Liu, C. G. Wasterlain, and S. S. Schreiber. 2002. Differential induction of p53 in immature and adult rat brain following lithium-pilocarpine status epilepticus. *Brain Res.* **928:**187–193.

Toggas, S. M., E. Masliah, E. M. Rockenstein, G. F. Rall, C. R. Abraham, and L. Mucke. 1994. Central nervous sys-tem damage produced by expression of the HIV-1 coat protein gp120 in transgenic mice. *Nature* **367:**188–193.

Tornatore, C., R. Chandra, J. Berger, and E. Major. 1994. HIV-1 infection of subcortical astrocytes in the pediatric central-nervous-system. *Neurology* **44:**481–487.

Trimmer, P. A., T. S. Smith, A. B. Jung, and J. P. Bennett, Jr. 1996. Dopamine neurons from transgenic mice with a knockout of the p53 gene resist MPTP neurotoxicity. *Neurodegeneration* **5:**233–239.

Trinh, E., A. L. Boutillier, and J. P. Loeffler. 2001. Regulation of the retinoblastoma-dependent Mdm2 and E2F-1 signaling pathways during neuronal apoptosis. *Mol. Cell. Neurosci.* **17:**342–353.

Tsai, K., Y. Hu, K. Macleod, D. Crowley, L. Yamasaki, and T. Jacks. 1998. Mutation of E2F1 suppresses apoptosis and inappropriate S phase entry and extends survival of Rb-deficient mouse embryos. *Mol. Cell* **2:**293–304.

Uberti, D., M. Belloni, M. Grilli, P. Spano, and M. Memo. 1998. Induction of tumour-suppressor phosphoprotein p53 in the apoptosis of cultured rat cerebellar neurones triggered by excitatory amino acids. *Eur. J. Neurosci.* **10:**246–254.

Valcour, V., C. Shikuma, B. Shiramizu, M. Watters, P. Poff, O. Selnes, P. Holck, J. Grove, and N. Sacktor. 2004. Higher frequency of dementia in older HIV-1 individuals: the Hawaii Aging with HIV-1 Cohort. *Neurology* **63:**822–827.

Vincent, I., G. Jicha, M. Rosado, and D. W. Dickson. 1997. Aberrant expression of mitotic cdc2/cyclin B1 kinase in degenerating neurons of Alzheimer's disease brain. *J. Neurosci.* **17:**3588–3598.

Vincent, I., M. Rosado, and P. Davies. 1996. Mitotic mechanisms in Alzheimer's Disease? *J. Cell Biol.* **132:**413–425.

Vogel, K. S., and L. F. Parada. 1998. Sympathetic neuron survival and proliferation are prolonged by loss of p53 and neurofibromin. *Mol. Cell. Neurosci.* **11:**19–28.

Vogelstein, B., D. Lane, and A. J. Levine. 2000. Surfing the p53 network. *Nature* **408:**307–310.

Wang, Y., M. G. White, C. Akay, R. A. Chodroff, J. Robinson, K. A. Lindl, M. A. Dichter, Y. Qian, Z. Mao, D. L. Kolson, and K. L. Jordan-Sciutto. 2007. Activation of cyclin-dependent kinase 5 by calpains contributes to human immunodeficiency virus-induced neurotoxicity. *J. Neurochem.* **103:**439–455.

Watanabe, H., S. Ohta, Y. Kumon, S. Sakaki, and M. Sakanaka. 1999. Increase in p53 protein expression following cortical infarction in the spontaneously hypertensive rat. *Brain Res.* **837:**38–45.

Watanabe, T., H. Huang, M. Nakamura, J. Wischhusen, M. Weller, P. Kleihues, and H. Ohgaki. 2002. Methylation of the p73 gene in gliomas. *Acta Neuropathol.* **104:**357–362.

Wiley, C. A., and C. Achim. 1994. Human immunodeficiency virus encephalitis is the pathological correlate of dementia in acquired immunodeficiency syndrome. *Ann. Neurol.* **36:**673–676.

Wiley, C. A., V. Soontornniyomkij, L. Radhakrishnan, E. Masliah, J. Mellors, S. A. Herman, P. Dailey, and C. L. Achim. 1998. Distribution of brain HIV load in AIDS. *Brain Pathol.* **8:**277–284.

Wullner, U., and T. Klockgether. 2003. Inflammation in Parkinson's disease. *J. Neurol.* **250**(Suppl. 1)**:**I35–I38.

Xiang, H., D. W. Hochman, H. Saya, T. Fujiwara, P. A. Schwartzkroin, and R. S. Morrison. 1996. Evidence for p53-mediated modulation of neuronal viability. *J. Neurosci.* **16:**6753–6765.

Xiang, H., Y. Kinoshita, C. M. Knudson, S. J. Korsmeyer, P. A. Schwartzkroin, and R. S. Morrison. 1998. Bax involvement in p53-mediated neuronal cell death. *J. Neurosci.* **18:**1363–1373.

Xie, Z., K. Sanada, B. A. Samuels, H. Shih, and L. H. Tsai. 2003. Serine 732 phosphorylation of FAK by Cdk5 is important for microtubule organization, nuclear movement, and neuronal migration. *Cell* **114**:469–482.

Yan, G. Z., and E. B. Ziff. 1995. NGF regulates the PC12 cell cycle machinery through specific inhibition of the Cdk kinases and induction of cyclin D1. *J. Neurosci.* **15**:6200–6212.

Yan, G. Z., and E. B. Ziff. 1997. Nerve growth factor induces transcription of the p21 WAF1/CIP1 and cyclin D1 genes in PC12 cells by activating the Sp1 transcription factor. *J. Neurosci.* **17**:6122–6132.

Yang, Y., D. S. Geldmacher, and K. Herrup. 2001. DNA replication precedes neuronal cell death in Alzheimer's disease. *J. Neurosci.* **21**:2661–2668.

Yang, Y., E. J. Mufson, and K. Herrup. 2003. Neuronal cell death is preceded by cell cycle events at all stages of Alzheimer's disease. *J. Neurosci.* **23**:2557–2563.

Yu, J., H. Zhang, J. Gu, S. Lin, J. Li, W. Lu, Y. Wang, and J. Zhu. 2004. Methylation profiles of thirty four promoter-CpG islands and concordant methylation behaviours of sixteen genes that may contribute to carcinogenesis of astrocytoma. *BMC Cancer* **4**:65.

Zhang, Y., R. McLaughlin, C. Goodyer, and A. LeBlanc. 2002. Selective cytotoxicity of intracellular amyloid beta peptide 1-42 through p53 and Bax in cultured primary human neurons. *J. Cell Biol.* **156**:519–529.

NEUROIMAGING
IN HIV INFECTION

The Spectrum of Neuro-AIDS Disorders:
Pathophysiology, Diagnosis, and Treatment
Edited by K. Goodkin et al.
©2008 ASM Press, Washington, DC

18

The Uses of Structural Neuroimaging in the Brain in HIV-1-Infected Patients

MAJDA M. THURNHER AND M. JUDITH DONOVAN POST

As the HIV/AIDS epidemic approaches the 20th anniversary of the first mysterious reports of people with the syndrome, researchers and clinicians continue to grapple with the complexities of the virus. An estimated 36 million people worldwide are currently living with HIV, and some 20 million people have already died. If the number of new infections continues at the current rate, even the most devastating impact that can be anticipated from current levels of infection will seem minor compared with that of the future.

HIV enters the central nervous system (CNS) early in the course of infection, and the virus resides primarily at the cellular level in microglia and macrophages. Cerebrospinal fluid (CSF) analysis has demonstrated that HIV can enter the CNS soon after exposure, even before antibodies are detectable in the blood. HIV has been detected in the brain as early as 15 days after accidental intravenous inoculation (Davis et al., 1992). More than a decade ago, it became clear that the neuron dysfunction or death that underlies the clinical symptoms of HIV/CNS disease could not result from direct infections of neurons. However, the mechanism of HIV-related brain injury remains poorly understood. The predominant pathogenesis is believed to involve the combined influences of both HIV infection and the activation of immune-competent cells and their subsequent release of toxins that lead to neuronal and astrocytic dysfunction (Rausch and Davis, 2001).

The brain may be affected by a variety of abnormalities in association with HIV infection. Knowledge of these abnormalities and their characteristic imaging features is important to neuroradiologists for detection and diagnosis and the initiation of appropriate treatment. Nowadays, patients with AIDS form a considerable part of routine neuroradiological work. The imaging modalities commonly used in patients with HIV/AIDS are computed tomography (CT) and magnetic resonance imaging (MRI). In addition, nuclear-medicine techniques, such as single-photon emission CT (SPECT) and positron emission tomography (PET), are also helpful.

This review attempts to describe the imaging findings associated with brain disorders in HIV-seropositive patients and the rationales for integrating neuroradiological techniques, including radionuclide techniques.

The spectrum of CNS abnormalities can be divided into three main categories: (i) HIV-associated lesions, (ii) opportunistic infections, and (iii) neoplasms.

HIV-ASSOCIATED CNS ABNORMALITIES

Like all viruses, HIV is a parasite that replicates within the living cells of the host. HIV has nine genes and belongs to the lentivirus genus of retroviruses. HIV infection of the CNS produces a range of cognitive, motor, and behavioral abnormalities (Arendt et al. 1990; Navia et al., 1986; Power et al., 1995; Price and Sidtis, 1990). The syndrome observed after infection with HIV has been designated HIV-associated dementia (HAD) (Rausch and Davis, 2001; Wesselingh et al., 1993). The prevalence of HAD was estimated in the early 1990s to be as high as 20 to 30% in those patients with advanced HIV disease and low CD4 counts. HAD is now probably the most common cause of dementia worldwide among people aged 40 or less. With the advent of potent combination antiretroviral therapy (highly active antiretroviral therapy [HAART]), the incidence of HAD has decreased to as low as 10.5% (Sacktor et al., 2001). The widespread implementation of HAART has resulted in a dramatic decrease in AIDS-related morbidity and mortality (Flexner, 1998). While the incidence of HAD appears to be declining, the prevalence of milder, yet debilitating, neuropsychological impairments may rise as individuals infected with HIV live longer. These findings support the hypothesis that HAART does not provide complete protection from the development of HAD.

The histopathological marker of the HIV-infected brain is the presence of multinucleated giant cells (MGC). Two

Majda M. Thurnher, Neuroradiology Section, Department of Radiology, Medical University of Vienna, Vienna, Austria. **M. Judith Donovan Post,** Neuroradiology, Department of Radiology, University of Miami Miller School of Medicine, Miami, FL 33136-1094.

neuropathological correlates of cerebral infection by HIV are MGC encephalitis and progressive diffuse leukoencephalopathy (Budka et al., 1987; Kleihues et al., 1985). MGC encephalitis and progressive diffuse leukoencephalopathy may be end points, with a morphological spectrum of HIV-induced changes in between.

The most common reported imaging finding is cerebral atrophy. The predominant pattern of atrophy may be central (ventricular dilatation), peripheral (sulcal dilatation), or mixed (central and peripheral) (Arendt et al., 1993; Bencherif and Rottenberg, 1998; Bursztyn et al., 1984; Elovaara et al., 1990; Levy et al., 1986; Post et al., 1985; Poutiainen et al., 1993). Levy et al. reported in their early CT study of 200 patients with AIDS that 37.5% of the patients presented with cerebral atrophy (Levy et al., 1986). Serial CT studies have demonstrated progression of the atrophy over time in patients with HAD. Jakobsen et al. reported cortical atrophy in one-third of 400 AIDS patients with neurological manifestations (Jakobsen et al., 1989). Studies with symptomatic patients showed cortical atrophy in 85% of the patients, which suggests that cortical atrophy may be relatively specific to patients with neuropsychological impairment. Aylward et al. found an association between HAD and specific gray matter volume reduction in the basal ganglia and posterior cortex, as well as with generalized volume reduction of white matter (Aylward et al., 1995). The total CSF volumes were significantly greater for HIV-positive patients with HAD than for HIV-positive patients without dementia.

White-matter lesions are the second most common MRI finding in patients with HAD (Fig. 1 and 2). The average frequency of white-matter lesions in patients with AIDS is 78%, with a range of 43% to 100% (Bencherif and Rottenberg, 1998). A review of the MRI images of 365 AIDS patients revealed signal abnormalites in the white matter in 31% of the patients (Olsen et al., 1988), with four patterns observed: diffuse, patchy, focal, and punctate. The white-matter lesions demonstrate high signal on T2-weighted MRI sequences and usually are isointense or minimally hypointense on T1-weighted MRI sequences. In contrast to HAD lesions, progressive multifocal leukoencephalopathy (PML) lesions usually have low signal on T1-weighted MRI sequences. Enhancement and mass effect are not present. Two distinct MRI patterns on T2-weighted image (WI) were observed, which allow a distinction between the two types of HAD: (i) diffuse, bilateral, and symmetric high-signal-intensity involvement of the white matter (butterfly-like) (Fig. 2); and (ii) bilateral, scattered, high-signal-intensity lesions in the white and gray matter (patchy) (Olsen et al., 1988). The appearance of MRI images most likely reflects an increase in the water content and the leakage of serum proteins resulting from altered vascular permeability, possibly related to the presence of circulating cytokines. High-signal-intensity lesions in the splenium of the corpus callosum and in the crura of the fornices have been reported within 6 months of the onset of cognitive impairment (Kieburtz et al., 1990). Prospective studies with long-term follow-up comparing asymptomatic with symptomatic patients have shown that the percentage of white-matter abnormalities significantly increases with disease progression (Cohen et al., 1992; Post et al., 1992, 1993).

Although MRI is the most sensitive imaging modality for depicting the effects of HIV in the brain, it is nevertheless not sensitive enough to show early pathologic involvement. Several authors have claimed that neuroimaging studies are relatively insensitive in the detection of early changes in the brain due to HIV infection. Compared to postmortem studies, MRI underestimated the presence of HIV-related lesions in the brain (Grafe et al., 1990). Fluid attenuated-inversion recovery (FLAIR) techniques have been shown to significantly improve the conspicuity of the lesions in the periventricular and subcortical locations (Thurnher et al., 1997b).

The data from recent studies suggest that proton MRI spectroscopy (^{1}H-MRS) could potentially be more sensitive in detecting early CNS involvement by HIV than MRI (Chang et al., 1995, 1999; Ernst et al., 2000; Jarvik

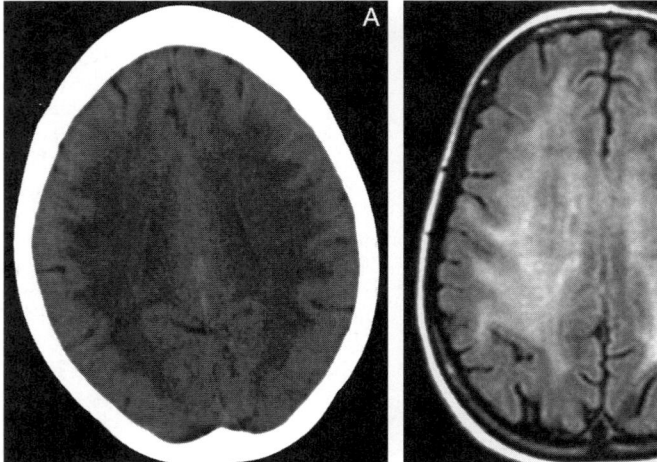

FIGURE 1 HIV-leukoencephalopathy in an HIV-positive patient presenting with dementia. (A) Precontrast axial CT scan showing marked bilateral hypodensity of the white matter. (B) Axial FLAIR (TR/TE/TI, 10,000/130/2,100). The MRI image demonstrates bilateral high-signal-intensity changes of the white matter without mass effect. Enhancement was not present on postcontrast T1-weighted MRI images (not shown).

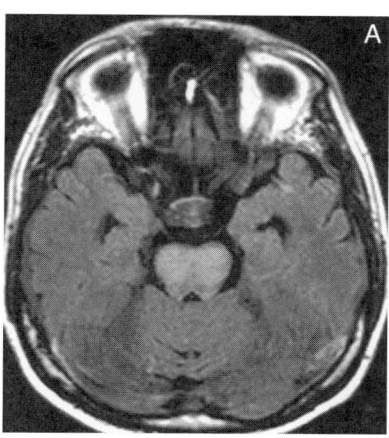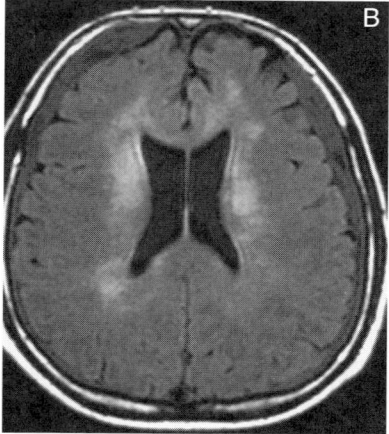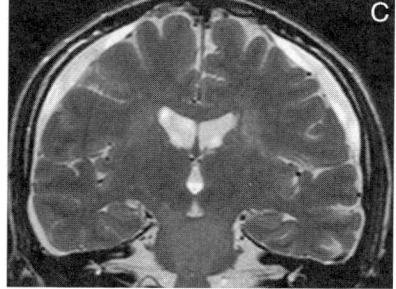

FIGURE 2 HIV-leukoencephalopathy in an HIV-positive female patient. (A) High-signal-intensity abnormality in the brainstem on axial FLAIR MRI image (TR/TE/TI, 10,000/130/2,100). The brainstem is not enlarged. (B and C) Axial FLAIR (TR/TE/TI, 10,000/130/2,100) and coronal T2-weighted MRI images showing high-signal-intensity abnormalities without mass effect in the white matter bilaterally. Note sparing of the subcortical fibers and dilatation of the ventricles, indicating associated atrophy. The lesions are iso- or hypointense on T1-weighted MRI images and show no enhancement on postcontrast images (not shown). In addition, bilateral subdural effusions are present.

et al., 1993; Laubenberger et al., 1996; Lopez-Villegas et al., 1997; Marcus et al., 1998; Moller et al., 1999; Otake et al., 1999; Salvan et al., 1997; Suwanwela et al., 2000; Tracey et al., 1996; Von Giesen et al., 2001). ^{1}H-MRS of the brain is a noninvasive study that is useful for certain aspects of cerebral biochemistry (Urenjak et al., 1993). Peaks of N-acetyl groups (N-acetylaspartate [NAA]), choline-containing compounds (Cho), and creatine plus phosphocreatine (Cr) are present in the spectrum. NAA is a marker for neuronal cell bodies (neuronal density). Creatinine represents the sum of creatine and phosphocreatine, with decrements also occurring with cell loss. The choline-to-creatinine ratio increases, a possible marker of membrane turnover. Determination of a myo-inositol (MI) peak is also possible using the short-echo-time technique. Elevated MI has been reported in cocaine abusers (Chang et al., 1997b), Alzheimer's disease (Klunk et al., 1992; Miller et al., 1993; Moats et al., 1994), and demyelination disorders, such as multiple sclerosis (Bruhn et al., 1994; Husted et al., 1994). The results of recent studies have shown that the metabolite pattern in patients with HAD indicates decreased NAA and elevated Cho and MI levels that are not observed in healthy subjects (Fig. 3) (a lower NAA/Cr ratio, an increased Cho/Cr ratio, and an increased MI/Cr ratio) (Chang et al., 1995, 1999a; Ernst et al., 2000; Jarvik et al., 1993; Laubenberger et al., 1996; Lopez-Villegas et al., 1997; Marcus et al., 1998; Moller et al., 1999; Otake et al., 1999; Salvan et al., 1997; Von Giesen et al., 2001). The findings indicate that diffuse brain involvement in AIDS can be marked not only by a loss of neurons, indicated by increased NAA levels, but also by increased MI levels. Ernst et al. recently reported an increased Cho/Cr ratio in the frontal white matter and in the basal ganglia, as well as an elevated MI/Cr ratio and MI concentrations in the basal ganglia (Ernst et al., 2000; Von Giesen et al., 2001). The results of the multicenter study of single-voxel MRS and magnetic-resonance spectroscopic imaging in individuals confirmed complementary roles of MRS in evaluating patients with HAD (Sacktor et al., 2005). Single-voxel

MRS showed elevated MI in early HAD, and magnetic-resonance spectroscopic imaging showed decreased NAA in mesial frontal gray matter in patients with psychomotor slowing compared with HIV$^+$ patients without psychomotor slowing.

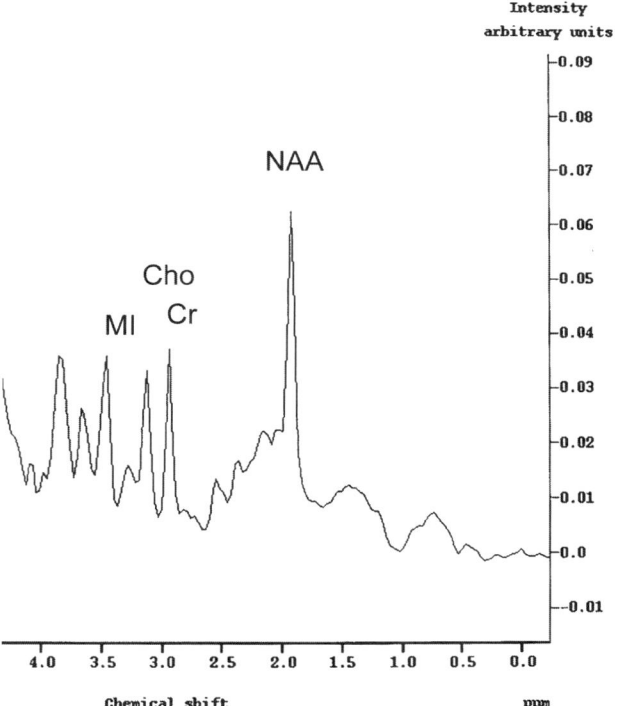

FIGURE 3 MRS in a symptomatic HIV-positive patient. A proton spectrum (TE, 23 ms; TR, 6,365 ms) from the voxel outlined from the frontal white matter shows slightly decreased NAA and increased MI, findings consistent with the early stage of HIV encephalitis.

Perfusion MRI (pMRI) can also detect abnormalities that correlate with disease severity in HAD. Ernst et al. evaluated the regional cerebral blood flow (rCBF) in 19 patients with early stages of HAD and correlated the results with those for 15 healthy seronegative subjects (Ernst et al., 2000). The patients with HAD had a statistically significant decrease in rCBF bilaterally in the inferior lateral frontal cortices and an increase in the posterior inferior parietal white matter. Because pMRI is faster and safer than nuclear medicine techniques, the authors suggested that pMRI could be used to monitor rCBF changes in HIV patients initially and during therapy.

Diffusion tensor imaging (DTI) is another promising MRI technique offering the possibility of measuring tissue anisotropy, thus providing details on tissue microstructure (Le Bihan et al., 2001; Ulug et al., 1999). Calculating the diffusion constant and anisotropy in the subcortical white matter and corpus callosum in patients with HIV, Filippi et al. recently found abnormalities despite normal-appearing white matter on conventional MRI images (Filippi et al., 2001). Patients with advanced HIV disease (a high viral load) had the highest diffusion constant elevations and the largest anisotropy decreases. The diffusion changes observed in the study by Filippi et al. may be a result of activation of inflammatory pathways in HIV infection of the brain. DTI did not correlate well with virological and immunological parameters in a recent study with 60 HIV-positive patients (Thurnher et al., 2005). No differences in fractional aniostropy (FA) were found between the different groups with regard to the CD4 T-lymphocyte count and viral-load level in plasma. The authors found a trend of FA reduction in the frontal white matter, the genu of the corpus callosum, and the hippocampi of the HIV$^+$ patients compared with healthy controls. The difference was statistically significant only for the genu of the corpus callosum. Future DTI studies comparing diffusion changes with MRS and virological and immunological parameters will be helpful in further understanding the alterations in the HIV-infected brain.

An increased knowledge of the pathogenesis of HIV, the development of sensitive measurements for such viral parameters as viral-load determinations, and the availability of new classes of antiretroviral drugs have profoundly improved the therapeutic management of HIV infection (Entning et al., 1998; Flexner, 1998; Tozzi et al., 1999; Von Giesen et al., 2000). Various combinations of drugs have been shown to increase CD4$^+$ lymphocyte counts and to decrease viral replication in plasma and lymph nodes to undetectable levels. The results of several recent studies (Chang et al., 1999b; DeSimone et al., 2000; Thurnher et al., 2000) suggest that MRI and MRS may help in the clinical management of patients with HAD who are receiving potent antiretroviral therapy and can be used to characterize changes due to HAART. A combination of antiretroviral drugs in patients with HAD may result in stabilization or even regression of white-matter signal intensity abnormalities observed on MRI images (Fig. 4) (Filippi et al., 1998; Thurnher et al., 2000). The progression of white-matter lesions on initial follow-up studies should not be mistaken for therapy failure, since the progression of MRI findings is likely the result of postinflammatory reactions due to immune reconstitutive effects after the initiation of HAART (DeSimone et al., 2000; Thurnher et al., 2000). Some other observations could also be important in understanding the discrepancies between the evolution of MRI findings and cognitive function in patients with HAD under HAART. The progression of cerebral atrophy was observed in all patients with

HAD who underwent HAART in one study, suggesting that despite potent therapy, the neuronal damage appears to progress without clinical manifestation (Thurnher et al., 2000).

OPPORTUNISTIC INFECTIONS

Viral Infections

CMV

Cytomegalovirus (CMV) is a member of the herpesvirus family; the infection in adults is a result of the reactivation of a latent infection, most commonly presented as mild infection mimicking mononucleosis. In immunocompromised patients, CMV can produce a variety of clinical syndromes. CMV infections have been described with increasing frequency in patients with AIDS (Morgello et al., 1987; Setinek et al., 1995). Chorioretinitis, gastrointestinal infection, pneumonitis, and neurological disease are the most common manifestations of CMV infection. Five distinct neurological syndromes due to CMV infection have been described: retinitis, myelitis/polyradiculopathy, diffuse micronodular encephalitis, ventriculoencephalitis, and mononeuritis multiplex.

Retinitis is one of the most common manifestations of CMV infection. Clinical diagnosis is based on funduscopic findings and recovery of the virus from any body site. Monette et al. have described MRI findings in one patient with late-stage CMV retinitis (Monette et al., 1992). Unenhanced T1-weighted MRI images showed thickening of the retinochoroid layer, with enhancement of the layer on postcontrast images.

In CMV-induced polyradiculopathy and myelitis, inflammation and axonal necrosis of the ventral and dorsal roots of the cauda equina are present (Behar et al., 1987). The diagnosis is based on clinical examination, CSF findings, and PCR. MRI reveals enlargement of the conus medullaris, clumping of the lumbosacral nerve roots, and leptomeningeal enhancement of the lower spinal cord (Talpos et al., 1991; Thurnher et al., 1997a).

Diffuse micronodular encephalitis histologically resembles HIV encephalitis. Small microglial nodules and inclusion-bearing cytomegalic cells are widely distributed in the cortex, basal ganglia, brain stem, and cerebellum. In an autopsy series of 30 cases of CMV encephalitis, 76% of the patients had microglial nodules containing inclusion-bearing cells and 24% had MV inclusions outside the nodules (Morgello et al., 1987). A distinct clinical syndrome of dementia associated with CMV has been described and compared with HAD (Holland et al., 1994). The two dementia syndromes differ in clinical presentation, course, associated electrolyte disturbances, and imaging findings. The most common imaging findings in patients with CMV encephalitis are cortical atrophy, periventricular enhancement, and diffuse white-matter abnormalities (Hassine et al., 1995; Post et al., 1986a). Generalized atrophy is the most commonly reported CT abnormality, but it is a nonspecific finding seen frequently in AIDS patients (Post et al., 1986a). Periventricular enhancement is also not diagnostic; it has been described in cases of lymphoma, toxoplasmosis, and other infections. White-matter disease occurs as a result of inflammation of the subependymal region and spread of the infection to the adjacent astrocytes of the white matter with infectious demyelination (Dorfman, 1973; Hawley et al., 1983). Hassine et al. found, in six patients with

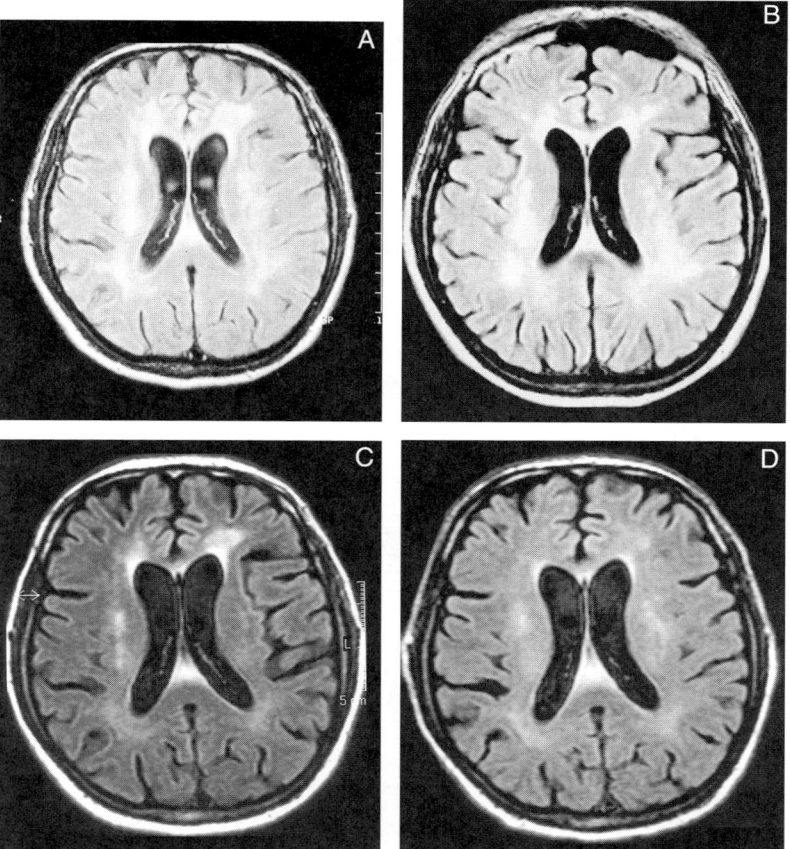

FIGURE 4 Patient with HIV encephalitis being treated with HAART. (A) Axial FLAIR-TSE (TR/TE/TI, 7,385/130/2,100) MRI image showing bilateral, symmetric, high-signal-intensity abnormalities in the periventricular white matter and white matter of the centrum semiovale. Additional widening of the sulci and ventricle is present. The patient had a high viral-load level in plasma and in the CSF and a low CD4+ T-lymphocyte count. The results of the neuropsychological examination were consistent with subcortical dementia. The diagnosis of HIV leukoencephalopathy was made, and combination antiretroviral therapy was started. (B) Nine months after the initiation of therapy, a follow-up FLAIR-TSE (TR/TE/TI, 7,385/130/2,100) MRI image shows progression of the white-matter SI abnormalities. (C) At 18 months after the initiation of HAART, a follow-up MRI scan shows interval decrease of the white-matter signal intensity abnormalities. (D) At 26 months after the initiation of the therapy, follow-up MRI scans show regression of the white-matter disease (not shown) and stabilization after 33 months.

pathologically confirmed CMV infection of the CNS, atrophy in three cases, subependymal nodular lesions without enhancement in two cases, and ventriculitis in one case (Hassine et al., 1995).

Patients with ventriculoencephalitis have a more acute onset, with death usually occurring quickly. Autopsies reveal periventriculitis, ependymal and subependymal necrosis, and associated inclusion-bearing CMV cells (Kalayjian et al., 1993; Salazar et al., 1995).

Rarely, cerebral mass lesions due to CMV can be observed in AIDS patients. In one study, two cases of cerebral mass lesions due to CMV were described (Dyer et al., 1995). In both cases, a large contrast-enhancing mass was seen in the frontal lobe with surrounding edema. Both patients described in the study died despite treatment. CMV should be considered in the differential diagnosis of mass lesions in AIDS patients with severe immune deficiency.

CMV infection can also be present as choroid plexitis. In one reported case, a contrast-enhanced CT scan showed marked enhancement of the slightly enlarged right plexus. MRI confirmed the findings and the absence of enhancement of ependyma (Guermazi et al., 1996). Infections of the choroid plexus are not common; nevertheless, CMV should be included among the causes of choroid plexitis in AIDS patients.

Infection of the CNS is difficult to diagnose while the patient is alive because CMV is difficult to culture from CSF. The recent development of the PCR technique has allowed isolation of CMV based on the presence of DNA within the CSF (Arribas et al., 1995). Discrimination between HIV- and CMV-associated CNS disease is often difficult using clinical and imaging findings. MRS could be useful in such cases. In one study, MRS was used to distingush HIV from CMV encephalitis (Wilkinson et al., 1996). The findings suggest that a larger choline signal and a smaller NAA signal could be inferred within the white-matter abnormalities due to HIV encephalitis/encephalopathy than in those due to CMV encephalitis.

PML

PML is a subacute opportunistic infection caused by *Polyomavirus* JC. The incidence of PML has greatly increased due to the AIDS epidemic, and 0.7 to 11% of HIV patients develop PML during the course of their illness (Berger and Concha, 1995; Thurnher et al., 1997c; Von Einsiedel et al., 1993). The histopathological hallmark of PML is demyelination with enlarged oligodendroglial nuclei and bizarre astrocytes. The disease is usually multifocal, and the lesions may occur in any location in the white matter, most often in the parieto-occipital region. Thalamic lesions

are frequently present, and the cerebellum and brainstem can also be involved. Posterior-fossa lesions are usually present simultaneously with supratentorial lesions, and in rare cases, PML may be limited to the posterior fossa (Kastrup et al., 2002). Although there are no significant pathological differences between patients with and without AIDS, in the AIDS population, more extensive disease with a necrotizing character was observed (Thurnher et al., 1997c).

The findings on MRI correlate very well with macroscopic changes. PML lesions are patchy, scalloped, high-signal-intensity lesions on T2-WI MRI images located in the white matter with extension along the white fibers (Fig. 5) (Whiteman et al., 1993; Thurnher et al., 1997c). Subcortical arcuate fibers are involved, mass effect is mild or absent, and peripheral, faint enhancement is a rare feature (Fig. 6) (Kotecha et al., 1998; Port et al., 1999; Wheeler et al., 1993;

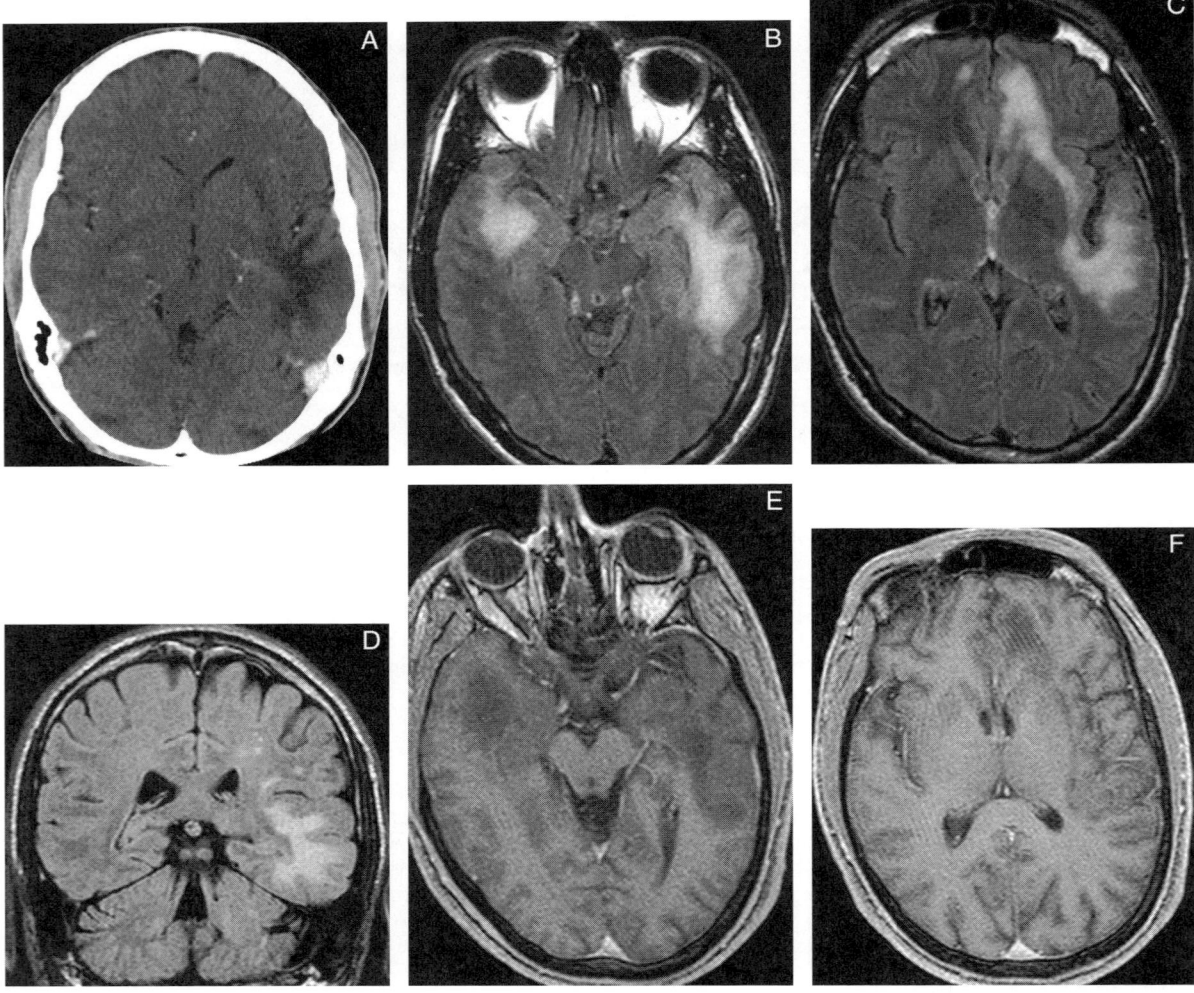

FIGURE 5 PML in an AIDS patient who presented at the emergency department with impaired consciousness. (A) Postcontrast CT scan of the brain showing a scalloped, nonenhancing, hypodense lesion in the left temporal lobe. (B to D) Axial and coronal FLAIR (TR/TE/TI, 6,000/100/2,000) MRI images showing a scalloped high-signal-intensity lesion located in the left temporal white matter with extension through the external capsule to the left frontal white matter. There is an additional lesion in the right temporal periventricular white matter. The subcortical fibers and cortex are also involved. There is no mass effect. (E and F) On postcontrast T1-weighted TFE (TR/TE/flip degree, 20/2.1/35°) MRI images, no enhancement is observed.

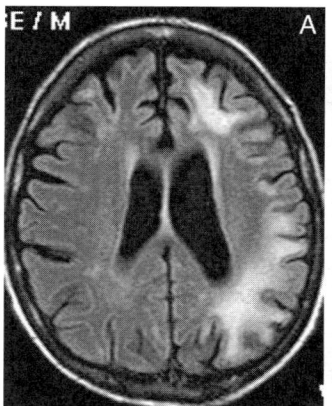 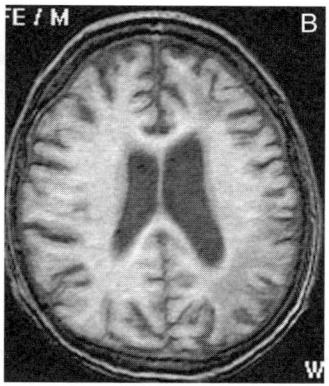 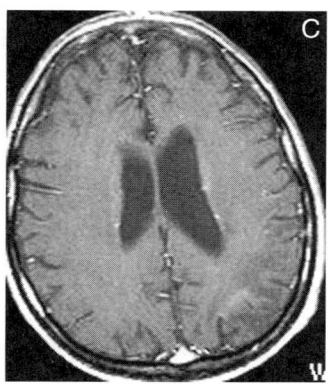

FIGURE 6 PML in an HIV-positive patient who responded well to HAART. (A) Scalloped high-signal-intensity lesions are demonstrated on an axial FLAIR (TR/TE/TI, 6,000/100/2,000) MRI image in the left frontal and parietal lobes. (B) The lesions have low signal on a T1-weighted TFE (TR/TE/flip degree, 20/2.1/35°) MRI image. (C) Faint peripheral enhancement is seen on a post-contrast T1-weighted TFE (TR/TE/flip degree, 20/2.1/35°) MRI image (unusual imaging feature in PML).

Woo et al., 1996). On T1-WI images, the PML lesions have low signal, in contrast to isointense HIV-associated lesions (Fig. 5 and 6) (Whiteman et al., 1993; Thurnher et al., 1997c).

A recent study demonstrated the existence of a significant difference between the magnetization transfer characteristics of PML lesions and white-matter lesions due to HAD in patients with AIDS (Ernst et al., 1999). The mean magnetization transfer ratio (MTR) of PML lesions was 26.1%, compared with 47.9% in HAD lesions in the study. The reported difference in MTR between PML- and HIV-associated lesions most likely reflects differences in pathophysiology and supports the fact that high MTR of normal white matter is due to the presence of myelinated axons. MRI with the magnetization transfer saturation technique as a noninvasive tool can be used to differentiate between PML- and HIV-related lesions in AIDS patients. A central area of marked hypointensity on T1-WI and hyperintensity on T2-WI MRI images was observed at follow-up, suggesting necrotic changes (Thurnher et al., 1997c). These findings are consistent with the low MTRs observed in PML lesions. Prominent necrotic changes in PML lesions in AIDS patients were also found in neuropathological studies (Kuchelmeister et al., 1993; Von Einsiedel et al., 1993).

1H-MRS was also used to image PML lesions, and the spectra were compared with those in normal brain parenchyma. The spectra of PML lesions were characterized by significantly reduced NAA, lactate presence, and increased choline and lipids (Chang et al., 1997a; Iranzo et al., 1999). A decrease in NAA is the result of axonal loss, and the presence of lactate is related to cellular hypoxia. The increase in choline and lipid may reflect an accumulation of myelin breakdown products.

201Tl brain SPECT has also been used in AIDS patients for differentiation of malignant lesions from lesions of infectious origin. In one study, combined gallium and thallium scans were performed on AIDS patients with focal brain lesions (Lee et al., 1999). Patients with PML had two different patterns: patients with positive gallium and negative thallium scans, and a second group with negative thallium and gallium scans. Some PML cases can, therefore, be mis-

taken for malignant lesions. Demyelination and destruction explain negative thallium and gallium scans. Positive gallium and negative thallium scans may be a result of coexisting pathology.

Without treatment, the prognosis for PML is usually poor, with death occurring after 2.5 to 4 months. Only a small number of cases have been reported to have a more benign clinical course (Berger et al., 1998). In one large prospective study of 48 AIDS patients with proven PML, except for mass effect, which was associated with shorter survival, no MRI abnormality was significantly correlated with patient survival (Post et al., 1999). Although at present there is no efficacious therapy for PML, recent studies have shown clinical and radiological improvement in patients with PML who underwent HAART (Baqi et al., 1997; De Luca et al., 1999; Happe et al., 1999; Giudici et al., 2000; Mayo et al., 1998; Miralles et al., 1998; Nicoli et al., 1991; Portegies et al., 1991; Tassie et al., 1999; Teofilo et al., 1998). In patients with prolonged survival regression or stabilization, MRI findings paralleled suppression of virus replication and immune response recovery (Fig. 7) (Baqi et al., 1997; Cardenas et al., 2001; Miralles et al., 1998; Shapiro et al., 2001; Thurnher et al., 2001a). In one study, initial worsening of the MRI findings with development of temporary contrast enhancement, mass effect, and edema was observed in patients who were long-term survivors (Collazos et al., 1999; Miralles et al., 2001; Thurnher et al., 2001a). This was probably a result of a posttreatment inflammatory reaction due to the immune reconstitutive effect. Atrophic changes and increased hypointensity on T1-WI images with concomitant low signal on FLAIR images in those patients represent leukomalacia and burned-out PML lesions (Fig. 7). In patients with no response, progressive disease can be recognized by increasing high signal on T2-WI and FLAIR images and increasing low signal on T1-WI images due to demyelination. About half of the AIDS patients with PML do not experience benefit from HAART. Tantisiriwat et al. showed that PML can also develop in AIDS patients who are undergoing HAART, making the interpretation of the imaging findings even more challenging (Tantisiriwat et al., 1999).

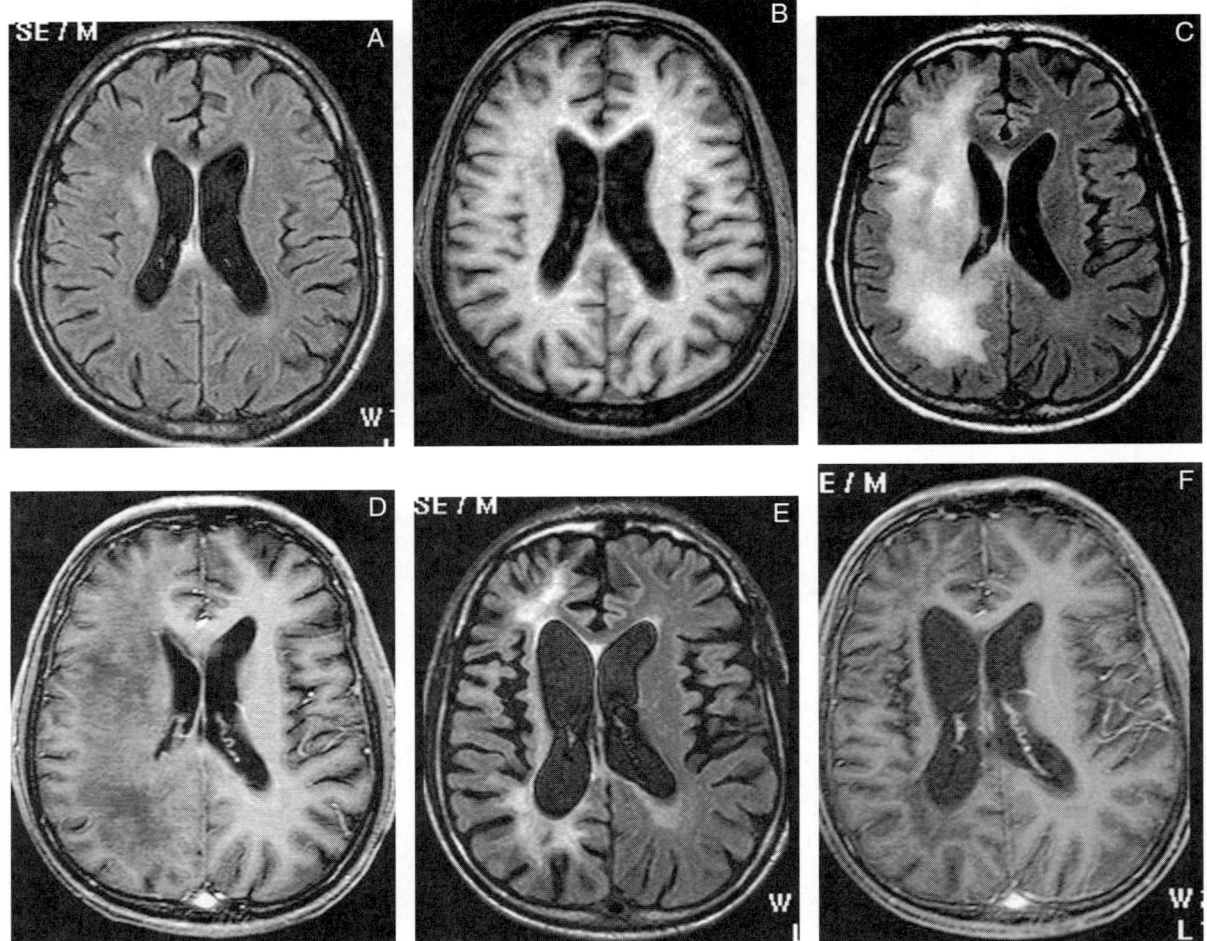

FIGURE 7 PML in an AIDS patient under HAART. (A) Initial FLAIR-TSE (TR/TE/TI, 7,373/130/2,100) MRI image showing a high-signal-intensity lesion in the right centrum semiovale. There is no mass effect. (B) The lesion has low signal on a T1-weighted TFE (TR/TE/flip degree, 10/3.5/10°) MRI image. Analysis of the CSF revealed positive PCR for JC virus, and HAART, including protease inhibitors, was initiated. (C and D) Two months after initiation of therapy, follow-up MRI images show progression of the disease with hyperintense white-matter abnormalities (C) extending to the entire white matter of the right side. Note the moderate mass effect with compression of the right lateral ventricle. (D) Postcontrast T1-weighted TFE (TR/TE/flip degree, 10/3.5/10°) MRI image showing low signal of the lesion but no enhancement. (E and F) Seven months later, subsequent MRI examination shows leukomalacia and atrophy of the right hemisphere and vacuo widening of the right lateral ventricle (E), indicating a burn-out process.

HSV

Infection with herpes simplex virus type 1 (HSV-1) appears in only 2% of autopsies of AIDS patients (Petito et al., 1986). In immunocompetent patients, the infection usually results in necrosis of the temporal lobe and the orbital surfaces of the frontal gyri with sparing of the basal ganglia. In the AIDS population, the involvement is more diffuse (Jordan and Enzmann, 1991). On MRI, high-signal-intensity lesions are observed on T2-WI images, with low signal on T1-WI images. The FLAIR technique has been reported to be even more sensitive than T2-WI in the detection of abnormalities due to HSV-1 infection, with the earliest imaging findings 48 h after the onset of symptoms. Early on, the enhancement is usually not present, and gyriform enhancement on enhanced T1-WI images can be observed

with disease progression (Jordan and Enzmann, 1991; Lizerbram and Hesselink, 1997).

Magnetization transfer suppression techniques with the administration of contrast enhancement have been shown to improve the detection of abnormalities associated with HSV-1 infection of the brain (Burke et al., 1996). Enhanced T1-WI sequences with MTC revealed a greater degree of disease involvement than was apparent on T2-WI or on T1-WI without magnetization transfer contrast (MTC) (Burke et al., 1996). This technique may be helpful in patients with an unclear diagnosis and atypical imaging findings.

On diffusion-weighted imaging (DWI), two distinct types of findings are characteristic of HSV-1 encephalitis: lesions similar to cytotoxic edema and lesions similar to vasogenic edema (Sener, 2001). The severity of the disease correlated well with the DWI findings in one study; the patients with lesions similar to cytotoxic edema had fulminating disease, while the others with lesions similar to vasogenic edema had a good outcome.

VZV

Varicella-zoster virus (VZV) causes chickenpox (varicella) in childhood, remains latent in the dorsal root ganglia, and may be reactivated decades later to produce shingles (zoster) in adults. Immunosuppressed patients may also develop encephalitis. In about 2% of AIDS autopsies, varicellazoster encephalitis is diagnosed by neuropathological examinations (Petito et al., 1986). CT is usually negative early on, and MRI reveals signal abnormalities in the brainstem and cortex (Fig. 8) (Tien et al., 1983). In one study, a case of proven chronic progressive VZV encephalitis in an AIDS patient was described (Gilden et al., 1988). MRI of the brain showed extensive necrosis of the basal ganglia and hydrocephalus in that case. A case of multifocal VZV leukoencephalitis was also described in an AIDS patient (Aygun et al., 1998). Multiple small, targetlike lesions coalescing into larger lesions were described on MRI images. However, there have been too few reported cases of VZV infections of the brain and MRI findings to know the full spectrum and characteristics of CNS abnormalities.

Bacterial Infections

Syphilis

Syphilis is a chronic infection that, when untreated, is expressed in three clinical stages: primary, secondary, and tertiary syphilis. About one-third of patients develop tertiary syphilis (Knox et al., 1976). Neurosyphilis can occur weeks and decades after initial infection. The course of the disease is accelerated in the AIDS population (Katz et al., 1993).

Most often, neurosyphilis is asymptomatic. Symptomatic neurosyphilis may present in two forms, parenchymal disease and a meningovascular form. Headache and vascular disease are characteristics of meningovascular neurosyphilis, which results in focal neurological deficits. Vascular occlusions, ischemia, and infarctions are consequences of

neurosyphilis-induced vasculitis. Heubner arteritis with involvement of the large and medium-size vessels is the common type, and Nissl-Alzheimer arteritis affects the small vessels (Bowen and Post, 1991). In 23% of the patients in one series of patients with syphilis, there was evidence of cerebral infarctions (Brightbill et al., 1995). The infarcts are located primarily in the basal ganglia and middle cerebral artery territory (Tien et al., 1992). Some reports of angiographic findings in vascular neurosyphilis include segmental constriction and occlusion of the supraclinoid carotid artery (Fig. 9) (Holland et al., 1986; Vatz et al., 1974). The stenoses in large arteries are concentric or asymmetric; small arteries show focal stenosis and aneurysmal dilatations. Areas of infarction are well demonstrated on MRI as a high-signal-intensity abnormality on T2-WI and FLAIR images with gyriform enhancement, indicating the subacute stage. Acute infarctions are better detected with the use of diffusion-weighted MRI images. MRI angiography (MRA) shows nicely and noninvasively the narrowing or occlusions of the vessels (Fig. 9).

Leptomeningeal disease is characterized pathologically by meningeal thickening and perivascular lymphocytic infiltrates. Nonspecific focal or diffuse enhancement observed on enhanced MRI images cannot be distinguished from meningitis of other origin.

Syphilitic gummas represent a parenchymal form of neurosyphilis, and they are a result of a cell-mediated response to *Treponema pallidum*. Spirochetes are rarely present in the lesion (Parker et al., 1985). Cortically located ring or nodular enhancing lesions with adjacent meningeal enhancement on MRI should raise a suspicion of syphilitic gumma. The cortical location and meningeal enhancement indicate the meningeal origin (Tien et al., 1992). On CT scans, the gummas are usually hyperintense, and on T2-WI images, high signal has been described. Application of a contrast agent is necessary for delineation of gummas, as well as meningeal abnormalities due to neurosyphilis.

Although symptomatic neurosyphilis is uncommon, in a young HIV-positive patient with ischemic events, meningeal disease, and/or cortically located enhancing lesions, neurosyphilis must be ruled out.

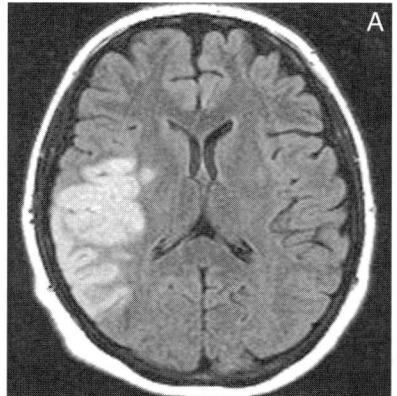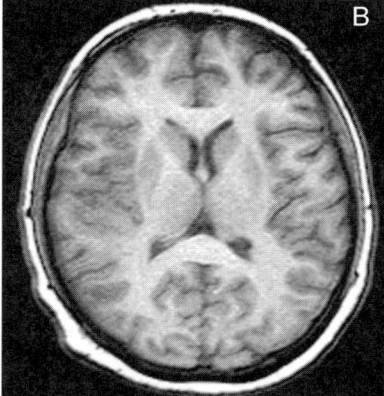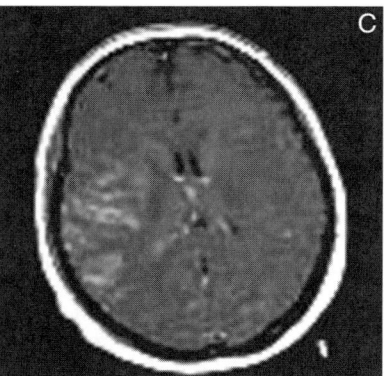

FIGURE 8 VZV encephalitis. (A) Axial FLAIR (TR/TE/TI, 7,383/130/2,100) MRI image showing high-signal-intensity abnormality of the cortex on the right side. (B) On a T1-weighted (TR/TE/flip degree, 8.4/2.8/10°) MRI image, swollen hypointense cortex can be observed. (C) Postcontrast T1-weighted SE (TR/TE, 500/15) MRI with MTC image demonstrating marked enhancement of the affected cortex.

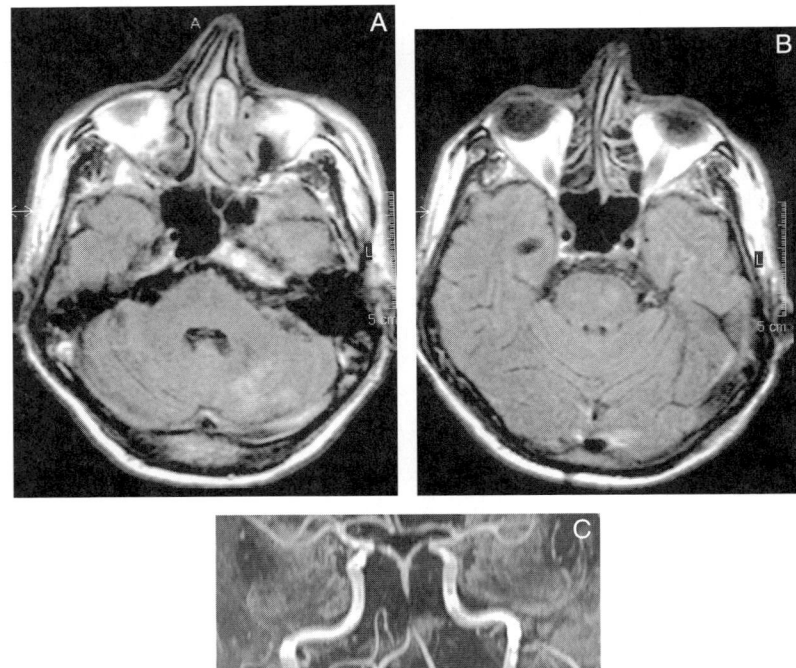

FIGURE 9 HIV-positive patient with meningovascular neurosyphilis. (A and B) Axial FLAIR-TSE (TR/TE/TI, 11,000/80/2,800) MRI images showing multiple hyperintense lesions in the left cerebellum and bilaterally in the brainstem. (C) Three-dimensional time-of-flight TFE MRA (TR/TE/flip degree, 22/2.9/20°) nicely demonstrating high-grade stenosis of the basilar artery. The combination of MRI findings of vascular lesions in the posterior fossa, narrowing of the basilar artery, and laboratory findings suggests vascular neurosyphilis.

Mycobacteria

The increased incidence of tuberculosis in developed countries is clearly related to the rise of AIDS. At present, about 30% of patients with tuberculosis are HIV positive; conversely, 5 to 9% of patients with AIDS develop tuberculosis (Centers for Disease Control and Prevention, 1987). Currently, AIDS is considered the main risk factor for the development of tuberculosis (Moreno et al., 1993). It is known that clinical manifestations, management, and epidemiology are altered in AIDS patients (Daley et al., 1992). HIV-positive patients may develop active tuberculosis by two different mechanisms: reactivation of a latent infection or rapid progression of a newly acquired infection (Daley et al., 1992; Moreno et al., 1993). Another important fact is that tuberculosis may appear in the early stages of immunodeficiency. The most striking clinical feature is the extremely high frequency of extrapulmonary involvement. About 10% of all AIDS patients with tuberculosis present with CNS disease (Berenguer et al., 1992; Bishburg et al., 1986).

Basically, tuberculous infection of the CNS results in tuberculous meningitis, which is characterized by a thick gelatinous exudate with a predilection for the meninges covering the base of the brain. Meningeal enhancement on enhanced CT and MRI images in the basal cisterns and over the convexity of the brain could be seen in approximately 36 to 61% of the cases (Fig. 10) (Kioumehr et al., 1994; Tayfun et al., 1995; Villoria et al., 1992, 1995; Whiteman et al., 1995).

Involvement of the vessels that course through the subarachnoid space by tuberculous inflammation results in narrowing and occlusions of the vessels and subsequent infarctions, usually located in the middle cerebral artery territory and small perforating arteries supplying the basal ganglia (Fig. 11) (Gupta et al., 1994). Diffusion-weighted MRI images are helpful in detecting early infarcts, and MRA has been reported to be very useful in showing the tuberculosis-induced vascular pathology (Gupta et al., 1994). Cerebral infarctions were seen in 36% of HIV-positive patients with intracranial tuberculosis in one study (Whiteman et al., 1995).

Associated ependymitis due to extension of the inflammation to the ventricular system can be recognized on CT/MRI images as abnormal enhancement of the ventricular ependyma. Communicating-type hydrocephalus is the most common complication in meningeal tuberculosis (Rovira et al., 1980). Villoria et al. reported hydrocephalus in 51% of patients in their series of 35 patients with AIDS-related CNS tuberculosis (Villoria et al., 1992).

Parenchymal forms of the tuberculous infection include tuberculomas, tuberculous abscesses, and focal tuberculous cerebritis. In the AIDS population, parenchymal involvement is not often seen. Tuberculous granulomas (tuberculomas) result from hematogenous spread of infection or from extension of meningitis into the parenchyma (Parker et al., 1985). Tuberculomas may be solitary or multiple and can be located anywhere in the brain, but predominantly in the supratentorial compartment (Villoria et al., 1992). The radiological features of tuberculomas depend on the maturity of the lesion. On CT, mature granulomas are ring-enhancing lesions. The "target sign" was first described as a pathognomonic feature

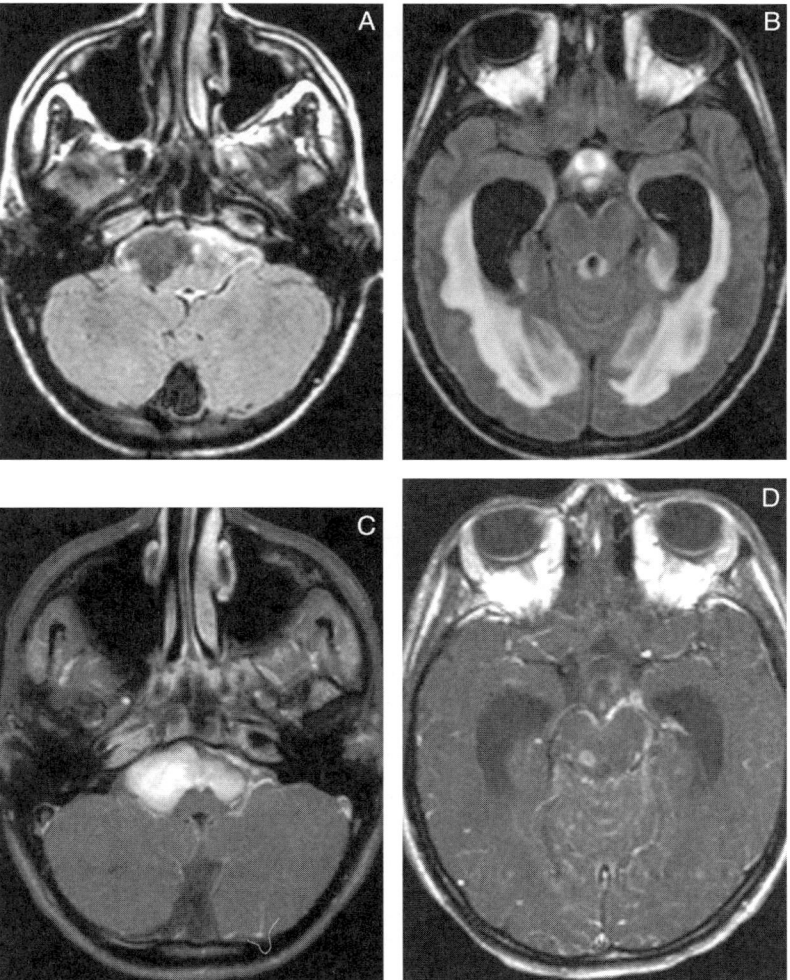

FIGURE 10 Tuberculous CNS infection in an AIDS patient. (A) Axial FLAIR-TSE (TR/TE/TI, 11,000/120/2800) MRI image showing low-signal abnormality in the right cerebellopontine angle region. (B) Axial FLAIR-TSE (TR/TE/TI, 11,000/120/2800) MRI image at a higher level demonstrating marked enlargement of the ventricular system, indicating hydrocephalus. (C and D) Contrast-enhanced T1-weighted TFE (TR/TE/flip degree, 20/1.9/35°) MRI images showing marked meningeal enhancement (tuberculous meningitis), homogeneous enhancement of the lesion in the right cerebellopontine angle (large tuberculoma), and ring-like enhancement of the lesion in the right midbrain (small tuberculoma).

for CNS tuberculoma (Welchman, 1979), representing central calcification or punctate enhancement surrounded by a zone of hypodensity and a rim of enhancement. Later reports have shown that the "target sign" on CT could be caused by other lesions as well, such as toxoplasmosis, lymphoma, or brain abscess (Bargallo et al., 1996). The tuberculomas appear isointense with a hyperintense ring on T1-WI MRI images and have variable signal on long echo time (TE) images (Fig. 10 and 12). Some tuberculomas are hypointense on T2-WI images. The possible explanation for the low signal of tuberculomas on T2-WI images is the presence of paramagnetic free radicals produced by macrophage activity (Sze and Zimmerman, 1988). Other tuberculomas have high signal on long TE images due to central liquefactive necrosis (Bowen and Post, 1991). Kim et al. compared MRI findings with pathologic features in tuberculomas and found that the outer

enhancing portion consisted of a layer of collagenous fibers, and inflammatory infiltrates showed on MRI as hypointense rings on T2-WI images; central caseation necrosis was recognized as iso- or hypointense on all pulse sequences (Kim et al., 1995). Healed tuberculomas do not enhance but may calcify. Recently, 52 intracranial tuberculomas were studied with magnetization transfer (MT) imaging, showing that the nonenhancing cores of tuberculosis have higher MTR than tumor necrosis or cysts (Pui and Ahmad, 2002). Tuberculosis cores with MTR were also higher in tuberculomas than in abscesses, which is likely related to the higher cell content. However, the diagnostic accuracy of MRI for MTR was only slightly improved in that study, and the differentiation of solitary tuberculoma from low-grade glioma was improved in five patients. With the use of MTR, multiple tuberculomas could be distinguished from metastatic disease in four patients.

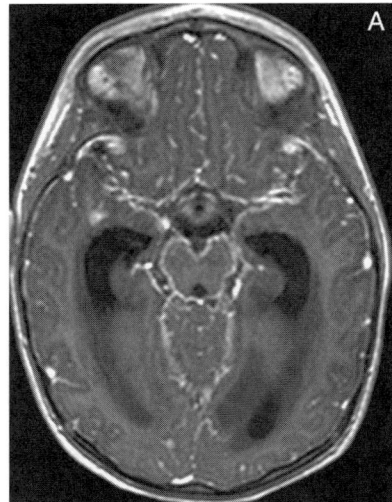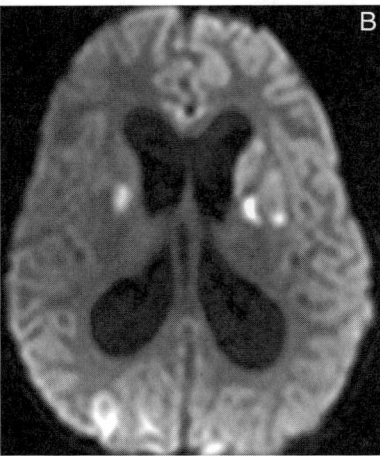

FIGURE 11 Tuberculous CNS infection with infarctions in a 50-year-old female patient. (A) Contrast-enhanced T1-weighted TFE (TR/TE/flip degree, 20/4.6/25°) MRI image in the axial plane showing extensive meningeal enhancement and enlargement of the ventricles, suggesting tuberculous meningitis with obstructive hydrocephalus. (B) On DWI (TR/TE/b value, 2,282/156/1,000 mm^2), high-signal-intensity abnormalities are demonstrated in the basal-ganglion region bilateral and in the right occipital cortex. On an apparent diffusion coefficient (ADC) map (not shown), low values were measured. The lesions were consistent with cytotoxic edema and infarctions. CSF analysis was consistent with tuberculosis.

A tuberculous abscess is a true pyogenic lesion that demonstrates an imaging appearance typical of pyogenic abscesses: hyperintense on T2-WI and hypointense on T1-WI MRI images. Typically, tuberculous abscesses are multiloculated and larger than tuberculomas and show ring-like enhancement (Fischl et al., 1985; Yang et al., 1987). Differentiation of tuberculous abscesses from pyogenic abscesses is important for patient management. A recent study has shown that with MRS combined with MT imaging it might be possible to distinguish the two enitities (Gupta et al., 1995, 2001). In that study, all pyogenic brain abscesses had lipid and lactate peaks and amino acid peaks. Patients with tuberculous abscesses had only lipid and lactate levels. The MT ratio from the wall of the pyogenic abscess was significantly higher than that from the tuberculous-abscess wall. In another series of 28 tuberculomas, lipid peaks were seen in 86% of the tuberculomas (Jayasundar et al., 1999). Large resonances of fatty acids at 1.3 ppm and 0.9 ppm, assigned to a methylene group, and terminal methyl groups of fatty acids described in tuberculomas are due to the high lipid content of caseous material (Gupta et al., 2001).

Focal tuberculous cerebritis is a rare form of tuberculosis characterized by intense gyral enhancement on CT scans (Jinkins, 1988). Calvarial tuberculosis is another rare manifestation of extrapulmonary tuberculosis. The presence of lytic lesions of the skull in a young individual in an area of endemicity should raise the suspicion of tuberculosis. Patankar et al. have described CT findings in five cases of tuberculosis of the calvarium (Patankar et al., 2000).

Nocardia

Less than 2% (0.3 to 1.8%) of all infections in AIDS patients are due to *Nocardia* (Utamchandani et al., 1994).

The most frequent *Nocardia* species is *Nocardia asteroides*, with pulmonary infection usually the primary type. In a study of 30 *Nocardia* infections in HIV-positive patients, 73% of the patients had pulmonary disease (Curry, 1980). CNS involvement is seen in 15 to 44% of the cases resulting from hematogenous spread of infection. Brain abscess is the most common manifestation of CNS *Nocardia* infection, with a very high mortality rate (80%) (Presant et al., 1973). Multiple or multiloculated ring-enhancing lesions with perifocal edema and mass effect are usually seen on enhanced CT scans (LeBlang et al., 1995). The MRI appearance of *Nocardia* abscesses is similar to that of other pyogenic brain abscesses (Fig. 13). The necrotic center is hyperintense on T2- and hypointense on T1-weighted MRI sequences. The capsule has high signal on T1- and low signal on T2-weighted MRI images and shows smooth peripheral enhancement on postcontrast images. Additional findings in CNS *Nocardia* infection are subependymal nodules and meningitis (LeBlang et al., 1995). In one study, 92% of AIDS patients with CNS *Nocardia* infection had associated meningeal disease. Five of the nine patients in the study had hydrocephalus, and clinical meningitis was present in three patients. Histological examination of small subependymal nodules, which were described in five patients, revealed inflammatory cells lining the ventricles, consistent with a ventriculitis/ependymitis with development of subependymal abscesses (LeBlang et al., 1995).

The results of the reported series suggested a strong correlation between patients who were intravenous drug abusers and *Nocardia* infection. Important clues to *Nocardia* infection are enhancing intraparenchymal lesions with additional subependymal nodules and evidence of meningitis.

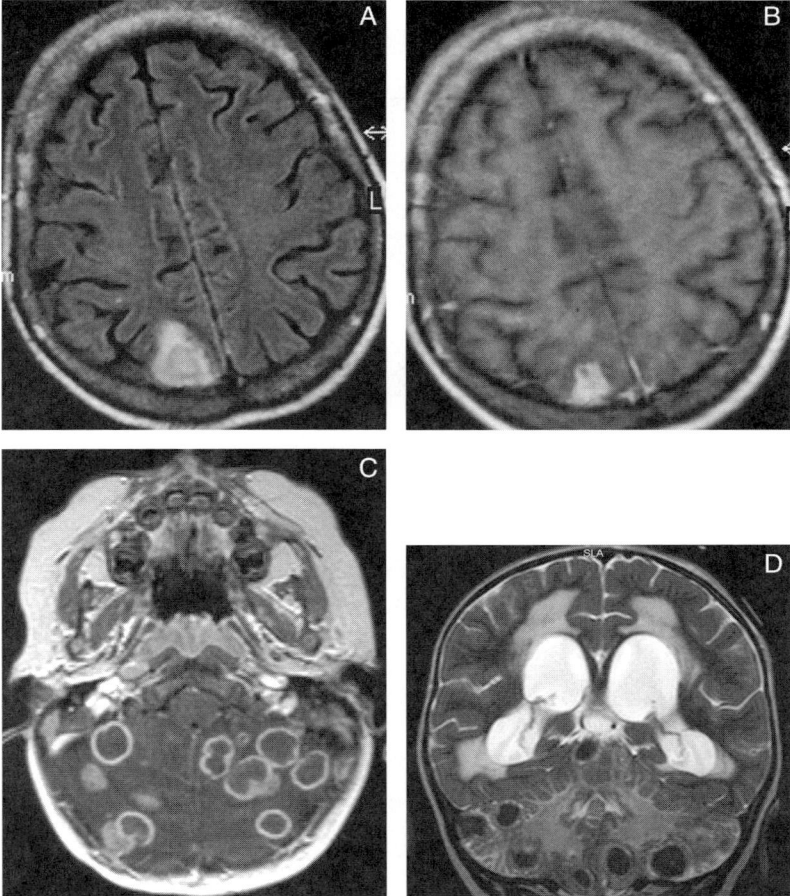

FIGURE 12 Multiple CNS tuberculomas with obstructive hydrocephalus. (A) Axial FLAIR-FSE (TR/TE/TI, 7000/150/2100) MRI image showing multiple low-signal-intensity lesions in the cerebellum bilateral. (B) On a nonenhanced T1-weighted TSE (TR/TE/flip degree, 20/4.6/25°) MRI image, the lesions have slightly higher signal than brain parenchyma. (C) Enhanced T1-weighted TSE (TR/TE/flip degree, 20/4.6/25°) MRI image demonstrating ring-like enhancement of the lesions. (D) Obstructive hydrocephalus with dilatation of the ventricular system is shown on a coronal T2-weighted MRI image. Note the marked low signal of tuberculomas. Brain biopsy revealed a diagnosis of tuberculous granuloma.

Fungal Infections

Cryptococcosis

CNS infection caused by the saprophytic yeast-like fungus *Cryptococcus neoformans* is the most common form of fungal infection in AIDS patients. The infection is a result of a newly acquired infection, with hematogenous dissemination of the infection from the lung to the CNS. Approximately 5 to 10% of patients with AIDS develop CNS cryptococcosis. Cryptococcal meningitis is the most common manifestation, in which the subarachnoid spaces are thickened and filled with multiple organisms and capsular material (Fetter et al., 1967). CT scans rarely show meningeal enhancement; enhanced T1-WI MRI images may demonstrate meningeal disease, but this is the exception rather than the rule (Arnder et al., 1996; Berkefeld et al., 1999). In a case of prominent meningeal enhancement on MRI, causes other than cryptococcosis should be considered first.

From the subarachnoid space, cryptococcus extends along the Virchow-Robin perivascular spaces into the basal ganglia, thalami, midbrain, and cerebellum. The Virchow-Robin spaces become dilated, without involvement of the brain parenchyma. On MRI images, widened perivascular spaces are recognized as multiple, bilateral, small round or oval lesions, usually located in the basal ganglia, which show high signal on T2-WI images and have signal slightly higher than the CSF on T1-WI MRI images (Fig. 14). The reason for the signal intensity characteristics is the mucoid content produced by the fungi. Perivascular spaces are anatomically outside the brain, inflammatory response is absent, there is no invasion of the brain parenchyma, and contrast enhancement is therefore always absent.

With disease progression, the dilated perivascular spaces become confluent, and cystic lesions, called "gelatinous pseudocysts" or "soap bubbles," develop. The lesions do not have a capsule and contain mucinous material and fungal organisms. Dentate nuclei have been shown to be frequently involved (Ruiz et al., 1997b). On MRI, the appearance does not differ from that of the dilated Virchow-Robin spaces, since mucinous material shortens the T1 relaxation time

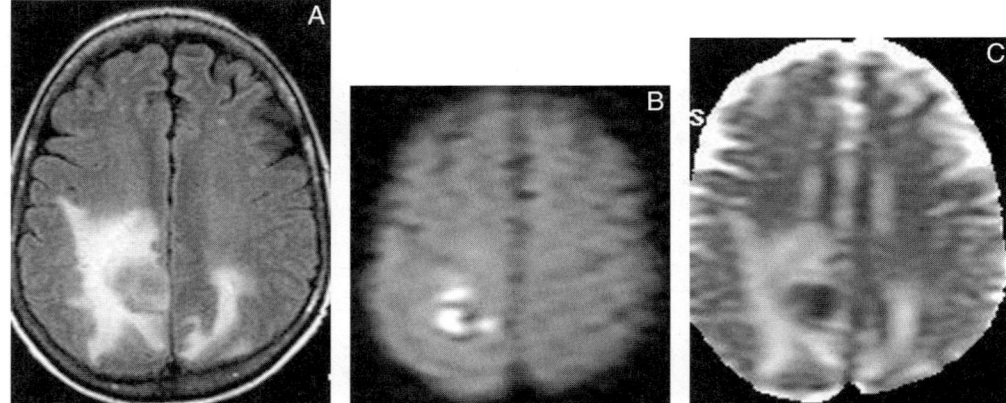

FIGURE 13 HIV-positive patient with a biopsy-proven *Nocardia* abscess. (A) Axial FLAIR-TSE (TR/TE/TI, 7,383/130/2,100) MRI image showing a lesion of intermediate signal intensity in the right parietal region. (B and C) High signal is present on trace DWI (TR/TE/b value, 2,286/83/1,000) (B) and low signal on an ADC map (C), indicating restricted diffusion in a bacterial abscess formation. Stereotactic biopsy confirmed the diagnosis of a *Nocardia* abscess of the brain.

and the lesions appear isointense to the cortex. Enhancement and mass effect are also absent.

Cryptococcoma is the only parenchymal form of cryptococcal CNS infection. The lesions result from the direct invasion of the brain by the fungus with the development of a granulomatous reaction. On CT, cryptococcomas are hypodense with high signal on T2-WI images and low signal on T1-WI MRI images. On enhanced images, the lesions usually demonstrate a ring-like or nodular enhancement and cannot be distinguished from granulomas of other ori-

gin. Recently, imaging findings with FLAIR and DWI of an intracerebral granuloma were described (Kamezawa et al., 2000). On FLAIR images, cryptococcoma showed signal higher than that of the CSF, and a mosaic pattern was observed on diffusion-weighted images, reflecting the inorganic structure of the lesion.

Recent experimental MRI spectroscopic studies performed on clinical isolates of *C. neoformans* have shown high concentrations of α,α-trehalose in cerebral cryptococcomas (Himmelreich et al., 2001).

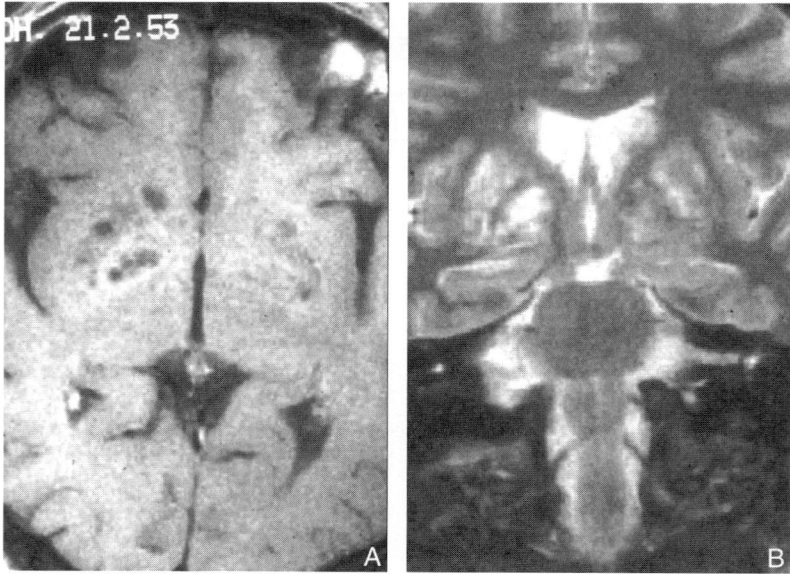

FIGURE 14 Dilated Virchow-Robin spaces in cerebral cryptococcosis (autopsy proven). Axial T1-weighted SE (TR/TE, 700/19) (A) and coronal T2-weighted MRI (TR/TE, 2,500/90) (B) images demonstrating small, cyst-like lesions bilaterally in the basal ganglia, representing dilated perivascular spaces filled with fungi. On an enhanced T1-weighted MRI image, no enhancement was observed (not shown).

Aspergillosis

Aspergillus is a frequent pathogen in the CNS, accounting for 18 to 28% of all fungal brain abscesses, and is the most common CNS complication following bone marrow transplantation (Miaux et al., 1995). *Aspergillus fumigatus* is the most common human pathogen. Because of the high mortality rate of 85 to 100% and difficulties in treating aspergillosis, it is important to raise suspicion early. Cerebral aspergillosis usually occurs after hematogenous dissemination from an extracerebral focus or is a result of contiguous spread of the infection from the paranasal sinuses. Meningitis, abscess, or granuloma; vascular invasion with thrombosis and infarction; and hemorrhage and aneurysm formation are manifestations of cerebral aspergillosis (Yuh et al., 1994).

Pathologically, hyphal elements invade cerebral vessels, resulting in thrombosis and infarctions. Sterile infarctions become septic when the fungus erodes the wall of the vessel with extension into the brain parenchyma, causing inflammatory reactions and necrosis. MRI is the method of choice in detecting cerebral infarctions due to aspergillosis. In addition, a recent study has shown that diffusion imaging allows early diagnosis of CNS aspergillosis (Kami et al., 1999). DWI revealed multiple signal intensity abnormalities consistent with infarctions while conventional MRI sequences were still normal (Kami et al., 1999). Intracerebral parenchymal lesions in aspergillosis have a central zone of hemorrhagic necrosis with sparse presence of fungi. On MRI, these lesions usually have low signal centrally or peripherally on T2-WI images (Fig. 15) (Yamada et al., 2000). Cox et al. showed that low peripheral signal is due to accumulation of fungi containing iron, magnesium, and manganese, as well as blood breakdown products (Cox et al., 1992). Low signal on T2-WI is not specific to aspergillosis, and it may be seen in tuberculomas, cysticercosis, etc. In one series, 14 of 36 lesions showed areas of low signal intensity located centrally, and in 8 of 36 lesions, low signal was present peripherally (Dietrich et al., 2001). Contrast enhancement is usually not present, depending on the severity of the immunocompetence (Fig. 15). Dietrich et al. observed faint enhancement in 15 of 36 lesions in patients with bone marrow transplantation and cerebral aspergillosis (Dietrich et al., 2001).

Parasitic Infections

Toxoplasmosis

Cerebral toxoplasmosis results from infection by an intracellular protozoan, *Toxoplasma gondii*. In the United States, 20 to 70% of adults are seropositive (Levy et al., 1985). After acute infection, the latent form, called encysted bradyzoites, remains in the tissues until there is a decline in immunity. Rupture of the cysts releases the free tachyzoite, which

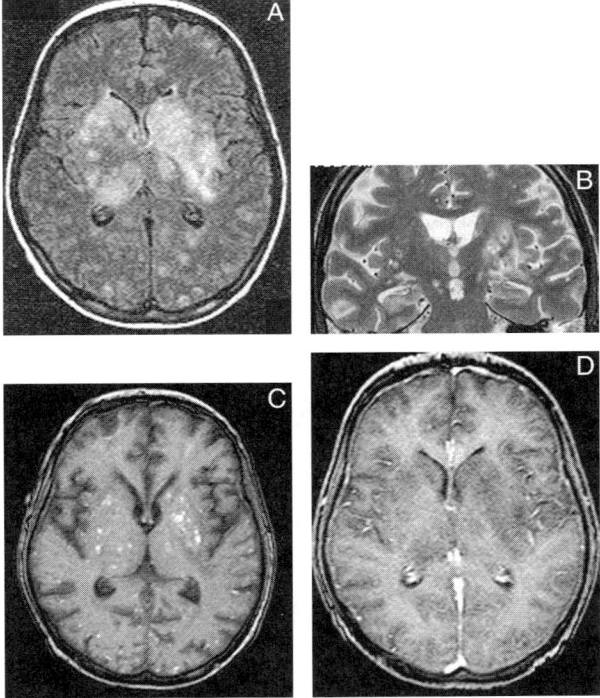

FIGURE 15 Cerebral aspergillosis in a patient after bone marrow transplantation. (A) Axial FLAIR-TSE (TR/TE/TI, 7,383/130/2,100) MRI image showing multiple hyperintense lesions in the basal-ganglion region and subcortical and cortical regions on both sides. (B) T2-weighted MRI image in the coronal plane demonstrating central low signal intensity of the lesions. (C) High signal intensities seen on T1-weighted (TR/TE/flip degree, 20/4.6/25°) image representing subacute hemorrhage. (D) No enhancement was observed on postcontrast T1-weighted (TR/TE/flip degree, 20/4.6/25°) MRI images. Necrotizing, hemorrhagic encephalitis due to the aspergillosis was found at the autopsy.

causes acute illness. Toxoplasma is found in 10 to 34% of all AIDS autopsies (Petito et al., 1986).

In AIDS patients, toxoplasma causes a necrotizing encephalitis, and the lesions have three well-defined zones: an avascular, necrotic center; an intermediate zone with intense inflammatory reaction; and a peripheral zone with the encystic form of toxoplasma (Post et al., 1983).

On nonenhanced CT scans, toxoplasma lesions are hypodense with edema and mass effect. Solid, nodular, or ring-enhancing lesions are typically observed on postcontrast studies. The most common locations are the basal ganglia and the corticomedullary junction. The number of detectable lesions significantly increases with a double-dose delayed technique (Post et al., 1985). Pathologic-radiologic correlation showed that the radiologic appearance correlates well with the pathology; the ring-enhancing lesions correlate with an inflammatory zone, the hypodense center correlates with an avascular necrosis, and edema correlates with the peripheral zone (Post et al., 1983).

On T1-WI MRI images, toxoplasma lesions have isointense to low signal centrally. The signal intensity on T2-WI images depends on the stage of the lesion, which could be iso-, hypo-, or hyperintense (Fig. 16 to 18 and Color Plate 8) (Brightbill et al., 1996; Post et al., 1986, 1988). Enhanced T1-WI images reveal ring or nodular enhancement (Fig. 16 to 18 and Color Plate 8).

Approximately 10 days after the initiation of antitoxoplasma therapy, a decrease in the number and size of the lesions with reduction in edema and mass effect should be observed on follow-up MRI examinations. Full resolution of the lesions may take 6 months (Levy et al., 1985), and healed foci may calcify or show changes consistent with leukomalacia. Lifelong maintenance of therapy is necessary, because discontinuation of treatment results in recurrence. Encysted forms of toxoplasma cannot be treated with therapy; thus, the toxoplasma is never entirely eradicated.

Based on imaging findings on conventional MRI sequences, cerebral toxoplasmosis cannot be distinguished

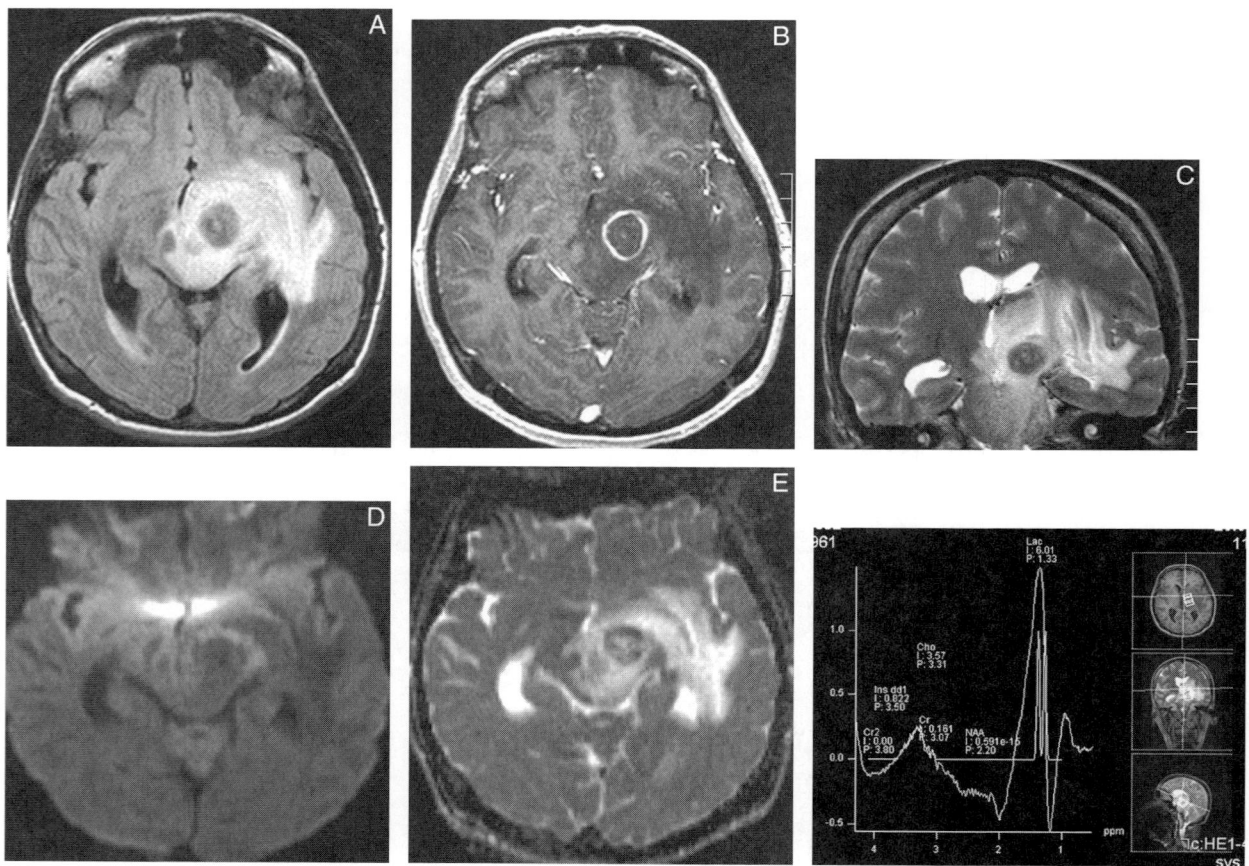

FIGURE 16 Cerebral toxoplasmosis in an HIV-positive individual. (A) Low-signal-intensity lesion with high-signal-intensity edema located in the left basal-ganglion region is shown on an axial FLAIR-TSE (TR/TE/TI, 11,000/140/2,800) MRI image. (B) The lesion shows ring enhancement after gadolinium injection on a T1-weighted TFE (TR/TE/flip degree, 20/1.8/35°) MRI image. (C) Low signal intensity of the lesion shown on a coronal T2-weighted MRI image. (D and E) On trace DWI, the lesion shows low signal (D), with mixed intensity on an ADC map (E). (F) Proton MRI spectrum acquired from a lesion demonstrating a large lipid/lactate peak and no NAA or choline peaks. The imaging findings on conventional MRI and MRI spectrum and the results of the FDG-PET (not shown) were consistent with toxoplasmosis. Ten days after the initiation of treatment, a follow-up MRI showed a decrease in size and enhancement of the lesion (not shown).

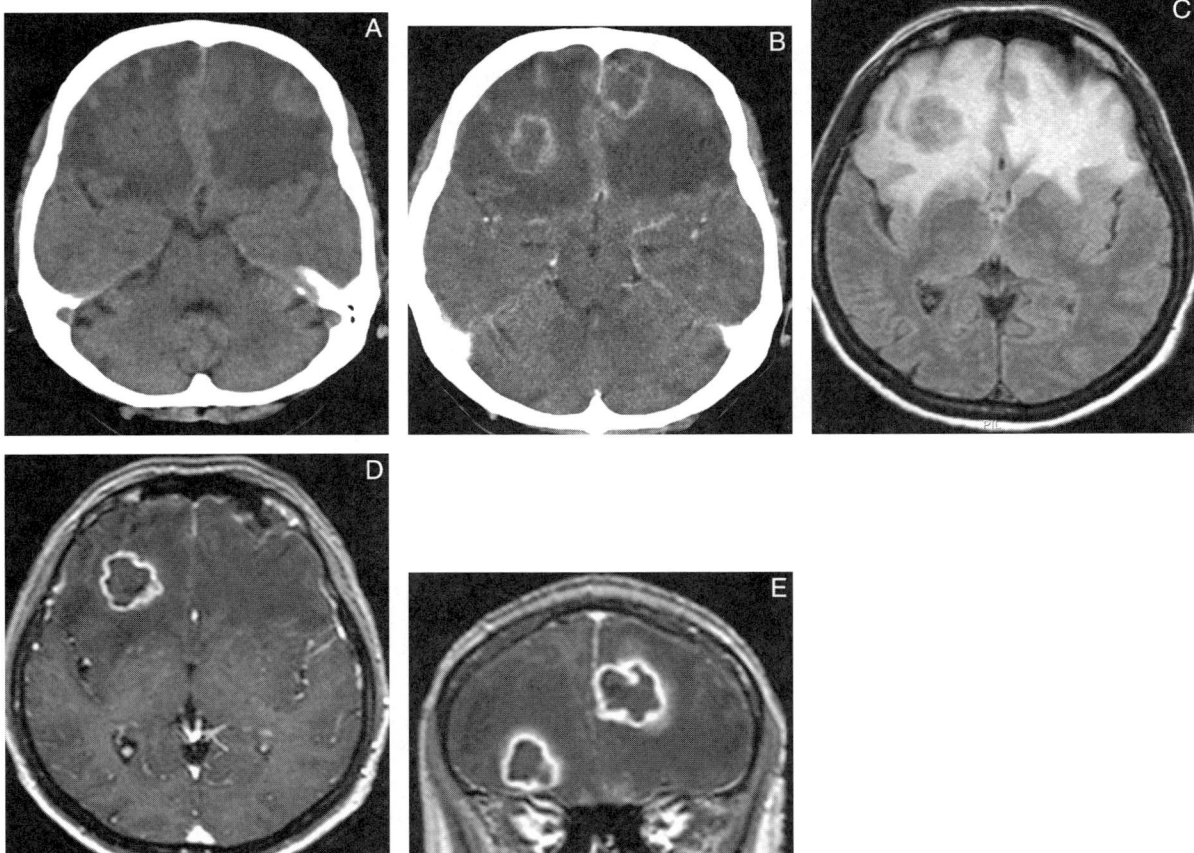

FIGURE 17 Cerebral toxoplasmosis in an HIV-positive patient. (A) Nonenhanced CT scan of the brain demonstrating bilateral hypodensity in the frontal lobes. (B) Postcontrast scan showing peripherally enhancing lesions with associated edema. (C) The lesions have low signal on an axial FLAIR MRI image (TR/TE/TI, 10,000/150/2,600). (D and E) Postcontrast T1-weighted TFE (TR/TE/flip degree, 10/3.4/10°) MRI images in the axial (D) and the coronal (E) planes demonstrating peripheral enhancement of the necrotic lesion surrounded by edema.

from primary cerebral lymphoma. Early reports about MRI findings of toxoplasmosis and lymphoma in AIDS patients describe solitary lesions, which suggest lymphoma, and multiple lesions, which suggest toxoplasmosis (Dina, 1991; Kupfer et al., 1990; Laissy et al., 1995b). Further studies have shown that the number of lesions, the signal intensities of the lesions, their locations, and their appearance on postcontrast images are not reliable factors in differentiating between the two entities. New MRI methods have been introduced to improve differentiation, such as MRS and pMRI.

The MRI spectroscopic pattern of toxoplasma lesions is nonspecific, consistent with anaerobic inflammation within the abscess (Fig. 16). In lymphoma, an increase of lactate and lipids, as well as an elevated choline peak, has been described. Chinn et al. have studied MRI spectra from 18 toxoplasma and 9 lymphoma lesions on 1.5 Tesla with an echo time of 135 ms (Chinn et al., 1995). Visual analysis in their study failed to differentiate between toxoplasma and lymphoma. An important variable for MRI spectra is the maturity of the lesions, as well as the presence of necrosis. At some stage, all intracranial processes destroy brain

parenchyma, and in AIDS patients, lymphomas are usually necrotic tumors. Therefore, necrotic lymphomas have compounds similar to those of a necrotic toxoplasma abscess. The presence of lipids is seen in both entities as a result of brain destruction. A relatively immature toxoplasma lesion will be more cellular, resulting in a spectrum with no lipid, increased Cho, and decreased NAA. It is crucial to place the voxel for spectroscopic analysis over the cellular portion of the lesion. In another series of 11 toxoplasma lesions and 8 lymphomas of the brain in AIDS patients, MRS was considered a potentially specific, noninvasive adjunctive method for differential diagnosis of focal brain lesions in AIDS (Chang et al., 1995; Miller et al., 1998). Toxoplasma was correctly diagnosed in 11/11 cases, and lymphoma in 8/8 cases. The lactate peak was greatest in lymphoma in the study. Although much work has been done, MRS must be seen as a valuable adjunctive tool and cannot replace conventional MRI in differentiating toxoplasmosis and lymphoma.

pMRI is another potential noninvasive method that may allow differentiation between toxoplasmosis and lymphoma in patients with AIDS. Prospective evaluation of 13 patients

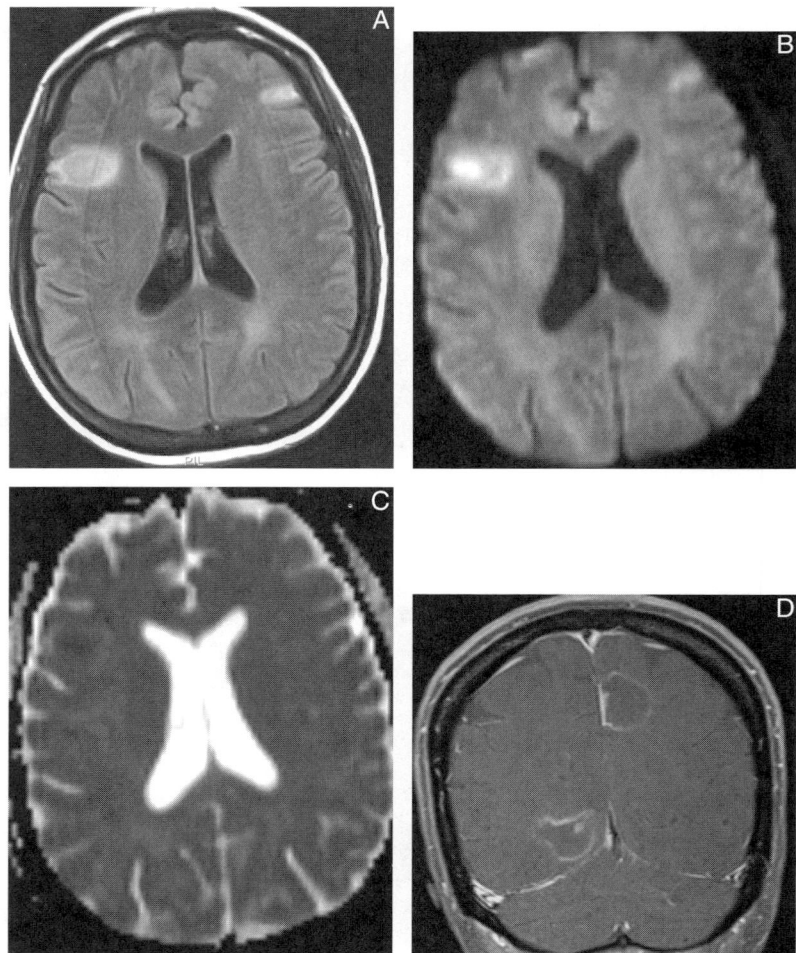

FIGURE 18 Cerebral toxoplasmosis in a 30-year-old female patient with AIDS. (A) Low-signal-intensity lesions with high-signal-intensity edema located in the right and left frontal lobes are shown on an axial FLAIR-TSE (TR/TE/TI, 11,000/140/2,800) MRI image. (B and C) On a trace DWI (B), the lesion located in the right frontal lobe has high signal intensity with a low ADC value (C), indicating restricted diffusion. (D) Coronal postcontrast T1-weighted TFE (TR/TE/flip degree, 10/3.4/10°) MRI image showing peripheral enhancement of the necrotic toxoplasma lesions.

with focal brain lesions by pMRI showed reduced regional cerebral blood volume (rCBV) in toxoplasma lesions and increased rCBV in lymphoma (Ernst et al., 1998). Reduced rCBV in toxoplasmosis is probably due to a lack of vasculature within the abscess, while the hypervascularity of lymphoma is the reason for increased rCBV in lymphoma.

The use of ^{201}Tl brain SPECT in AIDS patients has been proven to be very helpful in distinguishing toxoplasmosis from lymphoma (Miller et al., 1998; Ruiz et al., 1994). Thallium is a potassium analogue with uptake in active tissue, with a half-life of approximately 73 h (Ruiz et al., 1994). After intravenous administration, ^{201}Tl rapidly disappears from the blood, and increased activity is normally seen in the orbits, the base of the skull, the scalp, and the nasopharyngeal region. Normally, there is no uptake of ^{201}Tl in the brain. Positive ^{201}Tl brain SPECT is suggestive of CNS lymphoma, and negative uptake suggests infection (toxoplasmosis) in AIDS patients (Ruiz et al., 1994). A study of 37 patients with AIDS and focal brain lesions evaluated

with ^{201}Tl SPECT has shown the benefit of ^{201}Tl SPECT in differentiating between lymphoma and infectious lesions. All lymphomas in this series showed uptake of ^{201}Tl, in contrast to infections, which showed negative uptake (Ruiz et al., 1994). Contrary to the results of Ruiz et al., the results from a recent prospective study of 14 patients with AIDS and focal brain lesions suggest the inability of ^{201}Tl SPECT to differentiate lymphoma from toxoplasmosis (Licho et al., 2002). The accuracy was 57% in the study, with a positive predictive value of 43% and a negative predictive value of 71%. A combination of ^{201}Tl SPECT and toxoplasma serology may improve diagnostic accuracy for toxoplasmosis (Skiest et al., 2000). A combined approach with ^{201}Tl SPECT and Epstein-Barr virus DNA PCR in CSF provides high diagnostic accuracy for cerebral lymphoma (Antinori et al., 1999). Thallium and gallium scans were reviewed in 40 AIDS patients with focal brain lesions (Lee et al., 1999). All patients with lymphomas and gliomas had positive thallium and gallium scans. Patients with infections

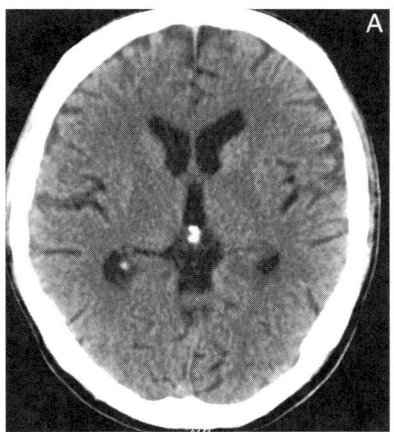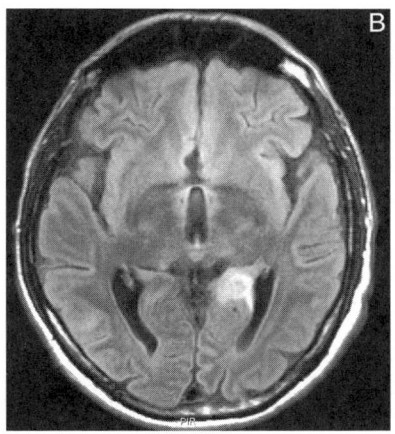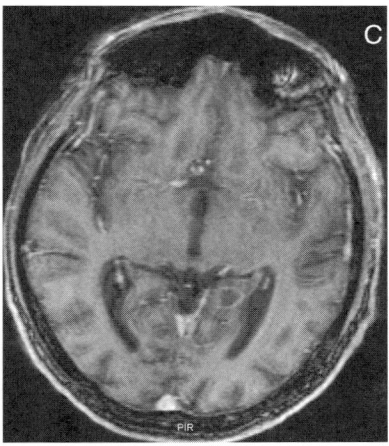

FIGURE 19 Non-Hodgkin's lymphoma in an HIV-positive patient. (A) Nonenhanced CT scan of the brain showing a hypodense lesion in the left occipital periventricular cortex. (B) Centrally low-signal-intensity lesion with high-signal-intensity edema on an axial FLAIR-TSE (TR/TE/TI, 11,000/140/2,800) MRI image. (C) A ring-like enhancing lesion on an axial postcontrast T1-weighted TFE (TR/TE/flip degree, 10/3.4/10°) MRI image. Two other lesions were also present (not shown). At the autopsy, lymphoma was confirmed.

(toxoplasmosis and tuberculosis, mycobacterial infection, or cryptococcosis) had positive gallium and negative thallium scans. Negative thallium and gallium scans were also seen in patients with infarcts.

The potential use of [18F]fluorodeoxyglucose (FDG)-PET in differentiating lymphoma from toxoplasmosis in AIDS patients has been also examined (Villringer et al., 1995). The results of the studies have shown that FDG-PET can accurately differentiate lymphoma from infections (Heald et al., 1996; Hoffmann et al., 1993). The standardized uptake values over cerebral lesions were much higher in lymphomas than in toxoplasma lesions (O'Doherty et al., 1997). In another study, the highest FDG uptake was found in patients with lymphoma (Villringer et al., 1995). Diagnostic problems may occur in cases of PML, in which high metabolic activity and FDG uptake may be found (Heald et al., 1996; Provinciali et al., 1988). Two cases of PML had high metabolic activity in a series of 18 AIDS patients and could not be differentiated from lymphoma.

In hospitals with SPECT/PET facilities, a thallium scan or an FDG scan in patients with AIDS and focal brain lesions allows a rapid evaluation of the brain and, combined with toxoplasma immunoglobulin G and Epstein-Barr virus DNA PCR in CSF, improves diagnostic accuracy.

NEOPLASTIC LESIONS

Lymphoma

Primary CNS lymphoma (PCNSL) is of major importance because of its increasing frequency, especially in immunocompromised patients (Ammassari et al., 1998; So et al., 1986). Up to 6% of all patients with AIDS develop high-grade lymphomas, almost always non-Hodgkin's type (Hainfellner and Budka, 1997). Multicentric lymphomas are a common finding, as solitary lesions, with a percentage between 41 and 81% (Ciricillo and Rosenblum, 1990; Dina, 1991; Goldstein et al., 1991; Thurnher et al., 2001c). The number of lesions on CT/MRI, however, does not allow

a definitive final diagnosis. On nonenhanced CT scans (Fig. 19), the lymphomas are usually hyperdense, while on MRI images, lymphomas may have low, high, or intermediate signal on both T1- and T2-weighted sequences (Fig. 20) (De La Blanchardière et al., 1997; Ferraresi et al., 1989; Goldstein et al., 1991; Laissy et al., 1995a; Poon et al., 1989; Schwaighofer et al., 1989). The enhancement is variable, but peripheral or ring enhancement is the most common pattern. Solid, homogeneous enhancement has been described in some CT series (Poon et al., 1989). Nonenhancing lymphomatous lesions have also been reported, as in one study in which 15 lymphomatous lesions in four patients with AIDS did not enhance (Thurnher et al., 2001c). Approximately 3.4% of PCNSL lesions show no enhancement in immunocompetent patients (Johnson et al., 1997), especially in those who receive steroids before imaging is performed. The diffuse form of lymphoma has also been described recently, presenting as nonenhancing, diffuse, white-matter lesions (Thurnher et al., 2001c). Differential diagnosis should include HIV encephalopathy and PML in such cases (Sieb et al., 1992). Lymphomas usually demonstrate a moderate degree of edema and mass effect, and marked edema with midline shift was observed in 25% of patients with AIDS and lymphoma in one series. The relatively mild mass effect in 53 to 75% of cases is due to the infiltrating nature of lymphoma (Cordoliani et al., 1992). Evidence of hemorrhage does not exclude PCNSL in AIDS patients, and 35% of untreated lymphomas were hemorrhagic in our series (Fukui et al., 1998; Thurnher et al., 2001c).

Lymphomatous involvement of the cranial vault in patients with AIDS is rare (Bhatia et al., 1997; Thurnher et al., 2001b). MRI revealed a large scalp enhancing lesion with bone destruction and an epidural component in the first HIV-positive patient in whom primary lymphoma of the cranial vault was described (Bhatia et al., 1997). Recently a published case of malignant lymphoma of the cranial vault was detected on CT/MRI scans, presenting as a large scalp lesion in the left frontoparietal region with extension through the bony calvarium, with an epidural component

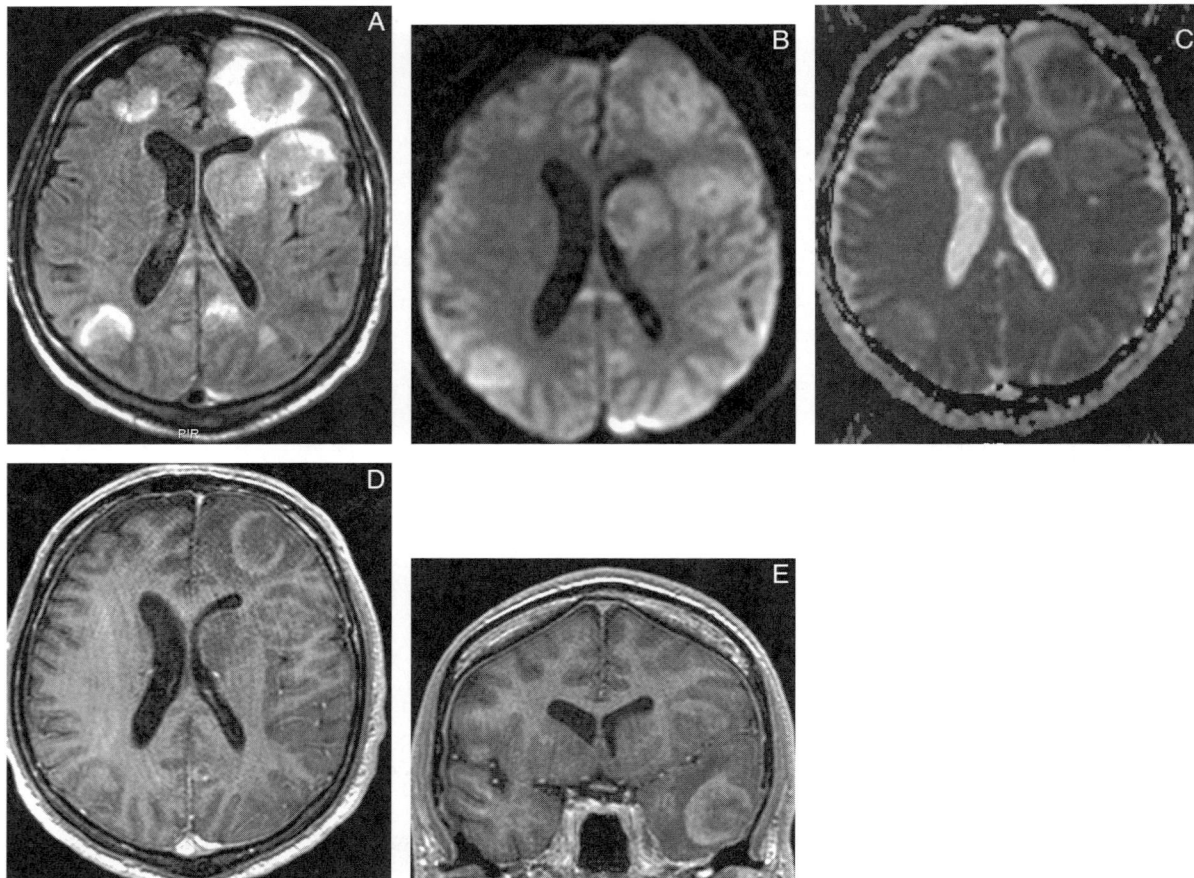

FIGURE 20 Multifocal CNS lymphoma in an HIV-positive patient. (A) Multiple hypointense lesions located in both hemispheres of the brain are shown on an axial FLAIR-TSE (TR/TE/TI, 11,000/140/2,800) MRI image. (B and C) On a trace DWI MRI image (B), the lesions have intermediate signal with low ADC values (C), indicating restricted diffusion due to the high cellularity of lymphoma lesions. (D and E) Peripherally enhancing lesions are demonstrated on axial (D) and coronal (E) postcontrast T1-weighted TFE (TR/TE/flip degree, 10/3.4/10°) MRI images.

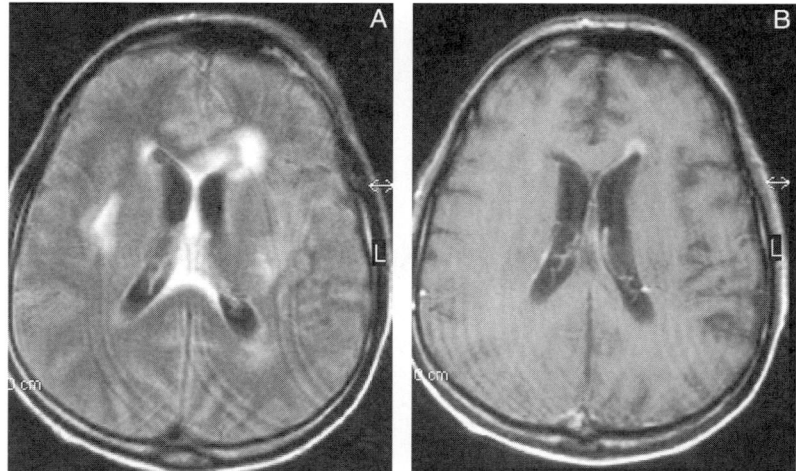

FIGURE 21 Periventricular lymphoma in a 30-year-old AIDS patient. (A) Axial FLAIR MRI image (TR/TE/TI, 10,000/150/2,600) showing hyperintense abnormality in the periventricular frontal white matter. (B) Postcontrast T1-weighted SE MRI image (TR/TE, 550/20) showing periventricular enhancement.

(Thurnher et al., 2001b). The lesion showed peripheral enhancement on postcontrast MRI images, and the epidural lesion demonstrated homogeneous enhancement. Although it is a rare entity, prominent soft tissue mass of the scalp associated with bone lesion and epidural mass in an HIV-positive patient should suggest lymphoma of the cranial vault.

Differentiation between lymphoma and toxoplasmosis in AIDS patients remains a diagnostic dilemma. The combination of a neuroradiological examination, a compatible radionuclide study, and CSF analysis (Epstein-Barr virus DNA) will certainly aid in correct diagnosis.

REFERENCES

Ammassari, A., G. Scoppettuolo, R. Murri, P. Pezzotti, A. Cingolani, C. Del Borgo, A. De Luca, A. Antinori, and L. Ortona. 1998. Changing disease patterns in focal brain lesion-causing disorders in AIDS. *J. Acquir. Immune Defic. Syndr. Hum. Retrovirol.* **18**:365–371.

Antinori, A., G. De Rossi, A. Ammassari, A. Cingolani, R. Murri, D. Di Giuda, A. De Luca, F. Pierconti, T. Taraglione, M. Scerrati, M. Larocca and L. Ortona. 1999. Value of combined approach with thallium-201 single-photon emission computed tomography and Epstein-Barr virus DNA polymerase chain reaction in CSF for the diagnosis of AIDS-related primary CNS lymphoma. *J. Clin. Oncol.* **17**:554–560.

Arendt, G., H. Hefter, C. Elsing, G. Strohmeyer, and H. Freund. 1990. Motor dysfunction in HIV-infected patients without clinically detectable central nervous deficit. *J. Neurol.* **237**:362–368.

Arendt, G., H. Hefter, E. Neuen-Jacob, S. Wist, H. Kuhlmann, G. Strohmeyer, and H. Freund. 1993. Electrophysiological motor testing, MRI findings and clinical course in AIDS patients with dementia. *J. Neurol.* **240**:439–445.

Arnder, L., M. Castillo, E. Heinz, J. Scatliff, and D. Enterline. 1996. Unusual pattern of enhancement in cryptococcal meningitis: in vivo findings with postmortem correlation. *J. Comput. Assist. Tomogr.* **20**:1023–1026.

Arribas, J., D. Clifford, C. Fichtenbaum, D. Commins, W. Powderly, and G. Storc. 1995. Level of cytomegalovirus (CMV) DNA in cerebrospinal fluid of subjects with AIDS and CMV infection of the central nervous system. *J. Infect. Dis.* **172**:527–531.

Aygun, N., D. Finelli, M. Rodgers, and R. Rhodes. 1998. Multifocal varicella-zoster virus leukoencephalitis in a patient with AIDS: MR findings. *Am. J. Neuroradiol.* **19**:1897–1899.

Aylward, E., P. Brettschneider, J. McArthur, G. Harris, T. Schleapfer, J. Henderer, P. Barta, A. Tien, and G. Pearlson. 1995. Magnetic resonance imaging measurement of gray matter volume reductions in HIV dementia. *Am. J. Psychiatry* **152**:987–994.

Baqi, M., W. Kucharczyk, and S. Walmsley. 1997. Regression of progressive multifocal leukoencephalopathy with highly active antiretroviral therapy. *AIDS* **11**:1526–1527.

Bargallo, J., J. Berenguer, J. Garcia-Barrionuevo, B. Ubeda, N. Bargallo, C. Cardenal, and J. Mercader. 1996. The "target-sign": is it a specific sign of CNS tuberculoma? *Neuroradiology* **38**:547–550.

Behar, R., C. Wiley, and J. McCutchan. 1987. Cytomegalovirus polyradiculoneuropathy in acquired immunodeficiency syndrome. *Neurology* **37**:557–561.

Bencherif, B., and D. Rottenberg. 1998. Neuroimaging of the AIDS dementia complex. *AIDS* **12**:233–244.

Berenguer, J., S. Moreno, F. Laguna, T. Vincente, M. Adrados, A. Ortega, J. Gonzalez-LaHoz, and E. Bouza. 1992. Tuberculous meningitis in patients infected with the human immunodeficiency virus. *N. Engl. J. Med.* **326**:668–672.

Berger, J., and M. Concha. 1995. Progressive multifocal leukoencephalopathy: the evolution of a disease once considered rare. *Neurovirology* **1**:5–18.

Berger, J., R. Levy, D. Flomenhoft, and M. Dobbs. 1998. Predictive factors for prolonged survival in acquired immunodeficiency syndrome-associated progressive multifocal leukoencephalopathy. *Ann. Neurol.* **44**:341–349.

Berkefeld, J., W. Enzensberger, and H. Lanferman. 1999. Cryptococcus meningoencephalitis in AIDS: parenchymal and meningeal forms. *Neuroradiology* **41**:129–133.

Bhatia, S., A. Smally, and P. Dekker. 1997. Primary non-Hodgkin's lymphoma of the cranial vault. *Clin. Oncol.* **9**:195–196.

Bishburg, E., G. Sunderama, L. Reichman, and R. Kapila. 1986. Central nervous system tuberculosis with the acquired immunodeficiency syndrome and its related complex. *Ann. Intern. Med.* **105**:210–213.

Bowen, B., and M. Post. 1991. Intracranial infection, p. 501–538. *In* S. W. Atlas (ed.), *Magnetic Resonance Imaging of the Brain and Spine.* Raven, New York, NY.

Brightbill, T., I. Ihmeidan, M. Post, J. Berger, and D. Katz. 1995. Neurosyphilis in HIV-positive and HIV-negative patients: neuroimaging findings. *Am. J. Nuroradiol.* **16**:703–711.

Brightbill, T., M. Post, G. Hensley, and A. Ruiz. 1996. MR of *Toxoplasma* encephalitis: signal characteristics on T2-weighted images and pathologic correlation. *J. Comput. Assist. Tomogr.* **20**:417–422.

Bruhn, H., J. Frahm, K. Merboldt, W. Hanicke, F. Hanefeld, H. Christen, B. Kruse, and H. Bauer. 1994. Multiple sclerosis in children: cerebral metabolic alterations monitored by localized proton magnetic resonance spectroscopy in vivo. *Ann. Neurol.* **32**:140–150.

Budka, H., G. Constanzi, S. Cristina, A. Lechi, C. Parravicini, R. Trabattoni, and L. Vago. 1987. Brain pathology induced by infection with the human immunodeficiency virus (HIV). *Acta Neuropathol.* **75**:185–198.

Burke, J., V. Mathews, A. Elster, J. Ulmer, F. McLean, and S. Davis. 1996. Contrast-enhanced magnetization transfer saturation imaging improves MR detection of herpes simplex encephalitis. *Am. J. Neuroradiol.* **17**:773–776.

Bursztyn, E., B. Lee, and J. Bauman. 1984. CT of acquired immunodeficiency syndrome. *Am. J. Neuroradiol.* **5**:711–714.

Cardenas, R., K. Cheng, and K. Sack. 2001. The effects of cidofovir on progressive multifocal leukoencephalopathy: an MRI case study. *Neuroradiology* **43**:379–382.

Centers for Disease Control and Prevention. 1987. Tuberculosis and acquired immunodeficiency syndrome—New York City. *MMWR Morb. Mortal. Wkly. Rep.* **36**:785–795.

Chang, L., T. Ernst, M. Leonido-Yee, I. Walot, and E. Singer. 1999a. Cerebral metabolite abnormalities correlate with clinical severity of HIV-1 cognitive motor complex. *Neurology* **52**:100–108.

Chang, L., T. Ernst, M. Leonido-Yee, M. Witt, O. Speck, I. Walot, and E. Miller. 1999b. Highly active antiretroviral therapy reverses brain metabolite abnormalities in mild HIV dementia. *Neurology* **53**:782–789.

Chang, L., T. Ernst, C. Tornatore, H. Aranow, R. Melchor, I. Walot, and E. Singer. 1997a. Metabolite abnormalities in progressive multifocal leukoencephalopathy: a proton magnetic resonance spectroscopy study. *Neurology* **48**:836–845.

Chang, L., C. M. Mehringer, T. Ernst, R. Melchor, H. Myers, D. Forney, and P. Satz. 1997b. Neurochemical alterations in asymptomatic abstinent cocaine users: a proton magnetic resonance spectroscopic study. *Biol. Psychiatry* **42**:1105–1114.

Chang, L., B. Miller, D. McBride, M. Cornford, G. Oropilla, S. Buchthal, F. Chiang, H. Aronow, C. Beck, and T. Ernst. 1995. Brain lesions in patients with AIDS: H-1 MR spectroscopy. *Radiology* **197**:525–531.

Chinn, R., I. Wilkinson, M. Hall-Craggs, M. Paley, R. Miller, B. Kendall, S. Newman, and M. Harrison. 1995. Toxoplasmosis and primary central nervous system lymphoma in HIV infection: diagnosis with MR spectroscopy. *Radiology* 197:649–654.

Ciricillo, S., and M. Rosenblum. 1990. Use of CT and MR imaging to distinguish intracranial lesions and to define the need of biopsy in AIDS patients. *J. Neurosurg.* 73:720–724.

Cohen, W. A., K. R. Maravilla, R. Gerlach, K. Claypoole, A. C. Collier, C. Marra, C. Maxwell, R. W. Coombs, W. T. Longstreth, Jr., B. D. Townes, et al. 1992. Prospective cerebral MR study of HIV seropositive and seronegative men: correlation of MR findings with neurologic, neuropsychologic, and cerebrospinal fluid analysis. *Am. J. Neuroradiol.* 13:1231–1240.

Collazos, J., J. Mayo, E. Martinez, and M. Blanco. 1999. Contrast-enhancing progressive multifocal leukoencephalopathy as an immune reconstitution event in AIDS patients. *AIDS* 13:1426–1428.

Cordoliani, Y., C. Derosier, C. Pharaboz, D. Jeanbourquin, H. Schill, and G. Cosnard. 1992. Primary cerebral lymphoma in patients with AIDS: MR findings in 17 cases. *Am. J. Radiol.* 159:841–847.

Cox, J., F. Murtagh, A. Wilfong, and J. Brenner. 1992. Cerebral aspergillosis: MR imaging and histopathologic correlation. *Am. J. Neuroradiol.* 13:1489–1492.

Curry, W. 1980. Human nocardiosis: a clinical review with selected case reports. *Arch. Intern. Med.* 140:818–826.

Daley, C., P. Small, G. Schecter, G. Schoolnik, R. McAdam, W. Jacobs, and P. Hopewell. 1992. An outbreak of tuberculosis with accelerated progression among persons with the human immunodeficiency virus. *N. Engl. J. Med.* 326:321–325.

Davis, L., B. Hjelle, V. Miller, D. Palmer, A. Llewellyn, T. Merlin, S. Young, R. Mills, W. Wachsman, and C. Wiley. 1992. Early viral brain invasion in iatrogenic human immunodeficiency virus infection. *Neurology* 42:1736–1739.

De La Blanchardière, A., P. Lesprit, J. M. Molina, A. M. Zagdanski, C. Hennequin, V. Garrait, J. M. Decazes, and J. Modai. 1997. Primary cerebral lymphoma in AIDS. Retrospective study of 20 patients. *Presse Med.* 26:940–944. (In French.)

De Luca, A., M. Giancola, A. Cingolani, A. Ammassari, L. Gillini, R. Murri, and A. Antinori. 1999. Clinical and virological monitoring during treatment with intrathecal cytarabine in patients with AIDS-associated progressive multifocal leukoencephalopathy. *Clin. Infect. Dis.* 28:624–628.

DeSimone, J., R. Pomerantz, and T. Babinchak. 2000. Inflammatory reactions in HIV-1-infected persons after initiation of highly active antiretroviral therapy. *Ann. Intern. Med.* 133:447–454.

Dietrich, U., M. Hettmann, M. Maschke, A. Doerfler, K. Schwechheimer, and M. Forsting. 2001. Cerebral aspergillosis: comparison of radiological and neuropathologic findings in patients with bone marrow transplantation. *Eur. Radiol.* 11:1242–1249.

Dina, T. 1991. Primary central nervous system lymphoma versus toxoplasmosis in AIDS. *Radiology* 179:823–828.

Dorfman, L. 1973. Cytomegalovirus encephalitis in adults. *Neurology* 23:136–143.

Dyer, J., M. French, and S. Mallal. 1995. Cerebral mass lesions due to cytomegalovirus in patients with AIDS: report of two cases. *J. Infect.* 30:147–151.

Elovaara, I., E. Poutiainen, R. Raininko, L. Valanne, A. Virta, S. L. Valle, J. Lähdevirta, and M. Iivanainen. 1990. Mild brain atrophy in early HIV infection: the lack of association with cognitive deficits and HIV-specific intrathecal immune response. *J. Neurol. Sci.* 99:121–136.

Entning, R., M. Hoetelmans, J. Lange, D. Burger, J. Beijnen, and P. Portegies. 1998. Antiretroviral drugs and the central nervous system. *AIDS* 12:1941–1955.

Ernst, T., L. Chang, M. Witt, H. Aronow, M. Cornford, I. Walot, and M. Goldberg. 1998. Cerebral toxoplasmosis and lymphoma in AIDS: perfusion MR imaging experience in 13 patients. *Radiology* 208:663–669.

Ernst, T., L. Chang, M. Witt, H. Aronow, I. Walot, M. Leonido-Yee, and E. Singer. 1999. Progressive multifocal leukoencephalopathy and human immunodeficiency virus-associated white matter lesions in AIDS: magnetization transfer MR imaging. *Radiology* 210:539–543.

Ernst, T., E. Itti, L. Itti, and L. Chang. 2000. Changes in cerebral metabolism are detected prior to perfusion changes in early HIV-CMC: a coregistered ^{1}H MRS and SPECT study. *J. Magn. Reson. Imaging* 12:859–865.

Ferraresi, S., D. Prosetti, C. Griffini, T. Motta, A. Signorelli, S. Pericotti, and V. Cassinari. 1989. Unusual radiological presentation of primary CNS lymphoma. *Ital. J. Neurol. Sci.* 10:583–586.

Fetter, B., G. Kintworth, and W. Hendy. 1967. *Mycoses of the Central Nervous System*, p. 87–123. Williams & Wilkins, Baltimore, MD.

Filippi, C., G. Sze, S. Farber, M. Shahmanesh, and P. Selwyn. 1998. Regression of HIV encephalopathy and basal ganglia signal intensity abnormality at MR imaging in patients with AIDS after initiation of protease inhibitor therapy. *Radiology* 206:491–498.

Filippi, C., A. Ulug, E. Ryan, S. Ferrando, and W. van Gorp. 2001. Diffusion-tensor imaging of patients with HIV and normal-appearing white matter on MR images of the brain. *Am. J. Neuroradiol.* 22:277–283.

Fischl, M., A. Pitchenik, and T. Spira. 1985. Tuberculous brain abscess and toxoplasma encephalitis in a patient with the acquired immunodeficiency syndrome. *JAMA* 256:362–366.

Flexner, C. 1998. HIV-protease inhibitors. *N. Engl. J. Med.* 338:1281–1292.

Fukui, M., B., Livstone, C. Meltzer, and R. Hamilton. 1998. Hemorrhagic presentation of untreated primary CNS lymphoma in a patient with AIDS. *Am. J. Radiol.* 170:1114–1115.

Gilden, D., R. Murray, M. Wellish, B. Kleinschmidt-DeMasters, and A. Vafai. 1988. Chronic progressive varicella-zoster virus encephalitis in an AIDS patient. *Neurology* 38:1150–1153.

Giudici, B., B. Vaz, S. Bossolasco, S. Casari, M. Brambilla, W. Luke, A. Lazzarin, T. Weber, and P. Cingue. 2000. Highly active antiretroviral therapy and progressive multifocal leukoencephalopathy: effects on cerebrospinal fluid markers of JC virus replication and immune response. *Clin. Infect. Dis.* 30:95–99.

Goldstein, J., B. Zeifer, C. Chao, F. Moser, D. Dickson, A. Hirschfeld, and L. Davis. 1991. CT appearance of primary CNS lymphoma in patients with acquired immunodeficiency syndrome. *J. Comput. Assist. Tomogr.* 15:39–44.

Grafe, M., G. Press, D. Berthoty, J. Hesselink, and C. Wiley. 1990. Abnormalities of the brain in AIDS patients: correlation of postmortem MR findings with neuropathology. *Am. J. Neuroradiol.* 11:905–911.

Guermazi, A., Y. Miaux, A. M. Zagdanski, and M. Laval-Jeantet. 1996. Choroid plexitis caused by cytomegalovirus in a patient with AIDS. *Am. J. Neuroradiol.* 17:1398–1399.

Gupta, R., S. Gupta, D. Singh, B. Sharma, A. Kohli, and R. Gujral. 1994. MR imaging and angiography in tuberculous meningitis. *Neuroradiology* 36:87–92.

Gupta, R., H. Poptani, A. Kohli, D. Chhabra, B. Sharma, and R. Gujral. 1995. In vivo localized proton magnetic spectroscopy of intracranial tuberculomas. *Indian J. Med. Res.* 101:19–24.

Gupta, R., D. Vatsal, N. Husain, S. Chawla, K. Prasad, R. Roy, R. Kumar, D. Jha, and M. Husain. 2001. Differentiation of tuberculous from pyogenic abscess with in vivo proton MR spectroscopy and magnetization transfer MR imaging. *Am. J. Neuroradiol.* **22**:1503–1509.

Hainfellner, J., and H. Budka. 1997. Neuropathology of human immunodeficiency virus-related opportunistic infections and neoplasms, p. 461–515. *In* J. R. Berger and R. M. Levy (ed.), *AIDS and the Nervous System*, 2nd ed. Lippincott-Raven Publishers, Philadelphia, PA.

Happe, S., M. Besselmann, P. Matheja, C. H. Rickert, G. Schuierer, D. Reichelt, and I. W. Husstedt. 1999. Cidofovir (vistide) in therapy of progressive multifocal leukoencephalopathy in AIDS. Review of the literature and report of 2 cases. *Nervenarzt* **70**:935–943. (In German.)

Hassine, D., F. Gray, R. Chekroun, P. De Truchis, E. Shouman-Claeys, and C. Vallée. 1995. CMV and VAV encephalitis in AIDS. *J. Neuroradiol.* **22**:184–192.

Hawley, D., J. Schaeffer, D. Schulz, and J. Muller. 1983. Cytomegalovirus encephalitis in acquired immunodeficiency syndrome. *Am. J. Clin. Pathol.* **80**:874–877.

Heald, A., J. Hoffman, J. Bartlett, and H. Waskin. 1996. Differentiation of central nervous system lesions in AIDS patients using positron emission tomography (PET). *Int. J. STD AIDS* **7**:337–346.

Himmelreich, U., T. Dzendrowskyj, C. Allen, S. Dowd, R. Malik, B. Shehan, P. Russel, C. Mountford, and T. Sorrell. 2001. Cryptococcomas distinguished from gliomas with MR spectroscopy: an experimental rat and cell culture study. *Radiology* **220**:122–128.

Hoffman, J. M., H. A. Waskin, T. Schifter, M. W. Hanson, L. Gray, S. Rosenfeld, and R. E. Coleman. 1993. FDG-PET in differentiating lymphoma from nonmalignant central nervous system lesions in patients with AIDS. *J. Nucl. Med.* **34**:567–575.

Holland, B., L. Perrett, and C. Mills. 1986. Meningovascular syphilis: CT and MR findings. *Radiology* **158**:439–442.

Holland, N. R., C. Power, V. P. Mathews, J. D. Glass, M. Forman, and J. C. McArthur. 1994. Cytomegalovirus encephalitis in acquired immunodeficiency syndrome (AIDS). *Neurology* **44**:507–514.

Husted, C., D. Goodin, J. Hugg, A. Maudsley, J. Tsuruda, S. de Bie, G. Fein, G. Matson, and M. Weiner. 1994. Biochemical alterations in multiple sclerosis lesions and normal-appearing white matter detected by in vivo ^{31}P and ^{1}H spectroscopic imaging. *Ann. Neurol.* **36**:157–165.

Iranzo, A., A. Moreno, J. Pujol, J. Marti-Fabregas, P. Domingo, J. Molet, J. Ris, and J. Cadafalch. 1999. Proton magnetic resonance spectroscopy pattern of progressive multifocal leukoencephalopathy in AIDS. *J. Neurol. Neurosurg. Psychiatry* **66**:520–523.

Jakobsen, J., C. Gyldensted, B. Brun, P. Bruhn, S. Helweg-Larsen, and P. Arlien-Soborg. 1989. Cerebral ventricular enlargement relates to neuropsychological measures in unselected AIDS patients. *Acta Neurol. Scand.* **79**:59–62.

Jarvik, J., R. Lenkinski, R. Grossman, J. Gomori, M. Schnall, and I. Frank. 1993. Proton MR spectroscopy of HIV-infected patients: characterization of abnormalities with imaging and clinical correlation. *Radiology* **186**:739–744.

Jayasundar, R., V. Singh, P. Raghunathan, K. Jain, and A. Banerji. 1999. Inflammatory granulomas: evaluation with proton MRS. *NMR Biomed.* **12**:139–144.

Jinkins, J. 1988. Focal tuberculous cerebritis. *Am. J. Neuroradiol.* **9**:121–124.

Johnson, B., E. Fram, P. Johnson, and R. Jacobowitz. 1997. The variable MR appearance of primary lymphoma of the central nervous system: comparison with histopathologic features. *Am. J. Neuroradiol.* **18**:563–572.

Jordan, J., and D. Enzmann. 1991. Encephalitis. *Neuroimag. Clin. N. Am.* **1**:17–38.

Kalayjian, R., M. Cohen, R. Bonomo, and T. Flanigan. 1993. Cytomegalovirus ventriculoencephalitis in AIDS: a syndrome with distinct clinical and pathologic features. *Medicine (Baltimore)* **72**:67–77.

Kamezawa, T., T. Shimozuru, M. Niiro, S. Nagata, and J. Kuratsu. 2000. MRI demonstration of intracerebral cryptococcal granuloma. *Neuroradiology* **42**:30–33.

Kami, M., I. Shirouzu, K. Mitani, S. Ogawa, T. Matsumura, Y. Kanda, T. Masumoto, Y. Saito, Y. Tanaka, K. Maki, H. Honda, S. Chiba, K. Ohtomo, H. Hirai, and Y. Yazaki. 1999. Early diagnosis of central nervous system aspergillosis with combination use of cerebral diffusion-weighted echoplanar magnetic resonance image and polymerase chain reaction of cerebrospinal fluid. *Intern. Med.* **38**:45–48.

Kastrup, O., M. Machke, H. Diener, and I. Wanke. 2002. Progressive multifocal leukoencephalopathy limited to the brain stem. *Neuroradiology* **44**:227–229.

Katz, D., J. Berger, and R. Duncan. 1993. Neurosyphilis, a comparative study of the effects of infection with human immunodeficiency virus. *Arch. Neurol.* **50**:243–249.

Kieburtz, K., L. Ketonen, A. Zettelmaier, L. Kentonen, M. Tuite, and E. Caine. 1990. Magnetic resonance imaging findings in HIV cognitive impairment. *Arch. Neurol.* **47**:643–645.

Kim, T., K. Chang, J. Goo, M. Kook, and M. Han. 1995. Intracranial tuberculoma: comparison of MR with pathologic findings. *Am. J. Neuroradiol.* **16**:1903–1908.

Kioumehr, F., M. Dadsetan, S. Rooholamini, and A. Au. 1994. Central nervous system tuberculosis: MRI. *Neuroradiology* **36**:93–96.

Kleihues, P., W. Lang, P. Burger, H. Budka, M. Vogt, R. Maurer, R. Luthy, and W. Siegenthaler. 1985. Progressive diffuse leukoencephalopathy in patients with acquired immune deficiency syndrome (AIDS). *Acta Neuropathol.* (Berlin) **68**:333–339.

Klunk, W. E., K. Panchalingam, J. Moossy, R. J. McClure, and J. W. Pettegrew. 1992. N-Acetyl-L-aspartate and other amino acid metabolites in Alzheimer's disease brain: a preliminary proton nuclear magnetic resonance study. *Neurology* **42**:1578–1585.

Knox, J., D. Musher, and N. Guzick. 1976. The pathogenesis of syphilis and related treponematoses, p. 249–259. *In* R. C. Johnson (ed.), *The Biology of Parasitic Spirochetes*. Academic Press, San Diego, CA.

Kotecha, N., M. George, T. Smith, F. Corvi, and N. Litofsky. 1998. Enhancing progressive multifocal leukoencephalopathy: an indicator of improved immune status. *Am. J. Med.* **105**:541–543.

Kuchelmeister, K., F. Gullotta, M. Bergmann, G. Angeli, and T. Masini. 1993. Progressive multifocal leukoencephalopathy (PML) in the acquired immunodeficiency syndrome (AIDS). A neuropathological autopsy study of 21 cases. *Pathol. Res. Pract.* **189**:163–173.

Kupfer, M., C. Zee, P. Colletti, W. Boswell, and R. Rhodes. 1990. MRI evaluation of AIDS related encephalopathy: toxoplasmosis vs lymphomas. *Magn. Reson. Imaging* **8**:51–57.

Laissy, J. P., R. Lebtahi, Y. S. Cordoliani, M. C. Henry-Feugeas, and E. Schouman-Claeys. 1995a. The diagnosis of primary cerebral lymphoma in AIDS. The contribution of imaging. *J. Neuroradiol.* **22**:207–217. (In French.)

Laissy, J.-P., P. Soyer, J. Tebboune, P. Gay-Depassier, E. Casalino, S. Lariven, A. Silbert, and Y. Menu. 1995b. Contrast enhanced fast MRI in differentiating brain toxoplasmosis and lymphoma in AIDS patients. *J. Comput. Assist. Tomogr.* **18**:714–771.

Laubenberger, J., D. Häussinger, S. Bayer, S. Theilemann, B. Schneider, A Mundinger, J. Hennig, and M. Langer. 1996. HIV-related metabolic abnormalities in the brain: depiction with proton MR spectroscopy with short echo time. *Radiology* **199**:805–810.

Le Bihan, D., J. F. Mangin, C. Poupon, C. A. Clark, S. Pappata, N. Molko, and H. Chabriat. 2001. Diffusion tensor imaging: concepts and applications. *J. Magn. Reson. Imaging* **13**:534–546.

LeBlang, S., M. Whiteman, M. Post, R. Uttamchanani, M. Bell, and J. Smirniotopolous. 1995. CNS nocardia in AIDS patients: CT and MRI with pathologic correlation. *J. Comput. Assist. Tomogr.* **19**:15–22.

Lee, V., V. Antonacci, S. Tilak, J. Fuller, and T. Cooley. 1999. Intracranial mass lesions: sequential thallium and gallium scintigraphy in patients with AIDS. *Radiology* **211**:507–512.

Levy, R., S. Rosenbloom, and L. Perrett. 1986. Neuroradiologic findings in AIDS: a review of 200 cases. *Am. J. Radiol.* **147**:977–983.

Levy, R. M., D. E. Bredesen, and M. L. Rosenblum. 1985. Neurological manifestation of the acquired immunodeficiency syndrome (AIDS): experience at UCSF and review of the literature. *J. Neurosurg.* **62**:475–495.

Licho, R., N. S. Litofsky, M. Senitko, and M. George. 2002. Inaccuracy of T1-201 brain SPECT in distinguishing cerebral infections from lymphoma in patients with AIDS. *Clin. Nucl. Med.* **27**:81–86.

Lizerbram, E., and J. Hesselink. 1997. Viral infections. *Neuroimag. Clin. N. Am.* **7**:261–180.

Lopez-Villegas, D., R. Lenkinski, and I. Frank. 1997. Biochemical changes in the frontal lobe of HIV-infected individuals detected by magnetic resonance spectroscopy. *Proc. Natl. Acad. Sci. USA* **94**:9854–9859.

Marcus, C., S. Taylor-Robinson, J. Sargentoni, J. Ainsworth, G. Frize, P. Easterbrook, S. Shaunak, and D. Bryant. 1998. [1]H MR spectroscopy of the brain in HIV-1-seropositive subjects: evidence for diffuse metabolic abnormalities. *Metab. Brain Dis.* **13**:123–136.

Mayo, J., J. Collazos, and E. Martinez. 1998. Progressive multifocal leukoencephalopathy following initiation of highly active antiretroviral therapy. *AIDS* **13**:1720–1722.

Miaux, Y., P. Ribaud, M. Williams, A. Guermazi, E. Gluckman, C. Brocheriou, and M. Laval-Jeantet. 1995. MR of cerebral aspergillosis in patients who have had bone marrow transplantation. *Am. J. Neuroradiol.* **16**:555–562.

Miller, B., R. Moats, T. Shonk, T. Ernst, S. Woolley, and B. Ross. 1993. Alzheimer disease: depiction of increased cerebral myo-inositol with proton MR spectroscopy. *Radiology* **187**:433–437.

Miller, R. F., M. A. Hall-Craggs, D. C. Costa, N. S. Brink, F. Scaravilli, S. B. Lucas, I. D. Wilkinson, P. J. Ell, B. E. Kendall, and M. J. Harrison. 1998. Magnetic resonance imaging, thallium-210 SPECT scanning, and laboratory analyses for discrimination of cerebral lymphoma and toxoplasmosis in AIDS. *Sex. Transm. Infect.* **74**:258–264.

Miralles, P., J. Berenguer, D. Garcia de Viedma, B. Padilla, J. Cosin, J. Lopez-Bernaldo deQuiros, S. Moreno, and E. Bouza. 1998. Treatment of AIDS-associated progressive multifocal leukoencephalopathy with highly active antiretroviral therapy. *AIDS* **12**:2467–2472.

Miralles, P., J. Berenguer, C. Lacruz, J. Cosin, J. Lopez, B. Padilla, L. Munoz, and D. Garcia de Viedma. 2001. Inflammatory reactions in progressive multifocal leukoencephalopathy after highly active antiretroviral therapy. *AIDS* **15**:1900–1902.

Moats, R., T. Ernst, T. Shonk, and B. Ross. 1994. Abnormal cerebral metabolite concentrations in patients with probable Alzheimer's disease. *Magn. Reson. Med.* **32**:110–115.

Moller, H., P. Vermathen, M. Lentschig, G. Schuierer, S. Schwarz, D. Weidermann, S. Evers, and I. Husstedt. 1999. Metabolic characterization of AIDS-dementia complex by spectroscopic imaging. *J. Magn. Reson. Imaging.* **9**:10–18.

Monette, R., D. Czarnecki, and B. Buggy. 1992. MR findings in an AIDS patient with cytomegalovirus retinitis. *Am. J. Radiol.* **158**:1176.

Moreno, S., J. Baraia-Etxaburu, E. Bouza, F. Parras, M. Perez-Tascon, P. Miralles, T. Vincente, J. Alberdi, J. Cosin, and D. Lopez-Gay. 1993. Risk for developing tuberculosis among anergic patients infected with HIV. *Ann. Intern. Med.* **119**:194–198.

Morgello, S., E. Cho, S. Nielsen, O. Devinsky, and C. Petito. 1987. Cytomegalovirus encephalitis in patients with acquired immunodeficiency syndrome: an autopsy study of 30 cases and a review of the literature. *Hum. Pathol.* **18**:289–97.

Navia, B., B. Jordan, and R. Price. 1986. The AIDS dementia complex. I. Clinical features. *Ann. Neurol.* **19**:517–524.

Nicoli, F., B. Chave, J. Peragut, and J. Gastaut. 1991. Efficacy of cytarabine in progressive multifocal leukoencephalopathy in AIDS. *Lancet* **339**:306.

O'Doherty, M., S. Barrington, M. Campbell, J. Lowe, and C. Bradbeer. 1997. PET scanning and the human immunodeficiency virus-positive patients. *J. Nucl. Med.* **38**:1575–1583.

Olsen, W., F. Longo, C. Mills, and D. Norman. 1988. White matter disease in AIDS: findings at MR imaging. *Radiology* **169**:445–448.

Otake, T., H. Mori, M. Morimoto, K. Miyano, N. Ueba, I. Oishi, N. Kunita, and T. Kurimura. 1999. Anti-HIV-1 activity of myo-inositol hexaphosphoric acid (IP6) and myo-inosytol hexasuljate (IS6). *Anticancer Res.* **19**:3723–3726.

Parker, J. C., Jr., and M. Dyer. 1985. Neurological infection due to bacteria, fungi, parasites, p. 632–703. *In* R. L. Davis and D. M. Robertson (ed.), *Textbook of Neuropathology*. Williams & Wilkins, Baltimore, MD.

Patankar, T., R. Varma, A. Krishnan, S. Prasad, K. Desai, and M. Castillo. 2000. Radiographic findings of tuberculosis of the calvarium. *Neuroradiology* **42**:518–521.

Petito, C., E. Cho, W. Lemann, B. Navia, and R. Price. 1986. Neuropathology of acquired immunodeficiency syndrome (AIDS): an autopsy review. *J. Neuropathol. Exp. Neurol.* **45**:635–646.

Poon, T., I. Matoso, V. Tcherkoff, I. Weitzner, and M. Gade. 1989. CT features of primary cerebral lymphoma in AIDS and non-AIDS patients. *J. Comput. Assist. Tomogr.* **13**:6–9.

Port, J., S. Miseljic, R. Lee, S. Ali, T. Nicol, W. Royal, and B. Chin. 1999. Progressive multifocal leukoencephalopathy demonstrating contrast enhancement on MRI and uptake of thallium-201: a case report. *Neuroradiology* **41**:895–898.

Portegies, P., P. Algra, C. Hollak, J. Prins, P. Reiss, J. Valk, and J. Lange. 1991. Response to cytarabine in progressive multifocal leukoencephalopathy in AIDS. *Lancet* **337**:680–681.

Post, M., G. Hensley, L. Moskowitz, and M. Fischl. 1986a. Cytomegalic inclusion virus encephalitis in patients with AIDS: CT, clinical, and pathologic correlation. *Am. J. Neuroradiol.* **7**:275–279.

Post, M. J., J. R. Berger, R. Duncan, R. M. Quencer, L. Pall, and D. Winfield. 1993. Asymptomatic and neurologically symptomatic HIV-seropositive subjects: results of long-term MR imaging and clinical follow-up. *Radiology* **188**:727–733.

Post, M. J., J. C. Chan, G. T. Hensley, T. A. Hoffman, L. B. Moskowitz, and S. Lippmann. 1983. Toxoplasma encephalitis in Haitian adults with acquired immunodeficiency syndrome: a clinical-pathological-CT correlation. *Am. J. Radiol.* **140**:861–868.

Post, M. J., S. J. Kursunoglu, G. T. Hensley, J. C. Chan, L. B. Moskowitz, and T. A. Hoffman. 1985. Cranial CT in acquired immunodeficiency syndrome: spectrum of diseases and optimal contrast enhancement technique. *Am. J. Neuroradiol.* **6**:743–754.

Post, M. J., B. E. Levin, J. R. Berger, R. Duncan, R. M. Quencer, and G. Calabro. 1992. Sequential cranial MR findings of asymptomatic and neurologically symptomatic HIV positive subjects. *Am. J. Neuroradiol.* **13**:359–370.

Post, M. J., J. J. Sheldon, G. T. Hensley, L. Soila, J. A. Tobias, J. C. Chan, R. M. Quencer, and L. B. Moskowitz.

1986b. Central nervous system disease in acquired immunodeficiency syndrome: prospective correlation using CT, MR imaging, and pathological studies. *Radiology* **158**:141–148.

Post, M. J., L. G. Tate, R. M. Quencer, G. T. Hensley, J. R. Berger, W. A. Sheremata, and G. Maul. 1988. CT, MR, and pathology in HIV encephalitis and meningitis. *Am. J. Radiol.* **151**:373–380.

Post, M. J., C. Yiannoutsos, D. Simpson, J. Booss, D. B. Clifford, B. Cohen, J. C. McArthur, and C. D. Hall. 1999. Progressive multifocal leukoencephalopathy in AIDS: are there any MR findings useful to patient management and predictive of patient survival? *Am. J. Neuroradiol.* **20**:1896–1906.

Poutiainen, E., I. Eloovara, R. Raininko, L. Hokkanen, S. Valle, J. Lahdevirta, and M. Livanainen. 1993. Cognitive performance in HIV-1 infection: relationship to severity of disease and brain atrophy. *Acta Neurol. Scand.* **87**:88–94.

Power, C., O. Selnes, J. Grim, and J. McArthur. 1995. HIV dementia scale: a rapid screening test. *J. Acquir. Immune Defic. Syndr. Hum. Retrovirol.* **8**:273–278.

Presant, C., P. Wiernik, and A. Serpick. 1973. Factors affecting survival in nocardiosis. *Am. Rev. Respir. Dis.* **108**:1444–1448.

Price, R., and J. Sidtis. 1990. Evaluation of the AIDS dementia complex in clinical trials. *J. Acquir. Immune Defic. Syndr* **3**:S51–S60.

Provinciali, L., M. Signorino, G. Ceravolo, and U. Pasguini. 1988. Onset of primary brain T-lymphoma simulating a progressive leukoencephalopathy. *Ital. J. Neurol. Sci.* **9**:377–381.

Pui, M., and M. Ahmad. 2002. Magnetization transfer imaging diagnosis of intracranial tuberculomas. *Neuroradiology* **44**:210–215

Rausch, D., and M. Davis. 2001. HIV in the CNS: pathogenic relationships to systemic HIV disease and other CNS disease. *J. Neurovirol.* **7**:85–96.

Rovira, M., F. Romero, O. Torrent, and B. Ibbara. 1980. Study of tuberculous meningitis by CT. *Neuroradiology* **19**:137–141.

Ruiz, A., M. Donovan Post, C. Bundschu, W. Ganz, and M. Georgiou. 1997a. Primary central nervous system lymphoma in patients with AIDS. *Neuroimag. Clin. N. Am.* **7**:281–296.

Ruiz, A., W. Ganz, M. Post, A. Camp, H. Landy, W. Mallin, and G. Sfakianakis. 1994. Use of thallium-201 brain SPECT to differentiate cerebral lymphoma from toxoplasma encephalitis in AIDS patients. *Am. J. Neuroradiol.* **15**:1885–1894.

Ruiz, A., M. Post, and C. Bundschu. 1997b. Dentate nuclei involvement in AIDS patients with CNS cryptococcosis: imaging findings with pathologic correlation. *J. Comput. Assist. Tomogr.* **21**:175–182.

Sacktor, N., R. Lyles, M. Skolasky, C. Kleeberger, O. Selnes, E. Miller, J. Becker, B. Cohen, J. McArthur, and Multicenter AIDS Cohort Study. 2001. HIV-associated neurologic disease incidence changes: multicenter AIDS cohort study, 1990–1998. *Neurology* **56**:257–260.

Sacktor, N., R. Skolaskiy, T. Ernst, X. Mao, O. Selnes, M. Pomper, L. Chang, K. Zhong, D. Shungu, K. Marder, D. Shibata, G. Schifitto, L. Bobo, and P. Barker. 2005. A multicenter study of two magnetic resonance spectroscopy techniques in individuals with HIV dementia. *J. Magn. Reson. Imaging* **21**:325–333.

Salazar, A., D. Podzamczer, R. Reñe, M. Santin, J. Perez, I. Ferrer, P. Fernandez-Viladrich, and F. Gudiol. 1995. Cytomegalovirus ventriculoencephalitis in AIDS patients. *Scand. J. Infect. Dis.* **27**:165–169.

Salvan, A., J. Vion-Dury, S. Confort-Gouny, F. Nicoli, S. Lamoureux, and P. Cozzone. 1997. Brain proton magnetic resonance spectroscopy in HIV-related encephalopathy: identification of evolving metabolic patterns in relation to dementia and therapy. *AIDS Res. Hum. Retrovir.* **13**:1055–1066.

Schwaighofer, B., J. Hesselink, G. Press, R. Wolf, M. Healy, and D. Berthoty. 1989. Primary intracranial CNS lymphoma: MR manifestations. *Am. J. Neuroradiol.* **10**:725–729.

Sener, R. 2001. Herpes simplex encephalitis: diffusion MR imaging findings. *Comput. Med. Imaging Graph.* **25**:391–397.

Setinek, U., E. Wondrusch, K. Jellinger, A. Streur, M. Drlicek, W. Grisold, and F. Lintner. 1995. Cytomegalovirus infection of the brain in AIDS: a clinicopathological study. *Acta Neuropathol. Berl.* **90**:511–515.

Shapiro, R., K. Mullane, L. Camras, C. Flowers, and S. Sutton. 2001. Clinical and magnetic resonance imaging regression of progressive multifocal leukoencephalopathy in an AIDS patient after intensive antiretroviral therapy. *J. Neuroimag.* **11**:336–339.

Sieb, J. P., D. van Roost, and L. Solymosi. 1992. Zerebrales B-Zell-Lymphom mit dem neuroradiologischen Bild einer multifokalen Leukoenzephalopathie. *Fortschr. Röntgenstr.* **156**:503–504.

Skiest, D., W. Erdman, W. Chang, O. Oz, A. Ware, and J. Fleckenstein. 2000. SPECT thallium-201 combined with *Toxoplasma* serology for the presumptive diagnosis of focal central nervous system mass lesions in patients with AIDS. *J. Infect.* **40**:274–281.

So, Y., J. Beckstead, and R. Davis. 1986. Primary central nervous system lymphoma in acquired immunodeficiency syndrome: a clinical and pathological study. *Ann. Neurol.* **20**:566–572.

Suwanwela, N., P. Phanuphak, K. Phanthumchinda, N. Suwanwela, J. Tantivatana, K. Ruxrungtham, J. Suttipan, S. Wangsuphachart, and M. Hanvanich. 2000. Magnetic resonance spectroscopy of the brain in neurologically asymptomatic HIV-infected patients. *Magn. Reson. Imaging* **18**:859–865.

Sze, G., and R. Zimmerman. 1988. The magnetic resonance imaging of infection and inflammatory disease. *Radiol. Clin. N. Am.* **26**:839–859.

Talpos, D., R. Tien, and J. Hesselink. 1991. Magnetic resonance imaging of AIDS-related polyradiculopathy. *Neurology* **41**:1522–1523.

Tantisiriwat, W., P. Tebas, D. Clifford, W. Powderly, and C. Fichtenbaum. 1999. Progressive multifocal leukoencephalopathy in AIDS receiving highly active antiretroviral therapy. *Clin. Infect. Dis.* **28**:1152–1154.

Tassie, J., J. Gasnault, M. Bentata, J. Deloumeaux, F. Boue, E. Billaud, and D. Costagliola. 1999. Survival improvement of AIDS-related progressive multifocal leukoencephalopathy in the era of protease inhibitors. *AIDS* **13**:1881–1887.

Tayfun, C., T. Uçöz, M. Ta ar, K. Ataç, O ur, T. Oztürk, and M. A. Yinanç. 1995. Diagnostic value of MRI in tuberculous meningitis. *Eur. Radiol.* **6**:380–386.

Teofilo, E., J. Gouveia, V. Brotas, and P. da Costa. 1998. Progressive multifocal leukoencephalopathy regression with highly active antiretroviral therapy. *AIDS* **12**:449.

Thurnher, M., M. Castillo, A. Stadler, A. Rieger B. Schmid, and P. Sundgren. 2005. Diffusion tensor MR imaging (DTI) of the brain in human immunodeficiency virus (HIV)-positive patients. *Am. J. Neuroradiol.* **26**:2275–2281.

Thurnher, M., M. Post, A. Rieger, C. Kleibl-Popov, C. Löwe, and E. Schindler. 2001a. Initial and follow-up MR imaging findings in AIDS-related progressive multifocal leukoencephalopathy treated with highly active antiretroviral therapy. *Am. J. Neuroradiol.* **22**:977–984.

Thurnher, M., R. Jinkins, and M. Post. 1997a. Diagnostic imaging of infections and neoplasms affecting the spine in patients with AIDS. *Neuroimag. Clin. N. Am.* **7**:341–357.

Thurnher, M., A. Rieger, C. Kleibl-Popov, and E. Schindler. 2001b. Malignant lymphoma of the cranial vault in an HIV-positive patient: imaging findings. *Eur. Radiol.* **11**:1506–1509.

Thurnher, M., A. Rieger, C. Kleibl-Popov, E. Schindler, U. Settinek, C. Henk, and C. Harberler. 2001c. Primary central nervous system lymphoma in AIDS: a wider spectrum of CT and MRI findings. *Neuroradiology* **43:**29–35.

Thurnher, M., E. Schindler, S. Thurnher, H. Pernerstorfer-Schön, C. Kleibl-Popov, and A. Rieger. 2000. Highly active antiretroviral therapy for patients with AIDS dementia complex: effect on MR imaging findings and clinical course. *Am. J. Neuroradiol.* **21:**670–678.

Thurnher, M., S. Thurnher, D. Fleischmann, A. Steuer, A. Rieger, T. Helbich, S. Trattnig, E. Schindler, and E. Hittmair. 1997b. Comparison of T2-weighted and fluid-attenuated inversion-recovery fast spin-echo MR sequences in intracerebral AIDS-associated disease. *Am. J. Neuroradiol.* **18:**1601–1609.

Thurnher, M., S. Thurnher, B. Mühlbauer, J. Hainfellner, A. Steuer, D. Fleischmann, S. Trattnig, H. Budka, and E. Schindler. 1997c. Progressive multifocal leukoencephalopathy in AIDS: initial and follow-up CT and MRI. *Neuroradiology* **39:**611–618.

Tien, R., G. Feldberg, and A. Osumi. 1983. Herpesvirus infections of the CNS: MR findings. *Am. J. Radiol.* **158:**1325–1328.

Tien, R., A. Gean-Marton, and A. Mark. 1992. Neurosyphilis in HIV carriers: MR findings in six patients. *Am. J. Radiol.* **158:**1325–1328.

Tozzi, V., P. Balestra, S. Galgani, P. Narciso, F. Ferri, G. Sabastiani, C. D'Amato, C. Africano, F. Pigorini, F. Pau, A. De Felici, and A. Benedetto. 1999. Positive and sustained effects of highly active antiretroviral therapy on HIV-1-associated neurocognitive impairment. *AIDS* **13:**1889–1897.

Tracey, I., C. Carr, A. Guimaraes, J. Worth, B. Navia, and R. Gonzalez. 1996. Brain choline-containing compounds are elevated in HIV-positive patients before the onset of AIDS dementia complex: a proton magnetic resonance spectroscopic study. *Neurology* **46:**783–788.

Ulug, A., D. Moore, A. Bojko, and R. Zimmerman. 1999. Clinical use of diffusion-tensor imaging for diseases causing neuronal and axonal damage. *Am. J. Neuroradiol.* **20:**1044–1048.

Urenjak, J., S. Williams, D. Gadian, and M. Noble. 1993. Proton nuclear magnetic resonance spectroscopy unambiguously identifies different neural cell types. *J. Neurosci.* **13:**981–989.

Utamchandani, R., G. Daikos, R. Reyes, M. Fischl, G. Dickinson, E. Yamaguchi, and M. Kramer. 1994. Nocardiosis in 30 patients with advanced human immunodeficiency virus infection. Clinical features and outcome. *Clin. Infect. Dis.* **18:**348–353.

Vatz, K., R. Scheibel, S. Keiffer, and K. Ansari. 1974. Neurosyphilis and diffuse cerebral angiography: a case report. *Neurology* **24:**472–476.

Villoria, F., F. Fortea, S. Moreno, L. Munoz, M. Manero, and C. Benito. 1995. MR imaging and CT of central nervous system tuberculosis in the patient with AIDS. *Radiol. Clin. N. Am.* **33:**805–820.

Villoria, M., J. de la Torre, F. Fortea, L. Munoz, T. Hernandez, and J. Alarcon. 1992. Intracranial tuberculosis in AIDS: CT and MRI findings. *Neuroradiology* **34:**11–14.

Villringer, K., H. Jager, M. Dichgans, S. Ziegler, J. Poppinger, M. Herz, C. Kruschke, S. Minoshima, H. Pfister, and M. Schwaiger. 1995. Differential diagnosis of CNS lesions in AIDS patients by FDG-PET. *J. Comput. Assist. Tomogr.* **19:**532–536.

Von Einsiedel, R., T. Fife, A. Aksamit, M. Cornford, D. Secor, U. Tomiyasu, H. Itabashi, and H. Vinters. 1993. Progressive multifocal leukoencephalopathy in AIDS: a clinicopathologic study and review of the literature. *J. Neurol.* **240:**391–406.

Von Giesen, H., H. Hefter, H. Jablonowski, and G. Arendt. 2000. HAART is neuroprophylactic in HIV-1 infection. *J. Acquir. Immune Defic. Syndr.* **23:**380–385.

Von Giesen, H., H. Wittsack, F. Wenserski, H. Koller, H. Hefter, and G. Arendt. 2001. Basal ganglia metabolite abnormalities in minor motor disorders associated with human immunodeficiency virus type 1. *Arch. Neurol.* **58:**1281–1286.

Welchman, J. 1979. Computerised tomography of intracranial tuberculomata. *Clin. Radiol.* **30:**567–573.

Wesselingh, S., C. Power, J. Glass, W. Tyor, J. McArthur, J. Farber, J. Griffin, and D. Griffin. 1993. Intracerebral cytokine messenger RNA expression in acquired immunodeficiency syndrome dementia. *Ann. Neurol.* **33:**576–582.

Wheeler, A. L., C. L. Truwit, B. K. Kleinschmidt-DeMasters, W. R. Byrne, and R. N. Hannon. 1993. Progressive multifocal leukoencephalopathy: contrast enhancement on CT scans and MR imaging. *Am. J. Radiol.* **161:**1049–1051.

Whiteman, M., L. Espinoza, M. J. Post, M. D. Bell, and S. Falcone. 1995. Central nervous system tuberculosis in HIV-infected patients: clinical and radiographic findings. *Am. J. Neuroradiol.* **16:**1319–1327.

Whiteman, M. L., M. J. Post, J. R. Berger, L. G. Tate, M. D. Bell, and L. P. Limonte. 1993. Progressive multifocal leukoencephalopathy in 47 HIV-seropositive patients: neuroimaging with clinical and pathologic correlation. *Radiology* **187:**233–240.

Wilkinson, I. D., R. F. Miller, M. N. Paley, K. A. Miszkiel, B. E. Kendall, M. A. Hall-Craggs, and M. J. Harrison. 1996. Cerebral proton magnetic resonance spectroscopy in cytomegalovirus encephalitis and HIV leukoencephalopathy/encephalitis. *AIDS* **10:**1443–1444.

Woo, H., A. Rezai, E. Knopp, H. Weiner, D. Miller, and P. Kelly. 1996. Contrast-enhancing progressive multifocal leukoencephalopathy: radiological and pathological correlations. Case Report. *Neurosurgery* **39:**1031–1035.

Yamada, K., G. Zoarski, M. Rothman, M. Zagardo, T. Nishimura, and C. Sun. 2000. An intracranial aspergilloma with low signal on T2-weighted images corresponding to iron accumulation. *Neuroradiology* **43:**559–561.

Yang, P., K. Reger, J. Seeger, R. Carmody, and R. Iacono. 1987. Brain abscess: an atypical CT appearance of CNS tuberculosis. *Am. J. Neuroradiol.* **8:**919–920.

Yuh, W. T., H. D. Nguyen, F. Gao, E. T. Tali, D. J. Fisher, N. A. Mayr, D. P. Mueller, Y. Sato, M. E. Trigg, and R. Gingrich. 1994. Brain parenchymal infection in bone marrow transplantation patients. CT and MR findings. *Am. J. Radiol.* **162:**425–430.

COLOR PLATES

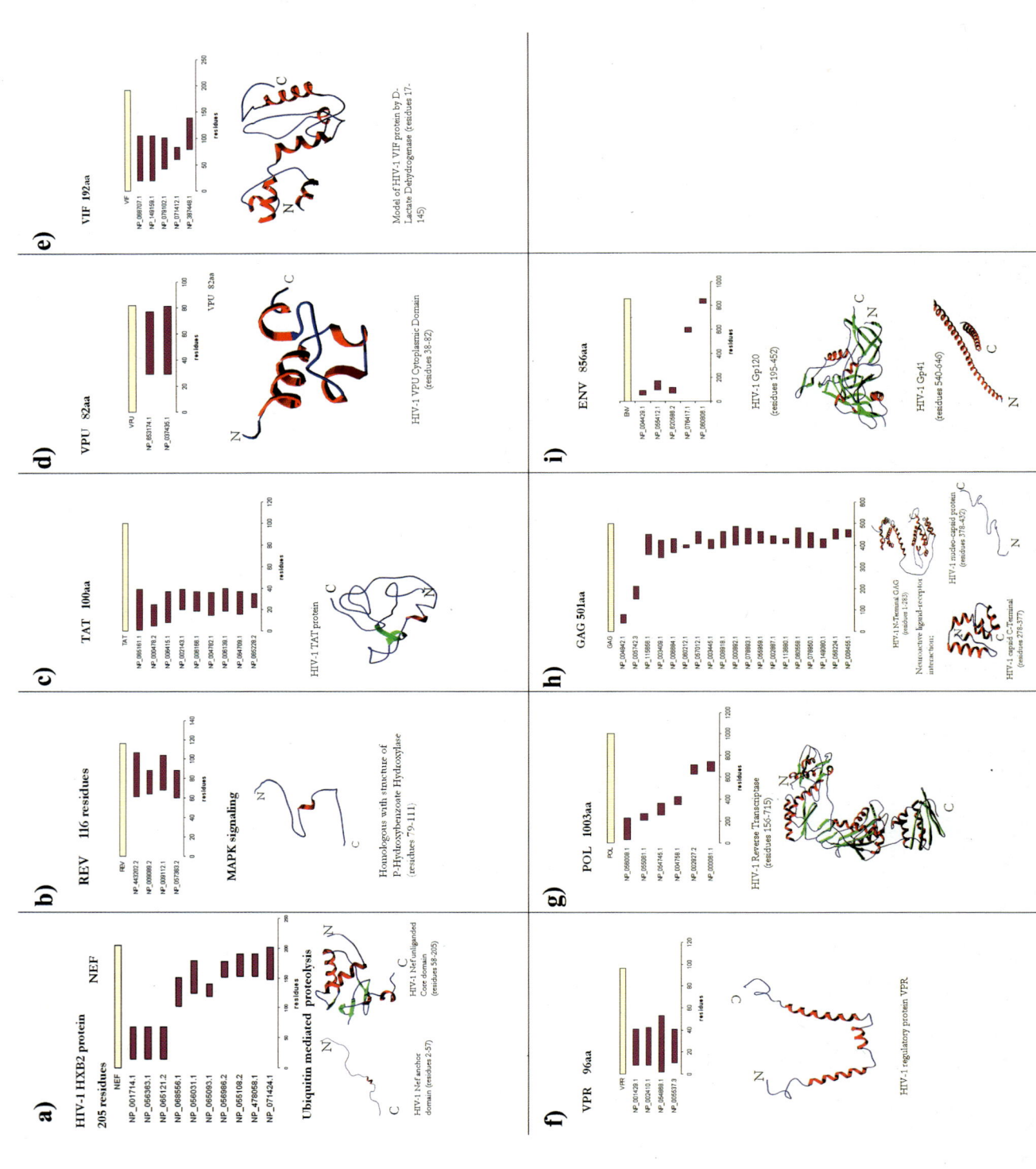

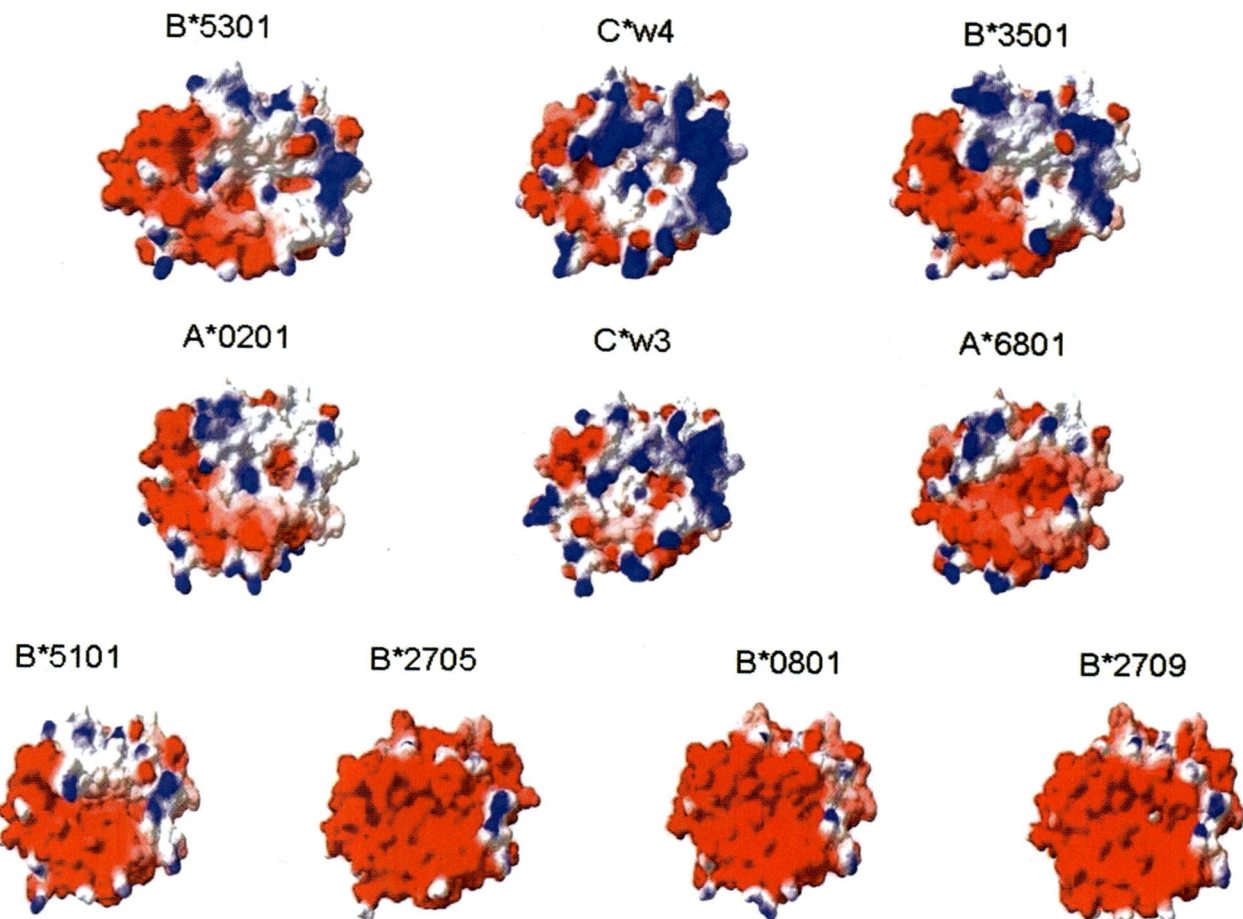

COLOR PLATE 2 (chapter 9)   The electrostatic distribution maps were calculated for each HLA allele structure (http://www.rcsb.org/pdb) using Coulomb's law as implemented in Deep View (Swiss PDB Viewer version 3.7). The electrostatic differences in the peptide binding groove between HLA alleles (A*0201, A*6801, B*0801, B*3501, B*5301, B*2705, B*2709, B*5101, C*w3, and C*w4) are shown. Red, electronegative; blue, electropositive; white, neutral.

COLOR PLATE 1 (chapter 9)   Segments of human HOMOLOGS (shaded bars) match different regions of HIV-1 proteins (open bars). The corresponding matching regions are mapped onto the known HIV-1 protein structures in red. aa, amino acids.

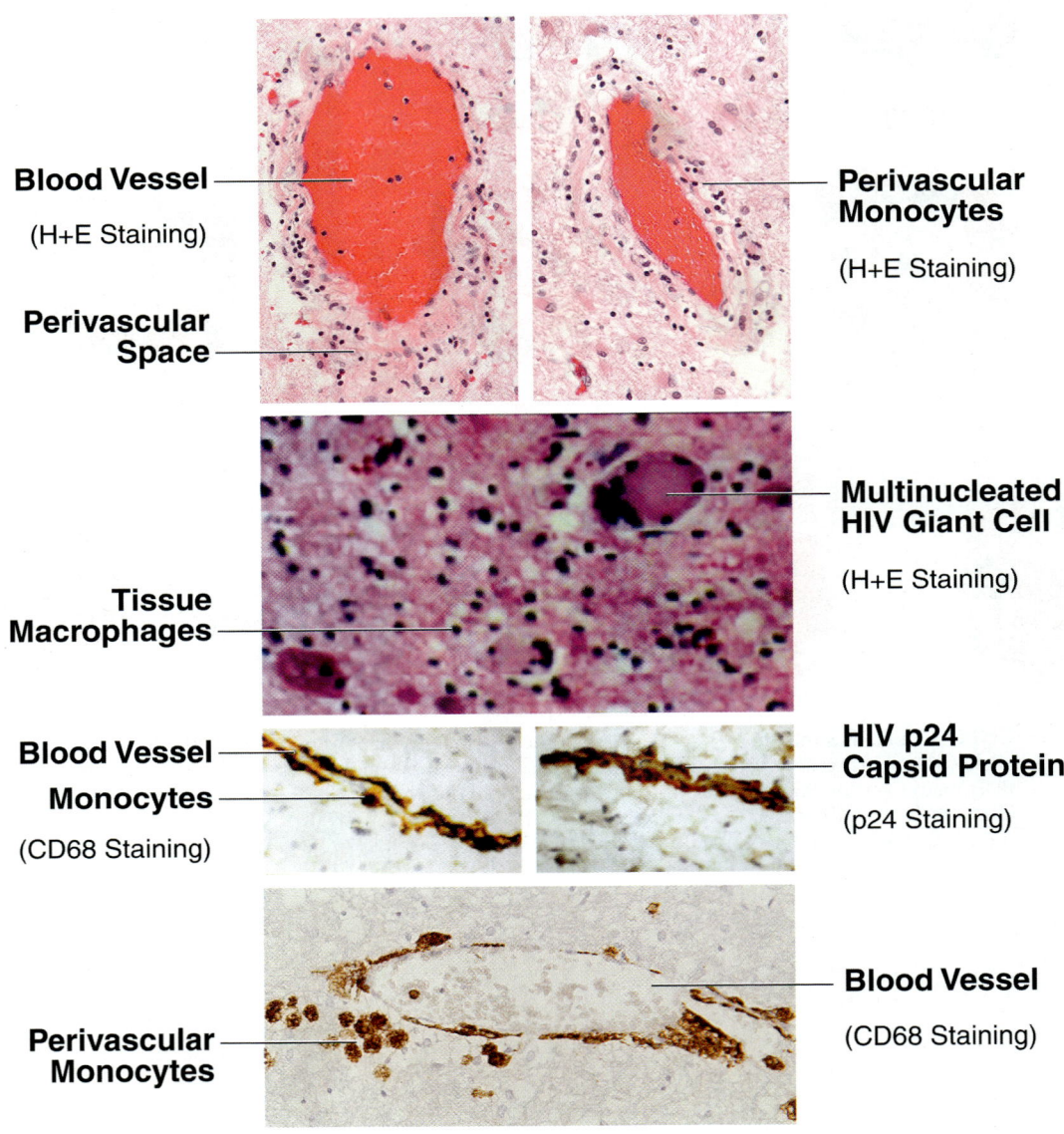

Blood Vessel

(H+E Staining)

Perivascular Space

Perivascular Monocytes

(H+E Staining)

Multinucleated HIV Giant Cell

(H+E Staining)

Tissue Macrophages

Blood Vessel

Monocytes

(CD68 Staining)

HIV p24 Capsid Protein

(p24 Staining)

Blood Vessel

(CD68 Staining)

Perivascular Monocytes

COLOR PLATE 3 (chapter 14) HIV encephalopathy is characterized by abundant perivascular monocytes/macrophages (CD68+) and tissue macrophages (CD68+) in the brain. Multinucleated HIV giant cells can also be present. HIV-infected (p24+) and uninfected monocytes/macrophages are found alongside blood vessels in the brain. H&E, hematoxylin and eosin.

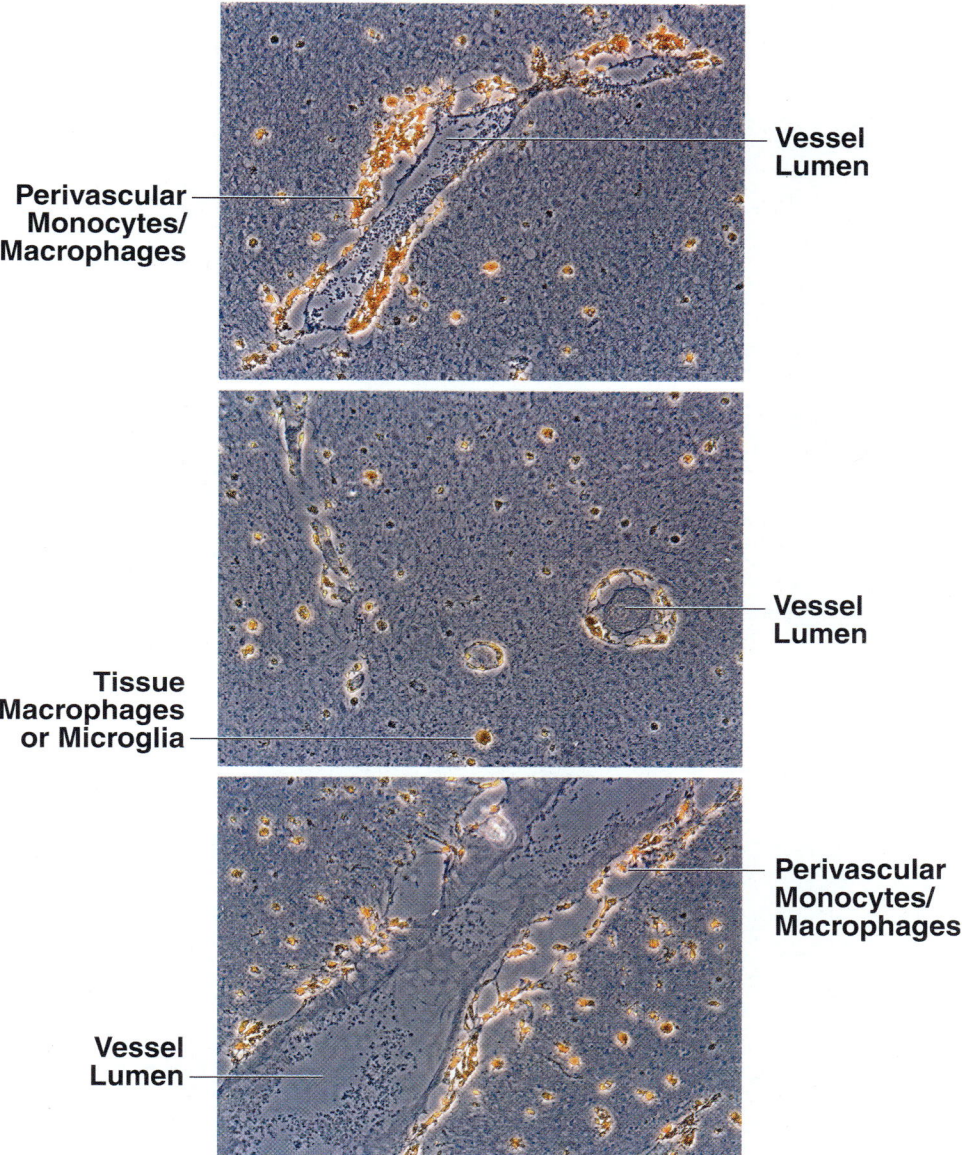

Vessel Lumen

Perivascular Monocytes/ Macrophages

Vessel Lumen

Tissue Macrophages or Microglia

Perivascular Monocytes/ Macrophages

Vessel Lumen

COLOR PLATE 4 (chapter 14) Phase-contrast microscopy of brain sections stained with hematoxylin and eosin shows perivascular monocytes/macrophages. Note the cross section of a blood vessel showing monocytes/macrophages surrounding the lumen.

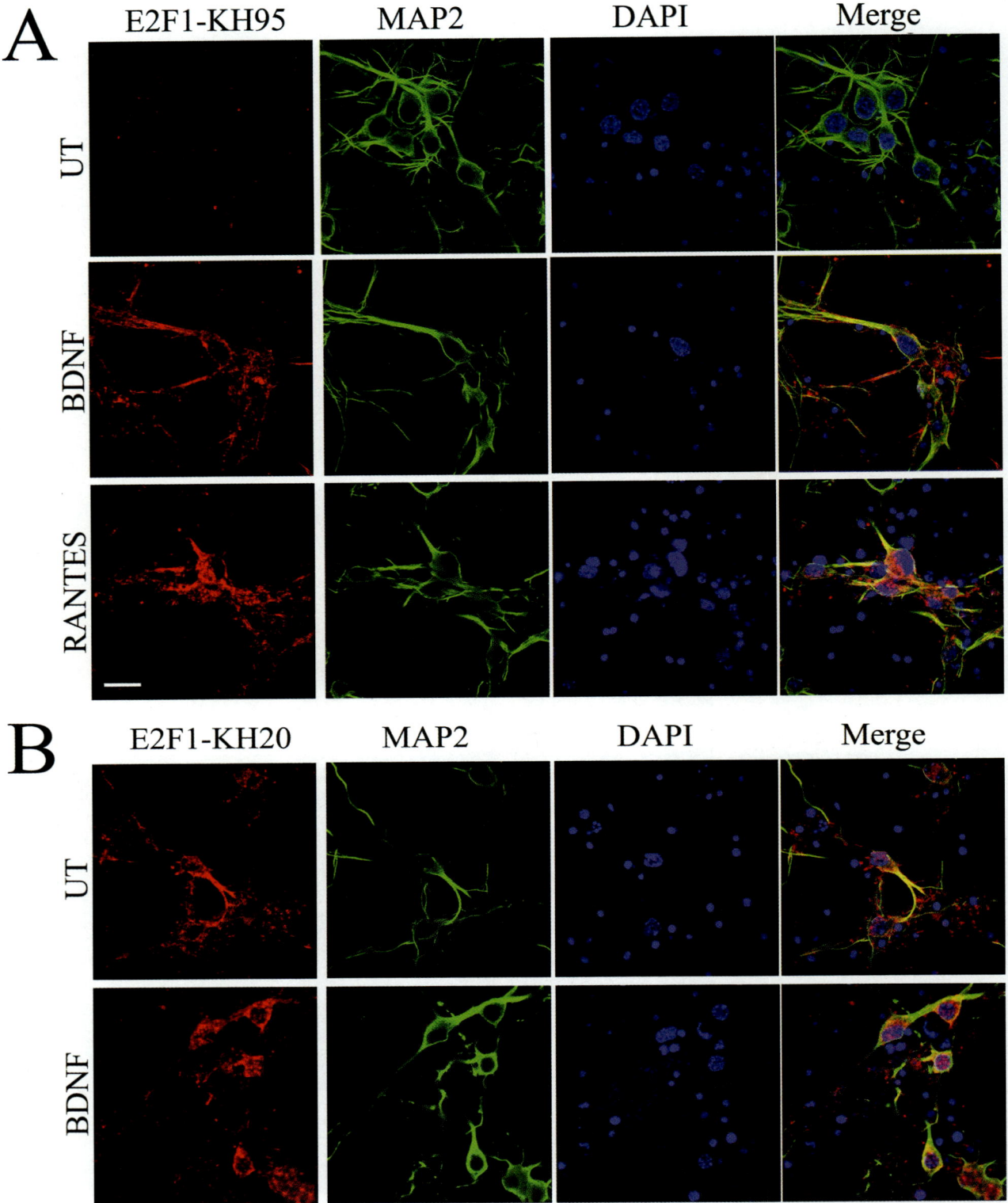

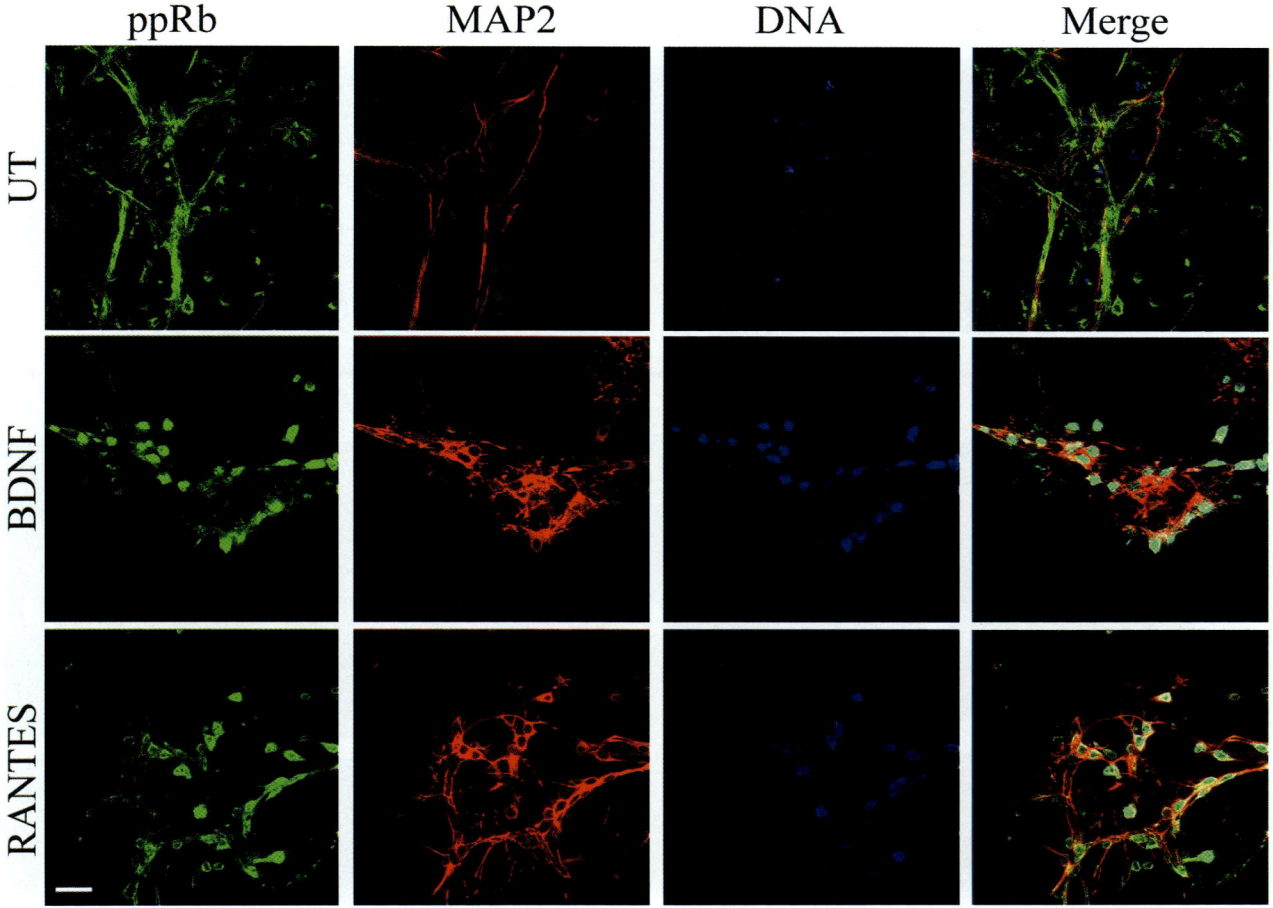

COLOR PLATE 6 (chapter 17) Trophic factors and chemokines induce increased ppRb in the nuclei of murine cortical neurons. Primary murine cortical cultures were grown for 7 days after plating and treated with 50 ng of BDNF/ml, or 50 ng of NGF/ml, or 100 ng of RANTES/ml, or 15 ng of MCP1/ml or left untreated (UT) for 24 h. Representative images from UT (row 1), BDNF-treated (row 2), and RANTES-treated (row 3) cultures are shown. Immunostaining for ppRb is shown in green (column 1). Neurons are labeled with anti-MAP2 antibody and are shown in red (column 2). Nuclear DNA is shown in blue (column 3). Merging of all three fluors is shown in column 4 (Merge). All images were captured by sequential triple-label immunofluorescent laser confocal microscopy using the same laser settings on the same day. These images are representative of more than 12 replicates of this experiment. Reprinted from *Experimental Neurology* (Strachan et al., 2005; Jordan-Sciutto et al., 2002b) with permission from the publisher.

COLOR PLATE 5 (chapter 17) Trophic factors and chemokines induce increased cytoplasmic staining of E2F1 in neurons. Primary murine cortical cultures were grown for 7 days after plating and treated with 50 ng of BDNF/ml, or 50 ng of NGF/ml, or 100 ng of RANTES/ml, or 15 ng of MCP1/ml or left untreated (UT) for 24 h. Representative images from UT (row 1), BDNF-treated (row 2), and RANTES-treated (row 3) cultures are shown. (A) Immunostaining for E2F1-KH95 is shown in red (column 1). Neurons are labeled with anti-MAP2 antibody and are shown in green (column 2). Nuclear DNA is shown in blue (column 3). Merging of all three fluors is shown in column 4 (Merge). (B) Immunostaining for E2F1-KH20 is shown in red (column 1). Neurons are labeled with anti-MAP2 antibody and are shown in green (column 2). Nuclear DNA is shown in blue (column 3). Merging of all three fluors is shown in column 4 (Merge). Colocalization between red and green appears yellow. All images were captured by sequential, triple-label immunofluorescent laser confocal microscopy using the same laser settings on the same day. These images are representative of more than 12 replicates of this experiment. Reprinted from *Experimental Neurology* (Strachan et al., 2005) with permission from the publisher.

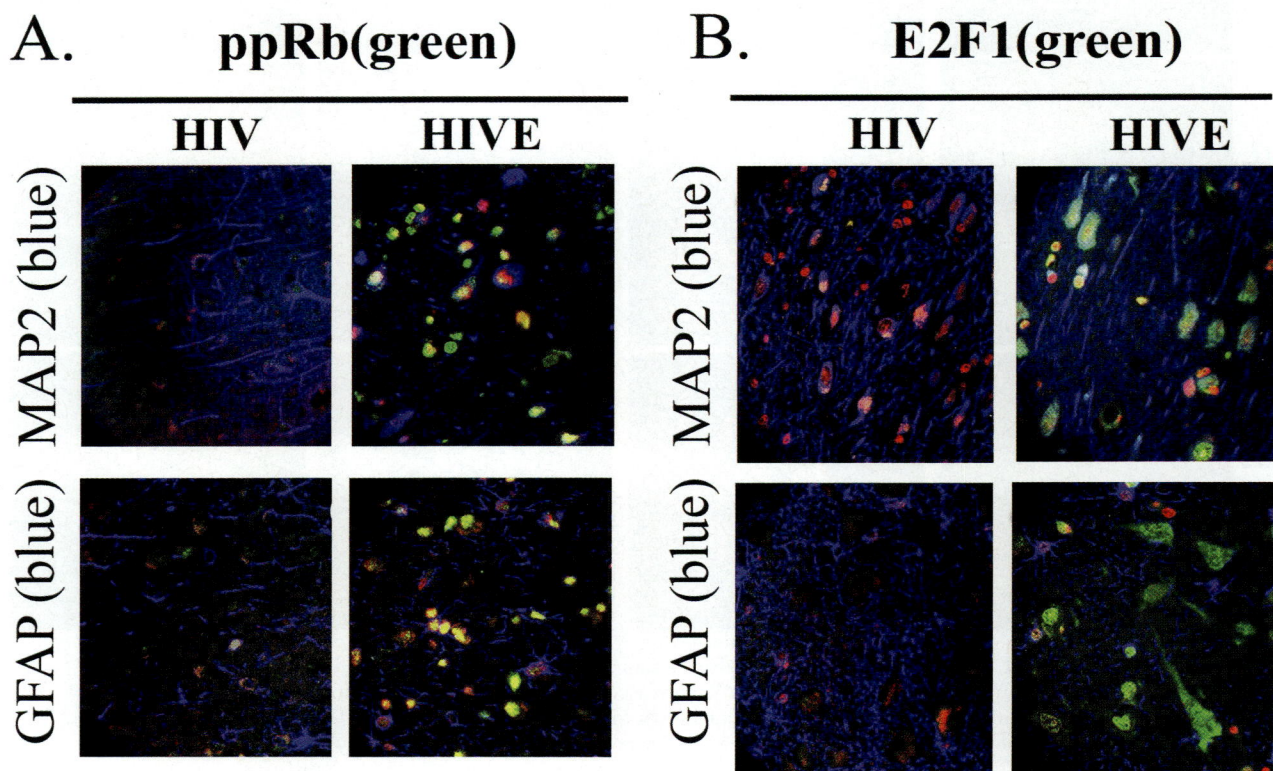

COLOR PLATE 7 (chapter 17) Immunostaining for ppRb and E2F1 in HIVE. (A) Using triple-label immunofluorescent laser confocal microscopy, immunostaining for the phosphor serine795 isoform of pRb [ppRb(green)] is nuclear (red) in hippocampal neurons stained for MAP2 (blue) as shown in patients with HIVE (top right panel). Cells from nonencephalitic, HIV-infected patients (HIV) do not exhibit abundant ppRb staining (top left panel). Similarly, glial fibrillary acidic protein (GFAP, bottom panels) staining astrocytes (blue) also exhibit increased ppRb staining (green) in nuclei (red) in HIVE, while minimal ppRb staining is seen in cells of HIV patients without encephalitis. Colocalization of red and green appears yellow. (B) Using triple-label immunofluorescent laser confocal microscopy, immunostaining for E2F1 (green) is predominantly cytoplasmic in hippocampal neurons stained for MAP2 (blue) as shown in patients with HIVE (top right panel). Cells from nonencephalitic, HIV-infected patients (HIV) do not exhibit appreciable E2F1 staining (top left panel). In a subset of neurons, E2F1 is both cytoplasmic and nuclear (red; top panels). GFAP (bottom panels) staining astrocytes (blue) do not exhibit abundant E2F1 staining (green) in the cytoplasm for HIV or HIVE patients. When staining is present, E2F1 colocalizes weakly with nuclei (red). Colocalization of red and green appears yellow, and colocalization of green and blue appears aquamarine. Reprinted from *Journal of Neuroscience* with permission from the publisher.

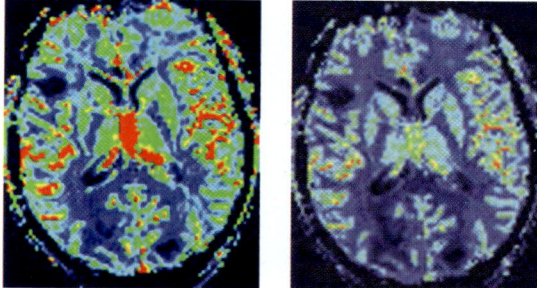

COLOR PLATE 8 (chapter 18) Cerebral toxoplasmosis in a 30-year-old female patient with AIDS. Low-signal-intensity lesions with high-signal-intensity edema located in the right and left frontal lobes are shown. On pMRI maps, both lesions have reduced CBF (left) and rCBV (right).

pMRI time course

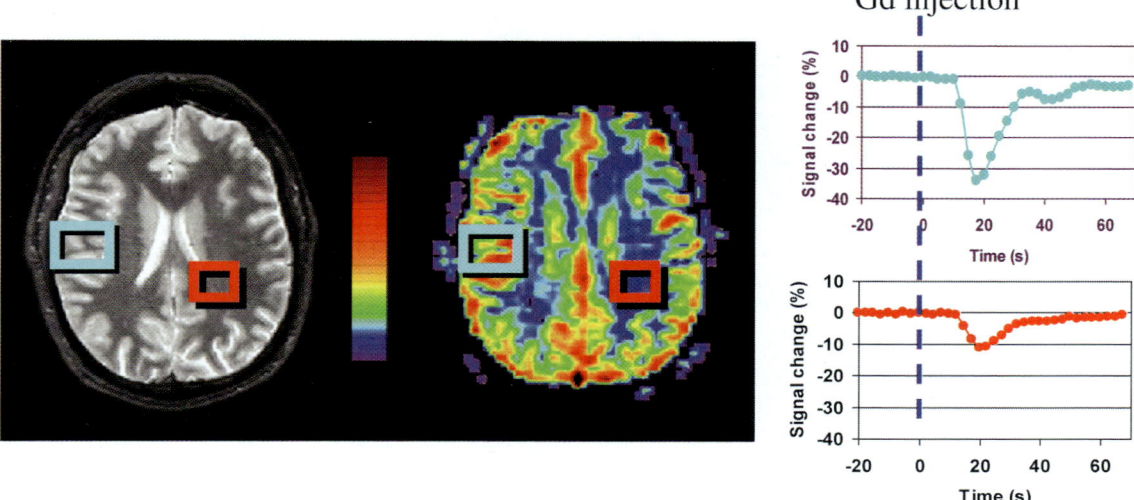

COLOR PLATE 9 (chapter 19) Example of signal-versus-time courses during a pMRI scan after bolus injection of a gadolinium-based contrast agent at time zero. The signal change in the gray-matter region (blue rectangles) is larger than that in the white-matter region (red rectangles) as a result of higher cerebral blood flow and volume in the gray matter. By analyzing the signal-versus-time course for each voxel of the pMRI scan, a map that reflects cerebral blood volume or blood flow can be calculated (right).

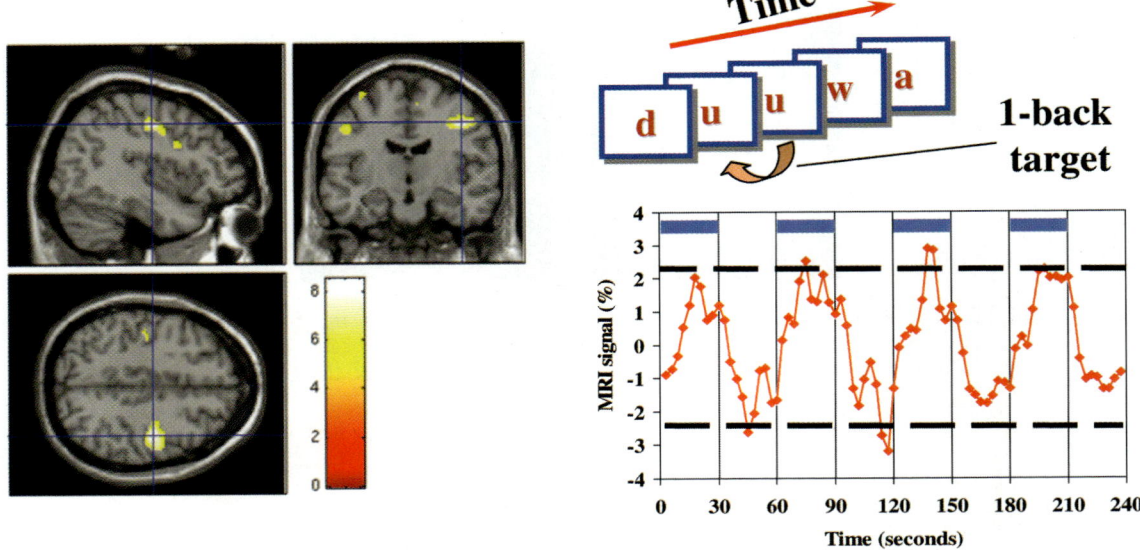

COLOR PLATE 10 (chapter 19) Example of a BOLD activation map and an fMRI time course in a healthy subject who was performing a one-back working-memory task. The subject was attending to a random sequence of alphabets on a computer display and was instructed to push a button whenever the current alphabet was the same as the previous one (one-back; activation periods). The activation periods and resting periods were alternated every 30 seconds. The BOLD signal in activated brain regions was increased during stimulus presentation (indicated by blue horizontal bars) and is represented as yellow overlays on a structural MRI. Of note, the signal change during brain activation was only a few percent, although the experiments were performed at high magnetic-field strength (4 T).

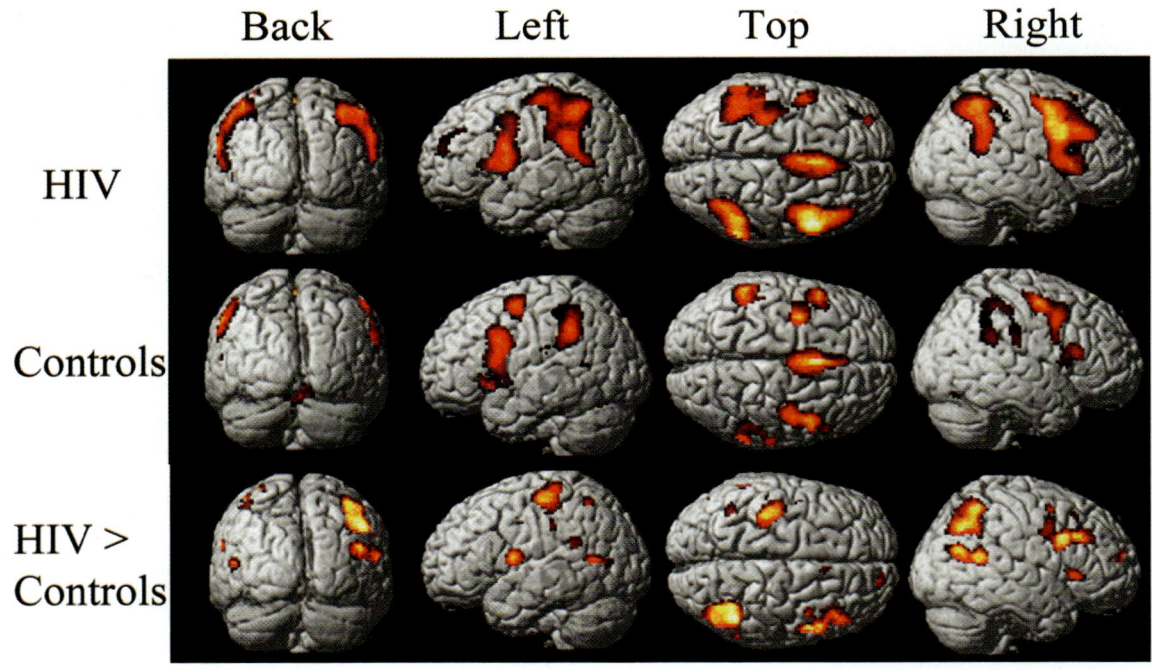

COLOR PLATE 11 (chapter 19) BOLD fMRI activation maps of healthy control subjects (middle row) and HIV patients (top row) who were performing the zero-back task. Activated brain regions are superimposed on several cortical representations. The bottom row shows brain areas that demonstrated significantly more activation in the HIV patients than in the control subjects.

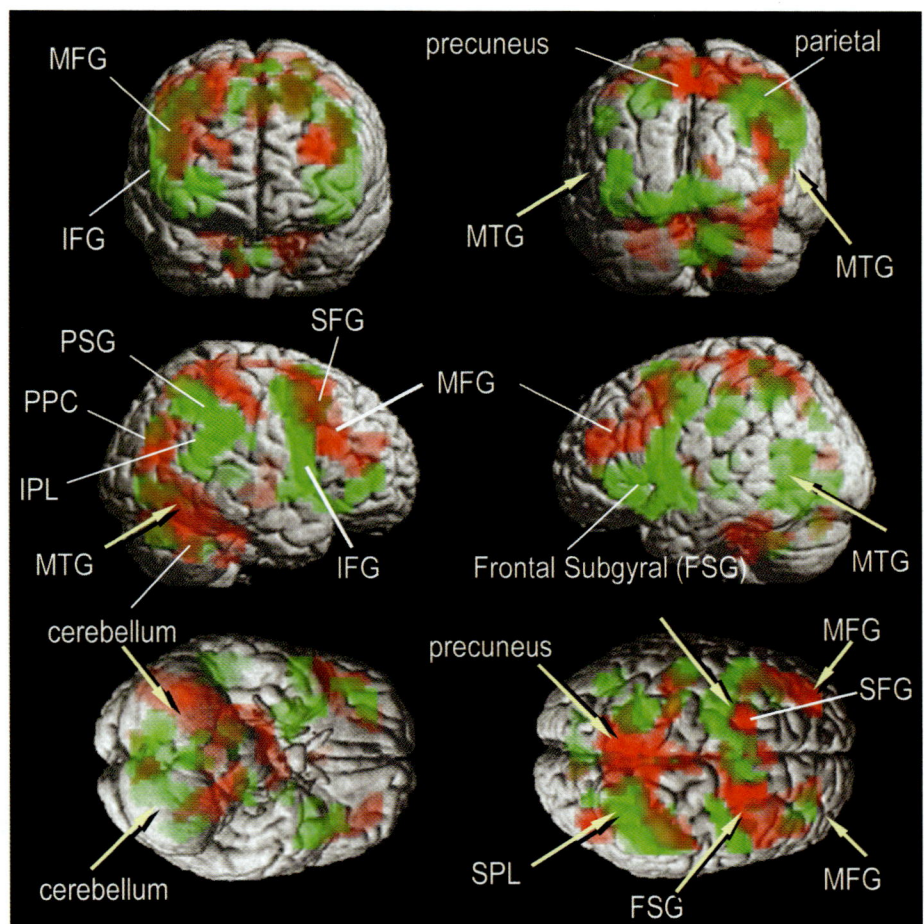

COLOR PLATE 12 (chapter 19) Neuroadaptation of the attention network in HIV patients. Surface-rendered maps show significantly reorganized brain activation pattern in HIV patients ($n = 18$) compared to seronegative (SN) control subjects ($n = 18$). The subjects were performing ball-tracking tasks that required visual attention (cluster level; P corrected > 0.05, cluster size > 100 voxels; voxel level T scores > 3.21; P uncorrected < 0.001 within the significant clusters). Note that regions where HIV was greater than SN (green) were typically adjacent or contralateral (yellow arrows) to regions where SN was greater than HIV (red). SFG, superior frontal gyrus; MFG, middle frontal gyrus; IFG, inferior frontal gyrus; PSG, parietal subgyral; FSG, frontal subgyral; SPL, superior parietal lobule; IPL, inferior parietal lobule; PPC, posterior parietal cortex; MTG, middle temporal gyrus.

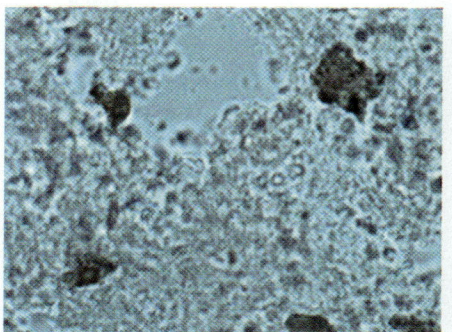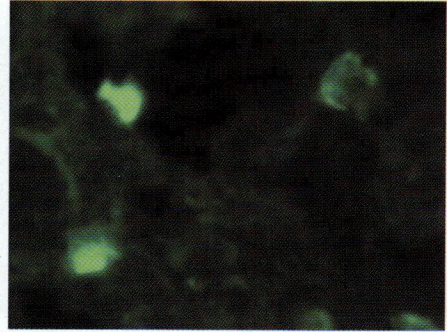

COLOR PLATE 13 (chapter 21)   Staining of cerebellum autopsy tissue with monoclonal anti-bodies against HCV NS3 and visualized with diaminobenzidine (Vectastain ABC kit, Vector Laboratories) is seen in the left panel. The same cells are positive when stained with fluorescein isothiocyanate-conjugated anti-CD68 monoclonal antibodies (right panel), implying that the cells harboring HCV belong to the macrophage/microglia lineage. This sample came from a 34-year-old HCV/HIV-coinfected IDU, who died of drug overdose (magnification, ×630).

The Spectrum of Neuro-AIDS Disorders:
Pathophysiology, Diagnosis, and Treatment
Edited by K. Goodkin et al.
©2008 ASM Press, Washington, DC

19

Functional Magnetic Resonance Imaging in HIV-Associated Dementia

THOMAS ERNST, DARDO TOMASI, AND LINDA CHANG

Neuroimaging studies can aid in the diagnosis of HIV-related brain diseases, as well as improve our understanding of the pathophysiology of HIV dementia. Because little is known about the neuroanatomical substrate underlying neuropsychological deficits in HIV brain injury, neuroimaging techniques that allow the evaluation of brain function in HIV patients are of particular interest. The ultimate goal of such "functional" neuroimaging studies is to improve the understanding of common cognitive deficits in HIV patients, such as decreased sustained attention, mental flexibility, general motor speed, and short-term and working memory (Grassi et al., 1999; Hinkin et al., 1996; Law et al., 1994; Martin et al., 1995; Miller et al., 1990; Selnes et al., 1994). Prior to the advent of noninvasive functional magnetic resonance imagery (fMRI) techniques, a variety of nuclear-medicine techniques, including positron emission tomography (PET) (Rottenberg et al., 1996) and single-photon emission computed tomography (SPECT) (Harris et al., 1994; Rosci et al., 1996), demonstrated alterations in cerebral blood flow and metabolism in the brains of HIV-infected individuals with and without cognitive deficits. Both cerebral blood flow and glucose metabolism are considered measures of brain "function," since these physiological processes are required for and associated with neuronal function. Furthermore, injured or dysfunctional brain areas typically show reduced blood flow or glucose consumption.

Over the past decade, several advanced MRI techniques have been developed that can noninvasively evaluate brain function and physiology, in particular, perfusion MRI (pMRI) and blood oxygenation level-dependent (BOLD) fMRI. pMRI can measure regional cerebral blood volume (rCBV) and blood flow (rCBF); the latter can also be measured by nuclear-medicine techniques. To date, only three studies have used pMRI to evaluate cerebral perfusion in

patients with HIV dementia (Chang et al., 2000; Tracey et al., 1998; Wenserski et al., 2003).

One of the disadvantages of past nuclear-medicine and pMRI studies is that brain "function" was evaluated at rest. In contrast, BOLD fMRI allows the direct observation of brain activation while subjects are performing cognitive tasks. This approach is analogous to performing a "stress test" for the brain. However, despite the large number of studies demonstrating cognitive deficits in HIV brain infection, there are few published studies utilizing BOLD fMRI to assess the neural substrate of cognitive abnormalities in HIV patients (Becker et al., 2005; Chang et al., 2001, 2004; Ernst et al., 2002). We will review some of the technical aspects of pMRI and BOLD fMRI, as well as the results of published studies of patients with HIV.

OVERVIEW OF PERFUSION fMRI

The most common pMRI technique uses dynamic MRI during a bolus injection of an intravascular, typically gadolinium-based MR contrast agent and is called "dynamic susceptibility contrast" (DSC) pMRI (Rosen et al., 1989). With susceptibility-weighted MRI sequences, the magnetic resonance (MR) signal in the brain changes due to the magnetic properties of the intravascular contrast agent (i.e., gadolinium) (Axel, 1980). The MR signal change in a given image element (voxel) is related to the amount (concentration) of contrast agent present. Following an intravenous bolus injection, the contrast agent travels to the brain via the heart, and the first noticeable change in the MR signal in the brain occurs approximately 10 s after injection (Color Plate 9). The maximum signal change is observed about 20 s after injection, indicating peaking of the intravascular gadolinium concentration. The signal intensity returns to baseline approximately 30 to 40 s postinjection.

For a typical DSC pMRI scan, a high-speed imaging sequence (such as echo planar imaging) is used to repeatedly scan the entire brain every few seconds immediately before and during, and for a brief period after, the bolus injection.

Thomas Ernst and Linda Chang, Department of Medicine, John A. Burns School of Medicine, University of Hawaii, Honolulu, HI 96813. **Dardo Tomasi,** Medical Department, Brookhaven National Laboratory, Upton, NY 11973.

The entire scan time is approximately 2 min. The rCBV and rCBF for each MRI voxel can be obtained from the amplitude and shape of the signal-versus-time curve. DSC pMRI is relatively robust, due to the short scan time and relatively large signal changes (typically 10% or more of the baseline signal) occurring during the first pass of the contrast agent (Color Plate 9). However, since it is difficult to determine absolute blood flow with DSC pMRI, the majority of studies report relative rCBV or rCBF. Furthermore, depending on the acquisition technique, the results may be weighted toward larger vessels (with gradient echo readouts) or capillaries (with spin echoes). Therefore, the interpretation of perfusion abnormalities on DSC MRI may present challenges.

An alternative approach to measuring cerebral perfusion with MRI is "arterial spin labeling" (ASL) (Detre et al., 1992; Williams et al., 1992). This noninvasive MRI technique can measure the absolute rCBF in one or more slices of interest. A radio frequency pulse is applied to the water molecules in arterial blood to invert the spins. After a brief delay, the inverted water spins reach the slice(s) of interest and freely diffuse through the capillary walls into the tissue in proportion to the rCBF. This causes a small decrease (~1%) in the MRI signal. An additional "control" image of the same slices is obtained without inverting the arterial blood. Tissue perfusion is related to the difference between the "control" and "inverted-spin" images. With certain assumptions, it is possible to calculate the absolute blood flow (Buxton et al., 1998; Detre et al., 1992). ASL scans obtain whole-brain rCBF values of typically 50 cm^3/100 g/min (Roberts et al., 1994), which is in general agreement with the results of nuclear-medicine studies.

pMRI STUDIES IN EARLY HIV BRAIN INJURY

Only three pMRI studies of HIV brain disease have been published; all were performed with the DSC bolus-tracking technique. In the first study, pMRI was used to evaluate the rCBV in 13 HIV-positive patients and 7 healthy control subjects (Tracey et al., 1998). The HIV patients showed increased relative rCBV in the deep gray matter and cortical gray matter. The deep-gray-matter abnormalities were more severe in patients with mild to moderate dementia (AIDS dementia complex [ADC] stage 1 or 2; $n = 9$) than in those with ADC stage 0 or 0.5. Increased rCBV in the deep gray matter was interpreted to reflect subcortical inflammatory changes and was in general agreement with prior PET findings of increased subcortical glucose metabolism during the early stages of HIV dementia (Rottenberg et al., 1987). In contrast, the increased rCBV on pMRI in the cortical gray matter was inconsistent with the findings of several previous nuclear-medicine studies that found decreased cortical perfusion in patients with HIV brain injury (Harris et al., 1994; Holman et al., 1992; Masdeu et al., 1991; Pohl et al., 1988; Rosci et al., 1996; Rottenberg et al., 1987, 1996; Schwartz et al., 1994). However, the pMRI study assessed rCBV, whereas the SPECT studies assessed cerebral blood flow. rCBF is related to regional neuronal activity (Raichle, 1987), while the relationship between rCBV and neuronal activity is less clear.

In a second pMRI study (Chang et al., 2000), the rCBF of 19 patients with early stages of HIV cognitive motor complex and 15 control subjects were compared. All but one HIV-positive subjects were treated with antiretroviral medications. In the HIV patients, rCBF was decreased bilaterally in the inferior lateral frontal cortices and in an inferior medial parietal region but increased bilaterally in the posterior inferior parietal white matter. rCBF abnormalities were associated with the CD4 count, plasma viral load, Karnofsky score, and HIV dementia scale; generally, more severe HIV brain disease was associated with reductions in the rCBF. The finding of decreased rCBF in the frontal cortex was consistent with previous findings from PET and SPECT studies, which also showed frontal hypoperfusion. It was speculated that increased perfusion in the parietal white matter might be related to reactive inflammatory processes or glial proliferation, which may be associated with higher blood flow.

The most recent study evaluated rCBF in three groups of HIV-positive subjects. Ten of the subjects had normal motor function, 8 had first-time psychomotor slowing, and 14 showed sustained psychomotor slowing (Wenserski et al., 2003). The rCBF in the basal ganglia was determined with DSC MRI and was expressed relative to that of normal-appearing occipital white matter. There was an overall difference in the basal ganglion rCBF among the three groups. Specifically, patients with first-time psychomotor slowing had significantly increased rCBF compared to those with sustained abnormalities. This finding is consistent with that of Tracey et al. (1998) and may reflect subcortical inflammatory changes.

In conclusion, MR studies showed resting perfusion abnormalities in patients with HIV infection. Two studies found increased relative perfusion in the deep gray matter of HIV patients during early stages of the disease, while another study demonstrated perfusion abnormalities in cortical regions (rCBF decreases) and also white matter (rCBF increases). pMRI may provide a good surrogate marker to assess the function of the resting brain in HIV patients. However, longitudinal studies will be required to validate the utility of pMRI in evaluating the HIV-infected brain. Furthermore, ASL techniques may help interpret changes in relative perfusion on DSC MRI studies, due to their ability to measure absolute rCBF.

OVERVIEW OF BOLD fMRI

BOLD Effect

fMRI allows the mapping of activated brain regions in the working brain (Bandettini et al., 1992; Frahm et al., 1993; Kim et al., 1993; Kwong et al., 1992; Ogawa et al., 1993; Turner et al., 1993). fMRI detects small MR signal changes associated with local increases in blood oxygenation in activated brain regions; this phenomenon is referred to as the BOLD effect (Ogawa et al., 1990).

The chain of events underlying BOLD fMRI is summarized in Fig. 1. Neural information processing via action potentials and neurotransmitters requires energy. Arterial blood supplies the oxygen (in the form of oxyhemoglobin) and glucose necessary for cerebral energy metabolism. Activation of brain regions causes a regional increase in glycolysis and blood flow (of oxygenated blood), which exceeds the local increase in oxygen consumption, leading to a net increase in the regional oxyhemoglobin concentration. Because oxyhemoglobin is less paramagnetic than deoxyhemoglobin, an increased oxyhemoglobin concentration in activated brain regions reduces microscopic distortions of the magnetic field. MRI sequences that are sensitive to microscopic-field homogeneity ("susceptibility" or "T2*" weighted) are able to detect these changes. For example, Color Plate 10 shows that the MRI signal increased in several brain regions of a control subject who was performing

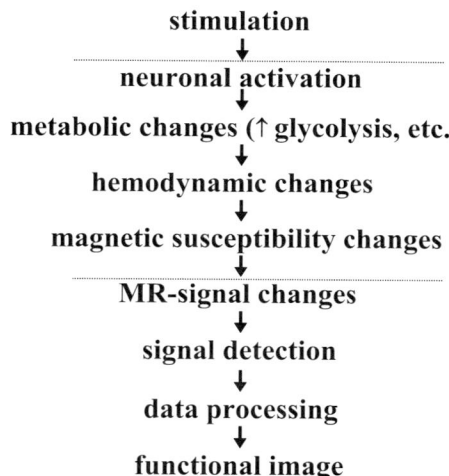

stimulation
↓
neuronal activation
↓
metabolic changes (↑ glycolysis, etc.)
↓
hemodynamic changes
↓
magnetic susceptibility changes
↓
MR-signal changes
↓
signal detection
↓
data processing
↓
functional image

FIGURE 1 Chain of events that link neuronal activation with BOLD signal changes on fMRI. Neuronal stimulation increases neuronal firing, which in turn leads to increased metabolism (glycolysis and oxygen consumption). These cellular events cause hemodynamic changes (increased transport of oxygenated blood to the activated regions), which alter the magnetic properties of the brain regions involved. The altered magnetic properties of the activated brain can be detected with susceptibility-weighted MR pulse sequences and analyzed to generate brain activation maps.

a working-memory task (activation periods) and returned to baseline during rest periods. Of note, the signal changes were on the order of a few percent, even on a high-field 4-T MRI scanner.

It is important to emphasize that the BOLD effect is not a direct measure of neural activity. Neural activity produces regional changes in cerebral blood flow, the cerebral metabolic rate of glucose consumption, the cerebral metabolic rate of oxygen consumption, and the cerebral blood volume. The BOLD signal is not a simple reflection of any one of these physiological parameters because it depends on changes in the balance between the rCBF and the cerebral metabolic rate of oxygen consumption.

Data Acquisition

Acquisition of MRI data for brain activation studies can be challenging. Because the BOLD signal change during brain activation is very small (typically a few percent) (Color Plate 10), even small amounts of subject motion may cause signal changes similar to those observed during brain activation. These motion-related signal changes may prevent the detection of BOLD signals. Conversely, task-related movements may erroneously increase fMRI signals and cause false brain activation.

While motion correction algorithms can remove some of the artifacts due to subject motion, even the best existing algorithms are unable to correct for movements much greater than 1 mm of translation or 1° of rotation. Online monitoring of motion makes it possible to repeat scans with excessive motion immediately (Caparelli et al., 2003). Even in the absence of subject motion, however, cardiac and respiratory pulsation effects cause signal fluctuations in fMRI time series, which limit the scan-to-scan reproducibility to approximately 1%. To minimize the influence of motion on fMRI scans, it is highly desirable to achieve the highest

acquisition rates. Therefore, ultrafast MRI techniques, such as echo planar imaging (Mansfield et al., 1977) or spiral scans (Glover and Lai, 1998), are used most commonly to acquire fMRI scans. These techniques can scan multiple slices covering the entire brain within a few seconds.

One of the most important variables to consider for fMRI acquisition is the echo time (TE), which characterizes the amount of "susceptibility weighting." Larger TE values increase the functional (BOLD) signal but simultaneously reduce the overall MR signal in the images. It can be shown that the contrast-to-noise ratio of fMRI data peaks when the TE equals the intrinsic T2*. Therefore, fMRI data are typically acquired at a TE of 50 ms at 1.5 T but at a TE of ~20 to 30 ms on higher-magnetic-field scanners (3 or 4 T). BOLD signals also increase with the magnetic-field strength, because higher field strengths magnify BOLD-related susceptibility effects. As a result, the BOLD signal is two to three times larger at 4 T than at 1.5 T (Gati et al., 1997; Kennan et al., 1994; Ogawa et al., 1993; Turner et al., 1993; Weisskoff et al., 1994).

Stimulus Presentation and Study Design

Most sensory systems can be evaluated with fMRI. Sensory stimuli, including visual (Iidaka et al., 2002; Katanoda et al., 2001; Peterson et al., 2002), olfactory (Sobel et al., 1997), tactile (Harrington et al., 2000), auditory (Hall et al., 2000; Newman et al., 2001), and even electrical stimulation, can lead to detectable brain activation. The most frequently used activation paradigms in human studies involve visual stimuli, which are presented to subjects via goggles or LCD projectors that are connected to computers outside the scanner room. To obtain reliable fMRI data, it is advisable to measure and ensure acceptable subject performance during the fMRI scans.

Many fMRI studies utilize a "block design," in which "task" and "rest" epochs are alternated repeatedly for defined durations (typically ≥30 s). Block designs provide robust activation and are relatively easy to analyze. However, due to the repetitive nature of block designs, subjects may fatigue and show training effects (Tomasi et al., 2004). These disadvantages of block designs may be avoided by the use of single-event designs, in which stimuli of short duration (typically only a few seconds) are presented in a pseudorandomized fashion. Compared to block designs, single-event experiments are more challenging in terms of data analysis, due to the more complicated nature of the stimulus presentation and the smaller signal changes resulting from the use of brief stimuli.

Data Analysis

The analysis of fMRI data sets is complex and has been reviewed extensively (Frackowiak et al., 1997; Friston et al., 1995a; Turner et al., 1998). The two most commonly used packages for fMRI analysis are SPM (Friston et al., 1995b) and AFNI (Cox, 1996). fMRI analyses typically involve the following major steps: (i) realignment of fMRI time series data to remove movement-related variance present in the data; (ii) spatial normalization to transform the image set into a standard stereotactic space, commonly that of Talairach and Tournoux (Talairach et al., 1988) (the use of a stereotactic space makes it possible to compare activation patterns across subjects); (iii) spatial smoothing to increase the signal-to-noise ratio and to eliminate interindividual structural differences in the stereotactic space; and (iv) statistical analysis and inference for modeling data and to extract statistical parameters from the measured BOLD responses (Frackowiak et al., 1997).

fMRI STUDIES IN HIV BRAIN DISEASE

fMRI Findings in Patients with Early HIV Dementia

Only a few BOLD-fMRI studies of HIV patients have been published (Becker et al., 2005; Chang et al., 2001, 2004; Ernst et al., 2002, 2003; Tomasi et al., 2005). The first study involved 11 HIV patients (average ADC stage, 0.5) and 11 age-, gender-, education-, and handedness-matched seronegative subjects (Chang et al., 2001). The subjects performed several working-memory tasks (zero-back, one-back, and two-back) that required different levels of attention and two tasks that additionally involved arithmetic skills (one-increment and two-increment tasks).

All of the tasks activated the lateral prefrontal cortex, the posterior parietal cortex, the supplementary motor area, and less consistently the caudate bilaterally (Color Plate 11). In seronegative subjects, brain activation increased with the more difficult tasks (e.g., from zero-back to one-back to two-back) on BOLD activation maps, as well as on the total activated brain volume (Fig. 2). This relationship between brain activation and task difficulty, or attentional load, probably reflects attentional modulation of neural circuits (Chang et al., 2001). It is well known that attention influences information processing in the brain by altering the firing rate of neurons that are sensitive to a specific attribute. For example, modulatory effects of attention

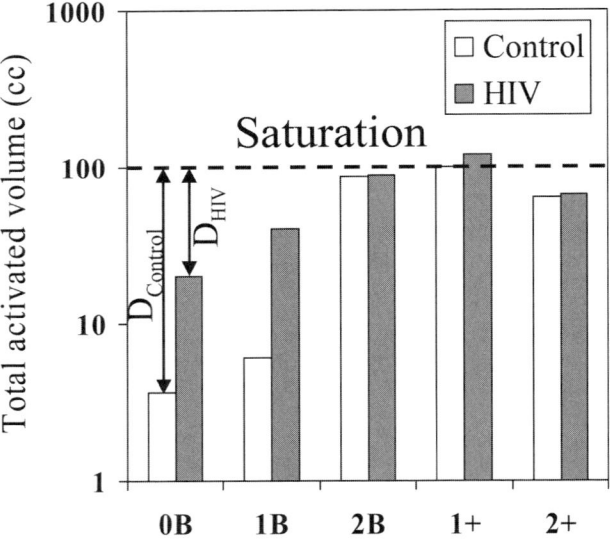

FIGURE 2 Activated brain volume on fMRI in HIV patients and control subjects who performed several cognitive tasks. The control subjects showed increasing activated brain volume with task difficulty for simpler tasks (e.g., from zero-back [0B] and one-back [1B]) but saturation of activated volume with more complex tasks (two-back [2B] and one- and two-increment [1+ and 2+]). The HIV patients showed marked increases in activated brain volume for the simpler tasks (0B and 1B) but a saturation volume on the more difficult tasks similar to that of the control subjects. As a result, the "dynamic range" (D) in activated brain volume (the ratio of largest to smallest activated volume) was markedly reduced in HIV patients (D_{HIV} = 5) compared to control subjects ($D_{Control}$ = 20). This reduced dynamic range in HIV may be interpreted as reduced "brain reserve" as a result of injury to the neural substrate due the HIV infection.

on neural activity have been demonstrated by single-cell recordings (Moran and Desimone, 1985), by event-related potentials (Mangun et al., 1993), by PET (Kawashima et al., 1995), and by fMRI (Courtney et al., 1997; Speck et al., 2000).

Compared to control subjects, the HIV patients showed increased regional activation (Fig. 2), as well as marked increases (over fivefold) in total activated volume, for the simpler tasks (zero-back and one-back), but not for the more difficult tasks (two-back and two-increment) (Fig. 2). These results suggest that HIV patients require greater activation of neural circuits, i.e., increased attentional modulation, to perform the simpler tasks to compensate for reduced efficiency of neural processing associated with the brain injury. In contrast, the activated volumes in HIV patients and control subjects reached a common saturation value for the other, more difficult tasks (Fig. 2). This suggests that on the more difficult tasks, all available network resources had been exhausted, and performance suffered. Thus, increased brain activation (usage of brain reserve) in the HIV patients is probably the direct neural correlate of the attentional problems that are common in HIV patients.

In a subsequent study, the relationship between BOLD signal strength and neurochemistry on proton MR spectroscopy was evaluated in 14 HIV-positive subjects (Ernst et al., 2003). All subjects had ADC stage 1 or lower. Higher BOLD signals in the posterior parietal and lateral prefrontal regions were associated with increased glial proton MR spectroscopy markers (choline-containing compounds, total creatine, and myoinositol) in the frontal white matter and basal ganglia. Conversely, no relationship was found between brain activation and the concentration of N-acetyl compounds, which reflect neuronal viability; this indicates that neuronal abnormalities may play a secondary role in impaired cognitive processing in early HIV brain injury (ADC ≤ 1). Altogether, the findings suggest that compensatory increases in attention and BOLD signals in the HIV-infected brain may be related to impaired neural processing due to inflammatory glial abnormalities.

fMRI Findings in HIV Patients without Cognitive Deficits

If the hypothesis that increased usage of the brain reserve network is related to HIV-associated brain injury is correct, then HIV patients who are asymptomatic might already be demonstrating increased brain activation to maintain normal function. Therefore, a second fMRI study was performed in 10 neurocognitively asymptomatic HIV patients to determine if fMRI could detect presymptomatic abnormalities on brain activation (Ernst et al., 2002). An extensive battery of neuropsychological tests was performed to ensure normal cognitive functioning in these patients compared to control subjects. Like the HIV patients with mild dementia, asymptomatic HIV patients showed greater BOLD signal changes and activated volumes, although only in the lateral prefrontal cortex.

These results suggest that mild brain injury is present even in HIV patients with normal cognitive function. However, the patients appear to be able to utilize their neural reserve networks to compensate for the impairments in neural processing. The limitation of these abnormalities primarily to the frontal lobe (the lateral prefrontal cortex) may be due to the fact that the frontostriatal system is often most severely affected in patients with HIV dementia (Barker et al., 1995; Kure et al., 1990; Power et al., 1993; Rottenberg et al., 1987). In particular, the dopaminergic system, which has a major role in regulating working-memory function in the prefrontal cortices (Goldman-Rakic, 1996), has been shown to be affected in patients with HIV dementia (Berger et al., 1994; Lopez et al., 1999; Wang et al., 2004).

The Effect of Increased Attentional Load on Brain Activation in HIV Patients

One recent fMRI study at 4 T used a "parametric" design to quantify the effect of varying attentional loads during a visual-attention task on brain activation in HIV patients (Chang et al., 2004). Eighteen HIV-positive and 18 control subjects were scanned while mentally tracking 2, 3, or 4 out of 10 randomly moving balls. Most of the HIV subjects had ADC stage 0.5 or 1 but were able to perform within the normal limits on the ball-tracking tasks. The tasks activated a visual-attention network that includes the dorsal parietal, bilateral prefrontal, and cerebellar regions (Jovicich et al., 2001). Compared to the control subjects, seropositive subjects showed greater activation in the right prefrontal and right parietal cortices (Color Plate 12); these are regions where the control subjects demonstrated clear increases in activation with cognitive load (i.e., the number of balls tracked). Conversely, seropositive subjects showed less activation in regions where the BOLD signal was minimally affected or even reduced with increasing load in the control subjects (Color Plate 12). These findings suggest a reorganization of the visual-attention network, in that HIV subjects appear to require increased usage of brain regions with "neural reserve capacity" to compensate for reduced efficiency in the normal attention network as a result of HIV brain injury.

The Effect of Acoustic Noise on Brain Activation in HIV-Positive Subjects

Since prior studies consistently demonstrated that HIV-infected subjects had attentional difficulties and required increased usage of neural reserve to perform tasks with higher attentional loads (Chang et al., 2004), HIV-infected subjects might have been more sensitive to interfering or distracting stimuli than HIV-negative subjects. Therefore, one study evaluated the effect of increased acoustic noise on BOLD signals while subjects performed a series of n-back working-memory tasks (Tomasi et al., 2005). Ten HIV-positive subjects (ADC stage 1) and 15 HIV-negative control subjects were scanned at 4 T. Acoustic noise was varied by 12 dB (i.e., fourfold) during the fMRI scan. HIV patients showed acoustic-noise-related increases in BOLD signals in the right cerebellum and in the left occipital and frontal cortices. In control subjects, however, louder acoustic noise increased BOLD signals in the left cerebellum and right occipital and prefrontal cortices. These findings were interpreted as interference of acoustic noise with normal attentional processing, leading to compensatory increases in brain activation. During acoustic interference, HIV-positive subjects appear to require usage of neural reserve (regions adjacent and contralateral to those activated in the control subjects) as an additional compensatory response.

fMRI in the Aging HIV-Infected Brain

Since the introduction of highly active antiretroviral therapy, HIV-infected persons are living significantly longer. Because aging, as well as HIV infection, may cause a cognitive decline, recent studies are focusing on the possible interaction between aging and HIV infection. One study used fMRI to study 27 patients with AIDS and 14 sero-

negative control subjects (Becker et al., 2005) in order to evaluate the effects of aging. Subjects performed a series of n-back working memory tasks ($n = 0$, 1, and 2) while being scanned in a 1.5-T scanner. Age was treated as a continuous variable. The zero-back task was used as the baseline condition; activation during the one-back and two-back tasks was contrasted with that during the zero-back task. Aging and HIV infection independently increased brain activation (two-back versus zero-back) in several areas of the frontal lobe. Furthermore, a statistically significant interaction was found between age and HIV status in the caudate nucleus, in that older HIV-positive subjects showed larger BOLD signals than the additive effects of serostatus or age alone. It was suggested that this finding indicates a synergistic effect of aging and HIV infection on brain function.

Current Limitations of fMRI Studies in HIV Brain Disease

As discussed above, few research studies have used fMRI to study neuropsychiatric diseases, including HIV dementia. To some degree, this scarcity of clinical fMRI studies may be due to the technical challenges associated with performing fMRI in patient populations. However, there are also several study design issues that render such studies difficult. First, various fMRI studies have demonstrated that the pattern and extent of brain activation with commonly used paradigms, including working-memory tasks, may depend on many variables, such as age, education, handedness, gender, and language skills (Peres et al., 2000; Ross et al., 1997; Speck et al., 2000). Additionally, activation on BOLD fMRI can be influenced by short-term practice effects (Tomasi et al., 2004), as well as the acoustic-noise level during the fMRI acquisition (Tomasi et al., 2005). Therefore, subject populations in clinical fMRI studies have to be matched carefully to control subjects for these potential confounding factors. However, clinical fMRI studies may show substantial intersubject variability in activation strength even if subjects are matched for all these variables. In contrast, the intrasubject reproducibility in consecutive trials is much better. Hence, longitudinal studies using fMRI may be useful for monitoring brain changes associated with changes in cognitive function.

Clinical fMRI studies may also be confounded by vascular and hemodynamic differences among groups. As outlined above, the exact size of the BOLD signal depends on an intricate balance between changes in cerebral blood flow, blood volume, and oxygen consumption during brain activation. Therefore, the alterations in cerebral resting perfusion in HIV patients described above (Chang et al., 2000; Harris et al., 1994; Tracey et al., 1998) might cause abnormal BOLD signals. It is difficult to assess the contributions of these vascular abnormalities to the findings with fMRI, however, since the effect of altered cerebral perfusion on BOLD signals is poorly understood.

Medication effects represent yet another potential confounding factor for fMRI studies in HIV patients, but no study has systematically evaluated the possible effect of antiretroviral medications or other potentially neuroactive medications that are often prescribed for HIV patients. In schizophrenic patients (Honey et al., 1999), as well as in patients with Parkinson's disease (Mattay et al., 2002), the BOLD signal is affected by medications that are used to treat these conditions (e.g., dopaminergic agents or dopamine-blocking agents). Unlike these medications, which specifically modulate the dopaminergic system and therefore may affect the microvasculature, antiretroviral medications would be less likely to affect cerebral perfusion. However, future fMRI studies should assess both perfusion and BOLD signal changes in the same HIV patients before and during antiretroviral treatment in order to evaluate the relationship between perfusion abnormalities and BOLD signal changes and to exclude the possibility that these medications might affect cerebral perfusion or the BOLD signal.

CONCLUSIONS AND FUTURE DIRECTIONS

Few functional or pMRI studies in patients with HIV brain injury have been published. The major findings from pMRI include frontal hypoperfusion, as well as subcortical gray-matter and parietal white-matter hyperperfusion. These regional perfusion abnormalities may reflect neuronal dysfunction or inflammatory changes. Hence, pMRI provides a macroscopic view of brain pathophysiology (i.e., cerebral perfusion) that is associated with the underlying neuropathology. On BOLD fMRI, HIV patients with mild dementia, and to a lesser degree those who are asymptomatic, require increased prefrontal brain activation while performing attention-requiring working-memory tasks, Increased activation on BOLD fMRI probably reflects the increased attention required by the patients to perform the working-memory tasks; this can be interpreted as increased usage of the brain reserve capacity to maintain normal performance. BOLD fMRI studies that assessed brain function with increasing cognitive loads under higher magnetic field strengths indeed confirmed such a neuroadaptive process, in that brain regions with reserve capacity are used extensively while the normal attention network is compromised in HIV patients with minor cognitive motor disorder.

The application of fMRI to study the neural correlate of cognitive deficits in HIV is still in its infancy. Future studies may utilize improved fMRI methods, such as single-trial paradigms, to minimize fatigue and practice effects and more complex paradigms, for instance, to separate activation due to attention from that due to working memory. Future studies also need to address the relationships between abnormal BOLD activation and clinical variables, such as immune markers, and/or neuroimaging markers of brain injury, such as metabolite concentrations on MR spectroscopy. Furthermore, fMRI has been applied to only a limited number of cognitive domains that might be affected by HIV brain disease (i.e., working memory in conjunction with attention). Since fMRI is exquisitely sensitive for detecting functional changes, it may be particularly useful for evaluating other early cognitive impairments that are common in HIV patients, such as sustained attention, mental flexibility, general motor speed, and short-term memory. For example, fMRI paradigms of the Stroop task or mental rotation (to evaluate mental flexibility), patterned finger tapping (fine-motor skills), and paced finger tapping (motor speed), all have been described in the literature, and many other neuropsychological tasks could be modified into fMRI paradigms. Finally, due to the highly reproducible intrasubject patterns of brain activation, fMRI holds great promise, not only for evaluating the extent of brain injury, but also for longitudinal clinical trials to monitor treatment effects in HIV-associated brain injury.

This work was supported by grants from NIDA (K24 DA16170 [L.C.] and K02 DA16991 [T.E.]) and NINDS (R01-NS38834).

REFERENCES

Axel, L. 1980. Cerebral blood flow determination by rapid-sequence computed tomography. *Radiology* **137**:679–686.

Bandettini, P. A., E. C. Wong, R. S. Hinks, R. S. Tikofky, and J. S. Hyde. 1992. Time course EPI of human brain function during task activation. *Magn. Reson. Med.* **25**:390–397.

Barker, P. B., R. R. Lee, and J. C. McArthur. 1995. AIDS dementia complex: evaluation with proton MR spectroscopic imaging. *Radiology* **195**:58–64.

Becker, J. T., S. Juengst, H. J. Aizenstein, J. Cochran, and O. L. Lopez. 2005. fMRI evidence of synergistic effects of AIDS and age on brain function. **64**:A245.

Berger, J. R., M. Kumar, A. Kumar, J. Fernandez, and B. Levin. 1994. Cerebrospinal fluid dopamine in HIV-1 infection. *AIDS* **8**:67–71.

Buxton, R., L. Frank, E. Wong, B. Siewert, S. Warach, and R. Edelman. 1998. A general kinetic model for quantitative perfusion imaging with arterial spin labeling. *Magn. Reson. Med.* **40**:383–396.

Caparelli, E. C., D. Tomasi, S. Arnold, L. Chang, and T. Ernst. 2003. k-Space based summary motion detection for functional magnetic resonance imaging. *Neuroimage* **20**:1411–1418.

Chang, L., T. Ernst, M. Leonido-Yee, and O. Speck. 2000. Perfusion MRI detects rCBF abnormalities in early stages of HIV-cognitive motor complex. *Neurology* **54**:389–396.

Chang, L., O. Speck, E. Miller, A. Braun, J. Jovicich, C. Koch, L. Itti, and T. Ernst. 2001. Neural correlates of attention and working memory deficits in HIV patients. *Neurology* **57**:1001–1007.

Chang, L., D. Tomasi, R. Yakupov, C. Lozar, S. Arnold, E. Caparelli, and T. Ernst. 2004. Adaptation of the attention network in human immunodeficiency virus brain injury. *Ann. Neurol.* **56**:259–272.

Courtney, S. M., L. G. Ungerleider, K. Keil, and J. V. Haxby. 1997. Transient and sustained activity in a distributed neural system for human working memory. *Nature* **386**:608–611.

Cox, R. W. 1996. AFNI: software for analysis and visualization of functional magnetic resonance neuroimages. *Comp. Biomed. Res.* **29**:162–173.

Detre, J. A., J. S. Leigh, D. S. Williams, and A. P. Koretsky. 1992. Perfusion imaging. *Magn. Reson. Med.* **23**:37–45.

Ernst, T., L. Chang, and S. Arnold. 2003. Increased glial markers predict increased working memory network activation in HIV patients. *Neuroimage* **19**:1686–1693.

Ernst, T., L. Chang, J. Jovicich, N. Ames, and S. Arnold. 2002. Abnormal brain activation on functional MRI in cognitively asymptomatic HIV patients. *Neurology* **59**:1343–1349.

Frackowiak, R. S. J., K. J. Friston, C. D. Frith, R. J. Dolan, and J. C. Mazziotta. 1997. *Human Brain Function*. Academic Press, San Diego, CA.

Frahm, J., K. D. Merboldt, and W. Hanicke. 1993. Functional MRI of human brain activation at high spatial resolution. *Magn. Reson. Med.* **29**:139–144.

Friston, K. J., J. Ashburner, J. B. Poline, C. D. Frith, and R. S. J. Frackowiak. 1995a. Spatial realignment and normalization of images. *Hum. Brain Mapp.* **2**:165–189.

Friston, K. J., A. P. Holmes, K. J. Worsley, J. B. Poline, C. D. Frith, and R. S. J. Franckowiak. 1995b. Statistical parametric maps in functional imaging: a general approach. *Hum. Brain Mapp.* **2**:189–210.

Gati, J. S., R. S. Menon, K. Ugurbil, and B. K. Rutt. 1997. Experimental determination of the BOLD field strength dependence in vessels and tissue. *Magn. Reson. Med.* **38**:296–302.

Glover, G. H., and S. Lai. 1998. Self-navigated spiral fMRI: interleaved versus single-shot. *Magn. Reson. Med.* **39**:361–368.

Goldman-Rakic, P. 1996. Regional and cellular fractionation of working memory. *Proc. Natl. Acad. Sci. USA* **93**:13473–13480.

Grassi, B., G. Graghentini, A. Campana, E. Grassi, S. Bertelli, P. Cinque, M. Epifani, A. Lazzarin, and S. Scarone.

1999. Spatial working memory in asymptomatic HIV-infected subjects. *J. Neuropsychiatry Clin. Neurosci.* **11**:387–391.

Hall, D. A., M. P. Haggard, M. A. Akeroyd, A. Q. Summerfield, A. R. Palmer, M. R. Elliott, and R. Bowtell. 2000. Modulation and task effects in auditory processing measured using fMRI. *Hum. Brain Mapp.* **10**:107–119.

Harrington, G. S., C. T. Wright, and J. Downs III. 2000. A new vibrotactile stimulator for functional MRI. *Hum. Brain Mapp.* **10**:140–145.

Harris, G. J., G. D. Pearlson, J. C. McArthur, S. Zeger, and N. D. LaFrance. 1994. Altered cortical blood flow in HIV-seropositive individuals with and without dementia: a single photon emission computed tomography study. *AIDS* **8**:495–499.

Hinkin, C. H., W. G. van Gorp, P. Satz, T. Marcotte, R. S. Durvasula, S. Wood, L. Campbell, and M. R. Baluda. 1996. Actual versus self-reported cognitive dysfunction in HIV-1 infection: memory-metamemory dissociations. *J. Clin. Exp. Neuropsychol.* **18**:431–443.

Holman, B. L., B. Garada, K. A. Johnson, J. Mendelson, E. Hallgring, S. K. Teoh, J. Worth, and B. Navia. 1992. A comparison of brain perfusion SPECT in cocaine abuse and AIDS dementia complex. *J. Nucl. Med.* **33**:1312–1315.

Honey, G., E. Bullmore, W. Soni, M. Varatheesan, S. Williams, and T. Sharma. 1999. Differences in frontal cortical activation by a working memory task after substitution of risperidone for typical antipsychotic drugs in patients with schizophrenia. *Proc. Natl. Acad. Sci. USA* **96**:13432–13437.

Iidaka, T., T. Okada, T. Murata, M. Omori, H. Kosaka, N. Sadato, and Y. Yonekura. 2002. Age-related differences in the medial temporal lobe responses to emotional faces as revealed by fMRI. *Hippocampus* **12**:352–362.

Jovicich, J., R. J. Peters, C. Koch, J. Braun, L. Chang, and T. Ernst. 2001. Brain areas specific for attentional load in a motion tracking task. *J. Cogn. Neurosci.* **13**:1048–1058.

Katanoda, K., K. Yoshikawa, and M. Sugishita. 2001. A functional MRI study on the neural substrates for writing. *Hum. Brain Mapp.* **13**:34–42.

Kawashima, R., B. T. O'Sullivan, and P. E. Roland. 1995. Positron-emission tomography studies of cross-modality inhibition in selective attentional tasks: closing the "mind's eye". *Proc. Natl. Acad. Sci. USA* **92**:5969–5972.

Kennan, R. P., J. Zhong, and J. C. Gore. 1994. Intravascular susceptibility contrast mechanisms in tissues. *Magn. Reson. Med.* **31**:9–21.

Kim, S. G., J. Ashe, K. Hendrich, J. M. Ellermann, H. Merkle, K. Ugurbil, and A. P. Georgopoulos. 1993. Functional magnetic resonance imaging of motor cortex: hemispheric asymmetry and handedness. *Science* **261**:615–617.

Kure, K., K. M. Weidenheim, W. D. Lyman, and D. W. Dickson. 1990. Morphology and distribution of HIV-1 gp41-positive microglia in subacute AIDS encephalitis. *Acta Neuropathol. (Berlin)* **80**:393–400.

Kwong, K. K., J. W. Belliveau, D. A. Chesler, I. E. Goldberg, R. M. Weisskoff, B. P. Poncelet, D. N. Kennedy, B. E. Hoppel, M. S. Cohen, R. Turner, H. M. Cheng, T. J. Brady, and B. R. Rosen. 1992. Dynamic magnetic resonance imaging of human brain activity during primary sensory stimulation. *Proc. Natl. Acad. Sci. USA* **89**:5675–5679.

Law, W. A., A. Martin, R. L. Mapou, T. L. Roller, A. M. Salazar, L. R. Temoshok, and J. R. Rundell. 1994. Working memory in individuals with HIV infection. *J. Clin. Exp. Neuropsychol.* **16**:173–182.

Lopez, O., G. Smith, C. Meltzer, and J. Becker. 1999. Dopamine systems in human immunodeficiency virus-associated dementia. *Neuropsychiatry Neuropsychol. Behav. Neurol.* **12**:184–192.

Mangun, G. R., S. A. Hillyard, and S. J. Luck. 1993. Electrocortical substrates of visual selective attention, p. 219–243.

In D. E. Meyer, and S. Kornblum (ed.), *Attention and Performance XIV*. MIT Press, Cambridge, MA.

Mansfield, P., and A. A. Maudsley. 1977. Planar spin imaging by NMR. *J. Magn. Reson.* **27**:101–119.

Martin, E., D. Pitrak, K. Pursell, K. Mullane, and R. Novak. 1995. Delayed recognition memory span in HIV-1 infection. *J. Int. Neuropsychol. Soc.* **1**:575–580.

Masdeu, J. C., A. Yudd, R. L. Van Heertun, M. Grundman, E. Hriso, R. A. O'Connell, D. Luck, U. Camli, and L. N. King. 1991. Single photon emission computed tomography in human immunodeficiency virus encephalopathy: a preliminary report. *J. Nucl. Med.* **32**:1471–1475.

Mattay, V., A. Tessitore, J. Callicott, A. Bertolino, T. Goldberg, T. Chase, T. Hyde, and D. Weinberger. 2002. Dopaminergic modulation of cortical function in patients with Parkinson's disease. *Ann. Neurol.* **51**:156–164.

Miller, E. N., O. A. Selnes, J. C. McArthur, P. Satz, J. T. Becker, B. A. Cohen, K. Sheridan, A. M. Machado, W. G. Van Gorp, and B. Visscher. 1990. Neuropsychological performance in HIV-1 infected homosexual men: the Multicenter AIDS Cohort Study (MACS). *Neurology* **40**:197–203.

Moran, J., and R. Desimone. 1985. Selective attention gates visual processing in the extrastriate cortex. *Science* **229**:782–784.

Newman, S. D., and D. Twieg. 2001. Differences in auditory processing of words and pseudo words: An fMRI study. *Hum. Brain Mapp.* **14**:39–47.

Ogawa, S., T. M. Lee, A. R. Kay, and D. W. Tank. 1990. Brain magnetic resonance imaging with contrast dependent on blood oxygenation. *Proc. Natl. Acad. Sci. USA* **87**:9868–9872.

Ogawa, S., R. S. Menon, D. W. Tank, S. G. Kim, H. Merkle, J. M. Ellermann, and K. Ugurbil. 1993. Functional brain mapping by blood oxygenation level-dependent contrast magnetic resonance imaging. A comparison of signal characteristics with a biophysical model. *Biophys. J.* **64**:803–812.

Peres, M., P. F. Van De Moortele, C. Pierard, S. Lehericy, P. Satabin, D. Le Bihan, and C. Y. Guezennec. 2000. Functional magnetic resonance imaging of mental strategy in a simulated aviation performance task. *Aviat. Space Environ. Med.* **71**:1218–1231.

Peterson, B. S., M. J. Kane, G. M. Alexander, C. Lacadie, P. Skudlarski, H. C. Leung, J. May, and J. C. Gore. 2002. An event-related functional MRI study comparing interference effects in the Simon and Stroop tasks. *Cogn. Brain Res.* **13**:427–440.

Pohl, P., G. Vogl, H. Fill, H. Rossler, R. Zangerle, and F. Gerstenbrand. 1988. Single photon emission computed tomography in AIDS dementia complex. *J. Nucl. Med.* **29**:1382–1386.

Power, C., P. A. Kong, T. O. Crawford, S. Wesselingh, J. D. Glass, J. C. McArthur, and B. D. Trapp. 1993. Cerebral white matter changes in acquired immunodeficiency syndrome dementia: alterations of the blood-brain barrier. *Ann. Neurol.* **34**:339–350.

Raichle, M. 1987. Circulatory and metabolic correlates of brain function in normal humans, p. 643–674. In V. Mountcastle, F. Plum, and S. Geiger (ed.), *Handbook of Physiology—the Nervous System*. American Physiological Society, Bethesda, Md.

Roberts, D., J. Detre, L. Bolinger, E. Insko, and J. S. Leigh, Jr. 1994. Quantitative magnetic resonance imaging of human brain perfusion at 1.5 T using steady-state inversion of arterial water. *Proc. Natl. Acad. Sci. USA* **91**:33–37.

Rosci, M. A., F. Pignorini, A. Bernabei, F. M. Pau, V. Volpini, D. E. Merigliano, and M. F. Meligrana. 1996. Methods for detecting early signs of AIDS dementia complex in asymptomatic subjects: a quantitative tomography study of 18 cases. *AIDS* **6**:1309–1316.

Rosen, B. R., J. W. Belliveau, and D. Chien. 1989. Perfusion imaging by nuclear magnetic resonance. *Magn. Reson. Q.* **5:**263–281.

Ross, M. H., D. A. Yurgelun-Todd, P. F. Renshaw, L. C. Maas, J. H. Mendelson, N. K. Mello, B. M. Cohen, and J. M. Levin. 1997. Age-related reduction in functional MRI response to photic stimulation. *Neurology* **48:**173–176.

Rottenberg, D. A., J. R. Moeller, S. C. Strother, J. J. Sidtris, B. A. Navia, V. Dhawan, J. Z. Ginos, and R. W. Price. 1987. The metabolic pathology of the AIDS dementia complex. *Ann. Neurol.* **22:**700–706.

Rottenberg, D. A., J. J. Sidtis, S. C. Strother, K. A. Schaper, J. R. Anderson, M. J. Nelson, and R. W. Price. 1996. Abnormal cerebral glucose metabolism in HIV-1 seropositive subjects with and without dementia. *J. Nucl. Med.* **37:**1133–1141.

Schwartz, R. B., A. L. Komaroff, B. M. Garada, M. Gleit, T. H. Doolittle, D. W. Bates, R. G. Vasile, and B. L. Holman. 1994. SPECT imaging of the brain: comparison of findings in patients with chronic fatigue syndrome, AIDS dementia complex, and major unipolar depression. *Am. J. Roentgenol.* **162:**943–951.

Selnes, O. A., and E. N. Miller. 1994. Development of a screening battery for the HIV-related cognitive impairment: the MACS experience, p. 176–187. *In* I. Grant, and A. Martin (ed.), *Neuropsychology of HIV Infection*. Oxford University Press, New York, NY.

Sobel, N., V. Prabhakaran, J. E. Desmond, G. H. Glover, E. V. Sullivan, and J. D. E. Gabrieli. 1997. A method for functional magnetic resonance imaging of olfaction. *J. Neurosci. Methods* **78:**115–123.

Speck, O., T. Ernst, J. Braun, C. Koch, E. Miller, and L. Chang. 2000. Gender differences in the functional organization of the brain for working memory. *Neuroreport* **11:**1–5.

Talairach, P., and J. Tournoux. 1988. *A Stereotactic Coplanar Atlas of the Human Brain*. Thieme, Stuttgart, Germany.

Tomasi, D., E. C. Caparelli, L. Chang, and T. Ernst. 2005. fMRI-acoustic noise alters brain activation during working memory tasks. *Neuroimage* **27:**377–386.

Tomasi, D., T. Ernst, E. C. Caparelli, and L. Chang. 2004. Practice-induced changes of brain function during visual attention: a parametric fMRI study at 4 Tesla. *Neuroimage* **23:**1414–1421.

Tracey, I., L. M. Hamberg, A. R. Guimaraes, G. Hunter, I. Chang, B. A. Navia, and R. G. Gonzales. 1998. Increased cerebral blood volume in HIV-positive patients detected by functional MRI. *Neurology* **50:**1821–1826.

Turner, R., A. Howseman, G. E. Rees, O. Josephs, and K. J. Friston. 1998. Functional magnetic resonance imaging of the human brain: data acquisition and analysis. *Exp. Brain Res.* **123:**5–12.

Turner, R., P. Jezzard, H. Wen, K. K. Kwong, D. LeBihan, T. Zeffiro, and R. S. Balaban. 1993. Functional mapping of the human visual cortex at 4 and 1.5 Tesla using deoxygenation contrast EPI. *Magn. Reson. Med.* **29:**277–279.

Wang, G., L. Chang, N. Volkow, F. Telang, J. Logan, T. Ernst, and J. Fowler. 2004. Decreased brain dopaminergic transporters in HIV-associated dementia patients. *Brain* **127:**2452–2458.

Weisskoff, R. M., C. S. Zuo, J. L. Boxerman, and B. R. Rosen. 1994. Microscopic susceptibility variation and transverse relaxation: theory and experiment. *Magn. Reson. Med.* **31:**601–610.

Wenserski, F., H. von Giesen, H. Wittsack, A. Aulich, and G. Arendt. 2003. Human immunodeficiency virus 1-associated minor motor disorders: perfusion-weighted MR imaging and H MR spectroscopy. *Radiology* **228:**185–192.

Williams, D. S., J. A. Detre, J. S. Leigh, and A. P. Koretsky. 1992. Magnetic resonance imaging of perfusion using spin inversion of arterial water. *Proc. Natl. Acad. Sci. USA* **89:**212–216.

The Spectrum of Neuro-AIDS Disorders:
Pathophysiology, Diagnosis, and Treatment
Edited by K. Goodkin et al.
©2008 ASM Press, Washington, DC

20

Magnetic Resonance Spectroscopy in HIV-Associated Brain Injury

LINDA CHANG, KAI ZHONG, AND THOMAS ERNST

Recent advances in neuroimaging techniques have enabled the noninvasive assessment of brain function and chemistry, which in turn has led to a better understanding of how neurological disorders may affect the brain. One of the more widely available techniques using commercial magnetic resonance (MR) scanners is proton MR spectroscopy (^{1}H-MRS). This technique has been used to identify chemical structures in vitro since the 1950s; however, its use to evaluate chemical concentrations in humans in vivo has been possible only for the past 20 years. ^{1}H-MRS has been applied to numerous clinical studies of HIV-associated brain injury, as well as opportunistic infections or neoplasms in patients with AIDS. Phosphorus (^{31}P) MRS, however, has been applied in only a few studies to evaluate high-energy phosphate metabolites in HIV-associated dementia.

Here, we describe the different methods used to perform MRS studies of patients with HIV infection, review the major findings from the studies, and identify future directions for clinical studies that may further elucidate the pathophysiology of HIV-associated brain injury, as well as discuss issues to consider in treatment monitoring.

TECHNICAL CONSIDERATIONS FOR MRS STUDIES IN HIV

^{1}H- and ^{31}P-MRS

A typical ^{1}H-MR spectrum has four major metabolite peaks (Fig. 1). The *N*-acetyl (NA) peak at 2.02 ppm includes the neuronal marker *N*-acetylaspartate (NAA) as a primary constituent (Birken et al., 1989). The creatine (CR) peak at 3.0 ppm consists of CR and phosphocreatine (PCr). The choline-containing compounds (CHO) resonate at 3.2 ppm and comprise soluble CHO, such as glycerophosphocholine, phosphocholine, and free choline (Miller et al., 1996). The *myo*-inositol (MI) peak at 3.56 ppm represents a putative glial marker (Brand et al., 1993). Other complex metabolite peaks that are visible on ^{1}H-MRS include the combination of glutamate and glutamine (2.1 to 2.7 ppm, with overlapping peaks) and gamma-acetyl butyric acid (GABA) (with peaks at 2.0 ppm and 3.0 ppm), which are measurable only with special editing techniques or special MR sequences. ^{1}H-MRS is especially valuable, since two of the major metabolites, the neuronal marker NAA and the glial marker MI, may provide in vivo evaluation of neuronal integrity and glial response in HIV-associated brain injury. In contrast, ^{31}P-MRS allows the measurement of phosphorus-containing compounds, including ATP, PCr, and inorganic phosphate (P_i), as well as a calculated pH (Fig. 2). These compounds are related to high-energy phosphate metabolism. ^{31}P-MRS was first applied to the study of HIV in 1989 but was viewed as less useful than ^{1}H-MRS due to the lower signal-to-noise ratio and the limited ability to measure only phosphate-containing compounds.

Metabolite Concentrations versus Metabolite Ratios

The majority of the MRS studies of HIV patients expressed the results as ratios between two metabolite peaks, for instance, as a ratio of NA to total CR or a ratio of NA to CHO. Total CR was most commonly used as an internal reference. The use of these "metabolite ratios" simplifies data analysis and eliminates some systematic or technical errors that might affect both metabolites in a ratio. However, the interpretation of metabolite ratios is intrinsically ambiguous because it is impossible to determine whether an abnormality in a metabolite ratio is due to a change in the numerator metabolite or the denominator metabolite, or both. Therefore, metabolite ratios can obscure underlying biological and physiological changes. For instance, using CR as a reference metabolite may yield ambiguous results, because the total CR concentration varies depending on the disease stage (Chang

Linda Chang and Thomas Ernst, Department of Medicine, Division of Neurology, John A. Burns School of Medicine, University of Hawaii, Honolulu, HI 96813. **Kai Zhong,** Department of Biomedical Magnetic Resonance, Institute for Experimental Physics, Otto-van-Guericke-University, Magdeburg, Germany.

¹H MRS from 1.5 Tesla   **¹H MRS from 4 Tesla**

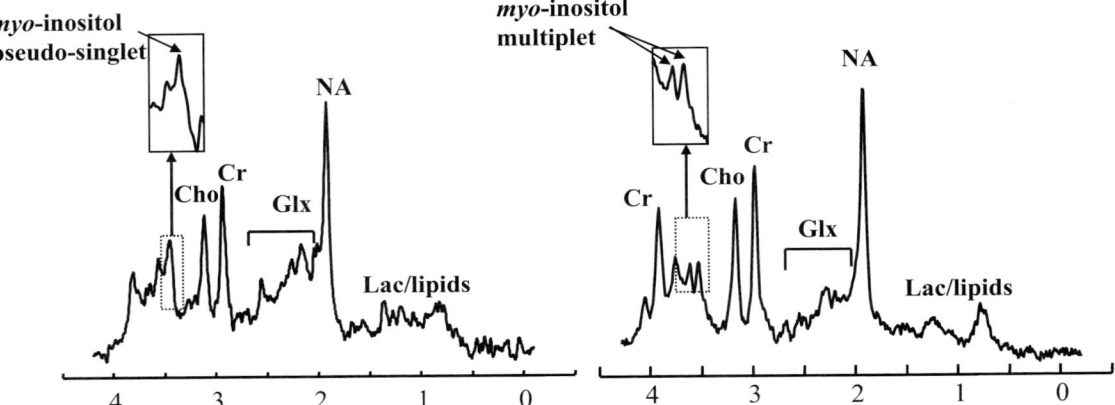

FIGURE 1 Typical ¹H-MR spectra acquired from a 1.5-T (left) and a 4-T (right) MR scanner; both used PRESS (TR/TE = 3,000/30 ms). The major metabolite peaks include an NA peak (2.02 ppm), glutamate and glutamine (Glx) (2.1 to 2.7 ppm), total CR (3.0 ppm), CHO (3.2 ppm), and occasional lactate (Lac) (1.3 ppm). Note that the MI peak(s) appears as a characteristic "pseudosinglet" at 1.5 T and as a multiplet at 4 T (insets); the difference demonstrates the better separation of the spectral peaks at higher magnetic-field strengths.

et al., 2002; Suhy et al., 2000) and age of the subject (5% increase per decade in normal white matter) (Chang et al., 1996; Suhy et al., 2000). This makes it difficult to interpret findings of abnormal metabolite ratios in HIV patients. For example, a mildly reduced NA/CR ratio in

patients with early stages of HIV dementia is commonly interpreted to reflect a decreased NA concentration; however, when the NA concentration is measured, it is usually found to be normal, whereas the CR concentration may be increased (Chang et al., 1999a).

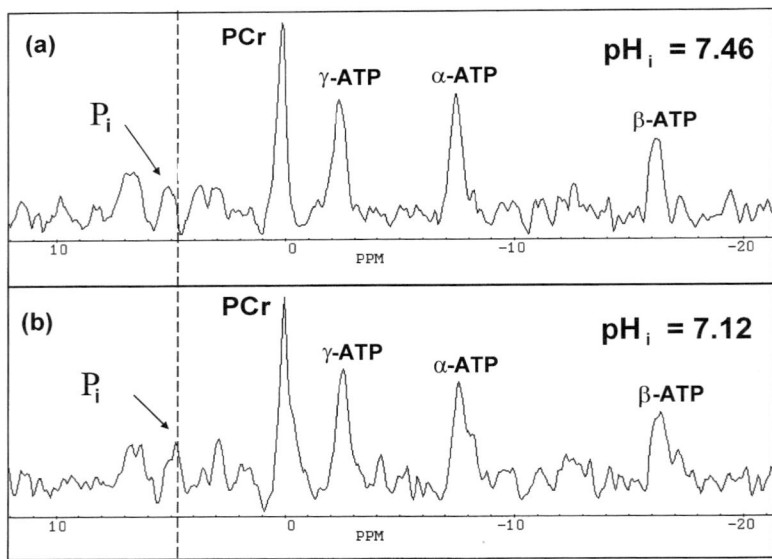

FIGURE 2 Selected ³¹P-MR spectra from the cerebellum in an HIV-infected patient (a) and a healthy volunteer (b), both acquired with a 4.1-T MR scanner. Each spectrum was selected in an 11.5-ml spectroscopic imaging voxel. PCr was used as an internal reference and was assigned a chemical shift of 0.0 ppm. The chemical shift of P_i versus PCr was used for pH determination. The spectra are shown with baseline correction. (Figure from Patton et al., 2001.)

To resolve the ambiguities associated with the use of metabolite ratios, the water signal from the brain parenchyma can be used as a reference signal (Barker et al., 1993). This approach can be used to determine the exact concentration of each metabolite in the human brain. In MRS, the metabolite signals are proportional to the total number of molecules in a unit volume (typically a few cubic centimeters, defined by the imaging methods). Since the water content in a unit volume is almost a constant, the use of the water signal as an internal spectral reference is a very good approach for measuring metabolite concentrations. Also, because the volume of interest and the MRS sequence for the water measurement are identical to those of the spectroscopic acquisition, many potential systematic errors are eliminated and the metabolite concentration measurement becomes very robust.

Another common problem in clinical MRS of dementia patients is the enlarged ventricles and sulci associated with brain atrophy, and since the cerebrospinal fluid (CSF) contains low concentrations of these major metabolites, it is important to eliminate the partial-volume (dilution) effect from the CSF in each MRS voxel. There are two solutions to this problem: (i) direct T_2 measurements of the water signal with a localized spectroscopy sequence to separate the brain water signal from that of the CSF (Ernst et al., 1993) and (ii) segmentation of MR images to quantify the gray/white matter and water content in the volume of interest; this method can be applied to both single-voxel spectroscopy and MRS imaging (MRSI) (Suhy et al., 2000). These two techniques yield similar results, as shown in recent studies of normal aging (Suhy et al., 2000; K. Zhong, L. Chang, D. Carasig, L. Zimmerman, and T. Ernst, Tenth *Ann. Meet. Int. Soc. Magn. Reson. Med.*, abstr. 2492, 2002). However, one should be very careful when comparing metabolite concentrations obtained from a localized MRS study with those obtained from an MRSI study, since the gray/white-matter composition and the water reference signals used in the two studies may be different.

Effect of Magnetic Field Strength

The majority of MRS studies in HIV patients were conducted on 1.5-T MR scanners. Only one ^{31}P-MRS study was performed on a 4-T scanner. Higher magnetic-field strengths generally yield higher signal intensities and better spectral separation; thus, the intrinsic error associated with the MRS measurement tends to be smaller. Preliminary studies in our laboratory showed that at 4 T, the intrasubject variability from single-voxel spectroscopy is only 4 to 5% for the major metabolites, including NAA, CR, and CHO, while the intersubject variability is approximately 6 to 9%. In contrast, at 1.5 T, the intrasubject variability is 6 to 7% while intersubject variability is 9 to 12%. The smaller variability at higher field strength suggests that a smaller sample size might suffice in clinical studies at the higher field strength than with the lower-field-strength scanners.

However, at higher field strength it may be more difficult to quantify metabolite peaks with a multiplet structure (e.g., MI, glutamate, and glutamine), which have lower peak heights. These multiplet peaks, along with the underlying macromolecules, can collapse into a "pseudosinglet" and therefore become more visible at lower field strength, such as the glutamate peak at 0.5 T (Antuono et al., 2001) and MI at 1.5 T (Fig. 1). Therefore, additional studies are needed to determine whether the higher-field-strength scanners

($\geq$3 T) are indeed more advantageous than the 1.5-T scanners for the evaluation of HIV brain injury.

Short TE versus Long TE

One of the most important MRS acquisition parameters is the "echo time" (TE), which characterizes the delay between spin excitation and data readout. Many early MRS studies of HIV were carried out at longer TEs (>100 ms), at which only the peaks of NA, CR, and CHO are visible in the spectrum. In contrast, more recent studies have often been conducted at short TEs of 20 to 35 ms. At short TEs, the major peaks, e.g., NAA, CR, CHO, MI, and Glx, and minor peaks, e.g., lactate and GABA, can all be measured with special sequences or editing techniques. Additionally, the contributions from macromolecules and lipids are also present at short TEs and may confound the major or minor metabolite signals. Therefore, improved spectral-analysis techniques are required to extract accurate metabolite concentrations from the "signal ensemble." Spectra can be fitted into the frequency domain (e.g., the LC model [Provencher, 1993]) and/or into the time domain (e.g., MRUI [http://www.mrui.uab.es/mrui/]). For interested readers, there are two excellent reviews on MRS quantitation methods using the frequency (Mierisova and Ala-Korpela, 2001) or time (Vanhamme et al., 2001) domain approach.

Single-Voxel MRS versus MRSI

MRS techniques can be divided into two groups: single-voxel, or localized, techniques and MRSI techniques. Localized MRS studies are performed with the point resolved spectroscopy (PRESS) technique or with the stimulated echo acquisition method. If implemented correctly, both of them provide relatively robust data acquisition and measurement of metabolite concentrations at short TEs. However, it is difficult to characterize the regional pattern of pathological changes with localized spectroscopy, since only a small selected volume (typically 2 to 8 ml) of the brain is evaluated at a time.

MRSI techniques can provide better assessment of different regional abnormalities than localized MRS, since an entire section, or multiple slices, of the brain can be imaged at once. However, MRSI intrinsically suffers from problems, such as magnetic susceptibility artifacts and point spread function dispersion. The former may lead to variations in the spectral line width across voxels and increase variability in the fitted peak areas. The latter can cause a dispersion of signal intensity across adjacent voxels and distort the true metabolite concentrations in those voxels. Larger imaging matrices can reduce the point spread function problem but may also make acquisition times unacceptably long. Furthermore, in order to avoid scalp lipid contamination of the metabolite signals, most MRSI studies use longer TEs (>100 ms) and evaluate only a single slice. Therefore, only the three major peaks (NAA, CR, and CHO) and a small cross section can be observed. More recently, advances in multislice short-TE MRSI with the use of higher-order shims yielded approximately 30% greater volume of brain tissue that could be shimmed, which leads to significant improvement in the homogeneity within specific areas of the brain, particularly those near the skull (Spielman et al., 1998). These advances may facilitate future MRS studies of HIV brain injury.

A recent study of HIV patients combined single-voxel spectroscopy and a multislice MRSI method. MRSI was performed at a TE of 270 ms to evaluate regional metabolite changes in NA, CR, and CHO throughout the brain, and localized spectroscopy at a 35-ms TE was used for additional metabolite quantitation of MI in a selected brain region (Sacktor et al., 2001). An optimized multislice MRSI at a short TE would be ideal for future studies of HIV brain injury or other neurological disorders.

¹H-MRS STUDIES OF HIV PATIENTS

MRS studies have been performed in both adult and pediatric patients with HIV infection, using localized MRS and MRSI techniques and long TEs, as well as short TEs, and before or after antiretroviral treatment. More recent studies have also evaluated HIV patients without neuropsychiatric symptoms or who are asymptomatic for cognitive deficits.

The majority of the studies used localized spectroscopy techniques (either PRESS or the stimulated echo acquisition method) and evaluated one to three brain regions. Earlier studies typically evaluated the parietal region, while the more recent studies evaluated frontal-lobe and basal-ganglion regions. Six studies used MRSI. The acquisition parameters for these studies varied widely. For single-voxel spectroscopy, the TEs varied from 20 ms to 270 ms. For MRSI, TEs were between 135 and 272 ms. In order to maximize the signal-to-noise ratio, earlier studies used larger voxels, 8 to 64 cm³ (Chong et al., 1993; McConnell et al., 1994; Menon et al., 1992); metabolite concentrations from these larger volumes typically contained combined signals derived from white matter, gray matter, and/or CSF. More recent MRS studies used smaller voxels (0.8 to 3 ml), which allowed white- and gray-matter regions to be evaluated separately.

³¹P-MRS in HIV Dementia

There are only a few published ³¹P-MRS studies of HIV-associated brain injury. The earliest study evaluated the brains of 12 HIV patients with an axial slice and found reduced PCr and ATP (Bottomley et al., 1990). Another study found that HIV patients had lower ATP/P_i and PCr/P_i ratios than the control group in the frontoparietal white matter (Deicken et al., 1991). Both the ATP/P_i and PCr/P_i ratios correlated negatively with the overall severity of neuropsychiatric impairment. These findings suggest that HIV brain infection might impair cellular oxidative metabolism. The third study evaluated the combined effects of alcohol and HIV in a large cohort and found that alcohol and HIV have cumulative effects on the reduction of PCr and phosphodiester (Meyerhoff et al., 1995). A fourth study conducted on a 4.1-T MR scanner found more alkaline pH in the cerebella of patients with HIV (Fig. 2); this finding suggests that HIV infection activates the astrocytic Na^+/H^+ exchanger (Patton et al., 2001). Taken together, these four studies demonstrate that ³¹P-MRS can provide an in vivo assessment of the high-energy metabolism and the pH in the brain, which may improve our understanding of the pathogenesis of HIV brain injury.

Metabolite Abnormalities in HIV Dementia and Changes with Disease Severity

The majority of ¹H-MRS studies reported a decreased NAA/CR ratio and a decreased NAA/CHO ratio in patients with HIV or AIDS. The same findings were reported regardless of whether the studies used single-voxel techniques with long TEs (Chong et al., 1993, 1994; Menon et al., 1990, 1992; Paley et al., 1996; Salvan et al., 1997a; Simone et al., 1998; Wilkinson et al., 1994) or short TEs (Chang et al., 1999a; English et al., 1997; Jarvik et al., 1993; Laubenberger et al., 1996; Paley et al., 1995; Tracey et al., 1996) or single-slice

(Lopez-Villegas et al., 1997; Marcus et al., 1998; Meyerhoff et al., 1993, 1994, 1996; Moller et al., 1999) or multislice (Barker et al., 1995) spectroscopic imaging. Most studies concurred that decreased NA/CR or NA/CHO ratios were more commonly observed in HIV patients with cognitive impairment, but not in those who were neurologically asymptomatic (Chang et al., 1999a; Chong et al., 1994; Laubenberger et al., 1996; Menon et al., 1992; Paley et al., 1996; Salvan et al., 1997a; Tracey et al., 1996). The decreased ratios were commonly interpreted as decreases in NAA, which is a neuronal marker, and were thought to imply neuronal loss in the HIV patients. However, studies that measured metabolite concentrations, rather than relying on ratios, generally found decreased NA, suggestive of neuronal loss, only at later stages of the disease and relatively normal NA levels during early stages of cognitive impairment (Barker et al., 1995; Chang et al., 1999a) or in those with mild or no cognitive deficits (Meyerhoff et al., 1999) (Fig. 3 and 4).

Another common finding in the brains of HIV patients is an increased CHO/CR ratio (Barker et al., 1995; Chang et al., 1999a; Chong et al., 1993; English et al., 1997; Jarvik et al., 1993; Marcus et al., 1998; Meyerhoff et al., 1999; Salvan et al., 1997a; Simone et al., 1998; Tracey et al., 1996). Elevated CHO might be associated with increased cellularity, since neuropathological studies have shown an increased number of macrophages and microglial cells in the brains of AIDS patients. Alternatively, higher CHO might be related to increased cell membrane breakdown and release of soluble CHO due to direct or indirect effects of HIV infection. Studies that evaluated metabolite concentrations indeed found elevated CHO in patients with minor cognitive motor disorder and even more so in those with AIDS dementia complex (ADC) (Fig. 3) (Barker et al., 1995; Chang et al., 1999a; Meyerhoff et al., 1999).

An elevated MI/CR ratio has also been reported in patients with various stages of HIV dementia (Chang et al., 1999a; Laubenberger et al., 1996; Lopez-Villegas et al., 1997; von Giesen et al., 2001). The elevation of the MI/CR ratio has been attributed to elevated MI, since it is present primarily in glial cells (Brand et al., 1993) and has the putative function of regulating the cellular osmotic environment and maintaining the cell volume (Graf et al., 1993). Therefore, glial activation, with glial hypertrophy, would be associated with elevated cytoplasmic MI. Measurements of MI concentrations in HIV patients further support this hypothesis, since MI levels increase with dementia severity (Fig. 3), especially in the frontal white matter, where glial activation has been observed in neuropathological studies (Power et al., 1993).

Although the CR peak is frequently used as an internal reference, total CR in patients infected with HIV may change depending on the disease stage and brain region. As mentioned above, prior reports observed a decreased NA/CR ratio (Jarvik et al., 1993; Menon et al., 1990; Meyerhoff et al., 1993; Paley et al., 1995), even in HIV patients who were neurologically asymptomatic (Suwanwelaa et al., 2000), and interpreted this as decreased neuronal marker NA due to neuronal damage. Studies that measured concentrations rather than ratios found that a decreased NA/CR ratio may be due to either a normal [NA] or a mildly decreased [NA], along with an elevated [CR], especially in the basal ganglia, during the cognitively asymptomatic stage (Chang et al., 1999a, 1999b). In the later stages of ADC, the [CR] is significantly elevated in the frontal lobe but decreased in the basal ganglia, along with a decreased [NA] (Chang et al., 2002). The elevated [CR] may also obscure concomitant

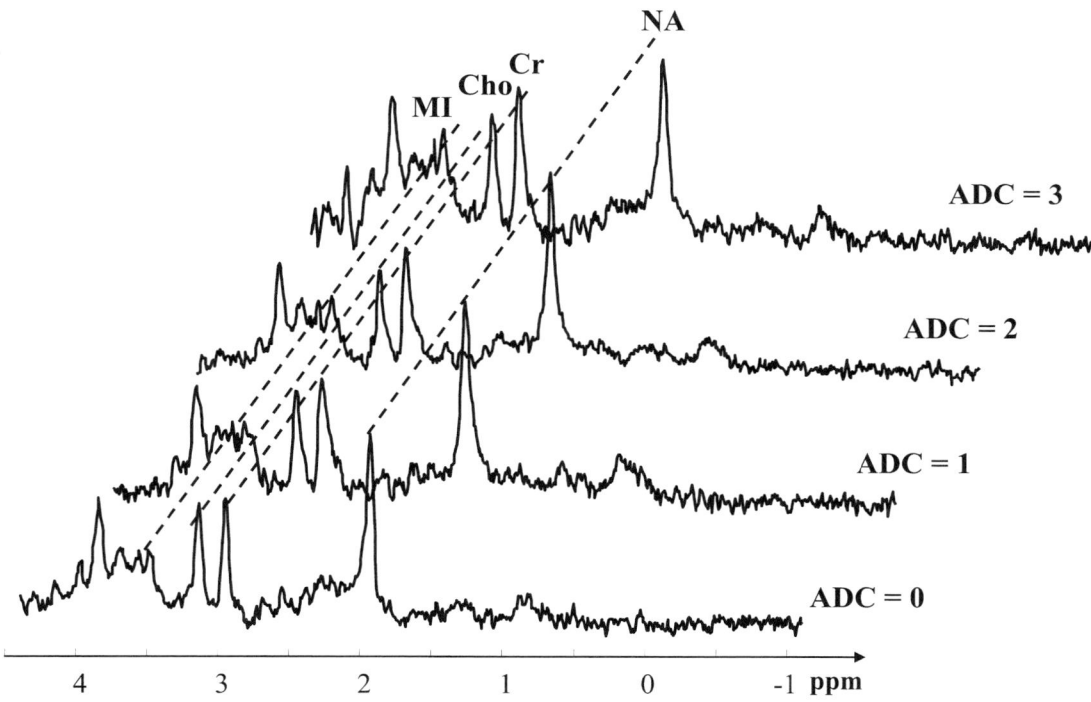

FIGURE 3 Metabolite changes dependent on ADC stages. Note that there is decreased NA only at stage 3 (ADC = 3) (severe dementia) and a relatively normal level of NA during the earlier stages of dementia. Note also the gradual increases in CR, CHO, and MI concentrations. All MR spectra were acquired on a 4-T MR scanner (PRESS sequence, TR/TE = 3,000/30 ms; 64 averages).

elevations in CHO and MI. This further emphasizes the importance of metabolite concentration measurements and that CR should not be used as an internal reference.

Investigators from one laboratory labeled a region of the MR spectrum as a "marker peak" (2.1 to 2.6 ppm), which "represents a combination of nonspecific amino acids and possibly myelin catabolites" (Jarvik et al., 1996). Since this region also contains overlapping peaks of glutamate/glutamine, which extend from 2.1 to 2.7 ppm, and a secondary peak from NAA, our ability to interpret the integrated value from this broad region is very limited. Future studies using different field strengths (i.e., a scanner with a higher magnetic-field strength) or special MRS sequences (e.g., two-dimensional MRS) may make it possible to further assess whether glutamate and glutamine levels are altered in HIV-associated brain injury.

Regional Variations in Metabolite Abnormalities

Limited by magnetic-susceptibility problems in evaluating the frontal brain regions, many of the earlier localized MRS studies evaluated the parietal or the occipital brain regions. Improvements in MRS techniques, such as adjustments of the slice order (Ernst and Chang, 1996), now allow the assessment of the frontal lobe and subcortical brain regions. Several localized MRS studies specifically evaluated metabolite changes in the frontal lobe and the subcortical regions, including the basal ganglia and the thalamus. An elevated CHO/CR or MI/CR ratio, as well as CHO and MI concentrations, have been observed in the frontal white matter of neuroasymptomatic HIV patients (English et al., 1997), whereas similar changes in the frontal gray matter and basal ganglia are present only in those with dementia (Chang

et al., 1999a; von Giesen et al., 2001). Another localized MRS study of asymptomatic HIV patients also found decreased NAA/CR and NAA/CHO ratios, without changes in the CHO/CR ratio, in both the centrum semiovale (white matter) and the thalamus; these findings are difficult to interpret, since they may be due to either decreased NA or concomitant increased CHO, CR, and MI or to changes in all of these variables (Suwanwelaa et al., 2000).

A more efficient approach to evaluating regional metabolite abnormalities in HIV patients is to use MRSI (Lopez-Villegas et al., 1997; Marcus et al., 1998; Meyerhoff et al., 1993, 1994, 1996, 1999; Moller et al., 1999). All except one of these studies utilized a single-slice approach and evaluated six to nine voxels in the slice in each subject. One study used a multislice approach and assessed four slices, with three or four voxels selected on each slice, totaling 11 brain regions (Barker et al., 1995). The findings from the long-TE (≥130-ms) spectroscopic-imaging studies are consistent with those observed using localized techniques, namely, a decreased NA/CR or NA/CHO ratio throughout the brain, primarily in those with more severe dementia, and an increased CHO/CR ratio in the majority of HIV patients, including those without cognitive deficits on neuropsychological testing (Meyerhoff et al., 1999). Therefore, the general consensus appears to be that metabolite abnormalities occur diffusely throughout the brain. However, with the multislice technique, spectroscopic-imaging maps illustrate higher CHO and lower NA levels in the frontal white matter of patients with ADC and primarily higher CHO levels without decreased NA in the frontal white-matter region in patients with only minor cognitive motor disorder (Fig. 4). Since these regional changes are not always evident on all

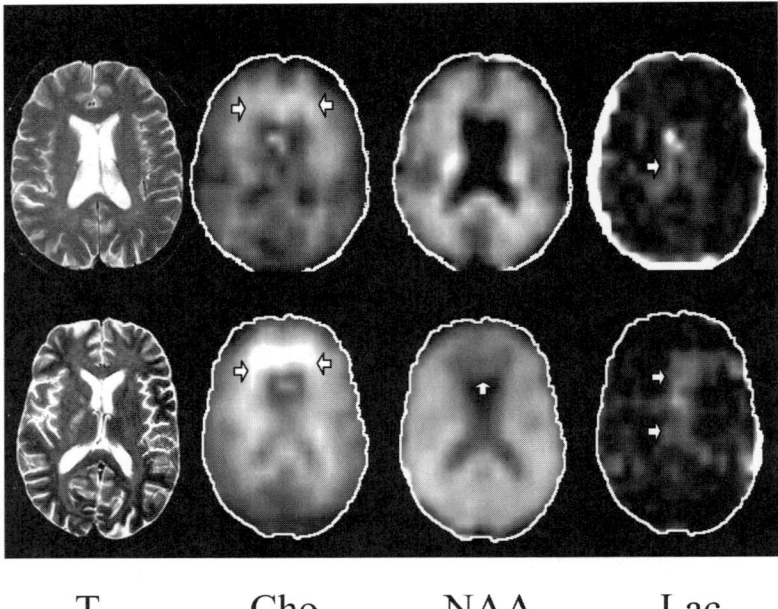

Mild Neurocognitive
Symptoms
58 years, CD4 300

AIDS Dementia
Complex
35 years, CD4 143

T_2 Cho   NAA   Lac

FIGURE 4 Characteristic metabolite maps from MRSI of two patients with HIV. The patient with mild cognitive motor disorder and a higher CD4 count had mildly elevated CHO in the frontal white-matter region with relatively normal NAA (top row), while the patient with ADC and a lower CD4 count had further elevation of CHO and decreased NAA in the frontal brain region. MRS images were acquired with a 1.5-T MR scanner; PRESS, TR/TE = 2 300/272 ms. (Courtesy of Peter Barker; modified from data presented in Barker et al., 1995.)

the slices, multislice MRSI may ensure a more comprehensive assessment of regional brain metabolite abnormalities. Furthermore, the only short-TE MRSI study specifically evaluated the frontal lobe and also found elevated MI/CR ratios in the white matter of neuroasymptomatic HIV patients, while ADC patients had normal MI/CR ratios in both gray and white matter and decreased NA/CR ratios in gray matter (Lopez-Villegas et al., 1997). These findings were later confirmed in a localized MRS study that found elevated CR and MI levels in the frontal white matter in patients without dementia and, to a greater extent, elevation of both CR and MI in those with dementia (Chang et al., 2002).

Reversal or Normalization of Metabolite Abnormalities in HIV after Antiretroviral Treatments

Prior to highly active antiretroviral therapy (HAART), several longitudinal MRS studies reported changes in metabolite ratios or levels in HIV patients during antiretroviral treatment. An early study followed seven HIV patients over 1 year and found that NA/CR ratios decreased in all subjects, although six of the subjects were treated with one to three antiretroviral medications (McConnell et al., 1994). This study contradicts three other small studies that followed HIV patients before and after antiretroviral treatment. One study followed five patients before and after the initiation of zidovudine (ZDV) treatment and found that the NA/(CR plus CHO plus CR) ratio improved (increased) 4 to 13 weeks after treatment, along with clinical improvement in four of five patients; however, two of the patients subsequently deteriorated, and their NA/(CR plus CHO plus CR) ratios also declined (Wilkinson et al., 1997b). Another study followed

11 patients after 1,000 mg/day of ZDV and found improvement only in those with an initially decreased NA/CR ratio but not in those with only elevated CHO/CR ratios (Salvan et al., 1997b). A third study of two pediatric patients found normalization of the initially decreased NA/CR ratio and disappearance of the lactate peaks 4 to 8 months after ZDV and ZDV plus didanosine. Since these studies relied on metabolite ratios, the changes in the NA/CR or NA/(CR plus CHO plus CR) ratio might in fact have been due to decreases in CR and CHO after treatment.

HAART has prolonged the survival and improved the quality of life of and significantly decreased the incidence of central nervous system AIDS-defining illnesses in patients infected with HIV (d'Arminio Monforte et al., 2000). The HIV load may be suppressed for long periods, and CD4 levels may increase significantly with HAART. However, the metabolite concentrations measured by MRS may be altered by HAART, either due to the treatment effects or due to possible neurotoxic effects of the medications. One study specifically evaluated HIV patients before and after HAART and found that those who tolerated HAART showed reversal of the initially increased MI concentration, and to a lesser degree the CHO concentration, toward normal levels in the frontal white matter and basal ganglia (Chang et al., 1999b). Another study followed a group of patients already on HAART over a period of 9 months and found that only those with cognitive impairment and lower NA/CR and higher MI/CR ratios initially showed improvement of the metabolite abnormalities (Stankoff et al., 2001). In order to better assess the time course of metabolite improvements in HIV patients, a recent study specifically recruited antiretroviral-naïve patients and followed them at 3, 6, and 9 months with CD4, plasma, and CSF viral-load measurements and MRS in three brain regions (Chang et al., 2001). This study found that although CD4, plasma, and CSF viral loads all improved rapidly, abnormalities in brain metabolites persisted after 3 months of HAART (Chang et al., 2000); initially elevated MI and CHO levels gradually improved between 6 and 9 months (Chang et al., 2001). Therefore, future medication trials using MRS metabolite measurements as surrogate markers should have follow-up evaluations 6 to 9 months after treatment.

Other studies using neuropsychological testing to evaluate cognitive improvements in HIV patients after HAART have found significant improvements in psychomotor speed at 6 months (Sacktor et al., 1999). Although several studies have shown that various regional metabolites on MRS correlate well with selected measures of neuropsychological tests (Chang et al., 2002; Lopez-Villegas et al., 1997; Meyerhoff et al., 1999), cognitive testing may be affected by mood disorders, education, or cultural influences. Therefore, the combination of cognitive testing and MRS might provide confirmatory and complementary information regarding treatment effects.

Presymptomatic Detection of Metabolite Abnormalities in HIV

The majority of the MRS studies compared HIV patients with mild or no cognitive deficits to those with definite diagnosis of ADC and found primarily elevated CHO/CR and MI/CR ratios during the early stages and additional decreased NA/CR ratios in later stages of ADC. However, some of these reports demonstrate conflicting findings. For example, some studies found no decreased NA/CR ratios (Marcus et al., 1998; Salvan et al., 1997a), while others reported decreased NA/CR ratios (Suwanwelaa et al., 2000; Wilkinson et al., 1997a) in asymptomatic HIV patients. Likewise, some observed elevated CHO/CR ratios in the white matter (Salvan et al., 1997a) or an elevated CHO level in the subcortical gray matter (Meyerhoff et al., 1999), while other studies found no change in CHO/CR ratios in those systemically asymptomatic (Wilkinson et al., 1997a), in CDC groups A and B (Moller et al., 1999), or in neurologically asymptomatic patients (Marcus et al., 1998; Suwanwelaa et al., 2000). Several studies even included careful assessments of cognitive function with neuropsychological tests to ensure the neuroasymptomatic status of the subjects (Chang et al., 2002; Jarvik et al., 1996; Meyerhoff et al., 1999). One possibility to explain these discrepant findings might be the medication status of the subjects, since two of the studies that found no change in CHO/CR ratios or CHO levels were performed in neuroasymptomatic subjects who were antiretroviral medication naïve (Chang et al., 2002; Suwanwelaa et al., 2000).

Since brain injury due to HIV might be partly mediated by cytokines and chemokines associated with systemic inflammation or central glial activation, the putative glial marker MI might be elevated during the earliest stages of the disease. Two short-TE MRS studies that evaluated neuroasymptomatic HIV patients found normal MI/CR ratios (Suwanwelaa et al., 2000; von Giesen et al., 2001), while a recent study found elevated MI and CR levels in those with normal cognitive function (Chang et al., 2002), which would lead to a normal MI/CR ratio. Therefore, measurement of the metabolite concentration, rather than the ratio, is particularly important in assessing subtle changes in the brain.

Furthermore, using short-TE MRS, a higher "marker peak"/CR ratio (Jarvik et al., 1996) has been observed, while another study found no change in the metabolite ratios (i.e., Glx/CR) in this frequency region of the MRS spectrum (Chang et al., 1999a; Marcus et al., 1998). Since the metabolites in this spectral region are particularly difficult to quantify and the presence of macromolecules might influence the quantification and baseline assessment, future studies are needed to further understand the significance of these reports.

Relationship between Brain Metabolites and Inflammatory Markers

Levels of inflammatory markers, such as the chemokine macrophage chemoattractant protein 1 (MCP-1), were found to be higher in patients with HIV-associated dementia than in those who were neuroasymptomatic (Conant et al., 1998). Therefore, inflammatory proteins might lead to brain injury. One study specifically evaluated the relationships between neurometabolites and MCP-1 in serum and CSF in HIV patients before and after antiretroviral treatment (Chang et al., 2004a). To minimize excess correlations, principal-component analyses (PCA) were used to group metabolites into those that were related to neurons (NA; glutamate plus glutamine) and those that were related to glia (including MI and CHO). A similar PCA approach has been applied to a large multicenter MRS data set of HIV patients to evaluate regional patterns of brain metabolite abnormalities (Yiannoutsos et al., 2004). HIV subjects were evaluated before and 3 months after HAART. CSF, but not serum, MCP-1 levels correlated inversely with the neuronal component (from PCA) prior to treatment. Conversely, after 3 months of HAART, the glial component (from PCA) correlated positively with CSF MCP-1 levels. These findings suggest that CSF MCP-1 levels are associated with neuronal dysfunction in untreated patients. However, after 3 months of HAART, systemic factors (the viral burden and systemically derived MCP-1) improved and were no longer related to neuronal dysfunction, but subjects with the strongest glial response in the brain continued to produce the highest levels of MCP-1. Further studies are needed to determine whether long-term treatment with HAART is associated with persistently elevated MCP-1 in the CSF and whether this might be related to further neuronal injury.

Effects of Aging on Brain Metabolites in HIV Patients

Normal aging and HIV infection both may lead to inflammatory changes and injury to the brain. Therefore, it is reasonable to assume that additive or interactive effects on brain metabolites may occur in the aging HIV population. One study evaluated 46 HIV patients naïve to antiretroviral medications and 58 seronegative (SN) control subjects using localized ^{1}H-MRS to assess brain metabolite abnormalities in three brain regions (frontal gray matter, frontal white matter, and basal ganglia) (Ernst and Chang, 2004). Compared to the SN controls, HIV-positive subjects showed additional and marked increases in the concentrations of the glial markers CHO (SN, +2%/decade; HIV, +10%/decade) and MI (SN, +3%/decade; HIV, +12%/decade) with aging in the frontal white matter. In the basal ganglia, the NA compounds NA and CR decreased with age only in the HIV patients (NA, −3.7%/decade; CR, −4%/decade). Analysis of covariance showed significant interaction effects between HIV and aging on the metabolites in the basal ganglia (NA, $P = 0.03$; CR, $P = 0.04$) and in the frontal white matter (interaction: CHO, $P = 0.002$; MI, $P = 0.007$). The investigators in this study concluded that in the basal ganglia, HIV infection appeared to induce neuronal damage or loss beyond that observed in normal aging. In the frontal white matter, HIV infection seemed to exacerbate glial activation beyond that observed in normal aging.

Data from a multicenter MRS study (AIDS Clinical Trials Group 700) provided additional confirmation of the interactive effect of age and HIV on brain metabolite abnormalities (Chang et al., 2004b). Three brain regions (frontal white matter, basal ganglia, and parietal cortex) were assessed in 100 HIV patients, mostly maintained on HAART (61 with ADC and 39 neuroasymptomatic), and 37 SN controls. Consistent with prior studies, the study found that glial activation (an elevated MI/CR ratio) in the white matter occurred during the neuroasymptomatic stages of HIV infection, whereas further inflammatory activity in the basal ganglia and neuronal injury in the white matter were associated with the development of cognitive impairment. As the effects of normal aging are similar to those of ADC (i.e., elevated CHO/CR and MI/CR ratios) (Chang et al., 1996; Schuff et al., 1999), the possible interaction between HIV and age was evaluated as part of the multivariate analysis model. A significant interaction between HIV and age was observed for the NA/CR ratio in the white matter, in that younger (<40 years), but not older, HIV subjects had lower NA/CR ratios than SN controls. Significant age effects on CHO/CR and MI/CR ratios (in both the basal ganglia and frontal white matter) were present that paralleled the HIV effects, suggesting additive rather than interactive effects on these metabolite ratios.

These two studies suggest that aging might further exacerbate neuronal injury in HIV patients. However, the additive or interactive effects on the glial markers (MI, CR, and CHO) might be different in younger versus older HIV patients and might depend on whether the HIV patients are treated with antiretroviral medications. Further studies of older HIV patients using a longitudinal, rather than a cross-sectional, approach are needed to further delineate the effects of aging in HIV patients.

MRS Abnormalities in Pediatric HIV Patients

Prior to perinatal prophylaxis with ZDV and other antiretroviral medications, approximately 20 to 40% of infants born to HIV-positive mothers were infected with HIV, and 20% developed HIV encephalopathy (Lobato et al., 1995). However, the incidence of vertical transmission of HIV has declined by two-thirds since the introduction of prophylactic treatment with ZDV during the perinatal period (Fiscus et al., 1996). Only five MRS studies have evaluated brain abnormalities in children infected with HIV. One study evaluated neonates born to HIV-positive mothers and found significantly lower NA/CR ratios, higher CHO/CR ratios, and higher "marker-region peak"/CR ratios than for neonate controls with HIV-negative mothers (Cortey et al., 1994), despite a low probability that these babies would develop AIDS. Therefore, the investigators postulated that the metabolite abnormalities might be related to the indirect effects of HIV, such as intrauterine growth retardation. Another study of 20 HIV-infected children found that the centrum semiovale showed increased lipid signals; 5 of these children with encephalopathy also showed decreased NA and increased MI relative to all the other metabolites (NA plus CR plus CHO plus Glx plus taurine plus MI) (Salvan et al., 1998). The largest series included 45 children with AIDS and found lower NA/CR ratios in those with

encephalopathy; however, children without encephalopathy showed normal NA/CR ratios but lower CHO/CR ratios in the basal-ganglion region (Lu et al., 1996). MRS was found to be more sensitive for detecting brain abnormalities than either structural MR imaging (MRI) or immunological testing. A report of two children with AIDS encephalopathy, furthermore, found that the initially decreased NA/CR ratio and presence of lactate in the basal ganglia improved (i.e., an increased NA/CR ratio and absence of lactate) after treatment with ZDV (Pavlakis et al., 1998).

A recent multivoxel MRS study by Keller et al. found that HIV-infected children ($n = 20$) had decreased CHO in the frontal white matter (Keller et al., 2004). However, those with high viral loads (>5,000 HIV RNA copies/ml) had decreased CHO, CR, and MI in the basal ganglia but higher CHO levels in the medial frontal gray matter. The most interesting finding from this study was that HIV-infected children do not show age-dependent increases in NAA but that MI increased with age in these HIV-infected children instead. The $\log_{10}$ plasma viral load also correlated positively with MI in the frontal white matter and with CHO in the medial frontal gray matter. Compared to controls, HIV patients had poorer spatial memory, and delayed spatial memory was correlated with CHO in the hippocampus. These data suggest that normal brain development may be affected in children infected with HIV at birth, which is particularly evidenced by the lack of age-related increases in the neuronal marker [NAA].

These few studies demonstrate that MRS may be particularly useful in the assessment and monitoring of children infected with HIV, since it is sensitive for assessing brain pathology, is useful for monitoring treatment effects, and is safe and clinically available. The study by Keller et al. further suggests that early, aggressive treatment of infants with HIV before development of encephalopathy is warranted.

MRS Studies in Preclinical Models of AIDS

One MRS study quantified NAA in brain extracts of control and simian immunodeficiency virus (SIV)-infected macaques, correlated these findings with histologic analyses, and found over 50% reduction of NAA in the SIV-infected animals compared with controls (Tracey et al., 1997). A significant decrease in NAA was also found in SIV-infected animals sacrificed in the acute stages of infection 9 or 10 days after inoculation with $SIV_{macYnef}$. Another study, conducted in the same laboratory, used a high-resolution magic angle spinning technique on snap-frozen specimens from the frontal cortical gray matter of SIV-infected macaques (Gonzalez et al., 2000). As early as 2 weeks postinfection, losses in NAA and calbindin (indicating neuronal injury and/or death) and decreases in synaptophysin immunoreactivity (indicating synaptodendritic injury) were detected, along with increases in glial fibrillary acid protein (indicating reactive gliosis). Cellular injury worsened progressively with increased time after infection. Furthermore, the CHO/CR ratio was increased shortly after SIV infection but decreased after 2 years. Similarly, reports of MRS studies of feline immunodeficiency virus (FIV)-infected cats demonstrated decreased NAA or NAA/CHO ratios in the frontal cortex 6 months after infection; the decreased NAA was correlated with the CD4 count, but not with the peripheral proviral load (Podell et al., 1999). Although the metabolite abnormalities in the animal models appear to occur in an accelerated time course, the findings are in general agreement with those in humans. Therefore, both SIV and FIV may provide useful models for understanding the neuropathogenesis of HIV dementia. MRS has an important role in the longitudinal assessment of in vivo and ex vivo brain pathology in these animal models.

SUMMARY, CONCLUSIONS, AND FUTURE DIRECTIONS

Numerous MRS studies have evaluated the effect of HIV infection on the brain. These studies included HIV patients who were neurologically asymptomatic and subjects at various stages of HIV dementia, as well as pediatric populations. The MRS findings ranged from subtle increases in MI in the white matter of neuroasymptomatic patients, indicating subclinical glial activation, to marked decreases in NA and increases in CHO and MI in patients with severe dementia, demonstrating additional neuronal damage or loss. The progressive metabolite changes with early glial activation and subsequent neuronal loss are consistent with those observed in neuropathology studies. Recent MRS studies further suggest that the level of CSF MCP-1 may affect the brain NA level or lead to neuronal injury.

The effects of antiretroviral treatments have also been evaluated in several small studies. Current approaches for monitoring treatment effects in HIV dementia are based on neuropsychological outcomes as primary measures. MRS has shown promise for providing additional surrogate markers to monitor treatment effects. Since several studies have shown good correlations between metabolites measured with MRS and neuropsychological performance, future clinical trials may benefit from using both MRS and neuropsychological testing for monitoring the effects of treatment. The sensitivity and specificity for treatment efficacy between MRS and neuropsychological testing, or a combination of the two, remain to be determined. As the population of HIV patients is aging and is kept on chronic maintenance antiretrovirals, the long-term effects of these medications on the brain and the potential interactive effects of HIV and aging on brain injury should be monitored and evaluated.

Many other neuroimaging techniques, including computed tomography, structural MRI, single-photon emission computed tomography (SPECT), positron emission tomography, and, more recently, functional MRI, have been applied to evaluate HIV-associated brain injury. However, few studies have directly compared or correlated in vivo MRS with these imaging modalities. Therefore, the relative sensitivities and specificities between these imaging techniques are difficult to assess. One study evaluated coregistered quantitative ^{1}H-MRS and quantitative ^{133}Xe-calibrated 99meta-technetium hexamethylpropylene amine oxime SPECT; despite a lack of correlation between regional cerebral blood flow (on SPECT) and metabolite concentrations (from MRS) in any of the brain regions evaluated, MRS was found to be more sensitive than SPECT for detecting early brain injury in HIV dementia (Ernst et al., 2000). Future studies using more than one neuroimaging modality for the same subjects are needed to determine the relative sensitivities and specificities of these techniques and may provide complementary information to further elucidate the pathogenesis of HIV brain injury.

Due to technical advances, earlier long-TE MRS studies are being replaced by short-TE MRS studies, and future MRS studies will likely involve spectroscopic imaging, two-dimensional MRS, or other novel MRS techniques to further assess regional changes and additional metabolites of interest (e.g., glutamate and GABA). In addition, both in vivo and ex vivo MRS studies in animal models of AIDS (e.g., SIV and FIV) should provide additional insights into the pathophysiology of HIV-associated dementia.

This work was supported by grants from NIDA (L.C., K24 DA16170; T.E., K02 DA16991) and NINDS (R01-NS38834).

REFERENCE

Antuono, P., J. Jones, Y. Wang, and S. Li. 2001. Decreased glutamate + glutamine in Alzheimer's disease detected in vivo with ^{1}H-MRS at 0.5 T. *Neurology* **56**:737–742.

Barker, P., B. Soher, S. Blackband, J. Chatham, V. Mathews, and R. Bryan. 1993. Quantitation of proton NMR spectra of the human brain using tissue water as an internal concentration reference. *NMR Biomed.* **6**:89–94.

Barker, P. B., R. R. Lee, and J. C. McArthur. 1995. AIDS dementia complex: evaluation with proton MR spectroscopic imaging. *Radiology* **195**:58–64.

Birken, D. L., and W. H. Oldendorf. 1989. N-Acetyl-L-aspartic acid: a literature review of a compound prominent in ^{1}H-NMR spectroscopic studies of brain. *Neurosci. Biobehav. Rev.* **13**:23–31.

Bottomley, P. A., C. J. Hardy, J. P. Cousins, M. Armstrong, and W. A. Wagle. 1990. AIDS dementia complex: brain high-energy phosphate metabolite deficits. *Radiology* **176**:407–411.

Brand, A., C. Richter-Landsberg, and D. Leibfritz. 1993. Multinuclear NMR studies on the energy metabolism of glial and neuronal cells. *Dev. Neurosci.* **15**:289–298.

Chang, L., T. Ernst, M. Leonido-Yee, I. Walot, and E. Singer. 1999a. Cerebral metabolite abnormalities correlate with clinical severity of HIV-cognitive motor complex. *Neurology* **52**:100–108.

Chang, L., T. Ernst, M. Leonido-Yee, M. Witt, O. Speck, I. Walot, and E. N. Miller. 1999b. Highly active antiretroviral therapy reverses brain metabolite abnormalities in mild HIV dementia. *Neurology* **53**:782–789.

Chang, L., T. Ernst, R. Poland, and D. Jenden. 1996. In vivo proton magnetic resonance spectroscopy of the normal human aging brain. *Life Sci.* **58**:2049–2056.

Chang, L., T. Ernst, C. St Hillaire, and K. Conant. 2004a. Antiretroviral treatment alters relationship between MCP-1 and neurometabolites in HIV patients. *Antivir. Ther.* **9**:431–440.

Chang, L., T. Ernst, M. Witt, N. Ames, J. Jocivich, O. Speck, M. Gaiefsky, I. Walot, and E. Miller. 2002. Relationships among cerebral metabolites, cognitive function and viral loads in antiretroviral-naïve HIV patients. *Neuroimage* **17**:1638–1648.

Chang, L., T. Ernst, M. Witt, J. Jocivich, I. Walot, M. DeSilva, N. Ames, N. Trivedi, and E. Miller. 2000. Cerebral metabolite abnormalities in antiretroviral-naïve HIV patients before and after HAART. *Neurology* **54**:S47.002.

Chang, L., P. Lee, C. Yiannoutsos, T. Ernst, C. Marra, T. Richards, D. Kolson, G. Schifitto, J. Jarvik, E. Miller, R. Lenkinski, G. Gonzalez, B. Navia, and the HIV MRS Consortium. 2004b. A multicenter in vivo proton-MRS study of HIV-associated dementia and its relationship to age. *Neuroimage* **23**:1336–1347.

Chang, L., M. Witt, E. Miller, J. Jovicich, N. Ames, W. Zhu, M. Gaiefsky, and T. Ernst. 2001. Cerebral metabolite changes during the first nine months of HAART. *Neurology* **56**:S63.001.

Chong, W. K., M. Paley, I. D. Wilkinson, M. A. Hall-Craggs, B. Sweeney, M. J. Harrison, R. F. Miller, and B. E. Kendall. 1994. Localized cerebral proton MR spectroscopy in HIV infection and AIDS. *Am. J. Neuroradiol.* **15**:21–25.

Chong, W. K., B. Sweeney, I. D. Wilkinson, M. Paley, M. A. Hall-Craggs, B. E. Kendall, J. K. Shepard, M. Beecham, R. F. Miller, I. V. Weller, S. P. Newman, and M. J. Harrison.

1993. Proton spectroscopy of the brain in HIV infection: correlation with clinical, immunologic and MR imaging findings. *Radiology* **188**:119–124.

Conant, K., A. Garzino-Demo, A. Nath, J. McArthur, W. Halliday, C. Power, R. Gallo, and E. Major. 1998. Induction of monocyte chemoattractant protein-1 in HIV-1 tat-stimulated astrocytes and elevation in AIDS dementia. *Proc. Natl. Acad. Sci. USA* **95**:3117–3121.

Cortey, A., J. G. Jarvik, R. E. Lenkinski, R. I. Grossman, I. Frank, and M. Deliveria-Papadopoulos. 1994. Proton MR spectroscopy of brain abnormalities in neonates born to HIV-positive mothers. *Am. J. Neuroradiol.* **15**:1853–1859.

d'Arminio Monforte, A., P. G. Duca, L. Vago, M. P. Grassi, and M. Moroni. 2000. Decreasing incidence of CNS AIDS-defining events associated with antiretroviral therapy. *Neurology* **54**:1856–1859.

Deicken, R. F., B. Hubesch, P. C. Jensen, D. Sappey-Marinier, P. Krell, A. Wisniewski, D. Vandenburg, R. Parks, G. Fein, and M. W. Weiner. 1991. Alterations in brain phosphate metabolite concentrations in patients with human immunodeficiency virus infection. *Arch. Neurol.* **48**:203–209.

English, C., M. Kaufman, J. Worth, S. Babb, C. Drebiing, B. Navia, and P. Renshaw. 1997. Elevated frontal lobe cytosolic choline levels in minimal or mild AIDS dementia complex patients: a proton magnetic resonance spectroscopy study. *Biol. Psychiatry* **41**:500–502.

Ernst, T., and L. Chang. 1996. Elimination of artifacts in short echo time ^{1}H MR spectroscopy of the frontal lobe. *Magn. Reson. Med.* **36**:462–468.

Ernst, T., and L. Chang. 2004. Effect of aging on brain metabolism in antiretroviral-naive HIV patients. *AIDS* **18**:S61–S67.

Ernst, T., E. Itti, L. Itti, and L. Chang. 2000. Changes in cerebral metabolism are detected prior to perfusion changes in early HIV-CMC: a coregistered ^{1}H MRS and SPECT study. *J. Magn. Reson. Imaging* **12**:859–865.

Ernst, T., R. Kreis, and B. D. Ross. 1993. Absolute quantitation of water and metabolites in the human brain. I: compartments and water. *J. Magn. Reson.* **B102**:1–8.

Fiscus, S., A. Adimora, V. Schoenbach, W. Lim, R. McKinney, D. Rupar, J. Kenny, C. Woods, and C. Wilfert. 1996. Perinatal HIV infection and the effect of zidovudine therapy on transmission in rural and urban counties. *JAMA* **275**:1483–1488.

Gonzalez, R., L. Cheng, S. Westmoreland, and K. Sakaie. 2000. Early brain injury in the SIV-macaque model of AIDS. *AIDS* **14**:2841–2849.

Graf, J., W. Guggino, and K. Turnheim. 1993. Volume regulation in transporting epithelia, p. 67–117. *In* F. Lang, and D. Häussinger (ed.), *Interactions in Cell Volume and Cell Function*. Springer-Verlag, Heidelberg, Germany.

Jarvik, J. G., R. E. Lenkinski, R. I. Grossman, J. M. Gomori, M. D. Schnall, and I. Frank. 1993. Proton MR spectroscopy of HIV-infected patients: characterization of abnormalities with imaging and clinical correlation. *Radiology* **186**:739–744.

Jarvik, J. G., R. E. Lenkinski, A. J. Saykin, A. Jaans, and I. Frank. 1996. Proton spectroscopy in asymptomatic HIV-infected adults: initial results in a prospective cohort study. *J. Acquir. Immune Defic. Syndr. Hum. Retrovirol.* **13**:247–253.

Keller, M., T. Venkatraman, A. Thomas, A. Deveikis, C. LoPresti, J. Hayes, N. Berman, I. Walot, S. Padilla, J. Johnston-Jones, T. Ernst, and L. Chang. 2004. Altered neurometabolite development in HIV-infected children: correlation with neuropsychological tests. *Neurology* **62**:1810–1817.

Laubenberger, J., D. Haussinger, S. Bayer, S. Thielemann, B. Schneider, A. Mundinger, J. Hennig, and M. Langer. 1996. HIV-related metabolic abnormalities in the brain: depiction with proton MR spectroscopy with short echo times. *Radiology* **199**:805–810.

Lobato, M., M. Caldwell, P. Ng, and M. Oxtoby. 1995. Encephalopathy in children with perinatally acquired human immunodeficiency virus infection. *J. Pediatr.* **126**:710–715.

Lopez-Villegas, D., R. E. Lenkinski, and I. Frank. 1997. Biochemical changes in the frontal lobe of HIV-infected individuals detected by magnetic resonance spectroscopy. *Proc. Natl. Acad. Sci. USA* **94**:9854–9859.

Lu, D., S. G. Pavlakis, Y. Frank, S. Bakshi, S. Pahwa, R. J. Gould, C. Sison, C. Hsu, M. Lesser, H. M, T. Barnett, and R. A. Hyman. 1996. Proton MR spectroscopy of the basal ganglia in healthy children and children with AIDS. *Radiology* **199**:423–428.

Marcus, C., S. Taylor-Robinson, J. Sargentoni, J. Ainsworth, G. Frize, P. Easterbrook, S. Shaunak, and D. Bryant. 1998. [1]H MR spectroscopy of the brain in HIV-1 seropositive subjects: evidence for diffuse metabolic abnormalities. *Metab. Brain. Dis.* **13**:123–136.

McConnell, J. R., S. Swindells, C. S. Ong, W. H. Gmeiner, W. K. Chu, D. K. Brown, and H. E. Gendelman. 1994. Prospective utility of cerebral proton magnetic resonance spectroscopy in monitoring HIV infection and its associated neurological impairment. *AIDS Res. Hum. Retrovir.* **10**:977–982.

Menon, D. K., J. G. Ainsworth, and I. J. Cox. 1992. Proton MR spectroscopy of the brain in AIDS dementia complex. *J. Comput. Assist. Tomogr.* **16**:538–542.

Menon, D. K., C. J. Baudouin, D. Tomlinson, and C. Hoyle. 1990. Proton MR spectroscopy and imaging of the brain in AIDS: evidence for neuronal loss in regions that appear normal with imaging. *J. Comput. Assist. Tomogr.* **16**:882–885.

Meyerhoff, D., C. Bloomer, V. Cardenas, D. Norman, M. Weiner, and G. Fein. 1999. Elevated subcortical choline metabolites in cognitively and clinically asymptomatic HIV+ patients. *Neurology* **52**:995–1003.

Meyerhoff, D., S. MacKay, N. Poole, and W. Dillon. 1994. N-Acetylaspartate reductions measured by ^{1}H MRSI in cognitively impaired HIV-seropositive individuals. *Magn. Reson. Imaging* **12**:653–659.

Meyerhoff, D., M. Weiner, and G. Fein. 1996. Deep gray matter structures in HIV infection: a proton MR spectroscopic study. *Am. J. Neuroradiol.* **17**:973–978.

Meyerhoff, D. J., S. MacKay, L. Bachman, N. Poole, W. P. Dillon, M. W. Weiner, and G. Fein. 1993. Reduced brain N-acetylaspartate suggests neuronal loss in cognitively impaired immunodeficiency virus-seropositive individuals: in vivo ^{1}H magnetic resonance spectroscopic imaging. *Neurology* **43**:509–515.

Meyerhoff, D. J., S. MacKay, D. Sappey-Marinier, R. Deicken, G. Calabrese, W. P. Dillon, M. W. Weiner, and G. Fein. 1995. Effects of chronic alcohol abuse and HIV infection on brain phosphorus metabolites. *Alcohol Clin. Exp. Res.* **19**:685–692.

Mierisova, S., and M. Ala-Korpela. 2001. MR spectroscopy quantitation: a review of frequency domain methods. *NMR Biomed.* **14**:247–259.

Miller, B. L., L. Chang, R. Booth, T. Ernst, M. Cornford, D. Nikas, D. McBride, and D. J. Jenden. 1996. In vivo ^{1}H MRS choline: correlation with in vitro chemistry/histology. *Life Sci.* **58**:1929–1935.

Moller, H., P. Vermathen, M. Lentschig, G. Schuierer, S. Schwarz, D. Wiedermann, S. Evers, and I. Husstedt. 1999. Metabolic characterization of AIDS dementia complex by spectroscopic imaging. *J. Magn. Reson. Imaging* **9**:10–18.

Paley, M., P. Cozzone, J. Alonso, J. Vion-Dury, S. Confort-Gouny, I. Wilkinson, W. Chong, M. Hall-Craggs, M. Harrison, J. Gili, A. Rovira, J. Capellades, I. Rio, I. Ocana, F. Nicoli, C. Dhiver, J. Gastaut, J. Gastaut, K. Wicklow, and R. Sauter. 1996. A multicenter proton magnetic spectroscopy study of neurological complications of AIDS. *AIDS Res. Hum. Retrovir.* **12**:213–222.

Paley, M., I. D. Wilkinson, M. A. Hall-Craggs, W. K. Chong, R. J. Chinn, and M. J. Harrison. 1995. Short echo time proton spectroscopy of the brain in HIV infection/AIDS. *Magn. Reson. Imaging* 13:871–875.

Patton, H., W. Chu, H. Hetherington, J. den Hollander, K. Stewart, J. Raper, B. Shelton, E. Benveniste, and D. Benos. 2001. Alkaline pH changes in the cerebellum of asymptomatic HIV-infected individuals. *NMR Biomed.* 14:12–18.

Pavlakis, S. G., D. Lu, Y. Frank, A. Wiznia, D. Eidelberg, T. Barnett, and R. A. Hyman. 1998. Brain lactate and N-acetylaspartate in pediatric AIDS encephalopathy. *Am. J. Neuroradiol.* 19:383–385.

Podell, M., K. Maruyama, M. Smith, K. Hayes, W. Buck, D. Ruehlmann, and L. Mathes. 1999. Frontal lobe neuronal injury correlates to altered function in FIV-infected cats. *J. Acquir. Immune Defic. Syndr.* 22:10–18.

Power, C., P. A. Kong, T. O. Crawford, S. Wesselingh, J. D. Glass, J. C. McArthur, and B. D. Trapp. 1993. Cerebral white matter changes in acquired immunodeficiency syndrome dementia: alterations of the blood-brain barrier. *Ann. Neurol.* 34:339–350.

Provencher, S. 1993. Estimation of metabolite concentrations from localized in vivo proton NMR spectra. *Magn. Reson. Med.* 30:672.

Sacktor, N., L. Bobo, M. Pomper, T. Ernst, K. Zhong, L. Chang, D. Shungu, X. Mao, K. Marder, D. Shibata, G. Schiffito, and P. Barker. 2001. A comparison of two magnetic resonance spectroscopy techniques in subjects with HIV-associated cognitive impairment: the NARC-005 study. *Neurology* 56:S63.002.

Sacktor, N., R. Lyles, R. Skolasky, D. Anderson, J. McArthur, G. McFarlane, O. Selnes, J. Becker, B. Cohen, J. Wesch, and E. Miller. 1999. Combination antiretroviral therapy improves psychomotor speed performance in HIV-seropositive homosexual men. Multicenter AIDS Cohort Study (MACS). *Neurology* 52:1640–1647.

Salvan, A., J. Vion-Dury, S. Confort-Gouny, F. Nicoli, S. Lamoureux, and P. Cozzone. 1997a. Brain proton magnetic resonance spectroscopy in HIV-related encephalopathy: identification of evolving metabolic patterns in relation to dementia and therapy. *AIDS Res. Hum. Retrovir.* 13:1055–1066.

Salvan, A., J. Vion-Dury, S. Confort-Gouny, F. Nicoli, S. Lamoureux, and P. Cozzone. 1997b. Cerebral metabolic alterations in human immunodeficiency virus related encephalopathy detected by proton magnetic resonance spectroscopy. Comparison using short and long echo times. *Invest. Radiol.* 32:485–495.

Salvan, A.-M., S. Lamoureux, G. Michel, S. Confort-Gouny, P. J. Cozzone, and J. Vion-Dury. 1998. Localized proton magnetic resonance spectroscopy of the brain in children infected with human immunodeficiency virus with and without encephalopathy. *Pediatr. Res.* 44:755–762.

Schuff, N., D. Amend, R. Knowlton, D. Norman, G. Fein, and M. Weiner. 1999. Age-related metabolite changes and volume loss in the hippocampus by magnetic resonance spectroscopy and imaging. *Neurobiol. Aging* 20:279–285.

Simone, I., F. Federico, C. Tortorella, C. Andreula, G. Zimatore, P. Giannini, G. Angarano, V. Lucivero, P. Picciola, D. Cazrrara, A. Bellacosa, and P. Livrea. 1998. Localised 1H-MR spectroscopy for metabolic characterisation of diffuse and focal brain lesions in patients infected with HIV. *J. Neurol. Neurosurg. Psychiatry* 64:516–523.

Spielman, D., E. Adalsteinsson, and K. Lim. 1998. Quantitative assessment of improved homogeneity using higher-order shims for spectroscopic imaging of the brain. *Magn. Reson. Med.* 40:376–382.

Stankoff, B., A. Tourbah, S. Suarez, E. Turell, J. Stievenart, C. Payan, A. Coutellier, S. Herson, L. Baril, F. Bricaire, V. Calvez, E. Cabanis, L. Lacomblez, and C. Lubetzki. 2001. Clinical and spectroscopic improvement in HIV-associated cognitive impairment. *Neurology* 56:112–115.

Suhy, J., W. Rooney, D. Goodkin, A. Capizzano, B. Soher, A. Maudsley, E. Waubant, P. Andersson, and M. Weiner. 2000. 1H MRSI comparison of white matter and lesions in primary progressive and relapsing-remitting MS. *Mult. Scler.* 6:148–155.

Suwanwelaa, N., P. Phanuphak, K. Phanthumchinda, N. Suwanwela, J. Tantivatana, K. Ruxrungtham, J. Suttipan, S. Wangsuphachart, and M. Hanvanich. 2000. Magnetic resonance spectroscopy of the brain in neurologically asymptomatic HIV-infected patients. *Magn. Reson. Imaging* 18:859–865.

Tracey, I., C. A. Carr, A. R. Guimaraes, J. L. Worth, B. A. Navia, and R. G. Gonzalez. 1996. Brain choline-containing compounds are elevated in HIV-positive patients before the onset of AIDS dementia complex: a proton magnetic resonance spectroscopic study. *Neurology* 46:783–788.

Tracey, I., J. Lane, I. Chang, B. Navia, A. Lackner, and R. Gonzalez. 1997. 1H magnetic resonance spectroscopy reveals neuronal injury in a simian immunodeficiency virus macaque model. *J. Acquir. Immune. Defic. Syndr. Hum. Retrovirol.* 15:21–27.

Vanhamme, L., T. Sundin, P. Hecke, and S. Huffel. 2001. MR spectroscopy quantitation: a review of time-domain methods. *NMR Biomed.* 14:233–246.

von Giesen, H., H. Wittsack, F. Wenserski, H. Koller, and G. Arendt. 2001. Basal ganglia metabolite abnormalities in minor motor disorder associated with human immunodeficiency virus type 1. *Arch. Neurol.* 58:1281–1286.

Wilkinson, I., R. Miller, K. Miszkiel, M. Paley, M. Hall-Craggs, T. Baldeweg, I. Williams, S. Carter, S. Newman, B. Kendall, J. Catalan, R. Chinn, and M. Harrison. 1997a. Cerebral proton magnetic resonance spectroscopy in asymptomatic HIV infection. *AIDS* 11:289–295.

Wilkinson, I. D., S. Lunn, K. A. Miszkiel, R. F. Miller, M. N. Paley, I. Williams, R. J. Chinn, M. A. Hall-Craggs, S. P. Newman, B. E. Kendall, and M. Harrison. 1997b. Proton MRS and quantitative MRI assessment of the short term neurological response to antiretroviral therapy in AIDS. *J. Neurol. Neurosurg. Psychiatry* 63:477–482.

Wilkinson, I. D., M. Paley, W. K. Chong, B. Sweeney, J. K. Shepherd, B. E. Kendall, M. A. Hall-Craggs, and M. J. Harrison. 1994. Proton spectroscopy in HIV infection: relaxation times of cerebral metabolites. *Magn. Reson. Imaging* 12:951–957.

Yiannoutsos, C., T. Ernst, L. Chang, P. Lee, T. Richards, C. Marra, D. Meyerhoff, J. Jarvik, D. Kolson, G. Schifitto, R. Ellis, S. Swindells, D. Simpson, E. Miller, R. Gonzalez, and B. Navia. 2004. Regional patterns of brain metabolites in AIDS dementia complex. *Neuroimage* 23:928–935.

HIV COMORBIDITIES

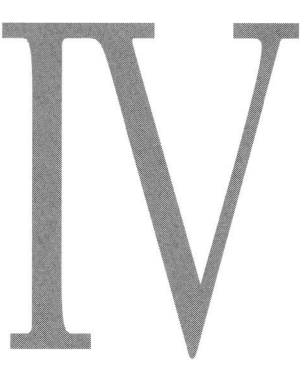

The Spectrum of Neuro-AIDS Disorders:
Pathophysiology, Diagnosis, and Treatment
Edited by K. Goodkin et al.
©2008 ASM Press, Washington, DC

21

Hepatitis C Virus: Variability, Extrahepatic Replication, and Neuroinvasion

MAREK RADKOWSKI, JONATHAN NASSERI, AND TOMASZ LASKUS

HCV EPIDEMIOLOGY AND BIOLOGY

Hepatitis C virus (HCV) is the major etiologic agent of parenterally transmitted non-A, non-B hepatitis (Choo et al., 1989; Kuo et al., 1989). In 75 to 85% of cases HCV infection persists indefinitely, leading to chronic hepatitis, cirrhosis, and hepatocellular carcinoma (Alter et al., 1992; Kiyosawa et al., 1990; Simonetti et al., 1992). However, since acute infection is typically mild, it is often unrecognized until the late-stage complications develop. Chronic HCV infection is quite common: estimates of its prevalence range between 0.3 and 4% for most parts of the world (Nishioka, 1994), and it constitutes an important cause of morbidity and mortality. The prevalence of anti-HCV in the United States is 1.8%, and approximately 2.7 million Americans carry the virus (Alter et al., 1999). Seeff et al. have recently reported on the long-term outcome in a cohort of patients infected through blood transfusion. A 25-year follow-up of the hepatitis C cases revealed viremia with chronic hepatitis in 38% of patients, viremia without chronic hepatitis in 39%, anti-HCV without viremia in 17%, and no residual HCV markers in 7%. Thirty-five percent of hepatitis C patients who were subjected to biopsies because of biochemically defined chronic hepatitis displayed cirrhosis, representing 17% of all those originally infected with HCV (Seeff et al., 2001).

Despite significant progress, the mechanisms behind HCV persistence are still unclear. The host usually mounts a vigorous humoral and cellular immune response; sera from infected humans were found to neutralize virus preparation inoculated into chimpanzees (Farci et al., 1994), and immunodominant B-cell sites have been identified within the envelope 2 (E2) glycoprotein as well as within the core region and nonstructural proteins (Cerino and Mondelli, 1991; Nasoff et al., 1991; Scarselli et al., 1995). Similarly, HLA class II-restricted (CD4[+]) and class I-restricted (CD8[+])

T-cell responses against a variety of viral polypeptides are generally demonstrable in vitro during chronic HCV infection (Botarelli et al., 1993; Ferrari et al., 1994; Hoffmann et al., 1995; Koziel et al., 1992, 1993; Schupper et al., 1993; Shirai et al., 1994). In a minority of HCV-positive individuals who clear HCV infection, viral clearance is associated with vigorous multispecific CD4 T-cell responses that are maintained, while "viral escape" is related to defective and narrow CD4 cell responses with continued dysregulation (Eckels et al., 2000; Gerlach et al., 1999). Studies of CD8-specific cytotoxic activity suggest great variability during chronic infection but vigorous cytotoxic T-lymphocyte (CTL) activity in those who clear HCV (Gruener et al., 2001; Koziel et al., 1993, 1995). However, it is clear that in spite of broad immune response HCV manages to escape eradication in the majority of infected individuals. Recent studies focusing on HCV survival strategies revealed that viral proteins may interfere with pathways of retinoid-acid-inducible gene I and Toll-like receptor 3, which constitute two major pathways of host defense triggered by viral nucleic acids. In particular, HCV seems to interfere at several different points with interferon (IFN) and IFN-stimulated gene signaling (Gale and Foy, 2005). A second powerful strategy employed by the virus is genetic variability resulting in the constant and dynamic development of variants capable of avoiding eradication by host defenses.

QUASISPECIES NATURE OF HCV

Like many other RNA viruses HCV is characterized by a high degree of genetic heterogeneity due to low viral RNA polymerase fidelity resulting from lack of proofreading 3' to 5' exonuclease activity (Choo et al., 1991; Domingo et al., 1985). As a consequence of high mutation and rapid turnover rates—it is estimated that 10^{12} virions may be produced and cleared each day (Neumann et al., 1998)—HCV circulates as a population of closely related but nonidentical genomes, referred to as quasispecies (Domingo et al., 1985; Martell et al., 1992; Steinhauer and Holland, 1987). It is

Marek Radkowski, Institute of Infectious Diseases, Warsaw Medical Academy, Warsaw, Poland. **Jonathan Nasseri and Tomasz Laskus,** St. Joseph's Hospital and Medical Center, Phoenix, AZ 85013.

assumed that at any given moment during the natural history of the infection the quasispecies distribution represents the best-fitting population that has established a status of equilibrium with host (Domingo et al., 1985).

However, the genetic heterogeneity is not uniform throughout the genome. The most highly conserved are the 5′ untranslated region (5′UTR) and the terminal part of the 3′ untranslated region (3′UTR), as their variability is constrained by the requirement for specific secondary structures. The capsid protein is the most conserved region of the viral single open reading frame, followed by sequences coding the nonstructural 3 (NS3) and nonstructural 5 B (NS5B) proteins, whereas the genes encoding the two envelope proteins E1 and E2 are the most heterogeneous parts of viral genome (Choo et al., 1991; Ogata et al., 1991; Okamoto et al., 1992). The N-terminal end of the E2 contains the most variable region of the entire genome and is called hypervariable region 1 (HVR1) (Hijikata et al., 1991; Weiner et al., 1991). The latter encodes a prominent B-cell epitope on the E2 envelope protein (Shirai et al., 1999), and its high mutation rate could contribute to the evasion of the host immune response (Scarselli et al., 1995; Weiner et al., 1991, 1992). The existence of multiple variants within quasispecies could be responsible for inefficient protective immunity: it was demonstrated in chimpanzees that persistent infection does not provide protection against subsequent infection with heterologous and even with homologous strains (Farci et al., 1992; Okamoto et al., 1994; Prince et al., 1992). The evidence that this is the case in humans is limited; however, Eyster et al. (1999) documented a common change of infecting HCV genotypes over time in high-risk patients with hemophilia. Similarly, it was shown that chronically infected patients can be superinfected with new HCV strains in the setting of blood transfusion whereby chronically infected patients were exposed to HCV-positive blood (Laskus et al., 2001) and in the setting of liver transplantation whereby patients with end-stage HCV-related liver disease received an organ from an infected donor (Laskus et al., 1996). Interestingly, the superinfecting strain often became dominant, eliminating or suppressing replication of the original virus below detection level. As the neutralizing antibodies are isolate specific, they may be ineffective against other variants present in the complex of quasispecies: in a chimpanzee challenge experiment a hyperimmune anti-HVR1 serum raised against the predominant strain present in the inoculum was able to neutralize the predominant clone but was ineffective against minor variants (Farci et al., 1994). Further evidence of the important role of humoral immune pressure in driving HVR1 variability is provided by the reported lack of genetic variations in patients with agammaglobulinemia (Kumar et al., 1994).

Nevertheless, it should be emphasized that a large part of HCV quasispecies studies come from experiments conducted with chimpanzees, in which the HCV infection may be profoundly different from that observed in humans. Thus, the baseline HCV replication in chimpanzees is typically very low, liver pathology is mild, and the virus itself shows very little variation in chronic infection (Bassett et al., 1999). Moreover, the immune response, particularly against E2, is weak (Choo et al., 1994). Chimpanzees may develop persistent infection despite the lack of viral quasispecies in the inoculum as documented by infection with monoclonal viruses derived from cDNA clones (Major et al., 1999). In addition, persistent viremia developed even when the infecting clone contained a deletion of the entire HVR1 (Forns et al., 2000).

HCV QUASISPECIES IN TRANSMISSION OF INFECTION

Several studies have reported that transmission of infection may be limited to a few variants present within the quasispecies population. Thus, viral populations found in children infected at birth were found to be more homogeneous than those in mothers (Kudo et al., 1997; Weiner et al., 1993). Similar results were reported from studies conducted with chimpanzees, in which only a few of the viral variants present in the inoculum would establish infection (Hijikata et al., 1995; Sugitani and Shikata, 1998). Also, in patients undergoing liver transplantation for HCV-related liver disease, the recurrent infection was characterized by a lower complexity (number of distinct viral variants) than that observed in the pretransplant viral population (Gretch et al., 1996; Martell et al., 1994). What determines this selective diminished complexity is unclear, but in the chimpanzee infection model it was suggested that the presence of antibodies to the HVR1 glycoprotein is protective and contributes toward the selective replication of "free" HCV (Kojima et al., 1994). This is compatible with observations that antibody-bound HCV particles were found in mothers who did not transmit infection to their offspring (Kudo et al., 1997). However, it should be emphasized that the issue of selective transmission is not settled, as the studies conducted so far are few and included a very limited number of subjects. Obviously, they often relate to very different situations in which different mechanisms may be operational: for example, during vertical transmission the infecting inoculum is probably too small to contain all the viral variants, whereas in liver transplantation the infection is undoubtedly massive but the issue is complicated by changed major histocompatibility complex type of the infected organ, which would alter the recognition of viral antigens, and by pharmacologically induced immunosuppression. The issue of quasispecies transmission is further complicated by the technical difficulties associated with quasispecies analysis. Thus, the most commonly used technique, i.e., sequencing of cloned PCR products, is prone to artificial polymorphism introduced during cloning due to preferential selection of genomes by *Escherichia coli* and is also influenced by sampling errors resulting from the typically small number of analyzed clones (Forns et al., 1997; Smith et al., 1997). Furthermore, the error rate of *Taq* DNA polymerase, which is estimated to be in the range of 0.2×10^4 to 2×10^4, ensures the presence of artifactual background variation whenever individual clones are analyzed (Smith et al., 1997).

We recently approached the issue of quasispecies transmission by employing heteroduplex mobility and single-strand conformational polymorphism assays, which circumvent many of the problems inherent in the analysis of cloned PCR products. In particular, the latter technique is very suitable for this kind of analysis because it can differentiate between sequences differing by a single nucleotide substitution and can at the same time identify minor variants constituting as little as 1.5 to 3% of the total population (Laskus et al., 2004b). The 3% detection sensitivity is equivalent to analyzing 99 clones per sample (confidence, 95%).

In the first of these studies, which was conducted with 15 patients infected through blood transfusion, in 10 (67%) recipients the posttransfusion E2/HVR1 quasispecies composition closely matched that found in the donor, whereas in 14 of 15 blood recipients all 5′UTR viral variants present in donors established infection in respective recipients. It is highly unlikely that this was due simply to passive transmission of donor virus, since this pattern persisted for at least several weeks. HCV is estimated to have a half-life of only a few hours in infected humans (Neumann et al., 1998), and in chimpanzee studies replication of HCV in the liver was demonstrated already a few days after infection (Farci et al., 1992; Shindo et al., 1992). Thus, the HCV RNA present in posttransfusion samples almost certainly represented actively replicating virus. The second study was conducted in the liver transplantation setting. Among 34 patients with end-stage HCV-related liver disease who received organs from uninfected patients, in 18 (53%) patients all variants present before transplantation established infection in the new organ (Arenas et al., 2004). The above studies support the notion that quasispecies equilibrium may be preserved from host to host.

HCV QUASISPECIES AND ACUTE INFECTION

A minority of patients can mount an effective immune response and clear the virus in the early phase of infection (Kenny-Walsh, 1999; Purcell, 1997). However, studies of the dynamics of HCV quasispecies in transmission and the natural course of infection from acute hepatitis to resolution or chronicity are extremely limited mainly due to difficulties in obtaining samples from patients during the early phase of primary infection and the lack of subsequent long-term follow-up. Securing samples from subjects who are the source of infection is even more difficult, as most new infections are currently associated either with intravenous drug use or with sexual exposure (Alter, 1999). Manzin et al. (1998) studied three acute hepatitis cases and found a different pattern of genetic evolution in each one. However, the mode of infection was different in each case, and altogether only 18 samples, drawn at 1- to 6-month intervals, were analyzed. More important, none of the studied cases cleared the virus. In another study Ray et al. (1999) compared 5 intravenous drug users (IDU) who cleared the viremia with 10 IDU who remained chronically infected. Patients who developed chronic hepatitis showed higher quasispecies complexity (number of viral variants) and a higher ratio of nonsynonymous (amino acid replacement) to synonymous (silent) nucleotide substitutions within the HVR1. However, only a single sample, drawn many months before or after detectable seroconversion, was analyzed, ensuring that the patients studied were at a different stage of infection. In addition, a small number of analyzed clones made the sampling error likely. So far the most extensive study of quasispecies in acute hepatitis is the one published by Farci et al. (2000). The analysis included three patients with acute resolving illness and six patients with acute hepatitis that progressed to chronicity. This study provided for the first time evidence that analysis of evolution of viral quasispecies during the acute phase could predict whether the infection will resolve or become chronic. Resolving hepatitis was characterized by homogeneous viral population and relative evolutionary stasis, whereas chronic infection was associated with genetic evolution within the first months of infection. However, the technique employed, i.e., sequencing of a limited number of clones from each sample (mean, 10.6), was not suitable to detect minor variants. In addition, only three to four samples from each case were studied, and the donor samples implicated in infection transmission were not available for analysis.

A unique opportunity to study natural HCV infection is provided by the Transfusion-Transmitted Viruses Study/ National Heart, Lung, and Blood Institute Repository. This prospective study of posttransfusion hepatitis was conducted in the years 1974 to 1980, when HCV was much more prevalent in the blood donor population. We analyzed 15 patients from the Transfusion-Transmitted Viruses Study, who were HCV negative at the time they received blood transfusions from HCV-infected donors (Laskus et al., 2004b). These cases were unique, as parental genomes from the actual infecting units of blood were defined and multiple follow-up samples were available from the infected recipient. Furthermore, in a late-term follow-up serum samples were collected from each infected patient 11 to 16 years after the original study (Seeff et al., 2001).

Analysis of seven patients with self-resolving hepatitis and eight patients who progressed to chronic infection revealed that in those patients who remained chronically infected the E2/HVR1 quasispecies underwent a series of dynamic changes, whereas in those who cleared infection, the quasispecies composition remained almost totally static. Importantly, the availability of numerous sequential samples allowed for determining the timing of changes. In our study the timing of viral clearance (mean and standard deviation, 14.0 ± 2.0 weeks; range, 7 to 24 weeks) coincided with the advent of quasispecies changes in those who remained chronically infected (mean and standard deviation, 13.1 ± 1.6 weeks; range, 8 to 22 weeks), suggesting that the mechanisms responsible for viral clearance and those driving E2/HVR1 quasispecies changes are the same. This is compatible with the primary role of immune pressure as the driving force behind quasispecies evolution in the E2/HVR1. In this scenario the immune host response is not strong enough to eliminate infection in a timely manner, thus allowing for the escape mutants to appear while rapid mutations could in turn constantly outpace the immune system. However, regardless of the underlying mechanism, the appearance of rapid changes in viral quasispecies composition seems to be predictive of ensuing chronic infection. Importantly, the chance for clearance of infection seems to be largely diminished after the initial acute phase: all patients who were found to be HCV RNA negative after 11 to 16 years cleared the infection within the first 7 to 24 weeks.

HCV INFECTION IN HIV-1-POSITIVE PATIENTS

HCV infection is common among HIV-positive patients, as the two pathogens share similar routes of transmission. In the United States and Europe, 13 to 43% of HIV-infected persons are also infected with HCV (Winnock et al., 2004), and this proportion is even higher among IDU. However, it seems that the interactions between the two pathogens are not confined to mere coexistence. First, HIV coinfection is likely to facilitate HCV spread: it was reported that dually HIV/HCV-infected mothers transmit HCV to infants at a much higher rate than mothers infected by HCV only (Granovsky et al., 1998; Thomas et al., 1998; Tovo et al., 1997). Similarly, horizontal, possibly sexual, transmission of HCV is more common in the HIV/HCV coinfection setting than in the setting of HCV monoinfection (Eyster et al., 1991). Second, HIV clearly accelerates the development of severe liver disease (Eyster et al., 1993; Garcia-Samaniego et al., 1997; Hanley et al., 1996; Ridzon et al., 1997). Paradoxically, recent reduction in mortality and morbidity among HIV-infected patients could have contributed to the emergence of HCV as a significant pathogen in this population (Monga et al., 1998). These negative effects of HIV on liver disease could be due to the increase of HCV replication in the setting of immunodeficiency. However, there is also evidence that HCV replication may be directly enhanced by the presence of HIV: HCV RNA levels were reported to be more closely associated with HIV RNA levels than with CD4+ T-cell counts (Thomas et al., 2001), and HIV seroconversion in HCV-infected patients is often associated with a burst of enhanced HCV replication (Beld et al., 1998). Furthermore, it was recently shown that concomitant HIV infection may facilitate HCV infection/replication in vitro (Laskus et al., 2004a).

HIV could also affect HCV quasispecies composition, and several studies suggest that there is a relationship between diversity of HCV and HIV disease progression. Thus, Mao et al. reported that HIV might affect HCV E2/HVR1 quasispecies by decreasing both complexity and the ratio of nonsynonymous to synonymous substitutions (Mao et al., 2001). Similar observations were reported by Toyoda et al. (1997). These effects could be related to HIV-induced immunosuppression and the ensuing lessening of selective pressure against HCV (Eckels et al., 2000; Farci et al., 2000).

There is emerging evidence that HCV infection may also negatively affect the course of HIV disease. Although some earlier studies suggested that the natural history of HIV infection is not influenced by concomitant HCV infection (Dorrucci et al., 1995; Wright et al., 1994), several recent reports found an association between HCV coinfection and progression of HIV disease (Lesens et al., 1999; Piroth et al., 1998; Sabin et al., 1997). In particular, a report from the Swiss cohort study, which included over 2,000 subjects, demonstrated that HIV/HCV-coinfected patients were more likely to develop AIDS-defining opportunistic infections than those infected with HIV only (Greub et al., 2000). Similar findings were reported in a large Italian study (De Luca et al., 2002) and recently among the Women's Interagency HIV-1 Study cohort patients (Kovacs et al., 2004). Among children with hemophilia, infection with HCV genotype 1 was associated with a lower CD4+ count and increased risk for progression to AIDS-related mortality (Yoo et al., 2005). The latter observation is interesting because genotype 1 and particularly genotype 1b were credibly associated with more severe chronic hepatitis, hepatocellular carcinoma, and rapid progression to cirrhosis and graft loss after liver transplantation (Gane et al., 1996; Nousbaum et al., 1995). However, Sulkowski et al. (2002) did not find any evidence that HCV infection substantially alters the risk of dying, developing AIDS, or responding immunologically to HAART. These discrepancies are difficult to sort out, particularly since the cohorts and their respective controls varied in demographics and epidemiologic background. In particular, HCV/HIV-coinfected patients are typically IDU, while HIV-monoinfected patients, who constitute the reference group, are usually infected through the sexual route. The nature of the above effects of HCV on HIV is unclear and could include immune activation secondary to HCV infection or intravenous drug use. However, some preliminary data in vitro suggest that concomitant HCV could inhibit HIV-induced apoptosis, thus perhaps delaying the elimination of HIV-infected cells. The latter study employed Daudi B-cell line expressing CD4, which is susceptible to both HIV and HCV infection (Kibler et al., 2003).

EXTRAHEPATIC REPLICATION OF HCV

HCV is a positive-strand RNA virus, which replicates through negative-strand RNA, the presence of which could be regarded as direct evidence of ongoing replication. However, strand-specific detection of RNA by reverse transcription-PCR, which is the most commonly applied technique for the detection of negative-strand RNA, is fraught with problems, as it has been demonstrated that it is prone to false priming of the incorrect strand or self-priming related to RNA secondary structures. These mispriming events can to a large extent be avoided by conducting cDNA synthesis at high temperature with thermostable enzyme Tth (Lanford et al., 1994). Several groups of researchers have detected HCV RNA-negative strand within peripheral blood mononuclear cells (PBMC), and it was also demonstrated that viral genomic sequences present in PBMC are often different from those found in serum and liver (Laskus et al., 1998a, 2000b; Lerat et al., 1998; Navas et al., 1998). These may occasionally belong to different genotypes altogether, and the latter phenomenon is likely to be the result of superinfection (Roque-Afonso et al., 2005). Furthermore, HCV RNA levels in the serum and PBMC do not correlate, which suggests differential regulation of viral replication at these compartments (Blackard et al., 2005). HCV RNA has also been detected in PBMC and hematopoietic progenitor cells by in situ hybridization (Samsonno et al., 1996). The presence of HCV replication was also documented in human hematopoietic cells inoculated into the severe combined immunodeficiency mice model (Bronowicki et al., 1998). Furthermore, it was reported that human T- and B-cell lines can support HCV infection, although at a low level (Nakajima et al., 1996; Shimizu et al., 1993). Importantly, the same minor quasispecies variants of HCV strain H77, which were selected in lymphoblastoid cells in vitro, were found to be replicating in vivo in PBMC of chimpanzees inoculated with the same parent strain (Shimizu et al., 1997). Within the population of PBMC, the cells harboring replicating virus have been identified primarily as monocytes/macrophages and B cells, although T cells can be infected as well, particularly in long-lasting infection (Bain et al., 2001; Ducoulombier et al., 2004; Laskus et al., 2000a). The above cells may manifest functional changes in chronic hepatitis C patients, although it is still unclear whether this is due directly to HCV infection. Thus, B-cell dysfunction is characterized by low-titer and delayed-onset antibody response and an increased frequency of naïve B cells (Chen et al., 1999; Ni et al., 2003), whereas monocyte-derived dendritic cells demonstrate impaired allostimulatory function (Auffermann-Gretzinger et al., 2001; Bain et al., 2001).

Some recent studies show that native human macrophages are susceptible to HCV infection in vitro (Caussin-Schwemling et al., 2001; Radkowski et al., 2004a). In our own study we demonstrated that after exposure to infectious sera in vitro, cultured macrophages can retain HCV RNA for 3 weeks, virus-negative-strand RNA is often detectable during this time, and the infecting strains may undergo changes, although it is unclear whether this is due to evolution or a successful growth of a minor variant already present in the infecting serum (Radkowski et al., 2004a). While the mere presence of HCV RNA in phagocytic cells could come, at least theoretically, from virions entrapped inside these cells or adsorbed on their surface, the presence of virus-negative strand and the occasional changes in viral sequence argue for the presence of genuine virus replication. HCV RNA-negative strand was detected only in a minority of cases; however, it is likely that the strand-specific assays are not sensitive enough to detect low-level extrahepatic replication. Indeed, in several studies they were found to be at least 1 log less sensitive than standard reverse transcription-PCR

(Lanford et al., 1994; Laskus et al., 1997). Importantly, in cells supporting HCV replication, negative RNA strands are generally detected at a lower level than positive strands (Lanford et al., 1994; Laskus et al., 1997).

Infected macrophages are likely to undergo functional changes. In one study exposure of primary macrophages to HCV-positive sera resulted in enhanced production of tumor necrosis factor alpha (TNF-α) and interleukin 8 (IL-8) and their respective mRNAs (Radkowski et al., 2004). TNF-α is a major component of the immune system involved in the control of virus infection through direct antiviral activity, usually in association with IFN-γ, and the induction of apoptosis (Herbein and O'Brien, 2000). It is made mainly by monocytes and macrophages, and its production was reported to increase when isolated human macrophages were infected with such RNA viruses as respiratory syncytial virus (Becker et al., 1991) or influenza A virus (Lehmann et al., 1996). Thus, production of TNF-α seems to be a natural response of macrophages to virus infection. IL-8 was originally described as a neutrophil chemotactic factor, but subsequent studies demonstrated its various effects on T cells and monocytes (Mukaida, 2000). There is growing evidence that infection with various viruses, or transfection with viral gene products, can induce IL-8 in different cells. For example, human cytomegalovirus (HCMV) infection can induce IL-8 production by concurrent activation of two distinct transcription factors, nuclear factor κB and activator protein-1 (Murayama et al., 1997); similar mechanisms of IL-8 gene transactivation were described for human T-cell leukemia virus type 1 Tax protein and hepatitis B virus X protein (Mahe et al., 1991; Mori et al., 1998). Interestingly, increased levels of IL-8 in serum were recently found in chronic hepatitis C patients (Polyak et al., 2001b), and the same group of researchers demonstrated that expression of HCV NS5A protein in human cells induces IL-8 mRNA and protein probably through a mechanism similar to that described previously for HCMV (Polyak et al., 2001a). Because monocytes are one of the main producers of IL-8 in vivo, they could be an important source of increased IL-8 levels in sera of chronic hepatitis C patients. Notably, IL-8 itself may directly promote virus replication. It was reported that IL-8 enhances HCMV and HIV-1 replication, probably by acting through its receptors CXCR1 (for HCMV) and CXCR1 and CXCR2 (for HIV-1) (Lane et al., 2001; Murayama et al., 1994). The effect on virus replication could also be indirect, as IL-8 was reported to reduce the antiviral activities of IFN-α. This inhibitory action on IFN-α antiviral activity was associated with reduced 2',5'-A oligoadenylate synthetase activity, a pathway well correlated with the antiviral action of IFN-α (Khabar et al., 1997). The latter mechanism has been postulated to promote HCV persistence and resistance to IFN therapy (Polyak et al., 2001a).

Infection of monocytes/macrophages by HCV is not unexpected, as these cells are known to be permissive to a wide range of viruses, including some other flaviviruses (Mogensen, 1979), and many RNA and DNA viruses are lymphotropic (Oldstone, 1996). HCV RNA in PBMC in the absence of HCV RNA in serum and concomitant absence of specific antibodies has been recently reported in a significant proportion of patients with chronic liver disease of unclear etiology (Castillo et al., 2004). While this by no means establishes an etiological connection between HCV and liver lesions present in these patients, it points to the likely existence of patients in whom the presence of HCV RNA in extrahepatic compartment is the only evidence of infection. The phenomenon of anti-HCV negativity despite the presence of HCV RNA in serum and/or PBMC may be due to the immaturity of the immune system, as it has been reported in infants born to HCV-infected mothers (Papaevangelou et al., 1998; Zanetti et al., 1995). However, an alternative explanation is that infection is at a low level and/or confined to PBMC, which could constitute an immunologically privileged site. It could be speculated that this form of infection is related to low-viral-load exposure. There may be similarities to other viral infections: exposure of woodchucks to a low load of woodchuck hepatitis virus was found to lead to low-level infection in PBMC but not in the liver, and specific antibodies did not develop (Michalak et al., 2004). A similar seronegative infection, in which the virus was detectable in the lymphatic system but not in the liver, was also documented to occur in vertical transmission of woodchuck hepatitis virus (Coffin and Michalak, 1999). Interestingly, chimpanzees challenged with low copy numbers of HCV were reported to develop cellular, but not humoral, immunity (Shata et al., 2003), and similar findings were recently reported among prospectively monitored high-risk human subjects (Post et al., 2004).

There is emerging evidence that HIV could facilitate HCV replication in vivo in the liver as well as at extrahepatic sites (Blackard et al., 2005; Daar et al., 2001; Laskus et al., 1998b; Sherman et al., 1993). It was recently shown that HIV coinfection may also facilitate HCV replication in vitro, either by rendering cells more susceptible to HCV infection or by increasing HCV replication (Laskus et al., 2004a). In that study monocytes/macrophages were collected from healthy donors, infected with HIV M-tropic molecular clone, and then exposed to HCV-positive sera. Preceding infection with HIV made the macrophages more susceptible to infection with HCV; in particular, HCV RNA-negative strand was detectable significantly more often in the setting of concomitant HIV infection. Importantly, the presence of NS3 was demonstrated by immunostaining in cells exposed to HCV-positive sera, and there was a highly significant positive correlation between the proportion of infected cells detectable by immunostaining and HCV RNA load in cell extracts. Furthermore, there was an increase in HCV RNA load in cell culture supernatant over the time of infection.

The positive correlation between HIV viral load at the time of HCV exposure and subsequent level of HCV replication suggests that HIV infection may increase the susceptibility of macrophages to HCV infection perhaps by activation of these cells. No such relationship was evident for HIV measured at 7 and 14 days, and high HIV replication could have even inhibited HCV replication at the late stage of infection, perhaps by taxing cell resources necessary for HCV replication. In the same study HIV infection was also found to facilitate HCV replication in a Daudi B-cell line with engineered CD4 expression. Importantly, in the same study it was also shown that the same cell may harbor both pathogens, which could facilitate close virus-virus interactions (Laskus et al., 2004a).

The mechanisms by which HIV could enhance extrahepatic HCV infection are still speculative, one possibility being that this effect is related to general immunosuppression. Accordingly, in one small study virus-negative strand was more common in PBMC from patients after liver transplantation than in patients before liver transplantation (Radkowski et al., 1998), and in a mouse model HCV replication was enhanced by the presence of immunodeficiency (Bronowicki et al., 1998). It has also been reported that removal of CD8$^+$ T cells results in increased HCV replication in PBMC cultures, which suggests that the innate immune system does exert some level of control over extrahepatic replication (Li et al., 2005). Another possibility is that extrahepatic HCV replication increase is related to HIV-induced cell activation. In support of such a possibility come observations that addition of pokeweed and phytohemagglutinin mitogens to PBMC cultures may significantly enhance HCV replication (Laskus et al., 2000a; Pham et al., 2004). However, HIV infection could also facilitate extrahepatic replication of HCV more directly. For example, the HIV tat protein is a strong transactivator, and a putative tat-binding motif was found in the NS4 region of HCV (Ferbeyre et al., 1997).

Facilitation of extrahepatic HCV replication by HIV could have clinical implications. In a recent study encompassing 75 HCV-infected women, 62 of whom were coinfected with HIV-1, local HIV viremia and the presence of HCV RNA in serum were the only independent predictors of HCV RNA in genital tract secretions. Significant (>600 IU/ml) HCV viremia in cervical lavage samples was present in 28% of HIV-coinfected women and in none of the HIV-negative women (Nowicki et al., 2005). Local interactions and possible coinfection of the same cells could perhaps explain the cotransmission of HIV with HCV reported in earlier mother-to-child transmission studies conducted before the introduction of HAART (Papaevangelou et al., 1998). However, after introduction of HAART, vertical transmission of HCV became rare. Interestingly, in the only published study analyzing the role of extrahepatic HCV replication in vertical transmission, the presence of both positive and negative viral strands in PBMC strongly correlated with transmission of infection to infants (Azzari et al., 2000). In light of the findings on the facilitating role of HIV for HCV macrophage infection, it is possible that children acquire infection from their mothers through infected cells, probably macrophages. This mechanism would be similar to perinatal transmission of HIV, which involves macrophage-tropic HIV-1 variants (Amedee et al., 1995; van't Wout et al., 1994). Cotransmission of both pathogens was also reported in sexual partners of HIV/HCV-coinfected hemophiliacs (Eyster et al., 1991).

The dynamic quasispecies nature of HCV could clearly facilitate viral adaptation to infect and replicate in various cells. Such changes could be relatively minor: for example, it has been demonstrated for lymphocytic choriomeningitis virus that strains differing by a single amino acid substitution, when inoculated together into a mouse, are competitively selected either by the liver and spleen or by neurons (Dockter et al., 1996). While the extent of viral changes necessary for successful colonizing of extrahepatic sites is unclear, it is intriguing that many sequences identified at nonliver sites share a common mutation in the 5'UTR (Forton et al., 2004; Laporte et al., 2000, 2003; Laskus et al., 1997, 2002; Lerat et al., 2000).

HCV genome translation starts at an internal ribosomal entry site (IRES) element, which comprises most of the 5'UTR and extends 12 to 30 nucleotides downstream of the initiation codon (Tsukiyama-Kohara et al., 1992; Wang et al., 1994). The importance of the 5'UTR in viral replication and translation is reflected by the fact that it is the most conserved region in the HCV genome, with a >85% homology between different viral strains (Bukh et al., 1992; Smith et al., 1995). Although IRES elements from different HCV genotypes and strains manifest differing translation efficiency in vitro (Buratti et al., 1997; Collier et al., 1998; Saiz et al., 1999), it is unclear at present whether these variations

affect clinical outcome (Thelu et al., 2004). It was shown that specific 5'UTR viral sequences harbored by monocyte-derived dendritic cells and macrophage/microglia may have lowered translational activity, which could result in lower viral replication and protein expression and could possibly facilitate viral persistence in these cells (Forton et al., 2004; Laporte et al., 2003). In addition, extrahepatic variants were also demonstrated to have low rates of nonsynonymous mutations in the hypervariable envelope region, which may suggest low immunologic pressure and/or low replication turnover, both of which could be conducive to viral persistence (Ducoulombier et al., 2004).

A recent study analyzing 5'UTR changes evolving during the natural course of transfusion-acquired hepatitis C and recurrent HCV infection after liver transplantation sheds some new light on the unexpected plasticity of this region. Functional effects of 5'UTR changes on IRES were analyzed using dual-luciferase reporter plasmid (Gallegos-Orozco et al., 2004). In that study the selection of 5'UTR variants seemed to follow two opposite patterns: in transfusion-acquired infection, low translation efficiency variants prevailed over the high-replicating variants, while in immunosuppressed liver transplant recipients, low translation efficiency variants were supplanted by high translation efficiency variants. Switching between high and low translation efficiency variants could represent a common mechanism aimed at adjusting viral replication to current host conditions and may be affected by the host immune status. Downregulation of viral replication could in effect lower antiviral immune response. There is evidence from the lymphocytic choriomeningitis virus infection model that low-replicating variants induce weaker CTL responses than more rapidly replicating strains (Bocharov et al., 2004). A direct relationship between the HCV replication kinetics and CTL response was also suggested by some human studies, although the number of patients analyzed so far is small (Thimme et al., 2001). Similarly, in the chimpanzee HCV infection model, an initial slow replication of infecting virus could predispose to subsequent chronic infection (Thimme et al., 2002).

Modern antiviral therapy is successful in approximately 50% of HCV-infected patients, resulting in clearance of HCV RNA from serum, which is usually accompanied by normalization of liver biochemical tests and improvement of liver histology (Lau et al., 1998; Lindsay, 2002). Currently accepted criteria for sustained virological response (SVR) require the patient to remain HCV RNA negative in serum for 6 months after termination of treatment when tested with an assay for which sensitivity is at least 100 viral copies/ml (Lindsay, 2002). Long-term virological outcome in patients with SVR has been analyzed only recently. Recurrence of infection, defined as reappearance of HCV RNA in serum, was found to be below 2% at 1 to 4 years after induction of SVR (McHutchison et al., 2001; Swain et al., 2001), although in one study in which patients were followed up for 3.5 to 8.8 years the relapse rate was as high as 8% (Reichard et al., 1999).

It is unclear whether ostensibly successful treatment of chronic hepatitis C or spontaneous clearance of infection results in sterilization, or whether low viral replication persists and is perhaps kept in check by cellular and humoral immune responses. Thus, the observation that specific antibodies and cellular immune response may persist for 2 decades after spontaneous resolution of acute hepatitis C could imply continuous antigen stimulation (Seeff et al., 2001; Takaki et al., 2000). In a recent report Pham et al. (2004) were able to amplify viral sequence from follow-up sera and/or PBMC in 11 of 11 SVR patients for up to 5 years after therapy. The majority of monocyte-derived dendritic cell cultures and mitogen-stimulated PBMC contained HCV RNA-negative strand as well. All those patients were HCV RNA negative in serum by commercial assays. In our recent study, only 2 of 17 patients were HCV RNA negative 40 to 109 months after SVR when tested in PBMC, liver, and serum by highly sensitive assays (Radkowski et al., 2004b). Viral HCV RNA sequences were detected in macrophage cultures from 11 patients (65%) and in lymphocyte cultures from 7 patients (41%).

It is currently unclear whether persistence of virus at extrahepatic sites could be responsible for treatment failures and whether patients could be reinfected by extrahepatic virus during or after therapy. However, in a recently published case report, an HCV-infected patient cleared the infection and subsequently experienced viral reactivation twice over the space of 8.5 years. Throughout that time the infecting viral strain remained virtually identical (Lee et al., 2005).

HCV EFFECT ON CNS

There have been a number of studies reporting that patients with chronic hepatitis C are likely to have significant changes in their physical and mental well-being, such as impairments in the quality of life, fatigue, depression, and musculoskeletal pain, and these symptoms are often more common in HCV-infected patients than in those with liver disease of other etiology (Barkhuizen et al., 1999; Foster, 1999; Kenny-Walsh, 1999; Singh, 1999). Functional complaints associated with HCV infection are often unrelated to the mode of acquisition of the infection or to the severity of liver disease but often remit following antiviral therapy (Bonkovsky and Woolley, 1999; Foster, 1999; Goh et al., 1999). However, there are other potential explanations for these symptoms, and numerous confounding factors such as emotional stress related to diagnosis may have affected these early findings. Nevertheless, there is more recent evidence that HCV infection is associated with cognitive dysfunction, which may be due to an underlying biological effect of HCV infection on cerebral function. Forton et al. (2002) found that patients with chronic hepatitis C were impaired in cognitive tasks. Moreover, impairments in power of concentration and speed of working memory were independent of a history of IDU, depression, or fatigue. The same researchers used proton magnetic-resonance spectroscopy (^{1}H MRS) and demonstrated elevations in basal ganglia and white matter of choline/creatine ratios in patients with mild hepatitis C, which were not present either in healthy volunteers or in patients with hepatitis B (Forton et al., 2001, 2002). These changes were unrelated to either hepatic encephalopathy or a history of IDU and were more pronounced in patients with cognitive impairment. It is of note that similar ^{1}H MRS abnormalities were found in patients with HIV infection, which suggests some similarities between the two pathogens with respect to CNS involvement (Marcus et al., 1998; Meyerhoff et al., 1999). Importantly, this pattern of ^{1}H MRS is different from that found in hepatic encephalopathy, which is characterized by depressed choline ratios (Taylor-Robinson, 2001). Findings suggestive of neurocognitive impairment were also reported by Kramer et al. (2002), who used P300 event-related potentials (a neurophysiologic measure of cognitive process) in a large cohort of patients with chronic HCV infection. In another study, which was conducted with abstinent methamphetamine

users, HCV infection was associated with reduced white-matter N-acetylaspartate, suggesting that the infection may worsen methamphetamine-associated neuronal injury (Taylor et al., 2004). The presence of MRS abnormalities consisting of increased choline and reduced N-acetylaspartate relative to controls was recently confirmed by another group of researchers (McAndrews et al., 2005). However, although HCV-infected patients showed poorer learning efficiency on neurocognitive testing, this effect was small. It is of note that the patients in the latter study were carefully screened to exclude potential other causes of cerebral dysfunction whereas illicit drug abuse, depression, anxiety related to diagnosis, ongoing IFN therapy, and liver cirrhosis could have been confounding factors of some other studies (Hilsabeck et al., 2002, 2003; Weissenborn et al., 2004). There is also evidence for subclinical motor effects of HCV infection. Electrophysiologic assessment of basal ganglia-mediated motor function revealed similar patterns of motor disturbances in HIV-positive and HCV-positive patients, which suggests common underlying pathogenetic mechanisms in these two different infections (von Giesen et al., 2004). Importantly, minor motor deficits are predictive of HIV-associated dementia (Sacktor et al., 1996). Additional evidence for a likely biological basis of cognitive dysfunction is provided by a recent report showing multiple gene expression differences in brain tissue between HCV-positive and HCV-negative patients (Adair et al., 2004).

Several studies indicate a possible impact of HCV on CNS function among HIV-infected cohorts. In one small sample, coinfected patients were more likely to show overall cognitive impairment than patients with exclusive HIV infection (Letendre et al., 2002). Distinct negative neurocognitive effects of HCV coinfection were recently documented in an advanced HIV cohort. HIV/HCV-coinfected patients were more likely to meet criteria for HIV-associated minor cognitive/motor disorder and HIV-associated dementia complex than HIV-positive HCV-negative patients despite similar CD4 and HIV RNA levels in both groups (Ryan et al., 2004). Another recent study analyzed 430 participants who either were healthy controls or had HCV infection, HIV infection, a history of methamphetamine dependence, or combinations of these factors (Cherner et al., 2005). Rates of global and of domain-specific neuropsychological impairment increased with the number of risk factors, and HCV serostatus was a significant predictor of performance both globally and in the areas of learning, abstraction, and motor skills, with trends in speeded information processing and delayed recall. However, HCV status did not affect attention/working memory or verbal fluency. In a study confined to women, Richardson et al. (2005) found that HCV-positive patients were significantly more likely to demonstrate abnormal results of neuropsychological testing and the combined effect of HCV and HIV was greater than either of these infections alone. However, neuropsychological impairment seemed to be moderated by age, and the relationship between HCV and neurocognitive abnormalities was significant only for those under 40 years of age. These studies point to the complexity of neurocognitive impairment in HIV/HCV-coinfected patients, in whose case cognitive impairment secondary to HCV infection should be taken into consideration.

Results of the above studies raise the possibility of direct HCV infection of CNS. HCV belongs to the *Flaviviridae* family, which includes well-known neurotropic viruses (e.g., West Nile, yellow fever, dengue, and tick-borne encephalitis viruses), and several reports have implicated

HCV as an occasional cause of CNS and peripheral nervous system pathologies (Bolay et al., 1996; Heckmann et al., 1999; Origgi et al., 1998). Viral sequences were also amplified directly from brain tissue from a patient diagnosed with progressive encephalomyelitis (Bolay et al., 1996). Moreover, HCV RNA was detected in cerebrospinal fluid (CSF) from both HIV-positive and HIV-negative patients (Maggi et al., 1999; Morsica et al., 1997). However, the presence of viral sequences in brain tissue could be the result of blood contamination and cannot be regarded as evidence for local HCV replication. In a recent study we detected negative-strand HCV RNA, which is viral replicative intermediary, in autopsy brain tissue of three of six HCV-infected patients, and in two of these patients there was evidence for viral brain compartmentalization as viral sequences amplified from the brain differed from those circulating in serum. Importantly, brain-derived HCV variants were found to be more closely related to the virus present in the lymphoid system than to the virus circulating in serum, as based on sequence analysis of two different viral regions (Radkowski et al., 2002). A close relationship between the HCV variants present in brain tissue and those present in lymph node was recently reported by another group of researchers. In their study Forton et al. (2004) found that 24% of 5'UTR sequences found in the brain tissue of the first patient and 55% of 5'UTR sequences amplified from the brain of the second patient were not represented in serum, suggesting their tissue derivation. Furthermore, there were phylogenetically distinct E2/HVR1 variants in both brains, and in one patient these unique sequences showed a close phylogenetic relationship to a lymphoid compartment. In the same study CNS-derived 5'UTR sequences were demonstrated to have reduced translation efficiency compared to sequences present in the serum and liver. The latter finding is compatible with the slow replication rate of brain HCV strains, which could theoretically elicit less immune response and thus favor viral latency at that site.

Which are the cells harboring HCV in the brain? Some preliminary data are provided by a recent study in which four basic brain cell types (macrophages/microglia, neurons, astrocytes, and oligodendrocytes) were separated by laser capture microscopy from autopsy brain tissue from two HCV-positive patients (Adair et al., 2004). HCV RNA-positive and -negative strands were consistently detected only in CD68+ cells (macrophage/microglia). In a different approach, brain tissue was stained with anti-NS3 monoclonal antibodies, and NS3-positive cells were separated by laser capture microscopy and phenotyped by amplification of cell-specific transcripts. Again, the analysis pointed to CD68+ cells as being infected by HCV. Additional evidence for HCV infection of CD68+ cells is shown in Color Plate 13. The same cerebellum autopsy tissue from a patient infected by both HCV and HIV was stained with anti-CD68+ fluorescein-conjugated monoclonal antibodies (right panel) and antibodies against HCV protein NS3 (left panel). The latter staining was visualized with diaminobenzidine. As seen, the same cells are positive under normal and UV light, indicating that they are both NS3 and anti-CD68 positive.

There remains the question as to how the HCV accesses the brain. A still largely hypothetical route for CNS infection could be provided by infected macrophages/monocytes, and perhaps also by B cells and T cells ("Trojan horse" mechanism). Although it was long believed that circulating leukocytes are excluded from the CNS, it is now known that all basic groups of leukocytes—T cells, B cells, macrophage/monocytes, and NK cells—have the ability to enter the brain under certain conditions (Hickey, 1999). Importantly, certain monocyte family members are constantly being replaced as part of normal physiology (Hickey et al., 1992; Unger et al., 1993), while the entry of T cells and B cells appears to be dependent only on the activation state of the leukocyte and not on CNS factors (Hickey et al., 1991; Knopf et al., 1998). In support of this hypothetical mechanism come observations on the presence of HCV in CSF from both HIV-positive and HIV-negative patients (Maggi et al., 1999; Morsica et al., 1997). In a more recent study, HCV RNA was found in the cellular fraction of CSF (8 of 13 patients), but viral sequences were rarely present in supernatants (2 of 13 patients) (Laskus et al., 2002). Importantly, in one-half of the patients in whom viral sequences could be amplified, the CSF-derived virus was closer to that found in PBMC than to that circulating in serum, which suggested that it was of lymphoid origin. In two of the latter patients sequences recovered from CSF and serum were classified as belonging to different genotypes altogether. However, they were compatible with the genotype present in PBMC. These findings strongly suggest that the virus found in CSF was derived from peripheral blood leukocytes and not serum. The presence of differing viral genotypes in serum and lymphoid compartments was also reported by others (Ducoulombier et al., 2004; Roque-Afonso et al., 2005) and was attributed to repeated superinfections among high-risk groups like IDUs.

A recent study provided some preliminary evidence for a possible biological basis of neuropsychiatric symptoms and cognitive impairment associated with HCV infection (Adair et al., 2005). In that study we analyzed samples of brain tissue obtained at autopsy from three HCV-positive patients and compared the pattern of gene expression with three HCV-negative control patients. Gene expression analysis, which was conducted using two independent techniques (differential display and reverse Northern hybridization), revealed a number of genes differentially expressed in the infected versus the uninfected patients. Only those genes that were up- or downregulated ≥1.8 times were considered to be differentially expressed.

A prominent finding in that study was downregulation of several oxidative phosphorylation genes in HCV-infected patients compared to controls. Oxidative phosphorylation, which is the primary source of energy in animal cells, occurs in mitochondria. In this process electrons are passed along a series of four respiratory enzyme complexes creating an electrochemical gradient, which in turn enables complex V (ATP synthase) to synthesize the energy carrier ATP (Saraste, 1999). As the brain is characterized by high aerobic metabolism, it is particularly susceptible to mitochondrial dysfunction (Nicholls and Budd, 2000; Orth and Schapira, 2001), and impairment of brain oxidative/energy metabolism has been suggested to be the proximate cause of many disorders that impair mentation (Blass, 2001). Moreover, alterations in brain energy metabolism could in turn induce disturbances in cellular calcium homeostasis and lead to generation of excess free radicals (Blass, 2001).

There is emerging evidence that HCV infection can affect mitochondria. During replication the HCV core protein is located on the mitochondrial outer membrane (Schwer et al., 2004), and it was reported that expression of core protein in cell lines leads to mitochondrial injury and oxidative stress (Okuda et al., 2002). Similarly, expression of HCV subgenomic replicon in Huh-7 cells leads to increase in oxidative stress as evidenced by induction of

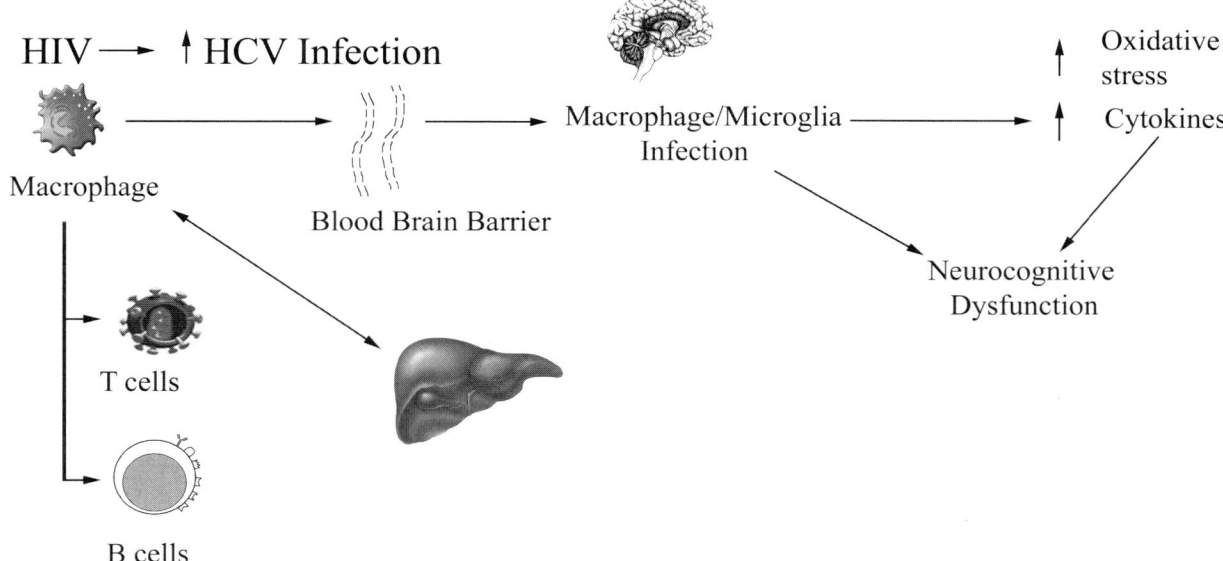

FIGURE 1 A working hypothesis regarding the effects of HCV on brain. HCV can infect PBMC, particularly macrophages, and this process is facilitated by concomitant HIV coinfection. Infected macrophages could cross the blood-brain barrier. Following the entry into the brain, infected macrophages release proinflammatory cytokines, which could induce alteration in brain function leading in turn to neurocognitive dysfunction. HCV infection may be also associated with oxidative stress, which could be due to release of reactive oxygen species by macrophages or to the direct effect of viral proteins on mitochondria.

cellular antioxidant response and increase in oxidative stress-induced proteins (Qadri et al., 2004). Induction of oxidative stress was also reported to be caused by NS5A protein, probably through disturbance of intracellular calcium homeostasis (Gong et al., 2001). However, downregulation of mitochondrial RNAs, including multiple oxidative phosphorylation genes, was found in fibroblasts exposed to H_2O_2, raising the possibility that it may represent a general mechanism by which cells protect themselves against oxidative stress (Crawford et al., 1997). Interestingly, oxidative stress commonly occurs in brain tissue of HIV-infected patients and could play an important role in the pathogenesis of neuroAIDS (Mollace et al., 2001). Although mitochondrial toxicity is commonly associated with antiretroviral therapy, there is evidence that HIV infection itself is associated with mitochondrial depletion, decreased activity of mitochondrial respiratory chain, and increased oxidative damage (Miro et al., 2004).

Another finding in our study was downregulation of multiple ribosomal protein genes, which could indicate reduced metabolic activities possibly secondary to deficiencies in oxidative phosphorylation. For example, translation, which is expensive in terms of metabolic energy, is inhibited when energy demands are not met as during cerebral ischemia (Althausen et al., 2001; Petrov et al., 2001). Interestingly, members of many different virus families inhibit the expression of host genes probably as a way of providing higher levels of cellular resources to be used for viral biosynthesis and to inhibit host antiviral responses (Lyles, 2000). Downregulation of a number of ribosomal protein genes was also reported in cells subjected to H_2O_2-induced oxidative stress, but the mechanism of this phenomenon remains unclear (Goswami et al., 2003).

Subsequent microarray analysis conducted on autopsy brain tissue material from eight HCV-positive subjects and five HCV-negative controls revealed increased expression of a number of TNF superfamily genes, several genes involved in apoptosis (e.g., Bax and MCL-1), and several genes suggesting macrophage (BLAME and CSF2RA) and immune activation (ICAM-3, ICAM-5, CRTAM, and CD74) (Adair et al., 2004). The latter changes suggest the presence of activated microglia/macrophages in brain in HCV-positive patients. Importantly, there was no change in expression of over 50 genes reported by others to be altered in hepatic encephalopathy (Desjardins et al., 2001; Song et al., 2002; Warskulat et al., 2002).

The above findings provide evidence for a possible biological basis of neuropsychiatric symptoms and cognitive impairment associated with HCV infection. However, it should be emphasized that differential display and particularly microarray data derived from analysis of brain tissue are difficult to interpret, as they represent a multitude of overlapping signals from a mixture of different cells. Thus, the results of gene expression analysis could vary depending on the proportion of different cell types in a given sample. To get insight into the possible effect of HCV infection on the brain, and particularly to elucidate the possible role of macrophages/microglia, it seems necessary to analyze the gene expression pattern in cells of uniform type. Judicious use of laser capture microscopy followed by analysis of gene expression patterns in isolated cells seems to be a logical method of choice.

The still hypothetical scenario connecting HCV infection and functional CNS is summarized in Fig. 1. HCV can infect PBMC, particularly macrophages, and this process is likely to be facilitated by concomitant HIV coinfection. Infected leukocytes could cross the blood-brain barrier

(Trojan horse phenomenon) in a process similar to that postulated for HIV-1 infection (Price et al., 1988; Zheng and Gendelman, 1997). Subsequently, there could be a secondary spread of HCV to permissive cells within the brain. The primary targets are brain microglia cells, which are essentially tissue resident macrophages of blood monocytic origin (Davis et al., 1994). Infected macrophages and microglia cells could release proinflammatory cytokines, such as TNF-α, IL-1, and IL-6, neurotoxins such as nitric oxide, and viral proteins, which could induce alteration in brain function leading in turn to neurocognitive dysfunction and depression (Capuron and Dantzer, 2003; Wilson et al., 2002). These effects may be enhanced by locally spread infection and activation of microglia cells and astrocytes (Aschner, 1998). HCV infection may be also associated with oxidative stress, which could be due to release of reactive oxygen species by macrophages or to the direct effect of viral proteins on mitochondria (Minagar et al., 2002; Okuda et al., 2002). A similar chain of events seems to be operational in HIV-1 infection (Kolson et al., 1998; Pulliam et al., 1991).

However, despite some similarities there is a fundamental difference between HIV-1 and HCV infections, as the latter does not progress into AIDS-type dementia. This could be due to the fact that HCV replication in macrophages occurs at a low level and is confined to a limited number of cells (Laskus et al., 2004a). It is also possible that the infection is not productive, infecting virions are not generated, and there is no local spread of infection. So far we have been unable to infect macrophages with the supernatants from infected cultures (our unpublished observations). Elucidation of the effect of HCV on brain is important, particularly in HIV/HCV-coinfected patients, since cognitive impairment in the latter group is generally attributed to HIV only.

REFERENCES

Adair, D., M. Radkowski, J. Jablonska, A. Pawelczyk, J. Wilkinson, J. Rakela, and T. Laskus. 2005. Differential display analysis of gene expression in brain from hepatitis C infected patients. *AIDS* 3(Suppl.):S145–S150.

Adair, D., J. Wilkinson, A. Scheck, M. Radkowski, J. Rakela, and T. Laskus. 2004. Differential display and micro-array analysis show differentially expressed genes in central nervous system in HCV infected patients and laser capture microscopy points to brain microglia as cells harboring HCV. *Hepatology* 40:433A.

Alter, M. J. 1999. Hepatitis C virus infection in the United States. *J. Hepatol.* 31:88–91.

Alter, M. J., D. Kruszon-Moran, O. V. Nainan, G. M. McQuillan, F. Gao, L. A. Moyer, R. A. Kaslow, and H. S. Margolis. 1999. The prevalence of hepatitis C virus infection in the United States, 1988 through 1994. *N. Engl. J. Med.* 341:556–562.

Alter, M. J., H. S. Margolis, K. Krawczynski, F. N. Judson, A. Mares, W. J. Alexander, P. Y. Hu, J. K. Miller, M. A. Gerber, R. E. Sampliner, E. L. Meeks, M. J. Beach, et al. 1992. The natural history of community-acquired hepatitis C in the United States. *N. Engl. J. Med.* 327:1899–1905.

Althausen, S., T. Mengesdorf, G. Mies, L. Olah, A. C. Nairn, C. G. Proud, and W. Paschen. 2001. Changes in the phosphorylation of initiation factor eIF-2alpha, elongation factor eEF-2 and p70 S6 kinase after transient focal cerebral ischaemia in mice. *J. Neurochem.* 78:779–787.

Amedee, A. M., N. Lacour, J. L. Gierman, L. N. Martin, J. E. Clements, R. Bohm, Jr., R. M. Harrison, and M. Murphey-Corb. 1995. Genotypic selection of simian immunodeficiency virus in macaque infants infected transplacentally. *J. Virol.* 69:7982–7990.

Arenas, J. I., J. F. Gallegos-Orozco, T. Laskus, J. Wilkinson, A. Khatib, C. Fasola, D. Adair, M. Radkowski, K. V. Kibler, M. Nowicki, D. Douglas, J. Williams, G. Netto, D. Mulligan, G. Klintmalm, J. Rakela, and H. E. Vargas. 2004. Hepatitis C virus quasi-species dynamics predict progression of fibrosis after liver transplantation. *J. Infect. Dis.* 189:2037–2046.

Aschner, M. 1998. Immune and inflammatory responses in the CNS: modulation by astrocytes. *Toxicol. Lett.* 102–103:283–287.

Auffermann-Gretzinger, S., E. B. Keeffe, and S. Levy. 2001. Impaired dendritic cell maturation in patients with chronic, but not resolved, hepatitis C virus infection. *Blood* 97:3171–3176.

Azzari, C., M. Resti, M. Moriondo, R. Ferrari, P. Lionetti, and A. Vierucci. 2000. Vertical transmission of HCV is related to maternal peripheral blood mononuclear cell infection. *Blood* 96:2045–2048.

Bain, C., A. Fatmi, F. Zoulim, J. P. Zarski, C. Trepo, and G. Inchauspe. 2001. Impaired allostimulatory function of dendritic cells in chronic hepatitis C infection. *Gastroenterology* 120:512–524.

Barkhuizen, A., H. R. Rosen, S. Wolf, K. Flora, K. Benner, and R. M. Bennett. 1999. Musculoskeletal pain and fatigue are associated with chronic hepatitis C: a report of 239 hepatology clinic patients. *Am. J. Gastroenterol.* 94:1355–1360.

Bassett, S. E., D. L. Thomas, K. M. Brasky, and R. E. Lanford. 1999. Viral persistence, antibody to E1 and E2, and hypervariable region 1 sequence stability in hepatitis C virus-inoculated chimpanzees. *J. Virol.* 73:1118–1126.

Becker, S., J. Quay, and J. Soukup. 1991. Cytokine (tumor necrosis factor, IL-6, and IL-8) production by respiratory syncytial virus-infected human alveolar macrophages. *J. Immunol.* 147:4307–4312.

Beld, M., M. Penning, V. Lukashov, M. McMorrow, M. Roos, N. Pakker, A. van den Hoek, and J. Goudsmit. 1998. Evidence that both HIV and HIV-induced immunodeficiency enhance HCV replication among HCV seroconverters. *Virology* 244:504–512.

Blackard, J. T., L. Smeaton, Y. Hiasa, N. Horiike, M. Onji, D. J. Jamieson, I. Rodriguez, K. H. Mayer, and R. T. Chung. 2005. Detection of hepatitis C virus (HCV) in serum and peripheral-blood mononuclear cells from HCV-monoinfected and HIV/HCV-coinfected persons. *J. Infect. Dis.* 192:258–265.

Blass, J. P. 2001. Brain metabolism and brain disease: is metabolic deficiency the proximate cause of Alzheimer dementia? *J. Neurosci. Res.* 66:851–856.

Bocharov, G., B. Ludewig, A. Bertoletti, P. Klenerman, T. Junt, P. Krebs, T. Luzyanina, C. Fraser, and R. M. Anderson. 2004. Underwhelming the immune response: effect of slow virus growth on CD8+-T-lymphocyte responses. *J. Virol.* 78:2247–2254.

Bolay, H., F. Soylemezoglu, G. Nurlu, S. Tuncer, and K. Varli. 1996. PCR detected hepatitis C virus genome in the brain of a case with progressive encephalomyelitis with rigidity. *Clin. Neurol. Neurosurg.* 98:305–308.

Bonkovsky, H. L., J. M. Woolley, et al. 1999. Reduction of health-related quality of life in chronic hepatitis C and improvement with interferon therapy. *Hepatology* 29:264–270.

Botarelli, P., M. R. Brunetto, M. A. Minutello, P. Calvo, D. Unutmaz, A. J. Weiner, Q. L. Choo, J. R. Shuster, G. Kuo, F. Bonino, et al. 1993. T-lymphocyte response to hepatitis C virus in different clinical courses of infection. *Gastroenterology* 104:580–587.

Bronowicki, J. P., M. A. Loriot, V. Thiers, Y. Grignon, A. L. Zignego, and C. Brechot. 1998. Hepatitis C virus persistence in human hematopoietic cells injected into SCID mice. *Hepatology* 28:211–218.

Bukh, J., R. H. Purcell, and R. H. Miller. 1992. Sequence analysis of the 5' noncoding region of hepatitis C virus. *Proc. Natl. Acad. Sci. USA* **89:**4942–4946.

Buratti, E., M. Gerotto, P. Pontisso, A. Alberti, S. G. Tisminetzky, and F. E. Baralle. 1997. In vivo translational efficiency of different hepatitis C virus 5'-UTRs. *FEBS Lett.* **411:**275–280.

Capuron, L., and R. Dantzer. 2003. Cytokines and depression: the need for a new paradigm. *Brain Behav. Immun.* 17(Suppl. 1):S119–S124.

Castillo, I., M. Pardo, J. Bartolome, N. Ortiz-Movilla, E. Rodriguez-Inigo, S. de Lucas, C. Salas, J. A. Jimenez-Heffernan, A. Perez-Mota, J. Graus, J. M. Lopez-Alcorocho, and V. Carreno. 2004. Occult hepatitis C virus infection in patients in whom the etiology of persistently abnormal results of liver-function tests is unknown. *J. Infect. Dis.* **189:**7–14.

Caussin-Schwemling, C., C. Schmitt, and F. Stoll-Keller. 2001. Study of the infection of human blood derived monocyte/macrophages with hepatitis C virus in vitro. *J. Med. Virol.* **65:**14–22.

Cerino, A., and M. U. Mondelli. 1991. Identification of an immunodominant B cell epitope on the hepatitis C virus nonstructural region defined by human monoclonal antibodies. *J. Immunol.* **147:**2692–2696.

Chen, M., M. Sallberg, A. Sonnerborg, O. Weiland, L. Mattsson, L. Jin, A. Birkett, D. Peterson, and D. R. Milich. 1999. Limited humoral immunity in hepatitis C virus infection. *Gastroenterology* **116:**135–143.

Cherner, M., S. Letendre, R. K. Heaton, J. Durelle, J. Marquie-Beck, B. Gragg, and I. Grant. 2005. Hepatitis C augments cognitive deficits associated with HIV infection and methamphetamine. *Neurology* **64:**1343–1347.

Choo, Q. L., G. Kuo, R. Ralston, A. Weiner, D. Chien, G. Van Nest, J. Han, K. Berger, K. Thudium, C. Kuo, et al. 1994. Vaccination of chimpanzees against infection by the hepatitis C virus. *Proc. Natl. Acad. Sci. USA* **91:**1294–1298.

Choo, Q. L., G. Kuo, A. J. Weiner, L. R. Overby, D. W. Bradley, and M. Houghton. 1989. Isolation of a cDNA clone derived from a blood-borne non-A, non-B viral hepatitis genome. *Science* **244:**359–362.

Choo, Q. L., K. H. Richman, J. H. Han, K. Berger, C. Lee, C. Dong, C. Gallegos, D. Coit, R. Medina-Selby, P. J. Barr, A. J. Weiner, D. W. Bradley, G. Kuo, and M. Houghton. 1991. Genetic organization and diversity of the hepatitis C virus. *Proc. Natl. Acad. Sci. USA* **88:**2451–2455.

Coffin, C. S., and T. I. Michalak. 1999. Persistence of infectious hepadnavirus in the offspring of woodchuck mothers recovered from viral hepatitis. *J. Clin. Investig.* **104:**203–212.

Collier, A. J., S. Tang, and R. M. Elliott. 1998. Translation efficiencies of the 5' untranslated region from representatives of the six major genotypes of hepatitis C virus using a novel bicistronic reporter assay system. *J. Gen. Virol.* **79:**2359–2366.

Crawford, D. R., Y. Wang, G. P. Schools, J. Kochheiser, and K. J. Davies. 1997. Down-regulation of mammalian mitochondrial RNAs during oxidative stress. *Free Radic. Biol. Med.* **22:**551–559.

Daar, E. S., H. Lynn, S. Donfield, E. Gomperts, M. W. Hilgartner, W. K. Hoots, D. Chernoff, S. Arkin, W. Y. Wong, and C. A. Winkler. 2001. Relation between HIV-1 and hepatitis C viral load in patients with hemophilia. *J. Acquir. Immune Defic. Syndr.* **26:**466–472.

Davis, E. J., T. D. Foster, and W. E. Thomas. 1994. Cellular forms and functions of brain microglia. *Brain Res. Bull.* **34:**73–78.

De Luca, A., R. Bugarini, A. C. Lepri, M. Puoti, E. Girardi, A. Antinori, A. Poggio, G. Pagano, G. Tositti, G. Cadeo, A. Macor, M. Toti, and A. D'Arminio Monforte. 2002. Coinfection with hepatitis viruses and outcome of initial antiretroviral regimens in previously naive HIV-infected subjects. *Arch. Intern. Med.* **162:**2125–2132.

Desjardins, P., M. Belanger, and R. F. Butterworth. 2001. Alterations in expression of genes coding for key astrocytic proteins in acute liver failure. *J. Neurosci. Res.* **66:**967–971.

Dockter, J., C. F. Evans, A. Tishon, and M. B. Oldstone. 1996. Competitive selection in vivo by a cell for one variant over another: implications for RNA virus quasispecies in vivo. *J. Virol.* **70:**1799–1803.

Domingo, E., E. Martinez-Salas, F. Sobrino, J. C. de la Torre, A. Portela, J. Ortin, C. Lopez-Galindez, P. Perez-Brena, N. Villanueva, R. Najera, et al. 1985. The quasispecies (extremely heterogeneous) nature of viral RNA genome populations: biological relevance—a review. *Gene* **40:**1–8.

Dorrucci, M., P. Pezzotti, A. N. Phillips, A. C. Lepri, G. Rezza, et al. 1995. Coinfection of hepatitis C virus with human immunodeficiency virus and progression to AIDS. *J. Infect. Dis.* **172:**1503–1508.

Ducoulombier, D., A. M. Roque-Afonso, G. Di Liberto, F. Penin, R. Kara, Y. Richard, E. Dussaix, and C. Feray. 2004. Frequent compartmentalization of hepatitis C virus variants in circulating B cells and monocytes. *Hepatology* **39:**817–825.

Eckels, D. D., H. Wang, T. H. Bian, N. Tabatabai, and J. C. Gill. 2000. Immunobiology of hepatitis C virus (HCV) infection: the role of CD4 T cells in HCV infection. *Immunol. Rev.* **174:**90–97.

Eyster, M. E., H. J. Alter, L. M. Aledort, S. Quan, A. Hatzakis, and J. J. Goedert. 1991. Heterosexual co-transmission of hepatitis C virus (HCV) and human immunodeficiency virus (HIV). *Ann. Intern. Med.* **115:**764–768.

Eyster, M. E., L. S. Diamondstone, J. M. Lien, W. C. Ehmann, S. Quan, J. J. Goedert, et al. 1993. Natural history of hepatitis C virus infection in multitransfused hemophiliacs: effect of coinfection with human immunodeficiency virus. *J. Acquir. Immune Defic. Syndr.* **6:**602–10.

Eyster, M. E., K. E. Sherman, J. J. Goedert, A. Katsoulidou, A. Hatzakis, et al. 1999. Prevalence and changes in hepatitis C virus genotypes among multitransfused persons with hemophilia. *J. Infect. Dis.* **179:**1062–1069.

Farci, P., H. J. Alter, S. Govindarajan, D. C. Wong, R. Engle, R. R. Lesniewski, I. K. Mushahwar, S. M. Desai, R. H. Miller, N. Ogata, and R. H. Purcell. 1992. Lack of protective immunity against reinfection with hepatitis C virus. *Science* **258:**135–140.

Farci, P., H. J. Alter, D. C. Wong, R. H. Miller, S. Govindarajan, R. Engle, M. Shapiro, and R. H. Purcell. 1994. Prevention of hepatitis C virus infection in chimpanzees after antibody-mediated in vitro neutralization. *Proc. Natl. Acad. Sci. USA* **91:**7792–7796.

Farci, P., A. Shimoda, A. Coiana, G. Diaz, G. Peddis, J. C. Melpolder, A. Strazzera, D. Y. Chien, S. J. Munoz, A. Balestrieri, R. H. Purcell, and H. J. Alter. 2000. The outcome of acute hepatitis C predicted by the evolution of the viral quasispecies. *Science* **288:**339–344.

Ferbeyre, G., V. Bourdeau, and R. Cedergren. 1997. Does HIV tat protein also regulate genes of other viruses present in HIV infection? *Trends Biochem. Sci.* **22:**115–116. (Letter.)

Ferrari, C., A. Valli, L. Galati, A. Penna, P. Scaccaglia, T. Giuberti, C. Schianchi, G. Missale, M. G. Marin, and F. Fiaccadori. 1994. T-cell response to structural and nonstructural hepatitis C virus antigens in persistent and self-limited hepatitis C virus infections. *Hepatology* **19:**286–295.

Forns, X., J. Bukh, R. H. Purcell, and S. U. Emerson. 1997. How *Escherichia coli* can bias the results of molecular cloning: preferential selection of defective genomes of hepatitis C virus during the cloning procedure. *Proc. Natl. Acad. Sci. USA* **94:**13909–13914.

Forns, X., R. Thimme, S. Govindarajan, S. U. Emerson, R. H. Purcell, F. V. Chisari, and J. Bukh. 2000. Hepatitis C virus lacking the hypervariable region 1 of the second envelope protein is infectious and causes acute resolving or persistent infection in chimpanzees. *Proc. Natl. Acad. Sci. USA* **97:**13318–13323.

Forton, D. M., J. M. Allsop, J. Main, G. R. Foster, H. C. Thomas, and S. D. Taylor-Robinson. 2001. Evidence for a cerebral effect of the hepatitis C virus. *Lancet* **358:**38–39.

Forton, D. M., P. Karayiannis, N. Mahmud, S. D. Taylor-Robinson, and H. C. Thomas. 2004. Identification of unique hepatitis C virus quasispecies in the central nervous system and comparative analysis of internal translational efficiency of brain, liver, and serum variants. *J. Virol.* **78:**5170–5183.

Forton, D. M., H. C. Thomas, C. A. Murphy, J. M. Allsop, G. R. Foster, J. Main, K. A. Wesnes, and S. D. Taylor-Robinson. 2002. Hepatitis C and cognitive impairment in a cohort of patients with mild liver disease. *Hepatology* **35:**433–439.

Foster, G. R. 1999. Hepatitis C virus infection: quality of life and side effects of treatment. *J. Hepatol.* **31:**250–254.

Gale, M., Jr., and E. M. Foy. 2005. Evasion of intracellular host defence by hepatitis C virus. *Nature* **436:**939–945.

Gallegos-Orozco, J. F., J. I. Arenas, K. Kibler, J. Wilkinson, D. Adair, M. Radkowski, H. Vargas, T. Laskus, and J. Rakela. 2004. Translation efficiency of hepatitis C 5'-untranslated region variants developing in transfusion acquired infection and in post-transplant recurrent hepatitis. *Hepatology* **40:**688A.

Gane, E. J., B. C. Portmann, N. V. Naoumov, H. M. Smith, J. A. Underhill, P. T. Donaldson, G. Maertens, and R. Williams. 1996. Long-term outcome of hepatitis C infection after liver transplantation. *N. Engl. J. Med.* **334:**815–820.

Garcia-Samaniego, J., V. Soriano, J. Castilla, R. Bravo, A. Moreno, J. Carbo, A. Iniguez, J. Gonzalez, F. Munoz, et al. 1997. Influence of hepatitis C virus genotypes and HIV infection on histological severity of chronic hepatitis C. *Am. J. Gastroenterol.* **92:**1130–1134.

Gerlach, J. T., H. M. Diepolder, M. C. Jung, N. H. Gruener, W. W. Schraut, R. Zachoval, R. Hoffmann, C. A. Schirren, T. Santantonio, and G. R. Pape. 1999. Recurrence of hepatitis C virus after loss of virus-specific CD4(+) T-cell response in acute hepatitis C. *Gastroenterology* **117:**933–941.

Goh, J., B. Coughlan, J. Quinn, J. C. O'Keane, and J. Crowe. 1999. Fatigue does not correlate with the degree of hepatitis or the presence of autoimmune disorders in chronic hepatitis C infection. *Eur. J. Gastroenterol. Hepatol.* **11:**833–838.

Gong, G., G. Waris, R. Tanveer, and A. Siddiqui. 2001. Human hepatitis C virus NS5A protein alters intracellular calcium levels, induces oxidative stress, and activates STAT-3 and NF-kappa B. *Proc. Natl. Acad. Sci. USA* **98:**9599–9604.

Goswami, S., N. L. Sheets, J. Zavadil, B. K. Chauhan, E. P. Bottinger, V. N. Reddy, M. Kantorow, and A. Cvekl. 2003. Spectrum and range of oxidative stress responses of human lens epithelial cells to H2O2 insult. *Investig. Ophthalmol. Vis. Sci.* **44:**2084–2093.

Granovsky, M. O., H. L. Minkoff, B. H. Tess, D. Waters, A. Hatzakis, D. E. Devoid, S. H. Landesman, A. Rubinstein, A. M. Di Bisceglie, and J. J. Goedert. 1998. Hepatitis C virus infection in the mothers and infants cohort study. *Pediatrics* **102:**355–359.

Gretch, D. R., S. J. Polyak, J. J. Wilson, R. L. Carithers, Jr., J. D. Perkins, and L. Corey. 1996. Tracking hepatitis C virus quasispecies major and minor variants in symptomatic and asymptomatic liver transplant recipients. *J. Virol.* **70:**7622–7631.

Greub, G., B. Ledergerber, M. Battegay, P. Grob, L. Perrin, H. Furrer, P. Burgisser, P. Erb, K. Boggian, J. C. Piffaretti, B. Hirschel, P. Janin, P. Francioli, M. Flepp, and A. Telenti. 2000. Clinical progression, survival, and immune recovery during antiretroviral therapy in patients with HIV-1 and hepatitis C virus coinfection: the Swiss HIV Cohort Study. *Lancet* **356:**1800–1805.

Gruener, N. H., F. Lechner, M. C. Jung, H. Diepolder, T. Gerlach, G. Lauer, B. Walker, J. Sullivan, R. Phillips, G. R. Pape, and P. Klenerman. 2001. Sustained dysfunction of antiviral CD8+ T lymphocytes after infection with hepatitis C virus. *J. Virol.* **75:**5550–5558.

Hanley, J. P., L. M. Jarvis, J. Andrews, R. Dennis, R. Lee, P. Simmonds, J. Piris, P. Hayes, and C. A. Ludlam. 1996. Investigation of chronic hepatitis C infection in individuals with haemophilia: assessment of invasive and non-invasive methods. *Br. J. Haematol.* **94:**159–165.

Heckmann, J. G., C. Kayser, D. Heuss, B. Manger, H. E. Blum, and B. Neundorfer. 1999. Neurological manifestations of chronic hepatitis C. *J. Neurol.* **246:**486–491.

Herbein, G., and W. A. O'Brien. 2000. Tumor necrosis factor (TNF)-alpha and TNF receptors in viral pathogenesis. *Proc. Soc. Exp. Biol. Med.* **223:**241–257.

Hickey, W. F. 1999. Leukocyte traffic in the central nervous system: the participants and their roles. *Semin. Immunol.* **11:**125–137.

Hickey, W. F., B. L. Hsu, and H. Kimura. 1991. T-lymphocyte entry into the central nervous system. *J. Neurosci. Res.* **28:**254–260.

Hickey, W. F., K. Vass, and H. Lassmann. 1992. Bone marrow-derived elements in the central nervous system: an immunohistochemical and ultrastructural survey of rat chimeras. *J. Neuropathol. Exp. Neurol.* **51:**246–256.

Hijikata, M., N. Kato, Y. Ootsuyama, M. Nakagawa, S. Ohkoshi, and K. Shimotohno. 1991. Hypervariable regions in the putative glycoprotein of hepatitis C virus. *Biochem. Biophys. Res. Commun.* **175:**220–228.

Hijikata, M., K. Mizuno, T. Rikihisa, Y. K. Shimizu, A. Iwamoto, N. Nakajima, and H. Yoshikura. 1995. Selective transmission of hepatitis C virus in vivo and in vitro. *Arch. Virol.* **140:**1623–1628.

Hilsabeck, R. C., T. I. Hassanein, M. D. Carlson, E. A. Ziegler, and W. Perry. 2003. Cognitive functioning and psychiatric symptomatology in patients with chronic hepatitis C. *J. Int. Neuropsychol. Soc.* **9:**847–854.

Hilsabeck, R. C., W. Perry, and T. I. Hassanein. 2002. Neuropsychological impairment in patients with chronic hepatitis C. *Hepatology* **35:**440–446.

Hoffmann, R. M., H. M. Diepolder, R. Zachoval, F. M. Zwiebel, M. C. Jung, S. Scholz, H. Nitschko, G. Riethmuller, and G. R. Pape. 1995. Mapping of immunodominant CD4+ T lymphocyte epitopes of hepatitis C virus antigens and their relevance during the course of chronic infection. *Hepatology* **21:**632–638.

Kenny-Walsh, E., et al. 1999. Clinical outcomes after hepatitis C infection from contaminated anti-D immune globulin. *N. Engl. J. Med.* **340:**1228–1233.

Khabar, K. S., F. Al-Zoghaibi, M. N. Al-Ahdal, T. Murayama, M. Dhalla, N. Mukaida, M. Taha, S. T. Al-Sedairy, Y. Siddiqui, G. Kessie, and K. Matsushima. 1997. The alpha chemokine, interleukin 8, inhibits the antiviral action of interferon alpha. *J. Exp. Med.* **186:**1077–1085.

Kibler, K., M. Radkowski, D. Adair, J. I. Arenas, J. Wilkinson, J. Rakela, and T. Laskus. 2003. HCV inhibition of HIV-induced apoptosis. *Hepatology* **38:**352A.

Kiyosawa, K., T. Sodeyama, E. Tanaka, Y. Gibo, K. Yoshizawa, S. Nakano, S. Furuta, Y. Akahane, K. Nishioka, R. H. Purcell, and H. J. Alter. 1990. Interrelationship of blood transfusion, non-A, non-B hepatitis and hepatocellular carcinoma: analysis by detection of antibody to hepatitis C virus. *Hepatology* **12:**671–675.

Knopf, P. M., C. J. Harling-Berg, H. F. Cserr, D. Basu, E. J. Sirulnick, S. C. Nolan, J. T. Park, G. Keir, E. J. Thompson, and W. F. Hickey. 1998. Antigen-dependent intrathecal antibody synthesis in the normal rat brain: tissue entry and local retention of antigen-specific B cells. *J. Immunol.* **161**:692–701.

Kojima, M., T. Osuga, F. Tsuda, T. Tanaka, and H. Okamoto. 1994. Influence of antibodies to the hypervariable region of E2/NS1 glycoprotein on the selective replication of hepatitis C virus in chimpanzees. *Virology* **204**:665–672.

Kolson, D. L., E. Lavi, and F. Gonzalez-Scarano. 1998. The effects of human immunodeficiency virus in the central nervous system. *Adv. Virus Res.* **50**:1–47.

Kovacs, A., W. Du, M. DeGiacomo, T. Shahidyazdani, D. Wright, and J. Nowicki. 2004. Impact of HCV viremia on HIV disease progression in women, abstr. MoPeB3343. *Abstr. 15th Int. AIDS Conf.* July 11–16, 2004, Bangkok, Thailand.

Koziel, M. J., D. Dudley, N. Afdhal, Q. L. Choo, M. Houghton, R. Ralston, and B. D. Walker. 1993. Hepatitis C virus (HCV)-specific cytotoxic T lymphocytes recognize epitopes in the core and envelope proteins of HCV. *J. Virol.* **67**:7522–7532.

Koziel, M. J., D. Dudley, N. Afdhal, A. Grakoui, C. M. Rice, Q. L. Choo, M. Houghton, and B. D. Walker. 1995. HLA class I-restricted cytotoxic T lymphocytes specific for hepatitis C virus. Identification of multiple epitopes and characterization of patterns of cytokine release. *J. Clin. Investig.* **96**:2311–2321.

Koziel, M. J., D. Dudley, J. T. Wong, J. Dienstag, M. Houghton, R. Ralston, and B. D. Walker. 1992. Intrahepatic cytotoxic T lymphocytes specific for hepatitis C virus in persons with chronic hepatitis. *J. Immunol.* **149**:3339–3344.

Kramer, L., E. Bauer, G. Funk, H. Hofer, W. Jessner, P. Steindl-Munda, F. Wrba, C. Madl, A. Gangl, and P. Ferenci. 2002. Subclinical impairment of brain function in chronic hepatitis C infection. *J. Hepatol.* **37**:349–354.

Kudo, T., Y. Yanase, M. Ohshiro, M. Yamamoto, M. Morita, M. Shibata, and T. Morishima. 1997. Analysis of mother-to-infant transmission of hepatitis C virus: quasispecies nature and buoyant densities of maternal virus populations. *J. Med. Virol.* **51**:225–230.

Kumar, U., J. Monjardino, and H. C. Thomas. 1994. Hypervariable region of hepatitis C virus envelope glycoprotein (E2/NS1) in an agammaglobulinemic patient. *Gastroenterology* **106**:1072–1075.

Kuo, G., Q. L. Choo, H. J. Alter, G. L. Gitnick, A. G. Redeker, R. H. Purcell, T. Miyamura, J. L. Dienstag, M. J. Alter, C. E. Stevens, et al. 1989. An assay for circulating antibodies to a major etiologic virus of human non-A, non-B hepatitis. *Science* **244**:362–364.

Lane, B. R., K. Lore, P. J. Bock, J. Andersson, M. J. Coffey, R. M. Strieter, and D. M. Markovitz. 2001. Interleukin-8 stimulates human immunodeficiency virus type 1 replication and is a potential new target for antiretroviral therapy. *J. Virol.* **75**:8195–8202.

Lanford, R. E., C. Sureau, J. R. Jacob, R. White, and T. R. Fuerst. 1994. Demonstration of in vitro infection of chimpanzee hepatocytes with hepatitis C virus using strand-specific RT/PCR. *Virology* **202**:606–614.

Laporte, J., C. Bain, P. Maurel, G. Inchauspe, H. Agut, and A. Cahour. 2003. Differential distribution and internal translation efficiency of hepatitis C virus quasispecies present in dendritic and liver cells. *Blood* **101**:52–57.

Laporte, J., I. Malet, T. Andrieu, V. Thibault, J. J. Toulme, C. Wychowski, J. M. Pawlotsky, J. M. Huraux, H. Agut, and A. Cahour. 2000. Comparative analysis of translation efficiencies of hepatitis C virus 5′ untranslated regions among intraindividual quasispecies present in chronic infection: opposite behaviors depending on cell type. *J. Virol.* **74**:10827–10833.

Laskus, T., M. Radkowski, A. Bednarska, J. Wilkinson, D. Adair, M. Nowicki, G. B. Nikolopoulou, H. Vargas, and J. Rakela. 2002. Detection and analysis of hepatitis C virus sequences in cerebrospinal fluid. *J. Virol.* **76**:10064–10068.

Laskus, T., M. Radkowski, J. Jablonska, K. Kibler, J. Wilkinson, D. Adair, and J. Rakela. 2004a. Human immunodeficiency virus facilitates infection/replication of hepatitis C virus in native human macrophages. *Blood* **103**:3854–3859.

Laskus, T., M. Radkowski, A. Piasek, M. Nowicki, A. Horban, J. Cianciara, and J. Rakela. 2000a. Hepatitis C virus in lymphoid cells of patients coinfected with human immunodeficiency virus type 1: evidence of active replication in monocytes/macrophages and lymphocytes. *J. Infect. Dis.* **181**:442–448.

Laskus, T., M. Radkowski, L. F. Wang, S. J. Jang, H. Vargas, and J. Rakela. 1998a. Hepatitis C virus quasispecies in patients infected with HIV-1: correlation with extrahepatic viral replication. *Virology* **248**:164–171.

Laskus, T., M. Radkowski, L. F. Wang, M. Nowicki, and J. Rakela. 2000b. Uneven distribution of hepatitis C virus quasispecies in tissues from subjects with end-stage liver disease: confounding effect of viral adsorption and mounting evidence for the presence of low-level extrahepatic replication. *J. Virol.* **74**:1014–1017.

Laskus, T., M. Radkowski, L. F. Wang, H. Vargas, and J. Rakela. 1997. Lack of evidence for hepatitis G virus replication in the livers of patients coinfected with hepatitis C and G viruses. *J. Virol.* **71**:7804–7806.

Laskus, T., M. Radkowski, L. F. Wang, H. Vargas, and J. Rakela. 1998b. The presence of active hepatitis C virus replication in lymphoid tissue in patients coinfected with human immunodeficiency virus type 1. *J. Infect. Dis.* **178**:1189–1192.

Laskus, T., L. F. Wang, M. Radkowski, H. Vargas, M. Nowicki, J. Wilkinson, and J. Rakela. 2001. Exposure of hepatitis C virus (HCV) RNA-positive recipients to HCV RNA-positive blood donors results in rapid predominance of a single donor strain and exclusion and/or suppression of the recipient strain. *J. Virol.* **75**:2059–2066.

Laskus, T., L. F. Wang, J. Rakela, H. Vargas, A. D. Pinna, A. C. Tsamandas, A. J. Demetris, and J. Fung. 1996. Dynamic behavior of hepatitis C virus in chronically infected patients receiving liver graft from infected donors. *Virology* **220**:171–176.

Laskus, T., J. Wilkinson, J. F. Gallegos-Orozco, M. Radkowski, D. M. Adair, M. Nowicki, E. Operskalski, Z. Buskell, L. B. Seeff, H. Vargas, and J. Rakela. 2004b. Analysis of hepatitis C virus quasispecies transmission and evolution in patients infected through blood transfusion. *Gastroenterology* **127**:764–776.

Lau, D. T., D. E. Kleiner, M. G. Ghany, Y. Park, P. Schmid, and J. H. Hoofnagle. 1998. 10-Year follow-up after interferon-alpha therapy for chronic hepatitis C. *Hepatology* **28**:1121–1127.

Lee, W. M., J. E. Polson, D. S. Carney, B. Sahin, and M. Gale, Jr. 2005. Reemergence of hepatitis C virus after 8.5 years in a patient with hypogammaglobulinemia: evidence for an occult viral reservoir. *J. Infect. Dis.* **192**:1088–1092.

Lehmann, C., H. Sprenger, M. Nain, M. Bacher, and D. Gemsa. 1996. Infection of macrophages by influenza A virus: characteristics of tumour necrosis factor-alpha (TNF alpha) gene expression. *Res. Virol.* **147**:123–130.

Lerat, H., S. Rumin, F. Habersetzer, F. Berby, M. A. Trabaud, C. Trepo, and G. Inchauspe. 1998. In vivo tropism of hepatitis C virus genomic sequences in hematopoietic cells: influence of viral load, viral genotype, and cell phenotype. *Blood* **91**:3841–3849.

Lerat, H., Y. K. Shimizu, and S. M. Lemon. 2000. Cell type-specific enhancement of hepatitis C virus internal ribosome entry site-directed translation due to 5′ nontranslated region substitutions selected during passage of virus in lymphoblastoid cells. *J. Virol.* **74**:7024–7031.

Lesens, O., M. Deschenes, M. Steben, G. Belanger, and C. M. Tsoukas. 1999. Hepatitis C virus is related to progressive liver disease in human immunodeficiency virus-positive hemophiliacs and should be treated as an opportunistic infection. *J. Infect. Dis.* **179:**1254–1258.

Letendre, S. L., M. Cherner, R. Ellis, and I. Grant. 2002. Individuals coinfected with hepatitis C (HCV) and HIV are more cognitively impaired than those infected with either virus alone. *J. Neurovirol.* **8:**27–28 (Abstract.)

Li, Y., X. Wang, S. D. Douglas, D. S. Metzger, G. Woody, T. Zhang, L. Song, and W. Z. Ho. 2005. CD8+ T cell depletion amplifies hepatitis C virus replication in peripheral blood mononuclear cells. *J. Infect. Dis.* **192:**1093–1101.

Lindsay, K. L. 2002. Introduction to therapy of hepatitis C. *Hepatology* **36:**S114–S120.

Lyles, D. S. 2000. Cytopathogenesis and inhibition of host gene expression by RNA viruses. *Microbiol. Mol. Biol. Rev.* **64:**709–724.

Maggi, F., M. Giorgi, C. Fornai, A. Morrica, M. L. Vatteroni, M. Pistello, G. Siciliano, A. Nuccorini, and M. Bendinelli. 1999. Detection and quasispecies analysis of hepatitis C virus in the cerebrospinal fluid of infected patients. *J. Neurovirol.* **5:**319–323.

Mahe, Y., N. Mukaida, K. Kuno, M. Akiyama, N. Ikeda, K. Matsushima, and S. Murakami. 1991. Hepatitis B virus X protein transactivates human interleukin-8 gene through acting on nuclear factor kB and CCAAT/enhancer-binding protein-like cis-elements. *J. Biol. Chem.* **266:**13759–13763.

Major, M. E., K. Mihalik, J. Fernandez, J. Seidman, D. Kleiner, A. A. Kolykhalov, C. M. Rice, and S. M. Feinstone. 1999. Long-term follow-up of chimpanzees inoculated with the first infectious clone for hepatitis C virus. *J. Virol.* **73:**3317–3325.

Manzin, A., L. Solforosi, E. Petrelli, G. Macarri, G. Tosone, M. Piazza, and M. Clementi. 1998. Evolution of hypervariable region 1 of hepatitis C virus in primary infection. *J. Virol.* **72:**6271–6276.

Mao, Q., S. C. Ray, O. Laeyendecker, J. R. Ticehurst, S. A. Strathdee, D. Vlahov, and D. L. Thomas. 2001. Human immunodeficiency virus seroconversion and evolution of the hepatitis C virus quasispecies. *J. Virol.* **75:**3259–3267.

Marcus, C. D., S. D. Taylor-Robinson, J. Sargentoni, J. G. Ainsworth, G. Frize, P. J. Easterbrook, S. Shaunak, and D. J. Bryant. 1998. 1H MR spectroscopy of the brain in HIV-1-seropositive subjects: evidence for diffuse metabolic abnormalities. *Metab. Brain Dis.* **13:**123–136.

Martell, M., J. I. Esteban, J. Quer, J. Genesca, A. Weiner, R. Esteban, J. Guardia, and J. Gomez. 1992. Hepatitis C virus (HCV) circulates as a population of different but closely related genomes: quasispecies nature of HCV genome distribution. *J. Virol.* **66:**3225–3229.

Martell, M., J. I. Esteban, J. Quer, V. Vargas, R. Esteban, J. Guardia, and J. Gomez. 1994. Dynamic behavior of hepatitis C virus quasispecies in patients undergoing orthotopic liver transplantation. *J. Virol.* **68:**3425–3436.

McAndrews, M. P., K. Farcnik, P. Carlen, A. Damyanovich, M. Mrkonjic, S. Jones, and E. J. Heathcote. 2005. Prevalence and significance of neurocognitive dysfunction in hepatitis C in the absence of correlated risk factors. *Hepatology* **41:**801–808.

McHutchison, J. G., G. Davis, L., R. Esteban-Mur, T. Poynard, M. H. Ling, J. J. Garaud, J. K. Albrecht, et al. 2001. Durability of sustained virologic response in patients with chronic hepatitis C after treatment with interferon alpha-2B alone or in combination with ribavirin. *Hepatology* **34:**244A. (Abstract.)

Meyerhoff, D. J., C. Bloomer, V. Cardenas, D. Norman, M. W. Weiner, and G. Fein. 1999. Elevated subcortical choline metabolites in cognitively and clinically asymptomatic HIV+ patients. *Neurology* **52:**995–1003.

Michalak, T. I., P. M. Mulrooney, and C. S. Coffin. 2004. Low doses of hepadnavirus induce infection of the lymphatic system that does not engage the liver. *J. Virol.* **78:**1730–1738.

Minagar, A., P. Shapshak, R. Fujimura, R. Ownby, M. Heyes, and C. Eisdorfer. 2002. The role of macrophage/

microglia and astrocytes in the pathogenesis of three neurologic disorders: HIV-associated dementia, Alzheimer disease, and multiple sclerosis. *J. Neurol. Sci.* **202:**13–23.

Miro, O., S. Lopez, E. Martinez, E. Pedrol, A. Milinkovic, E. Deig, G. Garrabou, J. Casademont, J. M. Gatell, and F. Cardellach. 2004. Mitochondrial effects of HIV infection on the peripheral blood mononuclear cells of HIV-infected patients who were never treated with antiretrovirals. *Clin. Infect. Dis.* **39:**710–716.

Mogensen, S. C. 1979. Role of macrophages in natural resistance to virus infections. *Microbiol. Rev.* **43:**1–26.

Mollace, V., H. S. Nottet, P. Clayette, M. C. Turco, C. Muscoli, D. Salvemini, and C. F. Perno. 2001. Oxidative stress and neuroAIDS: triggers, modulators and novel antioxidants. *Trends Neurosci.* **24:**411–416.

Monga, H. K., K. Breauz, M. C. Rodrigues-Barradas, and B. Yoffe. 1998. Increased HCV-related morbidity and mortality in HIV patients. *Hepatology* **28:**565A.

Mori, N., N. Mukaida, D. W. Ballard, K. Matsushima, and N. Yamamoto. 1998. Human T-cell leukemia virus type I Tax transactivates human interleukin 8 gene through acting concurrently on AP-1 and nuclear factor-kappaB- like sites. *Cancer Res.* **58:**3993–4000.

Morsica, G., M. T. Bernardi, R. Novati, C. Uberti Foppa, A. Castagna, and A. Lazzarin. 1997. Detection of hepatitis C virus genomic sequences in the cerebrospinal fluid of HIV-infected patients. *J. Med. Virol.* **53:**252–254.

Mukaida, N. 2000. Interleukin-8: an expanding universe beyond neutrophil chemotaxis and activation. *Int. J. Hematol.* **72:**391–398.

Murayama, T., K. Kuno, F. Jisaki, M. Obuchi, D. Sakamuro, T. Furukawa, N. Mukaida, and K. Matsushima. 1994. Enhancement human cytomegalovirus replication in a human lung fibroblast cell line by interleukin-8. *J. Virol.* **68:**7582–7585.

Murayama, T., Y. Ohara, M. Obuchi, K. S. Khabar, H. Higashi, N. Mukaida, and K. Matsushima. 1997. Human cytomegalovirus induces interleukin-8 production by a human monocytic cell line, THP-1, through acting concurrently on AP-1- and NF- kappaB-binding sites of the interleukin-8 gene. *J. Virol.* **71:**5692–5695.

Nakajima, N., M. Hijikata, H. Yoshikura, and Y. K. Shimizu. 1996. Characterization of long-term cultures of hepatitis C virus. *J. Virol.* **70:**3325–3329.

Nasoff, M. S., S. L. Zebedee, G. Inchauspe, and A. M. Prince. 1991. Identification of an immunodominant epitope within the capsid protein of hepatitis C virus. *Proc. Natl. Acad. Sci. USA* **88:**5462–5466.

Navas, S., J. Martin, J. A. Quiroga, I. Castillo, and V. Carreno. 1998. Genetic diversity and tissue compartmentalization of the hepatitis C virus genome in blood mononuclear cells, liver, and serum from chronic hepatitis C patients. *J. Virol.* **72:**1640–1646.

Neumann, A. U., N. P. Lam, H. Dahari, D. R. Gretch, T. E. Wiley, T. J. Layden, and A. S. Perelson. 1998. Hepatitis C viral dynamics in vivo and the antiviral efficacy of interferon-alpha therapy. *Science* **282:**103–107.

Ni, J., E. Hembrador, A. M. Di Bisceglie, I. M. Jacobson, A. H. Talal, D. Butera, C. M. Rice, T. J. Chambers, and L. B. Dustin. 2003. Accumulation of B lymphocytes with a naive, resting phenotype in a subset of hepatitis C patients. *J. Immunol.* **170:**3429–3439.

Nicholls, D. G., and S. L. Budd. 2000. Mitochondria and neuronal survival. *Physiol. Rev.* **80:**315–360.

Nishioka, K. 1994. Epidemiological studies on hepatitis C virus infection: detection, prevalence, exposure and prevention. *Intervirology* **37:**58–67.

Nousbaum, J. B., S. Pol, B. Nalpas, P. Landais, P. Berthelot, C. Brechot, et al. 1995. Hepatitis C virus type 1b (II) infection in France and Italy. *Ann. Intern. Med.* **122:**161–168.

Nowicki, M. J., T. Laskus, G. Nikolopoulou, M. Radkowski, J. Wilkinson, W. B. Du, J. Rakela, and A. Kovacs. 2005. Presence of hepatitis C virus (HCV) RNA in the genital tracts of HCV/HIV-1-coinfected women. *J. Infect. Dis.* **192:**1557–1565.

Ogata, N., H. J. Alter, R. H. Miller, and R. H. Purcell. 1991. Nucleotide sequence and mutation rate of the H strain of hepatitis C virus. *Proc. Natl. Acad. Sci. USA* **88:**3392–3396.

Okamoto, H., M. Kojima, S. Okada, H. Yoshizawa, H. Iizuka, T. Tanaka, E. E. Muchmore, D. A. Peterson, Y. Ito, and S. Mishiro. 1992. Genetic drift of hepatitis C virus during an 8.2-year infection in a chimpanzee: variability and stability. *Virology* **190:**894–899.

Okamoto, H., S. Mishiro, H. Tokita, F. Tsuda, Y. Miyakawa, and M. Mayumi. 1994. Superinfection of chimpanzees carrying hepatitis C virus of genotype II/1b with that of genotype III/2a or I/1a. *Hepatology* **20:**1131–1136.

Okuda, M., K. Li, M. R. Beard, L. A. Showalter, F. Scholle, S. M. Lemon, and S. A. Weinman. 2002. Mitochondrial injury, oxidative stress, and antioxidant gene expression are induced by hepatitis C virus core protein. *Gastroenterology* **122:**366–375.

Oldstone, M. B. 1996. Virus-lymphoid cell interactions. *Proc. Natl. Acad. Sci. USA* **93:**12756–12758.

Origgi, L., M. Vanoli, A. Carbone, M. Grasso, and R. Scorza. 1998. Central nervous system involvement in patients with HCV-related cryoglobulinemia. *Am. J. Med. Sci.* **315:**208–210.

Orth, M., and A. H. Schapira. 2001. Mitochondria and degenerative disorders. *Am. J. Med. Genet.* **106:**27–36.

Papaevangelou, V., H. Pollack, G. Rochford, R. Kokka, Z. Hou, D. Chernoff, B. Hanna, K. Krasinski, and W. Borkowsky. 1998. Increased transmission of vertical hepatitis C virus (HCV) infection to human immunodeficiency virus (HIV)-infected infants of HIV- and HCV-coinfected women. *J. Infect. Dis.* **178:**1047–1052.

Petrov, T., B. D. Underwood, B. Braun, S. S. Alousi, and J. A. Rafols. 2001. Upregulation of iNOS expression and phosphorylation of eIF-2alpha are paralleled by suppression of protein synthesis in rat hypothalamus in a closed head trauma model. *J. Neurotrauma* **18:**799–812.

Pham, T. N., S. A. MacParland, P. M. Mulrooney, H. Cooksley, N. V. Naoumov, and T. I. Michalak. 2004. Hepatitis C virus persistence after spontaneous or treatment-induced resolution of hepatitis C. *J. Virol.* **78:**5867–5874.

Piroth, L., M. Duong, C. Quantin, M. Abrahamowicz, R. Michardiere, L. S. Aho, M. Grappin, M. Buisson, A. Waldner, H. Portier, and P. Chavanet. 1998. Does hepatitis C virus co-infection accelerate clinical and immunological evolution of HIV-infected patients? *AIDS* **12:**381–388.

Polyak, S. J., K. S. Khabar, D. M. Paschal, H. J. Ezelle, G. Duverlie, G. N. Barber, D. E. Levy, N. Mukaida, and D. R. Gretch. 2001a. Hepatitis C virus nonstructural 5A protein induces interleukin-8, leading to partial inhibition of the interferon-induced antiviral response. *J. Virol.* **75:**6095–6106.

Polyak, S. J., K. S. Khabar, M. Rezeiq, and D. R. Gretch. 2001b. Elevated levels of interleukin-8 in serum are associated with hepatitis C virus infection and resistance to interferon therapy. *J. Virol.* **75:**6209–6211.

Post, J. J., Y. Pan, A. J. Freeman, C. E. Harvey, P. A. White, P. Palladinetti, P. S. Haber, G. Marinos, M. H. Levy, J. M. Kaldor, K. A. Dolan, R. A. Ffrench, A. R. Lloyd, and W. D. Rawlinson. 2004. Clearance of hepatitis C viremia associated with cellular immunity in the absence of seroconversion in the hepatitis C incidence and transmission in prisons study cohort. *J. Infect. Dis.* **189:**1846–1855.

Price, R. W., J. Sidtis, and M. Rosenblum. 1988. The AIDS dementia complex: some current questions. *Ann. Neurol.* **23:**S27–S33.

Prince, A. M., B. Brotman, T. Huima, D. Pascual, M. Jaffery, and G. Inchauspe. 1992. Immunity in hepatitis C infection. *J. Infect. Dis.* **165:**438–443.

Pulliam, L., B. G. Herndier, N. M. Tang, and M. S. McGrath. 1991. Human immunodeficiency virus-infected macrophages produce soluble factors that cause histological and neurochemical alterations in cultured human brains. *J. Clin. Investig.* **87:**503–512.

Purcell, R. 1997. The hepatitis C virus: overview. *Hepatology* **26:**11S–14S.

Qadri, I., M. Iwahashi, J. M. Capasso, M. W. Hopken, S. Flores, J. Schaack, and F. R. Simon. 2004. Induced oxidative stress and activated expression of manganese superoxide dismutase during hepatitis C virus replication: role of JNK, p38 MAPK and AP-1. *Biochem. J.* **378:**919–928.

Radkowski, M., A. Bednarska, A. Horban, J. Stanczak, J. Wilkinson, D. M. Adair, M. Nowicki, J. Rakela, and T. Laskus. 2004a. Infection of primary human macrophages with hepatitis C virus in vitro: induction of tumour necrosis factor-alpha and interleukin 8. *J. Gen. Virol.* **85:**47–59.

Radkowski, M., J. F. Gallegos-Orozco, J. Jablonska, T. V. Colby, B. Walewska-Zielecka, J. Kubicka, J. Wilkinson, D. Adair, J. Rakela, and T. Laskus. 2004b. Persistence of hepatitis C virus in patients successfully treated for chronic hepatitis C. *Hepatology* **41:**106–114.

Radkowski, M., L. F. Wang, H. E. Vargas, J. Rakela, and T. Laskus. 1998. Detection of hepatitis C virus replication in peripheral blood mononuclear cells after orthotopic liver transplantation. *Transplantation* **66:**664–666.

Radkowski, M., J. Wilkinson, M. Nowicki, D. Adair, H. Vargas, C. Ingui, J. Rakela, and T. Laskus. 2002. Search for hepatitis C virus negative-strand RNA sequences and analysis of viral sequences in the central nervous system: evidence of replication. *J. Virol.* **76:**600–608.

Ray, S. C., Y. M. Wang, O. Laeyendecker, J. R. Ticehurst, S. A. Villano, and D. L. Thomas. 1999. Acute hepatitis C virus structural gene sequences as predictors of persistent viremia: hypervariable region 1 as a decoy. *J. Virol.* **73:**2938–2946.

Reichard, O., H. Glaumann, A. Fryden, G. Norkrans, R. Wejstal, and O. Weiland. 1999. Long-term follow-up of chronic hepatitis C patients with sustained virological response to alpha-interferon. *J. Hepatol.* **30:**783–787.

Richardson, J. L., M. Nowicki, K. Danley, E. M. Martin, M. H. Cohen, R. Gonzalez, J. Vassileva, and A. M. Levine. 2005. Neuropsychological functioning in a cohort of HIV- and hepatitis C virus-infected women. *AIDS* **19:**1659–1667.

Ridzon, R., K. Gallagher, C. Ciesielski, M. B. Ginsberg, B. J. Robertson, C. C. Luo, and A. DeMaria, Jr. 1997. Simultaneous transmission of human immunodeficiency virus and hepatitis C virus from a needle-stick injury. *N. Engl. J. Med.* **336:**919–922.

Roque-Afonso, A. M., D. Ducoulombier, G. Di Liberto, R. Kara, E. Dussaix, D. Samuel, and C. Feray. 2005. Compartmentalization of hepatitis C virus genotypes between plasma and peripheral blood mononuclear cells. *J. Virol.* **79:**6349–6357.

Ryan, E. L., S. Morgello, K. Isaacs, M. Naseer, and P. Gerits. 2004. Neuropsychiatric impact of hepatitis C on advanced HIV. *Neurology* **62:**957–962.

Sabin, C. A., P. Telfer, A. N. Phillips, S. Bhagani, and C. A. Lee. 1997. The association between hepatitis C virus genotype and human immunodeficiency virus disease progression in a cohort of hemophilic men. *J. Infect. Dis.* **175:**164–168.

Sacktor, N. C., H. Bacellar, D. R. Hoover, T. E. Nance-Sproson, O. A. Selnes, E. N. Miller, G. J. Dal Pan, C. Kleeberger, A. Brown, A. Saah, and J. C. McArthur. 1996. Psychomotor slowing in HIV infection: a predictor of dementia, AIDS and death. *J. Neurovirol.* **2:**404–410.

Saiz, J. C., S. Lopez de Quinto, N. Ibarrola, F. X. Lopez-Labrador, J. M. Sanchez-Tapias, J. Rodes, and E. Martinez-Salas. 1999. Internal initiation of translation efficiency in different hepatitis C genotypes isolated from interferon treated patients. *Arch. Virol.* **144:**215–229.

Sansonno, D., A. R. Iacobelli, V. Cornacchiulo, G. Iodice, and F. Dammacco. 1996. Detection of hepatitis C virus (HCV) proteins by immunofluorescence and HCV RNA genomic sequences by non-isotopic in situ hybridization in bone marrow and peripheral blood mononuclear cells of chronically HCV-infected patients. *Clin. Exp. Immunol.* **103:**414–421.

Saraste, M. 1999. Oxidative phosphorylation at the fin de siecle. *Science* **283:**1488–1493.

Scarselli, E., A. Cerino, G. Esposito, E. Silini, M. U. Mondelli, and C. Traboni. 1995. Occurrence of antibodies reactive with more than one variant of the putative envelope glycoprotein (gp70) hypervariable region 1 in viremic hepatitis C virus-infected patients. *J. Virol.* **69:**4407–4412.

Schupper, H., P. Hayashi, J. Scheffel, S. Aceituno, T. Paglieroni, P. V. Holland, and J. B. Zeldis. 1993. Peripheral-blood mononuclear cell responses to recombinant hepatitis C virus antigens in patients with chronic hepatitis C. *Hepatology* **18:**1055–1060.

Schwer, B., S. Ren, T. Pietschmann, J. Kartenbeck, K. Kaehlcke, R. Bartenschlager, T. S. Yen, and M. Ott. 2004. Targeting of hepatitis C virus core protein to mitochondria through a novel C-terminal localization motif. *J. Virol.* **78:**7958–7968.

Seeff, L. B., F. B. Hollinger, H. J. Alter, E. C. Wright, C. M. Cain, Z. J. Buskell, K. G. Ishak, F. L. Iber, D. Toro, A. Samanta, R. L. Koretz, R. P. Perrillo, Z. D. Goodman, R. G. Knodell, G. Gitnick, T. R. Morgan, E. R. Schiff, S. Lasky, C. Stevens, R. Z. Vlahcevic, E. Weinshel, T. Tanwandee, H. J. Lin, and L. Barbosa. 2001. Long-term mortality and morbidity of transfusion-associated non-A, non-B, and type C hepatitis: a National Heart, Lung, and Blood Institute collaborative study. *Hepatology* **33:**455–463.

Shata, M. T., N. Tricoche, M. Perkus, D. Tom, B. Brotman, P. McCormack, W. Pfahler, D. H. Lee, L. H. Tobler, M. Busch, and A. M. Prince. 2003. Exposure to low infective doses of HCV induces cellular immune responses without consistently detectable viremia or seroconversion in chimpanzees. *Virology* **314:**601–616.

Sherman, K. E., J. O'Brien, A. G. Gutierrez, S. Harrison, M. Urdea, P. Neuwald, and J. Wilber. 1993. Quantitative evaluation of hepatitis C virus RNA in patients with concurrent human immunodeficiency virus infections. *J. Clin. Microbiol.* **31:**2679–2682.

Shimizu, Y. K., H. Igarashi, T. Kanematu, K. Fujiwara, D. C. Wong, R. H. Purcell, and H. Yoshikura. 1997. Sequence analysis of the hepatitis C virus genome recovered from serum, liver, and peripheral blood mononuclear cells of infected chimpanzees. *J. Virol.* **71:**5769–5773.

Shimizu, Y. K., R. H. Purcell, and H. Yoshikura. 1993. Correlation between the infectivity of hepatitis C virus in vivo and its infectivity in vitro. *Proc. Natl. Acad. Sci. USA* **90:**6037–6041.

Shindo, M., A. M. Di Bisceglie, R. Biswas, K. Mihalik, and S. M. Feinstone. 1992. Hepatitis C virus replication during acute infection in the chimpanzee. *J. Infect. Dis.* **166:**424–427.

Shirai, M., T. Arichi, M. Chen, T. Masaki, M. Nishioka, K. Ikeda, H. Takahashi, N. Enomoto, T. Saito, M. E. Major, T. Nakazawa, T. Akatsuka, S. M. Feinstone, and J. A. Berzofsky. 1999. T cell recognition of hypervariable region-1 from hepatitis C virus envelope protein with multiple class II MHC molecules in mice and humans: preferential help for induction of antibodies to the hypervariable region. *J. Immunol.* **162:**568–576.

Shirai, M., H. Okada, M. Nishioka, T. Akatsuka, C. Wychowski, R. Houghten, C. D. Pendleton, S. M. Feinstone, and J. A. Berzofsky. 1994. An epitope in hepatitis C virus core region recognized by cytotoxic T cells in mice and humans. *J. Virol.* **68:**3334–3342.

Simonetti, R. G., C. Camma, F. Fiorello, M. Cottone, M. Rapicetta, L. Marino, G. Fiorentino, A. Craxi, A. Ciccaglione, R. Giuseppetti, T. Stroffolini, and L. Pagliaro. 1992. Hepatitis C virus infection as a risk factor for hepatocellular carcinoma in patients with cirrhosis. A case-control study. *Ann. Intern. Med.* **116:**97–102.

Singh, N., T. Gayowski, M. M. Wagener, and I. R. Marino. 1999. Quality of life, functional status, and depression in male liver transplant recipients with recurrent viral hepatitis C. *Transplantation* **67:**69–72.

Smith, D. B., J. McAllister, C. Casino, and P. Simmonds. 1997. Virus 'quasispecies': making a mountain out of a molehill? *J. Gen. Virol.* **78:**1511–1519.

Smith, D. B., J. Mellor, L. M. Jarvis, F. Davidson, J. Kolberg, M. Urdea, P. L. Yap, P. Simmonds, et al. 1995. Variation of the hepatitis C virus 5′ non-coding region: implications for secondary structure, virus detection and typing. *J. Gen. Virol.* **76:**1749–1761.

Song, G., V. K. Dhodda, A. T. Blei, R. J. Dempsey, and V. L. Rao. 2002. GeneChip analysis shows altered mRNA expression of transcripts of neurotransmitter and signal transduction pathways in the cerebral cortex of portacaval shunted rats. *J. Neurosci. Res.* **68:**730–737.

Steinhauer, D. A., and J. J. Holland. 1987. Rapid evolution of RNA viruses. *Annu. Rev. Microbiol.* **41:**409–433.

Sugitani, M., and T. Shikata. 1998. Comparison of amino acid sequences in hypervariable region-1 of hepatitis C virus clones between human inocula and the infected chimpanzee sera. *Virus Res.* **56:**177–182.

Sulkowski, M. S., R. D. Moore, S. H. Mehta, R. E. Chaisson, and D. L. Thomas. 2002. Hepatitis C and progression of HIV disease. *JAMA* **288:**199–206.

Swain, M., E. J. Heathcote, L. M.Y., V. Bain, V. Feinman, M. Sherman, K. D. Kaita, E. Gane, K. Peltekian, and K. L. Lindsay. 2001. Long-lasting sustained virological response in chronic hepatitis C patients previously treated with 40 kD peginterferon alpha-2A (Pegasys). *Hepatology* **34:**330A. (Abstract.)

Takaki, A., M. Wiese, G. Maertens, E. Depla, U. Seifert, A. Liebetrau, J. L. Miller, M. P. Manns, and B. Rehermann. 2000. Cellular immune responses persist and humoral responses decrease two decades after recovery from a single-source outbreak of hepatitis C. *Nat. Med.* **6:**578–582.

Taylor, M. J., S. L. Letendre, B. C. Schweinsburg, O. M. Alhassoon, G. G. Brown, A. Gongvatana, and I. Grant. 2004. Hepatitis C virus infection is associated with reduced white matter N-acetylaspartate in abstinent methamphetamine users. *J. Int. Neuropsychol. Soc.* **10:**110–113.

Taylor-Robinson, S. D. 2001. Applications of magnetic resonance spectroscopy to chronic liver disease. *Clin. Med.* **1:**54–60.

Thelu, M. A., E. Drouet, M. N. Hilleret, and J. P. Zarski. 2004. Lack of clinical significance of variability in the internal ribosome entry site of hepatitis C virus. *J. Med. Virol.* **72:**396–405.

Thimme, R., J. Bukh, H. C. Spangenberg, S. Wieland, J. Pemberton, C. Steiger, S. Govindarajan, R. H. Purcell, and F. V. Chisari. 2002. Viral and immunological determinants of hepatitis C virus clearance, persistence, and disease. *Proc. Natl. Acad. Sci. USA* **99:**15661–15668.

Thimme, R., D. Oldach, K. M. Chang, C. Steiger, S. C. Ray, and F. V. Chisari. 2001. Determinants of viral clearance and persistence during acute hepatitis C virus infection. *J. Exp. Med.* **194:**1395–1406.

Thomas, D. L., J. D. Rich, P. Schuman, D. K. Smith, J. A. Astemborski, K. R. Nolt, and R. S. Klein. 2001. Multicenter evaluation of hepatitis C RNA levels among female injection drug users. *J. Infect. Dis.* **183:**973–976.

Thomas, S. L., M. L. Newell, C. S. Peckham, A. E. Ades, and A. J. Hall. 1998. A review of hepatitis C virus (HCV) vertical transmission: risks of transmission to infants born to mothers with and without HCV viraemia or human immunodeficiency virus infection. *Int. J. Epidemiol.* **27:**108–117.

Tovo, P. A., E. Palomba, G. Ferraris, N. Principi, E. Ruga, P. Dallacasa, A. Maccabruni, et al. 1997. Increased risk of maternal-infant hepatitis C virus transmission for women coinfected with human immunodeficiency virus type 1. *Clin. Infect. Dis.* **25:**1121–1124.

Toyoda, H., Y. Fukuda, Y. Koyama, J. Takamatsu, H. Saito, and T. Hayakawa. 1997. Effect of immunosuppression on composition of quasispecies population of hepatitis C virus in patients with chronic hepatitis C coinfected with human immunodeficiency virus. *J. Hepatol.* **26:**975–982.

Tsukiyama-Kohara, K., N. Iizuka, M. Kohara, and A. Nomoto. 1992. Internal ribosome entry site within hepatitis C virus RNA. *J. Virol.* **66:**1476–1483.

Unger, E. R., J. H. Sung, J. C. Manivel, M. L. Chenggis, B. R. Blazar, and W. Krivit. 1993. Male donor-derived cells in the brains of female sex-mismatched bone marrow transplant recipients: a Y-chromosome specific in situ hybridization study. *J. Neuropathol. Exp. Neurol.* **52:**460–470.

van't Wout, A. B., N. A. Kootstra, G. A. Mulder-Kampinga, N. Albrecht-van Lent, H. J. Scherpbier, J. Veenstra, K. Boer, R. A. Coutinho, F. Miedema, and H. Schuitemaker. 1994. Macrophage-tropic variants initiate human immunodeficiency virus type 1 infection after sexual, parenteral, and vertical transmission. *J. Clin. Investig.* **94:**2060–2067.

von Giesen, H. J., T. Heintges, N. Abbasi-Boroudjeni, S. Kucukkoylu, H. Koller, B. A. Haslinger, M. Oette, and G. Arendt. 2004. Psychomotor slowing in hepatitis C and HIV infection. *J. Acquir. Immune Defic. Syndr.* **35:**131–137.

Wang, C., P. Sarnow, and A. Siddiqui. 1994. A conserved helical element is essential for internal initiation of translation of hepatitis C virus RNA. *J. Virol.* **68:**7301–7307.

Warskulat, U., B. Gorg, H. J. Bidmon, H. W. Muller, F. Schliess, and D. Haussinger. 2002. Ammonia-induced heme oxygenase-1 expression in cultured rat astrocytes and rat brain in vivo. *Glia* **40:**324–336.

Weiner, A. J., M. J. Brauer, J. Rosenblatt, K. H. Richman, J. Tung, K. Crawford, F. Bonino, G. Saracco, Q. L. Choo, M. Houghton, et al. 1991. Variable and hypervariable domains are found in the regions of HCV corresponding to the flavivirus envelope and NS1 proteins and the pestivirus envelope glycoproteins. *Virology* **180:**842–848.

Weiner, A. J., H. M. Geysen, C. Christopherson, J. E. Hall, T. J. Mason, G. Saracco, F. Bonino, K. Crawford, C. D. Marion, K. A. Crawford, et al. 1992. Evidence for immune selection of hepatitis C virus (HCV) putative envelope glycoprotein variants: potential role in chronic HCV infections. *Proc. Natl. Acad. Sci. USA* **89:**3468–3472.

Weiner, A. J., M. M. Thaler, K. Crawford, K. Ching, J. Kansopon, D. Y. Chien, J. E. Hall, F. Hu, and M. Houghton. 1993. A unique, predominant hepatitis C virus variant found in an infant born to a mother with multiple variants. *J. Virol.* **67:**4365–4368.

Weissenborn, K., J. Krause, M. Bokemeyer, H. Hecker, A. Schuler, J. C. Ennen, B. Ahl, M. P. Manns, and K. W. Boker. 2004. Hepatitis C virus infection affects the brain-evidence from psychometric studies and magnetic resonance spectroscopy. *J. Hepatol.* **41:**845–851.

Wilson, C. J., C. E. Finch, and H. J. Cohen. 2002. Cytokines and cognition--the case for a head-to-toe inflammatory paradigm. *J. Am. Geriatr. Soc.* **50:**2041–2056.

Winnock, M., D. Salmon-Ceron, F. Dabis, and G. Chene. 2004. Interaction between HIV-1 and HCV infections: towards a new entity? *J. Antimicrob. Chemother.* **53:**936–946.

Wright, T. L., H. Hollander, X. Pu, M. J. Held, P. Lipson, S. Quan, A. Polito, M. M. Thaler, P. Bacchetti, and B. F. Scharschmidt. 1994. Hepatitis C in HIV-infected patients with and without AIDS: prevalence and relationship to patient survival. *Hepatology* **20:**1152–1155.

Yoo, T. W., S. Donfield, A. Lail, H. S. Lynn, and E. S. Daar. 2005. Effect of hepatitis C virus (HCV) genotype on HCV and HIV-1 disease. *J. Infect. Dis.* **191:**4–10.

Zanetti, A. R., E. Tanzi, S. Paccagnini, N. Principi, G. Pizzocolo, M. L. Caccamo, E. D'Amico, G. Cambie, L. Vecchi, et al. 1995. Mother-to-infant transmission of hepatitis C virus. *Lancet* **345:**289–291.

Zheng, J., and H. E. Gendelman. 1997. The HIV-1 associated dementia complex: a metabolic encephalopathy fueled by viral replication in mononuclear phagocytes. *Curr. Opin. Neurol.* **10:**319–325.

The Spectrum of Neuro-AIDS Disorders:
Pathophysiology, Diagnosis, and Treatment
Edited by K. Goodkin et al.
©2008 ASM Press, Washington, DC

22

Toxoplasmosis of the Central Nervous System

KATIA V. BROWN AND DANIEL J. SKIEST

Toxoplasma gondii is an obligate intracellular parasite present throughout the world. In immunocompromised individuals, especially those with AIDS, the organism has a predilection for the central nervous system (CNS), where it may cause a variety of clinical syndromes, encephalitis being the most common. In studies conducted in the era prior to the widespread use of highly active antiretroviral therapy (HAART), CNS toxoplasmosis was the most common cause of focal neurological disease in AIDS patients (Levy et al., 1985; McArthur, 1987). While the incidence of toxoplasmic encephalitis (TE) has decreased in patients treated with HAART and with appropriate anti-*Toxoplasma* prophylaxis, it still remains an important cause of morbidity and mortality. In recent years, in addition to the decreased incidence of TE, a number of advances have occurred in the diagnosis and management of TE. This chapter focuses on the pathogenesis, diagnosis, and management of CNS toxoplasmosis. The latest epidemiological trends are discussed, and special attention is given to recently developed diagnostic modalities including laboratory techniques and newer neuroimaging modalities. Current therapeutic and prophylactic guidelines are presented.

EPIDEMIOLOGY

The prevalence of *T. gondii* seropositivity throughout the world varies depending on the population being studied (Houff, 1997). The seroprevalence among HIV-infected patients reflects this geographic variability. It has been estimated that about 10 to 40% of AIDS patients in the United States are latently infected with *T. gondii*, while in Europe and Latin America the prevalence is estimated at 30 to 75% (Luft and Remington, 1988, 1992; Glatt, 1992; Grant et al., 1990; Zangerle et al., 1991; Israelski et al., 1993). The seroprevalence in a recent cohort of 2,628 U.S. women with HIV infection or at risk for HIV infection was 15.1% (Falusi et al., 2002). Factors associated with a higher seroprevalence rate

included age (≥50 years), birth outside the United States, and CD4 cell counts of 200 to 499 cells/μl (compared to counts of ≥500 cells/μl). This prevalence is consistent with findings of previous reports from the United States of seroprevalence in HIV-uninfected individuals (Jones et al., 2001). Other studies have found that the country of birth was strongly correlated with *Toxoplasma* seropositivity, as also was age (Glatt, 1992; Jones et al., 2001; Glatt, 2003).

Incidence

In the pre-HAART era approximately 5 to 47% of latently infected AIDS patients (mostly without antibiotic prophylaxis) eventually develop CNS toxoplasmosis (Grant et al., 1990; Zangerle et al., 1991; Cohen, 1999; Renold et al., 1992; Porter and Sande, 1992; Oksenhendler et al., 1994; Mariuz et al., 1997). In populations with widespread use of HAART and *Toxoplasma* prophylaxis the incidence is now reported to be lower in most but not all studies (Ledergerber et al., 1999; Olatinwo et al., 2001; San-Andrés et al., 2003; Abgrall et al., 2001; Jones et al., 1999; Ives et al., 2001; Maschke et al., 2000; Neuenburg et al., 2002). A recent Spanish study observed a cohort of 1,115 patients between 1989 and 1997. For the patients who adhered to antiretroviral therapy and to *Pneumocystis carinii* pneumonia (PCP) prophylaxis, an 18% annual risk reduction for CNS toxoplasmosis was observed (San-Andrés et al., 2003). Similarly, in a study aimed at assessing the incidence of TE before and after the availability of protease inhibitors, the incidence of TE decreased from 3.9 cases per 100 person-years to 1.0 case per 100 person-years (Abgrall et al., 2001). While there has clearly been a decline in HIV-related CNS pathology due to HAART as demonstrated by a recent study of 1,597 autopsies, the prevalence of CNS lesions from *Toxoplasma* remains relatively high in patients dying in the HAART era (~15%) (Vago et al., 2002).

PATHOGENESIS

Life Cycle

In cats, the definitive host, the complete life cycle (including a sexual and an asexual phase) occurs, while in intermediate hosts such as humans only the asexual (extraintestinal)

Katia V. Brown, Center for Infectious Diseases, McAllen, TX 78501.
Daniel J. Skiest, Division of Infectious Diseases, Baystate Medical Center, Springfield, MA 01199.

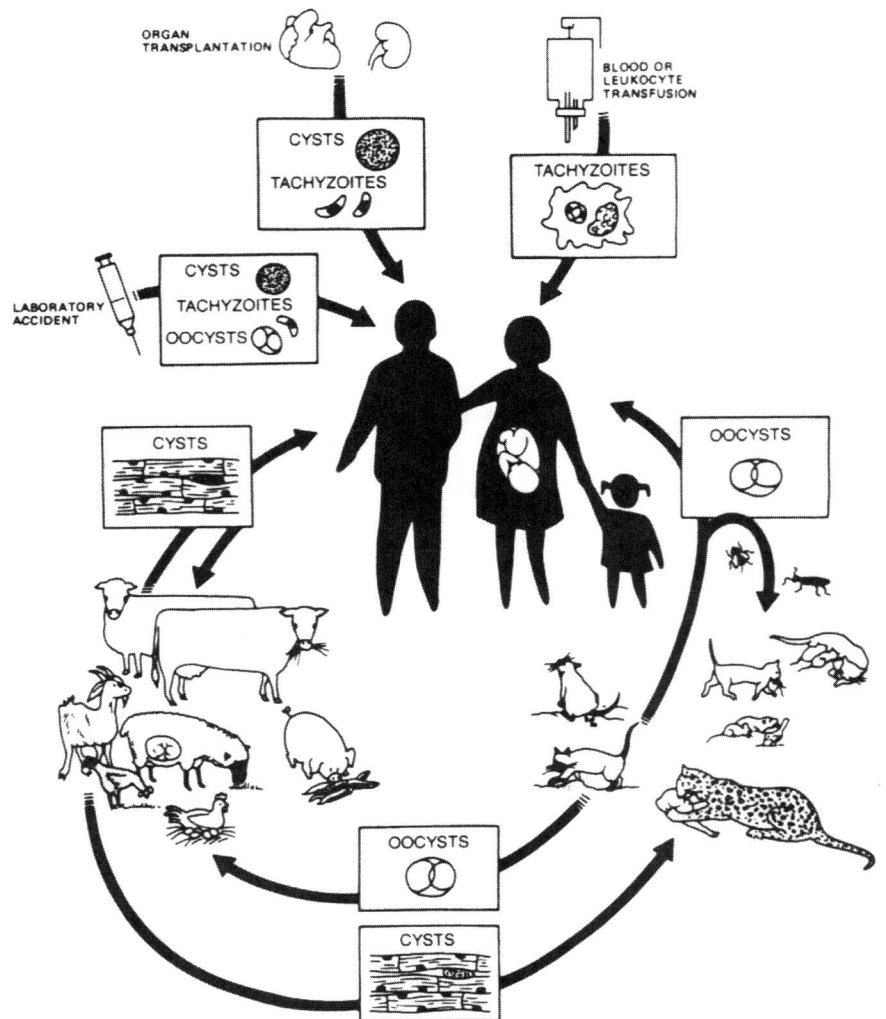

FIGURE 1 Life cycle of *T. gondii*. (Adapted with permission from Remington and McLeod, 1998.)

phase occurs (Fig. 1). Cats acquire infection by ingesting sporulated oocysts from food, soil, or water or from ingesting tissue cysts from contaminated food (e.g., muscle of an intermediate host). The oocysts are formed during an intraintestinal or sexual stage within the gut of the cat. Bradyzoites are released from tissue cysts, and sporozoites are released from oocysts (Dukes et al., 1997). After being released into the environment, and under certain favorable circumstances like a humid and warm climate, the oocysts have the ability to sporulate and remain infectious for as long as 1 to 1.5 years. Infection is more common in humid, temperate climates than in arid, hot climates (Jones et al., 2001).

Humans and other intermediate hosts may acquire the organism by ingestion of oocysts (excreted by cats) that contaminate soil, water, or cat litter or by ingestion of tissue cysts within undercooked meats such as pork and lamb. Recent studies indicate that the latter is the more common mode of acquisition (Renold et al., 1992). Less commonly, infection may occur transplacentally (when the mother is acutely infected during pregnancy) or rarely via a laboratory accident, blood transfusion, or organ transplantation

(D'Offizi et al., 2002; Parker and Holliman, 1992; Munir et al., 2000). After ingestion, sporozoites (from oocysts) or bradyzoites (from tissue cysts) are released into the gut, penetrate its wall, and invade cells. Within the cell vacuoles, asexual multiplication, or transformation of bradyzoites or sporozoites into tachyzoites, occurs until the cell ruptures, resulting in spread to adjacent cells. Phagocytosis of tachyzoites occurs with hematogenous dissemination throughout the host. There is a predilection for the brain, skeletal muscle, lymphatic tissue, and heart, although any mammalian cell can be infected. This represents the acute infection phase. In tissues tachyzoites aggregate until they form tissue cysts, which contain bradyzoites and are responsible for the disease's latent stage. The tissue cysts, which are able to persist for life in the host, are believed to have a preference for the CNS, where there is a relative lack of host defense (Chao et al., 1994). Animal studies have shown that there are intermittent cycles of cyst rupture, which may explain the persistence of antibody titers. Humans with intact cell-mediated immunity are able to limit replication of tachyzoites and prevent reactivation of tissue cysts, although the exact mechanism is still unknown. It has been postulated that the immunosuppressed state, e.g., in AIDS patients with low CD4 cell counts, allows proliferation of tachyzoites following disruption of tissue cysts (Suzuki, 2002a).

Approximately 20 to 50% of the seropositive AIDS population will develop TE as a result of reactivation of latent CNS infection (Sarciron and Gherardi, 2000). It appears that host factors and parasite virulence factors are important determinants of reactivation (Chao et al., 1994; Suzuki, 2002a). A number of alterations in cellular and immunological markers have been implicated in disease reactivation. Both CD4$^+$ and CD8$^+$ T cells are important in the host response to infection with *T. gondii*. The important role of CD4 cells in preventing disease reactivation is evident by the CD4$^+$-cell depletion at the time of presentation of AIDS patients with TE (CD4$^+$-cell population is usually <100/μl) (Renold et al., 1992; Porter and Sande, 1992; Hunter and Remington, 1994; Dannemann et al., 1992). There is experimental evidence that depletion of CD4$^+$ T cells results in inability to control *T. gondii* infection (Houff, 1997). In addition, CD8$^+$ cells, which are directly cytotoxic to infected cells, release protective cytokines, which inhibit *T. gondii* replication. Models utilizing immunocompetent and immunosuppressed animals have helped analyze these complex interactions between cytokines as well as suggesting a possible genetic basis for the susceptibility to *T. gondii* (Araujo and Slifer, 2003). In mice differences in genes coding for the major histocompatibility complex correlate with susceptibility to active CNS disease (Hunter and Remington, 1994; Johnson et al., 2002). There is evidence that in humans certain major histocompatibility complex class alleles (HLA-DQ3) may increase susceptibility to TE, while DQ1 may decrease susceptibility (reviewed by Suzuki, 2002b).

Several studies support the important role of cytokines in the immunopathogenesis of TE (Sarciron and Gherardi, 2000; Suzuki, 2002b; Däubener and Hadding, 1997). Gamma interferon (IFN-γ)-dependent cell-mediated immunity plays a major role in resistance to *T. gondii* in mice in both acute and chronic infection by promoting activation of macrophages to kill intracellular tachyzoites after infection (Suzuki, 2002b; reviewed by Hunter and Remington [1994] and Suzuki et al. [1988]). Macrophages and other cells including NK cells, lymphokine-activated killer cells, neutrophils, and monocytes have the ability to kill the organism (Hunter and Remington, 1994; Suzuki, 2002b). Macrophages inhibit parasite replication via production of oxygen free radicals and reactive nitrogen intermediates as well as other mechanisms (reviewed by Hunter and Remington, 1994). Dendritic cells of infected animals have been shown to be major producers of interleukin-12 (IL-12), which is important for the maintenance of IFN-γ production in T cells responsible for resistance to chronic infection. Other cytokines including tumor necrosis factor alpha may play a role in resistance to *T. gondii* infection (Sarciron and Gherardi, 2000; Hunter and Remington, 1994; Suzuki, 2002b; Däubener and Haddin, 1997).

In the CNS, microglial cells and possibly astrocytes are important in the local defense against *T. gondii*. Microglial cells prevent proliferation of tachyzoites in the brain (reviewed by Suzuki, 2002b). In contrast to the important role of cell-mediated immunity, it appears that although antibodies to *T. gondii* are rapidly elicited upon acute infection, significant protection is not conferred by this response (Fadul et al., 1995).

PATHOLOGY

CNS toxoplasmosis has been reported in 3 to 41% of AIDS autopsy cases (Neuenberg et al., 2002; Hainfellner and Budkha, 1997; Burns et al., 1991; Kure et al., 1991; Masliah et al., 2000). The lesions associated with toxoplasmosis vary in size, characteristics, and location (Laing et al., 1996). Postmortem neuropathologic evaluations of AIDS patients with CNS toxoplasmosis have shown that the gross appearance is influenced by the duration of disease and prior therapy (Burns et al., 1991). Although any part of the brain may be involved, lesions occur most commonly in the parietal and frontal lobes, the corticomedullary junction, and the basal ganglia. The temporal and occipital lobes, as well as the thalamus, cerebellum, pituitary gland, and brain stem, are less commonly involved. There is a predilection for the superficial and deep gray matter. The choroid plexus may be involved as well. One study found involvement of the choroid plexus in 53% of cases, including one case in which it was the only site of CNS infection (Falangola and Petito, 1993). Leptomeningeal involvement is uncommon, but there may be local inflammation if there is an underlying process involving the cortex. Spinal cord lesions may also occur but are relatively uncommon (6% in one autopsy series) (Strittmatter et al., 1992; Vyas and Ebright, 1996).

Grossly the appearance of lesions may vary from ill-defined areas of opaque or dusky coagulation necrosis with variable degrees of edema to frank abscesses (Farkash et al., 1986) (Fig. 2). Microscopically the lesions differ, depending on the stage of disease. Early lesions are characterized by small aggregates of microglia associated with (pseudo)cysts and/or free tachyzoites and variable mononuclear infiltrates, histiocytes, and plasma cells (Burns et al., 1991). Typical lesions of toxoplasmosis are characterized histopathologically by three zones (Post et al., 1983). The central area demonstrates an area of necrosis without blood vessels. This is surrounded by a region consisting of a mixed inflammatory infiltrate with perivascular cuffing by lymphocytes, plasma cells, and macrophages. Tachyzoites may be seen in this zone. Cysts (which appear as 2- to 4-μm basophilic organisms)

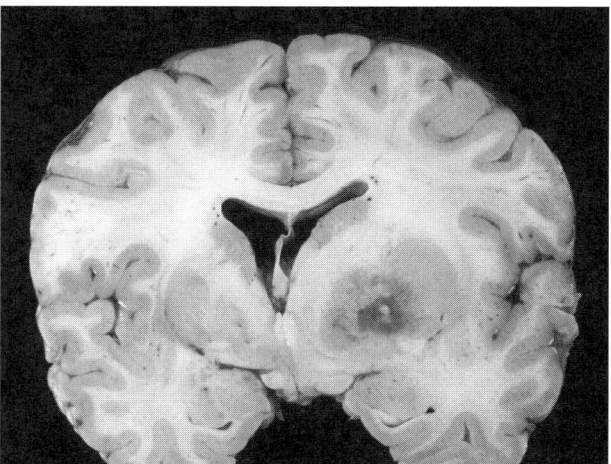

FIGURE 2 Postmortem brain showing a lesion of untreated toxoplasmosis involving the basal ganglia. There is significant surrounding edema and mass effect with compression of the ipsilateral ventricle. (Reprinted with permission from Rushing and Burns, 2001.)

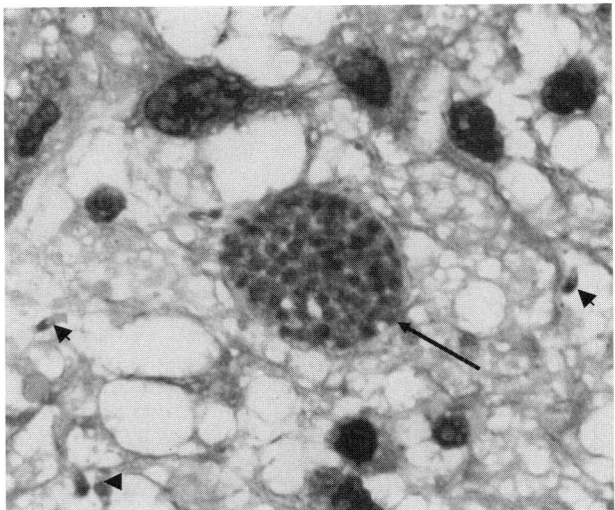

FIGURE 3 Giemsa stain (magnification, ×1,000) of brain biopsy specimen from a patient with CNS toxoplasmosis. Tissue cyst containing multiple bradyzoites (arrow). The surrounding area reveals numerous tachyzoites (arrowheads). (Photomicrograph is courtesy of Dennis Burns.)

may be found at the periphery of these lesions within the inflammatory infiltrate (Fig. 3) (Farkash et al., 1986). Vasculitis is common in the surrounding blood vessels with infiltration by neutrophils and often thrombosis. Areas of brain around the lesions are typically edematous and may be infarcted. One autopsy review found that tachyzoites were predominantly localized in the walls of hypertrophic arteries, suggesting that ischemic infarction plays a role in the pathogenesis of the disease (Huang and Chou, 1988). Staining with hematoxylin and eosin is relatively insensitive and may fail to detect organisms. Wright and Giemsa stains are useful in seeing organisms. Use of immunoperoxidase staining significantly increases diagnostic sensitivity (McArthur, 1998).

Less commonly, a diffuse form of encephalitis has been described in which the gross appearance of the brain is normal or atrophic. Histopathologically there are widespread microglial nodules, many of which contain cysts and/or tachyzoites throughout the brain (Renold et al., 1992; Hainfellner and Budkha, 1997; Post et al., 1983; Gray et al., 1989). Other uncommon pathologic findings include subependymal infection, ventriculitis, and microinfarction due to parasitic emboli (Hainfellner and Budkha, 1997).

Treated lesions appear to be better organized, with a well-defined area of central necrosis surrounded by macrophages and without significant surrounding edema. Organisms are fewer than in untreated infection. Reflecting the markedly impaired cell-mediated immunity that is characteristic of patients at risk for CNS toxoplasmosis, it is not uncommon to find concomitant AIDS-related CNS diseases along with cerebral toxoplasmosis in postmortem studies (Leport et al., 1988). In one series of 20 patients with TE, 8 patients had a concomitant diagnosis of either CNS lymphoma, HIV encephalitis, cytomegalovirus encephalitis, or a combination of these (Renold et al., 1992).

Although the brain is by far the most common organ involved in AIDS, involvement of almost every organ system has been described, including the heart, skeletal muscle, lungs, intestines, liver, and testes. Ocular involvement is characterized by necrotizing chorioretinitis but is relatively uncommon in AIDS patients (see below).

CLINICAL MANIFESTATIONS

Acute infection with *T. gondii* in the immunocompetent host is usually asymptomatic. Some experience a mononucleosis-like syndrome with cervical lymphadenopathy, fever, night sweats, malaise, pharyngitis, rash (usually maculopapular), hepatosplenomegaly, and a mild degree of atypical lymphocytosis. In the immunocompetent individual the above symptom complex is self-limited as the immune system controls infection and there are no further manifestations of toxoplasmosis.

In patients with AIDS, toxoplasmosis is almost always due to reactivation of previously acquired infection. Manifestations of toxoplasmosis in the AIDS population are primarily those of CNS dysfunction and usually reflect the multiple abscesses that are present. Accompanying pathology like cerebral edema or hemorrhage may affect the clinical presentation as well (Wijdicks et al., 1991). The onset of symptoms is generally subacute, lasting anywhere from 5 days to several weeks prior to diagnosis. More than two-thirds of patients present with focal signs and symptoms, which are often accompanied by signs of general CNS alteration (Table 1). The most common signs and symptoms are headache, fever, altered mentation, motor deficits, and seizures (Renold et al., 1992; Porter and Sande, 1992; Dannemann et al., 1988, 1992; Laing et al., 1996; Leport et al., 1988; Katlama et al., 1996b; Raffi et al., 1997; Wanke et al., 1987). Other findings include behavioral or neuropsychiatric changes, ataxia/cerebellar disturbance, cranial nerve palsies, visual field defects, and aphasia. Meningeal signs and symptoms are uncommon and are reported in approximately 10 to 16% of patients. Nystagmus, extrapyramidal symptoms, incontinence, and movement disorders have also been described (Sanchez-Ramos et al., 1989; Hamed et al., 1988). As many as 10% of patients present with a diffuse encephalitis without any visible focal lesions (Luft and Remington, 1992). Patients who present with diffuse cortical dysfunction with altered mentation usually exhibit focal neurologic deficits as the disease progresses. The diffuse encephalitic form can present acutely and follow a rapidly progressive course (Renold et al., 1992; Gray et al., 1989).

Brain stem lesions may present with oculomotor deficits and/or contralateral hemiplegia (Cohen, 1999). Other less common manifestations of CNS toxoplasmosis have been reported, including meningoencephalitis and ependymitis without parenchymal lesions (Caramello et al., 1993), obstructive hydrocephalus secondary to exudative ependymitis (Eggers et al., 1995), disseminated hemorrhagic encephalitis (Wijdicks et al., 1991), thalamic pain syndrome, bilateral opercular syndrome, panhypopituitarism, and the syndrome of inappropriate antidiuretic hormone secretion (Cohen, 1999).

More than a dozen cases of myelopathy secondary to *T. gondii* have been reported (Vyas and Ebright, 1996; Dal Pan and Berger, 1997). Most patients presented with signs of cord involvement, including motor deficits, particularly of the lower extremities; paraparesis; increased deep tendon reflexes; and sensory loss reflecting the spinal cord level involved. Other presentations include Babinski signs, back pain, urinary hesitancy, urinary and fecal incontinence,

TABLE 1 Clinical manifestations of CNS toxoplasmosis in AIDS

Clinical manifestation	No. (%) of patients with indicated symptoms as reported by:			
	Katlama et al., 1996b $n = 299$	Renold et al., 1992 $n = 86$	Porter and Sande, 1992 $n = 115$	Raffi et al., 1997 $n = 113$
Headache	187 (63)	42 (49)	63 (55)	62 (55)
Confusion	NA[a]	13 (15)	60 (52)	NA[a]
Fever	204 (68)	35 (41)	54 (47)	67 (59)
Hemiparesis/motor deficits	77 (51)[b]	42 (49)	45 (39)	55 (49)
Lethargy/coma	130 (43)	14 (16)	49 (43)	59 (52)
Psychomotor/behavioral disorders	NA[a]	32 (37)	49 (38)	NA[a]
Seizure	57 (19)	21 (24)	33 (29)	25 (22)
Cerebellar signs/ataxia	43 (15)[b]	8 (9)	34 (30)	NA[a]
Cranial nerve palsies	54 (29)[b]	15 (17)	32 (28)	14 (12)
Meningeal signs	NA[a]	14 (16)	11 (10)	NA[a]
Aphasia	79 (29)[b]	5 (6)	9 (8)	NA[a]
Visual disorder including visual field defects	18 (10)[b]	7 (8)	8 (7)	NA[a]
Focal signs	211 (71)	65 (76)	79 (69)	79 (70)

[a]NA, information not available or not stated.
[b]Based on 288 patients.

and conus medullaris syndrome (Dal Pan and Berger, 1997). In most patients, magnetic resonance image (MRI) abnormalities of the spinal cord characterized by intramedullary lesions with gadolinium enhancement are found. The majority of patients reported had concomitant brain lesions.

Ocular Toxoplasmosis

Chorioretinitis and the ocular findings associated with it may be present occasionally, but most patients with CNS toxoplasmosis, do not have associated eye disease. Only 3 of 86 patients with TE had retinitis in one series (Renold et al., 1992). However, of those patients who present with ocular toxoplasmosis, 29 to 63% have been reported to have concomitant brain involvement (Navia et al., 1986; Gagliuso et al., 1990; Cochereau-Massin et al., 1992). Patients may present with chorioretinitis, iridocyclitis, uveitis, or retinal detachment (Gagliuso et al., 1990; Cochereau-Massin et al., 1992; Holland et al., 1988). Bilateral disease is seen in 18 to 37% of patients (Gagliuso et al., 1990; Cochereau-Massin et al., 1992). Inflammation in the anterior chamber and vitreous is variable (Gagliuso et al., 1990; Cochereau-Massin et al., 1992; Holland et al., 1988). Funduscopic examination reveals yellow-white areas with fluffy borders. Retinal hemorrhage is uncommon. Histopathologically, the hallmark is a focal necrotizing chorioretinitis with associated surrounding vasculitis and varying degrees of vitritis or papillitis (Bottoni et al., 1990), but cases of diffuse chorioretinitis have been described (Parke and Font, 1986). Cysts and tachyzoites can be seen in the necrotic areas. These lesions are rarely associated with preexisting retinochoroidal scars, which supports the idea that it is a newly acquired infection rather than reactivation of congenital disease (Gagliuso et al., 1990; Holland et al., 1988). Diagnosis is based mainly on the funduscopic appearance and response to anti-*Toxoplasma* therapy (Gagliuso et al., 1990). The differential diagnosis includes cytomegalovirus retinitis and necrotizing retinitis due to herpes simplex virus or varicella zoster virus. Ocular toxoplasmosis generally responds to the same

regimens used for CNS toxoplasmosis (discussed below) (Gagliuso et al., 1990; Cochereau-Massin et al., 1992).

None of the clinical findings noted above are specific for toxoplasmosis; they may be encountered in patients with other opportunistic infections or tumors, especially primary CNS lymphoma (PCNSL), as well as progressive multifocal leukoencephalopathy (PML), cryptococcomas, tuberculomas, and even AIDS-associated dementia (Luft and Remington, 1992).

DIAGNOSIS

Definitive diagnosis of CNS toxoplasmosis can be made only by demonstration of the organism in brain biopsy or occasionally cerebrospinal fluid (CSF) specimens. In patients with advanced HIV disease, the morbidity associated with brain biopsy and the inaccessibility of some lesions have led to the acceptance of a presumptive diagnosis based on a combination of positive serology, compatible lesions on neuroimaging, and response to empiric anti-*Toxoplasma* therapy. However, in the era of HAART and toxoplasmosis prophylaxis, some have questioned the wisdom of empiric anti-*Toxoplasma* therapy in AIDS patients with a focal brain lesion, since the likelihood of *T. gondii* may be lower (Ammassari et al., 1998).

In the pre-HAART era the most important risk factors for development of TE were absolute CD4 cell count ($\leq$100 cells/μl), *T. gondii* antibody positivity, and lack of antibiotic prophylaxis (Grant et al., 1990; Renold et al., 1992; Abgrall et al., 2001; Raffi et al., 1997; Nascimento et al., 2001). The median CD4 cell count in most series of patients with TE ranges from ~13 to 78 cells/μl (Renold et al., 1992; Porter and Sande, 1992; Dannemann et al., 1992; Laing et al., 1996; Raffi et al., 1997; Nascimento et al., 2001; Katlama et al., 1996a, 1996b). These same risk factors remain important in the HAART era; lack of HAART is an additional risk factor (San-Andrés et al., 2003; Abgrall et al., 2001). TE is the AIDS-defining illness in one-third to one-half of patients (Dannemann et al., 1988, 1992; Wanke et al., 1987; Katlama et al., 1996a).

Tissue Culture

Although not used routinely, organisms can occasionally be isolated from the CSF or blood by using various tissue culture methods (Raffi et al,. 1997). However, this method takes several days and is not very sensitive for the diagnosis of TE in AIDS patients.

Specimens may be inoculated in tube or shell vial cell cultures. *T. gondii* is known to form a cytopathic effect characterized by plaques in tissue cultures in various cell lines (Israelski and Remington, 1988; Contini et al., 1995). Although it is seldom performed in practice, tissue culture is fairly sensitive and specific in cases of disseminated disease. Tissue culture is more accessible and provides results faster than traditional mouse inoculation, which may take up to 6 weeks, though the sensitivities of both have not been compared (Luft and Remington, 1988).

Serology

The primary utility of *Toxoplasma* serology in AIDS patients is to rule out infection in a patient with one or more focal parenchymal lesions and compatible clinical presentation. *Toxoplasma* immunoglobulin M (IgM) is generally not useful in the diagnosis of TE because it rises following acute infection and then falls rapidly. IgG antibodies develop within weeks of acute infection, peak at 1 to 2 months, and persist at lower levels indefinitely. Since most patients have TE as a result of reactivation of latent infection, most patients with TE have positive serum *Toxoplasma* IgG antibodies. The role of other serologic tests is limited. IgA and IgE *Toxoplasma* antibodies can be measured by enzyme-linked immunosorbent assay (ELISA) but are seldom found in AIDS patients with TE (Cohen, 1999).

Various methods are available for measuring *T. gondii* IgG antibodies including the Sabin-Feldman dye test (SFT), immunosorbent agglutination test, complement fixation, indirect hemagglutination (IHA), indirect fluorescent antibody (IFA), and ELISA. The SFT, first described in 1948, remains the reference test for serological diagnosis of *Toxoplasma* infection (Ashburn et al., 2001). Though highly sensitive and specific, this test, which measures total specific antibody, is complex and primarily available in research laboratories. Unfortunately, many of the other tests that are available in commercial kits have not been well standardized, resulting in relatively high false-positive and false-negative results. Agglutination tests have been found to result in high false-positive rates, and IHA and complement fixation detect antibodies produced at a later stage than those detected by SFT and IFA and thus are less sensitive (Porter and Sande, 1992; Wanke et al., 1987; Desmonts and Remington, 1980). In the clinical setting the most common methods used are the IFA and ELISA. ELISA is more sensitive and specific than IFA but may sometimes result in false positives (Mariuz et al., 1997). One study compared various *Toxoplasma* antibody methods in HIV-infected patients with and without TE. IgG titers were measured by different methods including SFT, direct agglutination, and IHA. The patients with TE had higher median SFT titers (1:256) than patients without TE (1:64) as well as higher median direct agglutination titers (1:14,580 versus 1:4,860) and IHA titers (1:2,048 versus 1:256) (Hellerbrand et al., 1996).

Given the high seroprevalence of toxoplasmosis, positive serology is not helpful in distinguishing reactivation from quiescent infection and is not very useful in ruling in active *Toxoplasma* infection. However, the absence of *Toxoplasma* IgG in serum strongly suggests an alternative diagnosis. In most studies absence of *Toxoplasma* IgG is associated with a negative predictive value of 94 to 97% (Grant et al., 1990; Renold et al., 1992; Raffi et al., 1997; Wanke et al., 1987; Israelski and Remington, 1988; Hellerbrand et al., 1996; Skiest et al., 2000). Obtaining serial titers has not been proven to be of benefit for AIDS patients, because although some have reported increases in IgG from baseline (less than fourfold) (Renold et al., 1992), titers do not reliably increase with disease reactivation (McArthur, 1987; Grant et al., 1990; Wong et al., 1984). Titers also do not decrease with treatment and thus are not helpful in assessing response to treatment. Obtaining baseline *Toxoplasma* IgG antibodies is helpful in identifying patients likely to benefit from antibiotic prophylaxis.

A few studies have noted higher rates of seronegative *Toxoplasma* IgG in patients diagnosed with TE (Porter and Sande, 1992; Laing et al., 1996; Wanke et al., 1987). One study found an unusually high percentage (16%) of seronegative patients for whom TE was diagnosed either histologically or presumptively based on typical neuroimaging and response to therapy (Porter and Sande, 1992). The reasons for these results are not clear but may reflect the methods used (IFA was used, which may be relatively insensitive), the fact that not all cases were confirmed histopathologically, or the fact that antibody titers may wane in some patients (Renold et al., 1992; Bretagne et al., 1993). In these situations, knowledge of prior serostatus in patients who present with a clinical picture compatible with TE may be useful. Despite these studies, most would agree that a negative IgG antibody titer in a patient with intracerebral mass lesions should suggest an alternative diagnosis. Recently, in vitro anti-*Toxoplasma* antibody production by peripheral blood mononuclear cells has been proposed as a surrogate marker of TE in patients with AIDS (Lacascade et al., 2000).

CSF Analysis

CSF analysis is usually of little diagnostic value in distinguishing patients with CNS toxoplasmosis from those with other causes of focal CNS process. The fluid cell count and chemistry vary widely, from a normal CSF to mild mononuclear or lymphocytic pleocytosis and variable elevations of the protein level. The glucose concentration may be normal or depressed (Renold et al., 1992; Wanke et al., 1987). Tachyzoites can rarely be seen in CSF.

Measurement of CSF *Toxoplasma* antibody is frequently performed but has not been studied extensively. In general, CSF antibody titers have been associated with a high specificity but sensitivity of only 35 to 75% (McArthur, 1987; Grant et al., 1990; Farkash et al., 1986; Wong et al., 1984; Contini et al., 1998; Potasman et al., 1988). When present, CSF antibody results need to be interpreted carefully, as it may reflect passive diffusion of antibody from the serum. An intrathecal antibody index can be calculated to distinguish passive from local antibody production (Israelski and Remington, 1988). Using the SFT, Potasman and colleagues found 100% specificity and 69% sensitivity for CSF IgG (Potasman et al., 1988). In one series a patient with TE had a rise in antibody titer to *Toxoplasma* in the CSF, while the serum antibody remained unremarkable (Wong et al., 1984). Thus, some suggest obtaining a CSF antibody titer when the clinical suspicion for TE is high, even in the absence of a significant serum titer.

PCR

In recent years the diagnosis of certain focal CNS processes, such as primary brain lymphoma, PML, cytomegalovirus, and tuberculosis, has been greatly aided by the development

TABLE 2 Results of CSF analyses by PCR for diagnosis of TE

Study	No. of samples	Patients with diagnosis of TE	Sensitivity (%)	Specificity (%)
d'Arminio-Monforte et al., 1997	20	5	0	100
Novati et al., 1994	82	35	42 (51)	100
Roberts and Storch, 1997	52	8	93 (88)	100
Schoondermark-van de Ven et al., 1993	20	13	65	100
Cingolani et al., 1996	88	18	33	100
Dupon et al., 1995	48	13	70	100
Joseph et al., 2002	68	12	67	100
Contini et al., 1998	31	11	90	88
Gianotti et al., 1997	58	37	16	100
Parmley et al., 1992	14	9	44	100

of PCR techniques (Cinque et al., 1997). DNA amplification-based techniques such as PCR have also been used to identify nucleic acids of *T. gondii* in biological samples; however, low sensitivity has limited routine use of *T. gondii* PCR. The most commonly used method to detect the parasite is nested PCR targeting the multicopy B1 gene of *T. gondii* (Contini et al., 1998). Several studies have attempted to determine the utility of PCR of serum and/or CSF samples in expediting the diagnosis of TE. In general, studies that utilized PCR of blood samples were associated with a low sensitivity (<30%) for patients with toxoplasmosis confined to the CNS (Lamoril et al., 1996; Pelloux et al., 1997).

Most studies evaluating the utility of CSF PCR have found relatively low sensitivity but excellent specificity (Table 2) (Contini et al., 1998; Cingolani et al., 1996; Dupon et al., 1995; Gianotti et al., 1997; Joseph et al., 2002; d'Arminio-Monforte et al., 1997; Novati et al., 1994; Schoondermark-van de Ven et al., 1993). Novati et al. reported a positive CSF PCR in 8 of 19 patients with a tissue culture-proven diagnosis of TE and in 10 of 16 patients with a presumptive TE diagnosis, for an overall sensitivity of 51%. No patients without TE had a positive CSF PCR (100% specificity) (Novati et al., 1994). A smaller study found the sensitivity of the CSF PCR to be 65% and specificity 100% (Schoondermark-van de Ven et al., 1993). None of the patients who were seronegative had a positive CSF PCR. Gianotti et al. found that *Toxoplasma* CSF PCR was associated with a sensitivity of only 16% in 33 patients with a presumptive diagnosis of TE (Gianotti et al., 1997). Antinori et al. found a CSF PCR to have a sensitivity of 50% and specificity of 100% (Antinori et al., 1997). Multiplex PCR for simultaneous detection of Epstein-Barr virus and *T. gondii* has been performed as well (Roberts and Storch, 1997). A recent small Peruvian study (Joseph et al., 2002) found a higher sensitivity (66%) of both serum and CSF PCRs, which could have been explained by the higher prevalence of toxoplasmosis in Peru. The sensitivity of CSF PCR decreases with treatment, and thus, if PCR is performed it should ideally be done prior to therapy or for patients who have received less than 1 week of therapy (Novati et al., 1994; Schoondermark-van de Ven et al., 1993; Antinori et al., 1997). Currently, CSF PCR cannot be routinely recommended for diagnosing TE because the reported sensitivity is only 50 to 60%. However, since the specificity is reported to be 97 to 100% (Cinque et al., 1997; Antinori et al., 1997), a positive result can confirm the diagnosis while a negative result does not rule it out.

Neuroimaging

While computed tomography (CT) and MRI are essential in making a presumptive diagnosis of TE, neither is reliably able to distinguish TE from other focal CNS processes, especially primary brain lymphoma (Skiest, 2002). In AIDS patients with CNS processes, MRI is the preferred neuroimaging modality. It is more sensitive than CT, may often reveal more lesions, and in some cases may show lesions when CT is normal (Porter and Sande, 1992; Ciricillo and Rosenblum, 1990). MRI is also more sensitive for lesions in the posterior fossa. Increasing the dose of the contrast and delayed imaging have been suggested as ways to increase the sensitivity of contrasted CT scans (Renold et al., 1992; Post et al., 1986).

Despite the lack of specificity there are certain radiographic characteristics that favor TE over CNS lymphoma. Typically, patients with TE have multiple rounded, hypodense, thick-walled lesions that enhance with contrast and are surrounded by edema on CT scan or MRI (Fig. 4).

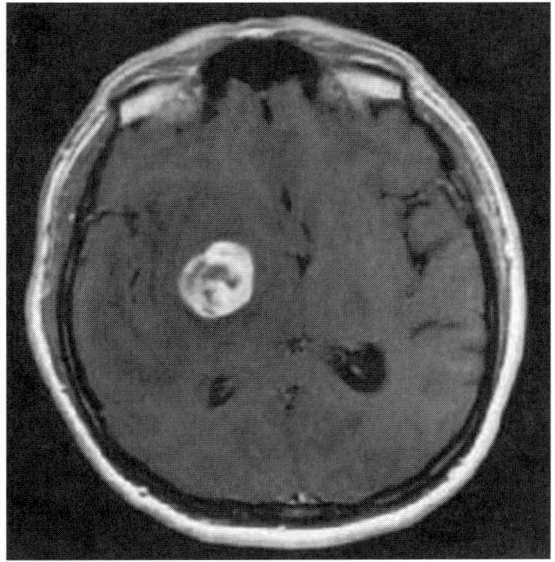

FIGURE 4 T1-weighted gadolinium-enhanced MRI revealing a large enhancing lesion of toxoplasmosis. There is surrounding edema and mass effect with midline shift.

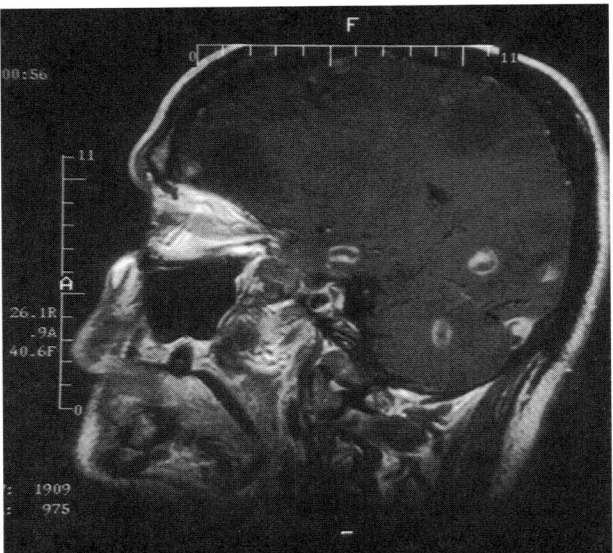

FIGURE 5 T1-weighted gadolinium-enhanced MRI revealing multiple ring-enhancing lesions of toxoplasmosis.

On T1-weighted MRI the lesions appear as focal areas of low signal intensity that are enhanced with gadolinium (often in a ring-enhancing pattern), whereas T2-weighted MRI lesions have a higher signal intensity that may be difficult to distinguish from the surrounding edema (Skiest, 2002). Mass effect is often demonstrated as well (Fig. 5). The lesions have a predilection for the corticomedullary junction and the basal ganglia (Levy et al., 1985; McArthur, 1987; Renold et al., 1992; Porter and Sande, 1992; Ciricillo and Rosenblum, 1990). None of these commonly seen features are specific. Although multiple lesions in the appropriate clinical setting suggest toxoplasmosis over CNS lymphoma (Ciricillo and Rosenblum, 1990), up to 27 to 43% of patients with TE may have a single lesion on imaging studies (McArthur, 1987; Renold et al., 1992; Porter and Sande, 1992; Luft et al., 1993; Gildenberg et al., 2000). Hemorrhagic lesions may occur as well (Walot et al., 1996). The locations of lesions adjacent to CSF pathways, e.g., periventricular as well as subependymal spread or ventricular encasement, are characteristic of PCNSL, rather than toxoplasmosis (Dina, 1991). The fact that some patients may have both disease processes at the same time further complicates the issue of distinguishing TE from PCNSL (McArthur, 1987; Renold et al., 1992; Gildenberg et al., 2000). Newer neuroimaging techniques developed in the past few years have improved the ability to diagnose TE and other focal CNS processes in AIDS patients.

CT scan and MRI are useful in the follow-up of lesions after initiation of therapy as well. The radiological resolution, manifested by decrease in mass effect and number of lesions, may lag behind the patient's clinical improvement, and it has been noted to occur anywhere from 2 weeks to 6 months, with the majority of lesions showing some resolution by day 14 of adequate therapy (Porter and Sande, 1992; Israelski and Remington, 1988). Calcifications may be seen at the site of treated infection.

Functional Neuroimaging

Thallium-201 single photon emission computed tomography (Tl-SPECT), fluorodeoxyglucose positron emission tomography (FDG-PET), and magnetic resonance spectroscopy have all been studied as methods to differentiate PCNSL from other causes of focal brain lesions, specifically toxoplasmosis. Unlike lymphoma cells, inflammatory lesions of the brain such as the ones produced by *T. gondii* do not take up thallium-201 on SPECT scintigraphy (Walot et al., 1996). Numerous studies have assessed the role of Tl-SPECT in the evaluation of mass lesions in AIDS (Skiest et al., 2000; Ruiz et al., 1994; O'Malley et al., 1994; Lorberboym et al., 1998; D'Amico et al., 1997; Antinori et al., 1999). In general, most have demonstrated a significantly higher uptake of thallium-201 in lesions due to lymphoma versus other causes (including toxoplasmosis). The reported sensitivity for a diagnosis of CNS lymphoma ranges from 55 to 100% (mean, 92%), and the specificity ranges from 76 to 100% (mean, 89%) (Skiest, 2002). Potential reasons for false-negative results include tumors causing insignificant alteration of the blood-brain barrier or small or low-grade lymphomas, which may not readily take up thallium. On the other hand, abnormally increased thallium uptake has been reported in nonneoplastic lesions, which may be due to the nature of the inflammatory process or to the subjective nature of visual interpretation (Kessler et al., 1998).

FDG-PET is a noninvasive method of measuring the metabolic activity of brain tissue by measuring the consumption of radiolabeled glucose in the affected regions. Malignant lesions like lymphoma have high metabolic activity and therefore high uptake of FDG, whereas infectious processes like toxoplasmic encephalitis have a lower metabolic activity. This has been confirmed in studies where FDG-PET accurately distinguished lymphoma from infectious lesions including toxoplasmosis with the exception of PML, which occasionally appears to be hypermetabolic (Heald et al., 1996; Pierce et al., 1995). The disadvantage of PET is its high cost and limited availability.

Magnetic resonance spectroscopy is a novel neuroimaging technique that is able to measure brain metabolites such as choline-containing compounds, *N*-acetyl aspartate, creatine, myoinositol, glutamate, lipids, and lactate, correlating metabolic alterations with underlying brain, neuronal, or myelin damage. Some studies have shown that toxoplasmic lesions have markedly elevated lactate and lipid peaks whereas lymphomas have produced elevated choline peaks and mildly to moderately elevated lactate and lipid levels (Chang et al., 1995); however, the sensitivity and specificity of this method have not been determined and other studies have been unable to document consistent findings or make an accurate distinction based on this imaging modality alone (Chinn et al., 1995).

Role of Brain Biopsy

Although the "gold standard" for the diagnosis of CNS toxoplasmosis remains brain biopsy, it is not routinely performed due to concerns about the risks. However, most studies have reported a relatively low complication rate. Published series of AIDS patients with focal CNS lesions undergoing brain biopsy have reported major morbidity of 0 to 12% (mean, ~4%) and mortality of 0 to 9% (mean, ~2%) (Skiest, 2002). Due to concerns about the procedure and the difficulty in obtaining a brain biopsy specimen, it has generally been reserved for the patients who fail to respond to empiric therapy, and the standard of care has been to treat empirically with anti-*Toxoplasma* therapy (Antinori, 1998). However, this strategy has not been rigorously studied, particularly with patients receiving HAART and toxoplasmosis

TABLE 3 Indications for brain biopsy in patients with AIDS and enhancing focal lesions[a]

Absence of clinical or radiographic improvement after 10 to 14 days of empiric anti-*Toxoplasma* therapy
Mass lesion in setting of negative *Toxoplasma* serology, and either negative Tl-SPECT (or PET) or negative EBV CSF PCR
Suspected coexisting infection
Atypical presentation
Spinal cord lesions in the setting of clinical suspicion of toxoplasmic myelitis and absence of brain lesions
Patient at risk for bacterial abscess

[a]Data from Grant et al., 1990; Luft and Remington, 1998; Skiest et al., 2000; and Vyas and Ebright, 1996.

prophylaxis, for whom the likelihood of toxoplasmosis may be lower. Additionally, TE in AIDS patients may occur concomitantly with other disease processes, complicating the issue of making a diagnosis (Luft and Remington, 1988; Renold et al., 1992; Gildenberg et al., 2000). Table 3 summarizes the indications to perform biopsy for the diagnosis of CNS mass lesions in patients with AIDS.

Due to the nonspecific nature of neuroimaging techniques and difficulty in distinguishing between TE and primary brain lymphoma, several groups have proposed diagnostic algorithms incorporating clinical features, serology, response to empiric anti-*Toxoplasma* therapy, neuroimaging findings, and CSF PCR for the diagnosis of the AIDS patient with a CNS mass lesion (Antinori, 1998; Antinori et al., 1997, 1999). At our institution, we employ an algorithm which incorporates *T. gondii* serology, Epstein-Barr virus (EBV) PCR in the CSF, and Tl-SPECT (Fig. 6). PET scanning can be substituted for SPECT scanning. According to this algorithm, if a patient presents with a focal brain lesion, *Toxoplasma* serology and EBV CSF PCR should be obtained and Tl-SPECT (or PET if available) performed. Patients with negative *Toxoplasma* serology, positive CSF EBV PCR, and positive SPECT, which is highly suggestive of lymphoma, generally undergo empiric brain irradiation or other treatment for lymphoma. Patients with positive *Toxoplasma* serology receive 14 days of anti-*Toxoplasma* therapy. Patients not improving clinically and radiographically at 2 weeks are referred for biopsy. Patients who do not meet these criteria are referred for brain biopsy.

TREATMENT

Treatment of CNS toxoplasmosis in patients with AIDS is successful in >70 to 90% of patients (McArthur, 1987; Renold et al., 1992; Porter and Sande, 1992; Dannemann et al., 1992; Luft et al., 1993). Nevertheless, therapeutic failures, relapses, and especially drug intolerance are not uncommon. Among patients who respond to therapy, approximately 85% of patients show clinical improvement by 1 week and 95% show radiographic improvement by day 14 of therapy (McArthur, 1987; Porter and Sande, 1992; Luft et al., 1993).

Treatment and prevention of TE are summarized in Table 4. Pyrimethamine and sulfadiazine remain the combination of choice for treatment of acute TE (Leport et al., 1988). Pyrimethamine, a folic acid antagonist that inhibits dihydrofolate reductase, and sulfadiazine, a competitive inhibitor of tetrahydrofolate synthetase, act synergistically to block folate metabolism in tachyzoites. However, neither drug is active against tissue cysts. Both drugs are generally well absorbed in the gastrointestinal tract and readily cross the blood-brain barrier, although pyrimethamine has been found to have erratic bioavailability (Luft and Remington, 1992). The recommended pyrimethamine dose is 100 to 200 mg

(loading dose) for 1 or 2 days followed by 50 to 75 mg/day, and the sulfadiazine dose is 4 to 8 g/day in four divided doses. Acute (induction) therapy should be given for 6 weeks (Mariuz et al., 1997). Folinic acid (leucovorin) is given at a dose of 10 to 25 mg/day to prevent bone marrow toxicity; it can be utilized by eukaryotic but not prokaryotic cells.

The pyrimethamine/sulfadiazine regimen has several potential adverse reactions. Side effects of sulfadiazine occur in 6 to 12% of patients, and this incidence may be higher in patients with AIDS (19 to 34%) (Behbahani et al., 1995). These include widely variable skin reactions from rash and urticaria to more severe reactions like Stevens-Johnson syndrome. Dermatologic reactions usually occur during the first weeks of treatment. Desensitization to sulfadiazine has been successful in patients with cutaneous reactions (Tenant-Flowers et al., 1991; McCabe and Oster, 1987; Caumes et al., 1995). Sulfadiazine may also cause crystalluria, hematuria, or nephrolithiasis leading to acute renal failure. Neuropsychiatric side effects of sulfadiazine like encephalopathy and psychoses have been described (Reboli and Mandler, 1992). Pyrimethamine has been associated with megaloblastic anemia, leukopenia, and thrombocytopenia as well as nausea and headache, and it has been shown to be teratogenic in animals (Luft and Remington, 1992; McCabe and Oster, 1987).

If the patient is unable to tolerate sulfa drugs, the combination of pyrimethamine and clindamycin is an acceptable alternative regimen (Dannemann et al., 1992; Katlama et al., 1996b). This regimen does not have activity against the cyst form of *T. gondii* either. Clindamycin, a drug with good oral absorption, likely acts by inhibition of protein synthesis. A randomized trial of 84 patients with TE in which the standard treatment of pyrimethamine/sulfadiazine was compared to pyrimethamine/clindamycin (at a dose of 1,200 mg intravenously every 6 h during the first 3 weeks followed by either 300 mg orally every 6 h or 450 mg every 8 h) found the two regimens to be equally efficacious with similar rates of adverse side effects (Dannemann et al., 1992). A larger randomized multicenter study which enrolled 299 patients had similar results (dose of clindamycin, 2.4 g daily divided in four doses); however, pyrimethamine/clindamycin appeared to be less effective than pyrimethamine/sulfadiazine for long-term relapse prevention (Katlama et al., 1996b). The side effects observed with clindamycin include pseudomembranous colitis, nausea, vomiting, neutropenia, and rash.

Although most patients can take one of the above treatment regimens, there are some patients who cannot tolerate these regimens. The activity of macrolide antimicrobials against *Toxoplasma* has been studied. These drugs, which have good oral absorption, have activity against the cyst form of the parasite. The efficacy of azithromycin in a murine model was demonstrated by Araujo et al. (1988). For humans there have been several reports of successful

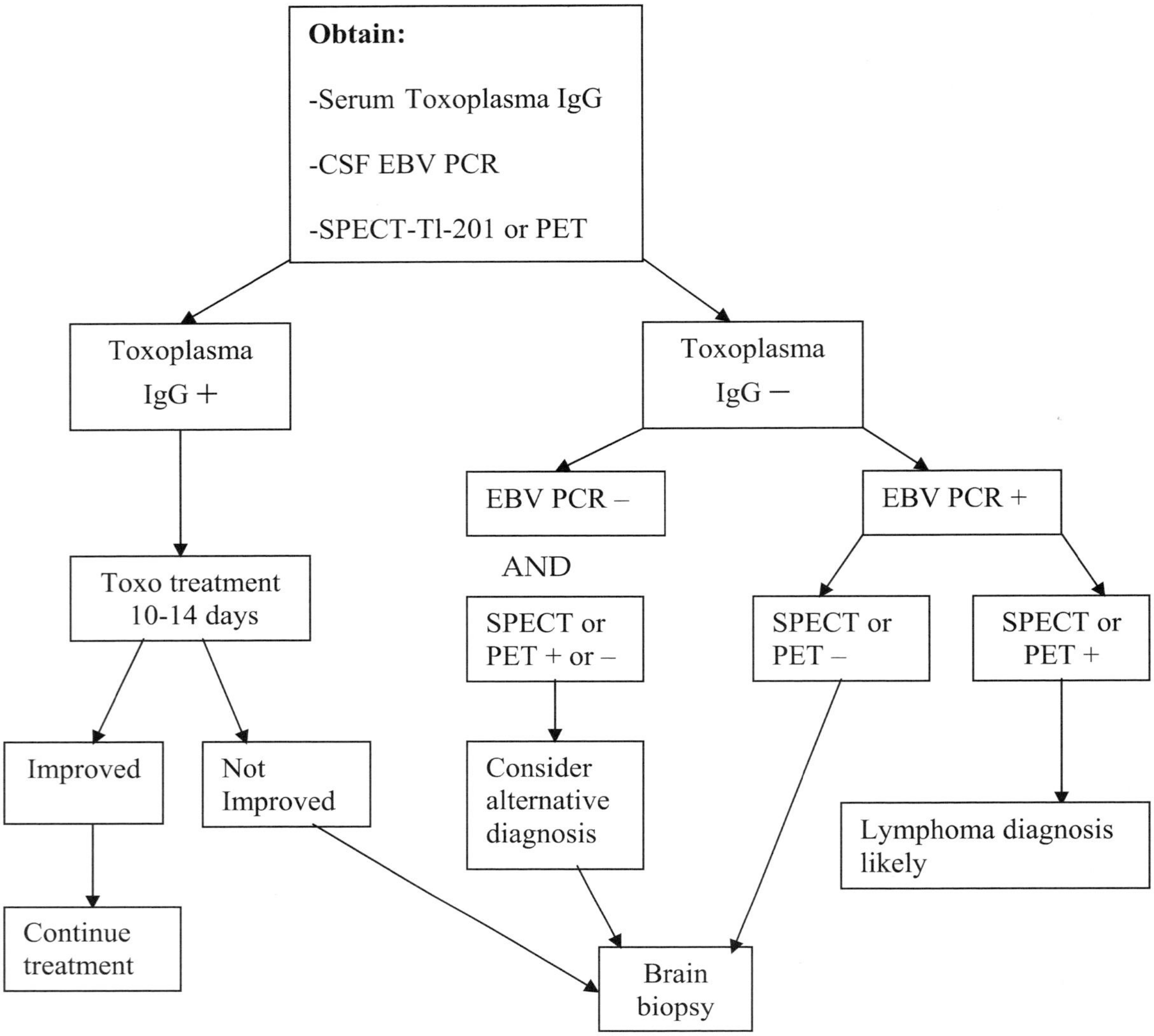

Obtain:

-Serum Toxoplasma IgG

-CSF EBV PCR

-SPECT-Tl-201 or PET

Toxoplasma IgG +

Toxoplasma IgG −

EBV PCR −

AND

SPECT or PET + or −

EBV PCR +

SPECT or PET −

SPECT or PET +

Toxo treatment 10-14 days

Consider alternative diagnosis

Lymphoma diagnosis likely

Improved

Not Improved

Brain biopsy

Continue treatment

FIGURE 6 Management algorithm for diagnosis of focal enhancing lesion(s) in an AIDS patient. SPECT-Tl-201, Tl-SPECT; PET, positron emission tomography with fluorodeoxyglucose.

initial therapy with azithromycin either alone or in combination with sulfadiazine, pyrimethamine, clindamycin, or doxycycline (Godofsky, 1994; Derouin et al., 1992; Jacobson et al., 2001; Nasta and Chiodera, 1997). In a small cohort of patients who received varying doses of azithromycin combined with pyrimethamine, the induction response rate was not better with higher doses of azithromycin (1,500 mg/day) (Jacobson et al., 2001); however, the rate of relapse was 47% after 30 weeks, which is much higher than the relapse rate reported with sulfadiazine and pyrimethamine. Azithromycin seems to be more active than other macrolides including roxithromycin or clarithromycin, but neither of these drugs should be used alone. Spiramycin, a macrolide widely utilized in Europe for the management of toxoplasmosis during pregnancy, is unavailable in the United States and has not been extensively tested for TE in AIDS (Fung and Kirschenbaum, 1996).

Atovaquone, a hydroxynaphthoquinone, has in vitro and in vivo activity against murine *T. gondii* (Araujo et al., 1991). A small randomized trial of atovaquone (1,500 mg twice per day) with pyrimethamine or sulfadiazine for treatment of TE showed that both regimens had a response at 6 weeks and were overall well tolerated (Chirgwin et al., 2002) with some failures observed. Atovaquone, at a dose of 750 mg orally four times per day, has been effective as suppressive therapy as well, either alone or in combination with pyrimethamine or clindamycin (Katlama et al., 1996a, Torres et al., 1997).

Other agents for which there are limited data include trimethoprim-sulfamethoxazole (TMP-SMX), trimetrexate, dapsone, doxycycline, and minocycline. TMP-SMX, which is used for primary prophylaxis of TE, has been used in limited numbers of patients (Luft and Remington, 1992). A randomized trial of 77 patients from Italy, which compared TMP-SMX to pyrimethamine and sulfadiazine, showed that the two regimens had similar efficacy (Torre et al., 1998). Trimetrexate is another potent inhibitor of dihydrofolate reductase with in vitro activity against *T. gondii*, but there is limited experience with this drug for treatment of TE (Masur et al., 1993). Dapsone, an inhibitor of

TABLE 4 Treatment and prophylaxis for acute CNS toxoplasmosis[a]

Line of treatment	Treatment		
	Acute TE (6 wks)	Suppressive[d]	Prophylaxis[b]
First Line	Pyrimethamine[c] 100–200 mg loading dose then 50–75 mg/day + sulfadiazine 1–2 g QID	Pyrimethamine[d] 25–50 mg/day + sulfadiazine 500–1000 mg QID	TMP/SMX DS QD
Alternative	Pyrimethamine (same as first line)[c] + clindamycin 600 mg IV or PO QID	Pyrimethamine[c] 25–50 mg/day + clindamycin 300–450 mg TID–QID	TMP/SMX SS QD
	Pyrimethamine (same as first line)[c] + azithromycin 900–1,200 mg/day[f]	Atovaquone 750 mg TID to QID with or without pyrimethamine[e] 25 mg/day[f]	Pyrimethamine[d] 50 mg weekly + dapsone 50 mg/day
	Pyrimethamine (same as first line)[c] + atovaquone 1,500 mg BID[f]	Pyrimethamine 25 mg + sulfadoxine 500 mg twice weekly[f, g]	Pyrimethamine[d] 75 mg weekly + dapsone 200 mg weekly
	Pyrimethamine (same as first line)[c] + TMP/SMX (5 mg/kg of TMP component) PO or IV Q6 h or (10 mg TMP/kg)/day[f]	TMP/SMX DS BID[f]	Atovaquone 750 mg BID with or without pyrimethamine[e] 25 mg/day[f]
	Pyrimethamine (same as first line)[c] + doxycycline 200–400 mg/day[f]		Pyrimethamine 25 mg + sulfadoxine 500 mg twice weekly[f, g]
	Minocycline 200 mg/day + clarithromycin 0.75–2 g/day[f] TMP/SMX (10 mg/kg of TMP component and 50 mg of SMX component)/day[f]		

[a] Abbreviations: BID, twice a day; TID, three times a day; QID, four times a day; QD, every day; DS, double strength; SS, single strength; IV, intravenously; PO, orally; /kg, per kilogram of body weight.
[b] Patients with CD4 T cells <100/mm^3 and positive *Toxoplasma* IgG.
[c] Folinic acid (10–25 mg/day) should be given with pyrimethamine to avoid toxicity to bone marrow.
[d] Folinic acid 25 mg weekly.
[e] Folinic acid (10 mg/day) should be given with pyrimethamine to avoid toxicity to bone marrow.
[f] Limited human data.
[g] Folinic acid twice 15 mg twice weekly.

dihydropteroate synthase, has been shown to be a potent sulfone against *T. gondii* with in vivo and in vitro synergism with pyrimethamine, but there are limited clinical data (Luft and Remington, 1992). Doxycycline and minocycline have also been used with limited success (Hagberg et al., 1993; Indorf and Pegram, 1994).

Corticosteroids should generally be withheld if possible for a patient with focal mass lesion(s) of undetermined etiology. Lesions due to lymphoma may show partial resolution with steroids. Thus, the clinician may be falsely reassured that the patient is responding to empiric anti-*Toxoplasma* therapy, when in fact the steroids are actually the cause for radiographic improvement.

Because of the recent understanding of the role of cytokines in the pathogenesis of TE, immunotherapy has been advocated as a promising therapeutic approach. Several studies of experimental TE in murine models have demonstrated decreased mortality of mice after treatment with IL-2 and IL-12 (Fung and Kirschenbaum, 1996; Sharma et al., 1985) as well as a protective role of IFN-γ in T-cell-deficient mice (Suzuki et al., 1991). The use of these therapies in humans has yet to be evaluated in appropriate clinical trials.

Maintenance Therapy

Even after clinical and radiographic improvement is achieved upon completion of acute illness treatment, relapse rates have been as high as 50 to 80% (Porter and Sande, 1992; Podzamczer et al., 1995). Therefore, maintenance therapy

with 25 to 50 mg of pyrimethamine per day and 2 to 4 g of sulfadiazine per day is required for all patients (Porter and Sande, 1992). In a study comparing daily administration of suppressive sulfadiazine (2 g/day) plus pyrimethamine (25 mg/day) to intermittent administration of the same doses 2 days per week, daily therapy had a lower relapse rate of 6% compared to 30% (Podzamczer et al., 1995, 2000). However, one study suggested that twice weekly dosing of pyrimethamine/sulfadiazine may be sufficient to prevent relapse of both TE and PCP (Ruf et al., 1993). Double-strength TMP-STX twice daily may be an alternative for maintenance therapy, but data are limited (Torre et al., 1998; Duval et al., 2004).

PROPHYLAXIS

Primary Prophylaxis

Primary chemoprophylaxis is indicated for *T. gondii*-seropositive individuals with <100 CD4 cells/μl (U.S. Public Health Service and Infectious Diseases Society of America, 2002). TMP/SMX, which also protects against *P. carinii*, is the prophylaxis of choice (U.S. Public Health Service and Infectious Diseases Society of America, 2002; Richards et al., 1995). The currently recommended dose is one double-strength tablet daily, but a few studies have suggested that lower doses are efficacious (Ribera et al., 1999). Thus, one TMP-SMX single-strength tablet per day may be used instead and may be better tolerated (U.S. Public Health Service and Infectious Diseases Society of America, 2002).

For patients intolerant of TMP-SMX, other options are available. An alternative regimen is the combination of pyrimethamine and a sulfadoxine, which proved to be safe and effective in preventing TE and PCP (Schurmann et al., 2002). Neither pyrimethamine nor daily dapsone alone is adequate for primary prophylaxis, but daily dapsone can be combined with once weekly pyrimethamine and is reasonably efficacious (Opravil et al., 1995; Leport et al., 1996). Atovaquone with or without pyrimethamine is another alternative for which there are some data supporting efficacy. Even though macrolide antimicrobials have activity against *T. gondii*, there is no evidence that these agents could be used for prophylaxis, and in fact, a failure of clarithromycin has been reported (Ruf et al., 1992).

Discontinuation of Prophylaxis

For patients who have not received HAART, primary prophylaxis and maintenance therapy need to be continued indefinitely due to the high risk of acute TE and relapse of TE, respectively. However, certain patients who respond well to HAART may be able to discontinue either primary prophylaxis or maintenance therapy. Several recent studies demonstrated that once a patient has responded to HAART and has achieved a CD4 count of >200 cells/μl for at least 3 to 6 months, it is safe to discontinue primary prophylaxis (U.S. Public Health Service and Infectious Diseases Society of America, 2002; Furrer et al., 2000; Mussini et al., 2000). Patients who took a protease inhibitor-containing regimen and who had immunologic response for a period of at least 3 months had a minimal risk of developing TE. The risk has not been evaluated for patients with CD4 T-cell counts between 100 and 200 cells/μl; therefore, if the CD4 T-cell count falls below these levels, prophylaxis needs to be reinitiated (U.S. Public Health Service and Infectious Diseases Society of America, 2002).

There are fewer data on the safety of interrupting maintenance therapy in TE, but it appears safe to do so for patients with a sustained CD4 cell count of >200 cells/μl for at least 6 months (U.S. Public Health Service and Infectious Diseases Society of America, 2002; Guex et al., 2000; Miro et al., 2000; Zeller et al., 2002; Soriano et al., 2000). Maintenance therapy was interrupted in 75 patients with toxoplasmosis, and only one relapse occurred when the CD4 count was >200 cells/μl (Kirk et al., 2002). In another study there were no recurrences in 27 patients who stopped maintenance therapy at a median CD4 cell count of 330 cells/μl (Miro et al., 2000). Occasional recurrences after discontinuation have been observed (Guex et al., 2000). If the decision is made to discontinue maintenance therapy, it is recommended that it be restarted if the CD4 cell count falls to <200 cells/μl (U.S. Public Health Service and Infectious Diseases Society of America, 2005; Benson et al., 2004).

REFERENCES

Abgrall, S., C. Rabaud, D. Costagliola, and Clinical Epidemiology Group of the French Hospital Database on HIV. 2001. Incidence and risk factors for toxoplasmic encephalitis in human immunodeficiency virus-infected patients before and during the highly active antiretroviral therapy era. *Clin. Infect. Dis.* **33:**1747–1755.

Ammassari, A., G. Scoppettuolo, R. Murri, P. Pezzotti, A. Cingolani, C. Del Borgo, A. De Luca, A. Antinori, and L. Ortona. 1998. Changing disease patterns in focal brain lesion-causing disorders in AIDS. *J. Acquir. Immune Defic. Syndr. Hum. Retrovirol.* **18:**365–371.

Antinori, A. 1998. Evaluation and management of intracranial mass lesions in AIDS: report of the Quality Standards Subcommittee of the American Academy of Neurology. *Neurology* **51:**1233–1234.

Antinori, A., A. Ammassari, A. De Luca, A. Cingolani, R. Murri, G. Scoppettuolo, M. Fortini, T. Tartaglione, L. Larroca, G. Zannoni, P. Cattani, R. Grillo, R. Roselli, M. Iacoangeli, M. Scerrati, and L. Ortona. 1997. Diagnosis of AIDS-related focal brain lesions: a decision-making analysis based on clinical and neuroradiologic characteristics combined with polymerase chain reaction assays in CSF. *Neurology* **48:**687–694.

Antinori, A., G. De Rossi, A. Ammassari, A. Cingolani, R. Murri, D. Di Giuda, A. De Luca, F. Piercontini, T. Tartaglione, M. Scerrati, L. M. Larocca, and L. Ortona. 1999. Value of combined approach with thallium-201 single-photon emission computed tomography and Epstein-Barr virus DNA polymerase chain reaction in CSF for the diagnosis of AIDS-related primary CNS lymphoma. *J. Clin. Oncol.* **17:**554–560.

Araujo, F., D. Guptill, and J. Remington. 1988. Azithromycin, a macrolide antibiotic with potent activity against *Toxoplasma gondii. Antimicrob. Agents Chemother.* **32:**755–757.

Araujo, F., J. Huskinson, and J. Remington. 1991. Remarkable in vitro and in vivo activities of the hydroxynaphthoquinone 566C80 against tachyzoites and tissue cysts of *Toxoplasma gondii. Antimicrob. Agents Chemother.* **35:**293–299.

Araujo, F., and T. Slifer. 2003. Different strains of *Toxoplasma gondii* induce different cytokine responses in CBA/Ca mice. *Infect. Immun.* **71:**4171–4174.

Ashburn, D., J. Chatterton, R. Evans, A. Joss, and D. Ho-Yen. 2001. Success in the Toxoplasma Dye Test. *J. Infect.* **42:**16–19.

Behbahani, R., M. Moshfeghi, and D. Baxter. 1995. Therapeutic approaches for AIDS-related toxoplasmosis. *Ann. Pharmacother.* **29:**760–768.

Benson, C., J. Kaplan, H. Masur, A. Pau, and K. Holmes. 2004. Opportunistic infections among HIV-infected adults and adolescents. *Morb. Mortal. Wkly. Rep.* **53:**1–112.

Bottoni, F., P. Gonnella, A. Autelitano, and N. Orzalesi. 1990. Diffuse necrotizing retinochoroiditis in a child with AIDS and toxoplasmic encephalitis. *Graefes Arch. Clin. Exp. Ophthalmol.* **228:**36–39.

Bretagne, S., F. Gray, and J. Costa. 1993. Central nervous system toxoplasmosis in AIDS. *N. Engl. J. Med.* **328:**1353–1354.

Burns, D., R. Risser, and C. White. 1991. The neuropathology of human immunodeficiency virus infection. *Arch. Pathol. Lab. Med.* **115:**1112–1124.

Caramello, P., B. Forno, A. Lucchini, A. Pollono, A. Sinicco, and P. Gioannini. 1993. Meningoencephalitis caused by *Toxoplasma gondii* diagnosed by isolation from cerebrospinal fluid in an HIV-positive patient. *Scand. J. Infect. Dis.* **25:**663–666.

Caumes, E., H. Bocquet, G. Guermonprez, O. Rogeaux, F. Bricaire, C. Katlama, and M. Gentilini. 1995. Adverse cutaneous reactions to pyrimethamine/sulfadiazine and pyrimethamine/clindamycin in patients with AIDS and toxoplasmic encephalitis. *Clin. Infect. Dis.* **21:**656–865.

Chang, L., B. Miller, D. McBride, M. Cornford, G. Oropilla, S. Buchthal, F. Chiang, H. Aronow, C. Beck, and T. Ersnt. 1995. Brain lesions in patients with AIDS: H-1 MR spectroscopy. *Radiology* **197:**525–531.

Chao, C., G. Gekker, S. Hu, and P. Peterson. 1994. Human microglial cell defense against *Toxoplasma gondii*. The role of cytokines. *J. Immunol.* **152:**1246–1252.

Chinn, R. J., I. D. Wilkinson, M. A. Hall-Craggs, M. N. Paley, R. F. Miller, B. E. Kendall, S. P. Newman, and M. J. Harrison. 1995. Toxoplasmosis and primary central nervous system lymphoma in HIV infection: diagnosis with MR spectroscopy. *Radiology* **197:**649–654.

Chirgwin, K., R. Hafner, C. Leport, J. Remington, J. Andersen, E. M. Bosler, C. Roque, N. Rajicic, V. McAuliffe, P. Morlat, D. T. Jayaweera, J. L. Vilde, and B. J. Luft. 2002. Randomized phase II trial of atovaquone with pyrimethamine or sulfadiazine for treatment of toxoplasmic encephalitis in patients with acquired immunodeficiency syndrome: ACTG 237/ANRS 039 Study. AIDS Clinical Trials Group 237/ Agence Nationale de Recherche sur le SIDA, Essai 039. *Clin. Infect. Dis.* **34:**1243–1250.

Cingolani, A., A. De Luca, A. Ammassari, R. Murri, A. Linzalone, R. Grillo, and A. Antinori. 1996. PCR detection of *Toxoplasma gondii* DNA in CSF for the differential diagnosis of AIDS-related focal brain lesions. *J. Med. Microbiol.* **45:**472–476.

Cinque, P., P. Scarpellini, L. Vago, A. Linde, and A. Lazzarin. 1997. Diagnosis of central nervous system complications in HIV-infected patients: cerebrospinal fluid analysis by the polymerase chain reaction. *AIDS* **11:**1–17.

Ciricillo, S., and M. Rosenblum. 1990. Use of Ct and MR imaging to distinguish intracranial lesions and to define the need for biopsy in AIDS patients. *J. Neurosurg.* **73:**720–724.

Cochereau-Massin, I., P. LeHoang, M. Lautier-Frau, E. Zerdoun, L. Zazoun, M. Robinet, P. Marcel, B. Girard, C. Katlama, C. Leport, et al. 1992. Ocular toxoplasmosis in human immunodeficiency virus-infected patients. *Am. J. Ophthalmol.* **114:**130–135.

Cohen, B. 1999. Neurologic manifestations of toxoplasmosis in AIDS. *Semin. Neurol.* **19:**201–211.

Contini, C., E. Fainardi, R. Cultrera, R. Canipari, F. Peyron, S. Delia, E. Paolino, and E. Granieri. 1998. Advanced laboratory techniques for diagnosing *Toxoplasma gondii* encephalitis in AIDS patients: significance of intrathecal production and comparison with PCR and ECL-western blotting. *J. Neuroimmunol.* **92:**29–37.

Contini, C., R. Romani, S. Magno, and S. Delia. 1995. Diagnosis of *Toxoplasma gondii* infection in AIDS patients by a tissue-culture technique. *Eur. J. Clin. Microbiol. Infect. Dis.* **14:**434–440.

Dal Pan, G., and J. Berger. 1997. Spinal cord disease in human immunodeficiency virus infection, p. 173–187. *In* J. Berger and R. Levy (ed.), *AIDS and the Nervous System*, 2nd ed. Lippincott-Raven, Philadelphia, PA.

D'Amico, A., C. Messa, A. Castagna, F. Zito, L. Galli, G. Pepe, A. Lazzarin, G. Lucignani, and F. Fazio. 1997. Diagnostic accuracy and predictive value of [201]T1 SPET for the differential diagnosis of cerebral lesions in AIDS patients. *Nucl. Med. Commun.* **18:**741–750.

Dannemann, B., D. Israelski, and J. Remington. 1988. Treatment of toxoplasmic encephalitis with intravenous clindamycin. *Arch. Intern. Med.* **148:**2477–2482.

Dannemann, B., J. A. McCutchan, D. Israelski, D. Antoniskis, C. Leport, B. Luft, J. Nussbaum, N. Clumeck, P. Morlat, J. Chiu, et al. 1992. Treatment of toxoplasmic encephalitis in patients with AIDS: a randomized trial comparing pyrimethamine plus clindamycin to pyrimethamine plus sulfadiazine. *Ann. Intern. Med.* **116:**33–43.

d'Arminio-Monforte, A., P. Clinque, L. Vago, A. Castagna, C. Gervasoni, M. Terreni, R. Novati, A. Gori, A. Lazzarin, and M. Moroni. 1997. A comparison of brain biopsy and CSF-PCR in the diagnosis of CNS lesions in AIDS patients. *J. Neurol.* **244:**35–39.

Däubener, W., and U. Hadding. 1997. Cellular immune reactions directed against Toxoplasma gondii with special emphasis on the central nervous system. *Med. Microbiol. Immunol.* **185:**195–206.

Derouin, F., R. Almadany, F. Chua, B. Rouveix, and J. Pocidalo. 1992. Synergistic activity of azithromycin and pyrimethamine or sulfadiazine in acute experimental toxoplasmosis. *Antimicrob. Agents Chemother.* **36:**997–1001.

Desmonts, G., and J. Remington. 1980. Direct agglutination test for diagnosis of *Toxoplasma* infection: method for increasing sensitivity and specificity. *J. Clin. Microbiol.* **11:**562–568.

Dina, T. 1991. Primary central nervous system lymphoma versus toxoplasmosis in AIDS. *Radiology* **179:**823–828.

D'Offizi, G., S. Topino, G. Anzidei, D. Frigiotti, and P. Narciso. 2002. Primary *Toxoplasma gondii* infection in a pregnant human immunodeficiency virus-infected woman. *Pediatr. Infect. Dis. J.* **21:**981–982.

Dukes, C., B. Luft, and D. Durack. 1997. Toxoplasmosis, p. 785–806. *In* W. Scheld, R. Whitley, and D. Durack (ed.), *Infections of the Central Nervous System*, 2nd ed. Lippincott-Raven, Philadelphia, PA.

Dupon, M., J. Cazenave, J. Pellegrin, J. Ragnaud, A. Cheyrou, I. Fischer, B. Leng, and J. Lacut. 1995. Detection of *Toxoplasma gondii* by PCR and tissue culture in cerebrospinal fluid and blood of human immunodeficiency virus-seropositive patients. *J. Clin. Microbiol.* **33:**2421–2426.

Duval, X., O. Pajot, V. Le Moing, P. Longuet, J. Ecobichon, F. Mentre, C. Leport, and J. Vidle. 2004. Maintenance therapy with cotrimoxazole for toxoplasmic encephalitis in the era of highly active antiretroviral therapy. *AIDS* **18:**1342–1344.

Eggers, C., A. Vortmeyer, and T. Emskötter. 1995. Cerebral toxoplasmosis in a patient with the acquired immunodeficiency syndrome presenting as obstructive hydrocephalus. *Clin. Neuropathol.* **14:**51–54.

Fadul, C., Y. Channon, and L. Kasper. 1995. Survival of immunoglobulin G-opsonized *Toxoplasma gondii* in nonadherent human monocytes. *Infect. Immun.* **63:**4290–4294.

Falangola, M., and C. Petito. 1993. Choroid plexus infection in cerebral toxoplasmosis in AIDS patients. *Neurology* **43:**2035–2040.

Falusi, O., A. French, E. Seaberg, P. Tien, D. Watts, H. Minkoff, E. Piessens, A. Kovacs, K. Anastos, and M. Cohen. 2002. Prevalence and predictors of *Toxoplasma* seropositivity in women with and at risk for human immunodeficiency virus infection. *Clin. Infect. Dis.* **35:**1414–1417.

Farkash, A., P. Maccabee, J. Sher, S. Landesman, and G. Hotson. 1986. CNS toxoplasmosis in acquired immune deficiency syndrome: a clinical-pathological-radiological review of 12 cases. *J. Neurol. Neurosurg. Psychiatr.* **49:**744–748.

Fung, H. B., and H. L. Kirschenbaum. 1996. Treatment regimens for patients with toxoplasmic encephalitis. *Clin. Ther.* **18:**1037–1056.

Furrer, H., M. Opravil, E. Bernasconi, A. Telenti, and M. Egger. 2000. Stopping primary prophylaxis in HIV-1-infected patients at high risk of toxoplasma encephalitis. Swiss HIV Cohort Study. *Lancet* **355:**2217–2218.

Gagliuso, D., S. Teich, A. Friedman, and J. Orellana. 1990. Ocular toxoplasmosis in AIDS patients. *Trans. Am. Ophthalmol. Soc.* **88:**63–86.

Gianotti, N., P. Cinque, A. Castagna, R. Novati, M. Moro, and A. Lazzarin. 1997. Diagnosis of toxoplasmic encephalitis in HIV-infected patients. *AIDS* **11:**1529–1530.

Gildenberg, P., J. Gathe, and J. Kim. 2000. Stereotactic biopsy of cerebral lesions in AIDS. *Clin. Infect. Dis.* **30:**491–499.

Glatt, A. 1992. *Toxoplasma gondii* serologies in patients with HIV infection. *Infect. Dis. Clin. Pract.* **1:**237–238.

Glatt, A. 2003. Toxoplasma seroprevalence rates. *Clin. Infect. Dis.* **36:**1203.

Godofsky, E. 1994. Treatment of presumed cerebral toxoplasmosis with azithromycin. *N. Engl. J. Med.* **330:**575–576.

Grant, I., J. Gold, M. Rosenblum, D. Niedzwiecki, and D. Armstrong. 1990. *Toxoplasma gondii* serology in HIV-infected patients: the development of central nervous system toxoplasmosis in AIDS. *AIDS* **4**:519–521.

Gray, F., R. Gherardi, E. Wingate, J. Wingate, G. Felenon, A. Gaston, A. Sobel, and J. Poirier. 1989. Diffuse "encephalitic" cerebral toxoplasmosis in AIDS. Report of four cases. *J. Neurol.* **236**:273–277.

Guex, A., A. Radziwill, and H. Bucher. 2000. Discontinuation of secondary prophylaxis for toxoplasmic encephalitis in human immunodeficiency virus infection after immune restoration with highly active antiretroviral therapy. *Clin. Infect. Dis.* **30**:602–603.

Hagberg, L., B. Palmertz, and J. Lindberg. 1993. Doxycycline and pyrimethamine for toxoplasmic encephalitis. *Scand. J. Infect. Dis.* **25**:157-160.

Hainfellner, J., and H. Budkha. 1997. Neuropathology of human immunodeficiency virus related opportunistic infections and neoplasms, p. 481–515. *In* J. Berger and R. Levy (ed.), *AIDS and the Nervous System*, 2nd ed. Lippincott-Raven, Philadelphia, PA.

Hamed, L., N. Schatz, and S. Galleta. 1988. Brainstem ocular motility defects and AIDS. *Am. J. Ophthalmol.* **106**:437–442.

Heald, A., J. Hoffman, J. Bartlett, and H. Waskin. 1996. Differentiation of central nervous system lesions in AIDS patients using positron emission tomography (PET). *Int. J. STD AIDS* **7**:337–346.

Hellerbrand, C., F. Goebel, and R. Disko. 1996. High predictive value of *Toxoplasma gondii* IgG antibody levels in HIV-infected patients for diagnosis of cerebral toxoplasmosis. *Eur. J. Clin. Microbiol. Infect. Dis.* **15**:869–872.

Holland, G. N., R. E. Engstrom, Jr., B. J. Glasgow, B. B. Berger, S. A. Daniels, Y. Sidikaro, J. A. Harmon, D. H. Fischer, D. S. Boyers, N. A. Rao, et al. 1988. Ocular toxoplasmosis in patients with the acquired immunodeficiency syndrome. *Am. J. Ophthalmol.* **106**:653–667.

Houff, S. 1997. Neuroimmunology of human immunodeficiency virus infection, p. 77–122. *In* J. Berger and R. Levy (ed.), *AIDS and the Nervous System*, 2nd ed. Lippincott-Raven, Philadelphia, PA.

Huang, T., and S. Chou. 1988. Occlusive hypertrophic arteritis as the cause of discrete necrosis in CNS toxoplasmosis in the acquired immunodeficiency syndrome. *Hum. Pathol.* **19**:1210–1214.

Hunter, C., and J. Remington. 1994. Immunopathogenesis of toxoplasmic encephalitis. *J. Infect. Dis.* **170**:1057–1067.

Indorf, A., and P. Pegram. 1994. Use of doxycycline in the management of a patient with toxoplasmic encephalitis. *AIDS* **8**:1633–1634.

Israelski, D., J. Chmiel, L. Poggensee, J. Phair, and J. Remington. 1993. Prevalence of *Toxoplasma* infection in a cohort of homosexual men at risk of AIDS and toxoplasmic encephalitis. *J. Acquir. Immune Defic. Syndr.* **6**:414–418.

Israelski, D., and J. Remington. 1988. Toxoplasmic encephalitis in patients with AIDS. *Infect. Dis. Clin. N. Am.* **2**:429–445.

Ives, N., B. Gazzard, and P. Easterbrook. 2001. The changing pattern of AIDS-defining illnesses with the introduction of highly active antiretroviral therapy (HAART) in a London clinic. *J. Infect.* **42**:134–139.

Jacobson, J., R. Hafner, J. Remington, C. Farthing, J. Holden-Wiltse, E. Bosler, C. Harris, D. Jayaweera, C. Rogue, B. Luft, and ACTG 156 Study Team. 2001. Dose-escalation, phase I/II study of azithromycin and pyrimethamine for the treatment of toxoplasmic encephalitis in AIDS. *AIDS* **15**:583–589.

Johnson, J. J., C. W. Roberts, C. Pope, F. Roberts, M. J. Kirisits, R. Estes, E. Mui, T. Krieger, C. R. Brown, J. Forman, and R. McLeod. 2002. In vitro correlates of Ld-restricted resistance to toxoplasmic encephalitis and their critical dependence on parasite strain. *J. Immunol.* **169**:966–973.

Jones, J., D. Hanson, M. Dworkin, D. Alderton, P. Fleming, J. Kaplan, and J. Ward. 1999. Surveillance for AIDS-defining opportunistic illnesses, 1992-1997. *MMWR CDC Surveill. Summ.* **48**:1–22.

Jones, J. L., D. Kruszon-Moran, M. Wilson, G. McQuillan, T. Navin, and J. McAuley. 2001. *Toxoplasma gondii* infection in the United States: seroprevalence and risk factors. *Am. J. Epidemiol.* **154**:357–365.

Joseph, P., M. M. Calderón, R. H. Gilman, M. L. Quispe, J. Cok, E. Ticona, V. Chavez, J. A. Jimenez, M. C. Chang, M. J. Lopez, and C. A. Evans. 2002. Optimization and evaluation of a PCR assay for detecting toxoplasmic encephalitis in patients with AIDS. *J. Clin. Microbiol.* **40**:4499–4503.

Katlama, C., B. Mouthon, D. Gourdon, D. Lapierre, and F. Rousseau. 1996a. Atovaquone as long-term suppressive therapy for toxoplasmic encephalitis in patients with AIDS and multiple drug intolerance. *AIDS* **10**:1107–1112.

Katlama, C., S. Wit, E. O'Doherty, M. Glabeke, and N. Clumeck. 1996b. Pyrimethamine-clindamycin vs. pyrimethamine-sulfadiazine as acute and long-term therapy for toxoplasmic encephalitis in patients with AIDS. *Clin. Infect. Dis.* **22**:268–275.

Kessler, L., A. Ruiz, M. Donovan Post, W. Ganz, A. Brandon, and J. Foss. 1998. Thallium-201 brain SPECT of lymphoma in AIDS patients: pitfalls and technique optimization. *AJNR Am. J. Neuroradiol.* **19**:1105–1109.

Kirk, O., P. Reiss, C. Uberti-Foppa, M. Bickel, J. Gerstoft, C. Pradier, F. Wit, B. Ledergerber, J. Lundgren, H. Furrer, and European HIV Cohorts. 2002. Safe interruption of maintenance therapy against previous infection with four common HIV-associated opportunistic pathogens during potent antiretroviral therapy. *Ann. Intern. Med.* **137**:239–250.

Kure, K., W. Lyman, R. Soeiro, K. Weidenheim, A. Hirano, and D. Dickson. 1991. Human immunodeficiency virus 1 infection of the nervous system: an autopsy study of 268 adult, pediatric, and fetal brains. *Hum. Pathol.* **22**:700–710.

Lacascade, C., A. Conge, V. Baillat, I. Pages, M. Huguet, J. Reynes, and J. Vendrell. 2000. In vitro anti-*Toxoplasma gondii* antibody production by peripheral blood mononuclear cells in the diagnosis and the monitoring of toxoplasmic encephalitis in AIDS-related brain lesions. *J. Acquir. Immune Defic. Syndr.* **25**:256–260.

Laing, R., P. Flegg, R. Brettle, C. Leen, and S. Burns. 1996. Clinical features, outcome and survival from cerebral toxoplasmosis in Edinburgh AIDS patients. *Int. J. STD AIDS* **7**:258–264.

Lamoril, J., J. Molina, A. Gouvello, Y. Garin, J. Deybach, J. Modai, and F. Derouin. 1996. Detection by PCR of *Toxoplasma gondii* in blood in the diagnosis of cerebral toxoplasmosis in patients with AIDS. *J. Clin. Pathol.* **49**:89–92.

Ledergerber, B., M. Egger, V. Erard, R. Weber, B. Hirschel, H. Furrer, M. Battegay, P. Vernazza, E. Bernasconi, M. Opravil, D. Kaufmann, P. Sudre, P. Francioli, and A. Telenti. 1999. AIDS-related opportunistic illnesses occurring after initiation of potent antiretroviral therapy: the Swiss HIV Cohort Study. *JAMA* **282**:2220–2226.

Leport, C., G. Chene, P. Morlat, B. Luft, F. Rousseau, S. Pueyo, R. Hafner, J. Miro, J. Aubertin, R. Salamon, and J. Vidle. 1996. Pyrimethamine for primary prophylaxis of toxoplasmic encephalitis in patients with human immunodeficiency virus infection: a double-blind, randomized trial. *J. Infect. Dis.* **173**:91–97.

Leport, C., F. Raffi, S. Matheron, C. Katlama, B. Regnier, A. Saimot, C. Marche, C. Vedrenne, and J. Vidle. 1988. Treatment of central nervous system toxoplasmosis with pyrimethamine/sulfadiazine combination in 35 patients with the acquired immunodeficiency syndrome. *Am. J. Med.* **84**:94–100.

Levy, R., D. Bredesen, and M. Rosenblum. 1985. Neurological manifestations of the acquired immunodeficiency syndrome

(AIDS): experience at UCSF and review of the literature. *J. Neurosurg.* **62:**475–495.

Lorberboym, M., F. Wallach, L. Estok, R. Mosesson, M. Sacher, C. Kim, and J. Machac. 1998. Thallium-201 retention in focal intracranial lesions for the differential diagnosis of primary lymphoma and nonmalignant lesions in AIDS patients. *J. Nucl. Med.* **39:**1366–1369.

Luft, B., and J. Remington. 1988. Toxoplasmic encephalitis. *J. Infect. Dis.* **157:**1–6.

Luft, B., and J. Remington. 1992. Toxoplasmic encephalitis in AIDS. *Clin. Infect. Dis.* **15:**211–222.

Luft, B. J., R. Hafner, A. H. Korzun, C. Leport, D. Antoniskis, E. M. Bosler, D. D. Bourland III, R. Uttamchandani, J. Fuhrer, J. Jacobson, et al. 1993. Toxoplasmic encephalitis in patients with the acquired immunodeficiency syndrome. *N. Engl. J. Med.* **329:**995–1000.

Mariuz, P., E. Bosler, and B. Luft. 1997. Toxoplasmosis, p. 641–659. *In* J. Berger, and R. Levy (ed.), *AIDS and the Nervous System,* 2nd ed. Lippincott-Raven, Philadelphia, PA.

Maschke, M., O. Kastrup, S. Esser, B. Ross, U. Hengge, and A. Hufnagel. 2000. Incidence and prevalence of neurological disorder associated with HIV since the introduction of highly active antiretroviral therapy (HAART). *J. Neurol. Neurosurg. Psychiatr.* **69:**376–380.

Masliah, E., R. DeTeresa, M. Mallory, and L. Hansen. 2000. Changes in pathological findings at autopsy in AIDS cases for the last 15 years. *AIDS* **14:**69–74.

Masur, H., M. A. Polis, C. U. Tuazon, D. Ogata-Arakaki, J. A. Kovacs, D. Katz, D. Hilt, T. Simmons, I. Feuerstein, B. Lundgren, et al. 1993. Salvage trial of trimetrexate-leucovorin for the treatment of cerebral toxoplasmosis in patients with AIDS. *J. Infect. Dis.* **167:**1422–1426.

McArthur, J. 1987. Neurologic manifestations of AIDS. *Medicine* **66:**407–437.

McArthur, J. 1998. Neurologic complications of HIV infection, p. 1123–1150. *In* B. Gorbach and J. G. Bartlett (ed.), *Infectious Diseases,* 2nd ed. W. B. Saunders, Philadelphia, PA.

McCabe, R., and S. Oster. 1987. Current recommendations and future prospects in the treatment of toxoplasmosis. *Drugs* **38:**973–987.

Miro, J., J. Lopez, and D. Podzamczer. 2000. Discontinuation of primary or secondary *Toxoplasma gondii* prophylaxis is safe in HIV-1-infected patients after immunological recovery with HAART. Final results of GESIDA 04/98-B study, abstr. L-16. *In Interscience Conference on Antimicrobial Agents and Chemotherapy,* Toronto, Ontario, Canada, 17–20 September 2000. American Society for Microbiology, Washington, DC.

Munir, A., M. Zaman, and M. Eltorky. 2000. *Toxoplasma gondii* pneumonia in a pancreas transplant patient. *South. Med. J.* **93:**614–617.

Mussini, C., P. Pezzotti, A. Govoni, V. Borghi, A. Antinori, A. d'Arminio Monforte, A. De Luca, N. Mongardo, M. C. Cerri, F. Chiodo, E. Concia, L. Bonazzi, M. Moroni, L. Ortona, R. Esposito, A. Cossariizza, and B. De Rienzo. 2000. Discontinuation of primary prophylaxis for *Pneumocystis carinii* pneumonia and toxoplasmic encephalitis in human immunodeficiency virus type I-infected patients: the changes in opportunistic prophylaxis study. *J. Infect. Dis.* **181:**1635–1642.

Nascimento, L., F. Stollar, L. Tavares, C. Cavasini, I. Maia, J. Cordeiro, and M. Ferreira. 2001. Risk factors for toxoplasmic encephalitis in HIV-infected patients: a case-control study in Brazil. *Ann. Trop. Med. Parasitol.* **95:**587–593.

Nasta, P., and S. Chiodera. 1997. Azithromycin for relapsing cerebral toxoplasmosis in AIDS. *AIDS* **11:**1188.

Navia, B., C. Petito, J. Gold, E. Cho, B. Jordan, and R. Price. 1986. Cerebral toxoplasmosis complicating the acquired immune deficiency syndrome: clinical and neuropathological findings in 27 patients. *Ann. Neurol.* **19:**224–238.

Neuenburg, J., H. Brodt, B. Herndier, M. Bickel, P. Bacchetti, R. Price, R. Grant, and W. Schlote. 2002. HIV-related neuropathology, 1985 to 1999: rising prevalence of HIV encephalopathy in the era of highly active antiretroviral therapy. *J. Acquir. Immune Defic. Syndr.* **31:**171–177.

Novati, R., A. Castagna, G. Morsica, L. Vago, G. Tambussi, S. Ghezzi, C. Gervasoni, C. Bisson, A. d'Arminio Monforte, and A. Lazzarin. 1994. Polymerase chain reaction for *Toxoplasma gondii* DNA in the cerebrospinal fluid of AIDS patients with focal brain lesions. *AIDS* **8:**1691–1694.

Oksenhendler, E., I. Charrea, C. Tournerie, M. Azihary, C. Carbon, and J. Aboulker. 1994. *Toxoplasma gondii* infection in advanced HIV infection. *AIDS* **8:**483–487.

Olatinwo, T., M. Herbowy, and R. Hewitt. 2001. Toxoplasmic encephalitis and primary lymphoma of the brain—the shift in epidemiology: a case series and review of the literature. *AIDS Read.* **2001:**444–449.

O'Malley, J., H. Ziessman, P. Kumar, B. Harkness, J. Tall, and P. Pierce. 1994. Diagnosis of intracranial lymphoma in patients with AIDS. Value of 201 T1 single-photon emission computed tomography. *Am. J. Roentgenol.* **163:**417–421.

Opravil, M., B. Hirschel, A. Lazzarin, A. Heald, M. Pechère, S. Rüttimann, A. Iten, J. von Overbeck, D. Oertle, G. Praz, et al. 1995. Once-weekly administration of dapsone/pyrimethamine vs. aerosolized pentamidine as combined prophylaxis for *Pneumocystis carinii* pneumonia and toxoplasmic encephalitis in human immunodeficiency virus-infected patients. *Clin. Infect. Dis.* **20:**531–541.

Parke, D., and R. Font. 1986. Diffuse toxoplasmic retinochoroiditis in a patient with AIDS. *Arch. Ophthalmol.* **104:**571–575.

Parker, S., and R. Holliman. 1992. Toxoplasmosis and laboratory workers: a case-control assessment of risk. *Med. Lab. Sci.* **49:**103–106.

Parmley, S. F., F. D. Goebel, and J. S. Remington. 1992. Detection of *Toxoplasma gondii* in cerebrospinal fluid from AIDS patients by polymerase chain reaction. *J. Clin. Microbiol.* **30:**3000–3002.

Pelloux, H., J. Dupouy-Camet, F. Derouin, J. Aboulker, and F. Raffi. 1997. A multicentre prospective study for the polymerase chain reaction detection of *Toxoplasma gondii* DNA in blood samples from 186 AIDS patients with suspected toxoplasmic encephalitis. *AIDS* **11:**1888–1890.

Pierce, M., M. Johnson, R. Maciunas, M. Murray, G. Allen, M. Harbison, J. Creasy, and R. Kessler. 1995. Evaluating contrast-enhancing brain lesions in patients with AIDS by using positron emission tomography. *Ann. Intern. Med.* **123:**594–598.

Podzamczer, D., J. Miro, E. Ferrer, J. Gatell, J. Ramon, E. Ribera, G. Sirera, A. Cruceta, H. Knobel, P. Domingo, R. Polo, M. Leyes, J. Cosin, M. Farinas, J. Arrizabalaga, J. Martinez-Lacasa, and F. Gudiol. 2000. Thrice-weekly sulfadiazine-pyrimethamine for maintenance therapy of toxoplasmic encephalitis in HIV-infected patients. *Eur. J. Clin. Microbiol. Infect. Dis.* **19:**89–95.

Podzamczer, D., J. Miro, F. Bolao, J. Gatell, J. Cosin, G. Sirera, P. Domingo, F. Laguna, J. Santamaria, and J. Verdejo. 1995. Twice-weekly maintenance therapy with sulfadiazine-pyrimethamine to prevent recurrent toxoplasmic encephalitis in patients with AIDS. *Ann. Intern. Med.* **123:**175–180.

Porter, S., and M. Sande. 1992. Toxoplasmosis of the central nervous system in the acquired immunodeficiency syndrome. *N. Engl. J. Med.* **327:**1643–1648.

Post, M., J. Chan, G. Hensley, T. Hoffman, L. Moskowitz, and S. Lippmann. 1983. Toxoplasma encephalitis in Haitian adults with acquired immunodeficiency syndrome: a clinical-pathologic-CT correlation. *Am. J. Roentgenol.* **140:**861–868.

Post, M., J. Sheldon, G. Hensley, K. Soila, J. Tobias, J. Chan, R. Quencer, and L. Moskowitz. 1986. Central nervous system disease in acquired immunodeficiency syndrome: prospective correlation using CT, MR imaging, and pathologic studies. *Radiology* **158**:141–148.

Potasman, I., L. Resnick, B. Luft, and J. Remington. 1988. Intrathecal production of antibodies against *Toxoplasma gondii* in patients with toxoplasmic encephalitis and the acquired immunodeficiency syndrome (AIDS). *Ann. Intern. Med.* **108**:49–51.

Raffi, F., J. Aboulker, C. Michelet, V. Reliquet, H. Pelloux, A. Huart, I. Poizot-Martin, P. Morlat, B. Dupas, J. Mussini, and C. Leport. 1997. A prospective study of criteria for the diagnosis of toxoplasmic encephalitis in 186 AIDS patients. *AIDS* **11**:177–184.

Reboli, A., and H. Mandler. 1992. Encephalopathy and psychoses associated with sulfadiazine in two patients with AIDS and CNS toxoplasmosis. *Clin. Infect. Dis.* **15**:556–557.

Remington, J., and R. McLeod. 1998. Toxoplasmosis, p. 1620–1640. *In* S. Gorbach, J. Bartlett, and N. Blacklow (ed.), *Infectious Diseases*, 2nd ed. Lippincott Williams and Wilkins, Philadelphia, PA.

Renold, C., A. Sugar, J. Chave, L. Perrin, J. Delavelle, G. Pizzolato, P. Burkhard, V. Gabriel, and B. Hirschel. 1992. Toxoplasma encephalitis in patients with the acquired immunodeficiency syndrome. *Medicine* **71**:224–239.

Ribera, E., A. Fernandez-Sola, C. Juste, A. Rovira, F. Romero, L. Armadans-Gils, I. Ruiz, I. Ocana, and A. Pahissa. 1999. Comparison of high and low doses of trimethoprim-sulfamethoxazole for primary prevention of toxoplasmic encephalitis in human immunodeficiency virus-infected patients. *Clin. Infect. Dis.* **29**:1461–1466.

Richards, F., J. Kovacs, and B. Luft. 1995. Preventing toxoplasmic encephalitis in persons infected with human immunodeficiency virus. *Clin. Infect. Dis.* **21**:S49–S56.

Roberts, T., and G. Storch. 1997. Multiplex PCR for diagnosis of AIDS-related central nervous system lymphoma and toxoplasmosis. *J. Clin. Microbiol.* **35**:268–269.

Ruf, B., D. Schurmann, and H. Pohle. 1992. Failure of clarithromycin in preventing toxoplasmic encephalitis in AIDS patients. *J. Acquir. Immune Defic. Syndr.* **5**:530–531.

Ruf, B., D. Schürmann, F. Bergmann, W. Schüler-Maué, T. Grünewald, H. J. Gottschalk, H. Witt, and H. D. Pohle. 1993. Efficacy of pyrimethamine/sulfadoxine in the prevention of toxoplasmic encephalitis relapses and *Pneumocystis carinii* pneumonia in HIV-infected patients. *Eur. J. Clin. Microbiol. Infect. Dis.* **12**:325–329.

Ruiz, A., W. Ganz, J. Donovan-Post, A. Camp, H. Landy, W. Mallin, and G. Sfakianakis. 1994. Use of Thallium-201 Brain SPECT to differentiate cerebral lymphoma from toxoplasma encephalitis in AIDS patients. *Am. J. Neuroradiol.* **15**:1885–1894.

Rushing, E. J., and D. K. Burns. 2001. Infections of the nervous system. *Neuroimaging Clin. N. Am.* **11**:1–13.

San-Andrés, F., R. Rubio, J. Castilla, F. Pulido, G. Palao, I. de Pedro, J. R. Costa, and A. del Palacio. 2003. Incidence of acquired immunodeficiency syndrome-associated opportunistic diseases and the effect of treatment on a cohort of 1115 patients infected with human immunodeficiency virus, 1989-1997. *Clin. Infect. Dis.* **36**:1177–1185.

Sanchez-Ramos, J., S. Factor, W. Weiner, and J. Marquez. 1989. Hemichorea-hemiballismus associated with acquired immune deficiency syndrome and cerebral toxoplasmosis. *Mov. Disord.* **4**:266–273.

Sarciron, M., and A. Gherardi. 2000. Cytokines involved in toxoplasmic encephalitis. *Scand. J. Immunol.* **52**:534–543.

Schoondermark-van de Ven, E., J. Galama, C. Kraaijeveld, J. van Druten, J. Meuwissen, and W. Melchers. 1993. Value of the polymerase chain reaction for the detection of *Toxoplasma gondii* in cerebrospinal fluid from patients with AIDS. *Clin. Infect. Dis.* **16**:661–666.

Schurmann, D., F. Bergmann, H. Albrecht, J. Padberg, T. Wunsche, T. Grunewald, M. Schurmann, M. Grobasch, M.

Vallee, B. Ruf, and N. Suttorp. 2002. Effectiveness of twice-weekly pyrimethamine-sulfadoxine as primary prophylaxis of *Pneumocystis carinii* pneumonia and toxoplasmic encephalitis in patients with advanced HIV infection. *Eur. J. Clin. Microbiol. Infect. Dis.* **21**:353–361.

Sharma, S., J. Hofflin, and J. Remington. 1985. In vivo recombinant interleukin 2 administration enhances survival against a lethal challenge with *Toxoplasma gondii. J. Immunol.* **135**:4160–4163.

Skiest, D. 2002. Focal neurological disease in patients with acquired immunodeficiency syndrome. *Clin. Infect. Dis.* **34**:103–115.

Skiest, D., W. Erdman, W. Chang, O. Oz, A. Ware, and J. Fleckenstein. 2000. SPECT Thallium-201 combined with *Toxoplasma* serology for presumptive diagnosis of focal central nervous system mass lesions in patients with AIDS. *J. Infect.* **40**:274–281.

Soriano, V., C. Dona, R. Rodriguez-Rosado, P. Barreiro, and J. Gonzalez-Lahoz. 2000. Discontinuation of secondary prophylaxis for opportunistic infections in HIV-infected patients receiving highly active antiretroviral therapy. *AIDS* **14**:383–386.

Strittmatter, C., W. Lang, O. Wiestler, and P. Kleihues. 1992. The changing pattern of human immunodeficiency virus-associated cerebral toxoplasmosis: a study of 46 postmortem cases. *Acta Neuropathol.* **83**:475–481.

Suzuki, Y. 2002a. Host resistance in the brain against *Toxoplasma gondii. J. Infect. Dis.* **185**:S58–S65.

Suzuki, Y. 2002b. Immunopathogenesis of cerebral toxoplasmosis. *J. Infect. Dis.* **186**:S234–S240.

Suzuki, Y., K. Joh, and A. Kobayashi. 1991. Tumor necrosis factor-independent protective effect of recombinant IFN-γ against acute toxoplasmosis in T-cell deficient mice. *J. Immunol.* **147**:2728–2733.

Suzuki, Y., M. Orellana, R. Schreiber, and J. Remington. 1988. Interferon-gamma: the major mediator of resistance against *Toxoplasma gondii. Science* **240**:516–518.

Tenant-Flowers, M., M. Boyle, D. Carey, D. Marriott, J. Harkness, R. Penny, and D. Cooper. 1991. Sulphadiazine desensitization in patients with AIDS and cerebral toxoplasmosis. *AIDS* **5**:311–315.

Torre, D., S. Casari, F. Speranza, A. Donisi, G. Gregis, A. Poggio, S. Ranieri, A. Orani, G. Angarano, F. Chiodo, G. Fiori, and G. Carosi. 1998. Randomized trial of trimethoprim-sulfamethoxazole versus pyrimethamine-sulfadiazine for therapy of toxoplasmic encephalitis in patients with AIDS. *Antimicrob. Agents Chemother.* **42**:1346–1349.

Torres, R., W. Weinberg, J. Stansell, G. Leoung, J. Kovacs, M. Rogers, and J. Scott. 1997. Atovaquone for salvage treatment and suppression of toxoplasmic encephalitis in patients with AIDS. *Clin. Infect. Dis.* **24**:422–429.

U.S. Public Health Service and Infectious Diseases Society of America. 2005. Guidelines for prevention of opportunistic infections. *Morb. Mortal. Wkly. Rep.* **51**(RR08):1–46.

Vago, L., S. Bonetto, M. Nebuloni, P. Duca, L. Carsana, P. Zerbi, and A. D'Arminio-Monforte. 2002. Pathological findings in the central nervous system of AIDS patients on assumed antiretroviral therapeutic regimens: retrospective study of 1597 autopsies. *AIDS* **16**:1925–1928.

Vyas, R., and J. Ebright. 1996. Toxoplasmosis of the spinal cord in a patient with AIDS: case report and review. *Clin. Infect. Dis.* **23**:1061–1065.

Walot, I., B. Miller, L. Chang, and C. Mehringer. 1996. Neuroimaging findings in patients with AIDS. *Clin. Infect. Dis.* **22**:906–919.

Wanke, C., C. U. Tuazon, A. Kovacs, T. Dina, D. O. Davis, N. Barton, D. Katz, M. Lunde, C. Levy, F. K. Conley, et al. 1987. *Toxoplasma* encephalitis in patients with acquired immune deficiency syndrome: diagnosis and response to therapy. *Am. J. Trop. Med. Hyg.* **36**:509–516.

Wijdicks, E., J. Borleffs, A. Hoepelman, and G. Jansen. 1991. Fatal disseminated hemorrhagic toxoplasmic encephalitis as the initial manifestation of AIDS. *Ann. Neurol.* **29:**683–686.

Wong, B., J. W. Gold, A. E. Brown, M. Lange, R. Fried, M. Grieco, D. Mildvan, J. Giron, M. Tapper, C. W. Lerner, et al. 1984. Central-nervous-system toxoplasmosis in homosexual men and parenteral drug abusers. *Ann. Intern. Med.* **100:**36–42.

Zangerle, R., F. Allerberger, P. Pohl, P. Fritsch, and M. Dierich. 1991. High risk of developing toxoplasmic encephalitis in AIDS patients seropositive to *Toxoplasma gondii. Med. Microbiol. Immunol.* **180:**59–66.

Zeller, V., C. Truffot, R. Agher, P. Bossi, R. Tubiana, E. Caumes, M. Jouan, F. Bricaire, and C. Katlama. 2002. Discontinuation of secondary prophylaxis against disseminated *Mycobacterium avium* complex infection and toxoplasmic encephalitis. *Clin. Infect. Dis.* **34:**662–667.

The Spectrum of Neuro-AIDS Disorders:
Pathophysiology, Diagnosis, and Treatment
Edited by K. Goodkin et al.
©2008 ASM Press, Washington, DC

23

Basic and Clinical Aspects of Human Cytomegalovirus Infection

ROBERT R. McKENDALL AND ALEX TSELIS

BRIEF HISTORICAL BACKGROUND

Enlarged cells bearing intranuclear inclusions resembling an "owl's eye" are a hallmark of cytomegalovirus (CMV) infection. In 1904 Jesionek and Kiolemenoglou (Jesionek and Kiolemenoglou, 1904) and also Ribbert (Ribbert, 1904) first observed such cells in multiple organs of a stillborn infant. They attributed the findings to a protozoan or syphilitic infection. In 1921 Lipschutz (Lipschutz, 1921) noted the similarity of the inclusions to the smaller ones in herpetic skin lesions. Goodpasture and Talbot (Goodpasture and Talbot, 1921) reported the cells to be similar to inclusion-bearing giant cells in the salivary glands of guinea pigs and proposed the term "cytomegalia." Shortly thereafter, Cole and Kuttner (Cole and Kuttner, 1926) postulated a viral etiology because a filtrate of inclusion-bearing salivary glands from mature guinea pigs could transmit the infection to younger animals. Soon, in 1932 Farber and Wolbach showed that 12% of infants dying of various causes had salivary gland intranuclear inclusions (Farber and Wolbach, 1932). In 1947, a report of two infants dying with cytomegalic inclusions in multiple organs was the first description of "cytomegalic inclusion disease" (Cappell and McFarland, 1947). The development of tissue culture methods led to the isolation of human CMV (HCMV) independently by three different laboratories in the mid-1950s (Weller, 1970).

Isolation of the virus led to the development of serologic diagnostic techniques, which in turn led to identifying a wider spectrum of human disease. Limited organ involvement in infants was recognized with reports of isolated hepatitis, chorioretinitis, or brain involvement (Bell and McCormick, 1981). In healthy adults Klemola and coworkers attributed an infectious mononucleosis-like syndrome and meningoencephalitis to CMV infection (Klemola and Kaariainen, 1965; Klemola et al., 1967). In 1968 CMV was found to be a rare cause of hepatitis in an otherwise healthy

individual (Carter, 1968). In 1972 interstitial pneumonitis (Klemola et al., 1972) and myocarditis (Tiula and Leinikki, 1972) were associated with CMV infectious mononucleosis. In 1977, sensorineural hearing loss was linked to perinatal CMV infection (Reynolds et al., 1974).

In the 1970s the expanding field of transplant medicine led to a wide variety of CMV diseases, both primary and reactivated. These included CMV mononucleosis, hepatitis, chorioretinitis, pneumonia, and encephalitis. The 1980s brought a similar story in the setting of the emerging disease AIDS. Here, retinitis, gastrointestinal disease, and nervous system infection predominated.

CMV VIROLOGY

CMV is an enveloped double-stranded DNA virus in the beta subgroup of the herpesvirus family. Mammals have strains that are species specific but share most biologic properties and significant nucleic acid homology. The large linear genome is 255 kbp, complex, and organized into unique short (US) and unique long (UL) segments, with a terminal repeat for each segment. The complete sequence contains 209 open reading frames coding for proteins of the core, capsid, tegument, matrix, envelope, and many others as yet unassigned as to structure or function.

Replication

Like all herpesviruses, the complex and highly coordinated replication strategy is divided into immediate-early (IE), delayed-early, and late gene expression. The earliest events in replication involve activation of host cellular protein kinases and cellular transcription factors and production of viral IE proteins (Albrecht et al., 1990), which regulate the later phases of replication. Next, CMV DNA polymerase and other proteins necessary to produce progeny viral genome appear. Finally, progeny viral DNA, capsid proteins, and envelope glycoproteins are synthesized, and new virus is assembled.

Primary Infection

Primary infection is usually asymptomatic and acquired by close contact at mucosal surfaces, including genitourinary,

Robert R. McKendall, Department of Neurology, Department of Microbiology and Immunology, University of Texas Medical Branch, Galveston, TX 77555. **Alex Tselis,** Department of Neurology, Wayne State University, Detroit, MI 48201.

respiratory, or upper gastrointestinal tracts. CMV replicates well in ductal epithelia, shedding virus into body secretions, including breast milk, providing an efficient transmission mechanism (Ho, 1991a, 1991b). Virus can also be acquired from seropositive donors through blood transfusions or organ transplantation. Fetal infection occurs transplacentally as a result of maternal viremia.

Following replication at the initial mucosal site, virus is systemically disseminated by infected circulating leukocytes. Virus is present in buffy coat cells in patients with CMV mononucleosis (Levin et al., 1979) and in transplant recipients (Wolf and Spector, 1993). In AIDS, infectious virus has been demonstrated in peripheral blood neutrophils, monocytes, and endothelial cells (Gerna et al., 1998). Infection of vascular endothelial cells ensues, followed by penetration of the parenchyma.

The distribution of virus after the initial local infection can be determined at autopsy, at least in hosts immunosuppressed enough to have disseminated CMV. Such studies show typical cytomegalic cells in bile duct, salivary gland, and bronchial epithelium, various epithelia of inner ear structures, Henle's loop, and proximal and distal tubules of the kidney and islet cells (Plachter et al., 1996; Sinzger and Jahn, 1996). Toorkey and Carrigan studied tissue from healthy seropositive patients who died of trauma and showed IE CMV antigens in kidney, lung, liver, spleen, and brain (Toorkey and Carrigan, 1989). Other organs with cytomegalic cells at autopsy include the eye, lung, liver, pancreas, ovaries, pituitary, adrenals, thyroid, brain, and skin (Plachter et al., 1996; Sinzger and Jahn, 1996). Ductal epithelium is a common secondary site of infection as stated above.

There is a wide tropism for neural cells. In fatal congenital CMV infection, inclusions appeared in neurons, glia, ependyma, choroid plexus, meninges, and vascular epithelium (Becroft, 1981). These findings are reproduced in animal models. In a murine model a recombinant murine CMV (mCMV) (with a reporter gene) was used to demonstrate that glia, microglia, endothelial cells, choroid plexus cells, ependyma, meningeal cells, and neurons were infected (van den Pol, 1999).

Viral shedding in urine, saliva, breast milk, and genital secretions occurs during the systemic dissemination phase of infection (Mocarski and Courcelle, 2001) and may persist for months in adults and sometimes for years in children, despite a vigorous immune response.

Latency

The acute infection clears, and viral shedding ends, with a slow rise in cell-mediated immunity. The virus is not eliminated but remains present as a latent or persistent infection in some sites and can reactivate to a replicative state. Latent infection is defined as the presence of viral DNA without the production of infectious virions. In persistent infection a low level of infectious virus is produced. No consensus molecular definition of latency exists (Hummel and Abecassis, 2002), but conceptually, in addition to evidence of viral DNA, there could be expression of some IE gene products with absence of late gene products or infectious virus. An example of this is the presence of latency-associated transcripts, which are a small number of IE transcripts, similar to what is seen in herpes simplex virus (HSV) infection, in naturally infected myeloid progenitor cells (Hahn et al., 1988).

Myeloid progenitor cells and peripheral blood monocytes (PBM) are important sites of HCMV latency. Myeloid progenitor cells are the precursor cells to granulocytes,

macrophages, and dendritic cells (Pass, 2001). Progenitor cells give rise to PBM that circulate and become tissue macrophages. PBM from seropositive healthy subjects harbor CMV DNA (Stanier et al., 1989; Bevan et al., 1991; Taylor-Wiedeman et al., 1991; Mendelson et al., 1996; Slobedman and Mocarski, 1999), but viral gene expression is limited to early genes only (Dankner et al., 1990; Ibanez et al., 1991; Taylor-Wiedeman et al., 1991). In granulocyte colony-stimulating factor-mobilized bone marrow or PBM from naturally infected autograft or allograft donors, rare cells (0.004 to 0.01%) are latently infected, expressing latency-associated transcripts (Hahn et al., 1988), and are mostly negative for CMV IE gene transcripts (Slobedman and Mocarski, 1999). B cells, T cells, and mature CD33 macrophages do not contain latency-associated transcripts. Similarly the frequency of latently infected PBMs in healthy seropositive subjects is only 0.01 to 0.12% (Soderberg-Naucler, 1997). Nevertheless, by using allogeneic stimulation of these cells, which promotes differentiation of monocytes, Soderberg-Naucler and others were able to isolate CMV from them (Soderberg-Naucler, 1997). The latently infected cells expressed dendritic cell markers (CD1a and CD83) and monocyte-macrophage lineage markers (CD14 and CD15). These data suggest a model of CMV persistence in which myelomonocytic progenitor cells in bone marrow maintain the latent infection and latently infected CD14$^+$ monocytes circulate in peripheral blood. In the presence of certain conditions, such as allogeneic stimulation or perhaps triggering by proinflammatory cytokines during intercurrent infection, reactivation of virus to productive infection occurs (Pass, 2001).

The distribution of other sites of human CMV latency is poorly understood. Tissues from healthy seropositive hosts, which have been shown to contain persistent CMV antigens or DNA, are candidate latency sites. Kidneys and hearts clearly harbor occult virus, as organs from CMV-seropositive, but not -seronegative, donors transplanted into seronegative recipients cause consistent seroconversion (83%) (Ho et al., 1975; Pollard et al., 1982). Other potential visceral sites include kidney, lung, liver, spleen, and brain (Toorkey and Carrigan, 1989), but whether the virus is latent or persistent in these organs is not clear.

The cell types that harbor latency have been partially determined. HCMV DNA has been shown to be present by PCR detection in CD14$^+$ PBM (Taylor-Wiedeman et al., 1991) and CD34$^+$ (Mendelson et al., 1996) and CD33$^+$ (Kondo et al., 1994) bone marrow cells. No infectious virus (but only CMV DNA) can be detected in PBM or bone marrow progenitor cells (Sissons et al., 2002), although transcription of CMV IE genes can be detected by reverse transcriptase PCR when cells from healthy seropositive subjects are treated with gamma interferon (IFN-γ) and granulocyte-macrophage colony-stimulating factor (Taylor-Wiedeman et al., 1994).

Human circulating endothelial cells in active HCMV infection harbor HCMV (Grefte et al., 1993), as do endothelial cells from patients dying of CMV disease. Human endothelial cells can be infected in vitro. CMV IE antigens in patients dying of trauma were widely detectable in endothelial cells in multiple organs (kidney, liver, spleen, lung, and brain), as well as in renal epithelial and Bowman's capsule cells, hepatocytes and Kupfer cells, splenic T cells and fibroblasts, alveolar epithelial cells, and macrophages (Toorkey and Carrigan, 1989). In the brain, endothelial cells and glial fibrillary acidic protein-positive astrocytes stained for CMV IE as well (Toorkey and Carrigan, 1989). Well-documented shedding of virus in human breast milk, urine, saliva, tears, semen, and cervical secretions, some of which occurs in healthy hosts (Ling et al., 2003), suggests that epithelial cells may harbor latent but reactivatable virus. However, in humans only for bone marrow and PBM is the evidence for latency good. If the rarity of latently infected cells in other organs and cell types approximates that seen in PBM and bone marrow progenitors, it may never be possible to gain adequate molecular evidence for true latency in these other sites. Nonetheless, it is clear that the viral burden, whether latent, persistent, or periodically reactivated, is substantial in healthy adults.

In murine models there is clearer evidence for latency in sites other than bone marrow and PBM. CMV DNA has been found in homogenates of brain and other organs (Collins et al., 1993). PCR in situ hybridization detects mCMV DNA in kidney, lung, liver, spleen, heart, and bone marrow cells from latently infected mice (Koffron et al., 1998). The bone marrow cell type was unidentified. In lung the cells were Mac-3-positive macrophages, and in all other organs the cells were PECAM-1 positive, indicating endothelial cells (Koffron et al., 1998). None of the cells contained IE transcripts.

Reactivation

Reactivation can occur under a variety of circumstances and also must be distinguished from reinfection or superinfection, which also has been demonstrated. Reactivation occurs in immunocompetent individuals, with asymptomatic viral shedding in urine, saliva, semen, and genital secretions, as well as in immunosuppressed patients, including solid organ and bone marrow transplant recipients and in AIDS patients, with the latter two having the highest frequency of reactivation. Most reactivations are asymptomatic but may result in clinical end-organ disease such as pneumonia, retinitis, encephalitis, or gastrointestinal disease. Nonimmunosuppressed patients with certain diseases or stress may exhibit reactivation, including those with sepsis, adult respiratory distress syndrome, critical illness in surgical intensive care units (Heininger et al., 2001), during space flight (Mehta et al., 2000), psoriasis (Asadullah et al., 1999), phenytoin hypersensitivity (Aihara et al., 2001), or periodontitis (Contreras and Slots, 1998; Slots and Contreras, 2000). Two of 56 critically ill surgical intensive care unit patients who were studied prospectively developed serious organ infection, and 20 of 56 had virus in blood or lower respiratory secretions (Heininger et al., 2001).

Reactivation triggers include whole-body irradiation, cytotoxic drugs, tumor necrosis factor alpha (TNF-α) in transplant patients, and antilymphocyte serum (Hummel and Abecassis, 2002). Cell differentiation also induces viral gene expression. Thus, treatment with granulocyte-macrophage colony-stimulating factor and hydrocortisone can induce monocytes from healthy seropositive subjects to express IE-1 transcripts, although no infectious virus is produced (Taylor-Wiedeman et al., 1994).

In transplant patients, the allogeneic response is a potent inducer of CMV reactivation, but concomitant immunosuppression confounds the picture. Recent elegant animal studies have elucidated the events in allogeneic reactivation. When latently infected murine allogeneic or syngeneic kidney was transplanted into nonimmunosuppressed recipients, extracts of RNA from allogeneic but not syngeneic kidney 2 days after transplant contained increased levels of IE-1 gene transcripts compared to nontransplanted latent controls (Hummel and Abecassis, 2002). This 2-day IE-1 gene expression in kidney was temporally associated with a strong activation of transcription factor nuclear factor kappa B (NF-κB) in allogeneic transplants and only weak activation in syngeneic transplants (Hummel and Abecassis, 2002). Another transcription factor, AP-1, was activated in both syngeneic and allogeneic transplants. AP-1 activation in syngeneic transplants has been attributed to ischemia/reperfusion injury. Both AP-1 and NF-κB are known to bind to the major IE promoter/enhancer that controls expression of both mouse and human CMV IE genes. Cytokine transcripts for TNF, interleukin-2 (IL-2), and IFN-γ but not IL-1 were induced in allogeneic but not syngeneic transplants. These cytokine transcripts appeared within 24 h of transplant and peaked at day 5 (Hummel and Abecassis, 2002). When TNF was injected directly into latently infected animals, activation of both AP-1 and NF-κB occurred in lung but only NF-κB activation occurred in kidney. Since IE gene expression was then observed only in the lung (Hummel and Abecassis, 2002), it appears that after transplant, the allogeneic response causes induction of cytokines, which in turn activate both transcription factors, which are required to induce IE gene expression in the kidney (Hummel and Abecassis, 2002).

Clinical studies support a role for TNF, showing a correlation between TNF levels and CMV reactivation in sepsis and transplantation (Hummel and Abecassis, 2002). Tong et al. (2001) showed that mean plasma TNF levels were much higher in renal transplant recipients with CMV disease than those without. Since CMV infection itself can induce TNF, they studied a patient group who had asymptomatic infection, evidenced by CMV DNA detectable in peripheral blood leukocytes (PBL) or plasma, and found that the TNF level was not increased. They suggested the high TNF level might be stimulating CMV replication through IE gene activation, which might increase the viral load and make disease more likely.

Immunology

Human sera contain antibodies to many (~25) CMV proteins (Landini and Michelson, 1988; Britt, 1991), but individuals vary. Nearly all have neutralizing antibodies which recognize gB (UL55) and gH (UL75) envelope proteins (Schoppel et al., 1997; Greijer et al., 1999). Other common targets are tegument protein pp150 (UL32) and pp52 (UL44), a nonstructural phosphoprotein which binds DNA, an IE gene product, pp72 (UL123), the tegument protein pp28 (UL99), and two matrix proteins, pp71 (UL82) and pp65 (UL83) (Pass, 2001). pp65 is an important target of CD8+ CTLs as well.

Substantial evidence indicates that antibody is important to prevent or ameliorate disease and spread of virus. Passively transferred antibody to gB in mice prevents lethal challenge (Pass, 2001), and treatment of renal transplant patients before transplantation with high-titer CMV immunoglobulin reduces the severity of disease in primary CMV infection (Snydman et al., 1987).

Natural killer (NK) cells may be important first responders in HCMV disease, but there are few direct data. Human NK cells in vitro can lyse CMV-infected target cells (Borysiewicz et al., 1985), and patients deficient of NK cells may have severe infections (Biron et al., 1989). In mice NK cell depletion results in more severe disease (Bukowski et al., 1984), and the NK-deficient beige mouse is more susceptible to CMV. A genetic locus, Cmv-1, which confers resistance on some adult mice strains, maps to the NK gene complex and may operate through the NK cell activation receptor Ly-49H (Scalzo et al., 1992; Brown et al., 2001).

T-lymphocyte responses in humans have been studied extensively because impairment of T-cell immunity strongly correlates with the severity of CMV disease (Pass, 2001). The dominant targets of CD4[+] T-cell responses are gB, gH, pp65 matrix protein, and IE proteins, while CD8[+] CTLs are directed primarily to IE1 (UL123), pp150 (UL32), pp65 (UL83), and gB (UL55) (Pass, 2001). The frequency of CD8[+] CTLs is highest for IE1 (Borysiewicz et al., 1988) and pp65 (Boppana and Britt, 1996). Limiting dilution studies show that the frequency of CMV-directed CD8[+] CTLs among all CD8 T cells is 1% (Wills, 1996). Studies of the clonotype of specific CD8[+] CTL T-cell receptors and studies using fluorochrome-labeled major histocompatibility complex (MHC) class I tetramers with CMV peptides have revealed the surprising finding that 1 to 4% of all CD8[+] T cells are directed at CMV proteins (Wills et al., 1999; Gillespie et al., 2000). In each seropositive subject, recognition by CTLs is limited to just a few peptides of each protein (Sissons et al., 2002). In fact the large circulating population of CD8[+] cells specific for a given peptide results from a massive expansion of a few individual T-cell clones which is maintained for years (Weekes, 1999).

The biologic importance of the T-cell-mediated immune response is clear. The most direct evidence for this in humans comes from adoptive transfer studies (Walter et al., 1995; Riddell and Greenberg, 1997). Bone marrow donor lymphocytes were stimulated in vitro with autologous CMV-infected fibroblasts and clones of CD3[+]CD8[+]CD4 CTLs. Infusion into bone marrow recipients prevented CMV viremia and disease in 14 patients, including 9 CMV-seronegative recipients who received marrow from CMV-seropositive donors (Walter et al., 1995).

Murine models have provided extensive evidence that the immune response limits local replication of CMV and dissemination (Redehase, 2000). T-lymphocyte suppression causes reactivation and dissemination of CMV in naturally infected mice. Adoptive transfer of CD8[+] CTLs protects mice from lethal challenge. CD4[+] lymphocyte production of IFN-γ restores CMV antigen presentation (Hengel et al., 1994). CD4[+] T-helper cell responses rather than CTLs are required to clear virus from salivary gland (Lucin et al., 1992).

CMV has a number of strategies to thwart the immune response ("immune evasion"). Four gene products (US2, US3, US6, and US11) down-regulate the expression of MHC class I molecules, thus reducing antigen presentation to CTLs (Sissons et al., 2002). pp65 (UL83 gene product), which has kinase activity, selectively blocks the presentation of IE1 peptides by phosphorylating it, thus eluding recognition by CTLs (Gilbert et al., 1996). HCMV also inhibits the expression of MHC class II, thus inhibiting initiation of cell-mediated immune reactions (Miller et al., 1998; Tomazin et al., 1999). NK cell recognition of CMV-infected cells may be thwarted by the UL 40 gene product of HCMV, which causes surface expression of HLA-E (Tomasec et al., 2000), a known inhibitor of NK cells. Other HCMV gene products which may be involved in NK or CTL immune reactivity have been described.

HCMV-infected cells exhibit upregulation of LFA-3 and ICAM-1 (Bodaghi et al., 1998). HCMV US28 encodes a protein that can bind chemokines CC and CX3C (Bodaghi et al., 1998) and act as a chemokine sink. Interestingly pUS28 can act as a coreceptor for HIV entry in vitro (Pleskoff et al., 1997). Other HCMV genes have been reported to code for chemokine and cytokine homologues (IL- 8 and IL-10) (Penfold et al., 1999; Kotenko et al., 2000). The significance of these molecules is an area of active research.

CMV EPIDEMIOLOGY

CMV infection is distributed worldwide. The seroprevalence of CMV ranges between 40 and 100% (Ho, 1990). Seropositivity rates in general increase with age and are higher in developing countries and in lower socioeconomic groups. The highest rates of conversion occur between 6 months and 2 years of age, and then the rate is about 1% per year (Borucki and Pollard, 1994). However, rates vary widely in specific groups of individuals (Pass, 2001). The overall seroconversion rate in healthy adults as reflected in blood donors is 1.5%. Other groups that have been studied are hospital employees (2%), day care workers in different cities (8 to 20%), pregnant middle-income women (2.5%) versus low-income women (6.8%), women in sexually transmitted disease clinics (37%), parents with a child 12 months old or younger who is known to be shedding CMV (47%), and parents of a 1.5- to 6-year-old child shedding CMV (13%). These rates indicate that spread is enhanced in settings where close contact with body fluids is expected, e.g., contact with care givers and sexual partners. Transmission between sexual partners has been proven by restriction enzyme analysis (Handfield et al., 1985). Virus has been isolated from toys and the hands of workers in day care centers (Hutto et al., 1986).

In HIV-infected individuals, 90% are seropositive for CMV (Drew et al., 1981), and most end-organ disease occurs in the context of advanced AIDS with CD4 counts below 100/mm[3], usually with culture-positive blood and urine (Caserta and Hall, 1998). The prevalence of CMV disease in adults with AIDS ranges between 23 and 60% based on autopsy studies (Morgello et al., 1987; Wiley and Nelson, 1988; Wilkes et al., 1988; Bylsma et al., 1995). Pathology attributed to CMV has been reported in 23 to 33% of brains and 40% of retinas of AIDS patients (Setinek et al., 1995; Bell, 1998; Caserta and Hall, 1998; Zelman and Mossakowski, 1998).

Reactivation of endogenous CMV secondary to the severe immunocompromise in these patients is assumed to be the cause of most of these diseases. However, there is clear evidence that reinfection occurs.

Autopsy studies of homosexual men with AIDS have shown that multiple strains of CMV can infect different tissues (Drew et al., 1984; Spector et al., 1984). Longitudinal serial isolates from homosexual men show that 29% have two or more strains and semen was the most common site of viral shedding (40%) (Leach et al., 1994).

Among AIDS patient groups, there are unexplained differences in the incidence of CMV disease. Thus, 28% of homosexual men develop CMV disease versus 15% of intravenous drug abusers (Jones et al., 1994).

SYSTEMIC CLINICAL MANIFESTATIONS

CMV Mononucleosis

CMV mononucleosis in an otherwise healthy adult presents with fever, lymphadenopathy, and a relative lymphocytosis. There may also be malaise, jaundice, hepatitis, or sweats. In a recent study of 124 patients the most frequent symptoms were malaise (67%), sweats (46%), and fever (46%) (Wreghitt et al., 2003). Features that distinguish this disease from Epstein-Barr virus mononucleosis are the rarity of pharyngitis, modest enlargement of lymph nodes and spleen, and a negative heterophile agglutinin test. Blood transfusion, prior to blood bank screening, was a proven source. The white cell count consists of 50% lymphocytes, and 10% are atypical lymphocytes. Transient immunologic aberrations occur, including mixed cryoglobulinemia, cold agglutinins, antinuclear antibodies, and rheumatoid factor. Abnormal liver function test results are common (69%).

The complications of CMV mononucleosis have been summarized elsewhere (Crumpacker and Wadhwa, 2005). Otherwise healthy hosts usually clear the infection without specific treatment. Interstitial pneumonia is the most severe complication of CMV mononucleosis and occurs in healthy or immunocompromised hosts. Respiratory distress may occur, and interstitial infiltrates on chest X ray are the primary findings. Hepatitis is common, mild, and usually asymptomatic in healthy hosts. Meningoencephalitis is very rare in healthy hosts. The spinal fluid shows a modest lymphocytosis, and CMV DNA may be detectable by PCR. Guillain-Barré syndrome was first associated with CMV infection in the 1970s, with about 10% of cases having high CMV immunoglobulin M antibody. Other rare complications of CMV infectious mononucleosis in normal hosts include myocarditis, thrombocytopenia, and hemolytic anemia. Skin rashes, usually associated with administration of ampicillin, also occur.

Immunocompromised hosts are at high risk of CMV infections. In 1,276 transplant patients the combined rate of CMV disease and asymptomatic shedding was 70% (Ho, 1991a, 1991b). CMV in immunocompromised hosts is clinically similar to CMV mononucleosis in healthy hosts (Hirsch, 2001), with atypical lymphocytosis, leukopenia, thrombocytopenia, and liver function test result abnormalities. End-organ complications are more common than in healthy hosts and include interstitial pneumonitis, hepatitis, retinitis, esophagitis, gastritis, colitis, adrenalitis, encephalitis, polyradiculomyelitis, and mononeuritis multiplex. These are most common in AIDS patients with CD4 cell counts below 50 to 100 cells per μl. For organ transplant patients, the risk factors for developing the more severe CMV complications include degree of immunosuppression, specific immunosuppressive therapy (higher risk with antithymocyte globulin), primary CMV infection (i.e., seronegative recipient), and type of organ transplanted, with bone marrow recipients being at highest risk. Often it is the transplanted organ that develops severe infection, particularly liver and lung transplants.

NEUROLOGIC MANIFESTATIONS OF CMV INFECTION IN HIV-INFECTED PATIENTS

CMV Encephalitis

Clinical Presentation

AIDS-associated CMV encephalitis presents in two clinical forms. One is a microglial nodule encephalitis, characterized by acute onset, confusion, delirium, and a relatively bland CSF formula; and the other is a ventriculoencephalitis, characterized by a slow progressive apathy, confusion, cranial nerve palsies, and occasionally a CSF formula of pleocytosis with a neutrophilic predominance and hypoglycorrhachia (Kalayjian et al., 1993; Grassi et al., 1998). (See below.) However, atypical presentations are possible.

CMV encephalitis can be difficult to distinguish from HIV dementia. In a retrospective case-control study, in which 14 autopsy-confirmed CMV cases were compared to 17 controls with HIV dementia (Holland et al., 1994), CMV encephalitis patients were found to have relatively more confusion, disorientation, apathy, withdrawal, and focal neurological signs and relatively less primitive reflexes than the HIV dementia controls.

Clinical characterization is confounded by other disease in the brain. In H. Vinters's series, 50% of the brains (Vinters et al., 1989) had other coexisting central nervous system (CNS) disease complicating the clinical-pathologic correlation. Fulminant systemic disease can obscure the effects of CMV in the brain (Hawley et al., 1983). It is possible that a few isolated inclusion-bearing cells or a few microglial nodules do not have much clinical effect (Navia et al., 1986). Indeed, among seven cases of microglial nodule encephalitis for which clinical data were available (Morgello et al., 1987), two patients were apparently without cognitive dysfunction, while five patients were demented. One patient, case 3 in the study by Moskowitz et al. (1984), developed lethargy, confusion, and a poor memory over several months. At autopsy he had a pure CMV microglial nodule encephalitis, with a few cytomegalic cells and no perivascular infiltrates.

Other presentations include hemispheral signs with heminumbness (Masdeu et al., 1988), seizures (Fuller et al., 1989), hallucinations (Fuller et al., 1989), prominent brain stem involvement (Fuller et al., 1989), multiple cranial neuropathies (Kenyon et al., 1998), and focal cerebellar lesions (Tselis and Lavi, 2000).

Abnormalities in serum electrolytes and osmolarity are well known to occur in AIDS-associated CMV encephalitis. In the study of Holland et al. (1994), patients were hyponatremic (53%), hypernatremic (30%), or normonatremic (15%). The HIV dementia controls all had normal electrolytes. Serum electrolytes are rarely reported in the literature, but abnormal electrolytes or osmolarity were reported for two of the seven cases studied by Kalayjian et al. (1993). Notably CMV adrenalitis, which can cause serum electrolyte abnormalities, is very commonly described in autopsy series. Thus, in the series of Morgello et al. (1987), 26 of 29 patients with CMV encephalitis had CMV adrenalitis.

Diagnosis

Diagnosis of CMV encephalitis can be difficult. In the older case reports, in HIV-negative patients, the diagnosis was made by a significant increase in anti-CMV antibodies between acute- and convalescent-phase sera in the context of a febrile encephalopathic illness (Parham et al., 1971; Chin et al., 1973; Back et al., 1977; Duchowny et al., 1979).

Viral Isolation

Isolation of CMV from blood or urine is common in systemic CMV infection, including those with evidence of encephalitis, but is not diagnostic of encephalitis, since this can occur in asymptomatic reactivation (Weller, 1971). Virus often cannot be cultured from the CSF, as in the following studies: Berman and Kim, 1994 (0 of 5 patients); Cohen, 1996 (0 of 7 patients); Kalayjian et al., 1993 (0 of 4 patients); but rare isolations have been reported (Edwards et al., 1985; Belec et al., 1990).

Serology

Anti-CMV antibody levels for the diagnosis of CMV encephalitis can be misleading. CMV antibody titers can fluctuate spontaneously. In one study, serial complement-fixing (CF) antibody titers from healthy donors were shown to fluctuate between significant and nondetectable titers in 22% of the cases, without known external cause (Waner et al., 1973). Two patients with biopsy-proved CMV encephalitis had no changes in the level of anti-CMV antibody (Philips et al., 1977). Neutralizing antibodies are more stable and more reliable for demonstrating previous exposure to CMV. Commercially, most CMV antibody tests measure binding of antibody to whole CMV virus, rather than using functional assays (such as neutralization or CF). Nevertheless, while serology can prove past or recent infection, it is of little use in proving the diagnosis of encephalitis.

Diagnosis by measuring the specific intrathecal immune response has been attempted. The CSF-to-serum ratio of CMV antibody was examined in three patients with presumed AIDS-associated CMV encephalitis (one confirmed by autopsy) and five HIV-positive patients with other neurological disease (none with autopsy) (Fiala et al., 1993). The results showed a trend towards slightly higher CSF/serum ratios for the CMV cases. This approach has not been developed further.

Brain Imaging

Imaging results range from normal to generalized atrophy, periventricular abnormalities, and focal, discrete lesions. Computed tomography (CT) of the brain can be normal or show only mild atrophy (Kalayjian et al., 1993). Ten patients with autopsy-proved CMV encephalitis all had abnormal CT scans, but only three had abnormalities specific for CMV. The pathology was often more extensive than the CT would indicate (Post et al., 1986).

Magnetic resonance imaging (MRI) scans are more sensitive but can still be normal or show only atrophy (Kalayjian et al., 1993; Holland et al., 1994; Arribas et al., 1996). The most common specific MRI finding in CMV encephalitis is increased periventricular signal on T2-weighted images and ependymal enhancement on T1-weighted images (Kalayjian et al., 1993). Both CT and MRI may reveal discrete white matter lesions (Post et al., 1986). Case reports have documented other abnormalities. A cerebellar hemisphere hypodensity on CT was shown to be a necrotizing leukoencephalopathy at autopsy (Tselis and Lavi, 2000). Small right frontal lobe lucencies on CT have been noted (Laskin et al., 1987). These contained cytomegalic cells, as well as cells staining with HSV-1 antigens. In an MRI scan (Masdeu et al., 1988), lesions were noted in the right internal capsule, right basis pontis, and left pontine tegmentum, with the first lesion showing necrosis admixed with cytomegalic cells on biopsy.

EEG

The electroencephalogram (EEG) in CMV encephalitis is nonspecific. In the pre-AIDS era, a 52-year-old man with sudden onset of headache, nausea, and lethargy showed slow left temporal activity. In the case of a 20-year-old woman with rapid onset of severe headache and confusion, followed by a seizure, serial EEGs showed an initial diffuse slowing evolving to left-sided focal "changes" and right temporal spikes (Philips et al., 1977).

CSF Findings

The CSF findings are highly variable. In one study, 2 of 13 CMV encephalitis patients had a pleocytosis, with 25 and 3,179 cells/mm³ (Holland et al., 1994). In another study, two CMV ventriculoencephalitis patients had cell counts of 10 and 50 cells/mm³. A substantial proportion of these cells were neutrophils. None of the CSFs from patients with microglial nodule encephalitis had pleocytosis (Grassi et al., 1998). Four of nine patients with ventriculoencephalitis had pleocytosis, including two with over 800 cells/mm³ (Arribas et al., 1995). It is noteworthy that neutrophilic pleocytosis can be seen in CMV encephalitis in both the normal and severely immunocompromised hosts.

Detection of CMV Nucleic Acid or Antigen in CSF

Recently, use of PCR to detect CMV DNA in CSF has been proposed as a means for diagnosing CMV encephalitis antemortem. Two reports document the use of PCR amplification of CMV DNA in the diagnosis of CMV encephalitis in four immunocompetent hosts (Studahl et al., 1992; Kanzaki et al., 1995).

In AIDS-associated CMV encephalitis, PCR methods have been more extensively studied. The sensitivity of PCR is high, but results are difficult to compare across studies due to the marked differences both in the population of patients studied in each series and in the PCR assay employed (Cinque et al., 1992; Gozlan et al., 1992; Wolf and Spector, 1992; Clifford et al., 1993; Fillet et al., 1993; Achim et al., 1994; Holland et al., 1994). The variability of results in these studies can be attributed to several factors.

First, the severity of disease varies from widespread ventriculoencephalitis to focal microglial nodules or isolated cytomegalic cells. Arribas et al. (1995) have hypothesized that the level of CMV DNA in the CSF of AIDS patients might correlate with the extent of CMV infection of the CNS. By subjecting serial dilutions of CSF to PCR, Arribas et al. found that only patients with ventriculoencephalitis had levels of CMV DNA higher than 10^3 genomes per μl of CSF. Only one sample was available from a patient with isolated cytomegalic cells obtained shortly (3 days) before death. This specimen had a level of CMV DNA of 10 to 100 genomes per 8 μl of CSF. The quantity of virus (measured in genomes per cell) appears to correlate with the presence of disease (Wildemann et al., 1998).

Second, both premortem and postmortem CSF samples have been looked at. Four studies (Cinque et al., 1992; Gozlan et al., 1992; Fillet et al., 1993; Holland et al., 1994) used only premortem CSF samples, one study used only postmortem CSF samples (Achim et al., 1994), and one study used both pre- and postmortem samples (Wolf and Spector, 1992). The study in which only postmortem samples were used showed a low specificity and differs from the other studies that used premortem samples and had much higher specificities. Results of CMV CSF PCR in samples obtained postmortem are not comparable with results obtained with premortem samples.

Third, there have been significant differences between the studies in specimen preparation and assay sensitivity. Analytic sensitivity of the different PCR assays varied between 1 (Achim et al., 1994) and 40 CMV genome copies (Gozlan et al., 1992). These differences in the analytic sensitivity are likely related to differences in CSF preparation, PCR target, PCR protocol, and method of detection of amplified products. These variations affect the clinical sensitivity of the PCR assay.

A potential pitfall of CMV CSF PCR is that its extreme sensitivity might detect latent nonreplicating virus in the CNS or CMV DNA in the CSF of patients with only minimal focal involvement (such as isolated cytomegalic cells within areas of normal brain parenchyma) (Cinque et al., 1992; Wolf and Spector, 1992).

This problem has been partially addressed with two new approaches. A PCR which detects mRNA transcripts for detection of the CMV pp67 late gene in the CSF has been shown to be 85 to 93% sensitive and 87 to 100% specific in AIDS-associated CMV encephalitis (Zhang et al., 2000; Bestetti et al., 2001). An antigen detection assay directed at the CMV pp65 matrix protein has been used to demonstrate pp65 in CSF leukocytes of HIV patients with painful peripheral neuropathy (Mastroianni et al., 1994) and in polyradiculopathy or encephalitis (Revello et al., 1994). Both of these results indicate that active CMV replication is present.

Other Diagnostic Tests

Monocyte chemotactic protein-1 has been shown to be elevated in the CSF of HIV-infected patients with CMV encephalitis at a significantly higher level than that of HIV-infected patients with primary intracerebral lymphoma, progressive multifocal leukoencephalopathy, and toxoplasma encephalitis (Bernasconi et al., 1996).

CMV Polyradiculomyelitis

CMV polyradiculomyelitis results from CMV infection of the peripheral nerves, nerve roots, and spinal cord in patients with advanced HIV disease. A single report documents an identical presentation in an apparently immunocompetent patient (Kabins et al., 1976).

CMV polyradiculomyelitis generally presents with pain and paresthesias in the lower extremities, followed by a subacute hypotonic weakness and areflexia in the legs, urinary retention, and sensory loss (Eidelberg et al., 1986; Behar et al., 1987; Mahieux et al., 1989; Cohen et al., 1993). CSF examination usually, but not always, shows a neutrophilic pleocytosis and hypoglycorrhachia (deGans et al., 1990; Miller et al., 1996). CMV PCR is positive in the CSF, while virus only occasionally can be cultured. Electromyography generally shows diffuse denervation in the lower extremities. Imaging studies show enhancement of the conus medullaris, cauda equina, and nerve roots as well as diffuse meningeal enhancement of the lumbar thecal sac (Bazan et al., 1991; Talpos et al., 1991).

Pathological findings in CMV polyradiculomyelitis recently have been reviewed (Kolson and Gonzalez-Scarano, 2001). CMV antigens without HIV antigens are present in the dorsal and ventral roots with focal nerve root inflammatory lesions. CMV infection is present within venular endothelial cells of the epineurium of the sural nerve and within the connective tissue of the dorsal root ganglia. Areas of inflammation contain polymorphonuclear cell infiltration, necrosis, and CMV infection of endoneurial cells. Overall ventral nerve root involvement is more common than dorsal root and ganglia involvement. Occasionally there is a cranial neuritis. Thus, this disease appears to result primarily from CMV infection of nerve roots.

CMV Mononeuritis Multiplex

CMV mononeuropathy multiplex generally presents with numbness and painful paresthesias in a multifocal distribution in upper and/or lower extremities. Over weeks to months there may be progression to a severe sensorimotor neuropathy. Most patients have CMV detectable in the CSF by PCR. The electromyography findings are typical of a mononeuropathy multiplex with multifocal axonopathy (Roullet et al., 1994).

The pathology has been studied in only a few cases (Kolson and Gonzalez-Scarano, 2001). CMV has been demonstrated in the astrocytes of the spinal cord and in macrophages, fibroblasts, and endoneurial cells in the superficial peroneal nerves. CMV inclusions have been observed in the brachial and tibial nerves of late-stage AIDS patients with a primarily demyelinating neuropathy (Morgello and Simpson, 1994). Roullet et al. (1994) reported improvement with anti-CMV treatment in 14 of 15 cases of late-stage AIDS-associated multifocal neuropathy. Though incomplete,

these data suggest that direct CMV infection plays a role in mononeuritis multiplex associated with AIDS.

Differential Diagnosis

In a patient with subacute encephalopathy and cranial nerve palsies or nystagmus, neutrophilic pleocytosis, increased CSF protein, and hypoglycorrhachia, CMV ventriculoencephalitis is very likely and can be confirmed by PCR detection of CMV DNA in the CSF. Similarly the patient with a painful hypotonic progressive paraparesis, neutrophilic CSF pleocytosis, and lumbar meningeal enhancement on MRI most likely has CMV polyradiculitis, which can be confirmed by CSF PCR. In contrast, for the AIDS patient with progressive encephalopathy, the differential diagnosis is broad and includes HIV-associated dementia, progressive multifocal leukoencephalopathy, primary CNS lymphoma, and cerebral toxoplasmosis.

PATHOLOGY

There is a broad pathological spectrum of CMV brain infection in AIDS. It ranges from the presence of isolated scattered cytomegalic cells, to scattered microglial nodules with or without inclusions, to widespread necrotizing ependymitis with periventricularly distributed cytomegalic cells, microglial nodules, and perivascular infiltrates, to vasculitis, and to necrotizing leukoencephalopathy (Vinters et al., 1989). In an autopsy study of 30 AIDS patients with CMV encephalitis, Morgello et al. (1987) distinguished five types of neuropathological findings: microglial nodules ($n = 30$), isolated inclusion-bearing cells ($n = 15$), focal parenchymal necrosis ($n = 4$), necrotizing ventriculoencephalitis ($n = 3$), and necrotizing radiculomyelitis ($n = 3$).

The pathology of CMV radiculomyelitis usually consists of inflammation and necrosis, with typical cytomegalic inclusion cells in the lumbosacral roots (especially the ventral roots) and motor neurons, conus medullaris, and cauda equina (Behar et al., 1987; Mahieux et al., 1989). CMV inclusion bodies may be found in both endothelial and endoneurial cells in the roots. Focal areas of vasculitis in the nerve roots are also seen (Eidelberg et al., 1986). CMV infection can simultaneously affect nerve roots and peripheral nerves (Grafe and Wiley, 1989).

The pathology of CMV neuropathy consists of multifocal inflammatory infiltrates (mostly with mononuclear cells and neutrophils) in the nerves, with associated necrosis. Cells with cytomegalic inclusions are seen (Said et al., 1991). Cases with disproportionate loss of myelin relative to axonal dropout have been described (Morgello and Simpson, 1994). Schwann cell infection with CMV has been reported (Grafe and Wiley, 1989).

PATHOGENESIS

Many factors are undoubtedly involved in the pathogenesis of the varied picture of CMV in the nervous system of AIDS patients. Most important among them is immunosuppression, since disseminated CMV infection and CMV encephalitis affect patients with severe immune deficiency, with CD4$^+$ cell counts of <100 cells/mm. Clearance of systemic CMV even in the immunocompetent patient is associated with the onset of cell-mediated immunity rather than with the presence of antibodies (van den Berg et al., 1992), and cell-mediated immunity is important in the control of CMV replication.

Humoral immunity seems to be less important in CMV disease. Disseminated CMV disease is not commonly seen in patients with agammaglobulinemia or hypogammaglobulinemia, in which infections with bacteria (Buckley, 1986) or mycoplasma (Roifman et al., 1986) occur. Also, apart from chronic enterovirus meningoencephalitis (McKinney et al., 1987), viral infections in hypo- and agammaglobulinemic patients are not different from those in otherwise healthy individuals (Buckley, 1986). Very rarely such patients have had encephalitis ascribed to measles virus and HSV (Lederman and Winkelstein, 1985), although most cases of encephalitis have been due to enteroviruses. Systemic infections (but not encephalitis) with a few other viruses have been described in patients with hypogammaglobulinemia, but not CMV (Lederman and Winkelstein, 1985). Therefore, hosts with deficits in humoral immunity appear to handle CMV as do intact hosts.

However, there are subtleties in the relative effectiveness of the two arms of immunity against CMV. For example, in one patient with thymoma and immunoglobulin deficiency (Kauffman et al., 1979), there was a noticeable inflammatory response in the brain, with perivascular hemorrhages and lymphocytic cuffs, even though microglial nodules were not seen. The patient had immunoglobulin deficiency and a selective nonresponsiveness of lymphocytes to CMV antigens, but other T-cell functions (formation of rosettes and mitogenic responsiveness to nonspecific and specific activators) were normal. Furthermore, CMV immunoglobulin has been useful in the prevention of CMV opportunistic infection in transplant patients (Emanuel et al., 1988; Emanuel, 1991), so humoral immunity may be subtly involved.

The broad spectrum of observed CNS disease in AIDS is likely related to a broader range of viral load secondary to the immunodeficiency. Different viral loads may induce qualitatively different pathologies. In a guinea pig CMV encephalitis model, the histopathology is predominantly that of a microglial nodule encephalitis, with some perivascular cuffing (Booss et al., 1989), as seen in almost all of the reported human cases. But when lower viral loads were studied, microglial nodules and cells with inclusions were the predominant result, while higher viral loads led to perivascular infiltrates and necrosis (Booss et al., 1989).

Equally important in influencing the pattern of CNS disease may be route of entry. A heuristic model of CMV infection in the CNS, which postulates an important role for route of entry, as well as viral burden, has been proposed (Tselis and Lavi, 2000). This model summarizes three basic pathological patterns of nervous system involvement in CMV disease, each of which can be viewed as part of a hierarchy in the severity of the pathology. The first pattern is diffuse multifocal CMV encephalitis. This may manifest as isolated inclusion-bearing cells, microglial nodule encephalitis, or focal parenchymal necrosis. The second pattern is CMV ventriculoencephalitis, or more descriptively, ventriculoependymoencephalitis. In this manifestation there may be ependymitis alone, ependymitis with subependymal involvement, or in the most severe cases, encephalitis with necrotizing periventricular lesions. The third pathological pattern is CMV radiculomyelitis, which may appear as CMV polyradiculitis or a necrotizing radiculomyelitis.

For CMV encephalitis Morgello et al. (1987) suggested five distinct neuropathological findings, described above. However, some of the pathological entities can be viewed as different parts of a spectrum of the same process (Tselis and Lavi, 2000). For example, the mildest form of multifocal encephalitis is that of isolated inclusion-bearing cells. In the microglial nodule form, there are usually inclusion-bearing cells in addition to the scattered microglial nodules.

Focal parenchymal necrosis is the most advanced form of this spectrum, since it usually contains necrosis in addition to microglial nodules and inclusion-bearing cells. Diffuse multifocal nodular encephalitis is different from ventriculoencephalitis and radiculomyelitis, because these are often seen in isolated forms, although occasionally more than one form occurs in one patient.

In otherwise healthy individuals and in non-AIDS immunosuppressed patients usually only diffuse multifocal nodular encephalitis is seen, mostly in its nonnecrotizing forms. In AIDS patients ventriculoencephalitis and radiculomyelitis are seen in addition to multifocal nodular encephalitis. The reason for that is not entirely clear, but it may in part be related to viral load or other factors discussed below.

The severity of the pathological picture is roughly reflected in the CSF abnormalities. Microglial nodule encephalitis usually presents with normal or slightly abnormal CSF. Pleocytosis, increased protein, and decreased glucose are usually correlated with diffuse multifocal necrotizing lesions or with ventriculoencephalitis and polyradiculomyelitis. It would be interesting to correlate viral quantity with type of disease process.

One may speculate (Tselis and Lavi, 2000) that the particular distribution of CMV CNS infection in any given patient depends on the mode of entry of the virus into the brain and the degree of disease depends on viral dose. Guinea pig models show that infection with a low viral dose of CMV results in inclusion-bearing cells and microglial nodule encephalitis while infection with a high viral dose results in more exuberant inflammation and necrosis (Booss and Kim, 1989; Booss et al., 1989). There are two possible modes of entry into the brain. One is through the choroid plexus, which would carry virus to diffuse through the CSF. The other is by passage through the blood-brain barrier (BBB), either through infection of endothelial cells or by passage of infected, activated lymphocytes or monocytes through the endothelium or through other, as yet poorly understood, means (Petito and Cash, 1992). There is no evidence that CMV can reach the CNS by transneuronal and interneuronal propagation, as proven for rabies, poliovirus, HSV, and varicella-zoster virus. It has been proposed that the choroid plexus mode of entry results in periventricular disease (Tselis and Lavi, 2000). A low transchoroid plexus viral dose results in a mild ependymitis, while a large dose would be more likely to cause necrotizing periventricular lesions.

The hematogenous-endothelial mode of entry is postulated to lead to diffuse disease. A small trans-BBB viral dose causes scattered inclusion-bearing cells and some microglial nodules, while a large trans-BBB viral dose results in focal parenchymal necrosis, microglial nodules, and inclusion-bearing cells. In addition, infection of endothelial cells by CMV may lead to vascular thrombosis and parenchymal necrosis and infarction, which may be a factor in the pathogenesis of the focal necrotizing forms of the disease (Wiley and Nelson, 1988). Similar mechanisms have been documented in CNS disease in mice caused by a murine leukemia virus (Park et al., 1993, 1994).

Recent elegant studies in an mCMV model confirm many of the pathogenetic postulates that have been suggested based on earlier animal models and human data (Reuter et al., 2003). These workers compared wild-type mCMV and a recombinant mCMV containing a green fluorescent protein reporter gene to study the conditions and mechanisms which influence CNS invasion and the pattern of CNS disease after different routes of peripheral infection in normal versus nude and SCID immunocompromised mice. Despite multiorgan systemic infection in all groups of mice, CNS invasion occurred only in the nude and SCID mice. It occurred late, only after 21 days postinoculation. SCID mice with the highest level of CMV in the brain had detectable but low frequencies of infected circulating MAC-3/CD45⁺ IL-2Rbeta/B220/CD3⁻ mononuclear cells beginning 14 days postinoculation, and these infected MAC-3 cells were found in infected brain foci. After 14 days, sera and PBL infection was detectable by PCR only on pooled specimens, indicating a very low level of viremia. Distinct infection foci were found in the CNS, in a nonsymmetrical multifocal pattern. Over time foci expanded locally. They often involved both neurons and glial cells. Forebrain, midbrain, and hindbrain were equally affected. The relative numbers of cells infected in the CNS were strongly correlated to the numbers of cells infected in systemic organs, indicating that a high level of peripheral infection promotes CNS infection. CNS invasion did not correlate with BBB leakage as detected by intravenous injection of horseradish peroxidase. Circumventricular organs, which lack tight junctions, stained with horseradish peroxidase, as they should, but no CMV was found in the same areas. Dissemination within the CNS was greatest when viral infection included the ventricular system or the meninges. Both peritoneal and intravenous routes of infection resulted in asymmetrical localized CNS infection. Intranasal infection of SCID mice led to local infection of the olfactory epithelium, but no neuronal/axonal spread to the olfactory bulb was detected.

This animal model recapitulates many of the conditions operant in AIDS patients. CMV CNS disease in AIDS occurs when CD4 cell counts are very low and tends to occur when there is a durable PBL viremia. The most frequent CNS manifestation of CMV infection in AIDS is the multifocal nodular encephalitis, which occurs in a multifocal nonsymmetrical pattern and shows expansion of foci. The more severe ventriculoencephalitis in AIDS is the result of ventricular infection and ependymitis.

These studies do not rule out the possibility that CNS CMV in AIDS might be the result of reactivation of CMV from sites of latent infection within the CNS. The SCID and nude mice were not latently infected in any organ. Most AIDS patients have generally acquired their CMV infection much earlier in life, and thus, some may have latent infection in the CNS. However, the murine studies clearly suggest that even an AIDS patient without latent CNS infection is at elevated risk for CNS invasion in the presence of a low CD4 count and reactivation of virus at peripheral latent site(s), leading to significant episodes of viremia of sufficient duration to cause CNS invasion (Reuter et al., 2003).

Other factors besides immunocompromise, viral load, and duration of viremia may also contribute in ways that are important pathogenetically. Viral strain differences, which have been described but not extensively studied, could affect several aspects of the pathogenetic potential in a given patient. Viral tropism selective for the choroid plexus, ependyma, or nerve roots is an obvious consideration. Differences in viral strain and the particular host immunogenetic makeup could translate into greater immunosuppressive effects or greater immune evasion induced by the virus itself.

Finally, synergistic interactions between CMV and HIV could also contribute to viral load in some patients. CMV can coinfect cells with HIV, and each genome can induce upregulation of protein synthesis and replication by the other (Nelson et al., 1988; Skolnik et al., 1988; Ho et al.,

1990). Coinfection by HIV and CMV of brain cells in vivo has been documented (Nelson et al., 1988). This is not unprecedented. A possible transactivation of a papovavirus promoter by HIV proteins has been suggested in cases with a combination of enhanced progressive multifocal leukoencephalopathy and HIV infection (Tada et al., 1990; Vazeux et al., 1990).

THERAPY

Presently available antiviral therapy clinically effective against CMV consists of four drugs: ganciclovir, valganciclovir, foscarnet, and cidofovir. Another drug, fomivirsen, which is an antisense inhibitor of CMV, has been approved for intravitreal injection to treat CMV retinitis (Vitravene Study Group, 2002).

Ganciclovir, a nucleoside analogue and homologue of acyclovir, is active against all members of the herpesvirus family in addition to CMV and has good CSF penetration (Fletcher et al., 1986). Ganciclovir is converted to an active phosphorylated triphosphate by a combination of CMV and cellular enzymes. The triphosphate then inhibits CMV DNA polymerase and becomes incorporated into nascent viral DNA, thus interfering with chain elongation. Ganciclovir is toxic to bone marrow and causes significant neutropenia in one-third of patients receiving it for CMV retinitis (Jabs et al., 1989). The clinical response of CMV encephalitis to ganciclovir alone is not impressive (Price et al., 1992; Arribas et al., 1996), and several cases of CMV encephalitis developing during maintenance ganciclovir treatment of CMV retinitis have been described (Berman and Kim, 1994).

Valganciclovir is a valine ester prodrug of ganciclovir with a much higher absorption into the bloodstream. Oral doses can produce drug levels in blood that are comparable to those obtained with intravenous ganciclovir. It has been as effective as intravenous ganciclovir in the treatment of CMV retinitis in AIDS patients. Toxicities are primarily neutropenia and thrombocytopenia.

Resistance to ganciclovir/valganciclovir has been recognized for about 15 years. Since activation of the drug requires phosphorylation by a CMV phosphotransferase, mutations in the UL97 gene that codes for this protein lead to resistance. Less often resistance has been associated with mutation in the viral DNA polymerase gene. Isolates resistant to ganciclovir have been reported in patients who died despite therapy.

Foscarnet is an analog of inorganic pyrophosphate, which at therapeutic concentrations reversibly binds to the pyrophosphate-binding site on viral DNA polymerases and reverse transcriptase, but not cellular DNA polymerases. It inhibits replication not only of all known herpesviruses but also of HIV (Chrisp and Clissold, 1991). Foscarnet has good CSF penetration, being found in concentrations of about 25% of those found in serum (Raffi et al., 1993). The CSF concentration was found to be higher when the meninges were inflamed in one study (Raffi et al., 1993), but not in another (Hengge et al., 1993). The main toxicity is renal and significant in one-half of treated patients (Chrisp and Clissold, 1991). CMV strains that are resistant to foscarnet have been recognized (Weinberg et al., 2003). They have mutations in the CMV DNA polymerase gene at codons that are different from those that confer resistance to ganciclovir.

Ganciclovir, valganciclovir, and foscarnet have efficacy in treating CMV retinitis, a complication of AIDS. In one two-armed study of AIDS patients with CMV retinitis, foscarnet therapy was compared to ganciclovir. Time to progression of the CMV retinitis and time to death were recorded. The drugs had equal efficacy in increasing time to progression, but survival was significantly better in the foscarnet group. The median survivals were 8.5 months in the ganciclovir group and 12.6 months in the foscarnet group. The reason for the improved survival is not clear, but foscarnet has greater anti-CMV efficacy and also has anti-HIV activity (SOCA Research Group, 1992; Dieterich et al., 1993). Valganciclovir has been shown to be equivalent to intravenous ganciclovir in CMV retinitis in AIDS patients on HAART (Martin et al., 2002).

Combination therapy with ganciclovir and foscarnet may have greater efficacy, since the drugs have synergistic antiviral effects in vitro (Freitas et al., 1989; Manischewitz et al., 1990; Enting et al., 1992). In an open-label study, AIDS patients with systemic CMV disease (retinitis, colitis, and esophagitis) which had progressed on both monotherapies were put on a combination of ganciclovir and foscarnet. Of a total of 10 patients, 9 had an objective response, and all patients tolerated the combination acutely (SOCA Research Group, 1992; Dieterich et al., 1993). In a phase I trial of ganciclovir and foscarnet given either concurrently or on alternate days to patients with CMV retinitis who had just completed a 14-day induction course of ganciclovir, those on concurrent therapy had more toxicity than the others, but less than those in previous studies (Jacobson et al., 1994). Survival and median time to progression were not statistically significantly different in the two arms of the study, although these were not primary outcome variables. The doses of the drugs in this study were less than those usually given for maintenance.

Cidofovir is a nucleoside analogue of cytosine. It requires phosphorylation by cellular but not viral enzymes to the active triphosphate, which then acts as an inhibitor of viral DNA polymerase. Cidofovir is licensed for use in CMV retinitis (Polis et al., 1995). It is highly nephrotoxic (Fletcher et al., 1986) and must be administered with probenecid to block uptake of the drug by the proximal convoluted tubule, which causes irreversible tubular necrosis. It also can cause ocular hypotony. There is one report of its successful use in AIDS-associated ventriculoencephalitis with both clinical improvement and reversion of CSF to CMV negative by PCR (Sadler et al., 1997).

The clinical response of CMV encephalitis to antiviral drugs is not known because there have been no controlled clinical trials. Anecdotal experience suggests that it is not dramatic, although there are individual cases of dramatic response to therapy. A survey of cases reported in the literature shows that the median survival of those treated was not very different from that of untreated patients (Tucker et al., 1985; Vital et al., 1985; Belec et al., 1990; Fiala et al., 1993; Kalayjian et al., 1993; Singh et al., 1993).

Therapy of AIDS-associated CMV neuropathy and radiculopathy appears to be more efficacious, with some response (which can take months) to therapy with ganciclovir and foscarnet, although failure of therapy has also been described (Cohen et al., 1993; Kim and Hollander, 1993). Painful peripheral neuropathy due to CMV appears to be much more responsive to anti-CMV drugs, with 14 of 15 patients showing "marked improvement" in one series (Roullet et al., 1994).

The degree of CNS penetration and the antiviral activity of the levels typically reached in the CNS are two important considerations in the use of these medications.

The published data are meager. Only one study examined levels of ganciclovir in CSF (Huang et al., 1992), and four studies examined levels of foscarnet in CSF (van den Berg et al., 1992; Hengge et al., 1993; Raffi et al., 1993). The concentration of drug necessary for suppression of viral replication varies widely, depending on the CMV strain and the cell lines that were used to study the drug. Most studies employ the 50% inhibitory concentration (IC_{50}), i.e., the drug concentration necessary to decrease plaque titer by 50%. CSF levels of foscarnet roughly overlap the IC_{50}s of various established viral strains as well as CMV clinical isolates (Wahren and Oberg, 1980; Eriksson et al., 1982; Mar et al., 1983; Smee et al., 1983; Rasmussen et al., 1984; Freitas et al., 1985; Plotkin et al., 1985; Andrei et al., 1991). However, ganciclovir may not reach CSF levels (based on five samples) adequate to suppress most strains of CMV at the doses used (Wiley and Nelson, 1988). For foscarnet, on the other hand, it appears that drug levels readily achievable in the CSF tend to be considerably higher than IC_{50}, and one might therefore expect foscarnet to be quite effective. This is based on 31 CSF samples (van den Berg et al., 1992; Hengge et al., 1993; Raffi et al., 1993). The CSF-to-plasma ratio of foscarnet varies from 0.13 to 0.68, with an average of 0.43 (Sjovall et al., 1989).

Furthermore, it is difficult to determine the sensitivity of brain virus to the drugs because isolation of virus from CSF is uncommon, so that measurement of IC_{50} by plaque reduction assays cannot be done.

CONCLUSIONS

CMV infection is extremely common in the general population and usually causes no illness or a self-limited mononucleosis-like illness, and only rarely does it cause significant end-organ disease. Only a few cases of CMV neurological disease have been reported. The virus is transmitted through mucosal exposure to virus and is distributed in the body through viremia. The virus establishes infection in multiple tissues with a latent reservoir in myeloid progenitor cells and PBM. With increasing immunosuppression, viral replication is reactivated and results in disease. The distribution of end-organ disease depends on a number of still poorly understood local circumstances, such as the presence of particular cytokines seen at sites of allograft rejection or other inflammatory processes. The source of the local infection is not known and may involve variable amounts of locally reactivated virus or implanted virus from viremia.

CMV infection is nearly universal among AIDS patients, and in the days before HAART was an important cause of morbidity and mortality. Involvement of the nervous system occurs at all levels and is usually a premortem event. CMV encephalitis has a broad clinical spectrum, which likely reflects the various routes and quantity of infection as discussed above. Clinically the disease can range from a progressive encephalopathy with cranial nerve palsies and a neutrophilic pleocytosis and hypoglycorrhachia to a subacute confusional state with a relatively normal CSF. The diagnosis is made by detection of CMV DNA in the CSF by PCR.

While systemic and retinal CMV infections are known to respond very well to ganciclovir and foscarnet, at least initially, the clinical response of AIDS-associated CMV encephalitis to antiviral drugs is poor. Peripheral nerve infection can present as a radiculopathy or mononeuropathy multiplex and may resemble other rapidly progressive neuropathies such as Guillain-Barré syndrome. Again detection of CMV in the CSF provides the crucial evidence to make the correct diagnosis. The response of peripheral nerve infection with CMV appears to be better than that of CNS disease, but this has not been studied in a controlled manner, and the natural history of this disease is unknown.

The impact of HAART on the natural history of HIV disease has been profound, and CMV infection of the nervous system has become increasingly rare, although it is still occasionally seen. The effect of HAART on established CMV disease in a treatment-naïve AIDS patient is unknown but presumably may be beneficial. One recent longitudinal study of 374 HIV-infected patients with a CD4 nadir of <100 cells/mm^3 showed that a CMV-positive status in the blood as determined by PCR was associated with an increased risk to an AIDS-defining disorder (2.22) and with mortality (4.14) (Deayton et al., 2004). Hence, the presence of CMV in the blood continues to identify a poor prognosis in the HAART era, and anti-CMV medication trials aimed at differentiating this result as a marker or as a possible disease determinant merit investigation.

REFERENCES

Achim, C., R. Nagra, R. Wang, J. Nelson, and C. Wiley. 1994. Detection of cytomegalovirus in cerebrospinal fluid autopsy specimens from AIDS patients. *J. Infect. Dis.* **169:**623–627.

Aihara, M., Y. Sugita, S. Takahashi, T. Nagatani, S. Arata, K. Takeuchi, and Z. Ikezawa. 2001. Anticonvulsant hypersensitivity syndrome associated with reactivation of cytomegalovirus. *Br. J. Dermatol.* **144:**1231–1234.

Albrecht, T., I. Boldogh, M. Fons, S. AbuBakar, and C. Deng. 1990. Cell activation signals and the pathogenesis of human cytomegalovirus. *Intervirology* **31:**68–75.

Andrei, G., R. Snoeck, D. Schols, and P. Gonbau. 1991. Comparative activity of selected antiviral compounds against clinical isolates of HCMV. *Eur. J. Clin. Microbiol. Infect. Dis.* **10:**1026–1033.

Arribas, J., D. Clifford, C. Fichtenbaum, D. Commins, W. Powderly, and G. Storch. 1995. Level of cytomegalovirus (CMV) DNA in cerebrospinal fluid of subjects with AIDS and CMV infection of the central nervous system. *J. Infect. Dis.* **172:**527–531.

Arribas, J., G. Storch, D. Clifford, and A. Tselis. 1996. Cytomegalovirus encephalitis. *Ann. Intern. Med.* **125:**577–587.

Asadullah, K., S. Prosch, H. Audring, J. Buttnerova, and H. Volk. 1999. A high prevalence of cytomegalovirus antigenaemia in patients with moderate to severe chronic plaque psoriasis: an association with systemic tumour necrosis factor alpha overexpression. *Br. J. Dermatol.* **141:**94–102.

Back, E., C. Hoglund, and H. Malmlund. 1977. Cytomegalovirus infection associated with severe encephalitis. *Scand. J. Infect. Dis.* **9:**141–143.

Bazan, C., C. Jackson, J. Jinkins, and R. Barohn. 1991. Gadolinium enhanced MRI in a case of cytomegalovirus polyradiculopathy. *Neurology* **41:**1522–1523.

Becroft, D. 1981. Prenatal cytomegalovirus infection: epidemiology, pathology and pathogenesis. *Persp. Pediatr. Pathol.* **6:**203–241.

Behar, R., C. Wiley, and J. McCutchan. 1987. Cytomegalovirus polyradiculopathy in acquired immune deficiency syndrome. *Neurology* **37:**557–561.

Bélec, L., F. Gray, J. Mikol, F. Scaravilli, C. Mhiri, A. Sobel, and J. Poirier. 1990. Cytomegalovirus (CMV) encephalo-myeloradiculitis and human immunodeficiency virus (HIV) encephalitis: presence of HIV and CMV co-infected multinucleated giant cells. *Acta Neuropathol.* **81:**99–104.

Bell, J. 1998. The neuropathology of adult HIV infection. *Rev. Neurol.* **154:**816–829.

Bell, W., and W. McCormick. 1981. *Neurologic Infections in Children.* W. B. Saunders, Philadelphia, PA.

Berman, S., and R. Kim. 1994. The development of cytomegalovirus encephalitis patients receiving ganciclovir. *Am. J. Med.* **96:**415–419.

Bernasconi, S., P. Cinque, G. Peri, S. Sozzani, A. Crociati, W. Torri, E. Vicenzi, L. Vago, A. Lazzarin, G. Poli, and A. Mantovani. 1996. Selective elevation of monocyte chemotactic protein-1 in the cerebrospinal fluid of AIDS patients with cytomegalovirus encephalitis. *J. Infect. Dis.* **174:**1098–1101.

Bestetti, A., C. Pierotti, M. Terreni, A. Zappa, L. Vago, A. Lazzarin, and P. Clinque. 2001. Comparison of three nucleic acid amplification assays of cerebrospinal fluid for diagnosis of cytomegalovirus encephalitis. *J. Clin. Microbiol.* **39:**1148–1151.

Bevan, I., R. Daw, P. Day, F. Ala, and M. Walker. 1991. Polymerase chain reaction for detection of human cytomegalovirus infection in a blood donor population. *Br. J. Haematol.* **78:**94–99.

Biron, C., K. Byron, and J. Sullivan. 1989. Severe herpesvirus infections in an adolescent without natural killer cells. *N. Engl. J. Med.* **320:**1731–1735.

Bodaghi, B., T. Jones, D. Zipeto, C. Vita, L. Sun, L. Laurent, F. Arenzana-Seisdedos, J. Virelizier, and S. Michelson. 1998. Chemokine sequestration by viral chemoreceptors as a novel viral escape strategy: withdrawal of chemokines from the environment of cytomegalovirus-infected cells. *J. Exp. Med.* **188:**855–866.

Booss, J., and J. Kim. 1989. Cytomegalovirus encephalitis: neuropathological comparison of the guinea pig model with the opportunistic infection in AIDS. *Yale J. Biol. Med.* **62:**187–195.

Booss, J., S. Winkler, B. Griffith, and J. Kim. 1989. Viremia and glial nodule encephalitis after experimental systemic cytomegalovirus infection. *Lab. Investig.* **61:**644–649.

Boppana, S., and W. Britt. 1996. Recognition of human cytomegalovirus gene products by HCMV-specific cytotoxic T cells. *Virology* **222:**293–296.

Borucki, M., and R. Pollard. 1994. Cytomegalovirus diseases, p. 323–338. *In* R. McKendall and W. Stroop (ed.), *Handbook of Neurovirology*, vol. 27. Marcel Dekker, New York, NY.

Borysiewicz, L., J. Hickling, S. Graham, J. Sinclair, M. Cranage, G. Smith, and J. Sissons. 1988. Human cytomegalovirus-specific cytotoxic T cells. A relative frequency of stage-specific CTL recognizing the 72 kD immediate early protein and glycoprotein B expressed by recombinant vaccinia viruses. *J. Exp. Med.* **168:**919–931.

Borysiewicz, L., B. Rodgers, S. Morris, S. Graham, and J. Sissons. 1985. Lysis of human cytomegalovirus infected fibroblasts by natural killer cells: demonstration of an interferon-independent component requiring expression of early viral proteins and characterization of effector cells. *J. Immunol.* **134:**2695–2701.

Britt, W. 1991. Recent advances in the identification of significant human cytomegalovirus-encoded proteins. *Transplant. Proc.* **23:**64–69.

Brown, M., A. Dokun, J. Heusel, H. Smith, D. Beckman, E. Blattenberger, C. Dubbelde, L. Stone, A. Scalzo, and W. Yokoyama. 2001. Vital involvement of a natural killer cell activation receptor in resistance to viral infection. *Science* **292:**934–937.

Buckley, R. 1986. Humoral immunodeficiency. *Clin. Immunol. Immunopathol.* **40:**13–24.

Bukowski, J., B. Woda, and R. Welsh. 1984. Pathogenesis of murine cytomegalovirus infection in natural killer cell-depleted mice. *J. Virol.* **52:**119–128.

Bylsma, S., C. Achim, C. Wiley, C. Gonzalez, B. Kuppermann, C. Berry, and W. Freeman. 1995. The predictive value of cytomegalovirus retinitis for cytomegalovirus encephalitis in acquired immunodeficiency syndrome. *Arch. Ophthalmol.* **113:**89–95.

Cappell, D., and M. McFarland. 1947. Inclusion bodies (protozoan-like cells) in the organs of infants. *J. Pathol. Bacteriol.* **59:**385–398.

Carter, A. 1968. Cytomegalovirus disease presenting as hepatitis. *Br. Med. J.* **3:**786.

Caserta, M., and C. Hall. 1998. Human herpesvirus infections of the central nervous system in patients with HIV infection, p. 467–485. *In* H. Gendelman, S. Lipton, L. Epstein, and S. Swindells (ed.), *The Neurology of AIDS.* Chapman and Hall, New York, NY.

Chin, W., R. Magoffin, J. Frierson, and E. Lennette. 1973. Cytomegalovirus infection: a case with meningoencephalitis. *JAMA* **225:**740–741.

Chrisp, P., and S. Clissold. 1991. Foscarnet: a review of its antiviral activity, pharmacokinetic properties and therapeutic use in immunocompromised patients with cytomegalovirus retinitis. *Drugs* **41:**104–129.

Cinque, P., L. Vago, M. Brytting, A. Castagna, A. Accordini, V. A. Sundqvist, N. Zanchetta, A. D. Monforte, B. Wahren, A. Lazzarin, et al. 1992. Cytomegalovirus infection of the central nervous system in patients with AIDS: diagnosis by DNA amplification from CSF. *J. Infect. Dis.* **166:**1408–1411.

Clifford, D., J. Buller, R. Mohammed, L. Robinson, and G. Storch. 1993. Use of polymerase chain reaction to demonstrate cytomegalovirus DNA in CSF of patients with human immunodeficiency virus infection. *Neurology* **43:**75–79.

Cohen, B. 1996. Prognosis and response to therapy of cytomegalovirus encephalitis and meningomyelitis in AIDS. *Neurology* **46:**444–450.

Cohen, B., J. McArthur, S. Grohman, B. Patterson, and J. Glass. 1993. Neurologic prognosis of cytomegalovirus polyradiculomyelopathy in AIDS. *Neurology* **43:**493–499.

Cole, R., and A. Kuttner. 1926. A filterable virus present in the submaxillary glands of guinea pigs. *J. Exp. Med.* **44:**855–873.

Collins, T., C. Pomeroy, and M. Jordan. 1993. Detection of latent cytomegalovirus DNA in diverse organs of mice. *J. Infect. Dis.* **168:**725–729.

Contreras, A., and J. Slots. 1998. Active cytomegalovirus infection in human periodontitis. *Oral Microbiol. Immunol.* **13:**225–230.

Crumpacker, C., and S. Wadhwa. 2005. Cytomegalovirus, p. 1786–1801. *In* G. L. Mandell, J. E. Bennett, and R. Dolin (ed.), *Principles and Practice of Infectious Disease,* 6th ed., vol. 2. Elsevier Churchill Livingstone, Philadelphia, PA.

Dankner, W., J. McCutchan, D. Richman, K. Hirata, and S. Spector. 1990. Localization of human cytomegalovirus in peripheral blood leukocytes by in situ hybridization. *J. Infect. Dis.* **161:**31–36.

Deayton, J. R., C. A. Sabin, M. A. Johnson, V. C. Emery, P. Wilson, and P. D. Griffiths. 2004. Importance of cytomegalovirus viraemia in risk of disease progression and death in HIV-infected patients receiving highly active antiretroviral therapy. *Lancet* **363:**2116–2121.

deGans, J., G. Tiessens, P. Portegies, H. Tutuarima, and D. Troost. 1990. Predominance of polymorphonuclear leukocytes in cerebrospinal fluid of AIDS patients with cytomegalovirus polyradiculomyelitis. *J. Acquir. Immune Defic. Syndr.* **3:**1155–1158.

Dieterich, D., M. Poles, E. Low, P. Mendez, R. Murphy, A. Addessi, J. Holbrook, K. Naughton, and D. Friedberg. 1993. Concurrent use of ganciclovir and foscarnet to treat cytomegalovirus infection in AIDS patients. *J. Infect. Dis.* **167:**1184–1188.

Drew, W., L. Mintz, R. Miner, M. Sands, and B. Ketterer. 1981. Prevalence of cytomegalovirus in homosexual men. *J. Infect. Dis.* **143:**188–192.

Drew, W., C. Sweet, R. Miner, and E. Mocarski. 1984. Multiple infections by cytomegalovirus in patients with acquired immunodeficiency syndrome: documentation by Southern blot hybridization. *J. Infect. Dis.* **150:**952–953.

Duchowny, M., L. Caplan, and G. Siber. 1979. Cytomegalovirus infection of the adult nervous system. *Ann. Neurol.* **5:**458–461.

Edwards, R., R. Messing, and R. McKendall. 1985. Cytomegalovirus meningoencephalitis in a homosexual man with Kaposi's sarcoma: isolation of CMV from CSF cells. *Neurology* **35:**560–562.

Eidelberg, D., A. Sotrel, H. Vogel, P. Walker, J. Kleefield, and C. Crumpacker. 1986. Progressive polyradiculopathy in acquired immune deficiency syndrome. *Neurology* **36:**912–916.

Emanuel, D. 1991. Uses of immunotherapy for control of human cytomegalovirus-associated diseases. *Transplant. Proc.* **23:**144–146.

Emanuel, D., I. Cunningham, K. Jules-Elyse, J. Brochstein, N. Kernan, J. Laver, D. Stover, D. White, A. Fels, and B. Polsky. 1988. Cytomegalovirus pneumonia after bone marrow transplant successfully treated with the combination of ganciclovir and high dose intravenous immune globulin. *Ann. Intern. Med.* **109:**777–782.

Enting, R., J. de Gans, P. Reiss, C. Jansen, and P. Portegies. 1992. Ganciclovir/foscarnet for cytomegalovirus meningoencephalitis in AIDS. *Lancet* **340:**559–560.

Eriksson, B., B. Oberg, and B. Wahren. 1982. Pyrophosphate analogues as inhibitors of DNA polymerases of cytomegalovirus, herpes simplex virus and cellular origin. *Biochim. Biophys. Acta* **696:**115–123.

Farber, S., and S. Wolbach. 1932. Intranuclear and cytoplasmic inclusions ("protozoan-like bodies") in the salivary glands and other organs of infants. *Am. J. Pathol.* **8:**123–135.

Fiala, M., E. Singer, W. Tourtellotte, J. Stewart, C. Schable, R. Rhodes, and H. Vinters. 1993. AIDS-Dementia complex complicated by cytomegalovirus encephalopathy. *J. Neurol.* **240:**223–231.

Fillet, A., C. Katlama, B. Visse, S. Camilleri, O. Rogeaux, and J. Huraux. 1993. Human CMV infection of the CNS; concordance between PCR detection in the CSF and pathological examination. *AIDS* **7:**1016–1018.

Fletcher, C., R. Sawchuk, B. Chinnock, P. de Miranda, and H. Balfour. 1986. Human pharmacokinetics of the antiviral drug DHPG. *Clin. Pharmacol. Ther.* **40:**281–286.

Freitas, V., E. Fraser-Smith, and T. Matthews. 1989. Increased efficacy of ganciclovir in combination with foscarnet against cytomegalovirus and herpes simplex virus type 2 in vitro and in vivo. *Antivir. Res.* **12:**205–212.

Freitas, V. R., D. F. Smee, M. Chernow, R. Boehme, and T. R. Matthews. 1985. Activity of 9-(1,3-dihydroxy-2-propoxymethyl)guanine compared with that of acyclovir against human, monkey and rodent cytomegaloviruses. *Antimicrob. Agents Chemother.* **28:**240–245.

Fuller, G., R. Guiloff, F. Scaravilli, and J. Harcourt-Webster. 1989. Combined HIV-CMV encephalitis presenting with brainstem signs. *J. Neurol. Neurosurg. Psychiatry* **52:**975–979.

Gerna, G., M. Zavattoni, F. Baldanti, M. Furione, L. Chezzi, M. Revello, and E. Percivalle. 1998. Circulating cytomegalic endothelial cells are associated with high human cytomegalovirus (HCMV) load in AIDS patients with late-stage disseminated HCMV disease. *J. Med. Virol.* **55:**64–74.

Gilbert, M., S. Riddell, B. Plachter, and P. Greenberg. 1996. Cytomegalovirus selectively blocks antigen processing and presentation of its immediate-early gene product. *Nature* **383:**720–722.

Gillespie, G., M. Wills, V. Appay, C. O'Callaghan, M. Murphy, and N. Smith. 2000. Functional heterogeneity and high frequencies of cytomegalovirus-specific CD8+ T lymphocytes in healthy seropositive donors. *J. Virol.* **74:**8140–8150.

Goodpasture, E., and F. Talbot. 1921. Concerning the nature of "protozoan-like" cells in certain lesions of infancy. *Am. J. Dis. Child.* **21:**415–421.

Gozlan, J., J.-M. Salord, E. Roullett, M. Baudrimont, F. Caburet, O. Picard, M. Meyohas, C. Duvivier, C. Jacomet, and J. Petit. 1992. Rapid detection of CMV DNA in CSF of AIDS patients with neurologic disorders. *J. Infect. Dis.* **166:**1416–1421.

Grafe, M., and C. Wiley. 1989. Spinal cord and peripheral nerve pathology in AIDS: the roles of cytomegalovirus and human immunodeficiency virus. *Ann. Neurol.* **25:**561–566.

Grassi, M., F. Clerici, C. Perin, A. D'Arminio-Monforte, L. Vago, M. Borella, R. Boldorini, and A. Mangoni. 1998. Microglial nodular encephalitis and ventriculoencephalitis in patients with AIDS: two distinct clinical patterns. *Clin. Infect. Dis.* **27:**504–508.

Grefte, A., M. van der Giessen, W. van Son, and T. The. 1993. Circulating cytomegalovirus (CMV)-infected endothelial cells in patients with an active CMV infection. *J. Infect. Dis.* **167:**270–277.

Greijer, A., J. van de Crommert, S. Stevens, and J. Middledorp. 1999. Molecular fine-specificity analysis of antibody responses to human cytomegalovirus and design of novel synthetic-peptide-based serodiagnostic assays. *J. Clin. Microbiol.* **37:**179–188.

Hahn, G., R. Jores, and E. Mocarski. 1988. Cytomegalovirus remains latent in a common precursor of dendritic and myeloid cells. *Proc. Natl. Acad. Sci. USA* **95:**3937–3942.

Handfield, H., S. Chandler, V. Caine, J. Meyers, L. Corey, E. Medeiros, and J. McDougall. 1985. Cytomegalovirus infection in sex partners: evidence for sexual transmission. *J. Infect. Dis.* **151:**344–348.

Hawley, D., J. Schaefer, D. Schalz, and J. Muller. 1983. Cytomegalovirus encephalitis in acquired immunodeficiency syndrome. *Am. J. Clin. Pathol.* **80:**874–877.

Heininger, A., G. Jahn, C. Engel, T. Notheisen, K. Unertl, and K. Hamprecht. 2001. Human cytomegalovirus infections in nonimmunosuppressed critically ill patients. *Crit. Care Med.* **29:**541–547.

Hengel, H., P. Lucin, S. Jonjic, T. Ruppert, and U. Koszinowski. 1994. Restoration of cytomegalovirus antigen presentation by gamma interferon combats viral escape. *J. Virol.* **68:**289–297.

Hengge, U., N. Brockmeyer, R. Malessa, U. Ravens, and M. Goos. 1993. Foscarnet penetrates the blood-brain barrier: rationale for therapy of cytomegalovirus encephalitis. *Antimicrob. Agents Chemother.* **37:**1010–1014.

Hirsch, M. 2001. Cytomegalovirus and human herpesvirus types 6, 7, and 8, p. 1111–1115. *In* E. Braunwald et al. (ed.), *Harrison's Principles of Internal Medicine,* 15th ed. McGraw-Hill, New York, NY.

Ho, M. 1990. Epidemiology of cytomegalovirus infections. *Rev. Infect. Dis.* **12:**S701–S710.

Ho, M. 1991a. Epidemiology of cytomegalovirus infection in man, p. 79–104. *In* W. B. Greenough and T. C. Merigan (ed.), *Cytomegalovirus: Biology and Infection.* Plenum Press, New York, NY.

Ho, M. 1991b. Human CMV in immunosuppressed patients, p. 249–300. *In* W. B. Greenough and T. C. Merigan (ed.), *Cytomegalovirus: Biology and Infection.* Plenum Press, New York, NY.

Ho, M., S. Suwansirikul, J. Dowling, L. Youngblood, and J. Armstrong. 1975. The transplanted kidney as a source of cytomegalovirus infection. *N. Engl. J. Med.* **293:**1109–1112.

Ho, W., J. Harouse, R. Rando, E. Gonczol, A. Srinivasan, and S. Plotkin. 1990. Reciprocal enhancement of gene expression and viral replication between human cytomegalovirus and human immunodeficiency virus-1. *J. Gen. Virol.* **71:**97–103.

Holland, N., C. Power, V. Mathews, J. Glass, M. Forman, and J. McArthur. 1994. CMV encephalitis in acquired immunodeficiency syndrome. *Neurology* **44:**507–514.

Huang, E., J. Benson, S. Huong, B. Wilson, and C. van der Horst. 1992. Irreversible inhibition of human cytomegalovirus replication by topoisomerase II inhibitor, etoposide: a new strategy for the treatment of human cytomegalovirus infection. *Antivir. Res.* **17:**17–32.

Hummel, M., and M. Abecassis. 2002. A model for reactivation of CMV from latency. *J. Clin. Virol.* **25:**S123–S136.

Hutto, C., E. Little, R. Ricks, J. Lee, and R. Pass. 1986. Isolation of cytomegalovirus from toys and hands in a day care center. *J. Infect. Dis.* **154:**527–530.

Ibanez, C., R. Schrier, P. Ghazal, C. Wiley, and J. Nelson. 1991. Human cytomegalovirus productively infects primary differentiated macrophages. *J. Virol.* **65:**6581–6588.

Jabs, D., C. Enger, and J. Bartlett. 1989. Cytomegalovirus retinitis and acquired immunodeficiency syndrome. *Arch. Ophthalmol.* **107:**75–80.

Jacobson, M., F. Kramer, Y. Bassiakos, T. Hooton, B. Polsky, H. Geheb, J. O'Donnell, J. Walker, J. Korvick, and C. van der Horst. 1994. Randomized phase I trial of two different combination foscarnet and ganciclovir maintenance therapy regimens for AIDS patients with cytomegalovirus retinitis: AIDS Clinical Trials Group Protocol 151. *J. Infect. Dis.* **170:**189–193.

Jesionek, A., and R. Kiolemenoglou. 1904. Uber einen Befund von protoenartigan. *Muench. Med. Wochenschr.* **51:**1905–1907.

Jones, J., D. Hanson, S. Chu, P. Fleming, D. Hu, and J. Ward. 1994. Surveillance of AIDS-defining conditions in the United States. *AIDS* **8:**1489–1493.

Kabins, S., R. Keller, S. Naraqi, and R. Peitchel. 1976. Viral ascending radiculomyelitis with severe hypoglycorrhachia. *Arch. Intern. Med.* **136:**933–935.

Kalayjian, R., M. Cohen, R. Bonomo, and T. Flanigan. 1993. Cytomegalovirus ventriculoencephalitis in AIDS: a syndrome with distinct clinical and pathological features. *Medicine* **72:**67–77.

Kanzaki, A., S. Yabuki, and N. Yuki. 1995. Bickerstaff's brainstem encephalitis associated with cytomegalovirus infection. *J. Neurol. Neurosurg. Psychiatry* **58:**260–261.

Kauffman, C., C. Linnemann, and M. Alvira. 1979. Cytomegalovirus encephalitis associated with thymoma and immunoglobulin deficiency. *Am. J. Med.* **67:**724–728.

Kenyon, L., H. Goldberg, D. Kolson, R. Collman, and E. Lavi. 1998. Case of the month: May 1998: a patient with HIV infection and multiple cranial neuritis. *Brain Pathol.* **8:**815–816.

Kim, Y., and H. Hollander. 1993. Polyradiculopathy due to cytomegalovirus: report of two cases in which improvement occurred after prolonged therapy and review of the literature. *Clin. Infect. Dis.* **17:**32–37.

Klemola, E., and L. Kaariainen. 1965. Cytomegalovirus as a possible cause of a disease resembling infectious mononucleosis. *Br. Med. J.* **2:**1099.

Klemola, E., L. Kaariainen, R. von Essen, K. Haltia, A. Koivuniemi, and C. von Bonsdorff. 1967. Further studies on cytomegalovirus mononucleosis in previously healthy individuals. *Acta Med. Scand.* **182:**311.

Klemola, E., R. Stenstrom, and R. von Essen. 1972. Pneumonia as a clinical manifestation of cytomegalovirus infection in previously healthy adults. *Scand. J. Infect. Dis.* **4:**7–10.

Koffron, A., M. Hummel, B. Patterson, S. Yan, D. Kaufman, J. Fryer, F. Stuart, and M. Abecassis. 1998. Cellular localization of latent murine cytomegalovirus. *J. Virol.* **72:**95–103.

Kolson, D., and F. Gonzalez-Scarano. 2001. HIV-associated neuropathies: role of HIV-1, CMV, and other viruses. *J. Periph. Nervous Syst.* **6:**2–7.

Kondo, K., H. Kaneshima, and E. Mocarski. 1994. Human cytomegalovirus latent infection of granulocyte-macrophage progenitors. *Proc. Natl. Acad. Sci. USA* **91:**11879–11883.

Kotenko, S., S. Saccani, L. Izotova, O. Mirochnitchenko, and S. Pestka. 2000. Human cytomegalovirus harbors its own unique IL-10 homolog (cmvIL-10). *Proc. Natl. Acad. Sci. USA* **97:**1695–1700.

Landini, M., and S. Michelson. 1988. Human cytomegalovirus proteins. *Prog. Med. Virol.* **35:**152–185.

Laskin, O., C. Stahl-Bayliss, and S. Morgello. 1987. Concomitant herpes simplex virus type 1 and cytomegalovirus ventriculoencephalitis in acquired immunodeficiency syndrome. *Arch. Neurol.* **44:**843–847.

Leach, C., R. Detels, K. Hennesey, Z. Liu, B. Visscher, J. Dudley, and J. Cherry. 1994. A longitudinal study of cytomegalovirus infection in human immunodeficiency virus type 1-seropositive homosexual men: molecular epidemiology and association with disease progression. *J. Infect. Dis.* **170:**293–298.

Lederman, H., and J. Winkelstein. 1985. X-linked agammaglobulinemia: an analysis of 96 patients. *Medicine* **64:**145–156.

Levin, M., C. J. Rinaldo, P. Leary, J. Zaia, and M. Hirsch. 1979. Immune response to herpesvirus antigens in adults with acute cytomegaloviral mononucleosis. *J. Infect. Dis.* **140:**851–857.

Ling, P., J. Lednicky, W. Keitel, D. Poston, Z. White, R. Peng, Z. Liu, S. Mehta, D. Pierson, C. Rooney, R. Vilchez, E. Smith, and J. Butel. 2003. The dynamics of herpesvirus and polyomavirus reactivation and shedding in healthy adults: a 14 month longitudinal study. *J. Infect. Dis.* **187:**1571–1580.

Lipschutz, R. 1921. Untersuchungen uber die Atiologie der. *Arch. Dermatol. Syphilol.* (Berlin) **136:**428–482.

Lucin, P., I. Pavic, B. Polic, S. Jonjic, and U. Koszinowski. 1992. Gamma interferon-dependent clearance of cytomegalovirus infection in salivary glands. *J. Virol.* **66:**1977–1984.

Mahieux, F., F. Gray, G. Fenelon, R. Gherardi, D. Adams, A. Guillard, and J. Poirier. 1989. Acute myeloradiculitis due to cytomegalovirus as the initial manifestation of AIDS. *J. Neurol. Neurosurg. Psychiatry* **52:**270–274.

Manischewitz, J., G. Quinnan, H. Lane, and A. Wittek. 1990. Synergistic effect of ganciclovir and foscarnet on cytomegalovirus replication in vitro. *Antimicrob. Agents Chemother.* **34:**373–375.

Mar, E., Y. Cheng, and E. Huang. 1983. Effect of 9-(1,3-dihydroxy-2-propoxymethyl) guanine on human cytomegalovirus replication in vitro. *Antimicrob. Agents Chemother.* **24:**518–521.

Martin, D., J. Sierra-Madero, S. Walmsley, R. Wolitz, K. Macey, P. Georgiou, C. Robinson, and J. Stempien. 2002. A controlled trial of valganciclovir as induction therapy for cytomegalovirus retinitis. *N. Engl. J. Med.* **346:**1119–1126.

Masdeu, J., C. Small, L. Weiss, C. Elkin, J. Llena, and R. Mesa-Tejada. 1988. Multifocal cytomegalovirus encephalitis in AIDS. *Ann. Neurol.* **23:**97–99.

Mastroianni, C., G. Sebastiani, F. Folgori, C. Ajassa, V. Vullo, and A. Volpi. 1994. Detection of cytomegalovirus-matrix protein (pp65) in leukocytes of HIV-infected patients with painful peripheral neuropathy. *J. Med. Virol.* **44:**172–175.

McKinney, R., S. Katz, and C. Wilfert. 1987. Chronic enteroviral meningoencephalitis in agammaglobulinemic patients. *Rev. Infect. Dis.* **9:**334–356.

Mehta, S., R. Stowe, A. Feiveson, S. Tyring, and D. Pierson. 2000. Reactivation and shedding of cytomegalovirus in astronauts during spaceflight. *J. Infect. Dis.* **182:**1761–1764.

Mendelson, M., S. Monard, P. Sissons, and J. Sinclair. 1996. Detection of endogenous human cytomegalovirus in CD34+ bone marrow progenitors. *J. Gen. Virol.* **77:**3099–3102.

Miller, D., B. Rahill, J. Boss, M. Lairmore, J. Durbin, W. Waldman, and D. Sedmak. 1998. Human cytomegalovirus inhibits major histocompatibility complex class II expression by disruption of the Jak/Stat pathway. *J. Exp. Med.* **187:**675–683.

Miller, R., J. Fox, P. Thomas, J. Waite, Y. Sharvell, B. Gazzard, M. Harrison, and N. Brink. 1996. Acute lumbosacral polyradiculopathy due to cytomegalovirus in advanced HIV disease: CSF findings in 17 patients. *J. Neurol. Neurosurg. Psychiatry* **61:**456–460.

Mocarski, E., and C. Courcelle. 2001. Cytomegaloviruses and their replication, p. 2629–2673. *In* B. N. Fields and D. M. Knipe (ed.), *Fields Virology*, 4th ed. Lippincott, Williams and Wilkins, Philadelphia, PA.

Morgello, S., E.-S. Cho, S. Nielsen, O. Devinsky, and C. Petito. 1987. Cytomegalovirus encephalitis in patients with acquired immunodeficiency syndrome: an autopsy study of 30 cases and a review of the literature. *Hum. Pathol.* **18:**289–297.

Morgello, S., and D. Simpson. 1994. Multifocal cytomegalovirus demyelinative polyneuropathy associated with AIDS. *Muscle Nerve* **17:**176–182.

Moskowitz, L., J. Gregorios, G. Hensley, and J. Berger. 1984. Cytomegalovirus-induced demyelination associated with acquired immunodeficiency syndrome. *Arch. Pathol. Lab. Med.* **108:**873–877.

Navia, B., E. Cho, C. Petito, and R. Price. 1986. The AIDS dementia complex. II. Neuropathology. *Ann. Neurol.* **19:**525–535.

Nelson, J., C. Reynolds-Kohlewr, M. Oldstone, and C. Wiley. 1988. HIV and CMV coinfect brain cells in patients with AIDS. *Virology* **165:**286–290.

Parham, T., E. Caul, S. Clarke, and A. Gibson. 1971. Cytomegalovirus meningoencephalitis. *Br. Med. J.* **2:**50.

Park, B., E. Lavi, K. Blank, and G. Gaulton. 1993. Intracerebral hemorrhages and syncytia formation induced by endothelial cell infection with a murine leukemia virus. *J. Virol.* **67:**6015–6024.

Park, B., E. Lavi, A. Stieber, and G. Gaulton. 1994. Pathogenesis of cerebral infarction and hemorrhage caused by a murine leukemia virus. *Lab. Investig.* **70:**78–85.

Pass, R. 2001. Cytomegalovirus, p. 2675–2705. *In* B. N. Fields and D. M. Knipe (ed.), *Fields Virology*, 4th ed. Lippincott, Williams and Wilkins, Philadelphia, PA.

Penfold, M., D. Dairaghi, G. Duke, N. Saederup, E. Mocarski, G. Kemble, and T. Schall. 1999. Cytomegalovirus encodes a potent alpha chemokine. *Proc. Natl. Acad. Sci. USA* **96:**9839–9844.

Petito, C., and K. Cash. 1992. Blood-brain barrier abnormalities in the acquired immune deficiency syndrome: immunohistochemical localization of serum proteins in postmortem brain. *Neurology* **32:**658–666.

Philips, C., L. Fanning, D. Gump, and C. Phillips. 1977. Cytomegalovirus encephalitis in immunologically normal adults: successful treatment with vidarabine. *JAMA* **238:**2299–2300.

Plachter, B., C. Sinzger, and G. Jahn. 1996. Cell types involved in replication and distribution of human cytomegalovirus. *Adv. Virus Res.* **46:**195–261.

Pleskoff, O., C. Treboute, A. Brelot, N. Heveker, M. Seman, and M. Alizon. 1997. Identification of a chemokine receptor encoded by human cytomegalovirus as a cofactor for HIV-1 entry. *Science* **276:**1874–1878.

Plotkin, S., W. Drew, D. Felsenstein, and M. Hirsch. 1985. Sensitivity of clinical isolates of human cytomegalovirus to 9-(1,3-dihydroxy-2-propoxymethyl) guanine. *J. Infect. Dis.* **152:**833–834.

Polis, M., K. Spooner, B. Baird, J. Manischewitz, H. Jaffe, P. Fisher, J. Falloon, R. Davey, J. Kovacs, and R. Walker.

1995. Anticytomegaloviral activity and safety of cidofovir in patients with human immunodeficiency virus infection and cytomegalovirus viruria. *Antimicrob. Agents Chemother.* **39:**882–886.

Pollard, R., A. Arvin, P. Gamberg, K. Rand, J. Gallagher, and T. Merigan. 1982. Specific cell-mediated immunity and infections with herpes viruses in cardiac transplant recipients. *Am. J. Med.* **73:**679–687.

Post, M., G. Hensley, L. Moskowitz, and M. Fischl. 1986. Cytomegalic inclusion virus encephalitis in patients with AIDS: CT, clinical and pathologic correlation. *Am. J. Neuroradiol.* **7:**275–280.

Price, T., R. Digioia, and G. Simon. 1992. Ganciclovir treatment of cytomegalovirus ventriculitis in a patient infected with human immunodeficiency virus. *Clin. Infect. Dis.* **15:**606–608.

Raffi, F., A.-M. Taburet, B. Ghaleh, A. Huart, and E. Singlas. 1993. Penetration of foscarnet into cerebrospinal fluid of AIDS patients. *Antimicrob. Agents Chemother.* **37:**1778–1780.

Rasmussen, L., P. Chen, J. Mullenax, and T. Merigan. 1984. Inhibition of human cytomegalovirus replication by 9-(1,3-dihydroxy-2-propoxymethyl) guanine alone and in combination with human interferons. *Antimicrob. Agents Chemother.* **26:**441–445.

Redehase, M. 2000. The immunogenicity of human and murine cytomegaloviruses. *Curr. Opin. Immunol.* **12:**390–396.

Reuter, J., D. Gomez, J. Wilson, and A. van den Pol. 2003. Systemic immune deficiency necessary for cytomegalovirus invasion of the mature brain. *J. Virol.* **78:**1473–1487.

Revello, M., A. Percivalle, A. Sarasini, F. Baldanti, M. Furione, and G. Gerna. 1994. Diagnosis of human cytomegalovirus infection of the nervous system by pp65 detection in polymorphonuclear leukocytes of cerebrospinal fluid from AIDS patients. *J. Infect. Dis.* **170:**1275–1279.

Reynolds, D. W., S. Stagno, K. G. Stubbs, A. J. Dahle, M. M. Livingston, S. S. Saxon, and C. A. Alford. 1974. Inapparent congenital cytomegalovirus infection with elevated cord IgM levels. Causal relation with auditory and mental deficiency. *N. Engl. J. Med.* **290:**291–296.

Ribbert, H. 1904. Uber protosoenartigen Zellen in der Niere einer. *Zentbl. Allg. Pathol. Pathol. Anat.* **15:**945–948.

Riddell, S., and P. Greenberg. 1997. T cell therapy of human CMV and EBV infection in immunocompromised hosts. *Rev. Med. Virol.* **7:**181–192.

Roifman, C., C. Rao, H. Lederman, S. Lavi, P. Quinn, and E. Gelfand. 1986. Increased susceptibility to mycoplasma infection in patients with hypogammaglobulinemia. *Am. J. Med.* **80:**590–594.

Roullet, E., V. Assuerus, J. Gozlan, A. Ropert, G. Said, M. Baudrimont, M. el Amrani, C. Jacomet, C. Duvivier, and G. Gonzales-Canali. 1994. Cytomegalovirus multifocal neuropathy in AIDS: analysis of 15 consecutive cases. *Neurology* **44:**2174–2182.

Sadler, M., S. Morris-Jones, M. Nelson, and B. Gazzard. 1997. Successful treatment of cytomegalovirus encephalitis in an AIDS patient using cidofovir. *AIDS* **11:**1293–1294.

Said, G., C. Lacroix, P. Chemouilli, C. Goulon-Goeau, E. Roullet, D. Penaud, T. de Broucker, G. Meduri, D. Vincent, and M. Torchet. 1991. Cytomegalovirus neuropathy in acquired immunodeficiency syndrome: a clinical and pathological study. *Ann. Neurol.* **29:**139–146.

Scalzo, A., N. Fitzgerald, C. Wallace, A. Gibbons, Y. Smart, R. Burton, and G. Shellam. 1992. The effect of the Cmv-1 resistance gene, which is linked to the natural killer cell gene complex, is mediated by natural killer cells. *J. Immunol.* **149:**581–589.

Schoppel, K., B. Kropff, C. Schmidt, R. Vornhagen, and M. Mach. 1997. The humoral immune response against human cytomegalovirus is characterized by a delayed synthesis of glycoprotein-specific antibodies. *J. Infect. Dis.* **175:**533–544.

Setinek, U., E. Wondrusch, K. Jellinger, A. Steuer, M. Drlicek, W. Grisold, and F. Lintner. 1995. Cytomegalovirus infection of the brain in AIDS: a clinicopathological study. *Acta Neuropathol.* **90:**511–515.

Singh, N., K. Anderegg, and V. Yu. 1993. Significance of hypoglycorrhachia in patients with AIDS and CMV encephalitis. *Clin. Infect. Dis.* **17:**283–284.

Sinzger, C., and G. Jahn. 1996. Human cytomegalovirus cell tropism and pathogenesis. *Intervirology* **39:**302–319.

Sissons, P., M. Bain, M. Wills, and J. Sinclair. 2002. Latency and reactivation of human cytomegalovirus. *J. Infect.* **44:**73–77.

Sjovall, J., S. Bergdahl, G. Movin, S. Ogenstad, and M. Saarimaki. 1989. Pharmacokinetics of foscarnet and distribution to CSF after intravenous infusion in patients with human immunodeficiency virus infection. *Antimicrob. Agents Chemother.* **33:**1023–1031.

Skolnik, P., B. Bozloff, and M. Hirsch. 1988. Bidirectional interactions between human immunodeficiency virus type 1 and cytomegalovirus. *J. Infect. Dis.* **157:**508–514.

Slobedman, B., and E. Mocarski. 1999. Quantitative analysis of latent human cytomegalovirus. *J. Virol.* **73:**4806–4812.

Slots, J., and A. Contreras. 2000. Herpesviruses: a unifying causative factor in periodontitis? *Oral Microbiol. Immunol.* **15:**277–280.

Smee, D., J. Martin, J. Verheyden, and T. Matthews. 1983. Antiherpesvirus activity of the acyclic nucleotide 9-(1,3-dihydroxy-2-propoxymethyl) guanine. *Antimicrob. Agents Chemother.* **23:**676–689.

Snydman, R., B. Werner, B. Heinze-Lacey, V. Berardi, N. Tilney, R. Kirkman, E. Milford, S. Cho, H. Bush, and A. Levey. 1987. Use of cytomegalovirus immune globulin to prevent cytomegalovirus disease in renal-transplant recipients. *N. Engl. J. Med.* **317:**1049–1054.

SOCA Research Group. 1992. Mortality in patients with the acquired immunodeficiency syndrome treated with either foscarnet or ganciclovir for cytomegalovirus retinitis. *N. Engl. J. Med.* **326:**213–220.

Soderberg-Naucler, C. 1997. Reactivation of human cytomegalovirus by allogeneic stimulation. *Cell* **91:**119.

Spector, S., K. Hirata, and T. Neuman. 1984. Identification of multiple cytomegalovirus strains in homosexual men with acquired immunodeficiency syndrome. *J. Infect. Dis.* **150:**953–956.

Stanier, P., D. Taylor, A. Kitchen, N. Wales, Y. Tryhorn, and A. Tyms. 1989. Persistence of cytomegalovirus in mononuclear cells in peripheral blood from blood donors. *Br. Med. J.* **299:**897–898.

Studahl, M., A. Ricksten, T. Sandburg, and T. Burgstrom. 1992. Cytomegalovirus encephalitis in four immunocompetent patients. *Lancet* **340:**1045–1046.

Tada, H., J. Rappaport, M. Lashgari, S. Amini, F. Wong-Staal, and K. Khalili. 1990. Transactivation of the JC virus late promoter by the tat protein of type 1 human immunodeficiency virus in glial cells. *Proc. Natl. Acad. Sci. USA* **87:**3479–3483.

Talpos, D., R. Tien, and J. Hesselink. 1991. Magnetic resonance imaging of AIDS-related polyradiculopathy. *Neurology* **41:**1996–1997.

Taylor-Wiedeman, J., P. Sissons, L. Borysiewicz, and J. Sinclair. 1991. Monocytes are a major site of persistence of human cytomegalovirus in peripheral blood mononuclear cells. *J. Gen. Virol.* **72:**2059–2064.

Taylor-Wiedeman, J., P. Sissons, and J. Sinclair. 1994. Induction of endogenous human cytomegalovirus gene expression after differentiation of monocytes from healthy carriers. *J. Virol.* **68:**1597–1604.

Tiula, E., and P. Leinikki. 1972. Fatal cytomegalovirus encephalitis infection in a previously healthy boy. *Scand. J. Infect. Dis.* **4:**57.

Tomasec, P., V. Braud, C. Rickards, M. Powell, B. McSharry, S. Gadola, V. Cerundolo, L. Borysiewicz, A. McMichael, and G. Wilkinson. 2000. Surface expression of HLA-E, an inhibitor of natural killer cells, enhanced by human cytomegalovirus gpUL40. *Science* **287:**1031.

Tomazin, R., J. Boname, N. Hegde, D. Lewinsohn, Y. Altschuler, T. Jones, B. Cresswell, J. Nelson, S. Riddell, and D. Johnson. 1999. Cytomegalovirus US2 destroys two components of the MHC class II pathway, preventing recognition by CD4+ cells. *Nat. Med.* **5:**1039–1043.

Tong, C., A. Bakran, H. Williams, L. Cuevas, J. Peiris, and C. Hart. 2001. Association of tumour necrosis factor alpha and interleukin 6 levels with cytomegalovirus DNA detection and disease after renal transplantation. *J. Med. Virol.* **64:**29–34.

Toorkey, C., and D. Carrigan. 1989. Immunohistochemical detection of an immediate early antigen of human cytomegalovirus in normal tissues. *J. Infect. Dis.* **160:**741–751.

Tselis, A., and E. Lavi. 2000. Cytomegalovirus infection of the adult nervous system, p. 109–137. *In* L. Davis and P. Kennedy (ed.), *Infectious Diseases of the Nervous System.* Butterworth-Heinemann, Boston, MA.

Tucker, T., R. Dix, C. Katzen, R. Davis, and J. Schmidley. 1985. CMV and HSV ascending myelitis in a patient with AIDS. *Ann. Neurol.* **18:**74–79.

van den Berg, A., W. van Son, R. Janssen, N. Brons, A. Heyn, A. Scholten-Sampson, S. Postma, M. van der Giessen, M. Tegzess, and L. de Leij. 1992. Recovery from cytomegalovirus infection is associated with activation of peripheral blood lymphocytes. *J. Infect. Dis.* **166:**1228–1235.

van den Pol, A. 1999. Cytomegalovirus cell tropism, replication, and gene transfer in brain. *J. Neurosci.* **19:**10948–10965.

Vazeux, R., M. Cumont, P. Girard, X. Nassif, C. Trotot, L. Marche, L. Matthiessen, C. Vedrenne, J. Mikol, and D. Henin. 1990. Severe encephalitis resulting from coinfection with HIV and JC virus. *Neurology* **40:**944–948.

Vinters, H., M. Kwok, H. Ho, K. Anders, U. Tomiyasu, W. Wolfson, and F. Robert. 1989. Cytomegalovirus in the nervous system of the acquired immunodeficiency syndrome patient. *Brain* **112:**245–268.

Vital, C., A. Vital, B. Vignoly, M. Dupon, J. Y. Lacut, G. Gbikpi-Benissan, and J. P. Carnaud. 1985. Cytomegalovirus encephalitis in a patient with acquired immunodeficiency syndrome. *Arch. Pathol. Lab. Med.* **109:**105–106.

Vitravene Study Group. 2002. A randomized controlled clinical trial of intravitreous fomivirsen for treatment of newly diagnosed peripheral cytomegalovirus retinitis in patients with AIDS. *Am. J. Ophthalmol.* **133:**467–474.

Wahren, B., and B. Oberg. 1980. Reversible inhibition of cytomegalovirus replication by phosphonoformate. *Intervirology* **14:**7–15.

Walter, E., P. Greenberg, M. Gilbert, R. Finch, K. Watanabe, E. Thomas, and S. Riddell. 1995. Reconstitution of cellular immunity against cytomegalovirus in recipients of allogeneic bone marrow by transfer of T cell clones from the donor. *N. Engl. J. Med.* **333:**1038–1044.

Waner, J., T. Weller, and S. Kevy. 1973. Patterns of cytomegaloviral complement-fixing antibody activity: a longitudinal study of blood donors. *J. Infect. Dis.* **127:**538–543.

Weekes, M. 1999. The memory cytotoxic T lymphocyte (CTL) response to cytomegalovirus infection contains individual peptide-specific CTL clones that have undergone extensive expansion in vivo. *J. Virol.* **73:**2099–2108.

Weinberg, A., D. Jabs, S. Chou, B. Martin, A. Weinberg, D. Jabs, S. Chou, B. Martin, N. Lurain, M. Foreman, C. Crumpacker, and Cytomegalovirus Retinitis and Viral Resistance Study Group and Adult AIDS Clinical Trials Group Cytomegalovirus Laboratories. 2003. Mutations conferring foscarnet resistance in a cohort of patients with acquired immunodeficiency syndrome and cytomegalovirus retinitis. *J. Infect. Dis.* **187:**777–784.

Weller, T. 1970. Cytomegalovirus. The difficult years. *J. Infect. Dis.* **122:**532–539.

Weller, T. 1971. The Cytomegaloviruses: ubiquitous agents with protean clinical manifestations. *N. Engl. J. Med.* **285:**203–214, 267–274.

Wildemann, B., J. Haass, N. Lynen, K. Stingele, and B. Storch-Hagenlocher. 1998. Diagnosis of cytomegalovirus encephalitis in patients with AIDS by quantitation of cytomegalovirus genomes in cells of cerebrospinal fluid. *Neurology* **50:**693–697.

Wiley, C., and J. Nelson. 1988. Role of human immunodeficiency virus and cytomegalovirus in AIDS encephalitis. *Am. J. Pathol.* **133:**73–81.

Wilkes, M., A. Fortin, J. Felix, and T. Godwin. 1988. Value of necropsy in acquired immunodeficiency syndrome. *Lancet* **ii:**85–88.

Wills, M. 1996. The human cytotoxic T lymphocyte (TCL) response to cytomegalovirus is dominated by structural protein pp65: frequency, specificity, and T cell receptor usage of pp65-specific CTL. *J. Virol.* **70:**7569–7579.

Wills, M. R., A. J. Carmichael, M. P. Weekes, K. Mynard, G. Okecha, R. Hicks, and J. G. Sissons. 1999. Human virus-specific CD8+ CTL clones revert from CD45ROhigh to CD45RAhigh in vivo: CD45RAhigh CD8+ T cells comprise both naive and memory cells. *J. Immunol.* **162:**7080–7087.

Wolf, D., and S. Spector. 1992. Diagnosis of human CMV CNS disease in AIDS patients by DNA amplification from CSF. *J. Infect. Dis.* **166:**1412–1415.

Wolf, D., and S. Spector. 1993. Early diagnosis of human cytomegalovirus disease in transplant recipients by DNA amplification in plasma. *Transplantation* **56:**330–334.

Wreghitt, T., E. Teare, O. Sule, R. Devi, and P. Rice. 2003. Cytomegalovirus infection in immunocompetent patients. *Clin. Infect. Dis.* **37:**1603–1606.

Zelman, I., and M. Mossakowski. 1998. Opportunistic infections of the central nervous system in the course of acquired immune deficiency syndrome (AIDS). Morphological analysis of 172 cases. *Folia Neuropathol.* **36:**129–144.

Zhang, F., S. Tetali, X. Wand, M. Kaplan, F. Cromme, and C. Ginocchio. 2000. Detection of human cytomegalovirus pp67 late gene transcripts in cerebrospinal fluid of human immunodeficiency virus type-1-infected patients by nucleic acid sequence-based amplification. *J. Clin. Microbiol.* **38:**1920–1925.

The Spectrum of Neuro-AIDS Disorders:
Pathophysiology, Diagnosis, and Treatment
Edited by K. Goodkin et al.
©2008 ASM Press, Washington, DC

24

Cryptococcosis and Other Fungal Infections of the Central Nervous System

ROGER J. BEDIMO AND DANIEL J. SKIEST

Fungal infections of the central nervous system (CNS) are an important cause of morbidity and mortality in HIV-infected patients. *Cryptococcus neoformans* is the most important fungal pathogen in AIDS patients throughout the world. Other important but less frequent fungal pathogens include *Histoplasma capsulatum*, *Coccidioides immitis*, *Aspergillus* spp., the zygomyces, *Blastomyces dermatitidis*, *Paracoccidioides brasiliensis*, and *Candida* spp. Histoplasmosis, coccidioidomycosis, paracoccidioidomycosis, and blastomycosis are limited to certain geographic areas, whereas the other pathogens are relatively ubiquitous.

In the developed world the incidence of invasive fungal infections has declined with the widespread use of highly active antiretroviral therapy (HAART); however, in the developing world, where the vast majority of HIV-infected individuals are not receiving HAART, these pathogens, especially *C. neoformans*, continue to cause significant morbidity and mortality. Major advances in the management of cryptococcosis in the past few years have led to significant improvements in mortality, but morbidity remains elevated. The optimal management of other, less common CNS fungal infections in AIDS is less well defined due to the paucity of controlled trials.

CRYPTOCOCCOSIS

First described by Stoddard and Cutler in 1916, cryptococcal meningitis had a worldwide but low incidence until the early 1980s (Gould and Gould, 1985). The advent of the worldwide AIDS pandemic led to a sharp increase in the number of cases of cryptococcosis. Although its incidence has decreased recently in the developed world, *C. neoformans* remains the most common cause of meningitis in AIDS. In much of the developing world *C. neoformans* remains an important cause of morbidity and mortality and is one of the most common AIDS-defining conditions.

Epidemiology

C. neoformans is the most common CNS fungal infection in AIDS patients. In the pre-HAART era the annual incidence of cryptococcosis was 17 to 66 cases per 1,000 persons with a prevalence of 5 to 10% in AIDS patients in the United States and Europe (Chuck and Sande, 1989; Selik et al., 1997; Currie and Casadevall, 1994; Dromer et al., 2004). The incidence in the United States began to decline even before the advent of HAART, probably at least in part because of the increased prophylactic use of fluconazole (Mirza et al., 2003; Moore and Chaisson, 1996; Powderly et al., 1995; Selik et al., 2002). Further decreases in cryptococcosis have paralleled the decline in other opportunistic complications observed in the HAART era (Dromer et al., 2004; Mirza et al., 2003; Ives et al., 2001; Sacktor et al., 2001; Kaplan et al., 2000; Holtzer et al., 1998). One study from San Francisco demonstrated a decline of 63% in cases of cryptococcal meningitis (Holtzer et al., 1998). In the multicenter AIDS cohort study from the United States, the incidence of cryptococcal meningitis decreased from 5.0 to 1.5 cases per 1,000 person-years in the HAART era (Sacktor et al., 2001). Mirza et al. reported similar rates in the HAART era: 2 to 7 cases per 1,000 person-years (Mirza et al., 2003). A recent study from France demonstrated a 46% decline in the post-HAART compared to the pre-HAART era (Dromer et al., 2004).

Prior studies have emphasized the importance of *C. neoformans* as an AIDS-defining condition. In series from the pre-HAART era it was the first AIDS-related illness in 26 to 75% of patients (Chuck and Sande, 1989; Clark et al., 1990; Kovacs et al., 1985). In a study from the 1990s cryptococcosis was the initial AIDS-defining illness in 39% of patients from Atlanta and Houston (Mirza et al., 2003). Cases occurring in the United States today are mostly confined to patients either not receiving, or poorly adherent with, HAART (Mirza et al., 2003), with an estimated incidence of 5 to 10% per year (Adeyemi et al., 2004). Several studies have observed a high rate of cryptococcosis among African-Americans (Mirza et al., 2003; Hajjeh et al., 1999).

The incidence of invasive cryptococcal disease is much higher in the developing world, particularly in Southeast

Roger J. Bedimo, Infectious Diseases Section, VA North Texas Health Care System, Dallas, TX 75216, and Division of Infectious Diseases, The University of Texas Southwestern Medical Center at Dallas, Dallas, TX 75390-9113. **Daniel J. Skiest,** Division of Infectious Diseases, Baystate Medical Center, Springfield, MA 01199.

Asia and Africa. In sub-Saharan Africa, cryptococcosis affects 15 to 30% of patients with AIDS and is a major cause of morbidity and mortality, accounting for 44% of HIV-related deaths in one study (Corbett et al., 2002). Cryptococcal meningitis was the AIDS-defining illness in 84 and 88% of HIV patients in studies from South Africa and Zimbabwe, respectively, and accounted for 45% of all laboratory-proven cases of meningitis in adults at one institution (Heyderman et al., 1998; Moosa and Coovadia, 1997).

Microbiology

C. neoformans, the causative organism of cryptococcosis, has a worldwide distribution. The genus Cryptococcus includes approximately 37 species; C. neoformans is the only species of cryptococcus known to be pathogenic. The organism is classified into four distinct serotypes (A, B, C, and D), based on the immunologic properties of its capsular polysaccharides. However, the commonly used classification is according to phenotypical, genetical, biochemical, and epidemiological characteristics, which lead to the identification of three varieties within the species C. neoformans: C. neoformans var. grubii (serotype A), C. neoformans var. gattii (serotypes B and C), and C. neoformans var. neoformans (serotype D) (Callejas et al., 1998; Levitz, 1991). C. neoformans var. gattii is found most commonly in soil associated with eucalyptus trees (Chakrabarti et al., 1997) and decaying wood (Lazera et al., 1998). It causes infection mostly in immunocompetent hosts. The other two varieties are found in soil contaminated by pigeon droppings. They affect mostly immunocompromised hosts. Virtually all HIV-associated cryptococcal infections are caused by C. neoformans var. neoformans.

The organism is an encapsulated, spherical yeast, which varies in size—typically 5 to 10 μm in diameter. It reproduces by asexual narrow-based budding. A sexual stage has been observed in vitro, but the asexual stage is what has been observed in nature and in vivo. In most cases, the organism is surrounded by a polysaccharide capsule, which is an important virulence factor (see below).

In the laboratory, C. neoformans grows on most fungal media (Sabouraud agar) without cycloheximide, which can inhibit growth. Optimal growth occurs at 30 to 35°C, usually within 2 to 5 days. The colonies are smooth, white to tan colored, and several millimeters in diameter. The polysaccharide capsule causes the colonies to have a mucoid appearance with prolonged incubation. Identification is based on typical morphology and routine biochemical tests: C. neoformans converts phenolic compounds to melanin, which can be detected when incubated with niger seed extract media, and is usually positive on a rapid urease test.

Pathogenesis and Pathology

The route of infection is inhalation of the organism from environmental sources, e.g., soil. As noted above, bird guano often contains high levels of C. neoformans. However, although there have been cases of patients noted to have been exposed to birds or bird droppings, in most cases no specific bird exposure is noted. In immunocompetent hosts, following inhalation and deposition of the unencapsulated yeast form (basidiospores) in the alveoli, a granulomatous response ensues, resulting in pulmonary granuloma formation. This response, in most healthy hosts, is usually sufficient to prevent further disease, and thus, most pulmonary cases are asymptomatic and resolve spontaneously. In immunocompromised hosts, e.g., AIDS patients, dissemination to the CNS and other organs may occur. The timing of dissemination is uncertain, e.g., during primary lung infection, or months to years later during reactivation resulting from immune suppression. In either case, the site most likely to be involved in invasive cryptococcosis is the CNS.

C. neoformans, a facultative intracellular pathogen, is capable of invasion and replication inside macrophages. C. neoformans has evolved elaborate mechanisms to overcome or circumvent successive steps of the host innate and adaptive immune response. Following human infection, the fungus generates a large polysaccharide capsule, which is the most important virulence factor and allows the fungus to resist phagocytosis. Organisms lacking the polysaccharide capsule have been shown to be less virulent in animals (Chang and Kwon-Chung, 1994). The capsule is composed of mannoprotein, galactoxylomannan, and glucuronoxylomannan. The last is the primary component and the primary antigenic determinant of serotype specificity. The size of the capsule can be regulated by local environmental factors such as pH, temperature, osmolarity, carbon dioxide concentration, and concentration of glucose and iron (McFadden and Casadevall, 2001; Granger et al., 1985). Mannoprotein-4 desensitizes the host to cryptococcal infection by inhibiting neutrophil migration (Coenjaerts et al., 2001). In addition to resisting phagocytosis, the capsular polysaccharide has numerous other effects that promote pathogenicity including depletion of complement, dysregulation of cytokine secretion, interference with antigen presentation, loss of receptors for tumor necrosis factor alpha, and enhancement of HIV replication (reviewed by Perfect [2005]). The capsule may also play a role in producing brain edema. As noted below, detection of the capsular polysaccharide in body fluids allows for a useful diagnostic test.

Besides the capsular polysaccharide, other important virulence factors include the phenoloxidase enzyme system, mannitol, the alpha mating type, and the ability to grow at body temperature (37°C) (McFadden and Casadevall, 2001). The phenoloxidase enzyme system, which functions in the production of melanin, is thought to protect the yeast from several aspects of the host immune response. In vitro studies using amoeba models suggest that after phagocytosis, melanin production protects the fungus from macrophage-produced reactive oxygen and nitrogen intermediates, allowing survival from oxidative stress and replication within the phagocytic cells (Casadevall et al., 2000).

In animal models, immunity to cryptococcal infection, as in many chronic fungal infections, is associated with a granulomatous inflammatory response, intact cell-mediated immunity, and a Th1 pattern of cytokine release. A recent study by Siddiqui et al. highlighted the importance of Th1 response on the outcome of cryptococcal meningitis in HIV (Siddiqui et al., 2005). Th1 cytokine levels in the cerebrospinal fluid (CSF) (interleukin-6, gamma interferon [IFN-γ], tumor necrosis factor alpha, and interleukin-8) were significantly higher in survivors than in nonsurvivors. Th1 cytokines were also negatively correlated with baseline cryptococcal CFU, as well as positively with the rate of fall in CSF cryptococcal colony counts (Siddiqui et al., 2005).

A unique feature of cryptococcal meningitis is the frequent elevation of intracranial pressure (ICP), which is associated with significant morbidity and mortality. The pathogenesis of raised ICP in cryptococcal meningitis is still incompletely understood. Patients with raised ICP usually do not have evidence of obstructive hydrocephalus or mass lesions (Malessa et al., 1994). Encapsulated cryptococcal organisms may cause mechanical outflow obstruction by blocking CSF flow to the arachnoid villi. Alternatively, the polysaccharide capsule may increase the osmolarity of

CSF and interstitial fluid, promoting fluid accumulation or retention (Graybill et al., 2000). Brain edema may sometimes also occur and is likely due to capsular polysaccharide that interferes with the normal flow of interstitial fluid into the subarachnoid space, as was found in brains of experimentally infected mice (Goldman et al., 1995) and brains of HIV patients with cryptococcal meningitis (Lee and Casadevall, 1996; Lee et al., 1996).

Clinical Features

Cryptococcal meningitis affects primarily patients with severely depressed immune function; most have a CD4 cell count of <75 cells/μl at the time of diagnosis. In the HAART era, a low CD4 cell count remains the most important risk factor for invasive cryptococcal disease (Dromer et al., 2004; Mirza et al., 2003; Sacktor et al., 2001; Kaplan et al., 2000; Adeyemi et al., 2004). In general, cryptococcal meningoencephalitis in HIV patients differs from disease in non-HIV-infected persons by the relative paucity of the inflammatory response, evidenced by low CSF pleocytosis, and consequently large fungal burdens as well as few mass lesions (Powderly, 1993).

In the majority of patients, the clinical presentation is that of a subacute meningitis or meningoencephalitis with involvement of the brain and meninges (Chuck and Sande, 1989). On average, patients have been symptomatic for 2 to 4 weeks when the diagnosis is made. The most common symptoms are fever, headache, and malaise (Chuck and Sande, 1989; Clark et al., 1990; Kovacs et al., 1985). Other symptoms include confusion, lethargy, and memory loss (Chuck and Sande, 1989; Rozenbaum and Concalves, 1994). Seizures are uncommon (Chuck and Sande, 1989). Classic signs and symptoms of meningitis are usually absent: nausea and vomiting are present in less than one-half of patients, and neck stiffness is present in only one-fifth (Chuck and Sande, 1989; Kovacs et al., 1985; Cox and Perfect, 1997; Zuger et al., 1986). Since the presentation can be subtle, e.g., absence of fever, only mild headache, or mild confusion, a high index of suspicion is required. Occasionally a more abrupt presentation can occur.

On physical examination, meningismus is often absent (in over three-quarters of patients), and focal neurologic deficits, lethargy, obtundation, personality changes, or memory loss is found in fewer than one-fifth (Chuck and Sande, 1989; Kovacs et al., 1985; Cox and Perfect, 1997).

Patients with AIDS often have evidence of infection outside the CNS including blood (50 to 64%), lungs (20 to 30%), skin, and eyes (Clark et al., 1990; Kovacs et al., 1985). Less commonly, there is evidence of involvement of the mouth, bone marrow, liver and spleen, lymph nodes, mediastinum, pericardium, peritoneum, gastrointestinal tract, and genitourinary tract including the prostate (Clark et al., 1990; Kovacs et al., 1985; Zuger et al., 1996; Bonacini et al., 1990). Some studies have suggested that asymptomatic prostatic infection may play a role in relapse of systemic disease following treatment. Cutaneous lesions, which may occur in several forms, can provide an important clue to diagnosis. Most commonly the lesions are umbilicated and may resemble those seen in molluscum contagiosum; however, other types of lesions have been described.

Complications

Increased ICP and its consequences (including vision loss, hearing disturbance, and other cranial neuropathies) are by far the most significant complication of cryptococcal meningitis (discussed below). Other less frequently observed complications include hydrocephalus, dementia, and cerebrovascular infarction or transient neurologic deficits (Leite et al., 2004; Qureshi et al., 1997).

Ocular disease may frequently accompany the diagnosis of meningitis. In a series from Africa, 76% of HIV-infected patients with cryptococcosis had an abnormal eye exam. Papilledema, due to elevated ICP, is the most frequent ocular finding and was noted in 32.5% of patients in one series (Kestelyn et al., 1993). Other ophthalmologic complications include cranial nerve palsies (especially the sixth nerve), optic atrophy, optic nerve infarction, chorioretinitis with or without vitritis, and optic neuritis (Kestelyn et al., 1993; Crump et al., 1992; Rex et al., 1993; Johnston et al., 1992; Keane, 1993). *C. neoformans* may involve the optic nerve directly in some cases. Visual loss may be irreversible. Aggressive early treatment of raised ICP along with antifungal therapy may lead to reversal of visual loss in some cases.

Diagnosis

Cryptococcal meningitis should be considered in an AIDS patient with any of the following symptoms: confusion, fever, headache, or lethargy, particularly if the most recent CD4 cell count is <100 cells/μl. Microbiologic confirmation is required either via fungal culture or detection of the polysaccharide capsular antigen. CNS imaging should also be done to assess for hydrocephalus, brain edema, and focal lesions.

Imaging

Cranial imaging studies (head computed tomography [CT] and magnetic resonance imaging [MRI]) are most commonly normal (Chuck and Sande, 1989; Graybill et al., 2000). When abnormal, the most common finding on head CT or MRI is brain atrophy, which reflects underlying HIV infection of the brain, rather than cryptococcal infection. Other occasional findings include abscess, mass lesions, edema, infarction, white-matter lesions, and meningeal enhancement (Chuck and Sande, 1989; Clark et al., 1990; Graybill et al., 2000). Cryptococcomas, focal lesions caused by intracerebral granulomas, are a rare finding in the AIDS patient (Sanchez-Portocarrero and Perez-Cecilia, 1997; Dismukes, 1993). Thus, in the AIDS patient with cryptococcal meningitis and focal lesions, other more common causes of CNS mass lesions, such as CNS lymphoma or toxoplasmosis, should be considered (Sanchez-Portocarrero and Perez-Cecilia, 1997; Skiest, 2002).

CSF Analysis

Due to the severely immunosuppressed state of many AIDS patients with cryptococcal meningitis, the CSF findings are often unremarkable or only modestly abnormal, reflecting the inability of the patient to mount an adequate immune response. CSF profiles may be normal in 7 to 59% of patients (Clark et al., 1990; Heyderman et al., 1998; Moosa and Coovadia, 1997). Thus, even if CSF analysis (protein, glucose, and cell counts) is normal, the CSF cryptococcal antigen and fungal culture should be ordered for any patient for whom the diagnosis is suspected.

The typical picture is that of a CSF lymphocytic pleocytosis with mild elevation of CSF protein. CSF glucose may be normal, or there may be mild to moderate hypoglychorrhachia (Chuck and Sande, 1989; Kovacs et al., 1985). CSF opening pressure is elevated to more than 200 mm H_2O in about 25 to 69% of patients with cryptococcal meningitis (Chuck and Sande, 1989; Zuger et al., 1986). As is discussed in the following sections, increased intracranial pressure has great therapeutic and prognostic implications.

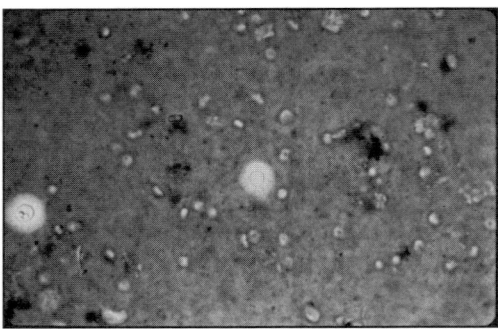

FIGURE 1 CSF India ink demonstrating large capsule. Slide courtesy of Paul M. Southern, The University of Texas Southwestern Medical Center at Dallas.

The India ink stain can be used to identify the yeast forms, but the sensitivity is only 74 to 88% and its interpretation requires a certain degree of expertise (Fig. 1) (Chuck and Sande, 1989; Clark et al., 1990; Kovacs et al., 1985). The "gold standard" in the diagnosis of cryptococcal meningitis is a positive CSF culture. As mentioned above the organism grows on routine fungal media.

Cryptococcal Antigen

Tests for cryptococcal polysaccharide antigen in CSF and blood have greatly aided in the diagnosis of cryptococcal infections. Antigen can be detected by latex agglutination or enzyme-linked immunoassay. The CSF cryptococcal antigen test (CRAG) has a sensitivity of 91 to 100% (Chuck

and Sande, 1989; Kovacs et al., 1985; Zuger et al., 1986). A titer of >1:8 is considered positive. False-positive results can occasionally be seen with titers of ≤1:8 and may be due to cross-reactivity to *Trichosporon beigelii* (McManus and Jones, 1985; Tanner et al., 1994). AIDS patients often have very high titers, which likely reflects the high fungal burden. High levels of CRAG have been associated with poor prognosis in AIDS patients.

The serum CRAG is also quite sensitive (range, 95 to 99%) (Chuck and Sande, 1989; Zuger et al., 1986; Saag et al., 2000) for invasive cryptococcal disease in AIDS including meningitis and is a good initial screening test in the patient with fever, headache, or other signs and symptoms suspicious of cryptococcal disease (Nelson et al., 1990). However, if clinical suspicion of meningitis is high, CSF analysis with fungal cultures should be performed even in the absence of a positive serum cryptococcal antigen.

CRAG positivity may precede disseminated disease in some patients (Manfredi et al., 1996). Whether routine serum CRAG screening is useful to detect cryptococcal disease in high-risk patients is controversial. While measurement of CRAG in CSF and serum is very useful diagnostically and in assessing prognosis, levels of serum CRAG have not been shown to be very useful in assessing response to therapy or in estimating likelihood of relapse. Serial CSF measurements have been somewhat more helpful (Clark et al., 1990; Powderly et al., 1994).

Antifungal Therapy

Antifungal therapy for cryptococcal meningitis significantly reduces morbidity and mortality. Therapy is generally administered in three phases: the induction phase

TABLE 1 Antifungal therapy for cryptococcal meningitis

Therapy	Duration	Comments
Induction therapy		
Amphotericin B deoxycholate 0.7–1.0 mg/kg/day + flucytosine (25 mg/kg every 6 h orally)	14 days	No mortality benefit from the addition of flucytosine to amphotericin B, but marginally associated with higher rate of CSF sterilization compared to amphotericin B alone
Amphotericin B deoxycholate (0.7–1.0 mg/kg/day)	14 days	
Liposomal amphotericin B (3–4 mg/kg/day)	14 days	Appears to be as efficacious as amphotericin B deoxycholate, but less toxic; however, experience is limited
Alternative induction therapy		
Fluconazole (400–800 mg/day)	10 weeks	Should be reserved for less severe disease. Associated with longer time to CSF sterilization than with amphotericin B
Fluconazole (400–800 mg/day) + flucytosine (25 mg/kg every 6 h)	6 weeks	Should be reserved for less severe disease. Associated with longer time to CSF sterilization than with amphotericin B
Consolidation therapy		
Fluconazole (400 mg per day)	8 weeks	
Itraconazole (200 mg twice per day)	8 weeks	In the largest published study itraconazole was associated with lower CSF sterilization rates than fluconazole, but clinical outcomes did not differ.
Maintenance therapy		
Fluconazole (200 mg per day orally)	Indefinite[a]	
Itraconazole (200 mg per day)	Indefinite[a]	Appears to be less efficacious than fluconazole, is less well tolerated, and has more drug interactions and unreliable oral bioavailability
Amphotericin B deoxycholate (1 mg/kg intravenously weekly)	Indefinite[a]	Associated with higher relapse rates

[a]May consider stopping maintenance therapy if patient remains asymptomatic and maintains CD4 cell count of >100 to 200 cells/μl in response to HAART. Restart maintenance if CD4 count subsequently declines.

(generally administered over 2 weeks), the consolidation phase (generally lasting 8 weeks), and the maintenance phase (indefinite unless significant immune reconstitution occurs) (Table 1).

Induction Therapy

Amphotericin B remains the mainstay of initial treatment of cryptococcal meningitis, based on cumulative experience and prospective studies. Most experts consider optimal initial therapy to be intravenous amphotericin B deoxycholate (0.7 to 1 mg/kg of body weight/day) plus oral flucytosine (100 mg/kg/day [divided into four doses per day]) for 2 weeks followed by consolidation and maintenance therapy with fluconazole. In a large multicenter trial addition of flucytosine (100 mg/kg/day) was found to have a marginal benefit in the rate of CSF sterilization at 14 days (51 versus 60%; $P = 0.06$) (Haubrich et al., 1994). However, the clinical outcome was not improved by the addition of flucytosine in this or prior studies (Chuck and Sande, 1989). A more recent study from Thailand found greater fungicidal activity with amphotericin B plus flucytosine than with amphotericin B alone (Brouwer et al., 2004). Flucytosine may result in leukopenia and thrombocytopenia, and levels should be monitored. Serum levels should be obtained 2 h after the dose is administered. Therapeutic levels are 30 to 80 µg/ml (Saag et al., 2000). For patients experiencing flucytosine toxicity, amphotericin

B should be used alone. Lower doses of amphotericin B deoxycholate (less than 0.7 mg/kg per day)—which were used in older studies—were associated with higher mortality and should not be used (Saag et al., 1992).

Liposomal amphotericin B (3 to 4 mg/kg/day) has been used successfully for induction and consolidation therapy. Efficacy appeared to be equivalent to conventional amphotericin B, and toxicity was lower. However, the number of patients studied to date is low (Coker et al., 1993; Leenders et al., 1997). Some authorities recommend performing a repeat spinal tap following the 2-week induction period to document sterilization of the CSF, which is an important prognostic factor (Fig. 2).

Fluconazole in Initial Therapy

Fluconazole is an attractive agent for use in cryptococcal meningitis. The drug has good in vitro activity, achieves good levels in the CSF, and is well tolerated. However, it is fungistatic rather than fungicidal. Several retrospective and prospective studies conducted in the 1990s suggested a role for fluconazole (400 to 800 mg per day) with or without flucytosine in the treament of cryptococcal meningitis. A small study found amphotericin B to be superior to fluconazole (Larsen et al., 1990). Subsequent studies found no significant difference in overall mortality due to cryptococcosis between patients treated with amphotericin and those treated with oral fluconazole (14 versus 18%; $P = 0.48$); but

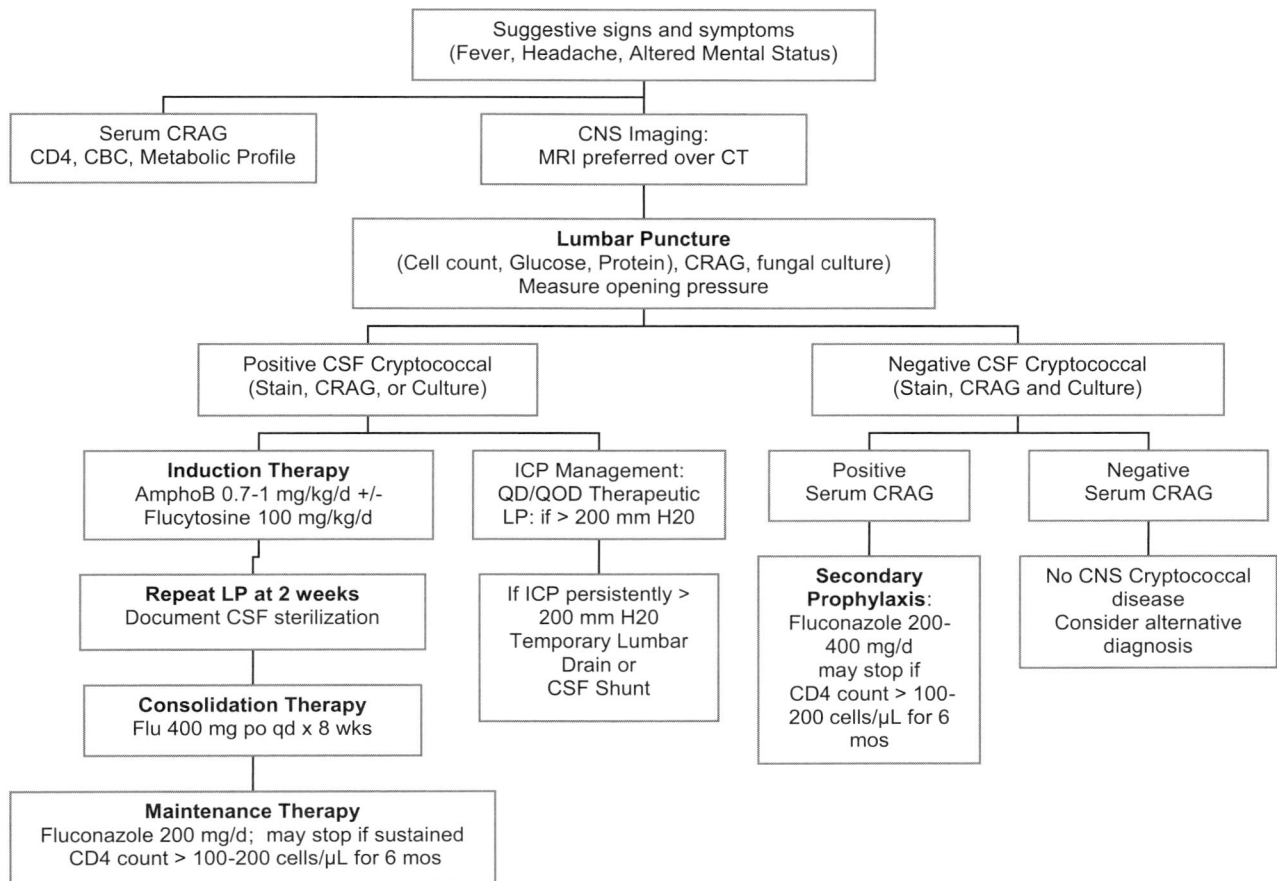

FIGURE 2 Algorithm for the diagnosis and management of cryptococcal meningitis in HIV.

fluconazole therapy was associated with a nonsignificantly longer time to CSF sterilization (45 versus 64 days) compared to amphotericin B (Saag et al., 1992). Fluconazole may be a reasonable option for patients with mild to moderate disease B (Saag et al., 1992; Haubrich et al., 1994). Fluconazole (400 to 800 mg/day) was also found to be effective when combined with flucytosine, but myelotoxicity and gastrointestinal side effects of this regimen are relatively high (Larsen et al., 1994).

Consolidation and Maintenance Therapy

Successful induction therapy with amphotericin B (with or without flucytosine) should be followed by consolidation therapy with fluconazole (400 mg/day) for 8 weeks and then chronic suppressive therapy (secondary prophylaxis or maintenance therapy) with fluconazole at 200 mg/day thereafter to prevent relapses. Several studies demonstrated the efficacy of this approach for the prevention of recurrent cryptococcal disease in AIDS patients (Bozzette et al., 1991; Powderly et al., 1992; Sugar and Saunders, 1988). Suppressive therapy should be for life unless the patient experiences significant immune recovery (see below).

Alternative maintenance/suppressive regimens for patients who cannot take fluconazole include weekly amphotericin B (1 mg/kg) or itraconazole (200 to 400 mg per day). Itraconazole is active in vitro against *C. neoformans*; however, unlike fluconazole, it has poor penetration of the blood-brain barrier and achieves low concentrations in the CSF. A prospective randomized, double-blinded trial demonstrated the superiority of fluconazole over itraconazole for prevention of cryptococcal meningitis relapse: relapse rate was 4% for fluconazole recipients compared to 23% for itraconazole recipients (Saag et al., 1999). Another study demonstrated a higher rate of CSF sterilization with fluconazole than with itraconazole (van der Horst et al., 1997). Similarly fluconazole was superior to intermittent amphotericin B (1 mg/kg per week) in preventing recurrent cryptococcal disease (Powderly et al., 1992). Thus, fluconazole remains the treatment of choice for consolidation and maintenance therapy.

Resistance

In vitro resistance to amphotericin B or fluconazole is rare but has been reported (Datta et al., 2003; Sar et al., 2004). Individual cases of azole resistance in patients failing therapy have also been reported (Alves et al., 1997; Armengou et al., 1996; Friese et al., 2001; Paugam et al., 1994). However, the correlation of in vitro susceptibility testing with clinical outcomes has not been well established. Thus, it is not clear what percentage of patients who fail fluconazole therapy clinically do so due to true in vitro resistance rather than because of poor host response.

New Antifungal Agents

Although current regimens are associated with lower mortality rates than those of earlier ones, which used relatively low doses of amphotericin B, newer agents are needed for those patients refractory to, or intolerant of, amphotericin B products. Voriconazole and posaconazole are newer azoles with good in vitro activity against *Cryptococcus*; however, clinical data are limited (Pfaller et al., 2004). The echinocandins, including caspofungin, do not have reliable activity against *Cryptococcus* spp. in vitro (Espinel-Ingroff, 1998; Verduyn Lunel and Rijs, 1997).

Adjuvant Therapy

IFN-γ

As noted above, the Th-1 cytokine response is important in the immune control of cryptococcal disease. Pappas et al. evaluated the safety and antifungal activity of adjuvant recombinant IFN-γ1b (rIFN-γ1b) in the treatment of acute cryptococcal meningitis in HIV (Pappas et al., 2004). Compared to patients receiving only amphotericin B (with or without flucytosine), addition of 100 or 200 mg of rIFN-γ1b thrice weekly was associated with a significantly higher rate of CNS sterilization at 2 weeks. Two-week culture conversion occurred in 13% of recipients of amphotericin with or without flucytosine, compared to 36 and 32% of recipients of 100 and 200 μg of adjuvant rIFN-γ1b, respectively. There was also a trend toward improved combined mycologic and clinical success in rIFN-γ1b recipients (26 versus 8%; $P = 0.078$). If further studies of this approach demonstrate a benefit of IFN-γ, it may be a useful addition to consider, particularly for patients with a poor prognosis.

Monoclonal Antibodies

Adjunctive passive immunotherapy with a monoclonal antibody directed against the capsular polysaccharide of *C. neoformans* was recently evaluated in successfully treated cryptococcal meningitis in HIV patients (Larsen et al., 2005). Administration of a single dose of monoclonal antibody was associated with a significant—up to threefold by week 3—but transient decline in serum cryptococcal antigen titers. Further studies of this therapy are warranted.

Discontinuation of Maintenance Therapy

As with other opportunistic infections, it appears that patients who have successfully completed a course of initial therapy for cryptococcosis remain free of clinical manifestations of the disease and have a sustained increase (≤6 months) in their CD4 cell counts to >100 to 200 cells/μl following HAART can safely discontinue maintenance therapy (U.S. Public Health Service/Infectious Diseases Society of America, 2001; Martinez et al., 2000; Vibhagool et al., 2003; Aberg et al., 2002). Some experts recommend performing a lumbar puncture to determine if the CSF is culture negative before stopping therapy even if patients have been asymptomatic; other experts do not believe this is necessary. However, it is important to restart secondary prophylaxis (e.g., fluconazole) if the CD4 count decreases to less than 100 cells/μl.

Management of Raised ICP

Several studies have demonstrated that ICP is common (affecting up to three-quarters of patients) in cryptococcal meningitis in AIDS (Chuck and Sande, 1989; Graybill et al., 2000; van der Horst et al., 1997; Saag et al., 1992; Denning et al., 1991). Failure to manage high ICP (as measured by elevated CSF opening pressure) appropriately is associated with neurologic complications including hearing loss, cranial neuropathies, visual disturbances, altered mentation, severe headache, papilledema, and retinal vein distention (Malessa et al., 1994; Graybill et al., 2000; Johnston et al., 1992; Keane, 1993; Denning et al., 1991; Shoham et al., 2005; Sun et al., 2004). Patients with raised ICP usually do not have evidence of obstructive hydrocephalus or mass lesions. Thus, following a head CT or MRI to rule out a mass lesion, measurement of CSF opening pressure should be performed for all patients with known or suspected cryptococcal meningitis. Since raised ICP may develop during treatment, some clinicians repeat measurement of opening pressure following induction therapy. In a study by Van der Horst et al., almost all (13 of 14) of the early deaths (defined as death within the first 2 weeks of therapy) and 40% of the deaths during weeks 3 to 10 were associated with elevated ICP (van der Horst et al., 1997).

Optimal treatment of elevated ICP has not been defined, but most authorities recommend repeated large-volume lumbar punctures. This may need to be done daily or every other day until the opening pressure is normal (<200 mm H_2O) or at 50% of the initial opening pressure and the patient is without symptoms (Graybill et al., 2000; Saag et al., 2000; Sun et al., 2004). If repeated lumbar punctures are not successful, a temporary lumbar drain or ventricular drain can be placed (Fessler et al., 1998). For patients with refractory elevated ICP or hydrocephalus despite appropriate antifungal therapy, CSF shunting should be considered (Graybill et al., 2000; Saag et al., 2000; Park et al., 1999).

The value of pharmacologic control of raised ICP with diuretics (such as acetazolamide or mannitol) or corticosteroids is uncertain. In one retrospective study corticosteroid use was associated with higher early mortality (Graybill et al., 2000). A study from Thailand showed that acetazolamide use did not improve the outcome of patients with acute CNS cryptococcosis and raised ICP (Newton et al., 2002). Based on the available data, we do not recommend use of these medications to treat high ICP.

IRIS

Numerous series have demonstrated a high rate of the immune reconstitution inflammatory syndrome (IRIS) in AIDS patients with cryptococcosis. Recent series found that the incidence of IRIS in patients with cryptococcal meningitis started on HAART was 10 to 33% (Lortholary et al., 2005; Shelburne et al., 2005a, 2005b). Although several syndromes have been described including recurrent meningitis, pneumonitis, lung nodules, lymphadenitis, abscesses, and cryptococcomas (Boelaert et al., 2004; Cattelan et al., 2004; Lanzafame et al., 1992; Rambeloarisoa et al., 2002), two presentations of IRIS predominate: CNS disease and lymphadenitis (Skiest et al., 2005). Typically the syndrome manifests in a previously highly immunosuppressed individual with an opportunistic infection (e.g., cryptococcosis) that is either previously diagnosed and partially treated or is occult at the time of HAART initiation and who sustains robust virologic and immunologic responses to therapy. Patients may have headaches and other CNS symptoms and/or exuberant lymphadenopathy at any location, most commonly mediastinal, cervical, or supraclavicular (Skiest et al., 2005). The time course for development of cryptococcal IRIS is variable. It has been reported to occur from a few days to 3 years after starting HAART (Lortholary et al., 2005; Shelburne et al., 2005a, 2005b; Skiest et al., 2005). CSF and other fluids or tissues may stain positive for yeast forms, but cultures are negative, indicating adequate control of the infection. CSF studies may reflect the enhanced inflammatory response with elevated protein and cell counts. Factors associated with a higher likelihood of a cryptococcal-infection-related IRIS include new HIV diagnosis, very low CD4 cell count, cryptococcemia, and HAART initiation within 1 to 2 months of cryptococcal diagnosis (Lortholary et al., 2005; Shelburne et al., 2005a, 2005b).

Management of cryptococcal IRIS usually consists of symptom control. In most cases HAART can be continued.

Some have advocated short courses of corticosteroids or nonsteroidal anti-inflammatory medications. However, the efficacy of these medications has not been proven. To prevent its occurrence, some experts recommend a delay between initiation of therapy for the opportunistic infection and that of HAART (>1 month for cryptococcal meningitis) (Shelburne et al., 2005a, 2005b). The efficacy of this strategy in reducing the incidence of the syndrome has not been conclusively proven, as no randomized studies have been conducted. Furthermore, the high morbidity associated with cryptococcal meningitis could potentially be lessened by early initiation of antiretroviral therapy, and there appears to be no increased mortality associated with the development of the immune reconstitution syndrome (Shelburne et al., 2005a, 2005b).

Prognosis

Untreated, cryptococcal meningitis is a fatal infection in patients with AIDS. Even with treatment, patients with a large fungal burden and poor host response may have poor outcomes. In U.S. studies conducted in the 1990s early mortality has been estimated at 6 to 15%, with 10 to 30% of patients dying before 10 weeks (van der Horst et al., 1997; Saag et al., 1992; Robinson et al., 1999). Mortality appears to be significantly higher in patients living in sub-Saharan Africa (Heyderman et al., 1998; Moosa and Coovadia, 1997).

Pretreatment factors independently associated with adverse early outcome include abnormal mental status (lethargy or obtundation); high CSF cryptococcal antigen titer (>1:1024); low CSF pleocytosis (CSF white blood cell count, <20/μl); hyponatremia; high opening pressure; positive CSF India ink stain; and positive cryptococcal blood culture or presence of extraneural sites of infection (Chuck and Sande, 1989; Clark et al., 1990; Zuger et al., 1986; Saag et al., 1992; Robinson et al., 1999) (Table 2). These factors have not been predictive of outcome in studies of patients from sub-Saharan Africa, however (Heyderman et al., 1998; Moosa and Coovadia, 1997). During antifungal therapy, the following have been identified as adverse prognostic indicators: cerebral edema, delayed CSF sterilization (defined as positive CSF culture at 2 weeks), failure to lower ICP, and concomitant cryptococcemia (Graybill et al., 2000; Saag et al., 2000; van der Horst et al., 1997; Shoham et al., 2005; Robinson et al., 1999; Pasqualotto et al., 2004).

Prevention

C. neoformans is found in the environment; thus, most patients are exposed to the fungus routinely and efforts to avoid exposure are not practical. Although pigeon droppings are known to concentrate cryptococcal organisms, there is no evidence that avoidance of contact with pigeon droppings is associated with a decreased risk for acquiring cryptococcosis.

TABLE 2 Prognostic factors associated with poor outcomes in cryptococcal meningitis

CSF CRAG, >1:1024
Altered mental status
CSF white blood cell count of <20 cells/μl
Extraneural site of infection (including positive blood culture)
High CSF opening pressure
Hyponatremia
Positive CSF India ink examination

Primary Prophylaxis of Cryptococcal Meningitis

Fluconazole and to a lesser extent itraconazole have been used effectively to prevent cryptococcal disease in high-risk patients. In the largest trial, the AIDS Clinical Trials Group conducted a prospective, randomized study of fluconazole (200 mg per day) versus clotrimazole troches for AIDS patients at risk for invasive fungal infections. Fluconazole was effective in reducing the number of patients diagnosed with invasive fungal infections, primarily cryptococcal disease (Powderly et al., 1995). Other studies have used doses of fluconazole ranging from 100 to 200 mg per day to 100 to 400 mg per week (Powderly et al., 1995; Manfredi et al., 1997; Chetchotisakd et al., 2004; Nightingale et al., 1992; McKinsey et al., 1999; Newton et al., 1995; Quagliarello et al., 1995; Singh et al., 1996a, 1996b). Itraconazole has also been shown to be effective for prevention of cryptococcal disease (McKinsey et al., 1999). The Mycoses Study Group conducted a prospective, randomized double-blind trial of itraconazole capsules versus placebo in patients with CD4 cell counts of <150 cells/μl. Receipt of itraconazole was associated with a statistically significant lower rate of cryptococcal disease (as well as histoplasmosis) than that seen with receipt of a placebo.

However, with the exception of a relatively small study from Thailand, no primary prophylaxis studies conducted to date have demonstrated an overall survival benefit. In the study that did demonstrate a survival benefit, the benefit was not due to a decreased rate of cryptococcal meningitis (Chetchotisakd et al., 2004). Due to the lack of survival benefit, concerns that ongoing fluconazole prophylaxis may result in fluconazole-resistant mucosal candidal infections, the relative infrequency of invasive cryptococcal disease, and the potential for CYP3A-mediated drug interactions, there has not been widespread enthusiasm for routine fluconazole prophylaxis and it is not routinely recommended by most experts (U.S. Public Health Service/Infectious Diseases Society of America, 2001). However, given the fact that the cost of fluconazole has recently decreased significantly and the fact that the frequency of resistant mucosal candidiasis appears to have diminished in the HAART era, consideration could be given to primary fluconazole prophylaxis for patients in whom the CD4 cell count is currently, and is expected to remain, <50 to 100 cells/μl (e.g., patients not on HAART or failing HAART), especially if the patient resides in a region of the world with high rates of cryptococcal disease and/or is at risk for additional invasive fungal infections such as candidiasis, histoplasmosis, or coccidioidomycosis.

OTHER FUNGAL INFECTIONS

Aspergillosis

CNS aspergillosis is a rare infection in patients with HIV. It is not clear whether HIV is an independent risk factor for invasive aspergillosis, since many patients concomitantly have other, well-established risk factors such as neutropenia, receipt of broad-spectrum antibiotics, and corticosteroid use (Denning, 1998; Holding et al., 2000; Minamoto et al., 1992; Pursell et al., 1992). Most cases occur in patients with low CD4 cell counts (<100 cells/μl) and/or a prior opportunistic infection (Holding et al., 2000; Pursell et al., 1992; Lortholary et al., 1993; Mylonakis et al., 2000). Injecting drug use may also be a risk factor for CNS aspergillosis (Minamoto et al., 1992). Infection with *Aspergillus fumigatus* is most common, but *Aspergillus flavus* and other species have been reported (Minamoto et al., 1992; Mylonakis et al., 2000; Tumbarello et al., 1997; Woods and Goldsmith, 1990).

The CNS is involved in ~10 to 30% of cases of invasive aspergillosis, making it the second or third most common site after the lungs and paranasal sinuses (Holding et al., 2000; Lortholary et al., 1993; Mylonakis et al., 2000). Involvement of the CNS can occur via bloodstream dissemination or direct extension from the paranasal sinuses. In one-fourth to one-third of cases in which the CNS is involved, it is the only site involved, while there is evidence of disseminated disease with multiorgan involvement in the remainder (Minamoto et al., 1992; Mylonakis et al., 2000; Woods and Goldsmith, 1990).

The clinical picture is most commonly that of a cerebral mass lesion. Occasionally patients present with the picture of a chronic meningitis, usually with subtle nonspecific signs and symptoms. The fungus has an affinity for blood vessels, which it readily invades. Thus, patients may present with signs and symptoms of an ischemic stroke. Involvement of the spinal cord has rarely been reported (Woods and Goldsmith, 1990). The most common presenting features are headache, altered mental status, and focal neurologic deficits including cranial nerves, and paresthesias (Mylonakis et al., 2000; Horgan and Powderly, 1997). Patients may have evidence of infection elsewhere, especially the lung and paranasal sinuses. CT or MRI scans may show one or more multiple hypodense lesions, which may enhance with contrast (Mylonakis et al., 2000). CSF is usually abnormal but is nonspecific, and aspergillus is rarely grown from CSF (Denning, 1998; Mylonakis et al., 2000). Definitive diagnosis requires a biopsy specimen showing evidence of branching septate hyphal elements, usually invading adjacent blood vessels, with a positive fungal culture. A presumptive diagnosis can be made if tissue obtained from extra-CNS sites, e.g., lung or sinuses, is positive for aspergillus. The recently licensed *Aspergillus* galactomannan assay may be useful for diagnosis of CNS *Aspergillus* infection. The test can be run on CSF as well as serum, although experience is limited (Klont et al., 2004).

The prognosis of HIV-infected patients with aspergillosis is very poor (Lortholary et al., 1993; Mylonakis et al., 2000; Tumbarello et al., 1997; Denning, 1996). In a review of published series the 3-month crude mortality rates of pulmonary, sinus, and cerebral aspergillosis were estimated at 86, 66, and 99%, respectively (Denning, 1996). In a recent study, median survival time after diagnosis of invasive aspergillosis (including CNS and extracranial sites) was 3 months; only 26% survived for 1 year (Holding et al., 2000). This is in part because the disease frequently goes unrecognized, with more than one-half of the cases diagnosed at autopsy (Mylonakis et al., 2000; Tumbarello et al., 1997; Khoo and Denning, 1994).

The poor response to treatment may partially reflect the low efficacy of conventional treatment. Until recently the treatment of choice was amphotericin B deoxycholate, with response rates reported to be <10% (Lortholary et al., 1993; Horgan and Powderly, 1997). Amphotericin B lipid preparations are now preferred over amphotericin B deoxycholate, because larger doses can be administered with less toxicity. Traditional second-line therapy is itraconazole, although lack of good CNS penetration has been a limitation. Voriconazole, a new azole, and caspofungin, an echinocandin, with good activity against aspergillus have recently been approved for aspergillus infections in immunosuppressed patients. Although experience with voriconazole in AIDS patients is limited, it should be considered in place of liposomal amphotericin or in the case of a patient failing liposomal amphotericin. As with other azoles, which inhibit cytochrome P450, drug interactions especially with antiretrovirals are potentially problematic. Caspofungin is another consideration for treatment of CNS aspergillosis in AIDS; however, data are very limited, and thus, at this time its use cannot be recommended. Data on combination antifungal therapy are also limited, but it should be considered for patients not responding to single-agent therapy. Surgical debridement should be considered in selected cases.

Zygomycosis

Infections with the zygomycetes have rarely been reported in HIV-positive patients. Most reported cases have occurred in patients with low CD4 cell counts. The usual predisposing conditions may not be present, although transient neutropenia may be present (Nagy-Agren et al., 1995). Intravenous drug use is the risk factor for HIV infection in most affected patients, and it is the likely portal of entry for the zygomycotic infection (Nagy-Agren et al., 1995; Van den Saffele and Boelaert, 1996).

The clinical course depends in large part on the predominant site of involvement and can be chronic and indolent or acute and fulminant, leading to rapid demise of the patient. The basal ganglia is the most common site of CNS involvement (Hopkins et al., 1994). Brain biopsy is usually needed for diagnosis. Both systemic antifungal therapy with high-dose amphotericin B ($\geq$1 mg/kg/day) or lipid amphotericin B ($\geq$5 mg/kg/day) and aggressive surgical debridement are essential for a successful outcome. However, even with aggressive treatment, mortality is high and is associated with sites of disease inaccessible to surgical debridement (Nagy-Agren et al., 1995).

Coccidioidomycosis

Coccidioidomycosis is endemic in the southwestern United States, northern Mexico, and other Sonoran desert regions. Among HIV-infected patients, its incidence has been estimated from 4% to as high as 25% in areas of endemicity (Ampel et al., 1993; Bronnimann et al., 1987). Woods et al. estimated the incidence of the disease in Arizona at 41 of 1,000 persons living with AIDS between 1995 and 1997 (Woods et al., 2000). Similar to other opportunistic infections, the incidence of coccidioidomycosis in the HAART era is declining (Woods et al., 2000).

The inhaled arthroconidia of C. immitis mature to form large (30- to 80-μm-diameter) spherules, each in turn releasing hundreds of endospores. Neutrophils are prominent in the lesions of coccidioidomycosis. Arthroconidia resist phagocytosis through their antiphagocytic surface, and only 20 to 30% of the ingested arthroconidia or endospores are killed. T-cell lymphokines are necessary to stimulate phagolysosomal fusion, and therefore fungal killing. Thus, AIDS patients with depressed cell-mediated immunity are at increased risk for invasive disease (Drutz and Huppert, 1983). Clinically apparent disease in HIV may be from either newly acquired infection or reactivation (Ampel, 2001). Among HIV-infected patients, the most important factor associated with the risk of developing clinically active coccidioidomycosis is a CD4 count of <250/μl (Ampel et al., 1993; Fish et al., 1990).

The clinical spectrum of coccidioidomycosis in HIV is wide. The most common manifestation is pulmonary disease followed by disseminated disease (most commonly meningeal, skin, lymph node, liver, and rarely bone joint) (Bronnimann et al., 1987; Fish et al., 1990; Singh et al., 1996b). In one series the CNS was the primary clinical manifestation of disease in 12% of HIV-infected patients (Fish et al., 1990). Patients with meningitis may have isolated CNS disease or concomitant pulmonary disease. The typical presentation is that of chronic meningitis, e.g., fever, headache, and confusion. CSF reveals lymphocytic pleocytosis (>50 cells/μl) and high protein levels. Hypoglycorrhachia may be present. Eosinophilic pleocytosis is sometimes present. Hydrocephalus may be a complication. Diagnosis is made by either a positive CSF complement fixation titer, positive serum complement fixation titer, or less commonly positive immunoglobulin M antibodies measured by immunodiffusion, or positive CSF fungal culture.

First-line therapy for disseminated C. immitis infection is with fluconazole or itraconazole (Deresinski, 2001; Stevens, 1995). Fluconazole (400 to 800 mg per day) is preferred over itraconazole for meningitis based on its good CNS penetration and more experience in the literature. Itraconazole (200 to 400 mg twice a day) has also been used successfully. Intravenous amphotericin B is not effective for CNS disease but can be given intrathecally for patients not responding to azole therapy. It is currently recommended that antifungal therapy for coccidioidomycosis in HIV infection be continued indefinitely due to the high rate of relapse (Ampel, 2004; Dewsnup et al., 1996; Galgiani et al., 2000).

Histoplasmosis

In areas of endemicity, 5 to 20% of HIV-infected persons develop disseminated histoplasmosis (Gutierrez et al., 2005; Wheat et al., 1990; Wheat and Kauffman, 2003). However, CNS disease is rare. In a recent study of 104 patients with histoplasmosis none was diagnosed with CNS disease (Gutierrez et al., 2005). CNS histoplasmosis in HIV often occurs in the setting of disseminated histoplasmosis, often as a relapse of previously treated disease, although isolated CNS disease has been described (Wheat and Kauffman, 2003; Saccente et al., 2003; Anaissie et al., 1988; Wheat et al., 2005). Most patients are profoundly immunosuppressed, with CD4 counts below 100 cells/μl (Wheat and Kauffman, 2003; Anaissie et al., 1988). The clinical features may include meningitis or one or more brain abscesses. Diagnosis is difficult for patients with isolated CNS histoplasmosis; the sensitivity and specificity of commonly used diagnostic tests are poor. The histoplasma antigen test may be elevated in the CSF, although a negative result does not rule out active CNS disease (Wheat et al., 2005). Positive results often require multiple specimens for testing including serum and CSF culture, antibody, antigen, and in some cases meninges or brain tissue (Wheat et al., 2005). Mortality is high despite appropriate antifungal therapy (Anaissie et al., 1988).

The optimal treatment for CNS histoplasmosis is unknown. Experts recommend the use of liposomal amphotericin B (3 to 5 mg/kg/day for 6 to 12 weeks), because it achieves higher concentrations in brain tissue than does the standard deoxycholate formulation and was a more effective treatment of non-CNS disseminated histoplasmosis in patients with AIDS (Wheat et al., 2005; Johnson et al., 2002). Following initial treatment with amphotericin, fluconazole (600 to 800 mg/day) or itraconazole (200 mg twice or three times daily) should be administered indefinitely. For patients who have completed 1 year of therapy and have experienced a good response to HAART (CD4 counts of >150 cells/μl) and with no evidence of ongoing disease, maintenance therapy may be stopped cautiously (Goldman et al., 2004).

Blastomycosis

Unlike other endemic fungal infections, AIDS does not appear to be a major risk factor for blastomycosis, as few cases have been reported (Bradsher, 1996); however, in AIDS patients with blastomycosis CNS involvement is common (40 to 46% of patients). Most patients have a CD4 cell count of <200 cells/μl (Pappas et al., 1992; Witzig et al., 1994). When CNS disease occurs, it is usually in the setting of disseminated blastomycosis (Pappas et al., 1992; Witzig et al., 1994). CNS disease may manifest as basilar meningitis or a brain mass/abscess. Diagnosis is made by culture of CSF or brain tissue or histopathology. The sensitivity of serologic testing for *B. dermatitidis* in HIV is low (Bradsher, 1996; Pappas et al., 1992).

Mortality for blastomycosis appears to be significantly higher in HIV-infected than in HIV-negative patients. In a series from the pre-HAART era 6 of 15 patients died less than 3 weeks after presentation (Pappas et al., 1992). Treatment for CNS blastomycosis is amphotericin B (0.7 to 1.0 mg/kg/day for a total dose of 1.5 to 2.5 g). Lipid amphotericin formulations are associated with lower toxicity and can be substituted for conventional amphotericin B. Amphotericin should be followed by long-term maintenance therapy with fluconazole (800 mg per day).

Paracoccidioidomycosis

P. brasiliensis is a dimorphic fungus found in Central and South America. In immunocompetent hosts, it causes acute pulmonary infections and cutaneous and/or mucosal lesions, as well as disseminated disease. Benard and Duarte reviewed clinical features of 75 published cases of paracoccidioidomycosis in HIV. HIV patients present with uncontrolled infection with lymphohematogenous dissemination, similar to the severe, acute form seen in immunocompetent patients (Benard and Duarte, 2000). Infection in HIV patients probably results from reactivated latent foci that in nonimmunocompromised hosts lead to the less severe chronic form, characterized by mucosal lesions. The CNS was involved in 14% of cases in a recent series (de Almeida et al., 2004). Two clinical presentations of CNS paracoccidioidomycosis can occur: mass lesions in the brain parenchyma (most cases) and meningitis (de Almeida et al., 2004; Elias et al., 2005). The most common finding on CT or MRI is a low-density lesion with ring enhancement. In most cases, diagnosis is made by identification of the organism from biologic specimens. The value of serologic diagnosis is controversial (Hamilton, 1998). Optimal treatment is not well established. Itraconazole is probably the drug of choice but co-trimoxazole has also been suggested (de Almeida et al., 2004; Elias et al., 2005).

Candidiasis

While mucosal and esophageal *Candida* infection is very common in HIV-infected patients, *Candida* infection of the CNS is rare. Two syndromes have been described: meningitis and parenchymal brain lesions in the form of microabscesses (Bruinsma-Adams, 1991; Casado et al., 1997; Ehni and Ellison, 1987; Levy et al., 1985; Sanchez-Portocarrero et al., 2000). Most HIV-infected patients with candida infection of the CNS have other known risk factors for disseminated candidiasis including intravenous drug use (Casado et al., 1997).

The most frequent symptoms are headache, fever, nuchal rigidity, and confusion, but an indolent course is also possible (Casado et al., 1997; Voice et al., 1994). The CSF usually shows a pleocytosis predominated by neutrophils and mononuclear cells, an elevated protein concentration, and a normal or low glucose concentration (Casado et al., 1997). CSF cultures were positive in 79% of patients with candida meningitis in one series (Casado et al., 1997), but large volumes may need to be cultured. Detection of the candida cell wall component, mannan, in CSF has recently been shown to be helpful in the diagnosis of candidal meningitis in non-AIDS patients, but experience is limited (Verduyn Lunel et al., 2004).

Candidal meningitis is associated with high morbidity and mortality in adults, estimated at 30 to 50% in small series (Casado et al., 1997; Voice et al., 1994). Treatment is not well standardized. Experts recommend amphotericin B and flucytosine followed by fluconazole. The duration of maintenance therapy with fluconazole is not well defined, however.

REFERENCES

Aberg, J., R. Price, D. Heeren, and B. Bredt. 2002. A pilot study of the discontinuation of antifungal therapy for disseminated cryptococcal disease in patients with acquired immunodeficiency syndrome, following immunologic response to antiretroviral therapy. *J. Infect. Dis.* **185**:1179–1182.

Adeyemi, O., J. Pulvirenti, S. Perumal, U. Mupiddi, B. Kohl, and T. Jezisek. 2004. Cryptococcosis in HIV-infected individuals. *AIDS* **18**:2218–2219.

Alves, S., J. Lopes, J. Costa, and C. Klock. 1997. Development of secondary resistance to fluconazole in *Cryptococcus neoformans* isolated from a patient with AIDS. *Rev. Inst. Med. Trop. Sao Paulo* **39**:359–361.

Ampel, N. 2001. Coccidioidomycosis among persons with human immunodeficiency virus infection in the era of highly active antiretroviral therapy (HAART). *Semin. Respir. Infect.* **16**:257–262.

Ampel, N. 2004. Combating opportunistic infections: coccidioidomycosis. *Expert Opin. Pharmacother.* **5**:255–261.

Ampel, N., C. Dols, and J. Galgiani. 1993. Coccidioidomycosis during human immunodeficiency virus infection: results of a prospective study in a coccidioidal endemic area. *Am. J. Med.* **94**:235–240.

Anaissie, E., V. Fainstein, T. Samo, G. Bodey, and G. Sarosi. 1988. Central nervous system histoplasmosis. An unappreciated complication of the acquired immunodeficiency syndrome. *Am. J. Med.* **84**:215–217.

Armengou, A., C. Porcar, J. Mascaro, and F. Garcia-Bragado. 1996. Possible development of resistance to fluconazole during suppressive therapy for AIDS-associated cryptococcal meningitis. *Clin. Infect. Dis.* **23**:1337–1338.

Benard, G., and A. Duarte. 2000. Paracoccidioidomycosis: a model for evaluation of the effects of human immunodeficiency virus infection on the natural history of endemic tropical diseases. *Clin. Infect. Dis.* **31**:1032–1039.

Boelaert, J., K. Goddeeris, L. Vanopdenbosch, and J. Casselman. 2004. Relapsing meningitis caused by persistent cryptococcal antigens and immune reconstitution after the initiation of highly active antiretroviral therapy. *AIDS* **18**:1223–1224.

Bonacini, M., J. Nussbaum, and C. Ahluwalia. 1990. Gastrointestinal, hepatic, and pancreatic involvement with *Cryptococcus neoformans* in AIDS. *J. Clin. Gastroenterol.* **12**:295–297.

Bozzette, S., R. Larsen, J. Chiu, et al. 1991. A placebo-controlled trial of maintenance therapy with fluconazole after treatment of cryptococcal meningitis in the acquired immunodeficiency syndrome. *N. Engl. J. Med.* **324**:580–584.

Bradsher, R. 1996. Histoplasmosis and blastomycosis. *Clin. Infect. Dis.* **22**:S102–S111.

Bronnimann, D., R. Adam, J. Galgiani, M. Habib, E. Peterson, B. Porter, and J. Bloom. 1987. Coccidioidomycosis in the acquired immunodeficiency syndrome. *Ann. Intern. Med.* **106:**372–379.

Brouwer, A., A. Rajanuwong, W. Chierakul, G. Griffin, R. Larsen, N. White, and T. Harrison. 2004. Combination antifungal therapies for HIV-associated cryptococcal meningitis: a randomised trial. *Lancet* **363:**1764–1767.

Bruinsma-Adams, I. 1991. AIDS presenting as *Candida albicans* meningitis: a case report. *AIDS* **5:**1268–1269.

Callejas, A., N. Ordonez, M. Rodriguez, and E. Castaneda. 1998. First isolation of *Cryptococcus neoformans* var. *gattii*, serotype C, from the environment in Colombia. *Med. Mycol.* **36:**341–344.

Casadevall, A., R. Rosas, and J. Nosanchuk. 2000. Melanin and virulence in *Cryptococcus neoformans. Curr. Opin. Microbiol.* **3:**354–358.

Casado, J., C. Quereda, J. Oliva, E. Navas, A. Moreno, V. Pintado, J. Cobo, and I. Corral. 1997. Candidal meningitis in HIV-infected patients: analysis of 14 cases. *Clin. Infect. Dis.* **25:**673–676.

Cattelan, A., M. Trevenzoli, L. Sasset, M. Lanzafame, U. Marchioro, and F. Meneghetti. 2004. Multiple cerebral cryptococcomas associated with immune reconstitution in HIV-1 infection. *AIDS* **18:**349–351.

Chakrabarti, A., M. Jatana, P. Kumar, L. Chatha, A. Kaushal, and A. Padhye. 1997. Isolation of *Cryptococcus neoformans* var. *gattii* from *Eucalyptus camaldulensis* in India. *J. Clin. Microbiol.* **35:**3340–3342.

Chang, Y., and K. Kwon-Chung. 1994. Complementation of a capsule-deficient mutation of *Cryptococcus neoformans* restores its virulence. *Mol. Cell. Biol.* **14:**4912–4919.

Chetchotisakd, P., S. Sungkanuparph, B. Thinkhamrop, P. Mootsikapun, and P. Boonyaprawit. 2004. A multicentre, randomized, double-blind, placebo-controlled trial of primary cryptococcal meningitis prophylaxis in HIV-infected patients with severe immune deficiency. *HIV Med.* **5:**140–143.

Chuck, S., and M. Sande. 1989. Infections with *Cryptococcus neoformans* in the acquired immunodeficiency syndrome. *N. Engl. J. Med.* **321:**794–799.

Clark, R., D. Greer, W. Atkinson, G. Valainis, and N. Hyslop. 1990. Spectrum of *Cryptococcus neoformans* infection in 68 patients infected with human immunodeficiency virus. *Rev. Infect. Dis.* **12:**768–777.

Coenjaerts, F., A. Walenkamp, P. Mwinzi, J. Scharringa, H. Dekker, J. van Strijp, R Cherniak, and I. Hoepelman. 2001. Potent inhibition of neutrophil migration by cryptococcal mannoprotein-4-induced desensitization. *J. Immunol.* **167:**3988–3995.

Coker, R., M. Viviani, B. Gazzard, B. Du Pont, S. Murphy, J. Atouguia, J. Champalimaud, and J. Harris. 1993. Treatment of cryptococcosis with liposomal amphotericin B (AmBisome) in 23 patients with AIDS. *AIDS* **7:**829–835.

Corbett, E. L., G. J. Churchyard, S. Charalambos, B. Samb, V. Moloi, T. C. Clayton, A. D. Grant, J. Murray, R. J. Hayes, and K. M. De Cock. 2002. Morbidity and mortality in South African gold miners: impact of untreated disease due to human immunodeficiency virus. *Clin. Infect. Dis.* **34:**1251–1258.

Cox, G., and J. Perfect. 1997. *Cryptococcus neoformans* var *neoformans* and *gattii* and *Trichosporon* species. *In* L. Edward (ed.), *Topley and Wilson's Microbiology and Microbial Infections*, 9th ed. Arnold Press, London, United Kingdom.

Crump, J., S. Elner, V. Elner, and C. Kauffman. 1992. Cryptococcal endophthalmitis: case report and review. *Clin. Infect. Dis.* **14:**1069–1073.

Currie, B., and A. Casadevall. 1994. Estimation of the prevalence of cryptococcal infection among patients infected with the human immunodeficiency virus in New York City. *Clin. Infect. Dis.* **19:**1029–1033.

Datta, K., N. Jain, S. Sethi, A. Rattan, A. Casadevall, and U. Banerjee. 2003. Fluconazole and itraconazole susceptibility of clinical isolates of *Cryptococcus neoformans* at a tertiary care centre in India: a need for care. *J. Antimicrob. Chemother.* **52:**683–686.

de Almeida, S., F. Queiroz-Telles, H. Teive, C. Ribeiro, and L. Werneck. 2004. Central nervous system paracoccidioidomycosis: clinical features and laboratorial findings. *J. Infect.* **48:**193–198.

Denning, D. 1996. Therapeutic outcome in invasive aspergillosis. *Clin. Infect. Dis.* **23:**608–615.

Denning, D. 1998. Invasive aspergillosis. *Clin. Infect. Dis.* **26:**781–803.

Denning, D., R. Armstrong, B. Lewis, and D. Stevens. 1991. Elevated cerebrospinal fluid pressures in patients with cryptococcal meningitis and acquired immunodeficiency syndrome. *Am. J. Med.* **91:**267–272.

Deresinski, S. 2001. Coccidioidomycosis: efficacy of new agents and future prospects. *Curr. Opin. Infect. Dis.* **14:**693–696.

Dewsnup, D., J. Galgiani, J. Graybill, M. Diaz, A. Rendon, G. Cloud, and D. Stevens. 1996. Is it ever safe to stop azole therapy for *Coccidioides immitis* meningitis? *Ann. Intern. Med.* **124:**305–310.

Dismukes, W. 1993. Management of cryptococcosis. *Clin. Infect. Dis.* **17:**S507–S512.

Dromer, F., S. Mathoulin-Pelissier, A. Fontanet, O. Ronin, B. Dupont, and O. Lortholary. 2004. Epidemiology of HIV-associated cryptococcosis in France (1985-2001): comparison of the pre- and post-HAART eras. *AIDS* **18:**555–562.

Drutz, D., and M. Huppert. 1983. Coccidioidomycosis: factors affecting the host-parasite interaction. *J. Infect. Dis.* **147:**372–390.

Ehni, W., and R. Ellison. 1987. Spontaneous *Candida albicans* meningitis in a patient with the acquired immune deficiency syndrome. *Am. J. Med.* **83:**806–807.

Elias J., A. dos Santos, C. Carlotti, B. Colli, A. Canheu, C. Matias, L. Furlanetti, R. Martinez, O. Takayanaqui, A. Sakamoto, L. Serafin, and L. Chimelli. 2005. Central nervous system paracoccidioidomycosis: diagnosis and treatment. *Surg. Neurol.* **63:**S13–S21.

Espinel-Ingroff, A. 1998. Comparison of in vitro activities of the new triazole SCH56592 and the echinocandins MK-0991 (L-743,872) and LY303366 against opportunistic filamentous and dimorphic fungi and yeasts. *J. Clin. Microbiol.* **36:**2950–2956.

Fessler, R., J. Sobel, L. Guyot, L. Crane, J. Vacquez, M. Szuba, and F. Diaz. 1998. Management of elevated intracranial pressure in patients with cryptococcal meningitis. *J. Acquir. Immune Defic. Syndr. Hum. Retrovirol.* **17:**137–142.

Fish, D. G., N. M. Ampel, J. N. Galgiani, C. L. Dols, P. C. Kelly, C. H. Johnson, D. Pappagianis, J. E. Edwards, R. B. Wasserman, R. J. Clark, et al. 1990. Coccidioidomycosis during human immunodeficiency virus infection. A review of 77 patients. *Medicine* (Baltimore) **69:**384–391.

Friese, G., T. Discher, R. Fussle, A. Schmalreck, and J. Lohmeyer. 2001. Development of azole resistance during fluconazole maintenance therapy for AIDS-associated cryptococcal disease. *AIDS* **15:**2344–2345.

Galgiani, J., N. Ampel, A. Catanzaro, R. Johnson, D. Stevens, P. Williams, et al. 2000. Practice guideline for the treatment of coccidioidomycosis. *Clin. Infect. Dis.* **30:**658–661.

Goldman, D., S. Lee, and A. Casadevall. 1995. Tissue localization of *Cryptococcus neoformans* glucuronoxylomannan in the presence and absence of specific antibody. *Infect. Immun.* **63:**3448–3453.

Goldman, M., R. Zackin, C. Fichtenbaum, D. Skiest, S. Koletar, R. Hafner, L. Wheat, P. Nyangweso, C. Yiannoutsos, C. Schnizlein-bick, S. Owens, J. Aberg, and AIDS Clinical Trials Group A5038 Study Group. 2004.

Safety of discontinuation of maintenance therapy for disseminated histoplasmosis after immunologic response to antiretroviral therapy. *Clin. Infect. Dis.* **38**:1485–1489.

Gould, P., and I. Gould. 1985. Cryptococcosis in Zimbabwe. *Trans. R. Soc. Trop. Med. Hyg.* **79**:67–69.

Granger, D., J. Perfect, and D. Durack. 1985. Virulence of *Cryptococcus neoformans*. Regulation of capsule synthesis by carbon dioxide. *J. Clin. Investig.* **76**:508–516.

Graybill, J. R., J. Sobel, M. Saag, C. van Der Horst, W. Powderly, G. Cloud, L. Riser, R. Hamill, W. Dismukes, et al. 2000. Diagnosis and management of increased intracranial pressure in patients with AIDS and cryptococcal meningitis. *Clin. Infect. Dis.* **30**:47–54.

Gutierrez, M., A. Canton, N. Sosa, E. Puga, and L. Talavera. 2005. Disseminated histoplasmosis in patients with AIDS in Panama: a review of 104 cases. *Clin. Infect. Dis.* **40**:1199–1202.

Hajjeh, R., L. Conn, D. Stephens, W. Baughman, R. Hamill, E. Graviss, P. Pappas, C. Thomas, A. Reingold, G. Rothrock, L. Hutwagner, A. Schuchat, M. Brandt, R. Pinner, et al. 1999. Cryptococcosis: population-based multistate active surveillance and risk factors in human immunodeficiency virus-infected persons. *J. Infect. Dis.* **179**:449–454.

Hamilton, A. 1998. Serodiagnosis of histoplasmosis, paracoccidioidomycosis and penicilliosis marneffei; current status and future trends. *Med. Mycol.* **36**:351–364.

Haubrich, R., D. Haghighat, S. Bozzette, J. Tilles, and J. McCutchan. 1994. High-dose fluconazole for treatment of cryptococcal disease in patients with human immunodeficiency virus infection. *J. Infect. Dis.* **170**:238–242.

Heyderman, R., I. Gangaidzo, J. Hakim, J. Miekle, A. Tawiza, P. Musvaire, V. Robertson, and P. Mason. 1998. Cryptococcal meningitis in human immunodeficiency virus-infected patients in Harare, Zimbabwe. *Clin. Infect. Dis.* **26**:284–289.

Holding, K., M. Dworkin, P. Wan, D. Hanson, R. Klevens, J. Jones, and P. Sullivan. 2000. Aspergillosis among people infected with human immunodeficiency virus: incidence and survival. *Clin. Infect. Dis.* **31**:1253–1257.

Holtzer, C., M. Jacobson, W. Hadley, L. Huang, H. Stanley, R. Montanti, M. Wong, and J. Stansell. 1998. Decline in the rate of specific opportunistic infections at San Francisco General Hospital, 1994–1997. *AIDS* **12**:1931–1933.

Hopkins, R., M. Rothman, A. Fiore, and S. Goldblum. 1994. Cerebral mucormycosis associated with intravenous drug use: three case reports and review. *Clin. Infect. Dis.* **19**:1133–1137.

Horgan, M., and W. Powderly. 1997. Aspergillosis. *J. Int. Assoc. Phys. AIDS Care* **3**:14–16.

Ives, N., B. Gazzard, and P. Easterbrook. 2001. The changing pattern of AIDS-defining illnesses with the introduction of highly active antiretroviral therapy (HAART) in a London clinic. *J. Infect.* **42**:134–139.

Johnson, P., L. Wheat, G. Cloud, M. Goldman, D. Lancaster, D. Bamberger, W. Powderly, R. Hafner, C. Kauffman, W. Dismukes, and U.S. National Institute of Allergy and Infectious Diseases Mycoses Study Group. 2002. Safety and efficacy of liposomal amphotericin B compared with conventional amphotericin B for induction therapy of histoplasmosis in patients with AIDS. *Ann. Intern. Med.* **137**:105–109.

Johnston, S., E. Corbett, O. Foster, S. Ash, and J. Cohen. 1992. Raised intracranial pressure and visual complications in AIDS patients with cryptococcal meningitis. *J. Infect.* **24**:185–189.

Kaplan, J., D. Hanson, M. Dworkin, T. Federick, J. Bertolli, M. Lindegren, S. Holmberg, and J. Jones. 2000. Epidemiology of human immunodeficiency virus-associated opportunistic infections in the United States in the era of highly active antiretroviral therapy. *Clin. Infect. Dis.* **30**:S5–S14.

Keane, J. 1993. Intermittent third nerve palsy with cryptococcal meningitis. *J. Clin. Neuroophthalmol.* **13**:124–126.

Kestelyn, P., H. Taelman, J. Bogaerts, A. Kagame, M. Abdel Aziz, J. Batungwanayo, A. Stevens, and P. Van de Perre. 1993. Ophthalmic manifestations of infections with *Cryptococcus neoformans* in patients with the acquired immunodeficiency syndrome. *Am. J. Ophthalmol.* **116**:721–727.

Khoo, S., and D. Denning. 1994. Invasive aspergillosis in patients with AIDS. *Clin. Infect. Dis.* **19**:S41–S48.

Klont, R., M. Mennink-Kersten, and P. Verweij. 2004. Utility of *Aspergillus* antigen detection in specimens other than serum specimens. *Clin. Infect. Dis.* **39**:1467–1474.

Kovacs, J. A., A. A. Kovacs, M. Polis, W. C. Wright, V. J. Gill, C. U. Tuazon, E. P. Gelmann, H. C. Lane, R. Longfield, G. Overturf, et al. 1985. Cryptococcosis in the acquired immunodeficiency syndrome. *Ann. Intern. Med.* **103**:533–538.

Lanzafame, M., M. Trevenzoli, G. Carretta, L. Lazzarini, S. Vento, and E. Concia. 1999. Mediastinal lymphadenitis due to cryptococcal infection in HIV-positive patients on highly active antiretroviral therapy. *Chest* **116**:848–849.

Larsen, R., S. Bozzette, B. Jones, D. Haghighat, M. Leal, D. Forthal, M. Bauer, J. Tilles, J. McCutchan, and J. Leedom. 1994. Fluconazole combined with flucytosine for treatment of cryptococcal meningitis in patients with AIDS. *Clin. Infect. Dis.* **19**:741–745.

Larsen, R., M. Leal, and L. Chan. 1990. Fluconazole compared with amphotericin B plus flucytosine for cryptococcal meningitis in AIDS. A randomized trial. *Ann. Intern. Med.* **113**:183–187.

Larsen, R., P. Pappas, J. Perfect, J. Aberg, A. Casadevall, G. Cloud, R. James, S. Filler, and W. Dismukes. 2005. Phase I evaluation of the safety and pharmacokinetics of murine-derived anticryptococcal antibody 18B7 in subjects with treated cryptococcal meningitis. *Antimicrob. Agents Chemother.* **49**:952–958.

Lazera, M., M. Cavalcanti, L. Trilles, M. Nishikawa, and B. Wanke. 1998. *Cryptococcus neoformans* var. *gattii*--evidence for a natural habitat related to decaying wood in a pottery tree hollow. *Med. Mycol.* **36**:119–122.

Lee, S., and A. Casadevall. 1996. Polysaccharide antigen in brain tissue of AIDS patients with cryptococcal meningitis. *Clin. Infect. Dis.* **23**:194–195.

Lee, S., D. Dickson, and A. Casadevall. 1996. Pathology of cryptococcal meningoencephalitis: analysis of 27 patients with pathogenetic implications. *Hum. Pathol.* **27**:839–847.

Leenders, A., P. Reiss, P. Portegies, K. Clezy, W. Hop, J. Hoy, J. Borleffs, T. Allworth, R. Kauffmann, P. Jones, F. Kroon, H. Verbrugh, and S. de Marie. 1997. Liposomal amphotericin B (AmBisome) compared with amphotericin B both followed by oral fluconazole in the treatment of AIDS-associated cryptococcal meningitis. *AIDS* **11**:1463–1471.

Leite, A., J. Vidal, F. Bonasser Filho, R. Nogueira, and A. Oliveira. 2004. Cerebral infarction related to cryptococcal meningitis in an HIV-infected patient: case report and literature review. *Braz. J. Infect. Dis.* **8**:175–179.

Levitz, S. 1991. The ecology of *Cryptococcus neoformans* and the epidemiology of cryptococcosis. *Rev. Infect. Dis.* **13**:1163–1169.

Levy, R., D. Bredesen, and M. Rosenblum. 1985. Neurological manifestations of the acquired immunodeficiency syndrome (AIDS): experience at UCSF and review of the literature. *J. Neurosurg.* **62**:475–495.

Lortholary, O., A. Fontanet, N. Memain, A. Martin, K. Sitbon, and F. Dromer. 2005. Incidence and risk factors of immune reconstitution inflammatory syndrome complicating HIV-associated cryptococcosis in France. *AIDS* **19**:1043–1049.

Lortholary, O., M. Meyohas, and B. Dupont. 1993. Invasive aspergillosis in patients with acquired immunodeficiency syndrome: report of 33 cases. *Am. J. Med.* **95:**177–187.

Malessa, R., M. Krams, U. Hengge, C. Weiller, V. Reinhardt, L. Volbracht, F. Rauhut, and N. Brockmeyer. 1994. Elevation of intracranial pressure in acute AIDS-related cryptococcal meningitis. *Clin. Investig.* **72:**1020–1026.

Manfredi, R., A. Mastroianni, O. Coronado, and F. Chiodo. 1997. Fluconazole as prophylaxis against fungal infection in patients with advanced HIV infection. *Arch. Intern. Med.* **157:**64–69.

Manfredi, R., A. Moroni, A. Mazzoni, A. Nanetti, M. Donati, A. Mastroianni, O. Coronado, and F. Chiodo. 1996. Isolated detection of cryptococcal polysaccharide antigen in cerebrospinal fluid samples from patients with AIDS. *Clin. Infect. Dis.* **23:**849–850.

Martinez, E., M. Garcia-Viejo, M. Marcos, J. Perez-Cuevas, J. Blanco, J. Mallolas, J. Miro, and J. Gatell. 2000. Discontinuation of secondary prophylaxis for cryptococcal meningitis in HIV-infected patients responding to highly active antiretroviral therapy. *AIDS* **14:**2615–2617.

McFadden, D., and A. Casadevall. 2001. Capsule and melanin synthesis in *Cryptococcus neoformans*. *Med. Mycol.* **39:**19–30.

McKinsey, D., L. Wheat, G. Cloud, M. Pierce, J. Black, D. Bamberger, M. Goldman, C. Thomas, H. Gutsch, B. Moskovitz, W. Dismukes, and C. Kauffman. 1999. Itraconazole prophylaxis for fungal infections in patients with advanced human immunodeficiency virus infection: randomized, placebo-controlled, double-blind study. *Clin. Infect. Dis.* **28:**1049–1056.

McManus, E., and J. Jones. 1985. Detection of a *Trichosporon beigelii* antigen cross-reactive with *Cryptococcus neoformans* capsular polysaccharide in serum from a patient with disseminated *Trichosporon* infection. *J. Clin. Microbiol.* **21:**681–685.

Minamoto, G., T. Barlam, and N. Vander. 1992. Invasive aspergillosis in patients with AIDS. *Clin. Infect. Dis.* **14:**66–74.

Mirza, S., M. Phelan, D. Rimland, E. Graviss, R. Hamill, M. Brandt, T. Gardner, M. Sattah, G. de Leon, W. Baughman, and A. Hajjeh. 2003. The changing epidemiology of cryptococcosis: an update from population-based active surveillance in 2 large metropolitan areas, 1992-2000. *Clin. Infect. Dis.* **36:**789–794.

Moore, R., and R. Chaisson. 1996. Natural history of opportunistic disease in an HIV-infected urban clinical cohort. *Ann. Intern. Med.* **124:**633–642.

Moosa, M., and Y. Coovadia. 1997. Cryptococcal meningitis in Durban, South Africa: a comparison of clinical features, laboratory findings, and outcome for human immunodeficiency virus (HIV)-positive and HIV-negative patients. *Clin. Infect. Dis.* **24:**131–134.

Mylonakis, E., M. Paliou, P. Sax, P. Skolnik, M. Baron, and J. Rich. 2000. Central nervous system aspergillosis in patients with human immunodeficiency virus infection. Report of 6 cases and review. *Medicine* **79:**269–280.

Nagy-Agren, S., P. Chu, G. Smith, H. Waskin, and F. Altice. 1995. Zygomycosis (mucormycosis) and HIV infection: report of three cases and review. *J. Acquir. Immune Defic. Syndr. Hum. Retrovirol.* **10:**441–449.

Nelson, M., M. Bower, D. Smith, C. Reed, D. Shanson, and B. Gazzard. 1990. The value of serum cryptococcal antigen in the diagnosis of cryptococcal infection in patients infected with the human immunodeficiency virus. *J. Infect.* **21:**175–181.

Newton, J., S. Tasker, W. Bone, E. Oldfield, P. Olson, M. Nguyen, and M. Wallace. 1995. Weekly fluconazole for the suppression of recurrent thrush in HIV-seropositive patients: impact on the incidence of disseminated cryptococcal infection. *AIDS* **9:**1286–1287.

Newton, P., H. Thai le, N. Tip, J. Short, W. Chierakul, A. Rajanuwong, P. Pitisuttithum, S. Chasombat, B. Phonrat, W. Maek-A-Nantawat, R. Teaunadi, D. Lalloo, and N. White. 2002. A randomized, double-blind, placebo-controlled trial of acetazolamide for the treatment of elevated intracranial pressure in cryptococcal meningitis. *Clin. Infect. Dis.* **35:**769–772.

Nightingale, S., S. Cal, D. Peterson, S. Loss, B. Gamble, D. Watson, C. Manzone, J. Baker, and J. Jockusch. 1992. Primary prophylaxis with fluconazole against systemic fungal infections in HIV-positive patients. *AIDS* **6:**191–194.

Pappas, P., B. Bustamante, E. Ticona, R. Hamill, P. Johnson, A. Reboli. A. Alberg, R. Hasbun, and H. Hsu. 2004. Recombinant interferon-gamma 1b as adjunctive therapy for AIDS-related acute cryptococcal meningitis. *J. Infect. Dis.* **189:**2185–2191.

Pappas, P., J. Pottage, W. Powderly, V. Fraser, C. Stratton, S. McKenzie, M. Tapper, H. Chmel, et al. 1992. Blastomycosis in patients with the acquired immunodeficiency syndrome. *Ann. Intern. Med.* **116:**847–853.

Park, M., D. Hospenthal, and J. Bennett. 1999. Treatment of hydrocephalus secondary to cryptococcal meningitis by use of shunting. *Clin. Infect. Dis.* **28:**629–633.

Pasqualotto, A., C. Bittencourt Severo, F. de Mattos Oliveira, and L. Severo. 2004. Cryptococcemia. An analysis of 28 cases with emphasis on the clinical outcome and its etiologic agent. *Rev. Iberoam. Micol.* **21:**143–146.

Paugam, A., J. Dupouy-Camet, P. Blanche, J. Gangneux, C. Tourte-Schaefer, and D. Sicard. 1994. Increased fluconazole resistance of *Cryptococcus neoformans* isolated from a patient with AIDS and recurrent meningitis. *Clin. Infect. Dis.* **19:**975–976.

Perfect, J. 2005. *Cryptococcus neoformans*, p. 2997–3012. *In* G. Mandell, J. Bennett, and R. Dolin (ed.), *Mandell, Douglas, and Bennett's Principles and Practice of Infectious Disease*, 6th ed. Elsevier, Churchill Livingstone, Philadelphia, PA.

Pfaller, M., S. Messer, L. Boyken, R. Hollis, C. Rice, S. Tendolkar, and D. Deikema. 2004. In vitro activities of voriconazole, posaconazole, and fluconazole against 4,169 clinical isolates of *Candida* spp. and *Cryptococcus neoformans* collected during 2001 and 2002 in the ARTEMIS global antifungal surveillance program. *Diagn. Microbiol. Infect. Dis.* **48:**201–205.

Powderly, W. 1993. Cryptococcal meningitis and AIDS. *Clin. Infect. Dis.* **17:**837–842.

Powderly, W., G. Cloud, W. Dismukes, and M. Saag. 1994. Measurement of cryptococcal antigen in serum and cerebrospinal fluid: value in the management of AIDS-associated cryptococcal meningitis. *Clin. Infect. Dis.* **18:**789–792.

Powderly, W., D. Finkelstein, J. Feinberg, P. Frame, W. He, C. van der Horst, S. L. Koletar, M. E. Eyster, J. Carey, H. Waskin, et al. 1995. A randomized trial comparing fluconazole with clotrimazole troches for the prevention of fungal infections in patients with advanced human immunodeficiency virus infection. *N. Engl. J. Med.* **332:**700–705.

Powderly, W., M. S. Saag, G. A. Cloud, P. Robinson, R. D. Meyer, J. M. Jacobson, J. R. Graybill, A. M. Sugar, V. J. McAuliffe, S. E. Follansbee, et al. 1992. A controlled trial of fluconazole or amphotericin B to prevent relapse of cryptococcal meningitis in patients with the acquired immunodeficiency syndrome. *N. Engl. J. Med.* **326:**793–798.

Pursell, K., E. Telzak, and D. Armstrong. 1992. Aspergillus species colonization and invasive disease in patients with AIDS. *Clin. Infect. Dis.* **14:**141–148.

Quagliarello, V., C. Viscoli, and R. Horwitz. 1995. Primary prevention of cryptococcal meningitis by fluconazole in HIV-infected patients. *Lancet* **345:**548–552.

Qureshi, A., R. Janssen, J. Karon, J. Weissman, M. Akbar, K. Safdar, and M. Frankel. 1997. Human immunodeficiency virus infection and stroke in young patients. *Arch. Neurol.* **54:**1150–1153.

Rambeloarisoa, J., D. Batisse, J. Thiebaut, J. Mikol, S. Mrejen, M. Karmochkine, M. Kazatchkine, L. Weiss, and C. Piketty. 2002. Intramedullary abscess resulting from disseminated cryptococcosis despite immune restoration in a patient with AIDS. *J. Infect.* **44:**185–188.

Rex, J., R. Larsen, W. Dismukes, G. Cloud, and J. Bennett. 1993. Catastrophic visual loss due to *Cryptococcus neoformans* meningitis. *Medicine* **72:**207–224.

Robinson, P., M. Bauer, M. Leal, S. Evans, P. Holtom, D. Diamond, J. Leedom, and R. Larsen. 1999. Early mycological treatment failure in AIDS-associated cryptococcal meningitis. *Clin. Infect. Dis.* **28:**82–92.

Rozenbaum, R., and A. Concalves. 1994. Clinical epidemiological study of 171 cases of cryptococcosis. *Clin. Infect. Dis.* **18:**369–380.

Saag, M. S., G. A. Cloud, J. R. Graybill, J. D. Sobel, C. U. Tuazon, P. C. Johnson, W. J. Fessel, B. L. Moskovitz, B. Weisinger, D. Cosmatos, L. Riser, C. Thomas, R. Hafner, and W. E. Dismukes. 1999. A comparison of itraconazole versus fluconazole as maintenance therapy for AIDS-associated cryptococcal meningitis. *Clin. Infect. Dis.* **28:**291–296.

Saag, M. S., R. J. Graybill, R. A. Larsen, P. G. Pappas, J. R. Perfect, W. G. Powderly, J. D. Sobel, W. E. Dismukes, et al. 2000. Practice guidelines for the management of cryptococcal disease. *Clin. Infect. Dis.* **30:**710–718.

Saag, M. S., W. G. Powderly, G. A. Cloud, P. Robinson, M. H. Grieco, P. K. Sharkey, S. E. Thompson, A. M. Sugar, C. U. Tuazon, J. F. Fisher, et al. 1992. Comparison of amphotericin B with fluconazole in the treatment of acute AIDS-associated cryptococcal meningitis. *N. Engl. J. Med.* **326:**83–89.

Saccente, M., R. McDonnell, L. Baddour, M. Mathis, and R. Bradsher. 2003. Cerebral histoplasmosis in the azole era: report of four cases and review. *South. Med. J.* **96:**410–416.

Sacktor, N., R. Lyles, R. Skolasky, C. Kleeberger, O. Selnes, E. Miller, J. Becker, B. Cohen, J. McArthur, and Multicenter AIDS Cohort Study. 2001. HIV-associated neurologic disease incidence changes: Multicenter AIDS Cohort Study, 1990-1998. *Neurology* **56:**257–260.

Sanchez-Portocarrero, J., and E. Perez-Cecilia. 1997. Intracerebral mass lesions in patients with human immunodeficiency virus infection and cryptococcal meningitis. *Diagn. Microbiol. Infect. Dis.* **29:**193–198.

Sanchez-Portocarrero, J., E. Perez-Cecilia, O. Corral, J. Romero-Vivas, and J. Picazo. 2000. The central nervous system and infection by *Candida* species. *Diagn. Microbiol. Infect. Dis.* **37:**169–179.

Sar, B., D. Monchy, M. Vann, C. Keo, J. Sarthou, and Y. Buisson. 2004. Increasing in vitro resistance to fluconazole in *Cryptococcus neoformans* Cambodian isolates: April 2000 to March 2002. *J. Antimicrob. Chemother.* **54:**563–565.

Selik, R., R. Byers, and M. Dworkin. 2002. Trends in diseases reported on U.S. death certificates that mentioned HIV infection, 1987-1999. *J. Acquir. Immune Defic. Syndr.* **29:**378–387.

Selik, R., J. Karon, and J. Ward. 1997. Effect of the human immunodeficiency virus epidemic on mortality from opportunistic infections in the United States in 1993. *J. Infect. Dis.* **176:**632–636.

Shelburne, S., J. Darcourt, A. White, S. Greenberg, R. Hamill, R. Atmar, and F. Visnegarwala. 2005a. The role of immune reconstitution inflammatory syndrome in AIDS-related *Cryptococcus neoformans* disease in the era of highly active antiretroviral therapy. *Clin. Infect. Dis.* **40:**1049–1052.

Shelburne, S., F. Visnegarwala, J. Darcourt, E. Graviss, T. Giordano, A. White, and R. Hamill. 2005b. Incidence and risk factors for immune reconstitution inflammatory syndrome during highly active antiretroviral therapy. *AIDS* **19:**399–406.

Shoham, S., C. Cover, N. Donegan, E. Fulnecky, and P. Kumar. 2005. *Cryptococcus neoformans* meningitis at 2

hospitals in Washington, D.C.: adherence of health care providers to published practice guidelines for the management of cryptococcal disease. *Clin. Infect. Dis.* **40:**477–479.

Siddiqui, A., A. Brouwer, V. Wuthiekanun, S. Jaffer, R. Shattock, D. Irving, J. Sheldon, W. Chierakul, S. Peacock, N. Day, N. White, and T. Harrison. 2005. IFN-gamma at the site of infection determines rate of clearance of infection in cryptococcal meningitis. *J. Immunol.* **174:**1746–1750.

Singh, N., M. Barnish, S. Berman, B. Bender, M. Wagener, M. Rinaldi, and V. Yu. 1996a. Low-dose fluconazole as primary prophylaxis for cryptococcal infection in AIDS patients with CD4 cell counts of < or = 100/mm^3: demonstration of efficacy in a positive, multicenter trial. *Clin. Infect. Dis.* **23:**1282–1286.

Singh, V. R., D. K. Smith, J. Lawerence, P. C. Kelly, A. R. Thomas, B. Spitz, and G. A. Sarosi. 1996b. Coccidioidomycosis in patients infected with human immunodeficiency virus: review of 91 cases at a single institution. *Clin. Infect. Dis.* **23:**563–568.

Skiest, D. J. 2002. Focal neurological disease in patients with acquired immunodeficiency syndrome. *Clin. Infect. Dis.* **34:**103–115.

Skiest, D. J., L. J. Hester, and R. D. Hardy. 2005. Cryptococcal immune reconstitution inflammatory syndrome: report of four cases in three patients and review of the literature. *J. Infect.* **51:**e289–e297.

Stevens, D. 1995. Coccidioidomycosis. *N. Engl. J. Med.* **332:**1077–1082.

Sugar, A., and C. Saunders. 1988. Oral fluconazole as suppressive therapy of disseminated cryptococcosis in patients with acquired immunodeficiency syndrome. *Am. J. Med.* **85:**481–489.

Sun, H., C. Hung, and S. Chang. 2004. Management of cryptococcal meningitis with extremely high intracranial pressure in HIV-infected patients. *Clin. Infect. Dis.* **38:**1790–1792.

Tanner, D., M. Weinstein, B. Fedorciw, K. Joho, J. Thorpe, and L. Reller. 1994. Comparison of commercial kits for detection of cryptococcal antigen. *J. Clin. Microbiol.* **32:**1680–1684.

Tumbarello, M., E. Tacconelli, L. Pagano, E. La Barbera, G. Morace, R. Cauda, G. Leone, and I. Ortona. 1997. Comparative analysis of prognostic indicators of aspergillosis in haematological malignancies and HIV infection. *J. Infect.* **34:**55–60.

U.S. Public Health Service/Infectious Diseases Society of America. 28 November 2001. *Guidelines for the Prevention of Opportunistic Infections in Persons Infected with Human Immunodeficiency Virus.* http://www.aidsinfo.nih.gov.

Van den Saffele, J., and J. Boelaert. 1996. Zygomycosis in HIV-positive patients: a review of the literature. *Mycoses* **39:**77–84.

van der Horst, C. M., M. S. Saag, G. A. Cloud, R. J. Hamill, J. R. Graybill, J. D. Sobel, P. C. Johnson, C. U. Tuazon, T. Kerkering, B. L. Moskovitz, W. G. Powderly, W. E. Dismukes, et al. 1997. Treatment of cryptococcal meningitis associated with the acquired immunodeficiency syndrome. *N. Engl. J. Med.* **337:**15–21.

Verduyn Lunel, F., and A. Rijs. 1997. In vitro susceptibility pattern of yeast blood culture isolates against standard and new antifungal drugs, p. 158. *In 37th Intersci. Conf. Antimicrob. Agents Chemother.* 28 Sept –to 1 Oct 1997, Toronto, Ontario, Canada.

Verduyn Lunel, F., A. Voss, E. Kuijper, L. Gelinck, P. Hoogerbrugge, K. Liem, B. Kullberg, and P. Verweij. 2004. Detection of the *Candida* antigen mannan in cerebrospinal fluid specimens from patients suspected of having *Candida* meningitis. *J. Clin. Microbiol.* **42:**867–870.

Vibhagool, A., S. Sungkanuparph, P. Mootsikapun, P. Chetchotisakd, S. Tansuphaswaswadikul, C. Bowonwat-anuwong, and A. Ingsatgit. 2003. Discontinuation of secondary prophylaxis for cryptococcal meningitis in human immunodeficiency virus-infected patients treated with highly active antiretroviral therapy: a prospective, multicenter, randomized study. *Clin. Infect. Dis.* **36:**1329–1331.

Voice, R., S. Bradley, J. Sangeorzan, and C. Kauffman. 1994. Chronic candidal meningitis: an uncommon manifestation of candidiasis. *Clin. Infect. Dis.* **19:**60–66.

Wheat, L., P. Connolly-Stringfield, R. Baker, M. Curfman, M. Eads, K. Isreal, S. Norris, D. Webb, and M. Zeckel. 1990. Disseminated histoplasmosis in the acquired immune deficiency syndrome: clinical findings, diagnosis and treatment, and review of the literature. *Medicine* **69:**361–374.

Wheat, L., and C. Kauffman. 2003. Histoplasmosis. *Infect. Dis. Clin. N. Am.* **17:**1–19.

Wheat, L., C. Musial, and E. Jenny-Avital. 2005. Diagnosis and management of central nervous system histoplasmosis. *Clin. Infect. Dis.* **40:**844–852.

Witzig, R., D. Hoadley, D. Greer, K. Abriola, and R. Hernandez. 1994. Blastomycosis and human immunodeficiency virus: three new cases and review. *South. Med. J.* **87:**715–719.

Woods, C., C. McRill, B. Plikaytis, N. Rosenstein, D. Mosley, D. Boyd, B. England, B. Perkins, N. Ampel, and R. Hajjeh. 2000. Coccidioidomycosis in human immunodeficiency virus-infected persons in Arizona, 1994-1997: incidence, risk factors, and prevention. *J. Infect. Dis.* **181:**1428–1434.

Woods, G., and J. Goldsmith. 1990. Aspergillus infection of the central nervous system in patients with acquired immunodeficiency syndrome. *Arch. Neurol.* **47:**181–184.

Zuger, A., E. Louie, R. Holzman, M. Simberkoff, and J. Rahal. 1986. Cryptococcal disease in patients with the acquired immunodeficiency syndrome. Diagnostic features and outcome of treatment. *Ann. Intern. Med.* **104:**234–240.

The Spectrum of Neuro-AIDS Disorders:
Pathophysiology, Diagnosis, and Treatment
Edited by K. Goodkin et al.
©2008 ASM Press, Washington, DC

25

Neurosyphilis in AIDS

JOSEPH R. BERGER AND AARON J. BERGER

HISTORICAL NOTE AND NOMENCLATURE

Syphilis was first recognized as a clinical entity at the turn of the 15th century, shortly after Columbus' crew returned to Spain in 1493 following their second voyage. Unlike the current disease, syphilis, referred to as the "Great Pox" or the "Evil Pox," was associated with mortality rates as high as 25% in its early stages. Its precise origin, whether arising from a spontaneous mutation in an endemic treponeme or whether originating in the Americas, remains a subject of considerable debate. Two pieces of evidence suggest the latter, namely, there is a paucity of evidence for a similar disease in pre-Columbian Europe and an abundance of evidence, chiefly syphilitic bone disorders, in the pre-Columbian Americas (Fleming, 1964).

In 1905, Schaudinn and Hoffmann identified the causative agent as an almost transparent, spiral-shaped organism that they labeled *Spirochaeta pallida*. The following year saw the introduction of dark-field microscopy by Landsteiner, which proved enormously helpful in studying the organism. During the following decade, the organism was observed in the meninges and brain. Successful serologic tests for syphilis employing a basic lipoidal antigen were first reported by Wasserman, Neisser, and Bruck in 1906; however, more than 40 years would elapse before the development of a specific treponemal test. The first of these tests to be employed was the *Treponema pallidum* immobilization test.

The treatment of syphilis until the last century was mostly ineffective, relying on heavy metals, such as mercury, arsenic, and bismuth, as well as fever therapy. In 1911, Ehrlich demonstrated that Salvarsan 606 was effective against syphilis, and Wagner-Jauregg received the Nobel Prize in 1917 for the introduction of malarial therapy. The modern treatment of syphilis begins in 1943 with Mahoney's introduction of penicillin.

ETIOLOGY

Syphilis is caused by the bacterium *Treponema pallidum*, a long, slender, coil-shaped organism that measures 6 to

Joseph R. Berger, Department of Neurology, University of Kentucky College of Medicine, Lexington, KY 40536. Aaron J. Berger, Yale University School of Medicine, New Haven, CT 06510.

15 μm in length but only 0.15 μm in width. Its narrow width is a dimension below the resolution of light microscopy. The organism has regular spirals numbering 5 to 20 and is actively motile, using a rotational screw-like activity, flexion, and back-and-forth motion. Electron microscopic studies reveal that the organism has an amorphous coat of mucopolysaccharides, an outer membrane, an electron-dense peptidoglycan layer, and a cytoplasmic membrane. Three flagella extending from each end of the organism are located between the outer membrane and the electron-dense layer. These flagella twist around the body of the organism and provide the spiral shape of the organism and its mode of locomotion.

T. pallidum belongs to one of five genera in the order *Spirochaetales*. Three of these genera are pathogenic to man, including *Treponema* (syphilis), *Leptospira* (leptospirosis), and *Borrelia* (tick- and louse-borne relapsing fever). The organisms responsible for endemic syphilis (*T. pallidum*), yaws (*T. pertenue*), and pinta ("*T. carateum*") are morphologically identical and antigenically similar. Extensive DNA homology has been demonstrated between these organisms.

Despite assertions to the contrary, *T. pallidum* is not an obligate anaerobe. It grows best in 3 to 5% O_2 and 5% CO_2 in H_2, but its cultivation in vitro is difficult. This fact, coupled with the exquisite fragility of the organism, has rendered its study difficult. Small mammals and primates have been used as animal models. The best animal model remains the rabbit, in which the disease closely parallels that in man. The organism invades interstitial spaces and chiefly proliferates there, with a doubling time of 30 to 33 h; however, it can be found intracellularly as well. The pathogen disseminates hematogenously.

BIOLOGICAL BASIS

Shortly after infection, a spirochetemia results with dissemination of *T. pallidum* to virtually any organ, including the central nervous system (CNS). Both humoral and cellular immune systems play a role in the ensuing infection. Antibodies to *T. pallidum* are detectable within 10 to 21 days of infection. The humoral response does not contain the infection but may affect the course of the disease. Cellular immunity appears to be effective in controlling the infection as evidenced by immunity during rechallenge. The degree of protection is directly proportional to the extent of the response. Impairment of cellular immunity due to drugs, pregnancy, AIDS, etc., appears to result in a more aggressive syphilitic infection than otherwise anticipated (see below).

Studies of cerebrospinal fluid (CSF) abnormalities occurring in association with early (primary or secondary) syphilis have detected abnormalities in 16 to 48% of cases. These results are suggestive of early invasion of the CNS by the organism. Several studies have confirmed the presence of viable treponemes in the CSF in these early stages of infection. Neurosyphilis is not believed to develop in the absence of CSF abnormalities. Merritt stated that "if the CSF is normal two or more years after infection, it will always remain so, and parenchymatous neurosyphilis will never develop." The converse, however, is not true. The presence of CSF abnormalities does not necessarily predict the development of neurosyphilis. In the Oslo study, 9.4% of the men and 5.0% of the women ultimately developed neurosyphilis (Clark and Danbolt, 1964), and in the Tuskegee study 4% of survivors had neurosyphilis after a 20-year follow-up, and 3% at 30 years (Rockwell et al., 1964). No satisfactory explanation has yet been proposed to account for the lack of universal invasion of the CNS by T. pallidum, nor is there an explanation for the absence of neurosyphilis in the majority of individuals who manifest CSF abnormalities indicative of CNS invasion.

The pathology of neurosyphilis is the consequence of the invasion of the CNS by T. pallidum and the associated immunological response. In syphilitic meningitis, the earliest neurologic complication of syphilis, invasion of the meninges by the spirochete, results in an infiltration of the meninges by lymphocytes and, to a lesser extent, plasma cells. This cellular infiltration may follow blood vessels into the brainstem and spinal cord along the Virchow-Robin spaces. Necrosis of the media and proliferation of the intima of small meningeal vessels accompany T. pallidum invasion of the vessel walls.

Late stages of neurosyphilis can be divided into meningovascular and parenchymatous disease. The inflammation observed in the former parallels that observed with syphilitic meningitis. The classical lesion is an endarteritis obliterans of medium and large vessels, first described by Huebner in 1874. This lesion is characterized by fibroblastic thickening of the intima and thinning of the media. Vasculitis in small vessels is referred to as Nissl-Alzheimer arteritis. Gummas of varying size, from microscopic to mass-producing lesions, may be observed. Pathologically, the gummas are thick, tough, rubbery lesions of fibrous trabecula with lymphocytic and plasma cell infiltration of the outer layers. Treponemes are seldom seen in the gumma.

Parenchymatous neurosyphilis is typified by tabes dorsalis and general paresis. The pathology of tabes dorsalis predominates in the dorsal roots and posterior columns of the lumbosacral and lower thoracic levels but is not confined to those areas. Variable lymphocytic infiltration of the meninges accompanies these degenerative changes. The predominant findings are believed to result from irreversible changes to the dorsal root fibers, but the exact pathogenesis of this disorder is not known. Typically, in general paresis the brain is atrophic and the meninges are thickened on pathological examination; however, the brain may appear grossly normal in a minority of cases. The cerebral cortex, striatum, and hypothalamus bear the brunt of the damage. The architecture of the cerebral cortex is disrupted, and neuronal loss accompanies astrocytic and microglial proliferation.

T. pallidum can be demonstrated in the cerebral cortex. Ependymal granulations are commonly observed, and the meningeal inflammation is chiefly composed of plasma cells. The specific mechanisms by which the spirochete results in these pathological changes in the CNS remain uncertain.

EPIDEMIOLOGY

The combination of the ready availability of penicillin and the sensitivity of the organism to this antibiotic has led to a widely held perception that syphilis in contemporary times is rare. The annual incidence of syphilis in the United States declined 18-fold from a peak of 72 cases per 100,000 in 1943 to 4 per 100,000 in 1956. The overall rate of primary and secondary syphilis in the United States was 2.1 per 100,000 in 2000 but saw a slight increase the following year, the first such increase since 1990 (Centers for Disease Control and Prevention, 2002a). In some areas of the country, e.g., particularly large urban areas, the incidence may be substantially higher than the national average (Centers for Disease Control and Prevention, 2002a). In Robeson County, NC, the rate of persons infected with syphilis was 73/100,000 for 2001 (Centers for Disease Control and Prevention, 2002a), 35 times the national average. In the 1970s, there was a clearly increased risk among homosexual and bisexual men; however, their adoption of safe sex techniques, with the advent of the AIDS era, resulted in a significant decline in the incidence of syphilis in this risk group. Groups that are currently at increased risk for syphilis include female prostitutes and crack cocaine abusers. The latter group is believed to have an increased risk due to the trading of sex for drugs and the lowering of inhibitions. The number of women with syphilis is rising at a rate disproportionate to that of men, and, not unexpectedly, there has been a substantial increase in the number of cases of congenital syphilis in the United States. Because of the higher rates of syphilis in the HIV-infected population, vigilance by increased surveillance for asymptomatic disease has been recommended (Winston et al., 2003). It is estimated that 20 to 70% of men who have sex with men in large urban areas may be coinfected with syphilis and HIV (Chan, 2005).

Neurosyphilis is surprisingly common in association with HIV infection. Prevalence rates of CSF Venereal Disease Research Laboratory (VDRL) test-reactive neurosyphilis have been reported to be between 1.0 and 2.0% for several large cohorts of HIV-seropositive individuals (Berger 1991; Holtom et al., 1992; Brandon et al., 1993). This prevalence rate is substantially higher if only patients with serological evidence of syphilis are included. In some HIV-infected populations, the prevalence rate of a reactive serum fluorescent treponemal antibody absorption test approaches 50% (Berger, 1991). In one study, 9.1% of HIV-infected patients undergoing lumbar puncture because of a reactive serology and having no history of recent treatment for syphilis had a reactive CSF VDRL test (Holtom et al., 1992). Neurosyphilis may be responsible for HIV-related neurologic manifestations in a significant minority of some populations, and neurosyphilis needs to be considered in the differential diagnosis of any HIV-infected person presenting with neurologic disease (Berger, 1991). Neurosyphilis in this population represents a potentially treatable and curable disorder.

CLINICAL MANIFESTATIONS

Syphilis has been referred to as "the great masquerader" due to the multiple and varied fashions in which it may present.

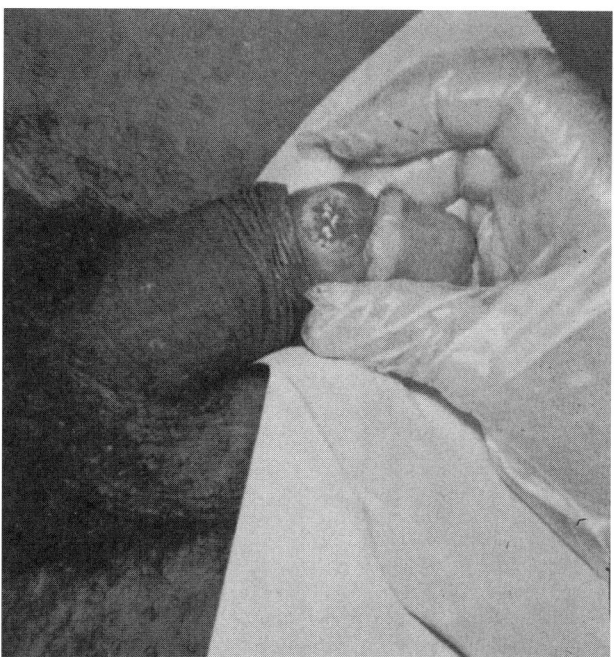

FIGURE 1   Penile chancre (reproduced from the USPHS files).

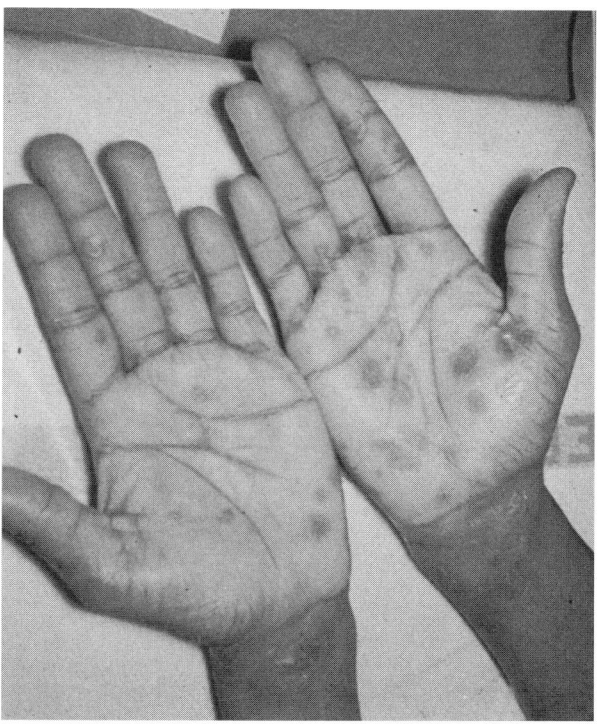

FIGURE 2   Maculopapular rash of secondary syphilis (reproduced from the USPHS files).

Infection with *T. pallidum* is divided into several stages. Primary syphilis is the initial manifestation of infection. It typically presents as an ulcerated, painless lesion with firm borders referred to as a chancre (Fig. 1) and develops at the site of epidermal or mucous membrane inoculation (penis, vulva, lips, tongue, etc.). The chancre is accompanied by regional adenopathy and generally appears about 3 weeks after infection, although the time to development ranges from 3 to 90 days, depending on the size of the inoculum. Although the lesion is a local manifestation, the spirochetes, even at this early stage, have disseminated systemically as evidenced by the ability to transmit syphilis by blood donation from incubating seronegative donors and the presence of detectable *T. pallidum* in the CSF of a substantial percentage of infected persons.

The features of secondary syphilis appear within 2 to 8 weeks following the appearance of the chancre and are attributable to the bacteremic phase of the illness. These secondary manifestations include a macular, maculopapular, or pustular rash that often involves the palms and soles (Fig. 2); mucous patches; and alopecia. Constitutional signs, diffuse adenopathy, iridocyclitis, hepatitis, periostitis, and arthritis often accompany the skin manifestations. A brisk immune response is observed, and immune complex deposition may lead to nephrotic syndrome. Symptomatic aseptic meningitis may occur in up to 5% of patients with secondary syphilis. The clinical manifestations of primary and secondary syphilis appear to be little affected by HIV infection (Rompalo et al., 2001).

Latent syphilis is defined as a quiescent phase of syphilis that precedes the development of tertiary complications. It is characterized by a positive serology and negative physical examination. The United States Public Health Service (USPHS) has divided latent syphilis into early (within 1 year of infection) and late (>1 year) stages to reflect the probability of recurrence of secondary syphilitic manifestations. It is recommended that late latent syphilis be treated for a longer duration, based on the notion that the biology of the spirochete evolves over time; *T. pallidum* is thought to develop a slower metabolism and a more prolonged dividing time (Centers for Disease Control and Prevention, 2002b).

Skin, osseous, cardiovascular, and neurologic complications are the chief characteristics of tertiary syphilis. The predominant manifestation of tertiary syphilis is gummas, which are granulomatous, nodular lesions that can be found in any organ. The major cardiovascular complication of tertiary syphilis is aortitis, which is due to infection of the vasa vasorum.

Patients with untreated syphilis may have a risk of tertiary syphilis that approaches 40%, though most studies suggest that the incidence of clinically recognized tertiary syphilis among untreated patients is closer to 25% (Rosahn, 1947). In the Oslo study of patients with untreated syphilis, 10% developed cardiovascular syphilis, 16% developed gummatous syphilis, and 6.5% developed symptomatic neurosyphilis (Clark and Danbolt, 1964). Clinically apparent neurologic complications of tertiary syphilis affect <10% of untreated patients.

Neurosyphilis is simply the occurrence of neurologic complications due to infection with *T. pallidum*. Neurosyphilis may occur during any stage of syphilis; therefore, it is incorrect to consider neurosyphilis a manifestation of tertiary syphilis. The spectrum of neurosyphilis is quite broad, and various forms of neurosyphilis may coexist in the same patient. The specific neurologic manifestations of syphilis are, in some respect, a function of the time from infection (Fig. 3). The spectrum of these neurological complications has changed somewhat over time. Tabes dorsalis was commonly observed in the preantibiotic era and is now rare. Studies from South Africa suggest that it is the only

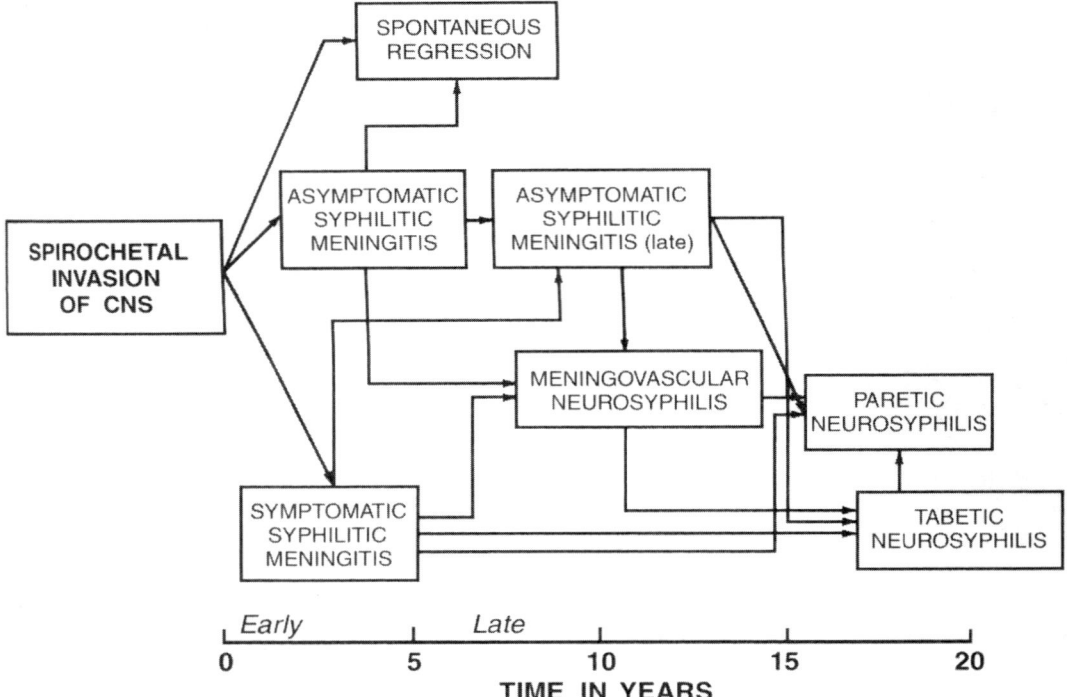

FIGURE 3 A timeline for the evolution of neurosyphilis. (Reproduced from Victor and Ropper, 2000.)

neurological manifestation of syphilis that has changed substantially over time (Timmermans and Carr, 2004).

The most common form of neurosyphilis currently diagnosed is asymptomatic neurosyphilis, typically as a consequence of lumbar puncture performed in neurologically normal individuals with serologic evidence of syphilis. The CSF reveals evidence of neurosyphilis, and these patients are at risk for developing symptomatic disease. Among the symptomatic disorders of neurosyphilis, the earliest manifestation is syphilitic meningitis (Fig. 4). The meninges are hemorrhagic and opacified as a consequence of syphilitic meningitis, which typically occurs within the first 12 months of infection and may accompany features of secondary syphilis. Although the majority of patients with CSF abnormalities occurring in association with secondary syphilis are neurologically asymptomatic, approximately 5% of all patients with secondary syphilis have an associated meningitis. Headaches, pain with neck flexion, impaired vision, cranial nerve palsies (chiefly, in descending order of frequency, nerves VII, VIII, VI, and II), hearing loss, tinnitus, and vertigo may be observed in isolation or in combination in upwards of 40% of patients with secondary syphilis. Encephalopathic features resulting from vascular compromise or increased intracranial pressure may be observed. These include confusion, lethargy, seizures, aphasia, and hemiplegia. Intractable seizures may, on rare occasion, be the initial manifestation of neurosyphilis (Phan et al., 1999). Acute sensorineural hearing loss and acute optic neuritis may occur in association with syphilitic meningitis or independently.

Meningovascular syphilis may affect the brain or spinal cord. It typically occurs 6 to 7 years after the initial infection but may occur as early as 6 months after the primary infection. Neurologic features are dependent on the area of the brain or spinal cord infarcted (Fig. 5). Many of the stroke eponyms, e.g., Weber's, Claude's, and Benedikt's syndromes, among others, were described in the 19th century in persons with meningovascular syphilis, as this disorder resulted in discrete lesions of the brainstem. The neurologic manifestations include aphasia, hemiparesis, hemianesthesia, diplopia, vertigo, dysarthria, and a variety of brainstem syndromes. Computed tomography and magnetic resonance imaging (MRI) of the brain are invaluable diagnostic aids.

A wide variety of spinal cord syndromes may be observed with syphilis (Table 1). The characteristic spinal cord syndrome associated with parenchymatous neurosyphilis is tabes dorsalis. This disorder usually has a latency of 15 to 30 years following infection. The most distinctive and often heralding symptom is shooting or lightning-like pains that typically affect the legs and abdomen. On occasion, these pains have been mistaken for surgical emergencies. Touch of the affected areas may serve as a trigger for the pain. Pupillary abnormalities are observed in over 90% of patients, with the hallmark abnormality being Argyll Robertson pupils: miotic, irregular pupils exhibiting light-near dissociation. The gait is ataxic with an associated foot-stomping character due to an associated impaired position sense. Romberg's test is positive. The impaired sensory perception also leads to the development of Charcot joints, painless swelling of joints, chiefly the knees, due to repeated trauma, and to perforating ulcers of the toes and soles of the feet. The impaired sense of deep pain may be demonstrated by its absence on squeezing the testicle (Pitre's sign), the ulnar nerve (Biernacki's sign), or Achilles tendon (Abadie's sign). Impotence and bladder dysfunction are expected. The lower extremity reflexes are absent. Optic atrophy and cranial

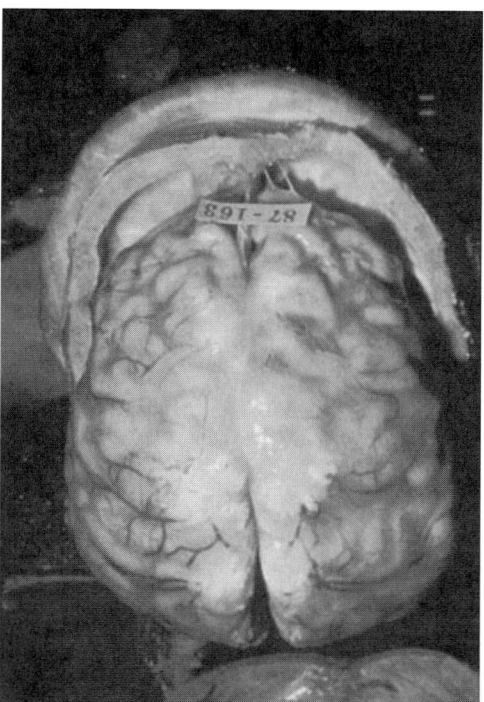

FIGURE 4 Syphilitic meningitis at autopsy in an AIDS patient.

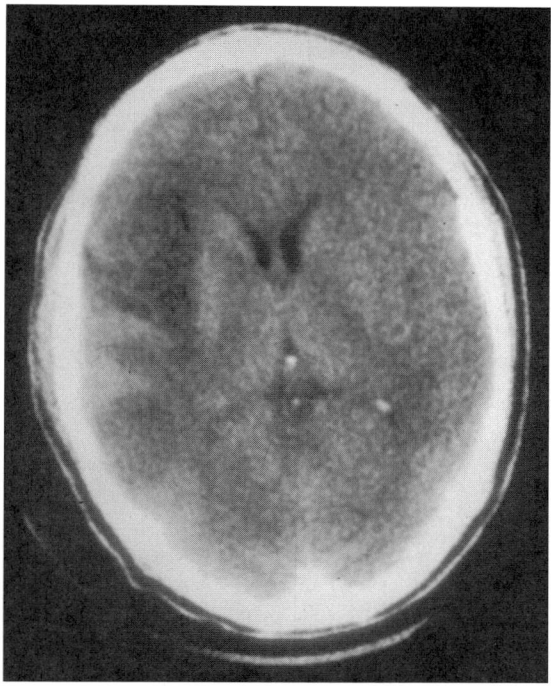

FIGURE 5 Meningovascular syphilis with right middle cerebral artery infarction.

nerve palsies are frequently observed. Tabes dorsalis has been mistakenly diagnosed as Miller Fisher syndrome, as it may present as a constellation of ophthalmoplegia, ataxia, and areflexia (Stepper et al., 1998). Paraparesis may also be seen as a consequence of syphilitic aortic dissection (Kellett et al., 1997). The spectrum of syphilitic spinal cord disease is quite diverse.

Syphilitic meningomyelitis is characterized by slowly progressive weakness and paresthesia of the lower extremities, with bowel and bladder incontinence and paraplegia eventually supervening. Examination reveals a spastic paraparesis or paraplegia with brisk lower extremity reflexes, loss of the superficial abdominal reflexes, and impaired sensory perception. Vibratory and position sense is typically disproportionately affected. Syphilitic transverse myelitis may also be observed, resulting in an acute onset of lower extremity paraplegia and sensory loss. Occasionally, the manifestations of this syndrome are more variable with asymmetrical

TABLE 1 Syphilis of the spinal cord[a]

Syphilitic meningomyelitis
Syphilitic spinal pachymeningitis
Spinal cord gumma
Syphilitic hypertrophic pachymeningitis
Spinal vascular syphilis
Syphilitic poliomyelitis
Tabes dorsalis
Miscellaneous
Syringomyelia
Syphilitic aortic aneurysm
Charcot vertebra with compression of the spinal cord

   [a]Modified from Berger, 1987.

findings noted, including a Brown-Sequard syndrome. An acute infarction of the anterior spinal artery results in paraplegia and loss of pain and temperature sensation below the level of the lesion with preservation of vibratory and position sense. The preceding spinal cord syndromes are manifestations of meningovascular syphilis.

General paresis is a manifestation of parenchymatous neurosyphilis and, like tabes dorsalis, usually develops after a long (15- to 30-year) hiatus from the time of infection. General paresis accounted for a substantial percentage of psychiatric illness in the preantibiotic era and, in a recent study from South Africa, was found in 1.3% of all patients being admitted for acute psychiatric care (Roberts et al., 1992). These patients display a wide variety of psychiatric disturbances, including emotional lability, paranoia, illusions, delusions of grandeur, hallucinations, and inappropriate behavior in addition to a progressive dementia. The diagnosis of neurosyphilis should be suspected in any middle-aged person exhibiting the new onset of a behavioral or psychiatric disorder (Lair and Naidech, 2004). Physical examination reveals tremors of the tongue, postural tremors of the extremities, hyperreflexia, hypomimetic facies, dysarthria, chorioretinitis, optic neuritis; and pupillary abnormalities, including Argyll Robertson pupils, are seen. Cranial MRI of patients with general paresis has demonstrated frontal and temporal atrophy, subcortical gliosis, and increased ferritin in the basal ganglia (Zifko et al., 1996).

Gummas of the nervous system are generally space-occupying lesions that result in progressive focal neurologic manifestations, seizures, headaches, and features of increased intracranial pressure (Fig. 6). A linear dural enhancement on MRI, similar to that observed with meningiomas, may be found with cerebral gummas (Inoue et al., 1995). Gummas affecting the spinal cord result in progressive quadriparesis

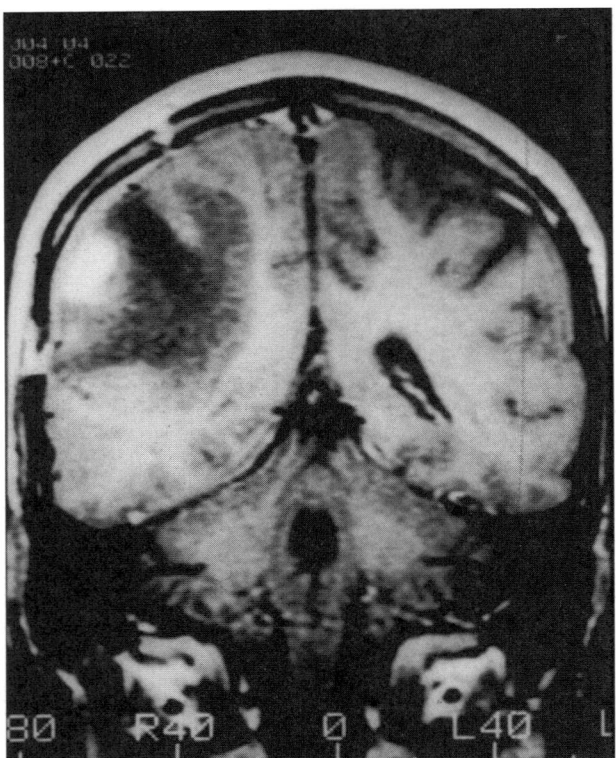

FIGURE 6 Cerebral gumma in neurosyphilis on MRI.

when located in the cervical area or result in progressive paraparesis when in the thoracic area.

An atypical form of neurosyphilis referred to as "modified neurosyphilis" has been attributed to the use of antibiotics for conditions other than syphilis in patients with unrecognized syphilis. This illness is characterized by a negative CSF VDRL test and clinical features that are outside the spectrum of classically described features of neurosyphilis. Whether modified neurosyphilis is a true clinical entity remains open to question.

HIV AND SYPHILIS

Concomitant HIV infection may result in a significant alteration of the natural history of neurosyphilis (Johns et al., 1987; Katz and Berger, 1989; Katz et al., 1993). The manifestations of syphilis may be not only more aggressive but also more difficult to treat in the setting of HIV infection (Berry et al., 1987; Musher et al., 1990; Katz et al., 1993). These observations suggest that the host's immune response is critical in controlling this infection. The inability of the HIV-infected patient to establish delayed hypersensitivity to *T. pallidum* may prevent secondary syphilis from evolving to latency or may cause a spontaneous relapse from a latent state. A more rapid development of neurosyphilis in HIV-infected individuals than would otherwise be expected may result from the impairment of delayed hypersensitivity. *T. pallidum* can be isolated from the CSF of HIV-seropositive patients with primary, secondary, and latent syphilis following currently recommended Centers for Disease Control and Prevention (CDC) penicillin therapy (Lukehart et al., 1988). Despite the associated immunosuppression, serum nontreponemal

titers at the time of presentation of neurosyphilis in the HIV-infected individual are typically high, averaging 1:128 (Katz et al., 1993; Flood et al., 1998).

In HIV infection, an acute, symptomatic, syphilitic meningitis during the course of secondary syphilis is not uncommon. A decrease in the latent period to the development of some neurosyphilitic manifestations, such as meningovascular syphilis and general paresis, has been suggested. Meningovascular syphilis within 4 months of primary infection despite the administration of accepted penicillin regimens (Johns et al., 1987) and the neurologic relapse of syphilis in HIV-infected individuals after appropriate doses of benzathine penicillin for secondary syphilis (Berry et al., 1987) have been reported. Other unusual manifestations of syphilis in association with HIV infection include unexplained fever (Chung et al., 1983), bilateral optic neuritis with blindness (Zambrano et al., 1987), vitritis (Kuo et al., 1998), Bell's palsy, and severe bilateral sensorineural hearing loss (Fernandez-Guerrero et al., 1988), syphilitic meningomyelitis (Berger, 1992), syphilitic polyradiculopathy (Lanska et al., 1988; Winston et al., 2005), and syphilitic cerebral gumma presenting as a mass lesion (Berger et al., 1992).

Certain ophthalmological and otolaryngological complications of syphilis occurring in the absence of neurologic disease may result in neurologic consultation. Although the characteristic ophthalmological abnormality of syphilis is the Argyll Robertson pupil, other conditions that can result from *T. pallidum* infection include interstitial keratitis, chorioretinitis, and optic atrophy. Syphilitic optic atrophy, which is commonly unilateral and may occur with or without an associated basilar meningitis, is notoriously difficult to treat effectively. Progression is observed in as many as 50% of patients despite treatment. Otitic syphilis is associated with hearing loss, either acute or gradually progressive in nature, and may occur in association with cochlear end organ damage (Darmstadt and Harris, 1989). Vertigo may also be a feature of this illness. Syphilitic eighth nerve dysfunction is largely recognized as a late manifestation of congenital syphilis but is also observed in acquired illness. In addition to these neurological and ophthalmological complications of syphilis occurring in association with HIV infection, aggressive syphilitic skin disorders may be observed as well (Liotta et al., 2000).

DIAGNOSTIC EVALUATION

The diagnosis of syphilis is dependent on serological study except in primary and secondary syphilis, during which *T. pallidum* can be demonstrated by the use of dark-field microscopy from skin and mucous membrane lesions. There are two categories of serological study: nontreponemal tests, which are flocculation tests using cardiolipin, lecithin, and cholesterol as antigen; and treponemal tests, which rely on specific treponemal cellular components as antigens. Nontreponemal tests include the VDRL, rapid plasma reagin, Wasserman, and Kolmer tests. Nontreponemal tests are not infrequently falsely positive. False-positive syphilis serological studies using these tests are common in the setting of intravenous drug abuse and hepatitis B, particularly in the HIV-infected population (Hernandez-Aguado et al., 1998). The treponemal tests include the fluorescent treponemal antibody absorption test, microhemagglutination assay, hemagglutination treponemal test for syphilis, and the treponemal immobilization test.

There is no "gold standard" for the diagnosis of neurosyphilis. Culturing the organism from the CSF is cumbersome and available in very few laboratories. The fragility of *T. pallidum* results in a low sensitivity of the test. Similarly, PCR assay for detection of *T. pallidum* remains experimental. Demonstrating the organism in the CSF does not reliably predict the subsequent development of neurosyphilitic manifestations, though the converse, a normal CSF, is a good indicator that neurosyphilis will not develop at a later point in time. A reactive VDRL test in the CSF is quite specific, with rare reports of false positivity, but the test is not sufficiently sensitive to exclude the diagnosis of neurosyphilis on the basis of a negative study. The serum VDRL is reactive in 72% of patients with primary syphilis, nearly 100% of patients with secondary syphilis, 73% of patients with latent syphilis, and 77% of patients with tertiary syphilis. Therefore, as many as one-quarter of patients with neurosyphilis are anticipated to have a negative serum VDRL test. Its frequency of reactivity appears to vary with the clinical form of neurosyphilis, and its presence in asymptomatic neurosyphilis may be substantially lower than in symptomatic disease. The CSF VDRL test is too insensitive to be relied on to exclude the diagnosis of neurosyphilis. In one study in which CSF was cultured in rabbit testicles, *T. pallidum* was isolated from CSF of 12 (30%) of 40 patients with primary and secondary syphilis, but the CSF VDRL test was reactive in only 4 (33%) of these 12 patients (Lukehart et al., 1988). Therefore, measures other than a reactive CSF VDRL test must be relied on to establish the diagnosis of neurosyphilis. The frequency with which this test is negative in the presence of neurosyphilis is not known but has been estimated to exceed 25%. In many respects, neurosyphilis is a diagnosis established on clinical grounds. To date, there is no consensus regarding diagnostic criteria, and the physician should probably refrain from rigid adherence to narrow guidelines in making the diagnosis.

A reactive serum treponemal test should be a prerequisite for diagnosing neurosyphilis. Neurosyphilis should be diagnosed for anyone with serologies reactive for a treponemal test occurring in association with a reactive CSF VDRL test. A diagnosis of neurosyphilis should be considered for patients with serological evidence of syphilis and one or more of the following abnormalities in their CSF: a mononuclear pleocytosis, an elevated protein, increased immunoglobulin G (IgG), or the presence of oligoclonal bands. Undoubtedly, neurosyphilis is overdiagnosed using these criteria. The CSF fluorescent treponemal antibody absorption (FTA-ABS) test has been suggested as a sensitive screening test for the presence of neurosyphilis (Davis and Schmitt, 1989). Carey and colleagues used the FTA-ABS test in a cross-sectional survey of hospitalized patients with serologic evidence of latent syphilis to conclude that the CSF abnormalities in 32% of HIV-seronegative persons and in 67% of HIV-seropositive persons were nonspecific in nature and not attributable to neurosyphilis (Carey et al., 1995). Small amounts of blood contamination of the CSF may give false-positive tests with the FTA-ABS test but not with the CSF VDRL test, which requires gross blood contamination of the CSF to be rendered falsely positive. Additionally, the FTA-ABS test is dependent on IgG antibody that may cross the blood-brain barrier to result in a false-positive test for neurosyphilis. The CSF fluorescent treponemal antibody-IgM test has been suggested as an alternative to avoid the latter possibility. Other CSF studies, not widely employed but believed to be diagnostically useful for neurosyphilis, are a treponemal pallidum hemagglutination (TPHA) test index of ≥100 (the TPHA index is CSF TPHA titers/CSF albumin × 10³/serum albumin) (where albumin is measured in milligrams per deciliter) and a TPHA-IgG index of ≥3 (the TPHA-IgG index is calculated as CSF TPHA-IgG titer/total CSF IgG divided by TPHA-IgG titer/total serum IgG). Newer-generation tests for syphilis and neurosyphilis, in particular those employing the PCR (Hay et al., 1990; Burstain et al., 1991) and monoclonal antibodies (Whang et al., 1992), may solve this dilemma but at this time require further study before widespread adoption.

Coinfection with HIV considerably complicates the interpretation of CSF abnormalities, as a mononuclear pleocytosis, increased protein, increased IgG, and the presence of oligoclonal bands may all attend HIV infection in the absence of neurosyphilis (Hollander, 1988). A schema has been proposed for the diagnosing of neurosyphilis in the face of HIV infection (Table 2).

Although not diagnostic of neurosyphilis, radiologic studies may be suggestive and are certainly helpful in excluding other pathologies. Radiologic manifestations of neurosyphilis include meningeal enhancement, hydrocephalus, gummas, periostitis, generalized cerebral atrophy, and stroke. Gummas appear as avascular, dura-based masses with surrounding edema that on MRI are characteristically isointense with gray matter on T1-weighted image and hyperintense on T2-weighted image. Dense contrast enhancement is usually observed. The T2-weighted hyperintense signal abnormalities of the parenchyma that may accompany cerebral atrophy in general paresis have been reported to resolve with treatment (Berbel-Garcia et al., 2004). Orbital periostitis typically involves the roof and supraorbital rim. These lesions may be hyperplastic, resulting in tender osteophytic nodules and exostoses (Harris et al., 1997). The periorbital inflammation can infiltrate the extraocular muscles and cranial nerves (Smith et al., 1990). MRI may also reveal multiple, bilateral, discrete white matter lesions involving deep periventricular and subcortical regions (Harris et al., 1997). Angiography of neurosyphilis is nonspecific. Large vessels may exhibit segmental constriction or occlusion (Harris et al., 1997). Smaller vessels, usually Sylvian branches of the middle cerebral artery, may display focal stenoses with or without adjacent dilatation (Harris et al., 1997). The sites of syphilitic brain lesions detected by MRI appear to correlate with psychiatric and cognitive symptoms (Russouw et al., 1997).

TABLE 2 Diagnosing neurosyphilis in the face of HIV infection

Definite neurosyphilis
  1. Positive blood treponemal serology, e.g., FTA-ABS, microhemagglutination assay for *T. pallidum*, etc.
  2. Positive CSF VDRL test

Probable neurosyphilis
  1. Positive blood treponemal serology
  2. Negative CSF VDRL test
  3. CSF mononuclear pleocytosis (>20 cells/mm³) or positive CSF protein (>60 mg/dl) with neurologic complications compatible with neurosyphilis, such as cranial nerve palsies, stroke, etc., or evidence of ophthalmological syphilis

Possible neurosyphilis
  1. Positive blood treponemal serology
  2. Negative CSF VDRL test
  3. CSF mononuclear pleocytosis (>20 cells/mm³) or positive CSF protein (>60 mg/dl) with no neurologic or ophthalmological complications compatible with syphilis

In a review of 35 patients with documented neurosyphilis (3 HIV seronegative and 32 HIV seropositive), Brightbill and colleagues found that 31% had normal brain imaging, 23% had cerebral infarction, and 20% had nonspecific cerebral white matter lesions. Cerebral gummas and extra-axial enhancement indicating meningitis were each noted in 2 (6%) of 35 patients, and arteritis was demonstrated in 2 (50%) of 4 patients undergoing either magnetic resonance angiography or conventional cerebral angiography (Brightbill et al., 1995).

PROGNOSIS AND COMPLICATIONS

The prognosis of neurologic complications of syphilis is dependent on the nature of the disorder. In general, those neurologic manifestations occurring early in syphilis, namely, asymptomatic neurosyphilis and syphilitic meningitis, are readily treatable and typically resolve without neurologic sequelae. Only a small minority of patients with the late neurologic manifestations of syphilis, such as general paresis and tabes dorsalis, however, show any improvement with penicillin therapy. Stabilization of the progressive neurologic disorder is generally the best that can be expected in these instances.

TREATMENT

T. pallidum is highly sensitive to penicillin, as was convincingly demonstrated by Mahoney in 1943. Despite 50 years of experience, however, the adequacy of currently recommended treatment regimens still remains questionable due to an absence of controlled, randomized, prospective studies for the optimal dose and duration of therapy in neurosyphilis. The treponemicidal level of penicillin is 0.03 μg/ml, and although the organism has been demonstrated to be capable of acquiring plasmids that produce penicillinase, there is no compelling evidence to suggest that it loses its efficacy in the treatment of *T. pallidum*. When penicillin levels become subtherapeutic, the spirochetes begin regenerating within 18 to 24 h. The Centers for Disease Control (1988) has recommended using 2.4 million U of benzathine penicillin intramuscularly at weekly intervals for 3 weeks in the treatment of neurosyphilis, but the recordable penicillin levels in the CSF during treatment fail to reach treponemicidal levels (Polnikorn et al., 1980). The concentration of penicillin in the CSF is typically unmeasurable, probably not exceeding 0.0005 μg/ml, which is 1 to 2% of the serum levels. Furthermore, viable treponemes have been recovered from the CSF of individuals at the completion of therapy (Tramont, 1976). Another "recommended" regimen is procaine penicillin, 600,000 U intramuscularly daily for 15 days. This regimen, too, may fail to achieve treponemicidal levels of penicillin in the CSF. Ideally, the treatment regimen for neurosyphilis should be 12 to 24 million U of crystalline aqueous penicillin administered intravenously daily (2 to 4 million U every 4 h) for a period of 10 to 14 days. This regimen generally requires hospitalization, but a prolonged hospitalization may be avoided for some reliable, well-motivated patients by placement of an indwelling catheter and home administration of penicillin after the first 24 to 48 h of therapy. The penicillin should be administered at no less than 4-h intervals to maintain the penicillin levels consistently at or above treponemicidal values and to avoid the subtherapeutic troughs that occur when it is administered at less frequent intervals. An alternative approach to the use of parenteral penicillin is the daily oral administration

of amoxicillin (3.0 g) and probenecid (0.5 g) administered twice daily for 15 days (Faber et al., 1983). This regimen achieves treponemicidal levels of amoxicillin in the CSF (Faber et al., 1983; Morrison et al., 1985).

For patients who are allergic to penicillin, erythromycin, 500 mg four times daily for a period of 30 days, has been recommended. Erythromycin does not diffuse readily into the brain and CSF, nor has its efficacy been demonstrated in the treatment of neurosyphilis. It has been associated with a high rate of treatment failures and, therefore, cannot be recommended in the treatment of neurosyphilis (Goldmeier and Hay, 1993). Oral therapy with tetracycline yields very low tetracycline concentrations in the CSF, and it, too, has unproven efficacy in the treatment of neurosyphilis. The successful uses of intravenous ceftriaxone, 2 g daily for 10 days (Hook et al., 1986), and oral doxycycline, 200 mg twice daily for 21 days (Yim et al., 1985), have been reported. These therapeutic regimens in individuals with established neurosyphilis and complicating HIV infection require further study; however, one study found a failure rate of 23% in HIV-infected patients with latent syphilis or asymptomatic neurosyphilis treated with ceftriaxone, typically administered as 1 g daily intravenously or intramuscularly over 10 to 14 days (Dowell et al., 1992).

The Jarisch-Herxheimer reaction is a systemic reaction to the rapid dissolution of treponemes occurring within several hours of the initiation of treatment. The disorder is characterized by the abrupt onset of fever and chills, headache, tachycardia, flushing, myalgias, and mild hypotension. Although many authorities advocate pretreatment with aspirin to ameliorate the symptoms of this disorder, acute brain infarction during the Jarisch-Herxheimer reaction has been observed in patients with meningovascular syphilis; therefore, some authorities recommend the administration of prednisone, 60 mg over the initial 24 h.

Determining the adequacy of therapy depends on careful follow-up of the patient. Conversion of the serum VDRL test or rapid plasma reagin test to nonreactive should occur within 1 year after treatment of primary syphilis, within 2 years after treatment of secondary syphilis, and within 5 years after treatment of latent syphilis. This delay to reversion from a seropositive status reflects the duration and severity of the illness. The presence of a persistently positive serum VDRL test or rapid plasma reagin test suggests either persistent infection, reinfection, or a biological false-positive test.

In patients with meningovascular syphilis, acute ischemic deficits have been treated successfully with tissue plasminogen activator (Han et al., 2004). As noted, the fixed neurologic deficits of neurosyphilis may fail to improve with treatment, and some abnormalities, such as tabes dorsalis and optic atrophy, may worsen despite adequate therapy. Resolution of CSF abnormalities is the best determinant for the adequacy of treatment. Examination of the CSF within several days of the institution of penicillin treatment may be confusing, as the CSF cell count may rise initially, particularly if accompanied by a Jarisch-Herxheimer reaction; however, the CSF should be examined at the termination of treatment to document a fall in cell count, and it should then be examined at 6-month intervals for 2 to 3 years. The cell count should return to normal within 1 year of treatment (usually 6 months), and the protein should return to normal within 2 years. The disappearance of the CSF VDRL test positivity typically parallels its resolution in the serum. The long hiatus to its eventual clearing makes it less useful for purposes of determining the adequacy of treatment than the CSF cell count or protein. However, the CSF VDRL test titers should not increase over time with effective therapy. A significant negative correlation between improvement in cognitive function and the CSF VDRL test titers 1 year following treatment suggests that the CSF VDRL titer is an indicator of continued *T. pallidum* infection (Roberts et al., 1992). Dependence on the CSF for determining the adequacy of treatment for neurosyphilis in HIV-infected individuals often yields inaccurate results, due to the frequency with which CSF abnormalities are detected with HIV infection alone. Other than reversion of a positive CSF VDRL test in those instances where it was initially present, a decline in a CSF pleocytosis may be of greatest value in monitoring the success of therapy. The potential for relapse of neurosyphilis following a course of "recommended" therapy suggests the potential need for secondary prophylaxis in treating neurosyphilis in the HIV-infected individual, as is employed in the management of some other CNS infections, such as toxoplasma encephalitis and cryptococcal meningitis. In a recent study of 100 HIV-infected military personnel with syphilis, 4 of 7 persons with a reactive CSF VDRL test relapsed following high-dose intravenous penicillin. Relapses were often observed more than 12 months after initial therapy (Malone et al., 1995). Other investigators, however, have found good clinical and serological responses to standard penicillin regimens in the HIV-infected population with syphilis (Bordon et al., 1999). In early syphilis, HIV-infected patients appear to respond serologically more frequently than those without HIV infection (Yinnon et al., 1996; Rolfs et al., 1997), but the presence of *T. pallidum* in the CSF did not predict treatment failure (Rolfs et al., 1997). The CDC has recommended that the initial therapy of intravenous aqueous penicillin be followed in HIV-infected individuals by weekly intramuscular injections of 2.4 million U of benzathine penicillin for 3 weeks. However, in light of lack of treponemicidal levels of penicillin with the latter and evidence that high-dose penicillin regimens are not consistently effective in patients infected with HIV (Gordon et al., 1994), a more logical course may be the administration of a 30-day course of doxycycline, 200 mg twice daily, following the completion of intravenous therapy. Although secondary prophylaxis is extensively employed, further studies are warranted before secondary prophylaxis or some permutation of it can be broadly recommended. A study of the addition of 10 days of amoxicillin and probenecid to standard penicillin therapy for early syphilis in HIV infection found no improvement with this "enhanced" regimen (Rolfs et al., 1997). HIV-seropositive patients should be carefully monitored for relapse of neurosyphilis for 2 or more years following initial treatment.

Otitic syphilis is relatively refractory to treatment regimens. Parenteral therapy is recommended for 6 weeks to 3 months with 12 to 24 million U of aqueous crystalline penicillin daily or oral therapy with 3.5 g of amoxicillin with 1.0 g of probenecid daily. Prednisone, 30 to 60 mg daily, is also recommended in combination with the antibiotic regimen for this disorder. Similarly, in the face of a progressive syphilitic optic neuritis, a trial of oral corticosteroids, e.g., prednisone, 60 mg daily, for 2 to 4 weeks with careful observation, is suggested.

For patients with hydrocephalus complicating neurosyphilis, CSF shunting has been recommended. However, resolution of syphilitic hydrocephalus following high-dose intravenous penicillin has been reported (Cosottini et al., 1997).

SUMMARY

Neurosyphilis is broadly defined as the occurrence of neurological complications due to infection with *T. pallidum*. It may occur during any stage of syphilis. Syphilitic meningitis is the earliest neurological complication of syphilis; late stages of neurosyphilis can be divided into meningovascular and parenchymatous disease. Neurosyphilis is surprisingly common in association with HIV infection, and it may be responsible for neurologic symptoms in a significant minority of some HIV populations. The manifestations of syphilis may be not only more aggressive but also, in some instances, more difficult to treat in the context of HIV infection. *T. pallidum* can be isolated from the CSF of HIV-seropositive patients with primary, secondary, and latent syphilis, even after CDC-recommended penicillin therapy. Acute, symptomatic, syphilitic meningitis during the course of secondary syphilis is not uncommon in association with HIV infection. Other unusual manifestations of syphilis in HIV infection include unexplained fever, bilateral optic neuritis with blindness, vitritis, Bell's palsy, severe bilateral sensorineural hearing loss, syphilitic meningomyelitis, syphilitic polyradiculopathy, and syphilitic cerebral gumma presenting as a mass lesion.

While the diagnosis of syphilis is relatively straightforward with serum tests for demonstration of treponeme or immune response to this pathogen, the diagnosis of neurosyphilis is more complicated. A reactive serum treponemal test should be a prerequisite for investigating neurosyphilis through prompt CSF studies. However, the diagnosis of neurosyphilis is also dependent on clinical findings. Efforts to develop newer-generation diagnostic tests, especially those employing PCR and monoclonal antibodies, promise to make the diagnosis of neurosyphilis less obscure. We recommend that the physician refrain from adherence to rigid guidelines in making a diagnosis, especially as coinfection with HIV complicates the picture.

The goal of neurosyphilis treatment is to reach treponemicidal levels of penicillin in the CSF. In patients who are allergic to penicillin, macrolide and tetracycline antibiotics may be used, though the efficacy of these regimens has not been fully studied. It is important to consider the Jarisch-Herxheimer reaction and treat patients with aspirin or prednisone as prophylaxis. The adequacy of therapy can be determined through patient follow-up. Conversion of the serum VDRL test or rapid plasma reagin test to nonreactive should occur within 1 year after treatment of primary syphilis, within 2 years after treatment of secondary syphilis, and within 5 years after treatment of latent syphilis. The best determinant of treatment adequacy for neurosyphilis is the resolution of CSF abnormalities, although it often yields inaccurate results in HIV patients because of irregularities due to HIV infection alone. HIV-seropositive patients should be monitored for neurosyphilis relapse for at least 2 years following treatment.

REFERENCES

Berbel-Garcia, A., J. Porta-Etessam, A. Martinez-Salio, M. Millan-Juncos, D. A. Perez-Martinez, R. A. Saiz-Diaz, and M. Toledo-Heras. 2004. Magnetic resonance image-reversible findings in a patient with general paresis. *Sex. Transm. Dis.* **31:**350–352.

Berger, J. R. 1987. Syphilis of the spinal cord, p. 491–538. *In* R. Davidoff (ed.), *The Handbook of the Spinal Cord,* vol. 5. Marcel-Dekker, New York, NY.

Berger, J. R. 1991. Neurosyphilis in human immunodeficiency virus type 1-seropositive individuals. A prospective study. *Arch. Neurol.* **48:**700–702.

Berger, J. R. 1992. Spinal cord syphilis associated with human immunodeficiency virus infection: a treatable myelopathy. *Am. J. Med.* **92:**101–103.

Berger, J. R., H. Waskin, L. Pall, G. Hensley, I. Ihmedian, and M. J. Post. 1992. Syphilitic cerebral gumma with HIV infection. *Neurology* **42:**1282–1287.

Berry, C. D., T. M. Hooton, A. C. Collier, and S. A. Lukehart. 1987. Neurologic relapse after benzathine penicillin therapy for secondary syphilis in a patient with HIV infection. *N. Engl. J. Med.* **316:**1587–1589.

Bordon, J., C. Martinez-Vazquez, J. de la Fuente-Aguado, B. Sopena, A. Ocampo-Hermida, J. Nunez-Torron, T. Rodriguez-Sousa, M. Alvarez-Fernandez, and T. del Blanco. 1999. Response to standard syphilis treatment in patients infected with the human immunodeficiency virus. *Eur. J. Clin. Microbiol. Infect. Dis.* **18:**729–732.

Brandon, W. R., L. M. Boulos, and A. Morse. 1993. Determining the prevalence of neurosyphilis in a cohort co-infected with HIV. *Int. J. STD AIDS* **4:**99–101.

Brightbill, T. C., I. H. Ihmeidan, M. J. Post, J. R. Berger, and D. A. Katz. 1995. Neurosyphilis in HIV-positive and HIV-negative patients: neuroimaging findings. *AJNR Am. J. Neuroradiol.* **16:**703–711.

Burstain, J. M., E. Grimprel, S. A. Lukehart, M. V. Norgard, and J. D. Radolf. 1991. Sensitive detection of *Treponema pallidum* by using the polymerase chain reaction. *J. Clin. Microbiol.* **29:**62–69.

Carey, L. A., M. J. Glesby, L. M. Mundy, E. M. Janis, and E. W. Hook III. 1995. Lumbar puncture for evaluation of latent syphilis in hospitalized patients. High prevalence of cerebrospinal fluid abnormalities unrelated to syphilis. *Arch. Intern. Med.* **155:**1657–1662.

Centers for Disease Control. 1988. Recommendations for diagnosing and treating syphilis in HIV-infected patients. *Morb. Mortal. Wkly. Rep.* **37:**600–608.

Centers for Disease Control and Prevention. 2002a. Primary and secondary syphilis—United States, 2000-2001. *Morb. Mortal. Wkly. Rep.* **51:**971–973.

Centers for Disease Control and Prevention. 2002b. Sexually transmitted diseases treatment guidelines 2002. *MMWR Recomm. Rep.* **51**(RR-6):1–78.

Chan, D. J. 2005. Syphilis and HIV co-infection: when is lumbar puncture indicated? *Curr. HIV Res.* **3:**95–98.

Chung, W. M., F. D. Pien, and J. L. Grekin. 1983. Syphilis: a cause of fever of unknown origin. *Cutis* **31:**537–540.

Clark, E., and N. Danbolt. 1964. The Oslo study of the natural course of untreated syphilis: an epidemiologic investigation based on a re-study of the Boeck-Bruusgard material. *Med. Clin. N. Am.* **48:**613–624.

Cosottini, M., M. Mascalchi, G. Zaccara, and G. Arnetoli. 1997. Reversal of syphilitic hydrocephalus with intravenous penicillin. *Can. J. Neurol. Sci.* **24:**343–344.

Darmstadt, G. L., and J. P. Harris. 1989. Luetic hearing loss: clinical presentation, diagnosis, and treatment. *Am. J. Otolaryngol.* **10:**410–421.

Davis, L. E., and J. W. Schmitt. 1989. Clinical significance of cerebrospinal fluid tests for neurosyphilis. *Ann. Neurol.* **25:**50–55.

Dowell, M. E., P. G. Ross, D. M. Musher, T. R. Cate, and R. E. Baughn. 1992. Response of latent syphilis or neurosyphilis to ceftriaxone therapy in persons infected with human immunodeficiency virus. *Am. J. Med.* **93:**481–488.

Faber, W. R., J. D. Bos, P. J. Rietra, H. Fass, and R. V. Van Eijk. 1983. Treponemicidal levels of amoxicillin in cerebrospinal fluid after oral administration. *Sex. Transm. Dis.* **10:**148–150.

Fernandez-Guerrero, M. L., C. Miranda, C. Cenjor, and F. Sanabria. 1988. The treatment of neurosyphilis in patients with HIV infection. *JAMA* **259:**1495–1496.

Fleming, W. 1964. Syphilis through the ages. *Med. Clin. N. Am.* **48:**587–612.

Flood, J. M., H. S. Weinstock, M. E. Guroy, L. Bayne, R. P. Simon, and G. Bolan. 1998. Neurosyphilis during the AIDS epidemic, San Francisco, 1985-1992. *J. Infect. Dis.* **177:**931–940.

Goldmeier, D., and P. Hay. 1993. A review and update on adult syphilis, with particular reference to its treatment. *Int. J. STD AIDS* **4:**70–82.

Gordon, S. M., M. E. Eaton, R. George, S. Larsen, S. A. Lukehart, J. Kuypers, C. M. Marra, and S. Thompson. 1994. The response of symptomatic neurosyphilis to high-dose intravenous penicillin G in patients with human immunodeficiency virus infection. *N. Engl. J. Med.* **331:**1469–1473.

Han, J. H., C. C. Lee, and R. S. Crupi. 2004. Meningovascular syphilis and improvement with tissue-plasminogen activator (T-PA). *Am. J. Emerg. Med.* **22:**426–427.

Harris, D. E., D. S. Enterline, and R. D. Tien. 1997. Neurosyphilis in patients with AIDS. *Neuroimaging Clin. N. Am.* **7:**215–221.

Hay, P. E., J. R. Clarke, D. Taylor-Robinson, and D. Goldmeier. 1990. Detection of treponemal DNA in the CSF of patients with syphilis and HIV infection using the polymerase chain reaction. *Genitourin. Med.* **66:**428–432.

Hernandez-Aguado, I., F. Bolumar, R. Moreno, F. J. Pardo, N. Torres, J. Belda, A. Espacio, et al. 1998. False-positive tests for syphilis associated with human immunodeficiency virus and hepatitis B virus infection among intravenous drug abusers. *Eur. J. Clin. Microbiol. Infect. Dis.* **17:**784–787.

Hollander, H. 1988. Cerebrospinal fluid normalities and abnormalities in individuals infected with human immunodeficiency virus. *J. Infect. Dis.* **158:**855–858.

Holtom, P. D., R. A. Larsen, M. E. Leal, and J. M. Leedom. 1992. Prevalence of neurosyphilis in human immunodeficiency virus-infected patients with latent syphilis. *Am. J. Med.* **93:**9–12.

Hook, E. W., III, S. A. Baker-Zander, B. L. Moskovitz, S. A. Lukehart, and H. H. Handsfield. 1986. Ceftriaxone therapy for asymptomatic neurosyphilis. Case report and Western blot analysis of serum and cerebrospinal fluid IgG response to therapy. *Sex. Transm. Dis.* **13**(Suppl. 3):S185–S188.

Inoue, R., S. Katayama, T. Kusakabe, T. Mori, and S. Hori. 1995. Cerebral gumma showing linear dural enhancement on magnetic resonance imaging case report. *Neurol. Med. Chir.* (Tokyo) **35:**813–817.

Johns, D. R., M. Tierney, and D. Felsenstein. 1987. Alteration in the natural history of neurosyphilis by concurrent infection with the human immunodeficiency virus. *N. Engl. J. Med.* **316:**1569–1572.

Katz, D. A., and J. R. Berger. 1989. Neurosyphilis in acquired immunodeficiency syndrome. *Arch. Neurol.* **46:**895–898.

Katz, D. A., J. R. Berger, and R. C. Duncan. 1993. Neurosyphilis. A comparative study of the effects of infection with human immunodeficiency virus. *Arch. Neurol.* **50:**243–249.

Kellett, M. W., G. R. Young, and N. A. Fletcher. 1997. Paraparesis due to syphilitic aortic dissection. *Neurology* **48:**221–223.

Kuo, I. C., M. A. Kapusta, and N. A. Rao. 1998. Vitritis as the primary manifestation of ocular syphilis in patients with HIV infection. *Am. J. Ophthalmol.* **125:**306–311.

Lair, L., and A. M. Naidech. 2004. Modern neuropsychiatric presentation of neurosyphilis. *Neurology* **63:**1331–1333.

Lanska, M. J., D. J. Lanska, and J. W. Schmidley. 1988. Syphilitic polyradiculopathy in an HIV-positive man. *Neurology* **38:**1297–1301.

Liotta, E. A., G. W. Turiansky, B. J. Berberian, V. I. Sulica, and M. M. Tomaszewski. 2000. Unusual presentation of secondary syphilis in 2 HIV-1 positive patients. *Cutis* **66:**383–386, 389.

Lukehart, S. A., E. W. Hook III, S. A. Baker-Zander, A. C. Collier, C. W. Critchlow, and H. H. Handsfield. 1988. Invasion of the central nervous system by *Treponema pallidum*: implications for diagnosis and treatment. *Ann. Intern. Med.* **109:**855–862.

Malone, J. L., M. R. Wallace, B. B. Hendrick, A. LaRocco, Jr., E. Tonon, S. K. Brodine, W. A. Bowler, B. S. Lavin, R. E. Hawkins, and E. C. Oldfield III. 1995. Syphilis and neurosyphilis in a human immunodeficiency virus type-1 seropositive population: evidence for frequent serologic relapse after therapy. *Am. J. Med.* **99:**55–63.

Morrison, R. E., S. M. Harrison, and E. C. Tramont. 1985. Oral amoxycillin, an alternative treatment for neurosyphilis. *Genitourin. Med.* **61:**359–362.

Musher, D. M., R. J. Hamill, and R. E. Baughn. 1990. Effect of human immunodeficiency virus (HIV) infection on the course of syphilis and on the response to treatment. *Ann. Intern. Med.* **113:**872–881.

Phan, T. G., E. R. Somerville, and S. Chen. 1999. Intractable epilepsy as the initial manifestation of neurosyphilis. *Epilepsia* **40:**1309–1311.

Polnikorn, N., R. Witoonpanich, M. Vorachit, S. Vejjajiva, and A. Vejjajiva. 1980. Penicillin concentrations in cerebrospinal fluid after different treatment regimens for syphilis. *Br. J. Vener. Dis.* **56:**363–367.

Roberts, M. C., R. A. Emsley, and G. P. Jordaan. 1992. Screening for syphilis and neurosyphilis in acute psychiatric admissions. *S. Afr. Med. J.* **82:**16–18.

Rockwell, D. H., A. R. Yobs, and M. B. Moore, Jr. 1964. The Tuskegee Study of Untreated Syphilis; the 30th year of observation. *Arch. Intern. Med.* **114:**792–798.

Rolfs, R. T., M. R. Joesoef, E. F. Hendershot, A. M. Rompalo, M. H. Augenbraun, M. Chiu, G. Bolan, S. C. Johnson, P. French, E. Steen, J. D. Radolf, S. Larsen, et al. 1997. A randomized trial of enhanced therapy for early syphilis in patients with and without human immunodeficiency virus infection. *N. Engl. J. Med.* **337:**307–314.

Rompalo, A. M., M. R. Joesoef, J. A. O'Donnell, M. Augenbraun, W. Brady, J. D. Radolf, R. Johnson, R. T. Rolfs, and the Syphilis and HIV Study Group. 2001. Clinical manifestations of early syphilis by HIV status and gender: results of the syphilis and HIV study. *Sex. Transm. Dis.* **28:**158–165.

Rosahn, P. 1947. Autopsy studies in syphilis. Information supplement #21. Washington DC: US Public Health Service Venereal Disease Division. *J. Vener. Dis.* **649**.

Russouw, H. G., M. C. Roberts, R. A. Emsley, and R. Truter. 1997. Psychiatric manifestations and magnetic resonance imaging in HIV-negative neurosyphilis. *Biol. Psychiatry* **41:**467–473.

Smith, J. L., S. F. Byrne, and C. R. Cambron. 1990. Syphiloma/gumma of the optic nerve and human immunodeficiency virus seropositivity. *J. Clin. Neuroophthalmol.* **10:**175–184.

Stepper, F., G. Schroth, and M. Sturzenegger. 1998. Neurosyphilis mimicking Miller-Fisher syndrome: a case report and MRI findings. *Neurology* **51:**269–271.

Timmermans, M., and J. Carr. 2004. Neurosyphilis in the modern era. *J. Neurol. Neurosurg. Psychiatry* **75:**1727–1730.

Tramont, E. C. 1976. Persistence of *Treponema pallidum* following penicillin G therapy. Report of two cases. *JAMA* **236:**2206–2207.

Victor, M., and A. H. Ropper. 2000. *Adams and Victor's Principles of Neurology*, 7th ed. McGraw-Hill, New York, NY.

Whang, K. K., M. G. Lee, W. Lew, and J. B. Lee. 1992. Production and characterization of monoclonal antibodies to *Treponema pallidum*. *J. Dermatol. Sci.* **4:**26–32.

Winston, A., D. Hawkins, S. Mandalia, F. Boag, B. Azadian, and D. Asboe. 2003. Is increased surveillance for asymptomatic syphilis in an HIV outpatient department worthwhile? *Sex. Transm. Infect.* **79:**257–259.

Winston, A., D. Marriott, and B. Brew. 2005. Early syphilis presenting as a painful polyradiculopathy in an HIV positive individual. *Sex. Transm. Infect.* **81:**133–134.

Yim, C. W., N. M. Flynn, and F. T. Fitzgerald. 1985. Penetration of oral doxycycline into the cerebrospinal fluid of patients with latent or neurosyphilis. *Antimicrob. Agents Chemother.* **28:**347–348.

Yinnon, A. M., P. Coury-Doniger, R. Polito, and R. C. Reichman. 1996. Serologic response to treatment of syphilis in patients with HIV infection. *Arch. Intern. Med.* **156:**321–325.

Zambrano, W., G. M. Perez, and J. L. Smith. 1987. Acute syphilitic blindness in AIDS. *J. Clin. Neuroophthalmol.* **7:** 1–5.

Zifko, U., D. Wimberger, K. Lindner, G. Zier, W. Grisold, and E. Schindler. 1996. MRI in patients with general paresis. *Neuroradiology* **38:**120–123.

The Spectrum of Neuro-AIDS Disorders:
Pathophysiology, Diagnosis, and Treatment
Edited by K. Goodkin et al.
©2008 ASM Press, Washington, DC

26

Progressive Multifocal Leukoencephalopathy in the Era of HAART

DAVID B. CLIFFORD

Progressive multifocal leukoencephalopathy (PML) is an important viral infection of the central nervous system that has attracted increasing attention in recent years because of the surge in incidence accompanying the epidemic of the human immunodeficiency virus (HIV). Over the past few decades, a considerable increase in knowledge about the biology of the JC virus (JCV) (Padgett et al., 1971), which causes PML, and increasing knowledge about immune function have expanded our understanding of PML (Major et al., 1992). However, efforts to directly treat this very serious infection remain frustrated, while patients continue to experience serious morbidity and mortality from its complications. It is hoped that increasing attention to the biology of this infection will encourage development of successful therapy in the coming year.

EPIDEMIOLOGY

JCV has been identified worldwide, and human infection appears to occur rather early in life. By adult life, a majority of people reveal immunologic evidence of JC virus exposure (Knowles et al., 2003; Stolt et al., 2003; Weber et al., 1997).

However, clinical manifestations of primary infection are not evident, and in almost all hosts the virus remains clinically silent throughout life, but it is well documented that healthy hosts often shed the virus, particularly in the urine. It is believed that the virus is often latent in the kidneys in healthy hosts.

A variety of tissues including brain, peripheral blood lymphocytes, and kidney are particularly prone to JC tropism, while variants may be recovered from lung, liver, gastrointestinal tract, spleen, lymph nodes, marrow, and urine. A recent classification of virus using data about insertions and deletions in the genome correlates some aspects of tissue specificity with viral sequences (Jensen and Major, 2001). However, the infection of B lymphocytes may be an important step in the spread of the virus to other regions of the

body, including the brain, as activated lymphocytes can traffic across the blood-brain barrier, introducing the virus to the brain (Aksamit et al., 1986). There is some controversy as to whether JCV may remain latent in the brain, with some reports discovering the virus in the CNS compartment at autopsy of elderly subjects (Mori et al., 1992), while others believe that the entry and replication in the brain are virtually always pathologic (Telenti et al., 1992).

Transformation to PML occurs when JCV infects oligodendrocytes with a lytic infection, resulting in demyelinating lesions. The name is appropriately descriptive, as the course of this disease after its initiation is classically progressive to death, causing neurological deterioration due to demyelinating lesions predominating in the white matter of the brain. Often foci of disease appear to progress by direct extension following white matter tracts in the brain. Gray matter involvement also occurs, as do spinal cord lesions. A recent description of apoptotic cell death may provide further ways to obstruct the progressive course of this disease (Richardson-Burns et al., 2002). This brain invasion with symptomatic demyelination virtually always takes place in immunodepressed hosts. Historically, the affected subjects had lymphoproliferative diseases (Astrom et al., 1958), often receiving aggressive chemotherapy in an effort to combat the underlying malignancy, or other conditions for which very long term immunosuppression occurs (Angelini et al., 2001), such as aggressive sarcoidosis, systemic lupus erythematosus (Kinoshita et al., 1998), or other autoimmune diseases (Rankin and Scaravilli, 1995; Katz et al., 1994; Scotton et al., 1998; Morgenstern and Pardo, 1995). The recent report of PML in the setting of natalizumab and rituximab therapy suggests that specific immune modulatory settings will continue to be potential risks for development of this disease (Kleinschmidt-DeMasters and Tyler, 2005; Langer-Gould et al., 2005; Van Assche et al., 2005; Yousry et al., 2006). In much of the developed world, a large majority of PML cases are now associated with HIV infection.

PATHOLOGY OF PML

The diagnosis of PML has typically been made on the basis of brain biopsy demonstrating classic findings associated

David B. Clifford, Forest and Melba Seay Professor of Clinical Neuropharmacology, Department of Neurology, Washington University School of Medicine, St. Louis, MO 63110.

with this disorder. On brain cutting, areas of white matter disease are evident, often affecting multiple areas of white matter in the same brain. White matter is affected by lytic infection of oligodendrocytes by JCV, accompanied by astrocytosis, with relative sparing of axons. Location of lesions may be at any point in white-matter-rich zones of the brain, but classic presentations include involvement in the posterior hemispheral white matter; in the cerebellum, where it often rapidly extends into the brainstem; and in deep frontal white matter.

Also evident on microscopic evaluation of lesions are enlarged astrocytes with large, bizarre lobulated hyperchromatic nuclei. Oligodendroglial cells are seen with basophilic nuclei that are enlarged and often contain inclusion bodies that may be identified on hematoxylin and eosin stained sections. Electron microscopy reveals 25- to 45-nm papovavirus-like virions in oligodendroglial cells primarily (Howatson et al., 1965). Immunohistochemical staining of the brains for capsid protein has been demonstrated to be useful in diagnosis of PML on brain tissue (Jochum et al., 1997). It is also possible to perform in situ PCR on tissue from the brain biopsy, which may be even more sensitive than traditional in situ hybridization, although specificity for PML in some but not all labs suffers with in situ hybridization (Vago et al., 1996; Perrons et al., 1996; Aksamit, 1993; Ueki et al., 1994).

The degree of inflammation associated with PML may vary, and speculation has surrounded the prognostic importance of this variable finding. In most cases, one striking aspect of this infection is the absence of inflammatory response. This correlates to a lack of mass effect in areas affected, so that the lesions do not appear to be mass lesions but rather to maintain the architecture or even appear slightly atrophied. This similarly corresponds to the absence of local breakdown in blood-brain barrier at the lesions and the lack of contrast enhancement in scans. In recent years, as PML has been identified during life and success in reversal of the immunodeficient state has occurred, it appears that there are cases where increasing immune function results in a greater degree of inflammation, and perhaps in a better prognosis. In HIV the development of immune reconstitution inflammatory syndrome has been associated with some quite severe cases of PML with brain swelling and death, so the spectrum of manifestations may vary over time with the inflammatory syndromes now seen (Vendrely et al., 2005; Berenguer et al., 2001; Cinque et al., 2001).

DIAGNOSIS OF PML

Identification of PML as the cause for progressing neurological disorders has undergone rapid evolution in recent years. Until quite recently, brain biopsy was absolutely required for the confident diagnosis of this condition, and recent controlled treatment trials have required biopsy (Hall et al., 1998). The widespread exposure to JCV has made peripheral immunological testing of virtually no value, and it is believed that rarely is the brain disease the result of primary infection. Similarly, shedding of JCV in the urine, or presence of circulating JCV, most commonly in lymphocytes, may be present in healthy hosts and is even more common in immunosuppressed individuals, making it of sadly little use in predicting that a brain problem may be JCV associated (Koralnik et al., 1999).

Clinical Setting

The clinical setting and presentation are important, however, in suggesting the possibility of this diagnosis. A focal neurological disorder progressing over days to weeks is typical of this illness. Most commonly motor manifestations bring the disease to light, with limb weakness, gait disturbance, and incoordination being common. Additional complaints include visual disturbance and cognitive changes (Berger et al., 1998b). Almost always, significant immunodeficiency is present when this disease develops, so the absence of an underlying immunodeficiency state would make the diagnosis almost unthinkable. HIV is the most common association at present. PML may be diagnosed with HIV infection in up to 4% of AIDS patients (Berger et al., 1998b). In most medical centers in the United States an overwhelming majority of PML cases are associated with HIV. The incidence of PML rises with declining CD4 counts, reflecting the importance of cell-mediated immunity in the pathophysiology of JCV infection in the host. In untreated HIV, it is typical for CD4 counts to be <200 cells/μl, but the range appears to be wider than is typical of most other opportunistic conditions seen in HIV infection. I have diagnosed definite PML in the presence of CD4 counts of >700 cells/μl, and as with several other opportunistic conditions, the mean CD4 counts at diagnosis appear to have risen since the advent of highly active antiretroviral therapy (HAART). Mean CD4 count was 53 (range 0 to 420) in the cytosine arabinoside trial (AIDS Clinical Trials Group 243) performed in the dual-nucleoside treatment era (Hall et al., 1998), while the more recent study of cidofovir in the HAART era has a baseline mean CD4 count of 124 cells/mm³ (Marra et al., 2002). The development of this condition in the setting of rather high CD4 counts in some cases suggests that disease-specific immunodeficiency probably exists, making highly important the efforts to define disease-specific immune parameters (Koralnik et al., 2001; Lima et al., 2007).

Clinical Presentation

Clinical presentations of PML are also helpful in suggesting the diagnosis. While the disease is often pathologically multifocal, in my experience it is most commonly clinically characteristic of a progressive focal disease. Nonlocalizing encephalopathy is not typical of PML, and encephalopathic presentations are rare enough to report separately (Zunt et al., 1997; Snyder et al., 2005). Instead, PML is typically an ideal disease for teaching localization of exam findings to students and residents because most often the historical and clinical presentation suggests clearly focal brain pathology. The actual presentation can be predicted by the pathologic localization of lesions. Common presentations include progressive asymmetric ataxia resulting from lesions of the cerebellum and its outflow, visual symptoms and signs resulting from brainstem and posterior hemispheral white matter involvement, and motor manifestations with long-tract disease suggesting a subacute upper motor neuron disease. Although one might expect aphasias to be less common since this is typically a subcortical process, lesions undercutting the speech cortex may present with progressive aphasic signs and symptoms. Spinal cord may be affected but is rarely the only, or major, site of PML.

Clinical presentation has several other useful characteristics that may be understood based on the knowledge of the pathology of this disease. While headaches occur in most people at times and are reported with PML as well, it is notable that headache is not frequently associated with the development of PML unless diplopia or other symptoms of the disease compound the tendency to develop headache. Infrequent association of headache with PML is probably because there is minimal inflammatory component pathologically and no increased pressure in the brain due to the development of this condition. The absence of headache contrasts with other inflammatory diseases or those that develop mass effect such as primary CNS lymphomas.

Imaging

Magnetic resonance (MR) brain scanning is very helpful in diagnosing PML (Hansman-Whiteman et al., 1993). The absence of definite white matter lesions, most clearly seen in T2 sequences of MR scans, should virtually eliminate this diagnosis from serious consideration. While pathologically multifocal, it is not rare for the imaging to demonstrate a single lesion in predominantly white matter regions of the brain. Other features that are very helpful include the observation that the lesions have little or no mass effect, unlike other similarly rapidly progressive complications of immunodeficiency, and that the lesions have little or no gadolinium contrast enhancement, corresponding to the rather intact blood-brain barrier. Recent reports have emphasized slight degrees of contrast enhancement (Kotecha et al., 1998; Wheeler et al., 1993) on brain scans, but even in these cases enhancement has not generally been as robust as is typical of other brain lesions with this rapid progression. In some reported cases with enhancement, unusually prominent inflammatory response has been seen in the PML lesions (Woo et al., 1996). Magnetic resonance spectroscopy may be helpful and is consistent with neuronal loss, breakdown of cell membrane and myelin, and increased glial activity in PML lesions (Chang et al., 1997; Iranzo et al., 1999). A recent report suggests prognostic value of elevated levels of myoinositol on magnetic resonance spectroscopy scans correlating to more inflammatory response and better prognosis (Katz-Brull et al., 2004). While computed tomography radiologic scans may detect areas of hypodensity, they are significantly less sensitive to MR lesions than MR scans.

Laboratory and CSF Evaluation

Analysis of the cerebrospinal fluid (CSF) has been complementary to examination and MR scanning and has improved the sensitivity and specificity to the point that in most cases, even for research purposes, a brain biopsy does not appear to be necessary. Routine CSF parameters are remarkable for their normalcy in cases of PML, most commonly being consistent with the underlying disease without further modification. Little or no additional cellular response is found in PML, the protein does not rise beyond what is anticipated for the underlying disease, and CSF glucose is normal. However, PCR detection of JCV-specific DNA has been found to be common and specific for PML in the setting of the above clinical presentation and appropriate MR lesions (Antinori et al., 1997; De Luca et al., 1996; Gibson et al., 1993; Hammarin et al., 1996; McGuire et al., 1995; Telenti et al., 1992; Weber et al., 1994b, 1994c). The sensitivity of JCV DNA detection in various labs does vary, so familiarity with the performance of the testing methodology used is critical. Most series in which specificity has been very high have less than perfect sensitivity, leaving 10 to 20% of cases negative on testing. In these cases, brain biopsy may be required, or clinical monitoring and repeat sampling of the CSF may result in detecting the condition subsequently. It is a concern that in the era of highly active HIV therapy, sensitivity of CSF PCR may be declining (Marzocchetti et al., 2005).

Developing the means of assessing the immune function may provide important ways to characterize this disease and follow the response to treatment. Thomas Weber and his colleagues have pioneered characterization of the humoral immune status of patients developing PML. PML patients have more frequent elevations of immunoglobulin G to VP1 in the CSF than do healthy controls. This has been suggested as an additional diagnostic test for PML (Weber et al., 1994a, 1997, 2001a, 2001b; Jochum et al.). Koralnik and colleagues are exploring the presence of cytotoxic T cells specific to JCV T or VP1 proteins and have found in HIV-positive patients improved prognosis with the presence of virus-specific cellular immune response (Koralnik et al., 2001; Koralnik, 2002; Lima et al., 2007). Gasnault recently evaluated anti-JCV $CD4^+$ T-cell response and found that this was present in subjects with JCV DNA excretion in urine and elevated CD4 counts but absent in the initial stages of clinical PML (Gasnault et al., 2002).

Differential Diagnosis

An interesting problem raising concern among neuro-AIDS experts has been the development of an increasing number of serious, undiagnosed white matter conditions in the setting of HAART. Neuro-AIDS centers in Italy have systematically followed presenting neurological conditions in HIV patients for some years and since the use of HAART have noted an increasing number of undiagnosed white matter lesions (Antinori et al., 2001). These fail to be consistent with PML due to negative JCV DNA in the CSF and have not uniformly been biopsied because they are not necessarily rapidly progressive. Since it is known that JCV DNA on PCR exam tends to decline and disappear in PML patients living long enough with successful HAART therapy (Clifford et al., 1999; De Viedma et al., 1999; Yiannoutsos et al., 1999), the notion that these represent a new form of PML has been considered. Pathologic evidence to date is lacking to ascertain if this is a plausible hypothesis, but given the uncertain performance of PCR diagnosis in the setting of recovering immune status, it remains a possible consideration. Another new, progressive white matter condition that has also been reported appears to be a much more disseminated leukoencephalopathy, consistent with escaping HIV encephalitis in HAART-treated patients (Langford et al., 2002). It is my experience that radiologists list PML in the differential of almost any extensive white matter condition, and thus, this too may be considered to be a form of PML, modified by the environment of HAART. However, the pathologic data in this case almost surely favor an HIV-associated cause rather than PML.

THERAPY FOR PML

Specific, effective therapy for PML has not yet been developed. Numerous obstacles have impeded the development of such therapy, yet it remains an important goal for clinical neuro-AIDS researchers. Unlike some other pathogens, PML continues to present in the era of HAART, often as a presenting complication of HIV-untreated patients, but sometimes in partially or even successfully treated patients (Clifford et al., 1998; Tantisiriwat et al., 1999). Because PML may progress to a fatal outcome or to disabling neurological status faster than immune reconstitution can be accomplished, many patients are suffering greatly from this condition. Were a specific therapy available to arrest the progress of the PML infection, this might allow time for redevelopment of successful immune responses to the infection.

Case reports of reversal of PML or a benign outcome are scattered throughout the literature, most commonly associated with efforts to reverse immunosuppression in patients. It has been well described that a significant minority, perhaps 10%, of PML patients may have a more prolonged course or achieve clinical stability, while the rest have tended to suffer a progressive course (Berger and Mucke, 1988; Berger et al., 1998b). However, HAART alone as it is currently applied remains deficient as therapy for PML (Enting and Portegies, 2000; Tantisiriwat et al., 1999; Weiner et al., 2000). Augmentation of therapy by speeding immune reconstitution or by a direct effect on the pathophysiology of JCV appears to be needed.

Cytosine Arabinoside

Numerous case reports of cytosine arabinoside (cytarabine) treatment associated with disease arrest were included in the literature through the years (Bauer et al., 1973; Berger and Mucke, 1988; Marriott et al., 1975; Blick et al., 1998; Steiger et al., 1993). Interest was further enhanced by series of cases treated intrathecally and intravenously showing unexpectedly good outcomes. An in vitro assay of JCV replication in astrocytes also demonstrated activity by cytosine arabinoside, while antiretrovirals showed no activity in this model (Hou and Major, 1998). The Neurologic AIDS Research Consortium and the AIDS Clinical Trials Group collaborated in a randomized trial using the most effective HIV therapy available at the time in all subjects (dual-nucleoside therapy, generally with the second drug added after virologic failure of the first drug, making this effectively monotherapy), using either intrathecal or intravenous cytosine arabinoside along with this therapy versus HIV therapy alone. The outcome demonstrated that in this setting cytosine arabinoside had no therapeutic benefit (Hall et al., 1998). While the study was necessary because of years of case reports suggesting its efficacy, and because it was in widespread clinical use at the time of the study, it is not surprising that the in vitro potential of cytosine arabinoside did not translate to an effective therapy, given the predicted drug penetration, which is probably inadequate either from the ventricular surfaces or from the blood. Recently, delivery of this drug via convection-enhanced infusion has been proposed (Levy et al., 2001). It is too early to know what the toxicity and efficacy of such an approach might be. Without such delivery, the addition of cytosine arabinoside to HAART also is reported to have no appreciable benefit (Enting and Portegies, 2000). Nonetheless, ongoing use particularly in non-HIV associated PML is reported with some indication of efficacy (Aksamit, 2001; Langer-Gould et al., 2005).

Cidofovir

With the elimination of routine use of cytosine arabinoside, attention was turned to cidofovir, an antiviral nucleotide that was developed for herpesviruses but showed a broad spectrum against several DNA viruses, including papova viruses (Blick et al., 1998; Gasnault et al., 1999; Portilla et al., 2000; Razonable et al., 2001). A pilot study was organized by Neurologic AIDS Research Consortium investigators that prospectively enrolled 24 PML patients in a study augmenting maximally effective antiretroviral therapy with intravenous cidofovir. The results were disappointing, with more than one-half of the patients dying by the end of the brief study, and most of the apparent benefit being associated with manifestation of HIV therapeutic responses (Marra et al., 2001, 2002). Although DeLuca et al. (2000) reported a potentially beneficial response to cidofovir in a retrospective Italian cohort, more recent continued analysis of this population is also reported to be less supportive of

this drug. Similarly, Gasnault reports no significant benefit observed in neurological outcome with the addition of cidofovir to HAART therapy (Gasnault et al., 2001). A recent meta-analysis failed to support use of cidofovir for PML.

Immune Reconstitution and the Immune Reconstitution Inflammatory Syndrome

The benefits of improved immune status, however, appear to be critical to achieving better clinical outcomes. Introduction of HAART has radically modified the prognosis of HIV-associated PML. In the post-HAART era, there are many subjects who appear to control the JCV infection with clinical stabilization, MR stabilization or improvement, and prolonged survival (Miralles et al., 1998; Berenguer et al., 2001; Dworkin et al., 1999; Cinque et al., 1998; Clifford et al., 1999; Gasnault et al., 1999; Giudici et al., 2000; Inui et al., 1999; Tassie et al., 1999). However, the best therapy available with HAART is still inadequate for approximately one-half of patients with PML (Enting and Portegies, 2000; Marra et al., 2001). Further, an increased inflammatory response early in therapy may either indicate beneficial response or be a pathologically dangerous conversion of the disease that will at least cause clinical exacerbation of the deteriorating course (Cinque et al., 2001; Miralles et al., 2001).

This longer survival of PML patients has complicated the ability of investigators to test alternative therapies directed at JCV itself. Since a relatively favorable outcome may be attained in more than one-half of subjects, pressure to randomly add highly toxic therapy becomes harder to recommend. A trial of topotecan, a topoisomerase inhibitor that may have efficacy against JCV, was stopped when efforts to enroll subjects in the trial for a somewhat toxic chemotherapeutic agent caused poor accrual to the trial, while substantial toxicity was seen (Dupont et al., 2001). Sadly, waiting to see what effect the antiretroviral therapy will achieve expends the critical time available to achieve early treatment of PML. It would seem that new surrogate markers of disease or prognosis will be required to more effectively plan studies. At present, low CD4 counts seem to have poor prognostic implications (Berger et al., 1998a; Dworkin et al., 1999), but perhaps humoral and/or cellular immune function analysis may further allow characterization of risks for progressive disease and define a population in whom distinct responses to therapeutic interventions might more reliably be tested (Du Pasquier et al., 2001; Weber et al., 2001b). JC viral load in the CSF may also be prognostic (De Luca et al., 1999; Taoufik et al., 2000; Yiannoutsos et al., 1999; Garcia et al., 2002). It seems that clinical stabilization in the course of PML is generally accompanied by clearing JC DNA from the CSF (Miralles et al., 1998). Better understanding of the changes in the virus that are associated with poor prognosis also is under consideration. It is reported that the presence of tandem repeats in plasma and especially CNS JCV regulatory region clones is associated with poor clinical outcome in patients with PML (Pfister et al., 2001).

IFN

Alpha interferon (IFN-α) is an agent for which observations of efficacy were probably confused by introduction of HAART. Early in the HIV epidemic an open-label trial failed to document likely benefit. However, in the era of early experience with HAART therapy, some series suggested that IFN-α might after all be making a clinical difference for PML patients (Huang et al., 1998). However, more recent analysis of this retrospective data set with attention to the impact of HAART fails to substantiate a convincing treatment effect for IFN-α (Geschwind et al., 2001).

Other Experimental Therapeutics

Future approaches to treatment of PML are clearly needed. Based on the observation that CD4 responses are important in the prognosis of the disease, early elevation of CD4 counts would appear to be potentially helpful. Interleukin-2 is being evaluated for its ability to raise circulating CD4 counts and has been considered as an intervention for PML, although it is recognized that functional CD4 count may not be increased, nor may the increase be in the site of disease. However, a few case reports support the possibility that administration of interleukin-2 could be beneficial (Przepiorka et al., 1997; Re et al., 1999). Splenectomy has also been reported to increase CD4 counts, and one case report describes a remission of PML following splenectomy and antiretroviral therapy (Power et al., 1997).

A recent observation that in vitro a subclass of serotonin receptors, the 5HT2a receptors, may play a role in the entry of JCV into cells has led to considerations of another approach to prevention or therapy. Atwood and colleagues (Elphick et al., 2004) report that antagonists to this receptor result in blocking infection. Since several approved drugs that are widely used are antagonists at this receptor, physicians have been interested in their potential to slow or limit the spread of PML. Whether sufficient changes of receptor density could be made to significantly control this disease remains an important clinical question, as does the dependence of this mechanism for spread of disease in vivo.

SUMMARY

PML remains an important challenge for clinicians and researchers. Increasing ability to detect and tract the activity of this ubiquitous virus will enhance our understanding of its pathobiology. It is encouraging that increasing worldwide attention is directed toward the biology of JCV, and active dialogue among investigators is being nurtured by regular international meetings. From this increasing base of knowledge, new approaches to early diagnosis and therapy may yet achieve vastly improved outcomes for our patients.

REFERENCES

Aksamit, A. J. 1993. Nonradioactive in situ hybridization in progressive multifocal leukoencephalopathy. *Mayo Clin. Proc.* **68:**899–910.

Aksamit, A. J. 2001. Treatment of non-AIDS progressive multifocal leukoencephalopathy with cytosine arabinoside. *J. Neurovirol.* **7:**386–390.

Aksamit, A. J., J. L. Sever, and E. O. Major. 1986. Progressive multifocal leukoencephalopathy: JC virus detection by in situ hybridization compared with immunohistochemistry. *Neurology* **36:**499–504.

Angelini, L., M. C. Pietrogrande, M. R. Delle Piane, F. Zibordi, P. Cinque, C. Maccagnano, and L. Vago. 2001. Progressive multifocal leukoencephalopathy in a child with hyperimmunoglobulin E recurrent infection syndrome and review of the literature. *Neuropediatrics* **32:**250–255.

Antinori, A., A. Ammassari, P. Cinque, L. Toma, A. Govoni, F. Soldani, M. L. Giancola, S. Grisetti, C. Pierotti, C. Fausti, M. G. Finazzi, T. Bini, B. Del Grosso, L. Cristiano, P. Corsi, G. Fasulo, M. Mena, G. Guaraldi, M. I. Arcidiacono, L. Monno, B. Gigli, G. C. Fibbia, M. Gentile, A. Mastroianni, F. Speranza, A. d'Arminio Monforte, G. Rezza, and G. Ippolito. 2001. Shift of prevalence and selected characteristics in HIV-1-related neurologic disorders in HAART era: data from Italian Register Investigative Neuro AIDS (IRINA), p. 45. *In 8th Conference on Retroviruses and Opportunistic Infections.* CROI, Alexandria, VA.

Antinori, A., A. Ammassari, A. De Luca, A. Cingolani, R. Murri, G. Scoppettuolo, M. Fortini, T. Tartaglione, L. M. Larocca, G. Zannoni, P. Cattani, R. Grillo, R. Roselli, M. Iacoangeli, M. Scerrati, and L. Ortona. 1997. Diagnosis of AIDS-related focal brain lesions: a decision-making analysis based on clinical and neuroradiologic characteristics combined with polymerase chain reaction assays in CSF. *Neurology* **48:**687–694.

Astrom, K. E., E. L. Mancall, and E. P. Richardson, Jr. 1958. Progressive multifocal leukoencephalopathy, a hitherto unrecognized complication of chronic lymphatic leukemia and Hodgkin's disease. *Brain* **81:**93–111.

Bauer, W. R., A. P. Truel, and K. P. Johnson. 1973. Progressive multifocal leukoencephalopathy and cytarabine. *JAMA* **226:**174–176.

Berenguer, J., P. Miralles, J. Arrizabalaga, E. Ribera, F. Dronda, J. Baraia, P. Domingo, M. Marquez, F. J. Rodriguez-Arrondo, F. Laguna, J. Rubio, J. López-Aldeguer, V. De Meguel, and Gesida 11/99 Study Group. 2001. Clinical course and prognostic factors of AIDS-associated progressive multifocal leukoencephalopathy (PML) in patients treated with HAART, p. 45. *In 8th Conference on Retroviruses and Opportunistic Infection.* CROI, Alexandria, VA.

Berger, J. R., R. M. Levy, D. Flomenhoft, and M. Dobbs. 1998a. Predictive factors for prolonged survival in acquired immunodeficiency syndrome-associated progressive multifocal leukoencephalopathy. *Ann. Neurol.* **44:**341–349.

Berger, J. R., and L. Mucke. 1988. Prolonged survival and partial recovery in AIDS-associated progressive multifocal leukoencephalopathy. *Neurology* **38:**1060–1065.

Berger, J. R., L. Pall, D. Lanska, and M. Whiteman. 1998b. Progressive multifocal leukoencephalopathy in patients with HIV infection. *J. Neurovirol.* **4:**59–68.

Blick, G., M. Whiteside, P. Griegor, U. Hopkins, T. Garton, and L. LaGravinese. 1998. Successful resolution of progressive multifocal leukoencephalopathy after combination therapy with cidofovir and cytosine arabinoside. *Clin. Infect. Dis.* **26:**191–192.

Chang, L., T. Ernst, C. Tornatore, H. Aronow, R. Melchor, I. Walot, E. Singer, and M. Cornford. 1997. Metabolite abnormalities in progressive multifocal leukoencephalopathy by proton magnetic resonance spectroscopy. *Neurology* **48:**836–845.

Cinque, P., S. Casari, and D. Bertelli. 1998. Progressive multifocal leukoencephalopathy, HIV and highly active antiretroviral therapy. *N. Engl. J. Med.* **339:**848–849.

Cinque, P., C. Pierotti, M. G. Vigano, A. Bestetti, C. Fausti, D. Bertelli, and A. Lazzarin. 2001. The good and evil of HAART in HIV-related progressive multifocal leukoencephalopathy. *J. Neurovirol.* **7:**358–363.

Clifford, D. B., and Neurological AIDS Research Consortium Study Team. 1998. Impact on highly active antiretroviral therapy on survival from progressive multifocal leukoencephalopathy in human immunodeficiency virus infection. *Neurology* **50:**A249.

Clifford, D. B., C. Yiannoutsos, M. Glicksman, D. M. Simpson, E. J. Singer, P. J. Piliero, C. M. Marra, G. S. Francis, J. C. McArthur, K. L. Tyler, A. C. Tselis, and N. E. Hyslop. 1999. HAART improves prognosis in HIV-associated progressive multifocal leukoencephalopathy. *Neurology* **52:**623–625.

De Luca, A., A. Cingolani, A. Linzalone, A. Ammassari, R. Murri, M. L. Giancola, G. Maiuro, and A. Antinori. 1996. Improved detection of JC virus DNA in cerebrospinal fluid for diagnosis of AIDS-related progressive multifocal leukoencephalopathy. *J. Clin. Microbiol.* **34:**1343–1346.

De Luca, A., M. L. Giancola, A. Ammassari, S. Grisetti, A. Cingolani, M. G. Paglia, A. Govoni, R. Murri, L. Testa, A. d'Arminio Monforte, and A. Antinori. 2000. Cidofovir added to HAART improves virological and clinical outcome in AIDS-associated progressive multifocal leukoencephalopathy. *AIDS* **14:**1–5.

De Luca, A., M. L. Giancola, A. Cingolani, A. Ammassari, L. Gillini, R. Murri, and A. Antinori. 1999. Clinical and virological monitoring during treatment with intrathecal cytarabine in patients with AIDS-associated progressive multifocal leukoencephalopathy. *Clin. Infect. Dis.* **28:**624–628.

De Viedma, D. G., R. Alonso, P. Miralles, J. Berenguer, M. Rodriguez-Créixems, and E. Bouza. 1999. Dual qualitative-quantitative nested PCR for detection of JC virus in cerebrospinal fluid: high potential for evaluation and monitoring of progressive multifocal leukoencephalopathy in AIDS patients receiving highly active antiretroviral therapy. *J. Clin. Microbiol.* **37:**724–728.

Du Pasquier, R. A., K. W. Clark, P. S. Smith, J. T. Joseph, J. M. Mazullo, U. De Girolami, N. L. Letvin, and I. J. Koralnik. 2001. JCV-specific cellular immune response correlates with a favorable clinical outcome in HIV-infected individuals with progressive multifocal leukoencephalopathy. *J. Neurovirol.* **7:**318–322.

Dupont, B., D. Fish, D. McGuire, W. Royal, E. Singer, K. Goodkin, D. Graden, H. Martino, S. Hearn, G. Ross, and R. Beckman. 2001. 21-day continuous infusion of Topotecan in AIDS-associated progressive multifocal leukoencephalopathy (PML), p. 223. *In 8th Conference on Retroviruses and Opportunistic Infections.* CROI, Alexandria, VA.

Dworkin, M. S., P. T. Wan, D. L. Hanson, J. L. Jones, and Adult & Adolescent Spectrum of HIV Disease Project. 1999. Progressive multifocal leukoencephalopathy: improved survival of human immunodeficiency virus-infected patients in the protease inhibitor era. *J. Infect. Dis.* **180:**621–625.

Elphick, G. F., W. Querbes, J. A. Jordan, G. V. Gee, S. Eash, K. Manley, A. Dugan, M. Stanifer, A. Bhatnagar, W. Kroeze, B. L. Roth, and W. J. Atwood. 2004. The human polyomavirus, JCV, uses serotonin receptors to infect cells. *Science* **306:**1380–1383.

Enting, R. H., and P. Portegies. 2000. Cytarabine and highly active antiretroviral therapy in HIV-related progressive multifocal leukoencephalopathy. *J. Neurol.* **247:**134–138.

Garcia, D., V. I. M. Diaz, P. Miralles, J. Berenguer, M. Marin, L. Munoz, and E. Bouza. 2002. JC virus load in progressive multifocal leukoencephalopathy: analysis of the correlation between the viral burden in cerebrospinal fluid, patient survival, and the volume of neurological lesions. *Clin. Infect. Dis.* **34:**1568–1575.

Gasnault, J., M. Kahraman, M. G. de Goër, J. F. Delfraissy, and Y. Taoufik. 2002. Analysis of anti-JC virus CD4+ T-cell response in healthy subjects and in HIV+ patients with or without progressive multifocal leukoencephalopathy, p. 317. *In 9th Conference on Retroviruses and Opportunistic Infections.* CROI, Alexandria, VA.

Gasnault, J., P. Kousignian, M. Kahraman, J. Rahoiljaon, S. Matheron, J. F. Delfraissy, and Y. Taoufik. 2001. Cidofovir in AIDS-associated progressive multifocal leukoencephalopathy: a monocenter observational study with clinical and JC virus load monitoring. *J. Neurovirol.* **7:**375–381.

Gasnault, J., Y. Taoufik, C. Goujard, P. Kousignian, K. Abbed, F. Boué, E. Dussaix, and J. F. Delfraissy. 1999. Prolonged survival without neurological improvement in patients with AIDS-related progressive multifocal leukoencephalopathy on potent combined antiretroviral therapy. *J. Neurovirol.* **5:**421–429.

Geschwind, M. D., R. I. Skolasky, W. S. Royal, and J. C. McArthur. 2001. The relative contributions of HAART and

alpha-interferon for therapy of progressive multifocal leukoencephalopathy in AIDS. *J. Neurovirol.* **7:**353–357.

Gibson, P. E., W. A. Knowles, J. F. Hand, and D. W. G. Brown. 1993. Detection of JC virus DNA in the cerebrospinal fluid of patients with progressive multifocal leukoencephalopathy. *J. Med. Virol.* **39:**278–281.

Giudici, B., B. Vaz, S. Bossolasco, S. Casari, A. M. Brambilla, W. Lüke, A. Lazzarin, T. Weber, and P. Cinque. 2000. Highly active antiretroviral therapy and progressive multifocal leukoencephalopathy: effects on cerebrospinal fluid markers of JC virus replication and immune response. *Clin. Infect. Dis.* **30:**95–99.

Hall, C. D., U. Dafni, D. Simpson, D. B. Clifford, P. E. Wetherill, B. Cohen, J. C. McArthur, H. Hollander, C. Yiannoutsos, E. Major, L. Millar, J. Timpone, and AIDS Clinical Trials Group 243 Team. 1998. Failure of cytarabine in progressive multifocal leukoencephalopathy associated with human immunodeficiency virus infection. *N. Engl. J. Med.* **338:**1345–1351.

Hammarin, A. L., G. Bogdanovic, V. Svedhem, R. Pirskanen, L. Morfeldt, and M. Grandien. 1996. Analysis of PCR as a tool for detection of JC virus DNA in cerebrospinal fluid for diagnosis of progressive multifocal leukoencephalopathy. *J. Clin. Microbiol.* **34:**2929–2932.

Hansman-Whiteman, M. L., M. J. Donovan Post, J. R. Berger, L. G. Tate, M. D. Bell, and L. P. Limonte. 1993. Progressive multifocal leukoencephalopathy in 47 HIV-seropositive patients: neuroimaging with clinical and pathologic correlation. *Radiology* **187:**233–240.

Hou, J., and E. O. Major. 1998. The efficacy of nucleoside analogs against JC virus multiplication in a persistently infected human fetal brain cell line. *J. Neurovirol.* **4:**451–456.

Howatson, A. F., M. Nagai, and G. M. ZuRhein. 1965. Polyoma-like virions in human demyelinating brain disease. *Can. Med. Assoc. J.* **93:**379–386.

Huang, S. S., R. L. Skolasky, G. J. Dal Pan, W. Royal III, and J. C. McArthur. 1998. Survival prolongation in HIV-associated progressive multifocal leukoencephalopathy treated with alpha-interferon: an observational study. *J. Neurovirol.* **4:**324–332.

Inui, K., H. Miyagawa, J. Sashihara, H. Miyoshi, K. Tanaka-Taya, T. Nishigaki, S. Teraoka, T. Mano, J. Ono, and S. Okada. 1999. Remission of progressive multifocal leukoencephalopathy following highly active antiretroviral therapy in a patient with HIV infection. *Brain Dev.* **21:**416–419.

Iranzo, A., A. Moreno, J. Pujol, J. Martí-Fàbregas, P. Domingo, J. Molet, J. Ris, and J. Cadafalch. 1999. Proton magnetic resonance spectroscopy pattern of progressive multifocal leukoencephalopathy in AIDS. *J. Neurol. Neurosurg. Psychiatry* **66:**520–523.

Jensen, P. N., and E. O. Major. 2001. A classification scheme for human polyomavirus JCV variants based on the nucleotide sequence of the noncoding regulatory region. *J. Neurovirol.* **7:**280–287.

Jochum, W., T. Weber, S. Frye, G. Hunsmann, W. Lüke, and A. Aguzzi. 1997. Detection of JC virus by anti-VP1 immunohistochemistry in brains with progressive multifocal leukoencephalopathy. *Acta Neuropathol.* **94:**226–231.

Katz, D. A., J. R. Berger, B. Hamilton, E. O. Major, and J. Donovan Post. 1994. Progressive multifocal leukoencephalopathy complicating Wiskott-Aldrich syndrome. *Arch. Neurol.* **51:**422–426.

Katz-Brull, R., R. E. Lenkinski, R. A. Du Pasquier, and I. J. Koralnik. 2004. Elevation of myoinositol is associated with disease containment in progressive multifocal leukoencephalopathy. *Neurology* **63:**897–900.

Kinoshita, M., K. Iwana, H. Shinoura, S. Aotsuka, and M. Sumiya. 1998. Progressive multifocal leukoencephalopathy resembling central nervous system systemic lupus erythematosus. *Clin. Exp. Rheumatol.* **16:**313–315.

Kleinschmidt-DeMasters, B. K., and K. L. Tyler. 2005. Progressive multifocal leukoencephalopathy complicating treatment with natalizumab and interferon beta-1a for multiple sclerosis. *N. Engl. J. Med.* **353:**369–374.

Knowles, W. A., P. Pipkin, N. Andrews, A. Vyse, P. Minor, W. G. Brown, and E. Miller. 2003. Population-based study of antibody to the human polyomaviruses BKV and JCV and the simian polyomavirus SV40. *J. Med. Virol.* **71:**115–123.

Koralnik, I. J. 2002. Overview of the cellular immunity against JC virus in progressive multifocal leukoencephalopathy. *J. Neurovirol.* **8:**59–65.

Koralnik, I. J., R. A. Du Pasquier, and N. L. Letvin. 2001. JC virus-specific cytotoxic T lymphocytes in individuals with progressive multifocal leukoencephalopathy. *J. Virol.* **75:**3483–3487.

Koralnik, I. J., J. E. Schmitz, M. A. Lifton, M. A. Forman, and N. L. Letvin. 1999. Detection of JC virus DNA in peripheral blood cell subpopulations of HIV-1-infected individuals. *J. Neurovirol.* **5:**430–435.

Kotecha, N., M. J. George, T. W. Smith, F. Corvi, and N. S. Litofsky. 1998. Enhancing progressive multifocal leukoencephalopathy: an indicator of improved immune status. *Am. J. Med.* **105:**541–543.

Langer-Gould, A., S. W. Atlas, A. W. Bollen, and D. Pelletier. 2005. Progressive multifocal leukoencephalopathy in a patient treated with natalizumab. *N. Engl. J. Med.* **353:**375–381.

Langford, T. D., S. L. Letendre, T. D. Marcotte, R. J. Ellis, J. A. McCutchan, I. Grant, M. E. Mallory, L. A. Hansen, S. Archibald, T. Jernigan, E. Masliah, and HNRC Group. 2002. Severe, demyelinating leukoencephalopathy in AIDS patients on antiretroviral therapy. *AIDS* **16:**1019–1029.

Levy, R. M., E. Major, M. J. Ali, B. Cohen, and D. Groothius. 2001. Convection-enhanced intraparenchymal delivery (CEID) of cytosine arabinoside (AraC) for the treatment of HIV-related progressive multifocal leukoencephalopathy (PML). *J. Neurovirol.* **7:**382–385.

Lima, M. A., A. Marzocchetti, P. Autissier, T. Tompkins, Y. Chen, J. Gordon, D. B. Clifford, R. T. Gandhi, N. Venna, J. R. Berger, and I. J. Koralnik. 2007. Frequency and phenotype of JC virus-specific CD8+ T lymphocytes in the peripheral blood of patients with progressive multifocal leukoencephalopathy. *J. Virol.* **81:**3361–3368.

Major, E. O., K. Amemiya, C. S. Tornatore, S. A. Houff, and J. R. Berger. 1992. Pathogenesis and molecular biology of progressive multifocal leukoencephalopathy, the JC virus-induced demyelinating disease of the human brain. *Clin. Microbiol. Rev.* **5:**49–73.

Marra, C. M., N. Rajicic, D. E. Barker, B. Cohen, D. Clifford, and ACTG 363 Team. 2001. Prospective pilot study of Cidofovir for HIV-associated progressive multifocal leukoencephalopathy (PML), p. 233. *In 8th Conference on Retroviruses and Opportunistic Infections.* CROI, Alexandria, VA.

Marra, C. M., N. Rajicic, D. E. Barker, B. A. Cohen, D. Clifford, M. J. D. Post, A. Ruiz, B. C. Bowen, M. L. Huang, J. Queen-Baker, J. Andersen, S. Kelly, S. Shriver, and ACTG 363 Team. 2002. A pilot study of cidofovir for progressive multifocal leukoencephalopathy in AIDS. *AIDS* **16:**1–7.

Marriott, P. J., M. D. O'Brien, I. C. K. MacKensie, and I. Janota. 1975. Progressive multifocal leukoencephalopathy: remission with cytarabine. *J. Neurol. Neurosurg. Psychiatry* **38:**205–209.

Marzocchetti, A., S. Di Giambenedetto, A. Cingolani, A. Ammassari, R. Cauda, and A. De Luca. 2005. Reduced rate of diagnostic positive detection of JC virus DNA in cerebrospinal fluid in cases of suspected progressive multifocal leu-

koencephalopathy in the era of potent antiretroviral therapy. *J. Clin. Microbiol.* **43:**4175–4177.

McGuire, D., S. Barhite, H. Hollander, and M. Miles. 1995. JC virus DNA in cerebrospinal fluid of human immunodeficiency virus-infected patients: predictive value for progressive multifocal leukoencephalopathy. *Ann. Neurol.* **37:**395–399.

Miralles, P., J. Berenguer, D. García de Viedma, B. Padilla, J. Cosin, J. C. Lopez-Bernaldo de Quirós, L. Muñoz, S. Moreno, and E. Bouza. 1998. Treatment of AIDS-associated progressive multifocal leukoencephalopathy with highly active antiretroviral therapy. *AIDS* **12:**2467–2472.

Miralles, P., J. Berenguer, C. Lacruz, J. Cosin, J. C. Lopez, B. Padilla, L. Muñoz, and D. García de Viedma. 2001. Inflammatory reactions in progressive multifocal leukoencephalopathy after highly active antiretroviral therapy. *AIDS* **15:**1900–1902.

Morgenstern, L. B., and C. A. Pardo. 1995. Progressive multifocal leukoencephalopathy complicating treatment for Wegener's granulomatosis. *J. Rheumatol.* **22:**1593–1595.

Mori, M., N. Aoki, H. Shimada, M. Tajima, and K. Kato. 1992. Detection of JC virus in the brains of aged patients without progressive multifocal leukoencephalopathy by the polymerase chain reaction and Southern hybridization analysis. *Neurosci. Lett.* **141:**151–155.

Padgett, B. L., G. M. ZuRhein, D. L. Walker, and R. J. Eckroade. 1971. Cultivation of papova-like virus from human brain with progressive multifocal leukoencephalopathy. *Lancet* **i:**1257–1260.

Perrons, C. J., J. D. Fox, S. B. Lucas, N. S. Brink, R. S. Tedder, and R. F. Miller. 1996. Detection of polyomaviral DNA in clinical samples from immunocompromised patients: correlation with clinical disease. *J. Infect.* **32:**205–209.

Pfister, L. A., N. L. Letvin, and I. J. Koralnik. 2001. JC virus regulatory region tandem repeats in plasma and central nervous system isolates correlate with poor clinical outcome in patients with progressive multifocal leukoencephalopathy. *J. Virol.* **75:**5672–5676.

Portilla, J., V. Boix, F. Román, S. Reus, and E. Merino. 2000. Progressive multifocal leukoencephalopathy treated with Cidofovir in HIV-infected patients receiving highly active anti-retroviral therapy. *J. Infect.* **41:**182–183.

Power, C., A. Nath, F. Y. Aoki, and M. Del Bigio. 1997. Remission of progressive multifocal leukoencephalopathy following splenectomy and antiretroviral therapy in a patient with HIV infection. *N. Engl. J. Med.* **336:**661–662.

Przepiorka, D., K. A. Jaeckle, R. R. Birdwell, G. N. Fuller, A. J. Kumar, Y. O. Huh, and I. McCutcheon. 1997. Successful treatment of progressive multifocal leukoencephalopathy with low-dose interleukin-2. *Bone Marrow Transplant.* **20:**983–987.

Rankin, E., and F. Scaravilli. 1995. Progressive multifocal leukoencephalopathy in a patient with rheumatoid arthritis and polymyositis. *J. Rheumatol.* **22:**777–779.

Razonable, R. R., A. J. Aksamit, A. J. Wright, and J. W. Wilson. 2001. Cidofovir treatment of progressive multifocal leukoencephalopathy in a patient receiving highly active antiretroviral therapy. *Mayo Clin. Proc.* **76:**1171–1175.

Re, D., S. Bamborschke, W. Feiden, R. Schröder, R. Lehrke, V. Diehl, and H. Tesch. 1999. Case report: progressive multifocal leukoencephalopathy after autologous bone marrow transplantation and alpha-interferon immunotherapy. *Bone Marrow Transplant.* **23:**295–298.

Richardson-Burns, S. M., B. K. Kleinschmidt-DeMasters, R. L. DeBiasi, and K. L. Tyler. 2002. Progressive multifocal leukoencephalopathy and apoptosis of infected oligodendrocytes in the central nervous system of patients with and without AIDS. *Arch. Neurol.* **59:**1930–1936.

Scotton, P. G., A. Vaglia, A. Carniato, and G. C. Marchiori. 1998. Progressive multifocal leukoencephalopathy in a patient with common variable immunodeficiency. *Clin. Infect. Dis.* **26:**215–216.

Snyder, M. D., G. A. Storch, and D. B. Clifford. 2005. Atypical PML leading to a diagnosis of common variable immunodeficiency. *Neurology* **64:**1661.

Steiger, M. J., G. Tarnesby, S. Gabe, J. McLaughlin, and A. H. V. Schapira. 1993. Successful outcome of progressive multifocal leukoencephalopathy with cytarabine and interferon. *Ann. Neurol.* **33:**407–411.

Stolt, A., K. Sasnauskas, P. Koskela, M. Lehtinen, and J. Dillner. 2003. Seroepidemiology of the human polyomaviruses. *J. Gen. Virol.* **84:**1499–1504.

Tantisiriwat, W., P. Tebas, D. B. Clifford, W. G. Powderly, and C. J. Fichtenbaum. 1999. Progressive multifocal leukoencephalopathy in patients with AIDS receiving highly active antiretroviral therapy. *Clin. Infect. Dis.* **28:**1152–1154.

Taoufik, Y., J. F. Delfraissy, and J. Gasnault. 2000. Highly active antiretroviral therapy does not improve survival of patients with high JC virus load in the cerebrospinal fluid at progressive multifocal leukoencephalopathy diagnosis. *AIDS* **14:**758–759.

Tassie, J. M., J. Gasnault, M. Bentata, J. Deloumeaux, F. Boué, E. Billaud, D. Costagliola, and Clinical Epidemiology Group from the French Hospital Database on HIV. 1999. Survival improvement of AIDS-related progressive multifocal leukoencephalopathy in the era of protease inhibitors. *AIDS* **13:**1881–1887.

Telenti, A., W. F. Marshall, A. J. Aksamit, J. D. Smilack, and T. F. Smith. 1992. Detection of JC virus by polymerase chain reaction in cerebrospinal fluid from two patients with progressive multifocal leukoencephalopathy. *Eur. J. Clin. Microbiol. Infect. Dis.* **11:**253–254.

Ueki, K., E. P. Richardson, J. W. Henson, and D. N. Louis. 1994. In situ polymerase chain reaction demonstration of JC virus in progressive multifocal leukoencephalopathy, including an index case. *Ann. Neurol.* **36:**670–673.

Vago, L., P. Cinque, E. Sala, M. Nebuloni, R. Caldarelli, S. Racca, P. Ferrante, G. R. Trabattoni, and G. Costanzi. 1996. JCV-DNA and BKV-DNA in the CNS tissue and CSF of AIDS patients and normal subjects. Study of 41 cases and review of the literature. *J. Acquir. Immune Defic. Syndr. Hum. Retrovirol.* **12:**139–146.

Van Assche, G., M. Van Ranst, R. Sciot, B. Dubois, S. Vermeire, M. Noman, J. Verbeeck, K. Geboes, W. Robberecht, and P. Rutgeerts. 2005. Progressive multifocal leukoencephalopathy after natalizumab therapy for Crohn's disease. *N. Engl. J. Med.* **353:**362–368.

Vendrely, A., B. Bienvenu, J. Gasnault, J. B. Thiebault, D. Salmon, and F. Gray. 2005. Fulminant inflammatory leukoencephalopathy associated with HAART-induced immune restoration in AIDS-related progressive multifocal leukoencephalopathy. *Acta Neuropathol.* **109:**449–455.

Weber, F., C. Goldmann, M. Krämer, F. J. Kaup, M. Pickhardt, P. Young, H. Petry, T. Weber, and W. Lüke.

2001a. Cellular and humoral immune response in progressive multifocal leukoencephalopathy. *Ann. Neurol.* **49:**636–642.

Weber, T., R. Beck, E. Stark, J. Gerhards, K. Korn, J. Haas, W. Lüer, and G. Jahn. 1994a. Comparative analysis of intrathecal antibody synthesis and DNA amplification for the diagnosis of cytomegalovirus infection of the central nervous system in AIDS patients. *J. Neurol.* **241:**407–414.

Weber, T., C. Trebst, S. Frye, P. Cinque, L. Vago, C. J. M. Sindic, W. J. Schulz-Schaeffer, H. A. Kretzschmar, W. Enzensberger, G. Hunsmann, and W. Lüke. 1997. Analysis of the systemic and intrathecal humoral immune response in progressive multifocal leukoencephalopathy. *J. Infect. Dis.* **176:**250–254.

Weber, T., R. W. Turner, S. Frye, W. Lüke, H. A. Kretzschmar, W. Lüer, and G. Hunsmann. 1994b. Progressive multifocal leukoencephalopathy diagnosed by amplification of JC virus-specific DNA from cerebrospinal fluid. *AIDS* **8:**49–57.

Weber, T., R. W. Turner, S. Frye, B. Ruf, J. Haas, E. Schielke, H. D. Pohle, W. Lüke, W. Lüer, K. Felgenhauer, and G. Hunsmann. 1994c. Specific diagnosis of progressive multifocal leukoencephalopathy by polymerase chain reaction. *J. Infect. Dis.* **169:**1138–1141.

Weber, T., F. Weber, H. Petry, and W. Luke. 2001b. Immune response in progressive multifocal leukoencephalopathy: an overview. *J. Neurovirol.* **7:**311–317.

Weiner, S. M., J. Laubenberger, K. Müller, J. Schneider, and W. Kreisel. 2000. Fatal course of HIV-associated progressive multifocal leukoencephalopathy despite successful highly active antiretroviral therapy. *J. Infect.* **40:**100–102.

Wheeler, A. L., C. L. Truwit, B. K. Kleinschmidt-DeMasters, W. R. Byrne, and R. N. Hannon. 1993. Progressive multifocal leukoencephalopathy: contrast enhancement on CT scans and MR images. *AJR Am. J. Roentgenol.* **161:**1049–1051.

Woo, H. H., A. R. Rezai, E. A. Knopp, H. L. Weiner, D. C. Miller, and P. J. Kelly. 1996. Contrast-enhancing progressive multifocal leukoencephalopathy: radiological and pathological correlations: case report. *Neurosurgery* **39:**1031–1035.

Yiannoutsos, C. T., E. O. Major, B. Curfman, P. N. Jensen, M. Gravell, J. Hou, D. B. Clifford, and C. D. Hall. 1999. Relation of JC virus DNA in the cerebrospinal fluid to survival in acquired immunodeficiency syndrome patients with biopsy-proven progressive multifocal leukoencephalopathy. *Ann. Neurol.* **45:**816–820.

Yousry, T. A., E. O. Major, C. Ryschkewitsch, G. Fahle, S. Fischer, J. Hou, B. Curfman, K. Miszkiel, N. Mueller-Lenke, E. Sanchez, F. Barkhof, E. W. Radue, H. R. Jäger, and D. B. Clifford. 2006. Evaluation of patients treated with natalizumab for progressive multifocal leukoencephalopathy. *N. Engl. J. Med.* **354:**924–933.

Zunt, J. R., R. K. Tu, D. M. Anderson, M. C. Copass, and C. M. Marra. 1997. Progressive multifocal leukoencephalopathy presenting as human immunodeficiency virus type 1 (HIV)-associated dementia. *Neurology* **49:**263–265.

The Spectrum of Neuro-AIDS Disorders:
Pathophysiology, Diagnosis, and Treatment
Edited by K. Goodkin et al.
©2008 ASM Press, Washington, DC

27

Epstein-Barr Virus Infection and Primary Central Nervous System Lymphoma

ALEX TSELIS AND ROBERT McKENDALL

BRIEF HISTORICAL BACKGROUND

The discovery of Epstein-Barr virus (EBV) is a fascinating medical detective story. An illness consisting of fever, malaise, pharyngitis, cervical lymphadenopathy, and splenomegaly had been described during the 19th and early 20th centuries by different physicians in Europe and was gradually differentiated from other febrile illnesses (Carter and Penman, 1969). This so-called glandular fever was found by Sprunt and Evans to be associated with a very high peripheral leukocytosis and was termed "infectious mononucleosis" (IM) by them (Sprunt and Evans, 1920). Shortly thereafter, Paul and Bunnell discovered that the sera of acute-phase IM patients strongly agglutinated sheep red blood cells (Paul and Bunnell, 1932). This gave rise to the Paul-Bunnell test, which is the basis of the modern IM slide tests. This reaction occurred only in the acute illness. Many attempts to isolate the pathogen responsible for IM failed.

In the late 1950s, Denis Burkitt, a British missionary surgeon in East Africa, noted a number of children with a very unusual jaw tumor (Burkitt, 1958). These patients frequently also had tumor deposits, soon identified as lymphoma, in multiple viscera. A survey of the geographical distribution of the prevalence of the tumor showed that it coincided with areas of high prevalence of malaria and some arboviral diseases. This suggested the possibility of a vector-borne disease. In 1961 Burkitt gave a talk about the disease on a visit back to London, and Anthony Epstein, a virologist with an interest in tumor viruses, was in the audience. An arrangement was made for tumor samples to be sent to Epstein's laboratory for further study. Neoplastic cells, immortalized and proliferating, were obtained from these samples, but conventional methods for isolation of a virus were fruitless. Electron microscopy, however, showed virions with the typical morphology of herpesviruses (Epstein et al., 1964).

Samples of the tumor were then sent to the laboratory of Werner and Gertrude Henle at the Children's Hospital of Philadelphia for further characterization. They found that antibodies to the virus were common in the general population and not especially more prevalent in cancer patients. In 1967 one of the technicians in the Henle laboratory, whose serum served as a negative control in their studies, became ill with infectious mononucleosis (diagnosed clinically and by the heterophile test). Her serum subsequently became highly seropositive (Henle et al., 1968). This was the first observation connecting EBV to infectious mononucleosis.

Epidemiologic studies followed, and the link between infectious mononucleosis and EBV was established. Many of these studies involved college students whose serum was banked and who were monitored for the development of IM. Only those seronegative were at risk for IM, and they all seroconverted, while those seropositive at baseline never developed IM (Evans et al., 1968). A large cohort study of African children also established the link between Burkitt's lymphoma and EBV (de Thé et al., 1978). Other diseases shown to be caused by EBV include posttransplant lymphoproliferative disorder (PTLD), nasopharyngeal carcinoma (NPC), and Hodgkin's disease. The link to NPC was uncovered by a survey of EBV titers in sera of patients with different diseases (Old et al., 1968). A group of patients with NPC had titers to EBV as high as those of Burkitt's lymphoma patients, and biopsy specimens of these lesions eventually showed that the carcinoma cells were latently infected with a single EBV clone.

In the early 1980s, AIDS patients were noted to have an unusually high incidence of B-cell lymphomas. Primary central nervous system (CNS) lymphomas (PCNSL) occurred in 5% of patients, a very high proportion for such an otherwise rare tumor, being monitored at an AIDS clinic in San Francisco (Ziegler et al., 1984; So et al., 1986).

VIROLOGY

EBV is a double-stranded DNA virus of 172 kbp. It is classified as a lymphocryptovirus in the gammaherpesvirus group. The viral genome is encased in an icosahedral capsid,

Alex Tselis, Department of Neurology, Wayne State University, Detroit, MI 48201. **Robert McKendall,** Department of Neurology, Department of Microbiology and Immunology, University of Texas Medical Branch, Galveston, TX 77555.

surrounded by an amorphous "tegument" (containing several nonstructural proteins of various functions), which is enclosed in a viral envelope. There are several intrinsic membrane proteins.

The viral genome is organized in a manner typical of the herpesviruses. The genome has a unique long segment and a unique short segment, in tandem, separated by a segment of multiple tandem repeats (6 to 12 of them) of a stretch of 3,071 bp. The unique long segment is further broken up into four smaller segments by tandem internal repeats (Kieff et al., 1982). This number of repeats is conserved in each strain of EBV and can be used for molecular epidemiologic tracing.

EBV infects a restricted number of cell types, including B and T lymphocytes, epithelial cells (in the oropharynx and in nasopharyngeal and gastric carcinoma cells), and smooth muscle cells. It is not known to infect neural cells such as neurons, oligodendrocytes, or astrocytes. B lymphocytes are immortalized by EBV. Ordinarily, B cells do not survive long in vitro. If infected with EBV, however, they form immortalized proliferating clones, known as lymphoblastoid cell lines. These have found a number of practical uses in the laboratory. Thus, Raji cells express a complement receptor and are used in assays of circulating immune complexes.

There are two main types of EBV infection, lytic and latent. In lytic infection the virus replicates in a permissive cell, lyses it, and is released to infect other cells. In latent infection, viral DNA is present in the cell, along with a limited number of viral proteins and RNA transcripts, but no active synthesis of virions occurs. There are several types of latency, to be discussed below. However, they share the property that the integrity of the cells is maintained. Viral replication also occurs in a lytic or latent manner. In lytic replication, DNA replication is specifically by a viral DNA polymerase and synthesis of virions proceeds as above. In latent replication, on the other hand, EBV DNA is replicated by host DNA polymerase, so that when a single lymphocyte with one EBV DNA genome undergoes mitosis, the product is two B lymphocytes, with two EBV genome copies, one allocated to each B cell (Colby et al., 1980).

The pattern of viral gene expression reflects either the lytic or the latent nature of infection and is thus highly regulated. In lytic infection, a coordinated expression of immediate early, early, and late genes, with production of regulatory proteins, viral DNA polymerase, and structural proteins, respectively, leads to the construction of fully mature virions, ready to be released and infect other cells. In latent infection, on the other hand, the virus is present in the nucleus of the cell as an episome (only rarely is the viral genome integrated directly into host chromosomes), and only a restricted set of genes are expressed, depending on the precise state of latency infection, or "latency program."

Latency-associated genes express several different proteins: Epstein-Barr nuclear antigen 1 (EBNA-1), EBNA-2, -3, -4, -5, and -6; LMP-1 and -2; the RNA transcripts EBV-encoded RNA 1 (EBER-1) and EBER-2; and transcripts from the BamHI A region of the genome. As stated above, there are several forms of latency expression (called latency programs) in latently infected B lymphocytes, depending on the immune status of the host. In normal carriers, only EBNA-1, EBERs, and BamHI A transcripts are expressed. EBNA-1 is relatively nonimmunogenic, and cells express this protein without being eliminated by the immune system. In patients with increasing immune deficiency, more latent proteins, with oncogenic properties, are expressed. Generally, the more immunosuppressed the host, the wider the spectrum of expression of the latency genes (Table 1).

TABLE 1 EBV latency expression

Latency program	EBV genes expressed	Clinical scenario
1	EBNA-1; EBERs; BamHI A	Normal carrier, Burkitt's lymphoma
2	EBNA-1; LMP-1 and -2; EBERs; BamHI A	H-L, T-cell lymphoma, NPC
3	EBNA-1, -2, -3, -4, -5, and -6; LMP-1 and -2; EBERs; BamHI A	EBV lymphoproliferative disease, IM, in vitro EBV-infected B lymphocytes
4	LMP-2; some EBNA-1	Circulating B cells

One may ask how EBV can be maintained in a latent or even low-level persistent state in the immunocompetent host. There are a variety of immune evasion strategies adopted by EBV (Cohen, 1997). Some of these are as follows. First, the virus codes for a protein which is an analog of interleukin-10 (IL-10), which interferes with gamma interferon (IFN-γ) synthesis. Second, the virus codes for another protein, which acts as a soluble receptor for colony-stimulating factor-1, thus decreasing the expression of IFN-α (with its antiviral effects) normally stimulated by colony-stimulating factor-1. Third, the presentation of EBNA-1, the dominantly expressed protein in type 1 latency, is inhibited. The protein contains a motif which renders the proteasomes, which degrade proteins to peptides presentable on major histocompatibility complex class I molecules to cytotoxic T cells, unable to degrade it properly. Fourth, EBV encodes several antiapoptotic proteins (Cohen, 2000).

EPIDEMIOLOGY

Infection with EBV is very common, usually occurring early in life, and is endemic in all human populations. The infection occurs even in populations that are geographically isolated, thus indicating that EBV is a fairly ancient virus. The virus is intermittently shed in saliva, and this suggests a likely route of infection. Indeed, Hoagland was the first to call IM the "kissing disease" (Hoagland, 1967). Infection tends to be asymptomatic or results in a mild febrile illness in young children but is more often symptomatic in young adults, with approximately 50% of infections resulting in the mononucleosis syndrome.

SYSTEMIC CLINICAL MANIFESTATIONS

Most acute infections with EBV in childhood are asymptomatic or are associated with a mild febrile illness indistinguishable from other childhood infections. In adolescents and young adults, IM is characterized by fever, sore throat, cervical lymphadenopathy, fatigue, and splenomegaly. Occasionally, single organ involvement (e.g., hepatitis or encephalitis) is prominent. There are occasional autoimmune manifestations, with hemolytic anemia, thrombocytopenia, arthralgias, rashes, and the development of serum autoantibodies. Most cases are self-limited. In some cases, however, infection is unusually severe and evolves into a chronic smoldering lymphoproliferative disease (chronic active EBV infection [CAEBV]), which can progress into a B-cell lymphoma, and occasionally a T-cell lymphoma.

Burkitt's lymphoma is a systemic, usually extranodal, lymphoma originally seen in African children in a sharply circumscribed geographical distribution coinciding with that of several arthropod-borne diseases, such as malaria. Classically, the disease consists of one or several localized masses, usually in the jaws, which enlarge relentlessly, and cause death by local compression of vital tissue. At autopsy, the tumors are generally located in multiple viscera, including the kidneys, liver, heart, lungs, and so forth. Burkitt's lymphoma often invades the nervous system and can result in brain parenchymal mass lesions and lymphomatous meningitis. The connection with EBV is very close in epidemic Burkitt's lymphoma in Africa, parts of South America, and New Guinea, but less so in North America and Europe. A prospective study of 42,000 African children in the West Nile district of Uganda from whom baseline EBV titers were obtained showed that those with high titers of EBV antibody were at greatest risk of developing the disease.

NPC is a tumor mostly present in Southeast Asia with an incidence of 30 to 80/100,000 in Southern China and rare elsewhere (incidence is below 1/100,000 in North America and Europe). The disease generally presents as a mass in the neck with enlargement and local involvement, which includes hearing problems, otitis media, nasal obstruction, and sinusitis, as well as dysphonia, dysphagia, and diplopia from neoplastic cranial nerve infiltration (Spano et al., 2003). The disease was first associated with EBV when a survey of sera from various cancer patients showed high titers in NPC patients. EBV DNA was found to be present in the neoplastic cells by zur Hausen (zur Hausen et al., 1970).

Hodgkin's lymphoma (HL) is a tumor consisting of a small number of neoplastic cells, Hodgkin cells (large atypical cells containing single nuclei) and Reed-Sternberg cells (large atypical cells containing several nuclei), which are closely related and are known as Hodgkin-Reed Sternberg (H-RS) cells. These cells are embedded in a reactive background consisting of lymphocytes, plasma cells, macrophages, neutrophils, eosinophils, and fibroblasts (Herbst, 1996). The disease generally presents with cervical lymphadenopathy, often along with systemic symptoms such as fever, night sweats, weight loss, and occasionally splenomegaly. Often there is mediastinal and retroperitoneal adenopathy, as well as bone marrow involvement, which may lead to a pancytopenia. Patients generally have deficient cell-mediated immunity, which renders them susceptible to viral and fungal infections. Advanced disease is associated with humoral immunodeficiency as well. The first indication of the relation between HL and EBV was the observation that those with clinical IM had a higher risk of developing HL than those not having symptomatic EBV infection (Hjalgrim et al., 2003). Furthermore, several cases of patients whose IM evolved into an HL have been reported. Finally, monoclonal EBV genomes have been detected in HL tissue samples.

T-cell lymphomas were found in a cohort of patients with severe, smoldering EBV infection (CAEBV). Three patients in this group developed a rapidly progressive systemic illness superimposed on their chronic illness and died (Jones et al., 1988). At autopsy, T-cell lymphoma was found. The conjunction of a rare neoplasm in the context of a rare disease (CAEBV) suggested an etiologic link, and EBV DNA was found in the T cells. This disease remains rare.

PATHOGENESIS OF DISEASE

The pathogenesis of EBV-related disease is most likely related to B-cell immortalization and proliferation and the immune reaction to that. Most of the time, the immune response is sufficient to easily control the proliferation and keep it controlled. This initial reaction, with the EBV-directed T cells "at war" with the EBV-infected B cells, and the associated bundle of inflammation and elaboration of cytokines form the acute illness. The eventual outcome essentially depends on the effectiveness of suppression of the lymphoproliferation. The vast majority of patients control this lymphoproliferation without much difficulty, but those with cell-mediated immune deficiency manifest a spectrum of disease.

In acute IM, a prominent leukocytosis appears in the blood, consisting of large atypical lymphocytes, which are activated T cells. Lymphoid tissues, where much of the disease process takes place, contain prominent proliferations of polymorphic lymphoid cells, some large cells with reactive morphology (immunoblasts) and others with plasmacytoid features. Macrophages may also be present and form granulomas. Other large atypical cells are seen which may resemble H-RS cells, although they display surface antigens different from those of true H-RS cells. In some cases, there is a profuse infiltration of T cells, especially in cases of IM with prominent visceral involvement.

Precisely how these proliferating B lymphocytes and their interaction with activated T cells cause tissue damage is not entirely clear, but a "bystander" mechanism is likely, with elaboration of a number of cytokines and chemokines in the actively affected tissues, both by the infected B cells themselves and by the local parenchyma and reactive infiltrating T cells (Niedobitek and Herbst, 2006). In some cases, acute IM is accompanied prominently by single organ involvement (e.g., hepatitis), and such cases may represent a situation in which the "battleground" between the proliferating B cells and T cells is focally prominent.

NEUROLOGICAL MANIFESTATIONS

There is a wide spectrum of neurological involvement in acute EBV infection. Aseptic meningitis is very common and likely underestimated. It is a typical meningitis, with headache, fever, photophobia, and a mild lymphocytic pleocytosis, which occurs in acute EBV mononucleosis, and resolves spontaneously.

Encephalitis is an uncommon manifestation of acute EBV infection but is well described. There is often (but not always) a febrile prodrome with the clinical features of IM (e.g., sore throat, cervical adenopathy, and splenomegaly). The clinical picture of the encephalitis is not especially different from that of any other viral encephalitis and includes fever, headache, delirium, seizures, and focal weakness. The precise pathogenesis of encephalitis due to EBV is not known and may be of different types, as stated above. There may be direct viral infections of cells in the CNS, most probably B lymphocytes, since neurons, astrocytes, and oligodendrocytes do not seem to be infected. Other cases of encephalitis associated with EBV are probably parainfectious forms of acute disseminated encephalomyelitis, although the peculiar mode of infection by EBV probably prevents a clear-cut distinction between infectious and postinfectious illness. Cerebellar ataxia also accompanies acute EBV mononucleosis, either coinciding with the acute illness or occurring shortly after. Serology is consistent with acute EBV infection, and cerebrospinal fluid (CSF) usually shows a very mild pleocytosis. Recovery occurs spontaneously over a few days or weeks, and relapses are quite rare. Acute transverse myelitis is a rare complication of EBV infection. The few cases ever reported with this showed slow but good improvement.

Other central manifestations of acute EBV infection include the peculiar Alice-in-Wonderland syndrome, in which there is a distortion in spatial perception, reminiscent of migrainous metamorphopsia, which is self-limited (Copperman, 1977; Eshel et al., 1987). Typically, this consists of several episodes, each lasting up to 30 min, occurring several times a day, of anxiety-provoking distortions of the size, shape, and orientation of objects in the patient's environment. Steroids and phenytoin were ineffective in the few cases in which they were tried. The symptoms resolved spontaneously within a few weeks. This parallel with migraine headaches continues with reported cases of unilateral headache with nausea and vomiting accompanied by contralateral hemiparesis, resolving several hours later (Baker et al., 1983; Leavell et al., 1986; Adamson and Gordon, 1992). The EBV serology in these cases was consistent with acute EBV infection.

Other manifestations include transient cranial nerve palsies, usually involving the facial nerve, resulting in unilateral or even bilateral Bell's palsy (Grose et al., 1973). Other cranial nerves, including the trigeminal, acoustic, and hypoglossal, have been involved, usually in the context of a febrile pharyngitis with cervical adenopathy and an EBV serological pattern typical of acute infection (Taylor and Parsons-Smith, 1969; DeSimone and Snyder, 1978).

Peripheral nerve involvement is relatively uncommon but is well described. Guillain-Barré syndrome has been associated with acute EBV infection, generally by coincidence of the illness with a positive heterophile test (Grose and Feorino, 1972). The pathology is typical for that of Guillain-Barré syndrome of any other kind. Episodes of painful shoulder leading to flaccidity of the ipsilateral arm, leading to the diagnosis of brachial plexopathy, have been described (Watson and Ashby, 1976). Several cases of gluteal pain, followed by lower extremity weakness severe enough to preclude ambulation, have been described, with an electromyographic diagnosis of lumbosacral plexopathy and acute EBV mononucleosis confirmed by a positive heterophile test. Most cases resolved, with restoration of normal or near-normal gait (Sharma et al., 1993).

EBV INFECTION IN IMMUNOCOMPROMISED AND HIV PATIENTS

EBV infection in the immunosuppressed patient is generally a result of reactivation of a latent infection, in which latently infected B cells are no longer prevented from proliferating. The cellular immune system is very efficient at suppressing such opportunistic lymphoproliferation, and only patients with severe prolonged cellular immunosuppression are likely to develop disease. Such lymphoproliferative disorders thus usually tend to occur in transplant and AIDS patients, although rarely patients with no obvious immunodeficiency are affected. PTLD occurs in 1 to 8% of patients, usually within the first year after transplant, and is usually preceded by an increase in viral burden in the blood, measured by quantitative PCR. Such an increase in viral burden also heralds other EBV-related neoplasms in high-risk populations (e.g., nasopharyngeal carcinoma in Southeast Asia).

EBV infection has a distinct spectrum of disease associations in the HIV-positive population. Titers of EBV antibodies increase in HIV-infected subjects, and as HIV disease progresses, titers to EBV viral capsid antigen (VCA) increase, while titers to EBV EBNA decrease. This may reflect a loss of control of EBV replication (either lytic or latent), and indeed EBV viral burden in the blood also increases in HIV infection. Interestingly, while high EBV loads in transplant patients are predictive of PTLD, this is not so in HIV patients.

Oral hairy leukoplakia is one of the earliest known EBV-caused diseases in HIV patients and consists of a painless whitish excrescence along the lateral borders of the tongue. It may occasionally be seen in other immunosuppressed patients. Microscopically, the lesions consist of epithelial thickening with squamous epithelial cells containing intranuclear inclusions. Some of these cells are balloonlike and have a ground glass appearance, with EBV detectable by immunohistochemistry and in situ PCR. Interestingly, both lytic and latent expression is present in the lesions. The nature of the lesion is poorly understood. Lymphoid interstitial pneumonitis is an EBV-associated disease of unclear nature.

As would be expected, opportunistic neoplasms are not rare in patients with HIV infection, and lymphomas are relatively common in this population. All types of lymphomas, both Hodgkin's and non-Hodgkin's, are seen, the latter category including immunoblastic lymphomas, large B-cell lymphomas, Burkitt's lymphomas, and primary effusion lymphomas. Overall, about 50% of HIV-associated lymphomas are EBV driven. Effusion lymphomas also frequently contain human herpesvirus 8, another member of the herpesvirus family. Some of these lymphomas have unexpected features. For instance, HIV-associated Burkitt's lymphomas, which are exclusively associated with EBV in the endemic African form of the disease, are less frequently EBV driven than other HIV-associated lymphomas. Also, HIV-associated HL can be present even in those with high CD4[+] T-cell counts.

Leiomyosarcoma is a rare tumor of smooth muscle usually seen in both adult and pediatric AIDS patients as well as transplant patients. EBV is found in almost all tumor cells, at a very high copy number, in a monoclonal episomal form.

DIAGNOSIS

The diagnosis of EBV-related disease must be planned thoughtfully, choosing appropriate methods to answer well-defined questions. Thus, a Monospot test, which detects the presence of heterophile antibodies (see below), is useful for confirming an acute primary EBV infection but does not help to diagnose CAEBV infection, oral hairy leukoplakia, or PCNSL. These require other modalities, such as biopsy, EBV viral load in the blood and CSF, etc.

In acute IM, most patients make antibodies which agglutinate sheep (and other animal, especially bovine and equine, but not human) red cells. This antibody is known to be mostly immunoglobulin M (IgM), but IgG and IgA fractions also have sheep cell agglutinating activity. Since this antibody is not directed toward EBV antigens, it is known as heterophile antibody. The original tests were crude and have been replaced by standardized extracts from beef red cells, which are available as slide tests that are sensitive, specific, and very easy to use. Heterophile antibodies are present only in acute EBV infection and are useful in demonstrating that a mononucleosis is caused by EBV or that some other febrile illness (like an encephalitis) is likely caused by EBV. However, not all cases of EBV mononucleosis are captured by the heterophile test, and an EBV panel may be needed.

More specific serological testing is available in the EBV panel, in which antibodies are measured against various

TABLE 2 Serology in EBV infection[a]

EBV status	VCA IgM	VCA IgG	EA	EBNA
Seronegative	−	−	−	−
Recent primary	+	+	+/−	−
Seropositive (remote infection)	−	+	+/−	+
IM	+	+	+	−
Reactivated infection	+/−	+++	+++	+

[a]−, no antibody; +/−, either positive or negative; +, detectable antibody; +++, high-titer antibody.

components of the virus, the lytic antigens VCA and early antigen (EA) and the latent antigens EBNA. Generally, the first antibody to appear in acute EBV infection, VCA-IgM, is IgM specific for the VCA complex. This is replaced within a few days to weeks by VCA-IgG. During the acute infection there is a transient rise in antibodies to EA, EA-IgG, which is generally considered a marker of active infection, although high titers can persist after resolution of the acute illness. Finally, as the acute infection resolves, IgG antibody to EBNA appears. This is a marker of remote infection. In the absence of a heterophile response in an illness thought likely to be EBV mononucleosis, the EBV panel can confirm or rule out involvement with this virus (Table 2).

In many situations, such as when solid lesions are present, particularly in lymphomas in immunosuppressed patients, which are suspected to be EBV driven, direct detection of EBV antigens in the abnormal tissue is possible. Thus, detection of a latency program expression confirms that a neoplasm is EBV driven. Such detection is accomplished by in situ hybridization for EBERs and immunostaining for LMP-1. The former is quite sensitive, since many copies (up to 106) are present in each cell, while the latter requires a careful search for positively staining lymphocytes.

PCNSL

PCNSL is an EBV-associated opportunistic neoplasm of the brain found in patients with very advanced HIV disease, having very low CD4$^+$ T-cell counts (usually <50/μl). This is the most common CNS manifestation of EBV infection in AIDS patients, although with the advent of highly effective combination antiretroviral therapy, the disease has become quite uncommon (Palella et al., 1998). As would be expected, the disease is aggressive, with a poor prognosis. Generally, survival is less than a month in untreated patients (see below).

The clinical presentation of PCNSL is as would be expected for an enlarging mass lesion, with focal deficits, headache, drowsiness, and occasionally seizures. Magnetic resonance imaging (MRI) generally shows ring-enhancing mass lesions which tend to be located in the deep gray structures of the brain and periventricularly in the ependyma and subependyma. Often these are single, but multifocal lymphoma is not uncommon, especially with autopsy, when most cases are multifocal. The main differential diagnosis is that of toxoplasmosis, but rarely bacterial abscesses, varicella-zoster virus leukoencephalitis, focal CMV encephalitis, and progressive multifocal leukoencephalopathy can resemble PCNSL.

The diagnosis of PCNSL depends on the demonstration of an enlarging mass lesion associated with EBV infection.

The diagnosis is suspected in a patient with progressive focal deficits whose brain MRI shows one or several ring-enhancing lesions in the deep gray structures of the brain or in the ependyma. Occasionally, pathologically proven PCNSL are nonenhancing, may show diffuse white matter involvement, or have spontaneous hemorrhages (Thurnher et al., 2001). Thus, MRI can suggest the possibility of the diagnosis but is nonspecific (Antinori et al., 1997). The workup then focuses on demonstrating that the mass is neoplastic and that it is associated with EBV infection.

The most direct way to diagnose this is to obtain tissue from biopsy of the mass. The morphology of the neoplastic B cells is variable but generally consists of large-cell, immunoblastic, and small noncleaved lymphoma cells (So et al., 1986). Almost all of these are high-grade, aggressive lymphomas (Camilleri-Broet et al., 1997). Virtually all HIV-associated PCNSL consist of neoplastic B cells which contain EBV with expression of latency markers (MacMahon et al., 1991). EBV is not detected in control specimens from HIV patients who had other opportunistic infections or from nonimmunosuppressed controls. The EBER in situ hybridization signal is found localized to tumor cells, thus demonstrating that the neoplastic B cells are infected by EBV. The B-cell nature of the cells requires confirmation of B-cell markers on the cell surface (e.g., by specific staining with the antibody L-26) (MacMahon et al., 1991). The presence of EBV is also demonstrated by appropriate detection of other latency markers such as LMP-1 by immunostaining. The latter requires a careful search for positively staining cells, since these are not numerous. At autopsy, most PCNSL are multifocal (So et al., 1986).

Less invasive methods of diagnosis are available, however. Detection of EBV in the CSF by PCR has been studied as a method of noninvasive diagnosis, because virtually all PCNSL in AIDS patients are EBV driven. A small prospective study comparing results of the biopsy method to those of CSF PCR for EBV found that the PCR was positive in all three cases of PCNSL in a series of AIDS patients and in no patient who had another diagnosis (d'Arminio Monforte et al., 1997). In a large retrospective series of 85 patients who died of AIDS, 17 of 17 patients with PCNSL had positive CSF PCRs for EBV, and only 1 of 68 who did not have PCNSL had a positive PCR, giving a sensitivity of 100% and specificity of 98.5% (Cinque et al., 1993).

Advanced imaging methods have been used to differentiate PCNSL from other mass lesions which may be typically found in this population. Several possibilities would include magnetic resonance spectroscopy (MRS), thallium-201 single photon emission tomography (SPECT), and labeled-fluorine fluorodeoxyglucose (FDG) positron emission tomography (PET) scans of the brain, since these are specifically sensitive to actively metabolizing tissue. Thallium-201 is a potassium analog that crosses the blood-brain barrier and is concentrated in neoplastic cells. FDG is a glucose analog that behaves similarly and has been used to detect systemic neoplasms (Bingham, 2002).

MRS has not been studied extensively in differentiating PCNSL from other brain lesions in AIDS patients. In one study, 26 patients with 35 lesions were studied by MRS, and PCNSL, toxoplasmosis, cryptococcoma, and progressive multifocal leukoencephalopathy were successfully differentiated by a somewhat complicated algorithm, comparing the peaks due to N-acetyl aspartate, choline, creatine, and myoinositol in each of the groups (Chang et al., 1995). This method of diagnosis has not been widely used.

Thallium-201 SPECT scanning was prospectively studied with 13 AIDS patients with intracranial masses (O'Malley et al., 1994). The relative intensity of the signals (the "uptake ratio") from the lesions was measured by the intensity in the lesion, divided by the intensity in normal tissue. For the six patients who had low uptake ratios and therefore were predicted to not have PCNSL, alternative diagnoses were established in all cases. As for the other seven patients, all had PCNSL except for one. In a meta-analysis of 10 studies of the utility of thallium scans in diagnosing PCNSL, with a total of 312 subjects, Skiest found an average sensitivity and specificity of 92 and 89%, respectively (Skiest, 2002).

FDG PET scanning is not a commonly available imaging modality. In a study of 11 AIDS patients with CNS lesions, the use of a very simple semiquantitative measure of FDG uptake by a lesion (grades 1 through 5, by eye) could predict very accurately whether a lesion was lymphoma (Hoffman et al., 1993). A quantitative analysis confirmed the results. In another study, 11 AIDS patients with brain lesions were studied by FDG PET scans. Four were diagnosed with PCNSL pathologically, and the other seven had other disease (some established indirectly) (Villringer et al., 1995). All of the PCNSL lesions had high uptake of FDG, while none of the others (six toxoplasmosis lesions and one tuberculoma) did. The technology of PET is rather elaborate, and the test is very expensive.

Combined diagnostic modalities are probably the best way to noninvasively diagnose PCNSL. A study of thallium-201 SPECT scan together with detection of EBV DNA in the CSF by PCR involving 31 AIDS patients with CNS lesions, 11 of whom had PCNSL, showed that the simultaneous presence of both increased uptake of thallium-201 by the lesion and a positive EBV DNA in the CSF by PCR was 100% sensitive and 100% specific for PCNSL in these patients (Antinori et al., 1999). The authors of the study suggested that biopsy was appropriate for discordant results.

HAART, CHEMOTHERAPY, AND RADIATION IN PCNSL

Treatment of PCNSL is difficult, and the overall prognosis is poor. The natural history of the disease is that of progressive deterioration to death within a few weeks to months. No definitive prospective randomized trials comparing various modes of antineoplastic therapy have been done.

Several broad approaches are possible. First would be immune reconstitution by treatment with highly active antiretroviral therapy (HAART), which would restore immune reactivity against latent EBV antigens that would eliminate EBV-driven neoplastic B cells. Second would be therapy directed against the neoplastic B cells themselves, as in any other form of cancer. Systemic chemotherapy can be used, as in patients with non-HIV-related PCNSL, but the concern is that since HIV patients with PCNSL are already severely immunosuppressed, this would be difficult to tolerate. Another directly antineoplastic approach would be that of cranial irradiation, which would be less likely to have the systemic toxicity of chemotherapy. Third, various other immunologic approaches have recently been explored for patients with various forms of lymphoma, especially PTLDs. These include cytokine and anticytokine therapy and the intriguing method of using EBV-specific HLA-matched cytotoxic T cells, expanded in vitro, in the treatment of PCNSL.

Restoration of immune function by suppressing HIV viral load has been reported in individual case reports and case series. In one case of PCNSL in an AIDS patient, a biopsy-proven diffuse large cell lymphoma was treated with a switch from an antiretroviral regimen containing two nucleoside reverse transcriptase inhibitors (NRTIs) to two other NRTIs and a protease inhibitor, after he declined radiation and chemotherapy. He gradually improved, and a repeat computed tomography scan several months later showed no evidence of disease (McGowan and Shah, 1998). In another AIDS patient, a biopsy of a frontal lobe mass showed a large cell lymphoma, and the CSF was positive for EBV. He was started on IL-2 (a T-cell growth factor), ganciclovir (which decreases lytic EBV replication), and highly active antiretroviral therapy (HAART) (two NRTIs and one protease inhibitor). Clinical improvement was evident within the next 10 days, and 6 months later the mass was considerably smaller on MRI (Aboulafia, 2002).

Several studies compared the effects of HAART and cranial irradiation on the course of HIV PCNSL. All of these studies are retrospective. In one, 29 patients with PCNSL were followed up (Hoffman et al., 2001). Twelve were treated with cranial radiation, and six received HAART. The others were treated with neither. Patients treated with HAART and those treated with radiation both had significantly longer survival than those not so treated. In another retrospective series of 25 patients diagnosed with HIV-related PCNSL, the median survival in 11 patients who did not receive HAART was 29 days, whereas 6 of 7 patients treated with HAART were alive at a median follow-up period of 667 days (Skiest and Crosby, 2003). Whole-brain radiation also provided a survival advantage. In a group of 55 patients with HIV-associated PCNSL, those treated with whole-brain irradiation survived longer than those who were not, with a mean survival of 134 versus 42 days (Baumgartner et al., 1990).

Some cases of PTLD have responded to IFN-α therapy. An 11-year-old child with PTLD in transplanted lung did not respond to reduction in immunosuppression and acyclovir but had dramatic improvement with IFN-α (Faro et al., 1996). In a larger open-label study of 19 patients with PTLD, 16 did not respond to local therapy. Fourteen of these patients received a daily dose of IFN-α (3×10^6 units/m² subcutaneously for 3 weeks or longer). Of these, eight had total regression of the tumor masses (Davis et al., 1998). There are limited data on the use of IFN-α in other AIDS-associated lymphomas, but there is a rationale for its use (Tossing, 1996). There are no systematic data on the use of IFN-α in AIDS-associated PCNSL.

A novel approach to the therapy of EBV-driven lymphoproliferative states most often seen in chronically immunosuppressed posttransplant patients is that of infusing EBV-specific cytotoxic T lymphocytes (autologous or HLA-matched heterologous) which would recognize EBV antigens in the context of major histocompatibility complex class I molecules in such a way as to lyse them. This comes closest to recapitulating the natural immunity preventing such lesions in the immunocompetent subject in the first place. This approach to the therapy of EBV-driven lymphoproliferation has been exploited in PTLD therapy, whereby EBV-specific cytotoxic T cells are generated and reinfused into the patient. The procedure involves separating lymphocytes from peripheral blood and serially exposing them to irradiated autologous lymphoblastoid cell lines as well as IL-2, a growth factor (Levitsky et al., 2001). Some success has been achieved in solid organ and hematopoietic stem cell transplant-associated PTLD (Straathof et al., 2003; Gottschalk et al., 2005). Whether this could be done with PCNSL is not known, since it is unclear how easily the cytotoxic T cells would penetrate the blood-brain barrier.

Other approaches are still at the theoretical level. One possibility is that of using monoclonal antibody that depletes B cells. One such has been rituximab, which is directed to the B-cell-specific antigen CD-20, and which is being used in B-cell lymphomas. The main difficulty would be whether there would be sufficient penetration of the blood-brain barrier to have a significant effect on the tumor (Rubenstein et al., 2003) and whether this would have an added immunosuppressive effect. Rituximab has been shown to possibly increase opportunistic infections in patients with HIV-associated systemic lymphoma (Spina et al., 2005). There are no data on the use of rituximab in PCNSL. IL-6 is a growth factor for B cells, and anti-IL-6 antibodies may potentially remove one support for neoplastic B cells. In one study of anti-IL-6 monoclonal antibodies in PTLD, 12 patients were treated: 5 had complete remissions, and 3 had partial remissions, with a single relapse (Haddad et al., 2001). Another possibility would be to use statins, which have effects other than inhibiting 3-hydroxy-3-methylglutaryl coenzyme A reductase, including interruption of the interaction of certain cell adhesion molecules interfering with lymphoproliferation. This has been shown to reduce the development of macroscopic tumors in severe combined immunodeficiency (SCID) mice who are injected intraperitoneally with EBV-transformed human lymphocytes (Cohen, 2005). Finally, latently infected B cells can be rendered susceptible to ganciclovir by induction of the synthesis of thymidine kinase by exposure of these cells to butyrate (Mentzer et al., 2001). The thymidine kinase phosphorylates ganciclovir in these cells, resulting in accumulation of high concentrations and interference with the cell's metabolism. This triggers apoptosis of these cells. In a series of six patients with refractory EBV-associated lymphoma or PTLD, dual treatment with nontoxic doses of arginine butyrate and ganciclovir was given. Four patients had complete responses, and one had a partial response (Mentzer et al., 2001). Two of three patients' pathologic specimens showed complete necrosis of their lymphoma.

CONCLUSION

Infection with EBV is common and lifelong in humans and rarely results in severe disease. Latent virus may be reactivated in certain situations of chronic immunosuppression, especially in transplant and AIDS patients, in whom the reactivation consists of proliferating latently EBV-infected B lymphocytes. A prominent aspect of such lymphoproliferation is involvement of the CNS, especially a primary lymphoma in the parenchyma of the brain. Treatment of such opportunistic neoplasms is difficult, and the prognosis is still not very good despite the progress that has been made in understanding these tumors. On the other hand, recent basic research has suggested a number of new approaches, and much clinical trial work remains to be done.

REFERENCES

Aboulafia, D. 2002. Interleukin-2, ganciclovir, and high-dose zidovudine for the treatment of AIDS-associated primary central nervous system lymphoma. *Clin. Infect. Dis.* **34:**1660–1662.

Adamson, D., and P. Gordon. 1992. Hemiplegia—a rare complication of acute Epstein-Barr virus (EBV) infection. *Scand. J. Infect. Dis.* **24:**79–80.

Antinori, A., A. Ammassari, A. De Luca, A. Cingolani, R. Murri, G. Scoppettuolo, M. Fortini, T. Tartaglione, K. M. Larocca, G. Zannoni, P. Cattani, R. Grillo, R. Roselli, M. Iacoangeli, M. Scerrati, and L. Ortona. 1997. Diagnosis of AIDS-related focal brain lesions: a decision-making analysis based on clinical and neuroradiologic characteristics combined with polymerase chain reaction assays in CSF. *Neurology* **48:**87–94.

Antinori, A., G. De Rossi, A. Ammassari, A. Cingolani, R. Murri, D. Di Giuda, A. De Luca, F. Pierconti, T. Tartaglione, M. Scerrati, L. M. Larocca, and L. Ortona. 1999. Value of combined approach with thallium-201 single-photon emission computed tomography and Epstein-Barr virus DNA polymerase chain reaction in CSF for the diagnosis of AIDS-related primary CNS lymphoma. *J. Clin. Oncol.* **17:**54–60.

Baker, F., G. S. Kotchmar, Jr., W. S. Foshee, and C. V. Sumaya. 1983. Acute hemiplegia of childhood associated with Epstein-Barr virus infection. *Pediatr. Infect. Dis. J.* **2:**36–38.

Baumgartner, J., J. Rachlin, J. H. Beckstead, T. C. Meeker, R. M. Levy, W. M. Wara, and M. L. Rosenblum. 1990. Primary central nervous system lymphomas: natural history and response to radiation therapy in 55 patients with acquired immunodeficiency syndrome. *J. Neurosurg.* **73:**206–211.

Bingham, J. 2002. Where can FDG-PET contribute most to anatomical imaging problems. *Br. J. Radiol.* **75**(Spec. no.): S32–S59.

Burkitt, D. 1958. A sarcoma involving the jaws in African children. *Br. J. Surg.* **46:**218–223.

Camilleri-Broet, S., F. Davi, J. Feuillard, D. Seilhean, J. F. Michiels, P. Brousset, B. Epardeau, E. Navratil, K. Mokhtari, C. Bourgeois, L. Marelle, M. Raphael, and J. J. Hauw. 1997. AIDS-related primary brain lymphomas: histopathologic and immunohistochemical study of 51 cases. *Hum. Pathol.* **28:**367–374.

Carter, R., and H. Penman. 1969. The early history of infectious mononucleosis and its relation to "glandular fever," p. 1–18. *In* R. Carter and H. Penman (ed.), *Infectious Mononucleosis.* Blackwell Scientific Publications, Oxford, United Kingdom.

Chang, L., B. L. Miller, D. McBride, M. Cornford, G. Oropilla, S. Buchthal, F. Chiang, H. Aronow, C. K. Beck, and T. Ernst. 1995. Brain lesions in patients with AIDS: H-1 MR spectroscopy. *Radiology* **197:**525–531.

Cinque, P., M. Brytting, L. Vago, A. Castagna, C. Parravicini, N. Zanchetta, A. D'Arminio Monforte, B. Wahren, A. Lazzarin, and A. Linde. 1993. Epstein-Barr virus DNA in cerebrospinal fluid from patients with AIDS-related primary lymphoma of the central nervous system. *Lancet* **342:**398–401.

Cohen, J. 1997. Epstein-Barr virus and the immune system. Hide and seek. *JAMA* **278:**510–513.

Cohen, J. 2000. Epstein-Barr virus infection. *N. Engl. J. Med.* **343:**481–492.

Cohen, J. 2005. HMG CoA reductase inhibitors (statins) to treat Epstein-Barr virus-driven lymphoma. *Br. J. Cancer* **92:**1593–1598.

Colby, B., J. Shaw, G. B. Elion, and J. S. Pagano. 1980. Effect of acyclovir on Epstein-Barr virus DNA replication. *J. Virol.* **34:**560–568.

Copperman, S. 1977. "Alice in Wonderland" syndrome as a presenting symptom of infectious mononucleosis in children. *Clin. Pediatr.* (Philadelphia) **16:**143–146.

d'Arminio Monforte, A., P. Cinque, L. Vago, A. Rocca, A. Castagna, C. Gervasoni, M. R. Terreni, R. Novati, A. Gori, A. Lazzarin, and M. Moroni. 1997. A comparison of brain biopsy and CSF-PCR in the diagnosis of CNS lesions in AIDS patients. *J. Neurol.* **244:**35–39.

Davis, C., B. L. Wood, D. E. Sabath, J. S. Joseph, C. Stehman-Breen, and V. C. Broudy. 1998. Interferon-alpha treatment of posttransplant lymphoproliferative disorder in recipients of solid organ transplants. *Transplantation* 66:1770–1779.

DeSimone, P., and D. Snyder. 1978. Hypoglossal nerve paralysis in infectious mononucleosis. *Neurology* 28:844–847.

de-The, G., A. Geser, N. E. Day, P. M. Tukei, E. H. Williams, D. P. Beri, P. G. Smith, A. G. Dean, G. W. Bronkamm, P. Feorino, and W. Henle. 1978. Epidemiological evidence for causal relationship between Epstein-Barr virus and Burkitt's lymphoma from Ugandan prospective study. *Nature* 274:756–761.

Epstein, M., B. Achong, and Y. M. Barr. 1964. Virus particles in cultured lymphoblasts from Burkitt's lymphoma. *Lancet* 15:702–703.

Eshel, G., A. Eyov, E. Lahat, and A. Brauman. 1987. Alice in Wonderland syndrome, a manifestation of acute Epstein-Barr virus infection. *Pediatr. Infect. Dis. J.* 6:68.

Evans, A., J. C. Niederman, and R. W. McCollum. 1968. Seroepidemiologic studies of infectious mononucleosis with EB virus. *N. Engl. J. Med.* 279:1121–1127.

Faro, A., G. Kurland, M. G. Michaels, P. S. Dickman, P. G. Greally, K. J. Spichty, B. B. Noyes, S. R. Boas, F. J. Fricker, J. M. Armitage, and A. Zeevie. 1996. Interferon alpha effects the immune response in post-transplant lymphoproliferative disorder. *Am. J. Respir. Crit. Care Med.* 153:1442–1447.

Gottschalk, S., C. Rooney, and H. E. Heslop. 2005. Posttransplant lymphoproliferative disorders. *Annu. Rev. Med.* 56:29–44.

Grose, C., and P. Feorino. 1972. Epstein-Barr virus and Guillain-Barre syndrome. *Lancet* ii:1285–1287.

Grose, C., P. Feorino, L. A. Dye, and J. Rand. 1973. Bell's palsy and infectious mononucleosis. *Lancet* ii:231–232.

Haddad, E., S. Paczesny, V. Leblond, J. M. Seigneurin, M. Stern, A. Achkar, M. Bauwens, V. Delmail, D. Debray, C. Duvoux, P. Hubert, B. Hurault de Ligny, J. Wijdenes, A. Durandy, and A. Fischer. 2001. Treatment of B-lymphoproliferative disorder with a monoclonal anti-interleukin-6 antibody in 12 patients: a multicenter phase 1-2 clinical trial. *Blood* 87:1680–1687.

Henle, G., W. Henle, and V. Diehl. 1968. Relation of Burkitt's tumor-associated herpes-type virus to infectious mononucleosis. *Proc. Natl. Acad. Sci. USA* 59:94–101.

Herbst, H. 1996. Epstein-Barr virus in Hodgkin's disease. *Semin. Cancer Biol.* 7:183–189.

Hjalgrim, H., J. Askling, K. Rostgaard, S. Hamilton-Dutoit, M. Frisch, J. S. Zhang, M. Madsen, N. Rosadhl, H. B. Konradsen, H. H. Storm, and M. Melbye. 2003. Characteristics of Hodgkin's lymphoma after infectious mononucleosis. *N. Engl. J. Med.* 349:1324–1332.

Hoagland, R. 1967. *Infectious Mononucleosis.* Grune and Stratton, New York, NY.

Hoffman, C., S. Tabrizian, E. Wolf, C. Eggers, A. Stoehr, A. Plettenberg, T. Buhk, H. J. Stellbrink, H. A. Horst, H. Jager, and T. Rosenkranz. 2001. Survival of AIDS patients with primary central nervous system lymphoma is dramatically improved by HAART-induced immune recovery. *AIDS* 15:2119–2127.

Hoffman, J. M., H. A. Waskin, T. Schifter, M. W. Hanson, L. Gray, S. Rosenfeld, and R. E. Coleman. 1993. FDG-PET in differentiating lymphoma from nonmalignant central nervous system lesions in patients with AIDS. *J. Nucl. Med.* 34:567–575.

Jones, J. F., S. Shurin, C. Abramowsky, R. R. Tubbs, C. G. Sciotto, R. Wahl, J. Sands, D. Gottman, B. Z. Katz, and J. Sklar. 1988. T-cell lymphomas containing Epstein-Barr viral DNA in patients with Epstein-Barr virus infections. *N. Engl. J. Med.* 318:733–741.

Kieff, E., T. Dambaugh, M. Heller, W. King, A. Cheung, V. van Santen, M. Hummel, C. Beisel, S. Fennewald, K. Hennessy, and T. Heineman. 1982. The biology and chemistry of Epstein-Barr virus. *J. Infect. Dis.* 146:506–517.

Leavell, R., C. G. Ray, P. C. Ferry, and L. L. Minnich. 1986. Unusual acute neurological presentations with Epstein-Barr virus infection. *Arch. Neurol.* 43:186–188.

Levitsky, V., T. Frisan, and M. Masucci. 2001. Generation of polyclonal EBV-specific CTL cultures and clones, p. 203–208. In J. Wilson and G. May (ed.), *Epstein-Barr Virus Protocols*, vol. 174. Humana Press, Totowa, NJ.

MacMahon, E., J. D. Glass, S. D. Hayward, R. B. Mann, P. S. Becker, P. Charache, J. C. McArthur, and R. F. Ambinder. 1991. Epstein-Barr virus in AIDS-related primary CNS lymphoma. *Lancet* 338:969–973.

McGowan, J., and S. Shah. 1998. Long-term remission of AIDS-related primary central nervous system lymphoma associated with highly active antiretroviral therapy. *AIDS* 12:952–954.

Mentzer, S., S. Perrine, and D. V. Faller. 2001. Epstein-Barr virus post-transplant lymphoproliferative disease and virus-specific therapy: pharmacological re-activation of viral target genes with arginine butyrate. *Transplant. Infect. Dis.* 3:177–185.

Niedobitek, G., and H. Herbst. 2006. Pathology of primary and persistent EBV infection, p. 59–78. In A. Tselis and H. Jenson (ed.), *Epstein-Barr Virus*. Taylor and Francis, New York, NY.

Old, L. J., E. A. Boyse, G. Geering, and H. F. Oettegen. 1968. Serologic approaches to the study of cancer in animals and in man. *Cancer Res.* 28:1288–1299.

O'Malley, J. P., H. A. Ziessman, P. N. Kumar, B. A. Harkness, J. G. Tall, and P. F. Poerce. 1994. Diagnosis of intracranial lymphoma in patients with AIDS: value of 201Tl single-photon emission computed tomography. *AJR Am. J. Roentgenol.* 163:412–421.

Palella, F., K. M. Delaney, A. C. Moorman, M. O. Loveless, J. Fuhrer, G. A. Satten, D. J. Aschman, and S. D. Holmberg. 1998. Declining morbidity and mortality among patients with advanced human immunodeficiency virus infection. *N. Engl. J. Med.* 338:853–860.

Paul, J., and W. Bunnell. 1932. The presence of heterophile antibodies in infectious mononucleosis. *Am. J. Med. Sci.* 183:191–194.

Rubenstein, J., D. Combs, J. Rosenberg, A. Levy, M. McDermott, L. Damon, R. Ignoffo, K. Aldape, A. Shen, D. Lee, A. Grillo-Lopez, and M. A. Shuman. 2003. Rituximab therapy for CNS lymphomas: targeting the leptomeningeal compartment. *Blood* 101:466–468.

Sharma, K., S. Sriram, T. Fries, H. J. Bevan, and W. G. Bradley. 1993. Lumbosacral radiculoplexopathy as a manifestation of Epstein-Barr virus infection. *Neurology* 43:2550–2554.

Skiest, D. 2002. Focal neurological disease in patients with acquired immunodeficiency syndrome. *Clin. Infect. Dis.* 34:103–115.

Skiest, D., and C. Crosby. 2003. Survival is prolonged by highly active antiretroviral therapy in AIDS patients with primary central nervous system lymphoma. *AIDS* 17:1787–1793.

So, Y., J. Beckstead, and R. L. Davis. 1986. Primary central nervous system lymphoma in acquired immune deficiency syndrome: a clinical and pathological study. *Ann. Neurol.* 20:566–572.

Spano, J., P. Busson, D. Atlan, J. Bourhis, J. P. Pignon, C. Esteban, and J. P. Armand. 2003. Nasopharyngeal carcinomas: an update. *Eur. J. Cancer* 39:2121–2135.

Spina, M., U. Jaeger, J. A. Sparano, C. Simonelli, M. Michieli, G. Rossi, E. Nigra, M. Barretta, C. Cattaneo, A. C. Rieger, E. Vaccher, and U. Tirelli. 2005. Rituximab plus infusional cyclophosphamide, doxorubicin, and etoposide in HIV-associated non-Hodgkin lymphoma: pooled results from 3 phase 2 trials. *Blood* 105:1891–1897.

Sprunt, T., and F. Evans. 1920. Mononuclear leucocytosis in reaction to acute infections (infectious mononucleosis). *Johns Hopkins Hosp. Bull.* 357:410–416.

Straathof, K., C. M. Bollard, C. M. Rooney, and H. E. Heslop. 2003. Immunotherapy for Epstein-Barr virus-associated cancers in children. *Oncologist* **8:**83–98.

Taylor, L., and G. Parsons-Smith. 1969. Infectious mononucleosis, deafness and facial paralysis. *J. Laryngol. Otol.* **83:**613–616.

Thurnher, M., A. Rieger, C. Kleibl-Popov, U. Settinek, C. Henk, C. Haberler, and E. Schindler. 2001. Primary central nervous system lymphoma in AIDS: a wider spectrum of CT and MRI findings. *Neuroradiology* **43:**29–35.

Tossing, G. 1996. Immunodeficiency and its relation to lymphoid and other malignancies. *Ann. Hematol.* **73:**163–167.

Villringer, K., H. Jager, M. Dichgans, S. Ziegler, J. Poppinger, M. Herz, C. Kruschke, S. Minoshima, H. W. Pfister, and M. Schwaiger. 1995. Differential diagnosis of CNS lesions in AIDS patients by FDG-PET. *J. Comput. Assist. Tomogr.* **19:**532–536.

Watson, P., and P. Ashby. 1976. Brachial plexus neuropathy associated with infectious mononucleosis. *Can. Med. Assoc. J.* **114:**758–759.

Ziegler, J. L., J. A. Beckstead, P. A. Volberding, D. I. Abrams, A. M. Levine, R. J. Lukes, P. S. Gill, R. L. Burkes, P. R. Meyer, C. E. Metroka, et al. 1984. Non-Hodgkin's lymphoma in 90 homosexual men. Relation to generalized lymphadenopathy and the acquired immunodeficiency syndrome. *N. Engl. J. Med.* **311:**565–570.

zur Hausen, H., H. Schulte-Holthausen, G. Klein, G. W. Henle, G. Henle, P. Clifford, and L. Santensson. 1970. EBV DNA in biopsies of Burkitt tumours and anaplastic carcinomas of the nasopharynx. *Nature* **228:**1056–1058.

28

Mood Disorders, Delirium, and Other Neurobehavioral Symptoms and Disorders in the HAART Era

STEPHEN J. FERRANDO AND TODD LOFTUS

Since the beginning of the HIV epidemic in the early 1980s, psychiatric, neuropsychiatric, and substance use disorders have been a central component of the landscape. These disorders increase the risk of acquiring HIV, can be reactive to the state of having an incurable and often fatal illness, and can be engendered by, or overlap with, central nervous system (CNS) complications of the infection and its treatments.

Although in the initial 15 years of the epidemic, HIV infection was uniformly fatal, the introduction of clinical HIV viral load monitoring and highly active antiretroviral therapy (HAART) in 1995 was accompanied by a dramatic decrease in HIV-associated morbidity and mortality (Palella et al., 1998). Consequently, while there remains no cure, living with HIV and maintenance therapy with HAART is now the norm rather than the exception. Nonetheless, living with HIV as chronic illness has presented its own challenges (Rabkin and Ferrando, 1997): HIV risk behavior has continued or increased in some communities; HAART may be associated with acute and long-term side effects that may require treatment modification or even cessation; adherence to HAART regimens may be problematic, resulting in treatment failure; and multiantiretroviral resistance has developed in a substantial minority of patients. All of these issues contribute to the ongoing importance of HIV-related psychiatric intervention and research.

In this chapter, we review of the epidemiology, diagnosis, and treatment of the major psychiatric aspects of HIV infection, in addition to somatic symptoms such as sleep disorder, fatigue, sexual dysfunction, and HIV-associated lipodystrophy, all of which have substantial quality of life impact. To the extent possible, we attempt to provide information that is clinically relevant and based on critical review of the latest medical literature.

Stephen J. Ferrando and Todd Loftus, New York-Presbyterian Hospital, Weill Medical College of Cornell University, New York, NY 10065.

EPIDEMIOLOGICAL OVERVIEW OF PSYCHIATRIC DISORDERS IN HIV INFECTION

From an epidemiological standpoint, reported prevalence rates of psychiatric and substance use disorders in the context of HIV depend on the setting and methods of assessment; however, regardless of setting, they are generally high relative to rates reported in the general population. In the HIV Cost and Services Utilization Study, well over one-half of a national probability sample of 2,864 HIV-infected patients screened positive for a current psychiatric disorder, including 36% for depression, 26.5% for dysthymia, 15.8% for generalized anxiety disorder, and 10.5% for history of panic attacks (Bing et al., 2001). Approximately 61% of these patients utilized some form of mental health or substance abuse treatment (Burnam et al., 2001). In a multisite mental health demonstration project, Acuff and colleagues (Acuff et al., 1999) found that 59% of patients sought mental health treatment for a major depression, 22% for dysthymia, 25% for generalized anxiety disorder, 14% for agoraphobia, 48% for a substance abuse disorder, and 22% for an alcohol disorder. In a cohort of HIV-infected homosexual/bisexual men without a history of injection drug use, Rabkin and colleagues (Rabkin et al., 1997) found rates for any current depressive disorder to be 10%; for any anxiety disorder, 11%; and for any noninjection drug or alcohol disorder, 11%. Among injection drug users in methadone maintenance treatment (MMT), Batki and colleagues (Batki et al., 1996) found 80% to be receiving psychiatric intervention: 42% for depression, 19% for cognitive disorders, 17% for insomnia disorders, 8% for anxiety disorder, 8% for psychotic disorders, and 2% for bipolar disorder. More than 70% of these patients were actively abusing illicit nonopioid drugs while in MMT, including cocaine, alcohol, benzodiazepines, and amphetamines. Finally, among patients medically hospitalized for complications of HIV/AIDS, Ferrando and colleagues (Ferrando et al., 1998b) found that 31% of patients had major depression, 19% had delirium and/or dementia,

19% had current substance abuse disorders, 16% had bipolar spectrum disorders, and 13% had anxiety disorders.

DEPRESSION

Depression is the most common psychiatric disorder for which HIV-infected individuals seek treatment. Lifetime rates of major depression in at-risk cohorts are as high as 50% (Rabkin et al., 1997). Rates of current depression among HIV-infected patients are at least twice that of the general population. The prevalence of current major depression found in studies utilizing structured diagnostic interviews ranges from 4 to 14%, depending on the setting and risk group studies (Rabkin et al., 1997); however, these rates may exceed 50% among HIV patients seeking psychiatric treatment (Acuff et al., 1999).

Most longitudinal studies have not found an increase in the rate of depression with advancing HIV illness stage. However, Lyketos and colleagues (Lyketos et al., 1996) noted a 43% increase in depressive symptoms 12 to 18 months prior to AIDS diagnosis. This increase was associated with earlier depressive symptoms, with the development of HIV-related symptoms, and with psychosocial stressors. Several studies have also investigated a potential link between baseline depressive symptoms and HIV illness progression or death, with mixed results. In one compelling study of a large cohort of HIV-infected women (HIV Epidemiology Research Study), Ickovics and colleagues (Ickovics et al., 2001) found an association between increased chronicity and severity of depression and decline in CD4$^+$ cell count and decreased survival. Such findings raise questions regarding the mechanism of the relationship between depression and illness progression and suggest that treatment of depression can improve survival.

The relationship of depressive symptoms to HAART has been investigated. Rabkin and colleagues (Rabkin et al., 2000a), in a longitudinal study of 173 HIV-infected men with symptomatic illness assessed semiannually after the initiation of therapy with HAART, observed a statistically significant but clinically modest reduction in measures of depression and hopelessness in the sample as a whole. Overall, this decline in distress was significantly correlated with increasing CD4$^+$ cell count, declining HIV symptoms, and improved social support. As seen in previous studies, physical symptoms were more strongly correlated to psychological distress than were laboratory findings (Rabkin et al., 2000a).

Depression and other factors, such as cognitive impairment, substance abuse, and poor social support, have been found to be a predictor of poor adherence to HAART. This poor adherence may be partially responsible for mediating the association between depression and poor HIV illness outcome.

Given the above findings on the prevalence and impact of depression in HIV, screening for, and treating, depression and other mental health and substance abuse issues are vital.

The diagnosis of depression in HIV-infected patients may be confounded by somatic symptoms common to depression and HIV illness itself, including fatigue, appetite loss, sleep disturbance, and difficulty with attention/concentration. However, most studies document that an inclusive approach to diagnosis is appropriate. There are several validated instruments for screening and diagnosing depression (Table 1). Each was developed with a particular purpose in mind; however, many of them can be found in the HIV research literature.

Because of the prevalence of depression in HIV, psychotherapeutic and psychopharmacological treatments for HIV-infected patients have been extensively researched. Most of this research has focused on psychopharmacological interventions. As with diagnosis, the psychopharmacological treatment of depression in HIV infection may be complicated by the somatic symptoms common to both disorders. In addition, the potential for antidepressants to interact with antiretroviral medications is important.

Fortunately, a substantial number of open-label and double-blind, placebo-controlled clinical trials of antidepressant treatment of depression in HIV have been conducted. In interpreting these studies, it is important to keep several issues in mind: studies have overrepresented homosexual/bisexual males and underrepresented women and intravenous drug users (IDUs); inclusion and outcome criteria for clinical response have varied; stage of HIV illness has varied; duration has ranged from 4 weeks to 1 year; in some studies, attrition rates have been high; there is often high placebo response, probably due to transient illness-related depressive

TABLE 1 Screening instruments for patients with depression

Screening instrument (reference)	Administration	No. of items	Comment
Beck Depression Inventory (Beck et al., 1961)	Self-report	20	Cognitive and somatic subscales; widely used clinically
Hamilton Rating Scale for Depression (Hamilton, 1960)	Clinician	17	Affective and vegetative symptom subscales; primarily used in depression treatment research
Center for Epidemiological Studies-Depression (Roberts and Vernon, 1983)	Self-report	20	Cognitive and somatic subscale; cut scores for clinically relevant symptoms; primarily used in epidemiological research
Patient Health Questionnaire-9 (Kroenke et al., 2001) depression module	Self-report	9	Extensively validated in primary-care settings; keyed to depression diagnostic criteria; other modules screen for somatic symptoms, anxiety disorders, substance abuse
Hospital Anxiety and Depression Scale (Zigmond and Snaith, 1983)	Self-report	7	Screens depression and anxiety; designed for use in medical settings; excludes somatic symptoms

symptoms experienced by persons with HIV; and, finally, whereas antidepressants have been studied in patients with symptomatic illness and AIDS on multiple HIV medications, few specific drug interaction studies have been conducted. A list of the conventional antidepressants that have been studied in HIV-infected patients is included in Table 2.

The earliest studies of antidepressant treatment in HIV infection employed the tricyclic antidepressant (TCA) imipramine. Rabkin and colleagues (Rabkin et al., 1994a), in a double-blind trial of imipramine (mean dose, 260 mg/day) versus placebo in 97 HIV-infected patients (39% with AIDS), reported a response rate of 74% for imipramine and 30% for placebo. Manning and colleagues (D. Manning, L. Jacobsberg, S. Erhart, Perry, and A. Frances, presented at the 7th International Conference on AIDS, 16 to 20 June 1990, San Francisco, CA) reported similar results, but with a higher placebo response rate. Anticholinergic, antihistaminic, antiadrenergic, and antimuscarinic side effects (e.g., constipation, dry mouth, drowsiness, headache, cognitive problems, dizziness, and sexual dysfunction) were more common in the imipramine group, contributing to significant attrition (30% of imipramine responders discontinued treatment at 6 months' follow-up). Response rates and adverse effects did not vary as a function of CD4$^+$ lymphocyte count. These studies reflect general concern regarding the use of tertiary amine tricyclic antidepressants (e.g., amitriptyline and imipramine) in HIV illness, although amitriptyline is commonly used in the treatment of HIV-associated neuropathic pain. If using a TCA for depression in HIV, most clinicians prefer secondary amines (e.g., desipramine, nortriptyline) and reserve their use for patients with asymptomatic illness. A final concern with TCAs is lethality in overdose, requiring close monitoring of suicide potential.

Concerns regarding TCA side effects and lethality have led to interest in the selective serotonin reuptake inhibitors

TABLE 2 Conventional and nonconventional antidepressants studied in HIV-infected patients

TCAs
  Imipramine[a]
  Desipramine
  Nortriptyline
SSRIs
  Fluoxetine[a]
  Sertraline[a]
  Paroxetine[a]
  Citalopram
Psychostimulants
  Dextroamphetamine[a]
  Methylphenidate
  Pemoline
Others
  Venlafaxine
  Nefazodone
  Buproprion
  Mirtazapine
  Modafinil
Nonconventional agents with antidepressant activity
  Testosterone[a]
  DHEA[a]
  S-Adenosylmethionine

[a]Medication for which there is double-blind trial evidence in HIV-infected patients.

(SSRIs) as first-line treatment of depression in HIV. Early open-label trials utilizing standard doses of fluoxetine, sertraline, and paroxetine for major depression across HIV illness stages produced encouraging response rates, ranging from 70 to 90%, with relatively few adverse effects and improvements in both affective and somatic depressive symptoms (Ferrando et al., 1997; Rabkin et al., 1994b). Subsequently, three double-blind, placebo-controlled comparison studies of SSRIs alone or SSRIs compared to tricyclics have been published. Rabkin and colleagues (Rabkin et al., 1999a), in a study including 84 men and 3 women (51% with AIDS), reported response rates of 74% for fluoxetine (mean dose, 37 mg/day) and 47% for placebo ($P < 0.05$), with similar dropout rates in both groups. The only side effect reported more for fluoxetine than for its placebo comparator was headache. Response rates and adverse effects did not differ as a function of CD4$^+$ lymphocyte count. Batki and colleagues (Batki et al., 1993) treated 15 HIV-infected opioid- and cocaine-dependent IDUs who had major depression with fluoxetine ($n = 7$) or a placebo ($n = 8$) and found significant reductions in depressive symptoms in the fluoxetine but not the placebo group. Elliott and colleagues (Elliott et al., 1998) reported a study including 68 men and 2 women (45 with AIDS), comparing paroxetine (mean dose, 34 mg/day), imipramine (mean dose, 163 mg/day), and placebo. Both drugs were superior to placebo at 6, 8, and 12 weeks of treatment. Imipramine was associated with significantly greater dropout than paroxetine or placebo (48, 20, and 24%, respectively) and with more dry mouth, postural hypotension, and palpitations. Zisook and colleagues (Zisook et al., 1998) reported a study comparing fluoxetine (36 mg/day) plus supportive group therapy to group therapy plus placebo in 47 HIV-infected asymptomatic or mildly symptomatic homosexual/bisexual men. The response after 8 weeks for the fluoxetine group was superior to that of the placebo group (64 versus 23%). Patients with more severe depression at baseline experienced the greatest benefit from fluoxetine. Adverse effects did not differ between the groups.

In a study mirroring the National Institute of Mental Health Collaborative Depression Treatment Study, Markowitz and colleagues (Markowitz et al., 1998) enrolled 65 HIV-infected men and 4 women (53% with major depression; 32% with AIDS) in a 16-week trial comparing interpersonal psychotherapy, cognitive behavioral therapy, supportive therapy with imipramine, and supportive therapy alone. Interpersonal therapy and supportive therapy with imipramine were superior to supportive therapy alone and cognitive behavioral therapy in ameliorating depressive symptoms and improving Karnofsky performance score (a measure of physical function). This study suggests that combining psychotherapy with medication may be the optimal approach to treating depression in HIV.

Two studies have specifically addressed the psychopharmacological treatment of depression in HIV-infected women. Schwartz and McDaniel compared fluoxetine ($n = 8$; mean dose, 20 mg/day) with desipramine ($n = 6$; mean dose, 100 mg/day) in women with AIDS. Response rates were 75% in the fluoxetine group and 50% in the desipramine group (Schwartz and McDaniel, 1999). Ferrando and colleagues treated 14 women with fluoxetine (average dose, 25 mg/day) and 4 women with sertraline (average dose, 62 mg/day) and observed response rates of 78% for fluoxetine and 75% for sertraline. Both study groups noted the difficulty of recruiting and retaining HIV-infected women in depression treatment studies (Ferrando et al., 1999). Among the barriers described were substance abuse, hesitancy to accept anti-depressant medication among individuals in recovery, child care and other family responsibilities, and suspicion regarding research and medication treatment for depression.

Mirtazapine, nefazodone, venlafaxine, and sustained-release bupropion have been studied in small open-label trials in patients with major depression and HIV infection (Currier et al., 2003; Elliott et al., 1999; Elliott and Roy-Byrne, 2000). All were associated with favorable response rates (more than 60 to 70%) and few adverse effects. One nefazodone-treated patient discontinued treatment due to a clinically significant interaction with ritonavir.

Psychostimulants have been studied for the treatment of depressed mood, fatigue, and cognitive impairment in the context of HIV infection, particularly in advanced illness and in situations where rapid onset of action is desirable. There are two open-label and two placebo-controlled studies addressing psychostimulant treatment of depression in HIV. Holmes and colleagues reported on the use of methylphenidate (20 to 90 mg/day) in 17 men with AIDS-related complex, with an 85% mood response rate (Holmes et al., 1989). Similarly, Wagner and colleagues reported on the use of dextroamphetamine (median dose, 10 mg/day) for 6 weeks in 19 men with AIDS, with a 95% mood response rate (Wagner et al., 1997). In a 2-week, double-blind trial, this same group treated 22 men with AIDS and major depression, subthreshold major depression, or dysthymia with either dextroamphetamine ($n = 11$; mean dose [± standard deviation], 22 ± 9 mg/day; range, 10 to 40 mg/day) or placebo ($n = 11$). Eight (73%) responded to dextroamphetamine, and three (27%) responded to placebo. Five patients on dextroamphetamine reported overstimulation, insomnia, or appetite suppression at some point during the trial; however, none discontinued treatment (Wagner and Rabkin, 2000). Finally, Breitbart and colleagues conducted a double-blind trial comparing methylphenidate (maximum dose, 60 mg/day), pemoline (maximum dose, 150 mg/day), and placebo in 144 HIV-infected patients (71% with AIDS) in the treatment of fatigue and found that improvement in fatigue was associated with improvement in subclinical depressive symptoms (Breitbart et al., 2001). This group also reported overstimulation to be more common with both psychostimulants than with placebo. Thus, psychostimulants appear to be efficacious in treating depressive symptoms in patients with advanced HIV, with relatively few intolerable side effects. Concern over abuse liability and tolerance may limit the use of these agents, particularly in substance abusers in early HIV infection. However, there are no published reports of abuse of prescription psychostimulants in HIV-infected patients who are under medical supervision.

Testosterone deficiency, with clinical symptoms of hypogonadism (depressed mood, fatigue, diminished libido, decreased appetite, and loss of lean body mass), is present in up to 50% of men with symptomatic HIV or AIDS (Rabkin et al., 1999b). Deficiency of adrenal androgens, particularly dehydroepiandrosterone (DHEA), is also common in both HIV-infected men and women and is associated with HIV disease progression and loss of lean body mass (Rabkin et al., 2006). The presence of these abnormalities has led to clinical interest in administering anabolic androgenic steroids, most commonly testosterone, to patients with HIV infection.

The most common screening test for testosterone deficiency is the measure of total serum testosterone (testosterone deficiency is defined as less than 300 to 400 ng/dl); however, serum-free (deficiency, less than 5 to 7 pcg/ml) and

bioavailable testosterone may be more accurate measures due to increase in sex hormone-binding globulin in late-stage HIV. For testosterone replacement, commonly used testosterone preparations include esterified depot testosterone (propionate, enanthate, and cypionate, generally initiated at 100 to 200 mg intramuscularly [i.m.] every 2 weeks; maximum, 400 mg i.m. weekly), skin patches (1 to 2 patches, 5 to 10 mg, to clean dry skin daily), and testosterone gel (1 to 4 packets, 25 to 100 mg, to clean dry skin daily), with the depot preparations being the least expensive and most studied. Patch and gel formulations may produce less variability in serum testosterone levels and, therefore, in target symptoms.

In an initial study of testosterone replacement therapy for libido, mood, energy, and body composition, Rabkin and colleagues treated 34 HIV-infected men (79% with AIDS) with low serum testosterone and major depression in an 8-week open-treatment phase (400 mg i.m. biweekly), followed by a placebo-controlled double-blind discontinuation phase (Rabkin et al., 1999b). In the open-treatment phase, mood response was 79%. In the placebo-controlled phase, response was maintained in the testosterone group but dropped to 13% in the placebo group. In a follow-up double-blind, placebo-controlled study of testosterone (400 mg i.m. biweekly) in 26 HIV-infected men with low serum testosterone and subclinical depressive disorders, 58% responded to testosterone compared to 18% for the placebo group (Rabkin et al., 2000c). Among reported side effects were irritability, tension, reduced energy, bossiness, hair loss, and acne; however, fewer than 5% dropped out due to adverse effects. Extreme irritability and assaultiveness ("roid rage") did not occur, most likely because the dose used for testosterone replacement therapy is different from supraphysiological dosing used illicitly for anabolic effects. Long-term adverse effects of testosterone replacement therapy in HIV-infected men include testicular atrophy and decreased volume of, and watery, ejaculate. There have been no reports of serious hepatotoxicity or prostate cancer; however, prostate-specific antigen levels should be monitored every 6 to 12 months in men aged more than 50 years.

DHEA, which has mild androgenic/anabolic effects and is a precursor to testosterone, has also been studied in a 12-week open-label trial (200 to 500 mg/day) with a 4-week placebo-controlled discontinuation phase in 30 men and 2 women with HIV (51% with AIDS) with subthreshold major depression, minor depression, and dysthymia (Rabkin et al., 2006). DHEA was associated with marked elevations in serum DHEA and DHEA-sulfate levels in all participants; in female participants, only increased testosterone was noted. Mood response was 79%; however, there was no difference between DHEA and placebo in the discontinuation phase. DHEA was associated with mild irritability and acne. A placebo-controlled trial of DHEA for depression in HIV is ongoing. Other steroid hormones, including nandrolone, oxandrolone, and androstenedione, have not been studied for their mood effects in HIV.

Saint-John's-wort has been used by depressed HIV-infected patients as an alternative to conventional antidepressants; however, it is a cytochrome P450 inducer and may reduce levels of protease inhibitors (PIs), so it is not recommended for use by HIV patients taking these agents. S-Adenosylmethionine has undergone a small open-label 8-week trial involving 15 HIV-infected patients with major depression, with results being consistent with other antidepressant agents. Thus, further investigation is warranted (K. Jones, R. Goldenberg, and I. Cerngul, presented at the

14th International AIDS Conference, 7 to 12 July 2002, Barcelona, Spain).

ANXIETY

Anxiety may be found in 11 to 25% of HIV-infected patients (Sewell et al., 2000). The most common manifestations are social phobia, agoraphobia, generalized anxiety disorder, and panic disorder. Prior traumatic life events are common to both men and women with HIV, and posttraumatic stress disorder symptoms have been found to be particularly prevalent among HIV-infected women attending HIV clinics (Martinez et al., 2002). Anxiety and depression are often comorbid. As with depression, anxiety presents prominently, if not predominantly, with somatic symptoms (e.g., hyperautonomic, cardiovascular, gastrointestinal, and neurologic), so that differential diagnostic considerations are central in the context of HIV. Finally, anxiety symptoms in HIV-infected patients have been found to correlate with increased fatigue, other HIV symptoms, and physical functional limitations (Sewell et al., 2000).

Rating scales to assess primary anxiety symptoms and disorders are listed in Table 3. While not included in the table, the Beck Depression Inventory, Hamilton Rating Scale for Depression, and Hospital Anxiety and Depression Scale have items that query anxiety symptoms.

Like depression, anxiety involves significant somatic symptoms, and attention to the potential organic etiologies of anxiety (i.e., substance abuse and withdrawal and cognitive disorders) is important prior to initiating treatment. Psychotherapeutic treatment of anxiety in HIV-infected patients includes psychotherapy, relaxation training, and counseling in stress reduction techniques. Caffeine, nicotine, and alcohol exacerbate anxiety, whereas physical activity tends to alleviate anxiety. The safety risk and abuse liability of benzodiazepines are the primary challenge in treating anxiety symptoms, particularly because patients often seek the immediate relief associated with these medications and see them as a long-term solution. Thus, it is important to employ a hierarchical approach to the treatment of anxiety in HIV-infected patients that involves the use of nonaddicting alternatives prior to utilizing a benzodiazepine. SSRIs are indicated for the treatment of chronic anxiety disorders, including generalized anxiety disorder, panic disorder, social phobia, obsessive compulsive disorder, and posttraumatic stress disorder. Buspirone, in doses of 10 to 60 mg/day, has been shown to be effective for treating anxiety symptoms in asymptomatic homosexual men and IDUs with HIV, is well tolerated, and has a low risk for drug interactions (Batki, 1990a; D. A. Hirsch, J. Fishman, P. Jacobsen, W. Breitbart, M. Emery, J. Schwimmer, and the Psychiatry Service, Memorial Sloan-Kettering Cancer Center, New York, NY, presented at the 7th International Conference on AIDS, 16 to 20 June 1990, San Francisco, CA).

Alternatives for more rapid anxiety relief include the antihistamines diphenhydramine (25 to 50 mg every day [q.d.] to three times a day [t.i.d.]) and hydroxyzine (10 to 50 mg q.d. to t.i.d.), sedating TCAs, and trazodone; however, use of many of these agents may be limited by sedating and anticholinergic side effects and risk in overdose. If a benzodiazepine is required, lorazepam (0.5 to 1.0 mg q.d. to q.i.d.) or clonazepam (0.25 to 1.0 mg q.d. to t.i.d.) are the most frequently used medications. Lorazepam has the advantage of having no active metabolites and nonoxidative metabolism but also has the disadvantages of a shorter half-life and requirement for more frequent dosing. In HIV patients with liver disease, lorazepam, oxazepam, and temazepam are preferred due to their oxidative metabolism. Benzodiazepines should be avoided in patients with cognitive impairment and delirium (Breitbart et al., 1996a).

MANIA

Manic symptomatology in HIV may be found in conjunction with primary bipolar illness or with HIV infection of the brain (HIV-associated mania). Assessing and treating HIV-associated mania may be different from mania not associated with HIV because HIV-associated mania has been differentiated from bipolar mania in a number of ways (Lyketsos et al., 1997). Descriptively, HIV-associated mania is found to be a late-onset, secondary affective illness associated with HIV infection of the brain, being less associated with a personal or family history of mood disorder. In addition, the symptomatology of HIV-associated mania may include more irritability, less hypertalkativeness, and more psychomotor slowing and cognitive impairment than primary bipolar mania. Given that HIV-associated mania is directly related to HIV brain infection, antiretroviral agents that penetrate cerebrospinal fluid may offer some protection from incident mania (Mijch et al., 1999). Indeed, despite scattered reports of manic or hypomanic symptoms being associated with antiretroviral medications (Kieburtz et al., 1991), since the advent of HAART, HIV-associated mania appears to be declining in incidence, consistent with the reduction in the incidence of HIV-associated dementia. Mania may appear in patients with AIDS who have mild cognitive impairment and is observed in both early- and late-stage disease.

Practice guidelines recommend lithium, valproic acid, or carbamazepine as standard therapy for a manic episode of bipolar affective illness (Work Group on Bipolar Disorder, 2003). However, in the context of HIV infection, there are particular considerations regarding their use, especially in later-stage illness. Lithium has a low therapeutic index, including a risk for neurotoxicity. Sodium valproate has been found to stimulate HIV-1 replication in vitro (Jennings and Romanelli, 1993). Carbamazepine may cause blood dyscrasias and may lower levels of PIs in serum. Further,

TABLE 3 Rating scales for patients with anxiety symptoms

Screening instruments	Administration	No. of items	Comments
State Trait Anxiety Inventory (Kendall et al., 1976)	Self-report	20	Assesses inherent (trait) and current (state) anxiety symptoms
PHQ, Anxiety Module (Spitzer et al., 1999)	Self-report	5	Assesses generalized anxiety, panic disorder, agoraphobia
Hamilton Rating Scale for Anxiety (Hamilton, 1959)	Clinician rating	14	Used primarily in psychopharmacology research

these medications require adherence to serum drug level monitoring.

There is relatively little research on the psychopharmacological treatment of HIV-associated mania. A case report on the use of lithium for HIV-associated mania in an AIDS patient showed control of symptoms at a dosage of 1,200 mg daily; however, significant neurotoxicity (cognitive slowing and fine tremor) occurred, leading to discontinuation (Tanquary, 1993). The most commonly used mood stabilizer for the treatment of HIV-associated mania has been valproic acid. One study showed that valproic acid, up to 1,750 mg daily, led to significant improvement in acute manic symptoms, at levels of >50 μg/liter in serum, with few adverse effects (Halman et al., 1993), and another reported clinical response at levels of 93 and 110 μg/liter in serum (Rach-Beisel and Weintraub, 1997). There have been three reports of valproic acid increasing HIV replication in vitro in a dose-dependent manner and one report of increased cytomegalovirus replication, perhaps mediated by alterations in intracellular glutathione, which is an important mediator of HIV replication (Jennings and Romanelli, 1993). The clinical relevance of these findings remains controversial, and to date, there are no reports of valproic acid causing elevations in viral load in vivo. Clearly, this issue warrants further investigation. Finally, there may be concern over hepatotoxicity associated with valporate use in HIV (Cozza et al., 2000).

Most recently, the anticonvulsant lamotrigine has received FDA approval for maintenance therapy in bipolar illness and may be useful for treating mania in HIV. This anticonvulsant requires careful upward dose titration due to risk of severe hypersensitivity; however, its safety has been documented in a study of treatment for peripheral neuropathy in HIV (Simpson et al., 2003). Finally, the anticonvulsant gabapentin, which is commonly used to treat HIV-associated peripheral neuropathy, may have mood stabilizing and sleep-enhancing properties; however, data to support its efficacy are limited.

Given the limitations of mood stabilizers, there has been interest in the use of atypical antipsychotics for HIV-associated mania. Risperidone (1 to 4 mg q.d.) in the treatment of HIV-related manic psychosis led to a significant decrease in the Young Mania Rating scale score (Singh and Catalan, 1994). There was no drug-induced leukopenia, nor were there significant drug-drug interactions with antiretroviral and other HIV disease medications, and no extrapyramidal signs were observed in the 10-day period of the study duration. Olanzapine may also play a role in the treatment of HIV-associated mania, and clinical experience suggests its effectiveness and safety.

Regarding benzodiazepine treatment, a case report on the use of clonazepam (2 mg orally [p.o.] t.i.d.) stated that the drug led to a rapid clinical response in control of HIV-associated manic symptoms, with the advantages of facilitating reduction of concurrent neuroleptic dosage and the absence of unacceptable side effects (Budman and Vandersall, 1990). Clonazepam may be a useful short-term adjuvant treatment due to its long half-life but (as with other benzodiazepines) is less useful as a maintenance treatment due to tolerance, dependence, and cognitive impairment.

In conclusion, limited information on the treatment of HIV-associated mania exists. While valproic acid has until recently been considered by clinicians to be the mood stabilizer of choice, serum valproate level, viral load, and hepatic function should be closely monitored. Newer anticonvulsants such as lamotrigine and gabapentin may show some

promise. The atypical neuroleptics, particularly risperidone and olanzapine, can be used for short-term stabilization while initiating a mood stabilizer or for longer-term treatment of patients who pose concerns regarding toxicity or poor adherence to drug level monitoring.

PSYCHOSIS

Accumulating evidence suggests that HIV infection may be directly linked to the onset of psychosis, which is defined by the onset of thought disorder, hallucinations, and delusions. Psychosis in HIV is most often seen as manifestation of substance intoxication and withdrawal, delirium, mood disorders with psychotic features, and schizophrenia. Estimates of the prevalence of new-onset psychosis in patients with HIV range from 0.5 to 15% (McDaniel, 2000). One study compared 20 HIV-infected patients with new-onset psychosis (and no prior psychotic episodes or current substance abuse) with 20 demographic and HIV illness-matched nonpsychotic patients. These investigators found that the former group showed a trend toward greater global neuropsychological impairment, were more likely to have a history of substance abuse, and had significantly higher mortality at follow-up, suggesting that psychotic patients had an increased CNS vulnerability to psychosis (Sewell et al., 1994a). Psychosis presumed secondary to antiretroviral medications has been reported (Foser et al., 2003); however, as with HIV-associated mania, antiretrovirals are much more likely to be protective in this regard (de Ronchi et al., 2000).

Patients with primary psychotic disorders such as schizophrenia and schizoaffective disorder are at increased risk for contracting HIV, especially with concurrent substance abuse (McKinnon et al., 2002). Once infected, such patients may have poor access to HIV care and may be at risk for poor adherence to care, unless provided with comprehensive supportive services including psychiatric treatment, housing, and community case management.

Psychosis associated with HIV disease can have multiple etiologies. New-onset psychosis is most often seen in the context of neurocognitive disorders, such as delirium, HIV-associated minor cognitive motor disorder, or HIV-associated dementia (also known historically as AIDS dementia complex and HIV encephalopathy) (Dana Consortium on Therapy for HIV, Dementia and Related Cognitive Disorders, 1996; Working Group of the American Academy of Neurology AIDS Task Force, 1991). However, psychosis in HIV may also be a manifestation of primary psychiatric disorders such as schizophrenia, mood disorders, or the result of substance abuse. Workup for psychosis in HIV-infected patients must rule out substance-induced and medical causes, prior to making a primary psychiatric diagnosis.

In general, treatment with antipsychotic medication requires awareness of HIV-infected patients' susceptibility to neuroleptic-induced extrapyramidal symptoms (EPS) as a result of HIV-induced neuronal damage to the basal ganglia. In fact, movement disorders (acute dystonia, parkinsonism, and ataxia) can be seen in advanced HIV disease in the absence of antipsychotic exposure. General recommendations include avoidance of high-potency D2 blocking agents, avoidance of depot neuroleptics, and the consideration that maintenance antipsychotic medication may not be necessary for the complete remission of newly onset or transient psychotic symptoms. Most clinicians prefer the use of atypical antipsychotics in this population.

A literature search on the use of antipsychotic medication in HIV/AIDS revealed six studies published since 1993; these studies described treatment of psychosis occurring in encephalopathic, schizophrenic, and manic patients. In terms of conventional antipsychotics, haloperidol (mean dose, 3 mg) was found to be effective in treating positive psychotic symptoms associated with HIV and schizophrenia but with a high incidence of EPS (Mauri et al., 1997; Sewell et al., 1994b). Thioridazine treatment (mean dose, 145 mg/day) resulted in similar benefit but no EPS (Sewell et al., 1994b).

In terms of atypical antipsychotic treatment, molindone (20 to 180 mg/day) was first reported to be beneficial for HIV-associated psychosis and agitation with minimal EPS (Fernandez and Levy, 1993). Clozapine (mean dose, 27 mg/day) was reported to be effective and generally safe in treating HIV-associated psychosis (including negative symptoms) in patients with prior drug-induced parkinsonism (Lera and Zirulnik, 1999).

However, clozapine must be used with caution in HIV-infected patients due to the risk of agranulocytosis, and it is contraindicated with ritonavir. Risperidone (mean dose, 3.3 mg/day) was reported to be effective in treating HIV-related psychotic and manic symptoms and was associated with mild sedation and sialorrhea but few EPS (Singh et al., 1997). Finally, there is one case report of use of olanzapine (10 to 15 mg/day) in a patient with AIDS and psychosis who developed EPS on risperidone and other neuroleptics (Meyer et al., 1998). This patient experienced akathisia on olanzapine that responded to treatment with propranolol.

Case reports have also described the use of risperidone (up to 6 mg/day) and clozapine in psychosis associated with HIV-associated dementia, both showing significant improvement in psychotic symptoms with minimal EPS (Dettling et al., 1998; Zilikis et al., 1998). A study of haloperidol, thioridazine, or lorazepam in the treatment of mildly to moderately delirious AIDS patients found low-dose haloperidol and chlorpromazine to be effective in treating symptoms of delirium, while lorazepam was ineffective and produced significant adverse effects (Breitbart et al., 1996a). Lorazepam was, however, reported to be useful in the treatment of AIDS-associated psychosis with catatonia (Scamvougeras and Rosebush, 1992).

In summary, psychosis occurs in HIV disease due to various etiologies. The few studies and case reports that have described pharmacologic treatment of psychosis in HIV disease suggest that antipsychotic medications can be effective, even in the setting of neurocognitive disorders. However, typical neuroleptic medications should be used in the lowest dose possible and for the shortest duration possible. Atypical antipsychotics are generally preferred due to their lower incidence of EPS.

DELIRIUM

Delirium is common among hospitalized HIV/AIDS patients. Most studies documenting rates of delirium were conducted in the pre-HAART era and were restricted to subsets of patients seen in psychiatric consultation. Nonetheless, point prevalence rates were relatively consistent, ranging from 12 to 29% (Ayuso Mateos et al., 1998; Bialer et al., 1996; O'Dowd and McKegney, 1990; Perry and Tross, 1984), and up to 65% of patients were reported to have some form of "organic mental disorder" that may overlap with delirium. Similarly, one study conducted in the HAART era, utilizing structured diagnostic interviews, documented

delirium in 19% of a sample of 40 HIV/AIDS medical inpatients (Ferrando et al., 1996).

Delirium in the HIV/AIDS patient is often superimposed on HIV-associated neurocognitive disorders, particularly dementia, and patients with these disorders are at increased risk for the development of delirium when medically hospitalized. The etiology of delirium in HIV/AIDS patients is generally multifactorial. Breitbart reported a mean of 12.6 medical complications in 30 delirious AIDS patients treated in the pre-HAART era, with the most common being hematological disorders (anemia, leukopenia, thrombocytopenia, and hypoalbuminemia) and infectious diseases (e.g., septicemia, systemic fungal infections, *Pneumocystis carinii* pneumonia, tuberculosis, and disseminated viral infections) (Breitbart et al., 1996a). Other potential etiologies include CNS opportunistic infections (see chapters 25–31, this volume); neuropsychiatric side effects of medications for HIV or its complications (e.g., efavirenz, ciprofloxacin, and interferons); drug interactions; substance intoxication or withdrawal (often with multiple concurrent substances); organ system failure (e.g., hepatitis and renal failure); hypoxemia; and metabolic derangements.

There are no data regarding specific or distinguishing symptom characteristics in delirium seen in HIV patients, and clinically the presentation is similar to that in other medically ill populations (Breitbart et al., 1996a). Both the hypoactive and hyperactive variants of delirium are seen, and in addition to cognitive disturbance, symptom manifestations include apathy, dysphoria, agitation, delusions, and hallucinations.

The diagnostic workup of delirium in HIV is focused on diagnosis and investigation of underlying etiologies. This should include complete blood count with differential serum chemistries (including liver and renal function tests, fasting glucose, and creatine phosphokinase), chest X ray, electrocardiogram, blood and urine cultures (if indicated), thyroid-stimulating hormone level, vitamins B_6 and B_{12} levels, and *Treponema pallidum* immunoglobulin G. Magnetic resonance imaging of the brain with gadolenium contrast is preferred over computed tomographic scan due to better visualization of subcortical and posterior fossa structures and focal lesions; however, it may be less feasible for the agitated patient. A lumbar puncture may also be obtained, if necessary under sedation with fluoroscopic guidance. Results are often nonspecific, but important tests include opening pressure, culture (viral, fungal, and mycobacterial), cell count, protein, neopterin, beta-2 microglobulin, and, if available, PCR testing for cytomegalovirus, Epstein-Barr virus, Jakob-Creutzfeldt virus, herpes simplex virus, and HIV-1.

The treatment of delirium in many respects overlaps with that of psychosis, discussed in the previous section. However, with delirious patients, treatment of the underlying medical cause is central. Symptomatic treatment includes psychoeducational, environmental, and psychopharmacological interventions. Psychoeducation regarding the risk and nature of delirium delivered to patients, their family, and the treatment team can be preventative and can result in earlier treatment and improved outcomes. Environmental interventions include titrating the level of stimulation, sitting the patient up, placing patients next to a window, frequent orientation, and placing familiar people and orienting objects in the room.

In terms of psychopharmacological treatment, most practitioners treat delirium with atypical antipsychotics, including olanzapine (available with dissolving oral preparation and i.m.), risperidone, quetiapine, and ziprasidone (available i.m.). However, the only double-blind clinical trial conducted to date involved halperidol, chlorpromazine, and lorazepam (Breitbart et al., 1996a). In this study, Breitbart et al. screened HIV medical inpatients for delirium. Thus, treatment was initiated early and when symptoms were mild to moderate in degree. Nonetheless, these patients were severely medically ill, as 9 (30%) of the 30 patients died within 1 week after completing the protocol. There were three important findings. First, haloperidol (mean dose, 2.8 mg per day for the acute phase and 1.4 mg per day for maintenance) and chlorpromazine (mean dose, 50 mg per day for the acute phase and 36.0 mg per day for maintenance) were equally efficacious. Second, the lorazepam arm (mean dose, 3.0 mg for the acute phase) was stopped early due to worsening of delirium symptoms, including oversedation, disinhibition, ataxia, and increased confusion. Thus, benzodiazepines should be used with extreme caution, if at all, and adjunctively with neuroleptics. Third, adverse effects in the antipsychotic arms were limited and included mild parkinsonian symptoms of decreased expressiveness, increased rigidity and tremor, and mild akathisia.

In sum, delirium is common in hospitalized HIV patients, who should be assessed frequently for early detection and treatment. A combination of psychoeducational, environmental, and pharmacological interventions, primarily with neuroleptic medications, will provide the best outcomes.

SLEEP DISORDERS

Sleep disorders, primarily insomnia disorders, are prevalent in the HIV-infected population. In a survey study of 115 HIV clinic patients, 73% endorsed insomnia. Patients with insomnia had significantly more cognitive impairment and greater levels of depression than did patients without sleep problems (Rubinstein and Selwyn, 1989; D. B. Clifford, presented at the 2nd International AIDS Society Conference on HIV Pathogenesis and Treatment, 13 to 16 July 2003, Paris, France). Other investigators have found that poor sleep quality in HIV-infected patients is associated with higher levels of depressive, anxiety, and physical symptoms, daytime sleepiness, and functional impairment (Nokes and Kendrew, 2001). In terms of antiretroviral medication, high efavirenz serum levels have been associated with the development of insomnia (Nunez et al., 2001) and with transient vivid dreams and insomnia in the early stages of treatment (Clifford, presented).

Polysomnographic study of patients with HIV compared to uninfected control subjects revealed HIV-infected patients to have longer sleep onset latency, shorter total sleep time, reduced sleep efficiency, more time spent awake, more time in stage 1 sleep, and decreased REM sleep latency, which correlated with increased levels of depression (Wiegand et al., 1991). All of the above findings suggest the commonality and broad differential diagnosis of sleep problems in the context of HIV infection, including CNS HIV infection.

Assessment of sleep disturbances may be done by using the Pittsburgh Sleep Quality Index (Buysse et al., 1989). This is a self-report instrument that assesses sleep quality and disturbances over a 1-month time interval. Nineteen individual items generate seven "component" scores: subjective sleep quality, sleep latency, sleep duration, habitual sleep efficiency, sleep disturbances, use of sleeping medication, and daytime dysfunction. The sum of scores for these seven components yields one global score.

Like other psychiatric symptoms, insomnia and other sleep disorders may be manifestations of the effects of HIV, HIV medications, active substance abuse, other psychiatric disorders, particularly depression and anxiety, or other factors, on the CNS. Thus, treatment of sleep disorders in HIV first entails addressing underlying or associated causes.

If vivid dreams occur in the context of efavirenz treatment, without evidence of other psychiatric disorder, patients should be reassured that this side effect generally resolves within days to weeks without discontinuation of efavirenz treatment. Further, the content of dreams should be queried, and patients should be reassured that violent or sexualized dreams are not uncommon and are generally not a manifestation of psychopathology.

As in the case of anxiety, psychopharmacological treatment of insomnia may be managed utilizing a hierarchical approach based on safety, abuse liability, and chronicity of symptoms. Generally, benzodiazepines and nonbenzodiazepine sedative hypnotics are indicated for short-term use only and should be avoided for patients with substance abuse histories. Other agents, such as sedating antidepressants, atypical antipsychotics, and anticonvulsants may be used with comorbid psychiatric symptoms.

SUBSTANCE USE DISORDERS

As emphasized in previous sections, substance abuse disorders figure prominently in the differential diagnosis and management of HIV. Of men living with AIDS in 2001, 32% were IDUs or men who have sex with men and who were also IDUs (Centers for Disease Control and Prevention, 2001). Women are at risk from heterosexual transmission of HIV from male IDU partners and bisexual partners. Since the epidemic began, 57% of AIDS cases among women have been attributed to IDU or sex with IDUs. Of new AIDS cases reported in 2000, AIDS associated with IDU accounted for 26% of cases among African-American and 31% among Hispanic adults and adolescents, compared with 19% of all cases among Caucasians (Anderson, 2001). Minority women are the largest growing group of the newly HIV-infected women. Children are at risk from vertical transmission of HIV from infected mothers; however, prenatal testing and treatment have decreased the number of children infected with HIV.

Practitioners in HIV treatment settings routinely face the clinical problems associated with substance abuse disorders. The treatment of individuals with the "triple diagnosis" of HIV, substance abuse, and psychiatric disorders has multiple levels of complexity stemming from distress and potentially poor adherence to medical treatment regimens (Batki, 1990b; Wall et al., 1995). Clinical samples of IDUs with HIV infection entering MMT reveal high rates of prior psychiatric morbidity, current distress, and suicidal ideation. While in MMT, up to 80% of these patients require psychiatric consultation for the treatment of depression, psychotic symptoms, anxiety, insomnia, cognitive impairment, and behavioral disinhibition, often with concurrent substance (cocaine, amphetamine, alcohol, and/or sedative-hypnotics) abuse (Batki et al., 1996). These co-occurring disorders may be associated with greater morbidity and mortality (Hu et al., 1995; Chaisson et al., 1995). These concerns have led to the development of integrated HIV, drug abuse, and psychiatric treatment services (Friedmann et al., 1999; Samet et al., 1995; Sorenson and Batki, 1992; Treatment Improvement Protocol, 2004).

Hepatitis C virus (HCV) infection is increasingly recognized as a significant comorbid condition that affects the clinical outcome of patients with substance abuse disorders and HIV disease (Sulkowski and Thomas, 2003). Coinfection is common, as HIV and HCV share routes of transmission, notably injection (Sorenson et al., 2002). HIV is a risk factor for accelerating the course of HCV, and conversely, HCV can worsen the outcome of HIV disease. HCV treatment involves the use of alpha interferon, which is associated with numerous neuropsychiatric adverse effects, most notably the onset or exacerbation of depression and other dysphoric symptoms (Dieperink et al., 2003). These psychiatric adverse effects can be successfully treated with antidepressant medications such as the SSRIs (Gleason et al., 2002; Kraus et al., 2002). Alcohol use is a highly significant cofactor in further increasing the morbidity and mortality associated with HCV infection, making abstinence from alcohol an important treatment goal in the individual with HCV infection (Bhattacharya and Shuhart, 2003).

Adherence to antiretroviral treatment is adversely affected by both substance use and psychiatric disorders (Arnsten et al., 2002; Ferrando et al., 1996; Turner et al., 2001). Interventions that appear to increase the likelihood of adherence among substance abusers with HIV disease include peer-driven support systems, on-site dispensing of HIV medications in substance abuse treatment programs, and individual medication management including directly observed therapy (Sorenson et al., 1998). Such interventions are helpful while administered but do not improve long-term adherence. Benzodiazepines should be reserved for short-term stabilization.

FATIGUE

Fatigue is common among patients with HIV/AIDS and may contribute to impairment in physical function and disability (Darko et al., 1992; Ferrando et al., 1998a; Perkins et al., 1995). The prevalence of fatigue reported in clinical samples is 2 to 27% in the early "asymptomatic" stages of HIV illness (Hoover et al., 1993; Kaslow et al., 1987; Palanicek et al., 1993; Vlahov et al., 1994) and 30 to 54% in symptomatic HIV-infected and AIDS patients (Darko et al., 1992; Palanicek et al., 1993; Vlahov et al., 1994). Fatigue is reported in conjunction with multiple AIDS-associated opportunistic infections (Cohen et al., 1994), wasting (Macallen et al., 1995), myopathy (Simpson and Bender, 1988), adrenal insufficiency (Piedrola et al., 1996), and hypogonadism (Rabkin et al., 1995). However, as one of the constitutional symptoms of HIV illness, fatigue often exists without apparent explanation.

Although fatigue is common in HIV illness, it is a nonspecific symptom that is difficult to define, and its meaning may vary between individuals and within a given individual over time. Fatigue has been defined as a reactive state, following a period of mental or physical exertion, which is characterized by a lessened capacity for work (Bates et al., 1995; Spraycar, 1995; Strauss, 1994); however, HIV-related fatigue is often reported by patients to be independent of exertion. Fatigue may comprise a multitude of symptoms and descriptors, such as weakness, listlessness, sleepiness, and low energy, and may have physiological and psychological components, most frequently depression. Rating scales used to measure fatigue reflect this multidimensionality (Chalder et al., 1993; Darko et al., 1992; Piper et al., 1989).

Two important unresolved issues regarding fatigue in HIV are its relationship to illness progression and to depression. Although fatigue has generally been found to be most prevalent in the latter stages of HIV, there are conflicting data regarding its association with immune suppression as measured by CD4+ lymphocyte count (Darko et al., 1992; Perkins et al., 1995; Piper et al., 1989). Furthermore, some investigators have suggested that fatigue in HIV illness may be a symptom of underlying depression (Perkins et al., 1995; Piper et al., 1989), whereas others maintain that it is a physical symptom that is independent of mood. Darko found that fatigue was more common among patients with more advanced HIV illness and that fatigue was associated with various laboratory measures, including CD4+ lymphocyte count, hematocrit, white blood cell, lactate dehydrogenase, and total globulin (Darko et al., 1992). Although they concluded that fatigue is an independent HIV symptom, they did not include measures of depression in their analyses. Perkins found that HIV-positive asymptomatic and HIV-negative men did not differ on degree of fatigue as measured by the fatigue subscale of the Profile of Mood States (Perkins et al., 1995). In this study, depressive symptoms and major depression, but not CD4 lymphocyte count, significantly predicted severity of fatigue, both at baseline and at 6-month follow-up, suggesting that fatigue is a manifestation of depression in early HIV illness. Likewise, Lyketsos et al., in a longitudinal study of depression as AIDS develops, found that fatigue and depressive symptoms were associated in close temporal proximity across HIV illness stages, and because neither depression nor fatigue was significantly correlated with immune or HIV illness measures, they concluded that fatigue is most likely a symptom of depression (Lyketsos et al., 1996).

PAIN

Pain in HIV-seropositive persons is widespread and associated with significant psychological and functional impairment (Breitbart, 1994; Breitbart et al., 1996b; Larue et al., 1997; Rosenfeld et al., 1996; Singer et al., 1993). Singer studied pain symptoms associated with HIV infection and found an association between the frequency of multiple pains and depressive symptoms (Singer et al., 1993). Breitbart et al. examined the medical characteristics of 438 ambulatory AIDS patients and found that over 60% reported frequent or persistent pain, and the "on average" pain intensity was in the moderate range (Breitbart et al., 1996b). The authors found that the presence of pain was significantly associated with a number of HIV-related symptoms and more functional impairment, reflecting greater physical debilitation. Pain was associated with interference with mood and enjoyment in life; this interference increased with the intensity of the pain. The impact of pain and pain intensity on psychological well-being and quality of life was further explored in a subsequent paper (Rosenfeld et al., 1996). The authors found that the patients with pain had significantly more depressive symptoms and psychological distress and were more hopeless than those without pain. Larue et al. looked at HIV patients at different stages of disease and found that those patients with significant pain reported lower quality of life than those with no pain and that significant pain had an independent negative impact on the HIV patient's quality of life after adjustment for treatment setting (Larue et al., 1997), stage of disease, fatigue, sadness, and depression.

Taken together, these studies suggest that pain in HIV disease is associated with depressive symptoms and has a negative effect on quality of life. Nonetheless, the question of comorbidity of pain and depression is confounded by the presence of physical symptoms common to both syndromes (Parham-Vetter, 1996; Perkins et al., 1995), such as disrupted sleep patterns, appetite changes, reduced activity, and decreased libido. Also, since depression inventories such as the Beck Depression Inventory and the Hamilton Depression Rating Scale include a number of somatic items, a question emerges as to whether high scores are related to the number of physical symptoms endorsed versus cognitive symptoms of depression, such as loss of pleasure and interest in life. Another question is whether HIV-infected patients with pain are physically sicker than those without pain and would therefore score higher on depression inventories that measure both physical and cognitive symptoms. Breitbart, for example, reports that, as with cancer, the prevalence of pain increases as disease progresses, with 25 to 30% of patients with early-stage HIV reporting pain, increasing to 50% in patients with late-stage HIV illness (Breitbart, 1996). McCormack et al., however, found that there did not appear to be a correlation between pain and severity of disease in HIV-infected patients, suggesting that pain in this population is nonspecific to the time course of the disease (McCormack et al., 1993). Lebovits et al. also found that pain in AIDS patients was not related to disease characteristics such as time since diagnosis (Lebovits et al., 1994).

INTERACTIONS BETWEEN ANTIRETROVIRAL MEDICATIONS AND PSYCHOTROPIC DRUGS

With the advent of nucleoside analog reverse transcriptase inhibitors (NRTIs) (e.g., zidovudine), nonnucleoside analog reverse transcriptase inhibitors (NNRTIs) (e.g., efavirenz), and PIs (e.g., indinavir) as part of HAART, there has been heightened interest in the issue of drug interactions in the context of HIV psychopharmacology. This is because PIs and NNRTIs are metabolized primarily by the cytochrome P450 3A4-microsomal enzyme isoform, with a secondary metabolic pathway being the 2D6 isoenzyme. The primary effect on these isoenzymes is inhibition by the PIs; however, enzyme induction has also been demonstrated in pharmacokinetic studies and is the predominant effect of the NNRTIs nevirapine and efavirenz. Another important issue is alteration of plasma proteins in HIV infection that may alter the free fraction of protein-bound drugs. Given that PIs, NNRTIs, and most psychotropic drugs are metabolized by, and may inhibit or induce, the same hepatic enzymes and are highly protein bound, clinically relevant drug interactions may result when these medications are combined. Fortunately, relatively few serious interactions have been reported in the literature, and this is reflected in general clinical experience.

However, fear over the potential for drug interactions may dissuade some clinicians from initiating needed psychotropic treatment for an HIV-infected patient.

There are important caveats in considering drug interactions between psychotropics and HIV medications. First, care should always be maintained when prescribing psychotropics with PIs and NNRTIs, and potential interactions should be investigated prior to initiating therapy. Second, in the absence of pharmacokinetic data, the in vivo direction of any potential drug interaction (i.e., enzyme inhibition or induction) can only be presumed. This is because drugs may inhibit or induce the same isoenzyme and because drugs may utilize more than one metabolic pathway. Third, an increase in the area under the plasma concentration curve (AUC) of a given drug does not necessarily translate into a clinically significant adverse effect. This depends primarily on the therapeutic index of the drug involved.

A modest but growing amount of pharmacokinetic and clinical data are available for interactions between antidepressants, sedative hypnotics, anticonvulsants, methadone, and antiretrovirals (Table 4). Most documented interactions between psychotropics and antiretrovirals involve ritonavir, which is the most powerful inhibitor of the cytochrome P450 3A enzyme isoform, but may also induce this enzyme and other isoenzymes and glucuronyltransferases. Thus, there are two antipsychotics (clozapine and pimozide) and several benzodiazepines that are contraindicated with concurrent ritonavir (Abbott Laboratories, 2001).

Regarding antidepressants, ritonavir has been documented to cause a 145% increase in the AUC of desipramine, suggesting the need for desipramine dose reduction and plasma level monitoring (Zilikis et al., 1998). Fluoxetine was associated with a 19% increase in the AUC of ritonavir; however, no alteration in ritonavir dosing has been suggested (Ouellet et al., 1998). Saint-John's-wort was associated with a decrease in the serum level of indinavir, which is of concern regarding viral suppression with this and other antiretrovirals (Elliott et al., 1999). Thus, Saint-John's-wort is not recommended for patients on concurrent antiretroviral therapy. As previously mentioned, concentrations of nefazodone in serum may be raised with PIs, so caution is encouraged in using this agent (Elliott et al., 1999). Bupropion was previously listed as contraindicated with ritonavir; however, this contraindication has been removed. Bupropion is metabolized by the 2B6 isoform, which is inhibited by ritonavir, efavirenz, and nelfinavir.

TABLE 4 Drug-drug interactions between psychotropic medications and antiretroviral medications

Type of medication	Action on levels of indicated medications in serum
Psychotropic	
St.-John's-wort	Decreases antiretroviral levels
Phenytoin	Decreases antiretroviral levels
Carbamazepine	Decreases antiretroviral levels
Nefazodone	Increases antiretroviral levels
Fluoxetine, norfluoxetine	Increases antiretroviral levels
Methadone	Increases zidovudine; decreases didanosine, stavudine
Antiretroviral	
Ritonavir	Increases TCAs, nefazodone, benzodiazepines, trazadone
Ritonavir, nelfinavir, efavirenz	Increases bupropion
Efavirenz, nevirapine, ritonavir	Decreases methadone

Regarding sedative hypnotic drugs, several benzodiazepines (clorazepate, diazepam, estazolam, flurazepam, midazolam, and triazolam) are listed as contraindicated with ritonavir, due to presumptive increase in serum levels of these sedatives (Abbott Laboratories, 2001). One study did show that ritonavir markedly impaired triazolam clearance (less than 4% control values) and augmented its sedative effects; however, this same study revealed that ritonavir had a nonsignificant effect on zolpidem metabolism (clearance, 78% of control values; half-life increased from 2 to 2.4 h) (Greenblatt et al., 2000b). Thus, the contraindication for zolpidem is questionable. There are conflicting pharmacokinetic data on alprazolam: one study revealed a 15 to 20% decrease in the AUC of alprazolam when coadministered with long-term ritonavir, while another reported a 41% reduction in alprazolam clearance and increased levels of sedation and performance impairment with short-term ritonavir (Greenblatt et al., 2000a).

Regarding methadone, there are numerous documented interactions with medications commonly used in the setting of HIV. These include rifampin (and to a lesser extent rifabutin) and the anticonvulsants dilantin and phenobarbital, all of which may lower serum methadone levels, leading to withdrawal symptoms and the need for increased methadone dosing. In terms of antiretrovirals, ritonavir has been associated with approximately 36% lowered AUC of methadone (A. Hsu, G. E. Granneman, G. Cao, L. Carothers, T. el-Shourbagy, P. Baroldi, K. Erdman, F. Brown, E. Sun, and J. M. Leonard, presented at the 5th Conference on Retroviruses and Opportunistic Infections, 1 to 5 February 1998, Chicago, IL) and the induction of withdrawal symptoms (Geletko and Erickson, 2000). Similarly, the initiation of nevirapine in formerly stable HIV-infected methadone patients led to significant withdrawal symptoms and negligible methadone levels in the sera of some patients (F. L. Altice, E. Cooney, and G. H. Friedland, presented at the 6th Conference on Retroviruses and Opportunistic Infections, 31 January to 4 February 1999, Chicago, IL). In general, given the magnitude of documented drug interactions, it is advisable to monitor serum methadone levels before and after the initiation of these PIs and NNRTIs, and it may be necessary to increase methadone dose by 25 to 30%. An in vitro study revealed that indinavir and saquinavir may inhibit methadone metabolism; however, this same study showed ritonavir to be a much more potent inhibitor, which is contrary to in vivo data mentioned above (Iribarne et al., 1998). Zidovudine, stavudine, and didanosine do not alter methadone levels; however, methadone may increase exposure to zidovudine (52% increase in AUC) (P. Jatlow, E. F. McCance-Katz, P. M. Rainey, and G. Friedland, presented at the 5th Conference on Retroviruses and Opportunistic Infections, 1 to 5 February 1998, Chicago, IL) and may decrease exposure to didanosine (63% decrease in AUC) and stavudine (25% decrease in AUC) (Rainey et al., 2000).

There is substantial concern over the use of the anticonvulsants carbamazepine, phenytoin, and phenobarbital in HIV infection due to their potential to induce PI metabolism and reduce PI levels in serum, leading to virologic failure (Bartt, 1998). One report associated carbamazepine with reduced plasma indinavir level and virologic failure in one patient (Hugen et al., 2000), and another report suggested that switching from phenytoin to valproate (which does not induce PI metabolism but may increase HIV replication) was associated with favorable virologic response in two-thirds of patients (Bartt, 1998). Further, ritonavir and nelfinavir may raise the levels of these anticonvulsants in serum into toxic ranges (Hugen et al., 2000). Because of these interactions, ritonavir, saquinavir, indinavir, and nelfinavir are not recommended for use with carbamazepine, phenytoin, and phenobarbital. However, valproic acid may also inhibit the glucuronidation of zidovudine, leading to increased zidovudine levels in plasma and cerebrospinal fluid, which may have positive implications for treating HIV-associated neurocognitive disorders (Akula et al., 1997; Lertora et al., 1994).

There are other serious drug interactions that are important to note. Serum levels of sildenafil, which is commonly used for the treatment of sexual dysfunction, may be raised by concurrent administration of ritonavir, saquinavir, and indinavir, resulting in potentially dangerous cardiovascular side effects (Merry et al., 1999; Muirhead et al., 2000). A similar interaction is expected for illicitly used inhaled nitrates ("poppers"). Thus, it is recommended that inhaled nitrates be avoided and that sildenafil be used in low doses (e.g., 25 mg) and with caution in patients receiving these PIs. Finally, other illicit drugs may have dangerous clinical interactions with PIs. Fatalities have been reported with concurrent use of methylenedioxymethamphetamine ("ecstasy"), methamphetamine, and ritonavir (Hales et al., 2000; Mirken, 1997).

PSYCHIATRIC ASPECTS OF HIV-ASSOCIATED LIPODYSTROPHY

HIV-associated lipodystrophy is an increasingly recognized complication of prolonged treatment with HAART that may have significant impact on the psychological well-being and quality of life of those affected. HIV-associated lipodystrophy consists of central lipohypertrophy and peripheral lipoatrophy with associated hypercholesterolemia, hypertriglyceridemia, and insulin resistance. Lipohypertrophy occurs as hypertrophy of the dorsocervical fat pad, circumferential expansion of the neck, breast enlargement, and abdominal visceral fat accumulation. Lipoatrophy occurs as peripheral fat wasting in the face, arms, legs, and buttocks (Carr et al., 1998, 1999; Safrin and Grunfeld, 1999).

Many studies have looked at the prevalence of HIV-associated lipodystrophy, but they have had inconsistent diagnostic criteria, study sample selection methods, study populations, and prevalence of other possible risk factors. The use of self-report methods, physician assessments, and imaging techniques such as computed tomographic scans varies among the available studies. Despite these differences, estimates of the prevalence of HIV-associated lipodystrophy range from approximately 35 to 50% of all HIV-infected patients in treatment with HAART and from 50 to 80% of those patients treated with PIs (Carr et al., 1999; Heath et al., 2001).

Particular groups may be at greater risk for developing HIV-associated lipodystrophy syndrome. Increasing age, length of HAART treatment, lower nadir CD4 count, use of PIs, and use of stavudine and lamivudine are associated with increased risk of developing lipodystrophy (Heath et al., 2001; Lichtenstein et al., 2001; Mauss et al., 2002). Whites and women may also be at increased risk compared to blacks and men, respectively. Studies show similar rates of lipodystrophy occurring with Asian and Caucasian patients (Paton et al., 2002). Although no study has looked for an association between neurocognitive deficits and lipodystrophy, the overlapping risk factors of increasing age and years of HAART treatment may indicate higher than otherwise expected rates of the disorders co-occurring.

The currently accepted model of HIV-related lipodystrophy syndrome involves the interaction of antiviral medications, HIV-1, and inflammatory cytokines (Kino and Chrousos, 2003). PIs have diverse effects on metabolism, including effects on lipid metabolism and insulin signal transduction (Jain et al., 2001; Murata et al., 2000; Schutt et al., 2000). It remains unclear which, if any, of these alterations causes significant clinical effects. However, it has been shown repeatedly that the use of PIs is associated with insulin resistance (Carr et al., 1999). NRTIs may cause mitochondrial toxicity with resulting muscle loss. NRTIs are DNA antimetabolites that inhibit the activity of DNA polymerase δ, which is responsible for the replication of mitochondrial DNA (Dalakas et al., 1990). It has been shown that at least one NRTI, zidovudine, causes a reduction in mitochondrial DNA in muscle tissue (Kino et al., 1999). HIV itself likely plays a role in the development of HIV-associated lipodystrophy syndrome. In particular, the HIV-1 accessory proteins Vpr and Tat have been shown to induce tissue hypersensitivity to glucocorticoids (Kino et al., 1999; Ledru et al., 2000). Elevated levels of cytokines such as tumor necrosis factor alpha have been demonstrated in AIDS patients with lipodystrophy syndrome (Diederich et al., 2000). Tumor necrosis factor alpha increases the activity of 11-β hydroxysteroid dehydrogenase-1, which catalyzes the conversion of inactive cortisone to active cortisol in the peripheral tissues (Escher et al., 1997; Seckl and Walker, 2001; Tomlinson et al., 2001). This creates a local environment of increased cortisol effect that could include insulin resistance. Taken collectively, the combined effects of medications, HIV-1 specific factors, and inflammatory cytokines produce the variable phenotype of the HIV-associated lipodystrophy syndrome (Tershakovec et al., 2004).

Examination of the impact of HIV-associated lipodystrophy on the quality of life and psychological well-being of those afflicted has produced variable results. Most studies have shown an overall impact on the quality of life for individuals affected by lipodystrophy, but the reaction to this syndrome appears to be complex and dependent on multiple factors. The progressive change in appearance may affect an individual's body image and self-esteem, interfere with daily functioning, and create concern regarding lipodystrophy as a marker of HIV disease (Mauss et al., 2002).

Particular groups may be vulnerable to the impact of lipodystrophy on quality of life in different ways. Both men and women are significantly impacted by lipodystrophy, but it remains unclear how their reactions may differ. Breast lipoaccumulation is of particular concern for women and has been shown to be associated with impaired psychosocial functioning (Blanch et al., 2004). Men with lipodystrophy were noted to have worsening mood on quality of life measurements (Blanch et al., 2002). There is some evidence that homosexual men may be at greater risk for impairment in psychological functioning when affected by lipodystrophy. Their perception of health status and confidence in relationships as well as sexual behavior are all affected. However, condom use does not appear to vary between homosexual men with and without lipodystrophy (Dukers et al., 2000). The unemployed and those in active psychiatric treatment who suffer from lipodystrophy have been noted to suffer more than those without lipodystrophy (Blanch et al., 2002). As a causal relationship could not be established, these groups may represent those negatively impacted by lipodystrophy through loss of employment, impaired work functioning, depression, and anxiety syndromes. The degree to which different body areas are affected is associated with the individual's reaction. Those with significant facial lipoatrophy are most likely to seek treatment. This reaction may indicate a higher level of distress associated with lipoatrophy of the face as a marker of HIV disease. Breast enlargement and abdominal weight gain are also associated with greater quality of life impact and can affect basic functions of daily living such as dressing and working (Blanch et al., 2004).

The extent to which lipodystrophy affects compliance with antiretroviral medications remains unknown, with some studies showing a significant association with nonadherence while others do not show a difference (Duran et al., 2001). Having had a serious medical illness related to HIV may increase acceptance of lipodystrophy as an unfortunate consequence of treatment and increase the likelihood of compliance (Power et al., 2003). This finding demonstrates the willingness of patients to endure this often disfiguring complication of treatment in order to continue the medication's life-saving benefits.

No specific treatment has been found to correct the underlying cause of HIV-associated lipodystrophy. Withdrawal of PIs has shown regression of the lipodystrophy in limited cases, leaving most treatment options to correcting the visible and metabolic changes and limiting the impact on quality of life.

Assessment for psychiatric conditions including depression and anxiety disorders should be a routine part of the evaluation of any patient with lipodystrophy. The impact of lipodystrophy on social and work functioning should also be questioned. Coexisting psychiatric conditions should be treated or referred for psychiatric consultation. The use of support groups for those affected by lipodystrophy may also be of benefit.

Cosmetic surgical procedures including liposuction to remove hypertrophied abdominal fat and using silicone or polylactic acid implants (New-Fill) to correct facial lipoatrophy have shown promise. Medications including human growth hormone, anabolic steroids, metformin, naltrexone, and combination DHEA and cyclo-oxygenase inhibitor may have some impact on the extent of lipodystrophy. Although no diet has demonstrated an ability to reverse the changes of lipodystrophy, nutritional counseling may help reduce confounding dietary problems that could worsen fat redistribution. Exercise may reduce abdominal fat.

SEXUAL DYSFUNCTION IN HIV-POSITIVE INDIVIDUALS

Sexual dysfunction is a common problem in the general population and may be even more prevalent in those infected with HIV (Hijazi et al., 2002). Lack of sexual interest (Brown and Rundell, 1990; Pace et al., 1990), avoidance or infrequent sexual intercourse, erectile dysfunction, premature or delayed ejaculation, anorgasmia, vaginismus, and dyspareunia represent some of the potential manifestations of sexual dysfunction in HIV. While many causes of HIV-associated sexual dysfunction overlap with those seen in the general population, there are several factors that are unique to the HIV-positive individual.

When evaluating the HIV patient with sexual dysfunction, it is important to note that, in the vast majority of cases, a combination of psychological and biological factors are likely to be responsible and that each factor needs to be addressed for resolution of the problem. A sample of the potential psychological and biological factors is given in Table 5.

TABLE 5 Potential psychological and biological etiologies for sexual dysfunction in HIV[a]

Psychological factors
  Predisposing
    Traumatic sexual experience
    Poor sex education
    Lifestyle problems
    Substance abuse
  Precipitating
    Expectations
    Depression
    Anxiety
    Relationship problems
    Loss of partner
  Maintaining
    Performance anxiety
    Diminished attraction
    Poor communication
    Fear of infecting others
Biological factors
  Endocrine
    Hypogonadism
    Hyperthyroidism
    Hypothyroidism
    Hyperprolactinemia
  Neurological
    CNS interference
    Spinal cord injury
  Cardiovascular
    Atherosclerosis
    Hypertension
    Hypercholesterolemia
  Infective
    Pelvic inflammatory disease
    Balanitis/vulvovaginitis
  Iatrogenic
    Drug related
    Drug interactions
    Radiotherapy
    Surgical

[a]Adapted from Hijazi et al., 2002.

Psychological factors commonly seen with HIV-infected patients include having a history of traumatic sexual experiences, anxiety, depression, reaction to lipodystrophy, interpersonal problems, substance abuse, fear of infecting a partner, or fear of being infected with resistant virus. Biological factors commonly seen include hypogonadism, fatigue, antidepressant-induced CNS interference, peripheral neuropathy, cardiovascular changes due to lipodystrophy, presence of other sexually transmitted diseases, antiretrovirals (Colson et al., 2002), and polypharmacy including PIs and antidepressants.

The evaluation of sexual dysfunction is based on information obtained through history, physical exam, and laboratory testing, which together should provide the treatment focus. It is of utmost importance for clinicians to take a thorough history of past and present sexual activity and to monitor it on an ongoing basis, with focus on both risk behavior and sexual function. Aside from routine laboratory testing, further evaluation may include serum testosterone, estrogen, thyroid, and prolactin hormone levels (Hijazi et al., 2002).

The treatment of some commonly encountered biological and psychological factors associated with sexual dysfunction is discussed below.

As discussed in the section on "Depression" above, hypogonadism is a common cause of sexual dysfunction in addition to low mood, fatigue, and weight loss in HIV-positive men (Rabkin et al., 1999b). Replacement therapy with testosterone, either through biweekly injections or gel preparations, has been shown to be safe and effective in treating low sexual desire and erectile dysfunction in HIV-positive men. In women, low estrogen levels can result in too little lubrication, vaginal epithelial atrophy, and dyspareunia. After consideration of the potential risks and benefits, estrogen replacement therapy may provide relief from these symptoms.

Male erectile dysfunction treatment has been advanced by the development of oral medication treatments that inhibit the enzyme phosphodiesterase-5 including sildenafil (Viagra), vardenafil (Lavitra), and tadalafil (Cialis). Potential side effects include headaches, vasodilation, diarrhea, and blue-tinged vision. Although sildenafil does not appear to affect levels of PIs, indinavir, saquinavir, and ritonavir significantly increase sildenafil levels (Hall and Ahmad, 1999). Therefore, sildenafil should be used with caution when combined with PIs. The lower starting dose of 25 mg should be used. All the phosphodiesterase-5 inhibitors are contraindicated for use with nitrates and may produce hypotension-induced cardiovascular events including myocardial infarction and cardiovascular accidents. In particular, patients should be educated regarding the potential serious cardiovascular risks of using amyl nitrate with the phosphodiesterase-5 inhibitors.

Premature ejaculation can be treated with SSRIs and/or with sex therapy.

Many psychological factors can be resolved through education and treatment by a compassionate primary care clinician. Simple interventions based on the particular situation, such as explaining normal expectations or suggesting placing a lock on the bedroom door to ensure privacy, often provide relief of symptoms. More complicated problems such as significant difficulties within a relationship, vaginismus, substance abuse, history of a traumatic sexual experience, or severe depression and anxiety disorders may benefit from referral to mental health providers.

It is important to note that in addition to treating the needs of the individual patient, the public health implications of treating sexual dysfunction in HIV-positive individuals need to be considered. Discussing issues including disclosure of HIV status, choice of partners (in particular, anonymous partners), drug and alcohol use during sex, barriers to condom use, and the presence of other sexually transmitted diseases can help reduce the spread of HIV while still allowing HIV-positive individuals to have satisfying sex lives.

REFERENCES

Abbott Laboratories. 2001. *Norvir®. Prescribing Information.* Abbott Laboratories, North Chicago, IL.

Acuff, C., J. Archambeqult, B. Greenberg, J. Hoeltzel, J. S. McDaniel, P. Meyer, C. Packer, F. J. Parga, M. B. Phillen, A. Ronhovde, M. Saldarriaga, M. J. W. Smith, D. Stroff, and D. Wagner. 1999. *Mental Health Care for People Living with or Affected by HIV/AIDS: a Practical Guide.* Research Triangle Institute, Research Triangle Park, NC.

Akula, S. K., A. B. Rege, A. W. Dreisbach, P. M. Dejace, and J. J. Lertora. 1997. Valproic acid increases cerebrospinal fluid zidovudine levels in a patient with AIDS. *Am. J. Med. Sci.* **313**:244–246.

Anderson, J. 2001. A guide to the clinical care of women with HIV/AIDS, 1st ed. http://hab.hrsa.gov/womencare.htm. Accessed 9 December 2003.

Arnsten, J. H., P. A. Demas, R. W. Grant, M. N. Gourevitch, H. Farzadegan, A. A. Howard, and E. E. Schoenbaum. 2002. Impact of active drug use on antiretroviral therapy adherence and viral suppression in HIV-infected drug users. *J. Gen. Intern. Med.* **17**:377–381.

Ayuso Mateos, J. L., C. Bayon Perez, J. Santo-Domingo Carrasco, J. de Salas Jimenez de Azcarate, and D. Olivares. 1998. Psychiatric aspects of patients with HIV infection in the general hospital. *Psychother. Psychosom.* **52**:110–113.

Bartt, R. 1998. An effect of anticonvulsants in antiretroviral therapy. Neuroscience of HV Infection. *J. Neurovirol.* **4**(Suppl.):S340.

Batki, S., S. Ferrando, L. Manfredi, J. London, J. Pattillo, C. Abbott, and R. Hartwig. 1996. Psychiatric disorders, drug use, and HIV disease in 84 injection drug users. *Am. J. Addict.* **5**:249–258.

Batki, S. L. 1990a. Buspirone in drug users with AIDS or AIDS-related complex. *J. Clin. Psychopharmacol.* **10**(Suppl. 3):S111–S115.

Batki, S. L. 1990b. Drug abuse, psychiatric disorders, and AIDS: dual and triple diagnosis. *West. J. Med.* **152**:547–552.

Batki, S. L., L. B. Manfredi, P. Jacob III, and R. T. Jones. 1993. Fluoxetine for cocaine dependence in methadone maintenance: quantitative plasma and urine cocaine/benzoylecgonine concentrations. *J. Clin. Psychopharmacol.* **13**:243–250.

Beck, A. T., C. H. Ward, M. Mendelson, J. Mock, and J. Erbaugh. 1961. An inventory for measuring depression. *Arch. Gen. Psychiatry* **4**:561–571.

Bhattacharya, R., and M. C. Shuhart. 2003. Hepatitis C and alcohol: interactions, outcomes, and implications. *J. Clin. Gastroenterol.* **36**:242–252.

Bialer, P., J. Wallack, S. Prenzlauer, L. Bogdonoff, and I. Wilets. 1996. Psychiatric comorbidity among hospitalized AIDS patients vs. non-AIDS patients referred for psychiatric consultation. *Psychosomatics* **37**:469–475.

Bing, E. G., M. A. Burnam, D. Longshore, J. A. Fleishman, C. D. Sherbourne, A. S. London, B. J. Turner, F. Eggan, R. Beckman, B. Vitiello, S. C. Morton, M. Orlando, S. A. Bozzette, L. Ortiz-Barron, and M. Shapiro. 2001. Psychiatric disorders and drug use among human immunodeficiency virus-infected adults in the United States. *Arch. Gen. Psychiatry* **58**:721–728.

Blanch, J., A. Rousaud, E. Martinez, E. De Lazzari, A. Milinkovic, J. M. Peri, J. L. Blanco, J. Laen, V. Navarro, G. Massana, and J. M. Gatell. 2004. Factors associated with severe impact of lipodystrophy on the quality of life of patients with HIV-1. *Clin. Infect. Dis.* **38**:1464–1470.

Blanch, J., A. Rousaud, E. Martinez, E. E. De Lazzari, J. M. Peri, A. Milinkovic, J. B. Perez-Cuevas, J. L. Blanco, and J. M. Gatell. 2002. Impact of lipodystrophy on the quality of life of HIV-1 infected patients. *J. Acquir. Immune Defic. Syndr.* **31**:404–407.

Breitbart, W. 1994. Pain management in the patient with AIDS. *Pain Manage.* **2**:1–9.

Breitbart, W. 1996. Pain management and psychosocial issues in HIV and AIDS. *Am. J. Hosp. Palliat. Care* **13**:20–29.

Breitbart, W., R. Marotta, M. M. Platt, H. Weisman, M. Derevenco, C. Grau, K. Corbera, S. Raymond, S. Lund, and P. Jacobson. 1996a. A double-blind trial of haloperidol, chlorpromazine, and lorazepam in the treatment of delirium in hospitalized AIDS patients. *Am. J. Psychiatry* **153**:231–237.

Breitbart, W., M. V. McDonald, B. Rosenfeld, S. D. Passik, D. Hewitt, H. Thaler, and R. K. Portenoy. 1996b. Pain in ambulatory AIDS patients. I. Pain characteristics and medical correlates. *Pain* **68**:315–321.

Breitbart, W., B. Rosenfeld, M. Kaim, and J. Funesti-Esch. 2001. A randomized, double-blind, placebo-controlled trial of psychostimulants for the treatment of fatigue in ambulatory patients with human immunodeficiency virus disease. *Arch. Intern. Med.* **161**:411–420.

Brown, G., and J. Rundell. 1990. Prospective study of psychiatric morbidity in HIV-seropositive women without AIDS. *Gen. Hosp. Psychiatry* **12**:30–35.

Budman, C. L., and T. A. Vandersall. 1990. Clonazepam treatment of acute mania in an AIDS patient. *J. Clin. Psychiatry* **51**:212.

Burnam, M. A., E. G. Bing, S. C. Morton, C. Sherbourne, J. A. Fleishman, A. S. London, B. Vitiello, M. Stein, S. A. Bozzette, and M. F. Shapiro. 2001. Use of mental health and substance abuse treatment services among adults with HIV in the United States. *Arch. Gen. Psychiatry* **58**:729–736.

Buysse, D. J., C. F. Reynolds III, T. H. Monk, S. R. Berman, and D. J. Kupfer. 1989. The Pittsburgh Sleep Quality Index: a new instrument for psychiatric practice and research. *Psychiatry Res.* **28**:193–213.

Carr, A., K. Samaras, S. Burton, M. Law, J. Freund, D. J. Chisholm, and D. A. Cooper. 1998. A syndrome of peripheral lipodystrophy, hyperlipidemia and insulin resistance in patients receiving HIV protease inhibitors. *AIDS* **12**:F51–F58.

Carr, A., K. Samaras, A. Thorisdottir, G. R. Kaufmann, D. J. Chisholm, and D. A. Cooper. 1999. Diagnosis, prediction, and natural course of HIV-1 protease-inhibitor-associated lipodystrophy, hyperlipidemia, and diabetes mellitus: a cohort study. *Lancet* **353**:2093–2099.

Centers for Disease Control and Prevention. 2001. HIV/AIDS surveillance report: December 2001, year-end edition, 13th ed. http://www.cdc.gov/hiv/stats/hasr1302.htm. Accessed 1 December 2003.

Chaisson, R. E., J. C. Keruly, and R. D. Moore. 1995. Race, sex, drug use, and progression of human immunodeficiency virus disease. *N. Engl. J. Med.* **333**:751–756.

Chalder, T., G. Berelowitz, T. Pawlikowska, L. Watts, S. Wessely, D. Wright, and E. P. Wallace. 1993. Development of a fatigue scale. *J. Psychosom. Res.* **37**:147–153.

Cohen, P. T., M. A. Sande, and P. A. Volberding (ed.). 1994. *The AIDS Knowledge Base*, 2nd ed. Little Brown, Boston, MA.

Colson, A. E., M. J. Keller, P. E. Sax, P. T. Pettus, R. Platt, and P. W. Choo. 2002. Male sexual dysfunction associated with antiretroviral therapy. *J. Acquir. Immune Defic. Syndr.* **30**:27–32.

Cozza, K. L., E. J. Swanton, and C. W. Humphreys. 2000. Hepatotoxicity with combination of valproic acid, ritonavir, and nevirapine: a case report. *Psychosomatics* **41**:452–453.

Currier, M. B., G. Molina, and M. Kato. 2003. A prospective trial of sustained-release bupropion for depression in HIV-seropositive and AIDS patients. *Psychosomatics* **44**:120–125.

Dalakas, M. C., I. Illa, G. H. Pezeshkpour, J. P. Laukaitis, B. Cohen, and J. L. Griffin. 1990. Mitochondrial myopathy caused by long-term zidovudine therapy. *N. Engl. J. Med.* **322**:1098–1105.

Dana Consortium on Therapy for HIV Dementia and Related Cognitive Disorders. 1996. Clinical confirmation of the American Academy of Neurology algorithm for HIV-1-associated cognitive/motor disorder. *Neurology* **47**:1247–1253.

Darko, D. F., J. A. McCutchan, D. F. Kripke, J. C. Gillin, and S. Golshan. 1992. Fatigue, sleep disturbance, disability, and indices of progression of HIV infection. *Am. J. Psychiatry* **149**:514–520.

de Ronchi, D., I. Faranca, P. Forti, G. Ravaglia, M. Borderi, R. Manfredi, and V. Volterra. 2000. Development of acute psychotic disorders and HIV-1 infection. *Int. J. Psychiatry Med.* 30:173–183.

Dettling, M., B. Muller-Oerlinghausen, and P. Britsch. 1998. Clozapine treatment of HIV-associated psychosis—too much bone marrow toxicity? *Pharmacopsychiatry* 31:156–157.

Diederich, S., C. Grossman, B. Hanke, M. Quinkler, M. Herrmann, V. Bahr, and W. Oelkers. 2000. In the search for specific inhibitors of human 11beta-hydroxysteroid-dehydrogenases (11beta-HSDs): chenodeoxycholic acid selectively inhibits 11beta-HSD-I. *Eur. J. Endocrinol.* 142:200–207.

Dieperink, E., S. B. Ho, P. Thuras, and M. L. Willenbring. 2003. A prospective study of neuropsychiatric symptoms associated with interferon-alpha-2b and ribavirin therapy for patients with chronic hepatitis C. *Psychosomatics* 44:104–112.

Dukers, N., I. G. Stolte, N. Albrecht, R. A. Coutinho, and J. B. F. deWit. 2000. The impact of experiencing lipodystrophy on the sexual behavior and well-being among HIV-infected homosexual men. *AIDS* 15:812–813.

Duran, S., M. Saves, B. Spire, V. Cailleton, A. Sobel, P. Carrieri, D. Salmon, J. P. Moatti, C. Leport, and the APROCO Study Group. 2001. Failure to maintain long-term adherence to highly active antiretroviral therapy: the role of lipodystrophy. *AIDS* 15:2441–2444.

Elliott, A. J., and P. P. Roy-Byrne. 2000. Mirtazapine for depression in patients with human immunodeficiency virus. *J. Clin. Psychopharmacol.* 20:265–267.

Elliott, A. J., J. Russo, K. Bergam, K. Claypoole, K. K. Uldall, and P. P. Roy-Byrne. 1999. Antidepressant efficacy in HIV-seropositive outpatients with major depressive disorder: an open trial of nefazodone. *J. Clin. Psychiatry* 60:226–231.

Elliott, A. J., K. K. Uldall, K. Bergam, J. Russo, K. Claypoole, and P. P. Roy-Byrne. 1998. Randomized, placebo-controlled trial of paroxetine versus imipramine in depressed HIV-positive outpatients. *Am. J. Psychiatry* 155:367–372.

Escher, G., I. Galli, B. S. Vishwanath, B. M. Frey, and F. J. Frey. 1997. Tumor necrosis factor alpha and interleukin 1beta enhance the cortisone/cortisol shuttle. *J. Exp. Med.* 186:189–198.

Fernandez, F., and J. K. Levy. 1993. The use of molindone in the treatment of psychotic and delirious patients infected with the human immunodeficiency virus. Case reports. *Gen. Hosp. Psychiatry* 15:31–35.

Ferrando, S., S. Evans, K. Goggin, M. Sewell, B. Fishman, and J. Rabkin. 1998a. Fatigue in HIV illness: relationship to depression, physical limitations, and disability. *Psychosom. Med.* 60:746–759.

Ferrando, S. J., J. D. Goldman, and W. E. Charness. 1997. Selective serotonin reuptake inhibitor treatment of depression in symptomatic HIV infection and AIDS: improvements in affective and somatic symptoms. *Gen. Hosp. Psychiatry* 19:89–97.

Ferrando, S. J., J. Rabkin, and J. Rothenberg. 1998b. Psychiatric disorders and adjustment of HIV and AIDS patients during and after medical hospitalization. *Psychosomatics* 39:214–215.

Ferrando, S. J., J. G. Rabkin, G. M. de Moore, and R. Rabkin. 1999. Antidepressant treatment of depression in HIV-seropositive women. *J. Clin. Psychiatry* 60:741–746.

Ferrando, S. J., T. L. Wall, S. L. Batki, and J. L. Sorensen. 1996. Psychiatric morbidity, illicit drug use and adherence to zidovudine (AZT) among injection drug users with HIV disease. *Am. J. Drug Alcohol Abuse* 22:475–487.

Foser, R., D. Olajide, and I. P. Everall. 2003. Antiretroviral therapy-induced psychosis; case report and brief review of the literature. *HIV Med.* 4:139–144.

Friedmann, P. D., J. A. Alexander, L. Jin, and T. A. D'Aunno. 1999. On-site primary care and mental health services in outpatient drug abuse treatment units. *J. Behav. Health Serv. Res.* 26:80–94.

Geletko, S. M., and A. D. Erickson. 2000. Decreased methadone effect after ritonavir initiation. *Pharmacotherapy* 20:93–94.

Gleason, O. C., W. R. Yates, M. D. Isbell, and M. A. Philipsen. 2002. An open-label trial of citalopram for major depression in patients with hepatitis C. *J. Clin. Psychiatry* 63:194–198.

Greenblatt, D. J., L. L. von Moltke, J. S. Harmatz, A. L. Durol, J. A. Graf, P. Mertzanis, J. L. Hoffman, and R. I. Shader. 2000a. Alprazolam-ritonavir interaction: implications for product labeling. *Clin. Pharmacol. Ther.* 67:335–341.

Greenblatt, D. J., L. L. von Moltke, J. S. Harmatz, A. L. Durol, J. P. Daily, J. A. Graf, P. Mertzanis, J. L. Hoffman, and R. I. Shader. 2000b. Differential impairment of triazolam and Zolpidem clearance by ritonavir. *J. Acquir. Immune Defic. Syndr.* 24:129–136.

Hales, G., N. Roth, and D. Smith. 2000. Possible fatal interaction between protease inhibitors and methamphetamine. *Antivir. Ther.* 5:19.

Hall, M. C., and S. Ahmad. 1999. Interaction between sildenafil and HIV-1 combination therapy. *Lancet* 353:2071–2072.

Halman, M. H., J. L. Worth, K. M. Sanders, P. F. Renshaw, and G. B. Murray. 1993. Anticonvulsant use in the treatment of manic syndromes in patients with HIV-1 infection. *J. Neuropsychiatry Clin. Neurosci.* 5:430–434.

Hamilton, M. 1959. The assessment of anxiety states by rating. *Br. J. Med. Psychol.* 32:50–55.

Hamilton, M. 1960. A rating scale for depression. *J. Neurol. Neurosurg. Psychiatry* 23:56–62.

Heath, K. V., R. S. Hogg, K. J. Chan, V. Harris Montessori, M. V. O'Shaughnessy, and J. S. Montaner. 2001. Lipodystrophy-associated morphological, cholesterol and triglyceride abnormalities in a population-based HIV/AIDS treatment database. *AIDS* 15:231–239.

Hijazi, L., R. Nandawani, and P. Kell. 2002. Medical management of sexual difficulties in HIV-positive individuals. *Int. J. STD AIDS* 13:587–592.

Holmes, V. F., F. Fernandez, and J. K. Levy. 1989. Psychostimulant response in AIDS-related complex patients. *J. Clin. Psychiatry* 50:5–8.

Hoover, D. R., A. J. Saah, H. Bacellar, R. Murphy, B. Visscher, R. Anderson, and R. A. Kaslow. 1993. Signs and symptoms of "asymptomatic" HIV-1 infection in homosexual men. *J. Acquir. Immune Defic. Syndr. Hum. Retrovirol.* 6:66–71.

Horberg, M., M. Silverberg, L. Hurley, G. Delorenze, and C. Quesenberry. 2008. Influence of prior antiretroviral experience on adherence and responses to a new highly active antiretroviral therapy regimens. *AIDS Patient Care STDs* 22:301–312.

Hu, D. J., R. Byers, Jr., P. L. Fleming, and J. W. Ward. 1995. Characteristics of persons with late AIDS diagnosis in the United States. *Am. J. Prev. Med.* 11:114–119.

Hugen, P. W., D. M. Burger, K. Brinkman, H. J. ter Hofstede, R. Schuurman, P. P. Koopmans, and Y. A. Hekster. 2000. Carbamazepine-indinavir interaction causes antiretroviral therapy failure. *Ann. Pharmacother.* 34:465–470.

Ickovics, J. R., M. E. Hamburger, D. Vlahov, E. E. Schoenbaum, P. Schuman, R. J. Boland, J. Moore, and the HIV Epidemiology Research Study Group. 2001. Mortality, CD4 cell count decline, and depressive symptoms among HIV-seropositive women: longitudinal analysis from the HIV Epidemiology Research Study. *JAMA* 285:1466–1474.

Iribarne, C., F. Berthou, D. Carlhant, Y. Dreano, D. Picart, F. Lohezic, and C. Riche. 1998. Inhibition of methadone and buprenorphine N-dealkylations by three HIV-1 protease inhibitors. *Drug Metab. Dispos.* 26:257–260.

Jain, R. G., E. S. Furfine, L. Pedneault, A. J. White, and J. M. Lenhard. 2001. Metabolic complications associated with antiretroviral therapy. *Antivir. Res.* **51**:151–177.

Jennings, H. R., and F. Romanelli. 1993. The use of valproic acid in HIV-positive patients. *Ann. Pharmacother.* **33**:1113–1116.

Kaslow, R. A., J. P. Phair, H. B. Friedman, D. Lyter, R. E. Solomon, J. Dudley, B. F. Polk, and W. Blackwelder. 1987. Infection with the human immunodeficiency virus: clinical manifestations and their relationship to immune deficiency. *Ann. Intern. Med.* **107**:474–480.

Kendall, P. C., A. J. Finch, Jr., S. M. Auerbach, J. F. Hooke, and P. J. Mikulka. 1976. The State-Trait Anxiety Inventory: a systematic evaluation. *J. Consult. Clin. Psychol.* **44**:406–412.

Kieburtz, K., A. E. Zettelmaier, L. Ketonen, M. Tuite, and E. D. Caine. 1991. Manic syndrome in AIDS. *Am. J. Psychiatry* **148**:1068–1070.

Kino, T., and G. P. Chrousos. 2003. AIDS-related insulin resistance and lipodystrophy syndrome. *Curr. Drug Targets Immune Endocr. Metabol. Disord.* **3**:111–117.

Kino, T., A. Gragerov, J. B. Kopp, R. H. Stauber, G. N. Pavlakis, and G. P. Chrousos. 1999. The HIV-1 virion-associated protein vpr is a coactivator of the human glucocorticoid receptor. *J. Exp. Med.* **189**:51–62.

Kraus, M. R., A. Schafer, H. Faller, H. Csef, and M. Scheurlen. 2002. Paroxetine for the treatment of interferon-alpha-induced depression in chronic hepatitis C. *Aliment. Pharmacol. Ther.* **16**:1091–1099.

Kroenke, K., R. L. Spitzer, and J. B. Williams. 2001. The PHQ-9: validity of a brief depression severity measure. *Am. Gen. Intern. Med.* **16**:606–613.

Larue, F., A. Fontaine, and S. M. Colleau. 1997. Underestimation and undertreatment of pain in HIV disease: a multicentre study. *BMJ* **314**:23–28.

Lebovits, A. H., G. Smith, M. Maignan, and M. Lefkowitz. 1994. Pain in hospitalized patients with AIDS: analgesic and psychotropic medications. *Clin. J. Pain* **10**:156–161.

Ledru, E., N. Christeff, O. Patey, P. de Truchis, J. C. Melchior, and M. L. Gougeon. 2000. Alteration of tumor necrosis factor-alpha T-cell homeostasis following potent antiretroviral therapy: contribution to the development of human immunodeficiency virus-associated lipodystrophy syndrome. *Blood* **95**:3191–3198.

Lera, G., and J. Zirulnik. 1999. Pilot study with clozapine in patients with HIV-associated psychosis and drug-induced parkinsonism. *Mov. Disord.* **14**:128–131.

Lertora, J. J., A. B. Rege, D. L. Greenspan, S. Akula, W. J. George, N. E. Hyslop, Jr., and K. C. Agrawal. 1994. Pharmacokinetic interaction between zidovudine and valproic acid in patients infected with human immunodeficiency virus. *Clin. Pharmacol. Ther.* **56**:272–278.

Lichtenstein, K. A., D. J. Ward, A. C. Moorman, K. M. Delaney, B. Young, F. J. Palella, Jr., P. H. Rhodes, K. C. Wood, and S. D. Holmberg; HIV Outpatient Study Investigators. 2001. Clinical assessment of HIV-associated lipodystrophy in an ambulatory population. *AIDS* **15**:1389–1398.

Lyketsos, C. G., D. R. Hoover, M. Guccione, M. A. Dew, J. E. Wesch, E. G. Bing, and G. J. Treisman. 1996. Changes in depressive symptoms as AIDS develops. *Am. J. Psychiatry* **153**:1430–1437.

Lyketsos, C. G., J. Schwartz, M. Fishman, and G. Treisman. 1997. AIDS mania. *J. Neuropsychiatry Clin. Neurosci.* **9**:277–279.

Macallen, D. C., C. Noble, C. Baldwin, S. A. Jebb, A. M. Prentice, W. A. Coward, M. B. Sawyer, T. J. McManus, and G. E. Griffin. 1995. Energy expenditure and wasting in human immunodeficiency virus infection. *N. Engl. J. Med.* **333**:83–88.

Markowitz, J. C., J. H. Kocsis, B. Fishman, L. A. Spielman, L. B. Jacobsberg, A. J. Fraces, G. L. Klerman, and S. W. Perry. 1998. Treatment of depressive symptoms in human immunodeficiency virus-positive patients. *Arch. Gen. Psychiatry* **55**:452–457.

Martinez, A., D. Israelski, C. Walker, and C. Koopman. 2002. Posttraumatic stress disorder in women attending human immunodeficiency virus outpatient clinics. *AIDS Patient Care STDs* **16**:283–291.

Mauri, M. C., L. Fabiano, S. Bravin, C. Ricci, and G. Invernizzi. 1997. Schizophrenic patients before and after HIV infection: a case-control study. *Encephale* **23**:437–441.

Mauss, S., M. Corzillius, E. Wolf, A. Schwenk, A. Adam, H. Jaeger, H. Knechten, J. Goelz, A. Goetzenich, and the DAGNA Lipantiretroviral Therapy Study Group. 2002. Risk factors for the HIV-associated lipodystrophy syndrome in a closed cohort of patients after 3 years of antiretroviral treatment. *HIV Med.* **3**:49–55.

McCormack, J., R. Li, D. Zarowny, and J. Singer. 1993. Inadequate treatment of pain in ambulatory HIV patients. *Clin. J. Pain* **9**:279–283.

McDaniel, J. S. 2000. Practice guideline for the treatment of patients with HIV/AIDS. *Am. J. Psychiatry* **157**:1–62.

McKinnon, K., F. Cournos, and R. Herman. 2002. HIV among people with chronic mental illness. *Psychiatr. Q.* **73**:17–31.

Merry, C., M. G. Barry, M. Ryan, M. Tjia Hennessy, V. A. Eagling, F. Mulcahy, and D. J. Back. 1999. Interaction of sildenafil and indinavir when co-administered to HIV-positive patients. *AIDS* **13**:F101–F107.

Meyer, J. M., J. Marsh, and G. Simpson. 1998. Differential sensitivities to risperidone and olanzapine in a human immunodeficiency virus patient. *Biol. Psychiatry* **44**:791–794.

Mijch, A. M., F. K. Judd, C. G. Lyketsos, S. Ellen, and A. Cockram. 1999. Secondary mania in patients with HIV infection: are antiretrovirals protective? *J. Neuropsychiatry Clin. Neurosci.* **11**:475–480.

Mirken, B. 1997. Danger: possibly fatal interactions between ritonavir and "ecstasy," some other psychoactive drugs. *AIDS Treat. Newsl.* **265**:5. (Abstract.)

Muirhead, G. J., M. B. Wulff, A. Fielding, D. Kleinermans, and N. Buss. 2000. Pharmacokinetic interactions between sildenafil and saquinavir/ritonavir. *Br. J. Clin. Pharmacol.* **50**:99–107.

Murata, H., P. W. Hruz, and M. Mueckler. 2000. The mechanism of insulin resistance caused by HIV protease inhibitor therapy. *J. Biol. Chem.* **275**:20251–20254.

Nokes, K. M., and J. Kendrew. 2001. Correlates of sleep quality in persons with HIV disease. *J. Assoc. Nurses AIDS Care* **12**:17–22.

Nunez, M., D. R. Gonzalez, L. Gallego, I. Jimenez-Nacher, J. Gonzalez-Lahoz, and V. Soriano. 2001. Higher efavirenz plasma levels correlate with development of insomnia. *J. Acquir. Immune Defic. Syndr.* **28**:399–400.

O'Dowd, M. A., and F. P. McKegney. 1990. AIDS patients compared with others seen in psychiatric consultation. *Gen. Hosp. Psychiatry* **12**:50–55.

Ouellet, D., A. Hsu, J. Qian, J. E. Lamm, J. H. Cavanaugh, J. M. Leonard, and G. R. Granneman. 1998. Effect of fluoxetine on pharmacokinetics of ritonavir. *Antimicrob. Agents Chemother.* **42**:3107–3112.

Pace, J., G. Brown, J. Rundell, S. Paolucci, K. Drexler, and S. McManis. 1990. Prevalence of psychiatric disorders in a mandatory screening program for infection with human immunodeficiency virus: a pilot study. *Mil. Med.* **155**:76–80.

Palella, F. J., K. M. Delaney, A. C. Moorman, M. O. Loveless, J. Fuhrer, G. A. Satten, D. J. Aschman, S. D. Holmberg, et al. 1998. Declining morbidity and mortality among patients with advanced human immunodeficiency virus infection. *N. Engl. J. Med.* **338**:853–860.

Palenicek, J., K. E. Nelson, D. Vlahov, N. Galai, S. Cohn, and A. J. Saah. 1993. Comparison of clinical symptoms of human immunodeficiency virus disease between intravenous drug users and homosexual men. *Arch. Intern. Med.* **153:**1806–1812.

Paton, N. I., A. Earnest, Y. M. Ng, F. Karim, and J. Aboulhab. 2002. Lipodystrophy in a cohort of human immunodeficiency virus-infected Asian patients: prevalence, associated factors, and psychological impact. *Clin. Infect. Dis.* **35:**1244–1249.

Perkins, D. O., J. Leserman, R. A. Stern, S. F. Baum, D. Liao, R. N. Golden, and D. L. Evans. 1995. Somatic symptoms of HIV infection: relationship to depressive symptoms and indicators of HIV disease. *Am. J. Psychiatry* **152:**1776–1781.

Perry, S., and S. Tross. 1984. Psychiatric problems of AIDS inpatients at The New York Hospital: preliminary report. *Public Health Rep.* **99:**200–205.

Piedrola, G., J. L. Casado, E. Lopez, A. Moreno, M. J. Perez-Elias, and R. Garcia-Robles. 1996. Clinical features of adrenal insufficiency in patients with acquired immunodeficiency syndrome. *Clin. Endocrinol.* **45:**97–101.

Piper, B. F., A. M. Lindsey, and M. J. Dodd. 1989. The development of an instrument to measure the subjective dimension of fatigue, p. 199–208. *In* S. Funk, E. Tornquist, M. Champagne, et al. (ed.), *Key Aspects of Comfort: Management of Pain, Fatigue, and Nausea.* Springer, New York, NY.

Power, R., H. L. Tate, S. M. McGill, and C. Taylor. 2003. A qualitative study of the psychosocial implications of lipodystrophy syndrome on HIV positive individuals. *Sex. Transm. Infect.* **79:**137–141.

Rabkin, J. G., and S. Ferrando. 1997. A "Second Life" agenda: policy and research issues raised by protease inhibitor treatment for people with HIV/AIDS. *Arch. Gen. Psychiatry* **54:**1049–1053.

Rabkin, J. G., S. J. Ferrando, L. B. Jacobsberg, and B. Fishman. 1997. Prevalence of axis I disorders in an AIDS cohort: a cross-sectional, controlled study. *Compr. Psychiatry* **38:**146–154.

Rabkin, J. G., S. J. Ferrando, S. H. Lin, M. Sewell, and M. McElhiney. 2000a. Psychological effects of HAART: a 2-year study. *Psychosom. Med.* **62:**413–422.

Rabkin, J. G., S. J. Ferrando, G. J. Wagner, and R. Rabkin. 2000b. DHEA treatment for HIV+ patients: effects on mood, androgenic and anabolic parameters. *Psychoneuroendocrinology* **25:**53–68.

Rabkin, J. G., M. McElhiney, R. Rabkin, P. McGrath, and S. J. Ferrando. 2006. DHEA effects on mild depression in HIV/AIDS: a placebo-controlled trial. *Am. J. Psychiatr.* **163:**59–66.

Rabkin, J. G., R. Rabkin, W. Harrison, and G. Wagner. 1994a. Effect of imipramine on mood and enumerative measures of immune status in depressed patients with HIV illness. *Am. J. Psychiatry* **151:**516–523.

Rabkin, J. G., R. Rabkin, and G. Wagner. 1994b. Effects of fluoxetine on mood and immune status in depressed patients with HIV illness. *J. Clin. Psychiatry* **55:**92–97.

Rabkin, J. G., R. Rabkin, and G. Wagner. 1995. Testosterone replacement therapy in HIV illness. *Gen. Hosp. Psychiatry* **17:**37–42.

Rabkin, J. G., G. Wagner, and R. Rabkin. 1994c. Effects of sertraline on mood and immune status in patients with major depression and HIV illness: an open trial. *J. Clin. Psychiatry* **55:**433–439.

Rabkin, J. G., G. J. Wagner, and R. Rabkin. 1999a. Fluoxetine treatment for depression in patients with HIV and AIDS: a randomized, placebo-controlled trial. *Am. J. Psychiatry* **156:**101–107.

Rabkin, J. G., G. J. Wagner, and R. Rabkin. 1999b. Testosterone therapy for human immunodeficiency virus-positive men with and without hypogonadism. *J. Clin. Psychopharmacol.* **19:**19–27.

Rabkin, J. G., G. J. Wagner, and R. Rabkin. 2000c. A double-blind, placebo-controlled trial of testosterone therapy for HIV-positive men with hypogonadal symptoms. *Arch. Gen. Psychiatry* **57:**141–147.

RachBeisel, J. A., and E. Weintraub. 1997. Valproic acid treatment of AIDS-related mania. *J. Clin. Psychiatry* **58:**406–407.

Rainey, P. M., G. Friedland, E. F. McCance-Katz, L. Andrews, S. M. Mitchell, C. Charles, and P. Jatlow. 2000. Interaction of methadone with didanosine and stavudine. *J. Acquir. Immune Defic. Syndr.* **24:**241–248.

Roberts, R. E., and S. W. Vernon. 1983. The Center for Epidemiologic Studies Depression Scale: its use in a community sample. *Am. J. Psychiatry* **140:**41–46.

Rosenfeld, B., W. Breitbart, M. V. McDonald, S. D. Passik, H. Thaler, and R. K. Portenoy. 1996. Pain in ambulatory AIDS patients. II. Impact of pain on psychological functioning and quality of life. *Pain* **68:**323–328.

Rubinstein, M. L., and P. A. Selwyn. 1989. High prevalence of insomnia in an outpatient population with HIV infection. *J. Acquir. Immune Defic. Syndr. Hum. Retrovirol.* **19:**260–265.

Safrin, S., and C. Grunfeld. 1999. Fat distribution and metabolic changes in patients with HIV infection. *AIDS* **13:**2493–2505.

Samet, J. H., M. D. Stein, and P. G. O'Connor. 1995. Models of medical care for HIV-infected drug users. *Subst. Abus.* **16:**131–139.

Scamvougeras, A., and P. I. Rosebush. 1992. AIDS-related psychosis with catatonia responding to low-dose lorazepam. *J. Clin. Psychiatry* **53:**414–415.

Schutt, M., M. Meier, M. Meyer, J. Klien, S. P. Aries, and H. H. Klein. 2000. The HIV-1 protease inhibitor indinavir impairs insulin signalling in HepG2 hepatoma cells. *Diabetologia* **43:**1145–1148.

Schwartz, J. A., and J. S. McDaniel. 1999. Double-blind comparison of fluoxetine and desipramine in the treatment of depressed women with advanced HIV disease: a pilot study. *Depress. Anxiety* **9:**70–74.

Seckl, J. R., and B. R. Walker. 2001. Minireview: 11beta-hydroxysteroid dehydrogenase type 1—a tissue-specific amplifier of glucocorticoid action. *Endocrinology* **142:**1371–1376.

Sewell, D. D., D. V. Jeste, J. H. Atkinson, R. K. Heaton, J. R. Hesselink, C. Wiley, L. Thal, J. L. Chandler, I. Grant, et al. 1994a. HIV-associated psychosis: a study of 20 cases. *Am. J. Psychiatry* **151:**237–242.

Sewell, D. D., D. V. Jeste, L. A. McAdams, A. Bailey, M. J. Harris, J. H. Atkinson, J. L. Chandler, J. A. McCutchan, I. Grant, et al. 1994b. Neuroleptic treatment of HIV-associated psychosis. *Neuropsychopharmacology* **10:**223–229.

Sewell, M. C., K. J. Goggin, J. G. Rabkin, S. J. Ferrando, M. C. McElhiney, and S. Evans. 2000. Anxiety syndromes and symptoms among men with AIDS: a longitudinal controlled study. *Psychosomatics* **41:**294–300.

Simpson, D. M., and A. N. Bender. 1988. Human immunodeficiency virus associated myopathy: analysis of 11 patients. *Ann. Neurol.* **24:**79–84.

Simpson, D. M., J. C. McArthur, R. Olney, D. Clifford, Y. So, D. Ross, B. J. Baird, P. Barrett, A. E. Hammer, and the Lamotrigine HIV Neuropathy Study Team. 2003. Lamotrigine for HIV-associated painful sensory neuropathies: a placebo-controlled trial. *Neurology* **60:**1508–1514.

Singer, E. J., C. Zorilla, B. Fahy-Charndon, S. Chi, K. Syndulko, and W. W. Tourtellotte. 1993. Painful symptoms reported by ambulatory HIV-infected men in a longitudinal study. *Pain* **54:**15–19.

Singh, A. N., and J. Catalan. 1994. Risperidone in HIV-related manic psychosis. *Lancet* **344:**1029–1030.

Singh, A. N., H. Golledge, and J. Catalan. 1997. Treatment of HIV-related psychotic disorders with risperidone: a series of 21 cases. *J. Psychosom. Res.* **42:**489–493.

Sorensen, J. L., and S. L. Batki. 1992. Methadone maintenance as a setting for treating drug abusers with HIV infection. *Psychol. Addict. Behav.* **6:**126–130.

Sorensen, J. L., A. Mascovich, T. L. Wall, D. DePhilippis, S. L. Batki, and M. Chesney. 1998. Medication adherence strategies for drug abusers with HIV disease. *AIDS Care* **10:**297–312.

Sorensen, J. L., C. L. Masson, and D. C. Perlman. 2002. HIV/hepatitis prevention in drug abuse treatment programs: guidance from research. *(NIDA) Sci. Pract. Persp.* **1:**4–11.

Spitzer, R. L., K. Kroenke, and J. B. Williams. 1999. Validation and utility of a self-report version of PRIME-MD: the PHQ primary care study. Primary Care Evaluation of Mental Disorders. Patient Health Questionnaire. *JAMA* **282:**1737–1744.

Spraycar, M. (ed.). 1995. *Stedman's Medical Dictionary*, 26th ed. Williams & Wilkins, Baltimore, MD.

Strauss, S. E. 1994. Chronic fatigue syndrome, p. 2798–2800. *In* K. J. Isselbacher, E. Braunwald, J. D. Wilson, et al. (ed.), *Harrison's Principles of Internal Medicine*, 13th ed. McGraw Hill, New York, NY.

Sulkowski, M. S., and D. L. Thomas. 2003. Hepatitis C in the HIV-infected patient. *Clin. Liver Dis.* **7:**179–194.

Tanquary, J. 1993. Lithium neurotoxicity at therapeutic levels in an AIDS patient. *J. Nerv. Ment. Dis.* **181:**518–519.

Tershakovec, A. M., I. Frank, and D. Rader. 2004. HIV-related lipodystrophy and related factors. *Atherosclerosis* **174:**1–10.

Tomlinson, J. W., J. Morre, M. S. Cooper, I. Bujalska, M. Shahmanesh, C. Burt, A. Strain, M. Hewison, and P. M. Stewart. 2001. Regulation of expression of 11beta-hydroxysteroid dehydrogenase type 1 in adipose tissue: tissue-specific induction by cytokines. *Endocrinology* **142:**1982–1989.

Treatment Improvement Protocol (TIP) Series 37 Consensus Panel. 2004. Substance abuse treatment for persons with HIV/AIDS. http://www.guideline.gov. Accessed 28 January 2004.

Turner, B. J., J. A. Fleishman, N. Wenger, A. S. London, M. A. Burnam, M. F. Shapiro, E. G. Bing, M. D. Stein, D. Longshore, and S. A. Bozzette. 2001. Effects of drug abuse and mental disorders on use and type of antiretroviral therapy in HIV-infected persons. *J. Gen. Intern. Med.* **16:**625–633.

Vlahov, D., A. Munoz, L. Solomon, J. Astemborski, A. Lindsay, J. Anderson, N. Galai, and K. E. Nelson. 1994. Comparison of clinical manifestations of HIV infection between male and female injecting drug users. *AIDS* **8:**819–823.

Wagner, G. J., J. G. Rabkin, and R. Rabkin. 1997. Dextroamphetamine as a treatment for depression and low energy in AIDS patients: a pilot study. *J. Psychosom. Res.* **42:**407–411.

Wagner, G. J., and R. Rabkin. 2000. Effects of dextroamphetamine on depression and fatigue in men with HIV: a double-blind, placebo-controlled trial. *J. Clin. Psychiatry* **61:**436–440.

Wall, T. L., J. L. Sorensen, S. L. Batki, K. L. Delucchi, J. A. London, and M. A. Chesney. 1995. Adherence to zidovudine (AZT) among HIV-infected methadone patients: a pilot study of supervised therapy and dispensing compared to usual care. *Drug Alcohol Depend.* **37:**261–269.

Wiegand, M., A. A. Moller, W. Schreiber, J. C. Krieg, and F. Holsboer. 1991. Alterations of nocturnal sleep in patients with HIV infection. *Acta Neurol. Scand.* **83:**141–142.

Work Group on Bipolar Disorder. 2003. Practice guideline for the treatment of patients with bipolar disorder (revision). http://www.psych.org/edu/cme/apacme/courses/course15/Bipolar2ePG.doc. Accessed 15 December 2003.

Working Group of the American Academy of Neurology AIDS Task Force. 1991. Nomenclature and research case definitions for neurologic manifestations of human immunodeficiency virus-type 1 (HIV-1) infection. *Neurology* **41:**778–785.

Zigmond, A. S., and R. P. Snaith. 1983. The hospital anxiety and depression scale. *Acta Psychiatr. Scand.* **67:**361–370.

Zilikis, N., I. Nimatoudis, V. Kiosses, and C. Ierodiakonou. 1998. Treatment with risperidone of an acute psychotic episode in a patient with AIDS. *Gen. Hosp. Psychiatry* **20:**384–385.

Zisook, S., J. Peterkin, K. J. Goggin, P. Sledge, J. H. Atkinson, and I. Grant. 1998. Treatment of major depression in HIV-seropositive men. *J. Clin. Psychiatry* **59:**217–224.

The Spectrum of Neuro-AIDS Disorders:
Pathophysiology, Diagnosis, and Treatment
Edited by K. Goodkin et al.
©2008 ASM Press, Washington, DC

29

Substance Use Disorders and Neuro-AIDS in the HAART Era

JEFFREY A. RUMBAUGH AND AVINDRA NATH

Human immunodeficiency virus (HIV) is transmitted via bodily fluids. One of the most common means of transmission, therefore, is via needle exchange among intravenous (IV) drug users. Approximately 2.5 million Americans use heroin, and in certain cities around the world, IV drug abuse has reached epidemic proportions. Up to 30% of injection drug users are HIV seropositive. Nearly one-half of the HIV-positive women in the United States contracted the infection via drug use. Furthermore, whereas rates of drug abuse fall off with age in the general HIV-seronegative population, this decline is not observed for HIV-seropositive adults, presumably because those individuals who continue to use drugs continue to contract HIV at a steady rate (Rabkin et al., 2004).

Yet, the interdependence of HIV and drug abuse does not stop merely at transmission. Drugs and HIV have synergistic effects on the function of brain and other organ systems. The addictive properties of many drugs of abuse are mediated through their effects on brain function, so it is not surprising that they might interact with HIV infection, which also affects brain function. Interestingly, one of the earliest studies to look at this issue found no significant differences in cognitive functioning between HIV-infected persons based on their history of drug abuse (Concha et al., 1997). However, all of the patients in this study were asymptomatic, perhaps making detection of a significant difference difficult. A later study, evaluating patients who presented with prominent psychomotor slowing, found that those with a history of injection drug use had more rapid neurologic progression (Bouwman et al., 1998). It is now apparent that, compared to HIV-positive patients who do not use drugs, HIV-positive drug abusers have more rapid progression to more severe forms of neurocognitive dysfunction, and in fact, some HIV-infected drug abusers may have an accelerated form of HIV dementia (Nath et al., 2001). Figure 1 depicts representative magnetic resonance imaging

(MRI) findings frequently seen in patients with coexistent HIV infection and drug abuse.

Recognizing the therapeutic implications of such potential interactions, many researchers have exerted a great deal of effort in studying possible mechanisms. Nevertheless, a clear understanding of the epidemiology, pathology, and molecular neuropathogenesis of drug abuse and HIV dementia has remained elusive. There are many aspects of the drug abuse epidemic which make these issues difficult to clarify. In particular, it is challenging to find a uniform patient population on which to base studies. Drug abusers often use more than a single drug, so it is difficult to separate out effects of different agents. Similarly, drug abusers may use different amounts of drugs at different frequencies, but dose effects may be significant. Current versus past drug use may also influence results of studies. Furthermore, drug abusers who are infected with HIV are often coinfected with other organisms, such as hepatitis C virus (HCV) (Murrill et al., 2002), making it difficult to differentiate interactions of HIV and drug abuse from interactions of HIV and HCV or interactions of HCV and drug abuse. Finally, active drug abuse is likely to influence a patient's ability to adhere to a HAART regimen, thereby speeding progression of HIV dementia, without invoking any direct interaction between the drugs and the virus.

In this chapter, we review the studies which provide evidence for a synergistic effect of drugs of abuse and HIV infection on brain function. Understanding the interactive mechanisms of this neurodegeneration is critical to our ability to optimize therapy for drug-abusing HIV-infected populations. We thus discuss the proposed underlying mechanisms of this combined neurotoxicity, the current state of knowledge about the role of HAART in this interaction, and implications for future research and therapeutic development.

DOPAMINERGIC SYSTEMS

The addictive properties of many common drugs of abuse, including cocaine, amphetamines, and opiates, are mediated,

Jeffrey A. Rumbaugh and Avindra Nath, Department of Neurology, Johns Hopkins University, Baltimore, MD 21287.

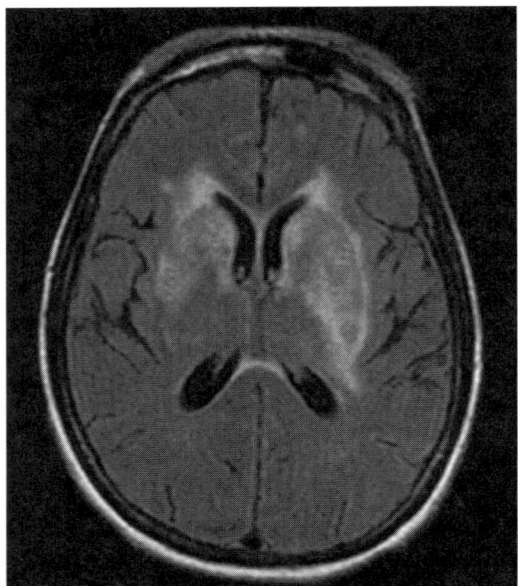

FIGURE 1 MRI scan of a patient with HIV infection who abused heroin and cocaine. This 51-year-old HIV-infected woman used cocaine several days per week and heroin on a regular basis. She was admitted to Johns Hopkins Hospital with the subacute onset of ataxia, postural instability, and severe dementia. Her CD4 cell count was 5 cells/mm³, and her plasma viral load was 436,000 copies/ml. MRI scan shows bilateral hyperintensities in the basal ganglia, without edema.

at least in part, by the dopaminergic system. It is therefore not surprising that they interact with HIV infection, which also affects the dopaminergic system.

HIV dementia patients are very sensitive to the adverse effects of neuroleptics, suggesting involvement of the dopamine system (Edelstein and Knight, 1987; Hollander et al., 1985; Hriso et al., 1991; Kieburtz et al., 1991; Mirsattari et al., 1998, 1999). For example, in one study, the response to neuroleptics of patients with HIV infection was compared to the response of psychotic patients without HIV infection. Controlling for mean neuroleptic dose and patient body weight, the HIV-infected patients had a two- to four-fold-increased risk of developing parkinsonian symptoms. Parkinsonian symptoms developed in 50% of HIV patients who received less than 4 mg of chlorpromazine per kg of body weight equivalents per day and in 78% of those who received more than 4 mg/kg per day (Hriso et al., 1991).

A specific predilection for damage to the dopaminergic system could help explain the parkinsonism frequently seen as a part of HIV dementia. Recent neuropathological and magnetic resonance spectroscopy evidence demonstrates neuronal loss in the basal ganglia in patients with HIV dementia (Berger and Arendt, 2000). Positron emission tomography studies demonstrate that patients with HIV dementia have lower dopamine transporter availability in their basal ganglia than nondemented HIV-positive patients (Wang et al., 2004). Compared to uninfected controls, rhesus monkeys with simian immunodeficiency virus (SIV) infection have decreased levels of dopamine, dopamine metabolites, and factors involved in the dopamine signaling pathways. This is true even at an asymptomatic stage, suggesting that the dopamine system is involved very early

on in infection (Jenuwein et al., 2004). Pathologically, SIV-infected monkeys also have decreased neuronal number, volume, and density in the globus pallidus and substantia nigra, with 10 to 50% loss of dopaminergic neurons in the substantia nigra (Marcario et al., 2004). Dopaminergic neurons seem particularly sensitive to the toxic effects of the HIV proteins, gp120 (Bennett et al., 1995) and Tat (Cass et al., 2003).

Cerebrospinal fluid (CSF) neurotransmitter levels provide a sensitive indication of the health of the associated neuronal system. Abnormalities can even be detected prior to symptom onset, giving a good indicator of incipient neurological disease (Hornykiewicz, 1998). The principal source of dopamine and its metabolites in the CSF is the dopaminergic system in the brain. CSF dopamine levels are thus a good reflection of the health of the dopaminergic system. In fact, CSF levels of the dopamine metabolite homovanillic acid are diminished in patients with AIDS but no dementia and more severely diminished in patients with HIV dementia (Berger et al., 1994; Larsson et al., 1991). Furthermore, a study of dopamine metabolites in the CSF of asymptomatic SIV-infected rhesus monkeys suggested increased dopamine turnover even in early stages of infection (Koutsilieri et al., 1997b).

One early autopsy study found that IV drug abusers with HIV infection had more severe neuronal damage and loss in the dopaminergic substantia nigra than HIV patients with no history of drug abuse (Reyes et al., 1991). More recently, we reported a patient with HIV dementia and a history of cocaine and methamphetamine use who developed a progressive resting tremor, dystonia, and athetoid movements (Nath et al., 2001). In subsequent sections of this chapter, we discuss the evidence that each of the drugs of abuse interacts with HIV infection through influences on the dopaminergic system and by other mechanisms as well.

OPIOIDS

The role of opioids in HIV dementia is perhaps better characterized than for any of the other drugs of abuse.

Neuropathology

Neuropathological studies have been performed extensively with a cohort of patients whose drug of choice was predominantly IV opiates. These patients seem to have an especially severe form of HIV encephalitis (HIVE) (Bell et al., 1998). They have more activated microglia, particularly in the thalamus, than do non-drug-abusing HIV-seropositive patients (Arango et al., 2004; Tomlinson et al., 1999), and more glial fibrillary acidic protein-positive reactive astrocytes in both gray and white matter than do HIV-negative drug users or HIV-seropositive drug users without HIVE (Anderson et al., 2003). The reactive astrocytes were numerous even in patients receiving treatment, suggesting that astrocytes serve as a reservoir for the HIV in this patient population (Anderson et al., 2003). Studies have not been able to demonstrate a significant effect of drug abuse on B-cell infiltrates into the brain of HIV-infected patients (Anthony et al., 2004).

Though the described pathological findings are convincing, the differences have not been consistently demonstrated. This difficulty is representative of the challenges inherent in this type of research, including differences in patient populations with respect to demographics and pattern of drug abuse.

Recent studies suggest that opiate use may also be associated with peripheral neuropathy in HIV-infected patients (Morgello et al., 2004), but this area has not been well studied.

Immune System Effects and HIV Replication

Opioids can be either pro- or anti-inflammatory depending on the particular opioid receptor and cell type that are affected. However, it is generally believed that the net consequence of opioid receptor activation is to suppress immune function, thereby contributing to worsening HIV complications.

This mechanism of interaction between opioids and HIV in worsening the effects of HIV has been termed the "opiate cofactor hypothesis" (Donahoe and Vlahov, 1998). Opioids can modulate HIV propagation in immune cells. Opioid drugs and HIV proteins act synergistically to destabilize immune function. Leukocytes express mu-, delta-, and kappa-opioid receptors, as well as endogenous opioid peptides such as enkephalins, and opioids can modulate neuroimmune function. The mechanisms of this modulation are complex and involve both direct and indirect effects on the peripheral nervous system, the central nervous system (CNS), and nonneural mechanisms (Bidlack, 2000; Chang et al., 1998; McCarthy et al., 2001; Mellon and Bayer, 1998). A recent study showed that morphine inhibits CD8-positive T-cell-mediated noncytotoxic anti-HIV activity in latently infected human immune cells, largely by interfering with a gamma interferon signaling pathway (Wang et al., 2005). Naltrexone blocked this morphine-induced inhibition. This study suggests that morphine impairs the anti-HIV function of the immune system.

The opioid system can have both positive and negative effects on HIV infection in immune cells. Probably due to the complexity of the system, the effects of opiates on SIV progression in nonhuman primates have not been clear (Donahoe, 2004). This confusion may have been resolved by a recent careful study, in which chronic morphine administration to SIV-infected monkeys clearly caused increased viral loads in plasma and CSF (Kumar et al., 2004). Another recent study demonstrated an increased SIV replication rate and an increased rate of mutation with development of zidovudine (AZT) resistance in morphine-dependent monkeys versus non-morphine-treated monkeys (Chuang et al., 2005). Mu receptor stimulation increases HIV expression in monocytic cells (Peterson et al., 1993, 1999), while kappa receptor activation has an inhibitory effect on HIV expression in both monocytic and lymphocytic cells (Chao et al., 1996, 2001; Peterson et al., 2001). Similar opposing effects of mu and kappa receptors have been noted in other systems as well (Bohn et al., 2000).

Opiates also have an effect on cytokine/chemokine signaling. Mu-opioid receptor activation increases expression of cytokine receptors that serve as coreceptors for HIV, including CCR3, CCR5, and CXCR4. Kappa-opioid receptor stimulation increases CCR2 expression but decreases CCR5 expression (Rogers and Peterson, 2003).

Opioid Effects on Neuronal Function

The intravenous heroin favored by drug abusers acts on the CNS after conversion to morphine, making morphine the most commonly used agent to study opiate effects in both in vivo and in vitro neurological model systems. Opioids are not generally intrinsically toxic, and morphine alone is rarely toxic to most neuronal types (Gurwell et al., 2001; Hauser et al., 2000). However, there are likely differences between a one-time, acute exposure, and chronic intermittent exposure. The chronic, intermittent opiate drug exposure that is typical of long-term drug abusers disrupts numerous second messenger cascades, alters patterns of gene activation, and increases oxidative stress (Hauser et al., 1998; Koob, 2000; Kreek and Koob, 1998), all of which may enhance the vulnerability of neurons to HIV infection. Mu-opioid drugs, including heroin, morphine, and fentanyl, can induce toxicity in cerebellar Purkinje cells (Hauser et al., 1994) and in the limbic system of rats at high dosages (Kofke et al., 1996). Fentanyl exacerbates the effects of ischemia-induced damage to the basal ganglia (Kofke et al., 1999), and morphine can induce apoptosis through a caspase-3-dependent pathway in primary human microglia and neurons (Hu et al., 2002).

As with the dichotomous effects of opioids on immune cells, opioids can have paradoxical neuroprotective and neurotoxic effects, depending on the target tissue, opioid receptor type, and pharmacodynamics of receptor activation. Opioid receptors interact with many different intracellular signaling pathways, and opioid receptor-effector coupling differs greatly among cell types (Hauser et al., 1998). Thus, depending on the experimental system under study, opioids have been shown to be protective (Hauser et al., 1999; Meriney et al., 1991; Polakiewicz et al., 1998). For example, in Chinese hamster ovary cells stably transfected with mu-opioid receptors, a selective mu-opioid receptor agonist stimulated antiapoptotic effectors via a phosphoinositide 3-kinase-dependent signaling cascade (Polakiewicz et al., 1998).

By contrast, nontoxic concentrations of opioids frequently synergize with toxic agents to exacerbate damage (Nair et al., 1997; Singhal et al., 1997, 1998, 1999; Yin et al., 1999). They augment the effects of nonopioid proapoptotic or proinflammatory signals, reducing cell viability either directly or indirectly through the further release of cytotoxic inflammatory intermediaries from immune cells (Goswami et al., 1998; Yin et al., 1997). For example, mu agonists enhance staurosporine or wortmannin-induced apoptosis in embryonic chick neurons and neuronal cell lines (Goswami et al., 1998). Significant neuronal cell death and oxidative stress occur in neuronal cell lines coexposed to supernatants from HIV-infected cells and morphine (Koutsilieri et al., 1997a, 1997b).

Interaction between opioids and the Tat protein may be the most important, or at least the best studied, viral protein-drug of abuse combination. Several lines of evidence have shown that this combination is synergistically toxic to neurons through direct action on neural targets, in both murine and human model systems. The neurodegenerative effects are dependent on the concentration of morphine and/or Tat that is used and can be reversed by opioid receptor antagonists, indicating that the synergistic toxicity is mediated through specific opioid receptors (Gurwell et al., 2001). Recent unpublished studies from our laboratories demonstrate that the enhanced toxicity is mediated by effects on mitochondria via activation of several signaling cascades involving Akt/PKB, PI-3 kinase, and caspases 1, 3, and 7. The neurons used in these experiments possess mu, delta, and/or kappa receptors, suggesting that the opioids can act on the neurons directly.

Limited studies of the interaction between opioids and gp120 have given conflicting results. One early study indicated that opioids can protect against the detrimental effects of gp120 (Stefano, 1999). However, a more recent study suggested that morphine potentiates gp120-induced neuronal apoptosis via an intracellular signaling pathway which is probably dependent on the presence of microglia in mixed glial-neuronal cell cultures (Hu et al., 2005).

Opioids also affect dopamine turnover, perhaps increasing the susceptibility of dopaminergic neurons to viral damage. Endogenous opioids and opioid drugs of abuse activate dopaminergic neurons through various mechanisms, which were the subject of a recent review (Kreek, 2001). Opioids disinhibit interneurons that synapse on dopaminergic neurons, such as in the ventral tegmental area, thus depleting dopamine. Opioids also alter cellular response to dopamine by altering expression of dopamine receptor subtypes. For example, opioid receptor activation increases D2 dopamine receptor binding sites in the rat striatum (Rooney et al., 1991) with considerable functional consequence (De Vries et al., 1999; Vanderschuren et al., 1999). The same study showed no effect of opioid receptor activation on D1 dopamine receptors (Rooney et al., 1991). Nevertheless, another study showed that repeated intermittent exposure to morphine increases D1 dopamine receptor-induced adenylyl cyclase activity in rat striatal neurons in vitro (Schoffelmeer et al., 1997). Not only are dopaminergic functions altered as part of the physiological development of tolerance and dependence to opiates, but also they are altered once again during drug withdrawal (Ammon-Treiber and Hollt, 2005; Koob, 2000). Thus, results of clinical or autopsy studies can vary significantly depending on the drug use history of the study population.

Opioids and Glial Function

Subpopulations of striatal astrocytes (Stiene-Martin et al., 1998) and microglia (Chao et al., 1996) express opioid receptors. In most experiments looking at neuronal function, including those using in vitro neuronal cultures, at least a small number of contaminating glia are present. It is thus difficult to exclude the possibility that some of the observed opiate-HIV actions on neurons are actually not direct actions but occur via glial intermediaries. Activated astrocytes and microglia can participate in various inflammatory processes. Additionally, any factor which affects astrocytes may disrupt their ability to perform their functions in support of neurons. Therefore, an interaction which affects these cells may have deleterious consequences for the development of HIV-associated dementia.

In fact, sustained exposure to morphine and Tat causes dysfunction and death of both glial precursors and astrocytes, mediated by mu-opioid receptors through the activation of caspase-3 (Khurdayan et al., 2004). Furthermore, recent studies have implicated astroglia as mediators for the proinflammatory effects of opiates in HIV-infected individuals. Combined opiate and Tat exposure synergistically destabilizes intracellular calcium, increases reactive oxygen species, and causes massive release of proinflammatory chemokines in cultured striatal astroglia (El-Hage et al., 2005). The released chemokines include monocyte chemoattractant protein-1 (MCP-1) and RANTES. MCP-1 triggers an influx of monocyte/macrophages and microglial activation. The recruitment of macrophages/microglia to the CNS in opiate-abusing HIV-infected patients would likely exaggerate neuronal dysfunction and death. Morphine also up-regulates expression of the HIV coreceptor CCR5 on normal human astrocytes (Mahajan et al., 2005a, 2005b) and exacerbates gp120-induced modulation of chemokine expression in a human astrocytoma cell line (Mahajan et al., 2005a, 2005b).

COCAINE

Autopsy studies also confirm injury to dopaminergic neurons in cocaine abusers (Wilson et al., 1996a, 1996b). Cocaine use has occasionally been associated with persistent choreoathetosis, tics, and seizures (Bartzokis et al., 1999a, 1999b; Pascual-Leone and Dhuna, 1990; Pascual-Leone et al., 1990; Weiner et al., 2001). Once again, Tat is probably an important contributor to neuronal damage in conjunction with cocaine (Cass et al., 2003). Cocaine synergizes with both Tat and gp120 to cause increased neurotoxicity (Turchan et al., 2001) (Fig. 2). However, in this study, only a small proportion of dopaminergic cells died, suggesting that other unidentified factors contribute to the susceptibility of neurons to the synergistic effects of HIV proteins and drugs of abuse.

Thus, the mechanism of neurotoxic synergism between HIV infection and cocaine remains unclear. At least in part, the mechanism seems to involve mitochondrial dysfunction (Turchan et al., 2001). Significant oxidative stress and neuronal cell death occur in neuronal cell lines coexposed to supernatants from HIV-infected cells and cocaine (Koutsilieri et al., 1997a, 1997b). Both cocaine and Tat seem to target the mitochondria and produce oxidative stress, which can ultimately lead to cell death. Cocaine decreases mitochondrial respiration and increases the production of reactive oxygen species in animals (Boess et al., 2000). Intrastriatal injections of Tat increase oxidative stress in an in vivo model (Aksenov et al., 2001), and in an in vitro model, Tat causes oxidative damage to neurons when it is released from glial cells (Chauhan et al., 2003). Furthermore, gp120 may also cause oxidative damage (Foga et al., 1997), though this is not as well studied as it is for Tat. Antioxidant compounds thus have therapeutic potential in preventing oxidative damage produced by cocaine and HIV interactions.

Another possible mechanism of cocaine-HIV interaction occurs at the blood-brain barrier. Several in vitro studies have demonstrated that HIV proteins can alter endothelial cell function (Andras et al., 2003; Pu et al., 2003; Toborek et al., 2003), and disruption of the blood-brain barrier has been confirmed in vivo in HIV-infected patients (Berger and Avison, 2004). An in vitro study showed that cocaine can enhance monocyte migration across the blood-brain barrier by inducing gene expression for adhesion molecules and other proteins important in remodeling of endothelial cells (Fiala et al., 1998, 2005). Cocaine also up-regulates a dendritic cell-specific CD4-independent HIV attachment receptor, called DC-SIGN, on dendritic cells and brain-derived endothelial cells, facilitating passage of infected dendritic cells through the blood-brain barrier (Nair et al., 2004, 2005). Cocaine may thus contribute to disruption of the blood-brain barrier, which in turn contributes to the development of HIV-related cognitive dysfunction. The combined effects of HIV and other drugs of abuse on the blood-brain barrier have not been studied.

METHAMPHETAMINE

Long-term methamphetamine use has been associated with neuronal damage through multiple case reports (Bartzokis et al., 1999b; Pascual-Leone and Dhuna, 1990; Pascual-Leone et al., 1990; Weiner et al., 2001). These reports are supported by studies of animal models, pathological specimens, and magnetic resonance spectroscopy brain imaging (Ernst et al., 2000; Wilson et al., 1996a, 1996b). A recent study suggests a complex interaction and even opposing effects on cerebral volume with methamphetamine and HIV infection. Neurocognitive impairment was associated with decreased cortical volumes in HIV-positive participants but with increased cortical volumes in methamphetamine-dependent participants

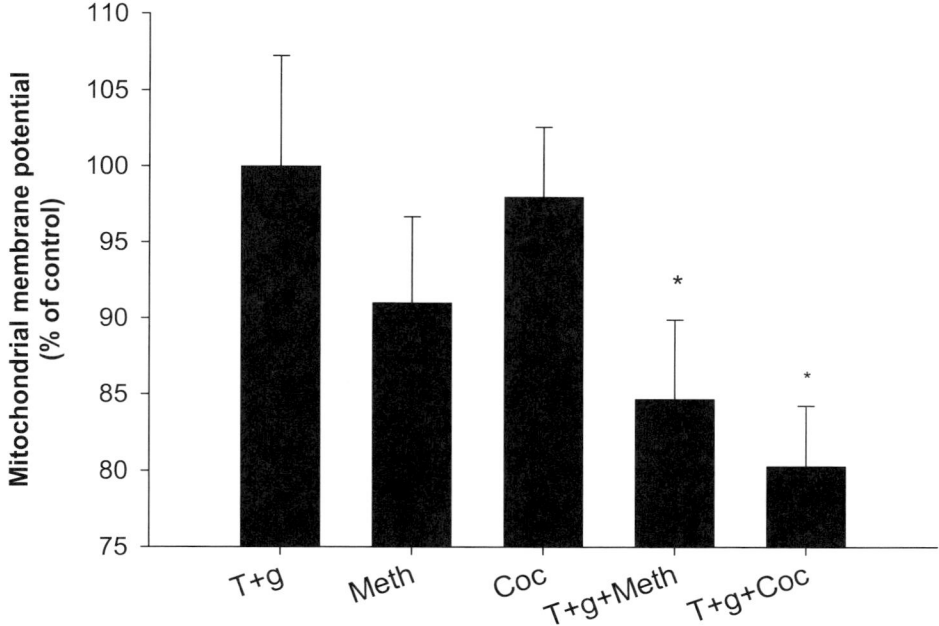

FIGURE 2   Synergistic neurotoxicity with HIV proteins and drugs of abuse. Human fetal neurons were incubated with HIV proteins gp120 (g) (30 pM) and Tat (T) (40 nM) at subneurotoxic dosages with or without methamphetamine (meth) (500 μM) or cocaine (16 μM). Changes in mitochondrial membrane potential were measured using JC-1 fluorescent dye. Synergistic neurotoxicity was noted as shown (modified from Turchan et al., 2001). Data are presented as mean + standard error of the mean and calculated as percentage of control. Untreated cells were used as control.

(Jernigan et al., 2005). Autopsy studies confirm injury to dopaminergic neurons (Wilson et al., 1996a, 1996b). Based on evidence from a rat model, interaction between the HIV Tat protein and methamphetamine, as well as other drugs of abuse, may be important to the damage in the dopaminergic system of the basal ganglia of patients with HIV dementia (Cass et al., 2003).

A severe microglial reaction has been found in methamphetamine-abusing patients with HIVE, compared to patients with HIVE who did not use methamphetamine. The methamphetamine users also demonstrated more pronounced loss of synaptophysin and calbindin immunoreactivity, suggesting greater damage to nonpyramidal neurons. However, the methamphetamine-using patients also had less gp41 staining, suggesting the presence of fewer HIV-infected macrophages/microglia, and clinically, they had less severe dementia but a higher frequency of ischemic events (Langford et al., 2003). MK-801 and dextromethorphan, which both inhibit microglial activation by Tat, were both able to prevent methamphetamine-induced neurotoxicity and damage to dopamine nerve terminals (Thomas and Kuhn, 2005).

Methamphetamine, like cocaine, synergizes with Tat and gp120 to cause increased neurotoxicity (Turchan et al., 2001) (Fig. 2), but again, the mechanism remains elusive. A recent in vivo study nicely demonstrated the synergism between methamphetamine and Tat (Maragos et al., 2002). Animals treated with methamphetamine alone showed only a 7% reduction in striatal dopamine levels, and Tat-treated animals showed only an 8% decline, but animals treated with both methamphetamine and Tat demonstrated a 65% reduction in striatal dopamine. This study might be particularly relevant, because the doses of methamphetamine and Tat used were equivalent to what might be seen in human disease. Subsequent microdialysis studies in the same animal model showed that the synergistic reduction in striatal dopamine is accompanied by significant decrease in dopamine release from the striatum (Cass et al., 2003). On the other hand, a recent magnetic resonance spectroscopy study evaluating subjects with and without HIV infection and with and without methamphetamine use history found only additive, not synergistic, effects on brain metabolites indicative of neuronal injury and glial activation (Chang et al., 2005).

As with cocaine, another possible mechanism for HIV-methamphetamine interaction is via oxidative stress. In one study (Flora et al., 2003), administration of either Tat or methamphetamine to mice increased markers of oxidative stress, including redox-regulated transcription factors, in cortical, striatal, and hippocampal brain regions. Furthermore, the DNA-binding activities of these transcription factors were greater in mice injected with both Tat and methamphetamine than in mice injected with either Tat or methamphetamine alone. The same study also suggested that Tat and methamphetamine may interact through changes in cell signaling and cytokine/chemokine expression. Mice treated with both agents had synergistic up-regulation of intercellular adhesion molecule-1 (ICAM-1), tumor necrosis factor alpha, and interleukin-1 beta gene expression compared to mice treated with either agent alone. Another study showed that Tat and methamphetamine interact to cause damage to calbindin immunoreactive nonpyramidal neurons by dysregulating mitochondrial calcium metabolism, associated with increased levels of oxidative stress (Langford et al., 2004).

MDMA

The effects of MDMA (methylenedioxymethamphetamine), or ecstasy, on the neuropathogenesis of HIV infection have not been studied. However, its use has been associated with high-risk sexual behavior, and fatal reactions in HIV-infected patients on protease inhibitors have been described. Some protease inhibitors such as ritonavir also inhibit the cytochrome P450 system in the liver, which leads to dangerously high levels of MDMA (Harrington et al., 1999). Prolonged MDMA use can have a variety of effects on the brain. These include down-regulation of dopaminergic and serotonergic transporters (Kindlundh-Högberg et al., 2007) and up-regulation of nicotinergic receptors (Garcia-Ratés et al., 2007). Since these neurotransmitter systems are also affected by HIV infection, it is important to determine the combined effects of MDMA and HIV on the brain.

CANNABINOIDS

The effect of cannabinoids on the disease course of HIV infection or the progression of HIV dementia remains largely unstudied. However, marijuana is frequently used by patients with HIV infection, with nearly 25% of these patients attending a public health clinic reporting its use for a variety of perceived benefits (Prentiss et al., 2004). Patients report improvement in appetite, muscle pain, nausea, anxiety, nerve pain, depression, and paresthesias (Woolridge et al., 2005). Further, cannabinoids do not have any known significant effect on antiretroviral efficacy (Kosel et al., 2002). Dronabinol, a commercially available form of delta(9)-THC, has been used successfully to increase appetite in patients with HIV wasting disease (Reiter, 1996). However, nearly 50% of all users reported associated memory deterioration (Woolridge et al., 2005).

The inhibitory effect of cannabinoids on reactive oxygen species, glutamate, and tumor necrosis factor suggests that they may be potent neuroprotective agents. Dexanabinol (HU-211), a synthetic cannabinoid, is currently being assessed in clinical trials for traumatic brain injury and stroke. The use of nonpsychoactive cannabinoids such as cannabidiol and dexanabinol may allow the dissociation of unwanted psychoactive effects from potential therapeutic benefits (Croxford, 2003).

ALCOHOL

Clinical Studies of Alcohol and HIV Infection

Though alcohol is not an injection drug, it is associated with increased HIV transmission, likely due to the risky behaviors of alcohol abusers (Weinhardt et al., 2001). Individuals who abuse alcohol often engage in high-risk sexual behavior (Baldwin et al., 2000; Stein et al., 2005). Also, like injection drugs, the interaction of alcohol and HIV likely extends beyond transmission. Alcohol compounds immunocompromise via direct immunotoxicity and nutritional deficiency (Dingle and Oei, 1997; Watzl and Watson, 1992) and thus may increase the risk of HIV-infected individuals for developing the immune-system-related complications of AIDS, including HIV dementia (Pillai et al., 1991; Tabakoff, 1994; Tyor and Middaugh, 1999). Further, in a simian model, alcohol intake has been shown to produce massive (30- to 85-fold) increases of HIV viral load in plasma and is associated with persistent HIV replication in brain (Kumar et al., 2005).

A small number of neurocognitive and neuroimaging studies have attempted and failed to demonstrate the link between alcohol abuse and worsened HIV dementia (Bornstein et al., 1993; Heaton et al., 1995). However, these studies typically were not properly controlled and did not compare alcoholic and nonalcoholic HIV-1-seropositive individuals (Basso and Bornstein, 2000). They also did not account for history of alcohol detoxification, a factor that can dramatically affect neuropsychological functioning (Craig and Mosier, 1978). Though these studies were therefore inconclusive, a recent study was more informative. It compared four groups of patients—with and without HIV infection and with and without a history of alcohol abuse—and demonstrated that HIV-infected individuals with a history of alcohol abuse were at greater risk for cognitive dysfunction than the other three groups. They found both additive and synergistic effects of previous alcohol abuse and HIV infection on cognition, depending on the specific cognitive domain being evaluated (Green et al., 2004). Another study showed reduced white matter concentrations of phosphodiester and phosphocreatine in HIV-infected patients with chronic alcohol usage, suggesting altered brain phospholipids and energy metabolites and demonstrating additive, but not synergistic, adverse metabolic effects of HIV and chronic alcohol abuse on brain function (Meyerhoff et al., 1995).

Alcohol Effects on Neuronal Function

The directly neurotoxic effects of chronic alcohol intake on CNS neurons have been well established. For example, chronic ethanol intake stimulates production of reactive oxygen species (Brooks, 1997), inhibits neuronal growth factors (Walker et al., 1993), and reduces cerebral glucose metabolism (Johnson-Greene et al., 1997). Chronic alcohol abuse in humans is associated with various neurological abnormalities, including impairment of executive function, even in the absence of Korsakoff's syndrome (Diamond and Messing, 1994). As with other drugs of abuse, it is thus not particularly surprising that there might be an interaction between alcohol acting on the CNS and HIV infection acting on the CNS, to worsen the effects of HIV-associated dementia.

Once again, many of the experiments looking at the synergistic effects of alcohol and HIV infection have focused on the interaction of this drug with Tat and/or gp120. It appears that this interaction is at least partly mediated through glutamate receptor systems (Chen et al., 2005; Self et al., 2004), like the N-methyl-D-aspartate (NMDA) receptor and the α-amino-3-hydroxy-5-methyl-4-isoxazole propionate (AMPA) receptor. Chronic alcoholism, as well as alcohol withdrawal, seems to activate these receptors (Littleton and Little, 1994), thus sensitizing them to the neurotoxic effects of Tat and gp120. Exposure of both primary neuronal cell cultures and animals to chronic alcohol increases the density and sensitivity of NMDA-type glutamate receptors in cortical and hippocampal neurons (Devaud and Morrow, 1999; Prendergast et al., 2000, 2004; Rudolph et al., 1998). This results in intracellular calcium elevations during alcohol withdrawal (Hu and Ticku, 1995), leading to neuronal death, which can be prevented using NMDA receptor antagonists (Ahern et al., 1994; Chandler et al., 1993; Prendergast et al., 2000). Pharmacological factors that increase the sensitivity of glutamatergic receptor systems promote HIV-1-related neurotoxicity (Epstein and Gelbard, 1999; Lipton, 1998; Nath and Geiger, 1998; Tyor and Middaugh, 1999). Thus, chronic ethanol exposure likely sensitizes the CNS to the neurotoxic effects of Tat and gp120, particularly during periods of alcohol withdrawal. Tat and alcohol also interact through production of oxidative stress, increased activity of redox-responsive transcription factors, and induction of inflammatory genes, including interleukin-1 beta and MCP-1 (Flora et al., 2005).

Alcohol abuse is also a well-established cause of peripheral neuropathy and thus may interact with HIV infection in causing peripheral neuropathy. The possibility of such an interaction has not been well studied.

ANABOLIC STEROIDS

Use of anabolic steroids is rapidly rising among the youth. Due to sharing of needles it has been implicated in transmission of HIV infection. These drugs may be prescribed to HIV-infected patients with wasting syndrome. These drugs also cause dependence. However, the effects of these drugs on the central nervous system have not been well studied. Recent studies suggest that these compounds may be detrimental to the brain and may impair repair processes since they inhibit neural progenitor cells (Brannvall et al., 2005). They also modulate dopaminergic and serotonergic pathways (Kurling et al., 2005), the consequences of which are not yet known.

DRUGS OF ABUSE AND HIV-ASSOCIATED PERIPHERAL NEUROPATHIES

The effects of drugs of abuse on the clinical course of HIV-associated peripheral neuropathies have not been well studied. It is an important topic, however, because opiates are frequently prescribed to treat the pain associated with HIV peripheral neuropathy and HIV patients frequently report the use of marijuana for treatment of pain as well. Studies to carefully evaluate the effects of the various drugs of abuse on the peripheral nervous system in HIV patients are therefore necessary and long overdue.

In one study, alcohol use was found to be an important contributory risk factor in the development of peripheral neuropathies in patients with HIV infection (Lopez et al., 2004). Another study reported a high incidence of peripheral neuropathy in HIV-seronegative IV drug abusers (25%), which was three to four times the reported frequency for HIV-seronegative persons in the general or male homosexual population. In the same study, peripheral neuropathy was present in 32% of HIV-seropositive patients. The peripheral neuropathy was axonal in nature and associated with increased age and alcohol use. It was asymptomatic in 80% of HIV-seronegative and 70% of HIV-seropositive patients (Berger et al., 1999).

THERAPEUTIC STRATEGIES

Substance Abuse and HIV Infection in the HAART Era

Highly active antiretroviral therapy (HAART) has significantly reduced rates of severe immunosuppression, thereby decreasing the incidence of severe forms of dementia. Nevertheless, the prevalence of dementia and other HIV-related neurocognitive dysfunction is actually rising due to the prolonged life span of HIV-infected individuals (Dore et al., 2003; McArthur et al., 2003; Neuenburg et al., 2002; Sacktor, 2002; Sacktor et al., 2002). Dementia also continues to be prominent in end-stage AIDS patients. A recent study demonstrated that 92% of HIV-infected outpatients who died between 1996 and 2001, after the introduction of HAART, were diagnosed with HIV dementia within 12 months of death (Welch and Morse, 2002). Another recent study comparing the neuropsychological performance of HIV-positive individuals with and without dementia and matched seronegative controls suggested that HAART has little effect on many cognitive domains and to see a memory benefit, a threshold of neuropsychological impairment must first be reached (Cysique et al., 2004).

Additionally, the agents used in HAART regimens consist of reverse transcriptase and protease inhibitors. There are no medications to target many of the mediators of neurotoxicity in HIV dementia, such as Tat and gp120, as discussed in this chapter. It is thus apparent that a reliance on HAART to control HIV dementia is not adequate. Consideration must also be given to neuroprotective and anti-inflammatory strategies (Gelbard, 1999; Turchan et al., 2003), and a clear understanding of the pathogenesis of neurotoxicity in HIV infection will guide rational development of such strategies. Elucidation of the neurotoxic mechanisms present in HIV-infected drug-abusing populations may provide additional therapeutic targets in this patient population. Alternatively, when the benefits of various neuroprotective therapies are demonstrated, understanding the important neuropathogenic mechanisms in this (or any) particular patient population will allow for selective design of the optimal therapeutic regimen.

Furthermore, pharmacological interactions may occur between drugs of abuse and antiretroviral therapies (Fabris et al., 2000; Flexner et al., 2001; Wynn et al., 2005). Additionally, active drug abuse decreases the ability of patients to strictly adhere to complex HAART regimens. Patients with neurocognitive impairment have even greater difficulty adhering to these regimens. Poor adherence allows viral escape by development of HAART-resistant mutations. For this reason, actively abusing HIV-infected individuals are frequently required to prove that they have discontinued drug use for a sustained time period before they are allowed access to HAART medications. These barriers make treatment of drug-abusing HIV-infected patients with cognitive impairment extremely challenging. However, stereotyping may lead to overemphasis on drug abuse as a barrier to adherence and underemphasis on non-drug-use-related obstacles and may contribute to unequal access of drug users to HAART compared to other HIV-positive populations (Ware et al., 2005).

A recent study showed that progression to AIDS and to all-cause mortality was greater even in noninjection drug users than in nonusers, and these differences were associated with lower utilization of HAART (Kapadia et al., 2005). In injection drug users, HAART utilization decreases mortality compared to nonutilization, though all injection drug users, with or without HAART utilization, have better survival in the HAART era than in the pre-HAART era (Vlahov et al., 2005). Among those patients who are able to adhere to a HAART regimen and maintain viral suppression for 24 months, former injection drug users had worse recovery of CD4 counts, suggesting that even former drug use impairs immunological recovery in HIV-positive patients (Dronda et al., 2004).

Studies on the molecular basis of addiction might enable us to identify pharmacological ways to prevent craving for drugs of abuse, assisting patients to abstain and gain access to HAART. Treatment strategies that have already been used with some success in this population include use of drugs with long half-lives and combination of several medications into a single pill, thus decreasing the number and frequency of pills which must be taken and creating a more simple regimen for this group to follow.

Interactions between Drugs of Abuse and Antiretroviral Drugs

Clinically significant interactions between drugs of abuse and antiretroviral drugs have been observed in a number of case reports (Antoniou and Tseng, 2002). Overdoses secondary to interactions between MDMA (ecstasy) or gamma-hydroxybutyrate and protease inhibitors have been reported. These interactions can be fatal (Henry and Hill, 1998). Protease inhibitors, particularly ritonavir, may inhibit metabolism of amphetamines, ketamine, lysergic acid diethylamide, and phencyclidine (Hales et al., 2000). Nevirapine and efavirenz induce methadone metabolism, which may lead to symptoms of opiate withdrawal (Stocker et al., 2004). A similar interaction may exist between methadone and the protease inhibitors ritonavir and nelfinavir, although the data are less consistent. Since opiate metabolism can be inhibited or induced by concomitant protease inhibitors, patients should be monitored for signs of toxicity and/or loss of analgesia.

Drug Abuse Intervention

By stopping the interactive mechanisms discussed in this chapter, it would seem reasonable that drug abstinence would halt or potentially reverse the synergistic progression of HIV-associated dementia in drug-abusing individuals. This possibility has not been well studied, however, and it may be that certain deleterious cascades, once initiated, are not easily reversed. Additionally, sustained abstinence is difficult to achieve. Thus, interventions that limit drug use or negate drug effects at the cellular or molecular level (Robinson and Berridge, 2000) appear promising. In heroin-abusing populations, methadone or buprenorphine treatment programs are likely to be beneficial by limiting and regulating opiate exposure. Furthermore, some of the detrimental effects of intravenous heroin abuse may be attributable to the high and/or fluctuating opiate levels seen in these patients (Kreek and Koob, 1998; Nestler and Aghajanian, 1997), while sustained, chronic exposure to more moderate dosages, as with methadone or buprenorphine treatment, may cause less toxicity. Protease inhibitors may reduce methadone levels requiring methadone dose adjustment in patients receiving both HAART and methadone (Stocker et al., 2004).

A recent report described a pilot program in which motivational interviewing and cognitive behavioral therapy was used to increase adherence to HAART and to decrease substance use in HIV-infected adults (Parsons et al., 2005). Though further study is needed, results suggest that this may be an effective strategy for addressing the complex connections between these two behaviors.

Antioxidants and Neuroprotectants

As discussed throughout this review, HIV proteins and drugs of abuse synergize to cause mitochondrial toxicity and generate oxidative stress in susceptible neurons, suggesting that antioxidants might protect HIV-infected drug-abusing patient populations from neurodegeneration. Antioxidants are especially promising because they are easily available as dietary supplements. Some novel compounds that have both antiretroviral and antioxidant properties are also under development (Turchan

et al., 2003). L-deprenyl is a medication of emerging interest for HIV-infected, drug-abusing populations. It is a specific monoamine oxidase B inhibitor but also has antioxidant effects, reduces the euphoric effects of cocaine, and normalizes blood flow in cocaine addicts. In preliminary studies, it has also been shown to slow the progression of HIV dementia (Bartzokis et al., 1999a).

Gonadal Hormones

Estrogen receptors are widely expressed in the brain (Gundlah et al., 2000). Estrogen deficiency has been implicated as a risk factor in the development of several neurodegenerative diseases (Manly et al., 2000; Saunders-Pullman et al., 1999; Slooter et al., 1999), and estrogen replacement may result in improvement of cognitive function (Asthana et al., 1999). Recent in vitro and in vivo studies demonstrated that 17β-estradiol and 5α-testosterone, at physiological and pharmacological concentrations, protected against the combined effects of Tat, gp120, methamphetamine, and cocaine (Corasaniti et al., 2005; Kendall et al., 2005; Russo et al., 2005; Turchan et al., 2001). Protection for both the estradiol and the testosterone was completely reversed by the estrogen receptor antagonist ICI 182,780, suggesting that the neuroprotective effect of both compounds is mediated through the estrogen receptor. Interestingly, no protection was seen at all with 17α-estradiol, and minimal protection was seen with dihydrotestosterone and progesterone, suggesting that not all gonadal compounds have the same therapeutic effects.

Overcoming Barriers to Treatment of Drug-Abusing Patients with HIV Dementia

Drug-abusing patients are poverty stricken, frequently have low motivation and self-esteem, and may have poor compliance with treatment for both drug abuse and HIV infection. Impairment of cognitive function leads to further challenges because of inability to remember appointments or to take medications. Hence, while it is critical that we develop drugs that are effective against the combined neurotoxic effects of HIV infection and drugs of abuse, attention is also necessary to develop new modes of delivery for these medications. Depot forms, injectables with long half-lives, therapeutic vaccines with HIV proteins that may decrease viral load, and delivery through food products are some possibilities that deserve further exploration.

CONCLUSIONS

Infection by HIV causes neuronal dysfunction and loss by numerous, interacting mechanisms. The addition of various drugs of abuse only adds to the complexity of these mechanisms. Recent research has exponentially increased our understanding, but much more work is needed. HIV-associated dementia in drug abusers results from a complex interplay of effects caused by viral proteins, the drugs of abuse, and host inflammatory mediators. Current HAART is inadequate to fully control the damage that these factors exert on brain cells. Our mechanistic understanding of HIV dementia has elucidated numerous therapeutic targets that we are only now beginning to exploit. Treatment of HIV-infected drug-abusing patients with cognitive impairment poses numerous challenges for the medical community. This will require not only drugs that can prevent the effects of both HIV and drugs of abuse on the brain but also the development of novel modes of drug delivery that do not require close monitoring and frequent dosing. Further work is needed to optimize and develop new strategies for the benefit of the drug-abusing population.

REFERENCES

Ahern, K., H. Lustig, and D. Greenberg. 1994. Enhancement of NMDA toxicity and calcium responses by chronic exposure of cultured cortical neurons to ethanol. *Neurosci. Lett.* **165**:211–214.

Aksenov, M., U. Hasselrot, A. Bansal, G. Wu, A, Nath, C. Anderson, C. Mactutus, and R. Booze. 2001. Oxidative damage induced by the injection of HIV-1 Tat protein in the rat striatum. *Neurosci. Lett.* **305**:5–8.

Ammon-Treiber, S., and V. Hollt. 2005. Morphine-induced changes of gene expression in the brain. *Addict. Biol.* **10**:81–89.

Anderson, C., G. Tomlinson, B. Pauly, F. Brannan, A. Chiswick, R. Brack-Werner, P. Simmonds, and J. Bell. 2003. Relationship of Nef-positive and GFAP-reactive astrocytes to drug use in early and late HIV infection. *Neuropathol. Appl. Neurobiol.* **29**:378–388.

Andras, I., H. Pu, M. Deli, A. Nath, B. Hennig, and M. Toborek. 2003. HIV-1 Tat protein alters tight junction protein expression and distribution in cultured brain endothelial cells. *J. Neurosci. Res.* **74**:255–265.

Anthony, I., D. Crawford, and J. Bell. 2004. Effects of human immunodeficiency virus encephalitis and drug abuse on the B lymphocyte population of the brain. *J. Neurovirol.* **10**:181–188.

Antoniou, T., and A. Tseng. 2002. Interactions between recreational drugs and antiretroviral agents. *Ann. Pharmacother.* **36**:1598–1613.

Arango, J., P. Simmonds, R. Brettle, and J. Bell. 2004. Does drug abuse influence the microglial response in AIDS and HIV encephalitis? *AIDS* **18**(Suppl. 1):S69–S74.

Asthana, S., S. Craft, L. Baker, M. Raskind, R. Birnbaum, C. Lofgreen, R. Veith, and S. Plymate. 1999. Cognitive and neuroendocrine response to transdermal estrogen in postmenopausal women with Alzheimer's disease: results of a placebo-controlled, double-blind, pilot study. *Psychoneuroendocrinology* **24**:657–677.

Baldwin, J., C. Maxwell, A. Fenaughty, R. Trotter, and S. Stevens. 2000. Alcohol as a risk factor for HIV transmission among American Indian and Alaska native drug users. *Am. Indian Alsk. Native Ment. Health Res.* **9**:1–16.

Bartzokis, G., M. Beckson, T. Newton, M. Mandelkern, J. Mintz, J. Foster, W. Ling, and T. Bridge. 1999a. Selegiline effects on cocaine-induced changes in medial temporal lobe metabolism and subjective ratings of euphoria. *Neuropsychopharmacology* **20**:582–590.

Bartzokis, G., M. Beckson, D. Wirshing, P. Lu, J. Foster, and J. Mintz. 1999b. Choreoathetoid movements in cocaine dependence. *Biol. Psychiatry* **45**:1630–1635.

Basso, M., and R. Bornstein. 2000. Neurobehavioural consequences of substance abuse and HIV infection. *J. Psychopharmacol.* **14**:228–237.

Bell, J., R. Brettle, A. Chiswick, and P. Simmonds. 1998. HIV encephalitis, proviral load and dementia in drug users and homosexuals with AIDS. Effect of neocortical involvement. *Brain* **121**:2043–2052.

Bennett, B., D. Rusyniak, and C. Hollingsworth. 1995. HIV-1 gp120-induced neurotoxicity to midbrain dopamine cultures. *Brain Res.* **705**:168–176.

Berger, A., H. Schaumburg, M. Gourevitch, K. Freeman, S. Herskovitz, and J. Arezzo. 1999. Prevalence of peripheral neuropathy in injection drug users. *Neurology* **53**:592–597.

Berger, J., and G. Arendt. 2000. HIV dementia: the role of the basal ganglia and dopaminergic systems. *J. Psychopharmacol.* **14**:214–221.

Berger, J., and M. Avison. 2004. The blood brain barrier in HIV infection. *Front. Biosci.* **9**:2680–2685.

Berger, J., M. Kumar, A. Kumar, J. Fernandez, and B. Levin. 1994. Cerebrospinal fluid dopamine in HIV-1 infection. *AIDS* **8**:67–71.

Bidlack, J. 2000. Detection and function of opioid receptors on cells from the immune system. *Clin. Diagn. Lab. Immunol.* **7**:719–723.

Boess, F., F. Ndikum-Moffor, U. Boelsterli, and S. Roberts. 2000. Effects of cocaine and its oxidative metabolites on mitochondrial respiration and generation of reactive oxygen species. *Biochem. Pharmacol.* **60**:615–623.

Bohn, L., M. Belcheva, and C. Coscia. 2000. Mu-opioid agonist inhibition of kappa-opioid receptor-stimulated extracellular signal-regulated kinase phosphorylation is dynamin-dependent in C6 glioma cells. *J. Neurochem.* **74**:574–581.

Bornstein, R., R. Fama, P. Rosenberger, C. Whitacre, M. Para, H. Nasrallah, and R. Fass. 1993. Drug and alcohol use and neuropsychological performance in asymptomatic HIV infection. *J. Neuropsychiatry Clin. Neurosci.* **5**:254–259.

Bouwman, F., R. Skolasky, D. Hes, O. Selnes, J. Glass, T. Nance-Sproson, W. Royal, G. Dal Pan, and J. McArthur. 1998. Variable progression of HIV-associated dementia. *Neurology* **50**:1814–1820.

Brannvall, K., N. Bogdanovic, L. Korhonen, and D. Lindholm. 2005. 19-Nortestosterone influences neural stem cell proliferation and neurogenesis in the rat brain. *Eur. J. Neurosci.* **21**:871–878.

Brooks, P. 1997. DNA damage, DNA repair, and alcohol toxicity—a review. *Alcohol Clin. Exp. Res.* **21**:1073–1082.

Cass, W., M. Harned, L. Peters, A. Nath, and W. Maragos. 2003. HIV-1 protein Tat potentiation of methamphetamine-induced decreases in evoked overflow of dopamine in the striatum of the rat. *Brain Res.* **984**:133–142.

Chandler, L., H. Newsom, C. Sumners, and F. Crews. 1993. Chronic ethanol exposure potentiates NMDA excitotoxicity in cerebral cortical neurons. *J. Neurochem.* **60**:1578–1581.

Chang, L., T. Ernst, O. Speck, and C. Grob. 2005. Additive effects of HIV and chronic methamphetamine use on brain metabolite abnormalities. *Am. J. Psychiatry* **162**:361–369.

Chang, S., G. Wu, N. Patel, E. Vidal, and M. Fiala. 1998. The effects of interaction between morphine and interleukin-1 on the immune response. *Adv. Exp. Med. Biol.* **437**:67–72.

Chao, C., G. Gekker, S. Hu, W. Sheng, K. Shark, D. Bu, S. Archer, J. Bidlack, and P. Peterson. 1996. Kappa opioid receptors in human microglia downregulate human immunodeficiency virus 1 expression. *Proc. Natl. Acad. Sci. USA* **93**:8051–8056.

Chao, C., G. Gekker, W. Sheng, S. Hu, and P. Peterson. 2001. U50488 inhibits HIV-1 expression in acutely infected monocyte-derived macrophages. *Drug Alcohol Depend.* **62**:149–154.

Chauhan, A., J. Turchan, C. Pocernich, A. Bruce-Keller, S. Roth, D. Butterfield, E. Major, and A. Nath. 2003. Intracellular human immunodeficiency virus tat expression in astrocytes promotes astrocyte survival but induces potent neurotoxicity at distant sites via axonal transport. *J. Biol. Chem.* **278**:13512–13519.

Chen, W., Z. Tang, P. Fortina, P. Patel, S. Addya, S. Surrey, E. Acheampong, M. Mukhtar, and R. Pomerantz. 2005. Ethanol potentiates HIV-1 gp120-induced apoptosis in human neurons via both the death receptor and NMDA receptor pathways. *Virology* **334**:59–73.

Chuang, Y., S. Suzuki, T. Chuang, T. Miyagi, L. Chuang, and R. Doi. 2005. Opioids and the progression of simian AIDS. *Front. Biosci.* **10**:1666–1677.

Concha, M., O. Selnes, D. Vlahov, T. Nance-Sproson, M. Updike, W. Royal, J. Palenicek, and J. McArthur. 1997. Comparison of neuropsychological performance between

AIDS-free injecting drug users and homosexual men. *Neuroepidemiology* **16**:78–85.

Corasaniti, M., D. Amantea, R. Russo, S. Piccirilli, A. Leta, M. Corazzari, G. Nappi, and G. Bagetta. 2005. 17beta-Estradiol reduces neuronal apoptosis induced by HIV-1 gp120 in the neocortex of rat. *Neurotoxicology* **26**:893–903.

Craig, J., and W. Mosier. 1978. Clinical and laboratory findings on admission to an alcohol detoxification service. *Int. J. Addict.* **13**:1207–1215.

Croxford, J. 2003. Therapeutic potential of cannabinoids in CNS disease. *CNS Drugs* **17**:179–202.

Cysique, L., P. Maruff, and B. Brew. 2004. Antiretroviral therapy in HIV infection: are neurologically active drugs important? *Arch. Neurol.* **61**:1699–1704.

Devaud, L., and A. Morrow. 1999. Gender-selective effects of ethanol dependence on NMDA receptor subunit expression in cerebral cortex, hippocampus and hypothalamus. *Eur. J. Pharmacol.* **369**:331–334.

De Vries, T., A. Schoffelmeer, R. Binnekade, and L. Vanderschuren. 1999. Dopaminergic mechanisms mediating the incentive to seek cocaine and heroin following long-term withdrawal of IV drug self-administration. *Psychopharmacology* (Berlin) **143**:254–260.

Diamond, I., and R. Messing. 1994. Neurologic effects of alcoholism. *West. J. Med.* **161**:279–287.

Dingle, G., and T. Oei. 1997. Is alcohol a cofactor of HIV and AIDS? Evidence from immunological and behavioral studies. *Psychol. Bull.* **122**:56–71.

Donahoe, R. 2004. Multiple ways that drug abuse might influence AIDS progression: clues from a monkey model. *J. Neuroimmunol.* **147**:28–32.

Donahoe, R., and D. Vlahov. 1998. Opiates as potential cofactors in progression of HIV-1 infections to AIDS. *J. Neuroimmunol.* **83**:77–87.

Dore, G., A. McDonald, Y. Li, J. Kaldor, and B. Brew. 2003. Marked improvement in survival following AIDS dementia complex in the era of highly active antiretroviral therapy. *AIDS* **17**:1539–1545.

Dronda, F., J. Zamora, S. Moreno, A. Moreno, J. Casado, A. Muriel, M. Perez-Elias, A. Antela, L. Moreno, and C. Quereda. 2004. CD4 cell recovery during successful antiretroviral therapy in naive HIV-infected patients: the role of intravenous drug use. *AIDS* **18**:2210–2212.

Edelstein, H., and R. Knight. 1987. Severe parkinsonism in two AIDS patients taking prochlorperazine. *Lancet* **ii**:341–342. (Letter.)

El-Hage, N., J. Gurwell, I. Singh, P. Knapp, A. Nath, and K. Hauser. 2005. Synergistic increases in intracellular Ca2+, and the release of MCP-1, RANTES, and IL-6 by astrocytes treated with opiates and HIV-1 Tat. *Glia* **50**:91–106.

Epstein, L., and H. Gelbard. 1999. HIV-1-induced neuronal injury in the developing brain. *J. Leukoc. Biol.* **65**:453–457.

Ernst, T., L. Chang, M. Leonido-Yee, and O. Speck. 2000. Evidence for long-term neurotoxicity associated with methamphetamine abuse: A 1H MRS study. *Neurology* **54**:1344–1349.

Fabris, P., G. Tositti, V. Manfrin, M. Giordani, A. Vaglia, A. Cattelan, and A. Carlotto. 2000. Does alcohol intake affect highly active antiretroviral therapy (HAART) response in HIV-positive patients? *J. Acquir. Immune Defic. Syndr.* **25**:92–93.

Fiala, M., A. Eshleman, J. Cashman, A. Lin, J. Lossinsky, V. Suarez, W. Yang, J. Zhang, W. Popik, E. Singer, F. Chiappelli, E. Carro, M. Weinand, M. Witte, and J. Arthos. 2005. Cocaine increases human immunodeficiency virus type 1 neuroinvasion through remodeling brain microvascular endothelial cells. *J. Neurovirol.* **11**:281–291.

Fiala, M., X. Gan, L. Zhang, S. House, T. Newton, M. Graves, P. Shapshak, M. Stins, K. Kim, M. Witte, and S. Chang. 1998. Cocaine enhances monocyte migration across the blood-brain barrier. Cocaine's connection to AIDS dementia and vasculitis? *Adv. Exp. Med. Biol.* **437**:199–205.

Flexner, C., V. Cargill, J. Sinclair, T. Kresina, and L. Cheever. 2001. Alcohol use can result in enhanced drug metabolism in HIV pharmacotherapy. *AIDS Patient Care STDs* **15**:57–58.

Flora, G., Y. Lee, A. Nath, B. Hennig, W. Maragos, and M. Toborek. 2003. Methamphetamine potentiates HIV-1 Tat protein-mediated activation of redox-sensitive pathways in discrete regions of the brain. *Exp. Neurol.* **179**:60–70.

Flora, G., H. Pu, Y. Lee, R. Ravikumar, A. Nath, B. Hennig, and M. Toborek. 2005. Proinflammatory synergism of ethanol and HIV-1 Tat protein in brain tissue. *Exp. Neurol.* **191**:2–12.

Foga, I., A. Nath, B. Hasinoff, and J. Geiger. 1997. Antioxidants and dipyridamole inhibit HIV-1 gp120-induced free radical-based oxidative damage to human monocytoid cells. *J. Acquir. Immune Defic. Syndr. Hum. Retrovirol.* **16**:223–229.

Garcia-Ratés, S., J. Camarasa, E. Escubedo, and D. Pubill. 2007. Methamphetamine and 3,4-methylenedioxymethamphetamine interact with central nicotinic receptors and induce their up-regulation. *Toxicol. Appl. Pharmacol.* **223**:195–205.

Gelbard, H. 1999. Neuroprotective strategies for HIV-1-associated neurologic disease. *Ann. N. Y. Acad. Sci.* **890**:312–313.

Goswami, R., S. Dawson, and G. Dawson. 1998. Cyclic AMP protects against staurosporine and wortmannin-induced apoptosis and opioid-enhanced apoptosis in both embryonic and immortalized (F-11kappa7) neurons. *J. Neurochem.* **70**:1376–1382.

Green, J., R. Saveanu, and R. Bornstein. 2004. The effect of previous alcohol abuse on cognitive function in HIV infection. *Am. J. Psychiatry* **161**:249–254.

Gundlah, C., S. Kohama, S. Mirkes, V. Garyfallou, H. Urbanski, and C. Bethea. 2000. Distribution of estrogen receptor beta (ERbeta) mRNA in hypothalamus, midbrain and temporal lobe of spayed macaque: continued expression with hormone replacement. *Brain Res. Mol. Brain Res.* **76**:191–204.

Gurwell, J., A. Nath, Q. Sun, J. Zhang, K. Martin, Y. Chen, and K. Hauser. 2001. Synergistic neurotoxicity of opioids and human immunodeficiency virus-1 Tat protein in striatal neurons in vitro. *Neuroscience* **102**:555–563.

Hales, G., N. Roth, and D. Smith. 2000. Possible fatal interaction between protease inhibitors and methamphetamine. *Antivir. Ther.* **5**:19. (Letter.)

Harrington, R., J. Woodward, T. Hooton, and J. Horn. 1999. Life-threatening interactions between HIV-1 protease inhibitors and the illicit drugs MDMA and gamma-hydroxybutyrate. *Arch. Intern. Med.* **159**:2221–2224.

Hauser, K., J. Foldes, and C. Turbek. 1999. Dynorphin A (1-13) neurotoxicity in vitro: opioid and non-opioid mechanisms in mouse spinal cord neurons. *Exp. Neurol.* **160**:361–375.

Hauser, K., J. Gurwell, and C. Turbek. 1994. Morphine inhibits Purkinje cell survival and dendritic differentiation in organotypic cultures of the mouse cerebellum. *Exp. Neurol.* **130**:95–105.

Hauser, K., M. Harris-White, J. Jackson, L. Opanashuk, and J. Carney. 1998. Opioids disrupt Ca2+ homeostasis and induce carbonyl oxyradical production in mouse astrocytes in vitro: transient increases and adaptation to sustained exposure. *Exp. Neurol.* **151**:70–76.

Hauser, K., A. Houdi, C. Turbek, R. Elde, and W. Maxson. 2000. Opioids intrinsically inhibit the genesis of mouse cerebellar granule neuron precursors in vitro: differential impact of mu and delta receptor activation on proliferation and neurite elongation. *Eur. J. Neurosci.* **12**:1281–1293.

Heaton, R., I. Grant, N. Butters, D. White, D. Kirson, J. Atkinson, J. McCutchan, M. Taylor, M. Kelly, R. J. Ellis, et al. 1995. The HNRC 500 — neuropsychology of HIV infection at different disease stages. *J. Int. Neuropsychol. Soc.* **1**:231–251.

Henry, J., and I. Hill. 1998. Fatal interaction between ritonavir and MDMA. *Lancet* 352:1751–1752.

Hollander, H., J. Golden, T. Mendelson, and D. Cortland. 1985. Extrapyramidal symptoms in AIDS patients given low-dose metoclopramide or chlorpromazine. *Lancet* ii:1186. (Letter.)

Hornykiewicz, O. 1998. Biochemical aspects of Parkinson's disease. *Neurology* 51:S2–S9.

Hriso, E., T. Kuhn, J. Masdeu, and M. Grundman. 1991. Extrapyramidal symptoms due to dopamine-blocking agents in patients with AIDS encephalopathy. *Am. J. Psychiatry* 148:1558–1561.

Hu, S., W. Sheng, J. Lokensgard, and P. Peterson. 2002. Morphine induces apoptosis of human microglia and neurons. *Neuropharmacology* 42:829-836.

Hu, S., W. Sheng, J. Lokensgard, and P. Peterson. 2005. Morphine potentiates HIV-1 gp120-induced neuronal apoptosis. *J. Infect. Dis.* 191:886–889.

Hu, X., and M. Ticku. 1995. Chronic ethanol treatment upregulates the NMDA receptor function and binding in mammalian cortical neurons. *Brain Res. Mol. Brain Res.* 30:347–356.

Jenuwein, M., C. Scheller, E. Neuen-Jacob, S. Sopper, T. Tatschner, V. ter Meulen, P. Riederer, and E. Koutsilieri. 2004. Dopamine deficits and regulation of the cAMP second messenger system in brains of simian immunodeficiency virus-infected rhesus monkeys. *J. Neurovirol.* 10:163–170.

Jernigan, T., A. Gamst, S. Archibald, C. Fennema-Notestine, M. Mindt, T. Marcotte, R. Heaton, R. Ellis, and I. Grant. 2005. Effects of methamphetamine dependence and HIV infection on cerebral morphology. *Am. J. Psychiatry* 162:1461–1472.

Johnson-Greene, D., K. Adams, S. Gilman, R. Koeppe, L. Junck, K. Kluin, S. Martorello, and M. Heumann. 1997. Effects of abstinence and relapse upon neuropsychological function and cerebral glucose metabolism in severe chronic alcoholism. *J. Clin. Exp. Neuropsychol.* 19:378–385.

Kapadia, F., J. Cook, M. Cohen, N. Sohler, A. Kovacs, R. Greenblatt, I. Choudhary, and D. Vlahov. 2005. The relationship between non-injection drug use behaviors on progression to AIDS and death in a cohort of HIV seropositive women in the era of highly active antiretroviral therapy use. *Addiction* 100:990–1002.

Kendall, S., C. Anderson, A. Nath, J. Turchan-Cholewo, C. Land, C. Mactutus, and R. Booze. 2005. Gonadal steroids differentially modulate neurotoxicity of HIV and cocaine: testosterone and ICI 182,780 sensitive mechanism. *BMC Neurosci.* 6:40–52.

Khurdayan, V., S. Buch, N. El-Hage, S. Lutz, S. Goebel, I. Singh, P. Knapp, J. Turchan-Cholewo, A. Nath, and K. Hauser. 2004. Preferential vulnerability of astroglia and glial precursors to combined opioid and HIV-1 Tat exposure in vitro. *Eur. J. Neurosci.* 19:3171–3182.

Kieburtz, K., L. Epstein, H. Gelbard, and J. Greenamyre. 1991. Excitotoxicity and dopaminergic dysfunction in the acquired immunodeficiency syndrome dementia complex. Therapeutic implications. *Arch. Neurol.* 48:1281–1284.

Kindlundh-Högberg, A., H. Schiöth, and P. Svenningsson. 2007. Repeated intermittent MDMA binges reduce DAT density in mice and SERT density in rats in reward regions of the adolescent brain. *Neurotoxicology* 28:1158–1169.

Kofke, W., R. Garman, R. Garman, and M. Rose. 1999. Opioid neurotoxicity: fentanyl-induced exacerbation of cerebral ischemia in rats. *Brain Res.* 818:326–334.

Kofke, W., R. Garman, R. Stiller, M. Rose, and R. Garman. 1996. Opioid neurotoxicity: fentanyl dose-response effects in rats. *Anesth. Analg.* 83:1298–1306.

Koob, G. 2000. Neurobiology of addiction. Toward the development of new therapies. *Ann. N. Y. Acad. Sci.* 909:170–185.

Kosel, B., F. Aweeka, N. Benowitz, S. Shade, J. Hilton, P. Lizak, and D. Abrams. 2002. The effects of cannabinoids on the pharmacokinetics of indinavir and nelfinavir. *AIDS* 16:543–550.

Koutsilieri, E., M. Gotz, S. Sopper, U. Sauer, M. Demuth, V. ter Meulen, and P. Riederer. 1997a. Regulation of glutathione and cell toxicity following exposure to neurotropic substances and human immunodeficiency virus-1 in vitro. *J. Neurovirol.* 3:342–349.

Koutsilieri, E., M. Gotz, S. Sopper, C. Stahl-Hennig, M. Czub, V. ter Meulen, and P. Riederer. 1997b. Monoamine metabolite levels in CSF of SIV-infected rhesus monkeys (*Macaca mulatta*). *Neuroreport* 8:3833–3836.

Kreek, M. 2001. Drug addictions. Molecular and cellular endpoints. *Ann. N. Y. Acad. Sci.* 937:27–49.

Kreek, M., and G. Koob. 1998. Drug dependence: stress and dysregulation of brain reward pathways. *Drug Alcohol Depend.* 51:23–47.

Kumar, R., A. Perez-Casanova, G. Tirado, R. Noel, C. Torres, I. Rodriguez, M. Martinez, S. Staprans, E. Kraiselburd, Y. Yamamura, J. Higley, and A. Kumar. 2005. Increased viral replication in simian immunodeficiency virus/simian-HIV-infected macaques with self-administering model of chronic alcohol consumption. *J. Acquir. Immune Defic. Syndr.* 39:386–390.

Kumar, R., C. Torres, Y. Yamamura, I. Rodriguez, M. Martinez, S. Staprans, R. Donahoe, E. Kraiselburd, E. Stephens, and A. Kumar. 2004. Modulation by morphine of viral set point in rhesus macaques infected with simian immunodeficiency virus and simian-human immunodeficiency virus. *J. Virol.* 78:11425–11428.

Kurling, S., A. Kankaanpaa, S. Ellermaa, T. Karila, and T. Seppala. 2005. The effect of sub-chronic nandrolone decanoate treatment on dopaminergic and serotonergic neuronal systems in the brains of rats. *Brain Res.* 1044:67–75.

Langford, D., A. Adame, A. Grigorian, I. Grant, J. McCutchan, R. Ellis, T. Marcotte, and E. Masliah. 2003. Patterns of selective neuronal damage in methamphetamine-user AIDS patients. *J. Acquir. Immune Defic. Syndr.* 34:467–474.

Langford, D., A. Grigorian, R. Hurford, A. Adame, L. Crews, and E. Masliah. 2004. The role of mitochondrial alterations in the combined toxic effects of human immunodeficiency virus Tat protein and methamphetamine on calbindin positive-neurons. *J. Neurovirol.* 10:327–337.

Larsson, M., L. Hagberg, A. Forsman, and G. Norkrans. 1991. Cerebrospinal fluid catecholamine metabolites in HIV-infected patients. *J. Neurosci. Res.* 28:406–409.

Lipton, S. 1998. Neuronal injury associated with HIV-1: approaches to treatment. *Annu. Rev. Pharmacol. Toxicol.* 38:159–177.

Littleton, J., and H. Little. 1994. Current concepts of ethanol dependence. *Addiction* 89:1397–1412.

Lopez, O., J. Becker, M. Dew, and R. Caldararo. 2004. Risk modifiers for peripheral sensory neuropathy in HIV infection/AIDS. *Eur. J. Neurol.* 11:97–102.

Mahajan, S., R. Aalinkeel, J. Reynolds, B. Nair, S. Fernandez, S. Schwartz, and M. Nair. 2005a. Morphine exacerbates HIV-1 viral protein gp120 induced modulation of chemokine gene expression in U373 astrocytoma cells. *Curr. HIV Res.* 3:277–288.

Mahajan, S., S. Schwartz, R. Aalinkeel, R. Chawda, D. Sykes, and M. Nair. 2005b. Morphine modulates chemokine gene regulation in normal human astrocytes. *Clin. Immunol.* 115:323–332.

Manly, J., C. Merchant, D. Jacobs, S. Small, K. Bell, M. Ferin, and R. Mayeux. 2000. Endogenous estrogen levels and Alzheimer's disease among postmenopausal women. *Neurology* 54:833–837.

Maragos, W., K. Young, J. Turchan, M. Guseva, J. Pauly, A. Nath, and W. Cass. 2002. Human immunodeficiency virus-1 Tat protein and methamphetamine interact synergistically to impair striatal dopaminergic function. *J. Neurochem.* 83:955–963.

Marcario, J., K. Manaye, K. SantaCruz, P. Mouton, N. Berman, and P. Cheney. 2004. Severe subcortical degeneration in macaques infected with neurovirulent simian immunodeficiency virus. *J. Neurovirol.* **10**:387–399.

McArthur, J., N. Haughey, S. Gartner, K. Conant, C. Pardo, A. Nath, and N. Sacktor. 2003. Human immunodeficiency virus-associated dementia: an evolving disease. *J. Neurovirol.* **9**:205–221.

McCarthy, L., M. Wetzel, J. Sliker, T. Eisenstein, and T. Rogers. 2001. Opioids, opioid receptors, and the immune response. *Drug Alcohol Depend.* **62**:111–123.

Mellon, R., and B. Bayer. 1998. Evidence for central opioid receptors in the immunomodulatory effects of morphine: review of potential mechanism(s) of action. *J. Neuroimmunol.* **83**:19–28.

Meriney, S., M. Ford, D. Oliva, and G. Pilar. 1991. Endogenous opioids modulate neuronal survival in the developing avian ciliary ganglion. *J. Neurosci.* **11**:3705–3717.

Meyerhoff, D., S. MacKay, D. Sappey-Marinier, R. Deicken, G. Calabrese, W. P. Dillon, M. W. Weiner, and G. Fein. 1995. Effects of chronic alcohol abuse and HIV infection on brain phosphorus metabolites. *Alcohol Clin. Exp. Res.* **19**:685–692.

Mirsattari, S., M. Berry, J. Holden, W. Ni, A. Nath, and C. Power. 1999. Paroxysmal dyskinesias in patients with HIV infection. *Neurology* **52**:109–114.

Mirsattari, S., C. Power, and A. Nath. 1998. Parkinsonism with HIV infection. *Mov. Disord.* **13**:684–689.

Morgello, S., L. Estanislao, D. Simpson, A. Geraci, A. DiRocco, P. Gerits, E. Ryan, T. Yakoushina, S. Khan, R. Mahboob, M. Naseer, D. Dorfman, and V. Sharp. 2004. HIV-associated distal sensory polyneuropathy in the era of highly active antiretroviral therapy: the Manhattan HIV Brain Bank. *Arch. Neurol.* **61**:546–551.

Murrill, C., H. Weeks, B. Castrucci, H. Weinstock, B. Bell, C. Spruill, and M. Gwinn. 2002. Age-specific seroprevalence of HIV, hepatitis B virus, and hepatitis C virus infection among injection drug users admitted to drug treatment in 6 US cities. *Am. J. Public Health* **92**:385–387.

Nair, M., S. Mahajan, S. Schwartz, J. Reynolds, R. Whitney, Z. Bernstein, R. Chawda, D. Sykes, R. Hewitt, and C. Hsiao. 2005. Cocaine modulates dendritic cell-specific C type intercellular adhesion molecule-3-grabbing nonintegrin expression by dendritic cells in HIV-1 patients. *J. Immunol.* **174**:6617–6626.

Nair, M., S. Schwartz, S. Mahajan, C. Tsiao, R. Chawda, R. Whitney, B. Don Sykes, and R. Hewitt. 2004. Drug abuse and neuropathogenesis of HIV infection: role of DC-SIGN and IDO. *J. Neuroimmunol.* **157**:56–60.

Nair, M., S. Schwartz, R. Polasani, J. Hou, A. Sweet, and K. Chadha. 1997. Immunoregulatory effects of morphine on human lymphocytes. *Clin. Diagn. Lab. Immunol.* **4**:127–132.

Nath, A., and J. Geiger. 1998. Neurobiological aspects of HIV infections: neurotoxic mechanisms. *Prog. Neurobiol.* **54**:19–33.

Nath, A., W. Maragos, M. Avison, F. Schmitt, and J. Berger. 2001. Accelerated HIV dementia with methamphetamine and cocaine use. *J. Neurovirol.* **7**:66–71.

Nestler, E., and G. Aghajanian. 1997. Molecular and cellular basis of addiction. *Science* **278**:58–63.

Neuenburg, J., H. Brodt, B. Herndier, M. Bickel, P. Bacchetti, R. Price, R. Grant, and W. Schlote. 2002. HIV-related neuropathology, 1985 to 1999: rising prevalence of HIV encephalopathy in the era of highly active antiretroviral therapy. *J. Acquir. Immune Defic. Syndr.* **31**:171–177.

Parsons, J., E. Rosof, J. Punzalan, and L. Di Maria. 2005. Integration of motivational interviewing and cognitive behavioral therapy to improve HIV medication adherence and reduce substance use among HIV-positive men and women: results of a pilot project. *AIDS Patient Care STDs* **19**:31–39.

Pascual-Leone, A., and A. Dhuna. 1990. Cocaine-associated multifocal tics. *Neurology* **40**:999–1000.

Pascual-Leone, A., A. Dhuna, I. Altafullah, and D. Anderson. 1990. Cocaine-induced seizures. *Neurology* **40**:404–407.

Peterson, P., G. Gekker, S. Hu, J. Lokensgard, P. Portoghese, and C. Chao. 1999. Endomorphin-1 potentiates HIV-1 expression in human brain cell cultures: implication of an atypical mu-opioid receptor. *Neuropharmacology* **38**:273–278.

Peterson, P., G. Gekker, J. Lokensgard, J. Bidlack, A. Chang, X. Fang, and P. Portoghese. 2001. kappa-Opioid receptor agonist suppression of HIV-1 expression in CD4(+) lymphocytes. *Biochem. Pharmacol.* **61**:1145–1151.

Peterson, P., G. Gekker, R. Schut, S. Hu, H. Balfour, and C. Chao. 1993. Enhancement of HIV-1 replication by opiates and cocaine: the cytokine connection. *Adv. Exp. Med. Biol.* **335**:181–188.

Pillai, R., B. S. Nair, and R. R. Watson. 1991. AIDS, drugs of abuse and the immune system: a complex immunotoxicological network. *Arch. Toxicol.* **65**:609–617.

Polakiewicz, R., M. Schieferl, A. Gingras, N. Sonenberg, and M. Comb. 1998. mu-Opioid receptor activates signaling pathways implicated in cell survival and translational control. *J. Biol. Chem.* **273**:23534–23541.

Prendergast, M., B. Harris, J. Blanchard, S. Mayer, D. Gibson, and J. Littleton. 2000. In vitro effects of ethanol withdrawal and spermidine on viability of hippocampus from male and female rat. *Alcohol Clin. Exp. Res.* **24**:1855–1861.

Prendergast, M., B. Harris, P. Mullholland, J. Blanchard, D. Gibson, R. Holley, and J. Littleton. 2004. Hippocampal CA1 region neurodegeneration produced by ethanol withdrawal requires activation of intrinsic polysynaptic hippocampal pathways and function of N-methyl-D-aspartate receptors. *Neuroscience* **124**:869–877.

Prentiss, D., R. Power, G. Balmas, G. Tzuang, and D. Israelski. 2004. Patterns of marijuana use among patients with HIV/AIDS followed in a public health care setting. *J. Acquir. Immune Defic. Syndr.* **35**:38–45.

Pu, H., J. Tian, G. Flora, Y. Lee, A. Nath, B. Hennig, and M. Toborek. 2003. HIV-1 Tat protein upregulates inflammatory mediators and induces monocyte invasion into the brain. *Mol. Cell. Neurosci.* **24**:224–237.

Rabkin, J., M. McElhiney, and S. Ferrando. 2004. Mood and substance use disorders in older adults with HIV/AIDS: methodological issues and preliminary evidence. *AIDS* **181**:S43–S48.

Reiter, G. 1996. The HIV wasting syndrome. *AIDS Clin. Care* **8**:89–91, 93, 96.

Reyes, M., F. Faraldi, C. Senseng, C. Flowers, and R. Fariello. 1991. Nigral degeneration in acquired immune deficiency syndrome (AIDS). *Acta Neuropathol.* **82**:39–44.

Robinson, T. E., and K. C. Berridge. 2000. The psychology and neurobiology of addiction: an incentive-sensitization view. *Addiction* **95**(Suppl. 2):S91–S117.

Rogers, T., and P. Peterson. 2003. Opioid G protein-coupled receptors: signals at the crossroads of inflammation. *Trends Immunol.* **24**:116–121.

Rooney, K., R. Armstrong, and R. Sewell. 1991. Increased dopamine receptor sensitivity in the rat following acute administration of sufentanil, U50,488H and D-Ala2-D-Leu5-enkephalin. *Naunyn Schmiedebergs Arch. Pharmacol.* **343**:458–462.

Rudolph, J., J. Lemasters, and F. Crews. 1998. Effects of chronic ethanol exposure on oxidation and NMDA-stimulated neuronal death in primary cortical neuronal cultures. *Alcohol Clin. Exp. Res.* **22**:2080–2085.

Russo, R., M. Navarra, J. Maiuolo, D. Rotiroti, G. Bagetta, and M. Corasaniti. 2005. 17beta-Estradiol protects SH-SY5Y cells against HIV-1 gp120-induced cell death: evidence for a role of estrogen receptors. *Neurotoxicology* **26**:905–913.

Sacktor, N. 2002. The epidemiology of human immunodeficiency virus-associated neurological disease in the era of highly active antiretroviral therapy. *J. Neurovirol.* 8(Suppl. 2): 115–121.

Sacktor, N., M. McDermott, K. Marder, G. Schifitto, O. Selnes, J. McArthur, Y. Stern, S. Albert, D. Palumbo, K. Kieburtz, J. De Marcaida, B. Cohen, and L. Epstein. 2002. HIV-associated cognitive impairment before and after the advent of combination therapy. *J. Neurovirol.* 8:136–142.

Saunders-Pullman, R., J. Gordon-Elliott, M. Parides, S. Fahn, H. Saunders, and S. Bressman. 1999. The effect of estrogen replacement on early Parkinson's disease. *Neurology* 52:1417–1421.

Schoffelmeer, A., F. Hogenboom, and A. Mulder. 1997. Kappa1- and kappa2-opioid receptors mediating presynaptic inhibition of dopamine and acetylcholine release in rat neostriatum. *Br. J. Pharmacol.* 122:520–524.

Self, R., P. Mulholland, B. Harris, A. Nath, and M. Prendergast. 2004. Cytotoxic effects of exposure to the human immunodeficiency virus type 1 protein Tat in the hippocampus are enhanced by prior ethanol treatment. *Alcohol Clin. Exp. Res.* 28:1916–1924.

Singhal, P., A. Kapasi, K. Reddy, N. Franki, N. Gibbons, and G. Ding. 1999. Morphine promotes apoptosis in Jurkat cells. *J. Leukoc. Biol.* 66:650–658.

Singhal, P., K. Reddy, N. Franki, V. Sanwal, and N. Gibbons. 1997. Morphine induces splenocyte apoptosis and enhanced mRNA expression of cathepsin-B. *Inflammation* 21:609–617.

Singhal, P., P. Sharma, A. Kapasi, K. Reddy, N. Franki, and N. Gibbons. 1998. Morphine enhances macrophage apoptosis. *J. Immunol.* 160:1886–1893.

Slooter, A., J. Bronzova, J. Witteman, C. Van Broeckhoven, A. Hofman, and C. van Duijn. 1999. Estrogen use and early onset Alzheimer's disease: a population-based study. *J. Neurol. Neurosurg. Psychiatry* 67:779–781.

Stefano, G. 1999. Substance abuse and HIV-gp120: are opiates protective? *Arch. Immunol. Ther. Exp.* 47:99–106.

Stein, M., D. Herman, E. Trisvan, P. Pirraglia, P. Engler, and B. Anderson. 2005. Alcohol use and sexual risk behavior among human immunodeficiency virus-positive persons. *Alcohol Clin. Exp. Res.* 29:837–843.

Stiene-Martin, A., R. Zhou, and K. Hauser. 1998. Regional, developmental, and cell cycle-dependent differences in mu, delta, and kappa-opioid receptor expression among cultured mouse astrocytes. *Glia* 22:249–259.

Stocker, H., G. Kruse, P. Kreckel, C. Herzmann, K. Arasteh, J. Claus, H. Jessen, C. Cordes, B. Hintsche, F. Schlote, L. Schneider, and M. Kurowski. 2004. Nevirapine significantly reduces the levels of racemic methadone and (R)-methadone in human immunodeficiency virus-infected patients. *Antimicrob. Agents Chemother.* 48:4148–4153.

Tabakoff, B. 1994. Alcohol and AIDS—is the relationship all in our heads? *Alcohol Clin. Exp. Res.* 18:415–416.

Thomas, D., and D. Kuhn. 2005. MK-801 and dextromethorphan block microglial activation and protect against methamphetamine-induced neurotoxicity. *Brain Res.* 1050:190–198.

Toborek, M., Y. Lee, H. Pu, A. Malecki, G. Flora, R. Garrido, B. Hennig, H. Bauer, and A. Nath. 2003. HIV-Tat protein induces oxidative and inflammatory pathways in brain endothelium. *J. Neurochem.* 84:169–179.

Tomlinson, G., P. Simmonds, A. Busuttil, A. Chiswick, and J. Bell. 1999. Upregulation of microglia in drug users with and without pre-symptomatic HIV infection. *Neuropathol. Appl. Neurobiol.* 25:369–379.

Turchan, J., C. Anderson, K. Hauser, Q. Sun, J. Zhang, Y. Liu, P. Wise, I. Kruman, W. Maragos, M. Mattson, R. Booze, and A. Nath. 2001. Estrogen protects against the synergistic toxicity by HIV proteins, methamphetamine and cocaine. *BMC Neurosci.* 2:3–13.

Turchan, J., C. Pocernich, C. Gairola, A. Chauhan, G. Schifitto, D. Butterfield, S. Buch, O. Narayan, A. Sinai, J. Geiger, J. Berger, H. Elford, and A. Nath. 2003. Oxidative stress in HIV demented patients and protection ex vivo with novel antioxidants. *Neurology* 60:307–314.

Tyor, W., and L. Middaugh. 1999. Do alcohol and cocaine abuse alter the course of HIV-associated dementia complex? *J. Leukoc. Biol.* 65:475–481.

Vanderschuren, L., G. Wardeh, T. J. De Vries, A. H. Mulder, and A. Schoffelmeer. 1999. Opposing role of dopamine D1 and D2 receptors in modulation of rat nucleus accumbens noradrenaline release. *J. Neurosci.* 19:4123–4131.

Vlahov, D., N. Galai, M. Safaeian, S. Galea, G. Kirk, G. Lucas, and T. Sterling. 2005. Effectiveness of highly active antiretroviral therapy among injection drug users with late-stage human immunodeficiency virus infection. *Am. J. Epidemiol.* 161:999–1012.

Walker, D., M. Heaton, N. Lee, M. King, and B. Hunter. 1993. Effect of chronic ethanol on the septohippocampal system: a role for neurotrophic factors? *Alcohol Clin. Exp. Res.* 17:12–18.

Wang, G., L. Chang, N. Volkow, F. Telang, J. Logan, T. Ernst, and J. Fowler. 2004. Decreased brain dopaminergic transporters in HIV-associated dementia patients. *Brain* 127:2452–2458.

Wang, X., N. Tan, S. Douglas, T. Zhang, Y. Wang, and W. Ho. 2005. Morphine inhibits CD8+ T cell-mediated, noncytolytic, anti-HIV activity in latently infected immune cells. *J. Leukoc. Biol.* 78:772–776.

Ware, N., M. Wyatt, and T. Tugenberg. 2005. Adherence, stereotyping and unequal HIV treatment for active users of illegal drugs. *Soc. Sci. Med.* 61:565–576.

Watzl, B., and R. Watson. 1992. Role of alcohol abuse in nutritional immunosuppression. *J. Nutr.* 122:733–737.

Weiner, W., A. Rabinstein, B. Levin, C. Weiner, and L. Shulman. 2001. Cocaine-induced persistent dyskinesias. *Neurology* 56:964–965.

Weinhardt, L., M. Carey, K. Carey, S. Maisto, and C. Gordon. 2001. The relation of alcohol use to HIV-risk sexual behavior among adults with a severe and persistent mental illness. *J. Consult. Clin. Psychol.* 69:77–84.

Welch, K., and A. Morse. 2002. The clinical profile of end-stage AIDS in the era of highly active antiretroviral therapy. *AIDS Patient Care STDs* 16:75–81.

Wilson, J., K. Kalasinsky, A. Levey, C. Bergeron, G. Reiber, R. Anthony, G. Schmunk, K. Shannak, J. Haycock, and S. Kish. 1996a. Striatal dopamine nerve terminal markers in human, chronic methamphetamine users. *Nat. Med.* 2:699–703.

Wilson, J., A. Levey, C. Bergeron, K. Kalasinsky, L. Ang, F. Peretti, V. Adams, J. Smialek, W. Anderson, K. Shannak, J. Deck, H. Niznik, and S. Kish. 1996b. Striatal dopamine, dopamine transporter, and vesicular monoamine transporter in chronic cocaine users. *Ann. Neurol.* 40:428–439.

Woolridge, E., S. Barton, J. Samuel, J. Osorio, A. Dougherty, and A. Holdcroft. 2005. Cannabis use in HIV for pain and other medical symptoms. *J. Pain Symptom Manage.* 29:358–367.

Wynn, G., K. Cozza, M. Zapor, G. Wortmann, and S. Armstrong. 2005. Med-psych drug-drug interactions update. Antiretrovirals, part III: antiretrovirals and drugs of abuse. *Psychosomatics* 46:79–87.

Yin, D., R. Mufson, R. Wang, and Y. Shi. 1999. Fas-mediated cell death promoted by opioids. *Nature* 397:218. (Letter.)

Yin, D., X. Ren, Z. L. Zheng, L. Pu, L. Z. Jiang, L. Ma, and G. Pei. 1997. Etorphine inhibits cell growth and induces apoptosis in SK-N-SH cells: involvement of pertussis toxin-sensitive G proteins. *Neurosci. Res.* 29:121–127.

SPECIAL POPULATIONS AND NEURO-AIDS

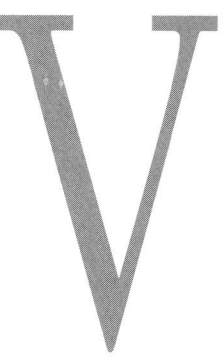

The Spectrum of Neuro-AIDS Disorders:
Pathophysiology, Diagnosis, and Treatment
Edited by K. Goodkin et al.
©2008 ASM Press, Washington, DC

30

Ethnicity and Neuro-AIDS Conditions in the HAART Era

LOYDA M. MELENDEZ, RAUL MAYO-SANTANA,
CARLOS LUCIANO, AND VALERIE WOJNA

The nature of neurocognitve impairment associated with HIV has changed, after the introduction of highly active antiretroviral therapy (HAART), to more subtle forms, requiring the establishment of new definitional criteria. This has precipitated a new suggested algorithm to assist in standardized diagnostic classification of HIV-associated neurocognitive disorders (HAND) (Antinori et al., 2007). Ethnic, gender, education or literacy, genetic, and age factors may contribute to different manifestations of HIV-1 cognitive impairment; consequently they should be considered or controlled in the research design. There is a need to develop culturally sensitive instruments that correctly identify cognitive impairment in different ethnic groups. Significant progress has been made toward identification of protein biomarkers associated with HIV-related cognitive impairment in macrophages and cerebrospinal fluid (CSF) from HIV-infected women (Laspiur et al., 2007; Rozek et al., 2007). However there is a need to validate these studies in larger numbers of samples from different ethnic groups and with both genders to detect possible differences associated with these factors. Regarding the viral clades or subtypes, additional studies are needed to confirm their distribution in the world, as it has become more diverse after 20 years of the epidemic. Their worldwide distribution in relation to cognitive impairment shows divergent results requiring further confirmation. Additional studies are needed for clades other than B, such as C, which circulates in the countries where the epidemic is most devastating. This clade predominantly infects macrophages, which are important reservoirs for HIV and major players in the development of brain inflammation during HIV dementia. We have found that distal sensory polyneuropathy (DSP), another HIV-associated neurological complication, is highly prevalent in both pediatric/adolescent and adult Puerto Rican/Latino patients and that, similar to what has been described in other groups from the mainland United States, the introduction of HAART has altered the association of HIV infection with HIV DSP. With the increased longevity of patients with HIV-1 infection, we also observed that aging is a powerful modifying factor in the frequency and severity of neuropathy.

Ethnicity, sex/gender, and age factors were not a special focus of interest during the early phase of the AIDS epidemic within the United States, since at that time, Caucasian men who have sex with men (MSMs) were the population group that became identified as having lifestyles that placed them at higher risk of acquiring HIV-1 infection. Thus, early neurological and neuropsychological studies were conducted mostly among homosexual and bisexual men. However, as HIV-1 infection grew and spread quite rapidly, affecting other groups and manifesting diversified risk factors, researchers started reporting demographic background in their study cohorts, including ethnicity and sex. Data analyses were increasingly performed with controls, mostly for age, education, and intellectual levels. HIV-1 infection demographic profiles changed by addressing specialized populations, including ethnic minorities, women, children, and the elderly. Neurological complications of HIV-1 infection in African-Americans, Hispanics, Asians, and "other" ethnic minorities were explored at that time. Later, women and, recently, children and the elderly, have been increasingly studied, and the composition and design of studies have changed accordingly, with new cohorts established. Nevertheless, there are still few investigations that have centered on ethnicity, sex/gender, or age as independent variables. Special population cohorts are still understudied. Minorities, such as Native Americans and Asian-Americans, are still amalgamated as "other." Thus, it is reasonable to conclude that little is known about the spectrum of neurological and neurocognitive manifestations of HIV-1 infection among special populations and ethnic groups.

Loyda M. Melendez, Department of Microbiology and Medical Zoology, NeuroAIDS Program, UPR, MSC, SNRP, University of Puerto Rico, Medical Sciences Campus, San Juan, PR 00936-5067. **Raul Mayo-Santana, Carlos Luciano, and Valerie Wojna,** Departments of Physical Medicine and Division of Neurology, NeuroAIDS Program, UPR, MSC, SNRP, University of Puerto Rico, Medical Sciences Campus, San Juan, PR 00936-5067.

The number of minority communities with AIDS is increasing (CDC, 2003, 2004). This increase has been observed within the United States, as well as in regions like the Caribbean, the Pacific Islands, Africa, and India (Quinn and Overbaugh, 2005). The spectrum of HIV-1 infection has evolved from a group of MSM and intravenous-drug users (IDU) to heterosexual transmission affecting other groups, such as women and the elderly (Quinn and Overbaugh, 2005; Valcour et al., 2004a). In the United States, HIV-1 infection is currently the second leading cause of death among women aged 25 to 44 and shows the highest incidence rates among African-Americans and Hispanics (CDC, 2003, 2004).

Recently, the neurological spectrum of HIV-1 infection has been divided into the eras before and after HAART. Antiretroviral (ARV) therapy has had a direct impact on patient survival and the clinical manifestations of neurological complications. In the pre-HAART era, the most common neurological complications were HIV encephalitis, cytomegalovirus infection, toxoplasmosis, cryptococcus infection, and progressive multifocal leukoencephalopathy (Masliah et al., 2000). In those communities where HAART is available, there has been a change in the neurological manifestations of HIV-1. The widespread use of HAART and the increased survival of HIV-1-infected patients have influenced the clinical manifestations of HIV-1-associated dementia (HAD). Thus, in the HAART era, HAD presents in a milder form, with mixed phenotypes (subcortical and cortical features), higher CD4 cell count, and lower levels of the previously established HAD biomarkers, like tumor necrosis factor alpha (TNF-α), neopterin, β_2-microglubulin, and plasma and CSF viral loads, which are no longer useful to monitor HAD (Gonzalez-Scarano and Martin-Garcia, 2005; McArthur, 2004; Saha and Pahan, 2003; Sevigny et al., 2004; Stein et al., 1997).

We have observed improvement in the neurological complications of HIV-1 infection after the advent of HAART; however, not all the HIV-1-infected populations have access to this treatment. These special populations continue to present with opportunistic brain infections, and the associated increased morbidity and mortality, as the most devastating neurological complication of HIV-1 infection. For example, in Haiti, where HAART was introduced in 2003, 25% of deaths among AIDS patients were related to opportunistic brain infections (Severe, 2005). In order to understand the AIDS epidemic among special populations, increased efforts have been directed to determine if genetic aspects affect the clinical neurological manifestations of HIV-1 infection in different ethnic groups. It has been found that age, genetic factors, and gender may play roles in the development of neurological complications of HIV-1 infection. For example, the Aging Cohort of HIV-1-infected elderly in Hawaii observed that the odds of meeting HAD criteria were higher than in a younger group (Valcour et al., 2004a). Likewise, host factors, such as Apo E4 (Cutler et al., 2004; Valcour et al., 2004b) and monocyte chemoattractant protein 1 (MCP-1) (Gonzalez et al., 2002, 2005), have been associated with HAD. Gender has become an important factor for study and exploration in HIV research, since women are now affected in increasing numbers (Quinn and Overbaugh, 2005). Among the women infected with HIV-1 in the United States, the largest increase has been in non-Caucasian women (CDC, 2003; Wortley and Fleming, 1997). Several cohorts of HIV-1-infected women have been established: CDC-sponsored HIV Epidemiology Research Study (HERS), the Women's Interagency HIV Study (WIHS), and the Puerto Rico NeuroAIDS Cohort (PRNAC) of HIV-1-infected women. In addition, women have been singled out for gender studies in already-established cohorts: the UCLA/Drew Women and Family Project and the Dana Consortium cohort. Data generated from the PRNAC indicate that women may represent an even higher proportion of those with HIV-associated cognitive impairment when compared with HIV-seropositive men from other cohorts (Wojna et al., 2006).

PATHOPHYSIOLOGY OF HIV DEMENTIA

HAD

A spectrum of neurological and psychiatric manifestations of disease follows progressive HIV-1 infection of the brain and is termed HAD. Among adults, clinical symptoms begin with forgetfulness, apathy, and motor impairments. Such neurological problems progress, often rapidly (within weeks to months), to hallucinations, delirium, coma, and ultimately death (Janssen et al., 1991; Marder et al., 1996; Navia et al., 1986b). A multinucleated giant-cell encephalitis, which is often correlated with neuronal loss, alterations in dendritic arbor, and decreased synaptic density, is the pathological correlate of HAD and is termed HIV-1 encephalitis. The depletion of CD4$^+$ T lymphocytes that occurs with advanced HIV-1 infection can affect disease progression in the brain and is associated with clinical neurological dysfunction typified by a subcortical dementia (Everall et al., 1994; Janssen et al., 1991; Marder et al., 1996; Navia et al., 1986b; Wiley et al., 1991). Importantly, all the pathological and clinical aspects of the disease process result, in whole or in part, from HIV-1 infection of the brain and perivascular macrophages and a subsequent induced brain immune activation response (Ardila-Ardila et al., 2003; Kim et al., 2003; Moses et al., 1993; Nath et al., 1995; Ranki et al., 1995; Tornatore et al., 1991; Williams et al., 2001). HAART has diminished the incidence of HAD but has not eliminated the development of cognitive impairment (Sacktor et al., 2001). In 2003 the incidence rate of HAD began to increase, suggesting that there may be some escape from the effects of HAART. In the North-Eastern AIDS Dementia Cohort, the prevalence of HAD or minor cognitive-motor disorder (MCMD) remained high (37%) among those with advanced HIV/AIDS, even with HAART (McArthur, 2004). Several studies indicated that cognitive deficits in HIV-1-infected individuals under HAART are not likely to remain static (McArthur, 2004). Transitions can occur with high frequency, either from normal cognitive function to MCMD to HAD or from MCMD or HAD to milder cognitive dysfunctions (McArthur, 2004).

Role of Monocytes/Macrophages in HAD

It has been demonstrated that the number of immune-competent macrophages is correlated with HAD and not the absolute levels of virus in the brain (Anderson et al., 2002; Elkabes et al., 1996; Gartner, 2000; Gonzalez-Scarano and Martin-Garcia, 2005; Heese et al., 1998; Kim et al. 2003; Williams et al., 2001). Moreover, as in other neurodegenerative disorders, the macrophage appears to be a major source of neurotoxins that affect neural function. Interestingly, under steady-state conditions, macrophages act as scavenger and sentinel cells, nonspecifically eliminating foreign material and secreting trophic factors critical for maintenance of the central nervous system (CNS) microenvironment (Elkabes et al., 1996; Heese et al., 1998). However, during disease, such as HAD, the normal protective functions of the macrophage are transformed (Soontornniyomkij et al., 1998; Zheng et al., 1999). This is likely the critical pathogenic event that leads to neuronal injury during HIV-1 disease. Once infected with HIV-1, macrophage populations are predisposed to immune activation (Kaul and Lipton, 1999; Nath et al., 1999; Zheng et al., 1999). In this way, macrophages become "primed" for subsequent activation by proinflammatory cytokines, chemokines, or T-cell-expressed immune modulatory factors (Gendelman et al., 1997). The combination of viral infection and immune activation in macrophages ultimately results in the production of significant quantities of neurotoxins and in neuronal demise (Gendelman et al., 1997; Kaul and Lipton, 1999; Zheng et al., 1999).

The mechanisms by which monocytes migrate to the brain have been elucidated. A subset of monocytes (CD14/CD69/CD16) that is correlated with dementia emerges during progressive HIV-1 infection (Pulliam et al., 1997). The majority of the CD14/CD16 antigen-positive macrophages are identified in microglial nodules and in the perivascular infiltrate that colocalizes with HIV-1 p24-expressing cells (Fischer-Smith et al., 2001). These cells, along with a restricted infection by astrocytes (Messam and Major, 2000), represent the predominant cell types infected by virus in the CNS. The above-mentioned studies have been performed mostly in male cohorts. In studies of monocyte phenotypes from minority populations, such as the female Hispanic cohort during the post-HAART era, after adjusting for age, education, CD4 cell counts, and viral load using a generalized linear-equation model, we found that the percentage of $CD14^+/CD16^+$ monocytes increased significantly with the degree of cognitive impairment. Our data indicate that monocyte activation occurs in early stages of cognitive impairment and remains elevated in patients who are using HAART (Melendez, 2006).

How do these peripheral blood monocytes infiltrate into brain tissue? Evidence shows that infiltration is facilitated by endothelial and monocyte/macrophage-derived nitric oxide and gelatinase B activity (Nottet, 1999). Chemokines produced within the brain regulate the traffic of infiltrating monocytes and lymphocytes through the brain parenchyma. Lymphocytes infected with HIV-1 induce dysregulation of monocyte function. In addition, endothelial cells and macrophages produce monocyte-attracting cytokines, such as MCP-1, during their first interactions with HIV-1-infected monocytes/macrophages, thus promoting an additional influx of phagocytes into the brain (Nottet, 1999). Excessive infiltration of monocytes into the brain is accompanied by endothelial damage, resulting in the loss of tight junctions and disruption of the blood-brain barrier (BBB) (the BBB disruption is more frequent in AIDS patients with dementia than in AIDS patients without dementia and seronegative controls [Avison et al., 2003; Power et al., 1993]) and in elevated levels of MCP-1, RANTES, MIP-1α, MIP-1β, and interleukin-8 chemokines in the CSF of HAD patients. MCP-1 was correlated with the CSF viral load and the severity of dementia in the pre-HAART era, increasing over time in patients with disease progression (Kelder et al., 1998). The increased level of chemokines and adhesion molecules in the disrupted BBB promoted the entry of more monocytes from peripheral blood. In recent studies, several additional macrophage markers have been associated with inflammation induced by HIV-1. Matrix metalloproteinase 9, a known neurotoxin, has been shown to be down-regulated in macrophages upon HIV-1 infection (Ciborowski et al., 2004). Amyloid precursor protein was found to be expressed in $CD16^+$ monocytes and brain macrophages, possibly influencing the ability of monocytes to cross the endothelium of the BBB (Vehmas et al., 2004). However, the surface expression of this protein is more an indicator of cellular activation than a possible biomarker

for HAD. Sialoadhesin, a protein that binds sialic acid that is not normally found in monocytes, is present in monocytes of HIV-1-infected patients with high viral loads under HAART (Pulliam et al., 2004). This protein could also play a role in facilitating the migration of monocytes across the BBB. Taken together, these findings support the role of monocytes and their differentiated counterparts, macrophages, in HIV-1-induced inflammatory response in neuronal damage and their importance in finding biomarkers in this cell population.

Several macrophage proteins have been described in the CSF or brain tissue of patients with HAD. They include amyloid precursor protein (Vehmas et al., 2004); chemokines, such as fractalkine (Cotter et al., 2002); cytokines, like TNF-α (Saha and Pahan, 2003); and interleukin-18 (von Giesen et al., 2004). However, none of these proteins has been shown to be predictive of HAD development in the post-HAART era. It is possible that patients with HAD who receive HAART have additional proteins that could be important in early diagnosis.

Host Genetics in HAD

The role of host factors in HAD has been illustrated by finding genetic mutations associated with the disease. Polymorphisms in TNF-α codon 308 (Quasney et al., 2001) and MCP-1 (Gonzalez et al., 2002) have been correlated with HAD. The latest studies utilizing adult (European-, African-, and Hispanic-American) and child cohorts for the mutant allele for monocyte chemoattractant protein-1 (MCP-1-2578G) indicated an association of this allele with a 4.5-fold-increased risk of HAD, resulting in increased serum levels of MCP-1 (Gonzalez et al., 2002). Since chemokine receptors are HIV-1 coreceptors, gene polymorphisms have been studied for association with HIV progression and cognitive impairment. The CCR2 chemokine receptor allele (CCR2-V64I) was associated with progression to cognitive impairment in 121 HIV patients (Singh et al., 2004). However, results demonstrated no association between plasma and CSF viral loads and progression to cognitive impairment. More recently, a low CCL3-L1 (the gene encoding the beta chemokine MIP-1α, a natural ligand of the CCR5 coreceptor) copy number was associated with enhanced HIV-1 susceptibility (Gonzalez et al., 2005). It remains to be determined if this allele is associated with progression to cognitive impairment. Apolipoprotein E (APOE) is an essential element in the metabolism and transport of serum lipids and is involved in cholesterol metabolism within the brain. Genetic polymorphisms in APOE have been associated with the prevalence of HAD and neuropathy (Corder et al., 1998). Recent studies of brain tissue belonging to a population of homosexual men from the pre-HAART era with no history of drug abuse categorized APOE polymorphisms into APOE3/4, -3/3, and -4/4 in order to study their effects in lipid metabolism. There was increased dysregulated lipid and sterol metabolism in HAD patients with the APOE4 genotype (Cutler et al., 2004). In the post-HAART era, a recent study of the Hawaii Aging with HIV Cohort showed an independent risk of HAD related to APOE4 in older participants (odds ratio = 2.898 [range, 1.031 to 8.244]), but not in younger participants (odds ratio = 0.373 [0.054 to 1.581]) (Valcour et al., 2004b). Differences in the genetic control of the immune system may influence an individual's risk for HAD, as is the case for other neurological conditions, such as Alzheimer's disease. Moreover, all of these studies were done predominantly in men, and it is unknown if these markers will show association with cognitive impairment in women.

Biomarkers for HAD

Despite advances that have been made in elucidating the neuropathogenesis of HIV-1, few tests are available that can diagnose the development or monitor the progression of HAD. Detailed neurological and cognitive examinations, as well as assessment of viral replication in the CSF, are currently used to monitor patients. Inflammatory mediators that were correlated with HAD, such as CSF β_2-microglobulin, neopterin levels, the cytokine TNF-α (Stein et al., 1997), nitric oxide (Boje, 2004), platelet-activating factor (Gelbard et al., 1994), quinolinic acid (Heyes et al., 1991), matrix metalloproteinases (Conant et al., 1999), and other inflammatory neurotoxins, decreased with HAART (Gendelman et al., 1998). Radiologic markers, such as magnetic resonance imaging and magnetic resonance spectroscopy, have been shown to be sensitive to the brain injury that occurs in HAD (Avison et al., 2003). At present, studies using this technique to evaluate the possibility of early biomarkers of HAD are ongoing. However, the techniques require sophisticated data analysis, and many are practical only in a specialized research center. In the context of these changes in the post-HAART era, there is a need to develop new biomarkers to identify and monitor HIV-associated neurocognitive disorders (Antinori et al., 2007).

Proteomics and HAD

The field of proteomics has evolved in such a way that, instead of detecting a particular protein in a clinical sample, all the proteins present in that sample can be detected and compared among groups of patients with different conditions. Surface-enhanced laser desorption ionization time of flight (SELDI-TOF) (Ciphergen, Inc., Freemont, CA [now BioRad]) protein chip mass spectrometry has been successfully employed in the biomarker discovery of proteins induced in tissue macrophages by HIV (Carlson et al., 2004; Ciborowski et al., 2004; Enose et al., 2005; Vehmas et al., 2004). A SELDI-TOF spectrum is a graphic representation of TOF, which is directly related to the molecular mass of an ion generated by the proteins of the sample tested. Preliminary studies by our group have demonstrated differences in the protein profiles in macrophages from HIV-infected women with cognitive impairment (Luo et al., 2003; Wojna et al., 2004a). The profile of certain protein peaks resolved upon HAART treatment (Luo et al., 2003; Wojna et al., 2004a). A combination of protein peaks in macrophage fingerprinting provided increased sensitivity and specificity for diagnostic studies of HIV minor cognitive impairment (Luo et al., 2003). More recently, in CSF proteomics studies (high-performance liquid chromatography fractionation, SELDI-TOF protein chip mass spectrometry, and tandem mass spectrometry) of the cohort of Hispanic women, we have found unique protein peaks associated with HIV cognitive impairment despite being in combined antiretroviral therapy (Laspiur et al., 2007). Some of these protein peaks were different from those in a similar study of a predominantly male population from the mainland United States (Berger et al., 2005). In further studies for identification with tandem mass spectrometry, we found 38 proteins in the CSF of women with HIV cognitive impairment. They were related to cell signaling, structural function, and antioxidant activities. Similar findings were obtained from six samples of CSF from the women's cohort using a different proteomics approach (depletion of the most abundant proteins and

two-dimensional gel electrophoresis and imaging, followed by tandem mass spectrometry) (Rozek et al., 2007). In this study, several different proteins were encountered in the Hispanic female cohort compared to CSF samples from the National NeuroAIDS Tissue Consortium. Additional studies are required in more diverse and larger groups to confirm if these important differences are due to ethnic or gender differences.

HIV Subtypes and Variants Associated with Studies from Outside the United States

HIV-1 plays an important role in macrophages and HAD (Gendelman et al., 2005). CCR5, and to a lesser extent CXCR4 and CCR3, chemokine cell receptors are used as coreceptors for HIV-1 envelope binding to the CNS (Albright et al., 1999; Gorry et al., 2002; Yi et al., 2003). HIV-1 envelope gp120 and supernatants from infected macrophages cause a broad range of neurotoxicities independent of virus replication abilities (Power et al., 1998). Specific envelope and long terminal repeat sequences were found more frequently in individuals with dementia (Boni et al., 1993; Burdo et al., 2004; Ross et al., 2001). These sequences may confer different biological properties and the ability to produce neuronal toxicity in vitro (Zhang et al., 2003) or to stimulate the production of proinflammatory cytokines (Khanna et al., 2000). Virus isolates from the peripheral blood of Hispanic women with cognitive impairment appear to use predominantly the CXCR4 coreceptor (Nieves et al., 2007). However, the few peripheral blood virus isolates from women with cognitive impairment that infected macrophages induced proteins associated with signaling, redox, and structural functions (Toro et al., 2007), as has been observed in studies of the CSF of the same patients.

HIV strains have a high degree of genetic diversity as a result of multiple introductions of genetically diverse simian viruses into humans (Hahn et al., 2000), the high error rate of reverse transcriptase (Preston et al., 1998), and the fast turnover of virions in HIV-infected individuals (Ho et al., 1995). Phylogenetic analyses performed on HIV envelope sequences and comparisons of numerous strains of HIV-1 isolated from diverse geographic regions have revealed three distinct groups of viruses, M (main), N (new), and O (outlier). Each of these groups must have arisen from separate cross-species transmission of simian immunodeficiency virus from chimpanzees (Gao et al., 1999; Peeters and Sharp, 2000). Group M is the most highly represented worldwide and has been responsible for more than 90% of reported HIV/AIDS cases to date, while groups O and N are endemic to west-central Africa. To classify the prevalent group of M viruses in the global AIDS epidemic, phylogenetic analyses of HIV-1 Env and Gag sequences have revealed nine distinct subtypes, or clades (A to D, F to H, J, and K) (reviewed in Liner et al., 2007). In addition, viral recombinants of these clades are common and result from transmission by individuals with multiple coexisting infections (Arroyo et al., 2005; Kijak and McCutchan, 2005). The greatest diversity has been found in Africa, which is the source of the epidemic. However, A and C are the most common clades in Africa, while clade B is the most common in the Americas, European countries, and Australia. It is also observed in the Middle East and Asia. Clade C is common in southern and eastern Africa, India, Nepal, and China, accounting for over 49% of infections worldwide (Liner et al., 2007). Studies of HIV clades in the Caribbean have revealed that, although clade B predominates in the region, other clades, such as C, B/D recombinants, H, A, and F, have been found in

St. Lucia, Antigua (Vaughan et al., 2003), Cuba (Gomez et al., 2001), Barbados (Roth et al., 1997), and Puerto Rico (Flores et al., 1999). This unusual diversity of clades found in the Caribbean could have been introduced from Africa.

Most studies of the effects of viral diversity in HIV neuropathogenesis and drug resistance have been done on clade B-infected individuals, as that is the predominant virus in the Western world. Research on drug resistance among the different HIV-1 subtypes has been contradictory (Liner et al., 2007). Since the CNS is a compartment protected against penetration by ARVs, the role of HIV clades in HIV CNS penetration is an important concern in the era of HAART.

Recent studies of the roles of ethnicity and HIV clades have been directed toward understanding HIV clade C, the most common virus where the epidemic is most devastating. Clade C virus is a macrophagetropic virus, the most common virus isolated from brain tissue in HIV-1 dementia, which suggests a higher incidence of the disease. These recent studies are from India and Africa, where the incidence and prevalence of HIV-1 dementia are still unknown. One neuropathological study done on 15 cases in India reported increased infectivity of HIV-1 clade C in the brain, including the parenchyma, choroid plexus, and meninges, despite the absence of giant cells (Mahadevan et al., 2007). This study suggested that even when patients are treated for opportunistic infections they are at increased risk of HIV dementia because of increased viral infection in the brain. Two recent studies characterized the cognitive function of HIV-1 clade C-infected patients in India. One of them applied neuropsychological tests to 119 adults stratified by CD4 counts, with no ARV therapy, and matched for gender, age, and education with HIV-1-seronegative controls (Gupta et al., 2007). They found that the group with CD4 cell counts of <200 cells/ml had the highest rate of impairment in working memory. They also found that the prevalence of HIV dementia in clade C-infected individuals was similar to that in ARV-naïve clade B infections in the Western world. However, the second study of 48 clade C-infected individuals characterized for cognitive function using the International HIV Dementia Scale found that in the AIDS group whose CD4 counts were <200 cells/ml, 35% scored below 10 on the test, while among HIV-1-seronegative controls, only 10% scored <10 (Riedel et al., 2006). The authors concluded that the prevalence of HIV dementia in the Indian population may be higher. One study was done in Africa with 506 HIV-infected individuals with a male/female ratio of 1.2:1, 84% of whom had CD4 cell counts of <200 cells/ml and 75% had neurological illness (Modi et al., 2007). However, we could not determine the effect of clade C, as most patients had opportunistic infections, predominantly tuberculosis (46%), and thus, we concluded that the neurological disease was mainly an effect of immunosuppression. Additional studies are necessary in this part of the world to follow HIV-infected patients for cognitive function after excluding opportunistic infections, which require additional therapies for this population.

One study done with in vitro HIV infection of macrophages using isolates from different clades revealed that clade C viruses exhibited decreased glutamate production and neurotoxicity compared to clade B viruses (Zheng et al., 2007). This suggests that clade C viruses may not be promoting higher neuropathology that could be linked to dementia. Additional studies will be necessary to understand the roles of clades and HAD.

HIV Neurocognitive Impairment among Special Groups

The presence of neurocognitive impairment in HIV-1-infected individuals, which varies from subtle, mild deficits (e.g., asymptomatic with subclinical neuropsychological deficits) to MCMD to HAD, is one of the common neurological, neuropsychological, and neuropsychiatric complications of HIV-1 infection (Goodkin et al., 1997; A. Nath and J. C. McArthur, presented at the Annual Meeting of the American Academy of Neurology, 10 June 2005). HAD was characterized very early (in the pre-HAART era) as a subcortical dysfunction marked by prominent psychomotor slowing and consistent absence of cortical symptoms (e.g., language deficits). Its manifestation and severity have been clearly associated with advanced stages of HIV-1 disease (Navia et al., 1986a, 1986b; Price and Brew, 1988). In the post-HAART era, the clinical and neuropsychological characterization of HAD has followed a frontal-subcortical pattern (Navia and Rostasy, 2005) or a frontostriatal dysfunction (Carey et al., 2006). The incidence of HAD has decreased with the advent of combined ARV therapies, but its prevalence has increased due to improved longevity of HIV-1-infected patients (McArthur, 2004; Sacktor et al., 2002; Selnes, 2005). Likewise, the temporal progression of the dementia (i.e., slow or stable) has been modified (McArthur, 2004). Subtle neuropsychological impairment and MCMD have remained significant causes of morbidity (Janssen et al., 1989; Sacktor et al., 2002), and HAD has been found to be an independent factor in time to death (Sevigny et al., 2007). Milder forms of neurocognitive impairment may represent early effects of HIV-1 infection in the brain and may have roles as predictors of HAD (Cherner et al., 2002; Grant et al., 2005; Mayeux et al., 1993; Sacktor et al., 1996; Antinori et al., 2007). In addition, the issues of HAART's incomplete protection against neurological damage and its neurotoxicity effects appear to play an important role in these alterations (McArthur, 2004). Due to the phenotypic changes of HIV-associated neurocognitive deficits, the National Institute of Mental Health and the National Institute of Neurological Diseases and Stroke charged a working group to review the definitional criteria of HAD (see chapter 1, this volume). This group recommends the inclusion of the term "asymptomatic neurocognitive impairment."

As is known, cultural background and educational level affect performance in psychological and neuropsychological tests. Therefore, it is important to make efforts to assess or control for the effects of demographic variables on individual test performance in order to distinguish the manifestations of brain dysfunction from those variations pertaining to membership in a particular socioeducational group (Ardila et al., 1992). The critical question of appropriate test population-based norms, particularly for special population groups, is addressed by pertinent demographic correction or adjustment and by homogenization of samples or normalization through the inclusion of proper control or reference groups. In addition, it seems pertinent to address the influence of sex/gender factors in performance on neuropsychological tests and the possible differences in brain function by sex (Matthews, 1992). Gender, considered as a nonphysiological component of sex, has generally been ignored in neuropsychological research (Matthews, 1992). Gender in HIV-1 infection research has been shown to be related to variables such as differential access to health services (Cook et al., 2004) and adherence to treatment (Jones et al., 2003; Ricart et al., 2002). The role played by systems of social and family support (Silberstein et al., 1987; Wohl et al., 2003), which are considered highly relevant for the understanding of HIV-1 disease progression and survival rates (Morgello et al., 2002), are also influenced by gender. Psychosocial factors (e.g., intellectual functioning, age, and somatic symptoms of depression) have been found to be predictors of HIV-1 disease progression and survival (Farinpour et al., 2003). Premorbid differences in intellectual level must also be taken into account, since performance on neuropsychological tests seems to be highly correlated with measures of intelligence (Goldstein and Shelly, 1972). This issue was raised very early in HIV neurocognitive research (Saykin et al., 1988; Selnes et al., 1990). Sex/gender differences concerning affective moods, either as they interact with immunosuppression levels or as an emotional reaction to HIV-1 disease, have occasionally been addressed (Cook et al., 2002, 2004). However, some early studies expressed concern about the role of depression as a determinant in HIV disease progression (Lyketsos et al., 1993; Vedhara et al., 1999). The influence of depression on neuropsychological test performance as a confounding variable is well recognized (Newman and Sweet, 1986). With respect to the factor of age, it is well known that the neuropsychological evaluation of children and adolescents (Cohen et al., 1992) and the elderly (La Rue, 1992; Valdois et al., 1990) raises specific testing and research issues and concerns (see chapter 33, this volume). Ethnicity has been increasingly recognized as an important demographic variable that must be addressed in HIV-1 research.

One of the first neuropsychological studies that specifically addressed the factor of ethnicity was carried out prospectively with asymptomatic men and women at risk for HIV-1 infection in a methadone program in New York City (Silberstein et al., 1987). The study found evidence of cognitive impairment early in the course of HIV-1 infection. The ethnic groups included were Caucasian (26%), African-American (27%), and Hispanic (47%). Seropositive Hispanic persons perceived more family support than did seronegative Hispanic persons, while no differences were found among the African-American group. However, since neuropsychological norms were not available for the ethnic population studied, no such comparisons were made. Several neuropsychological studies, some of them longitudinal, were conducted with only or mostly African-American men with HIV-1 infection (Durvasula et al., 2000; Martin et al., 2001; Richardson et al., 1999; Selnes et al., 1992, 1997), but no significant demographic differences were found or reported. One longitudinal study in 1992 with the AIDS-linked-to-intravenous-experience (ALIVE) cohort of mostly African-American men (75 to 80%) and large samples of HIV-1-seropositive persons, -seronegative persons, and IDU found that age and education were the most important predictors of test performance; neuropsychological measures did not vary by HIV-1 serostatus (Concha et al., 1992). A report of the Multicenter AIDS Cohort Study (MACS) of mostly Caucasian (~87 to 91%) homosexual and bisexual men found that the prevalence of neurocognitive deficits increased monotonically with advancing age but was larger for African-Americans and individuals with lower educational levels (Satz et al., 1993). The authors suggested that low education might reflect an indirect index of lower cognitive reserve capacity (i.e., a risk factor) in cases of early HIV-1 infection. A series of HIV-1 neurocognitive studies with mostly Caucasian men reported ethnicity background, but none found significant differences in terms of age, sex, education, intellectual level, or ethnicity (Basso and Bornstein, 2000; Carey et al., 2004; Miller et al., 1990; Rosenberger et al., 1993; Sacktor et al., 2005). In

other studies with the same population, comparison groups were well matched on those variables (Beason-Hazen et al., 1994) or balanced demographically (Price et al., 1999). Some studies with few women also recognized the importance of reporting or controlling by ethnicity (Becker et al., 1995; Cherner et al., 2002). In general, in HIV-1 dementia scale studies (e.g., HIV dementia scale [HDS] and Memorial Sloan Kettering), with the participation of diverse ethnic groups, did not reveal significant differences in terms of age, sex/gender, or ethnicity (Bouwman et al., 1998; Davis et al., 2002; Dougherty et al., 2002; Power et al., 1995).

Some studies with the Dana Consortium (Columbia, Hopkins, and Rochester Universities) and Northeastern AIDS Dementia Consortium cohorts have reported ethnicity but either have not analyzed the data by that factor (Dana Consortium, 1996; Schifitto et al., 2001) or have not found significant differences after adjusting for age, education, sex, and ethnicity (Sacktor et al., 2002). One longitudinal study with the Dana Consortium cohort reported an important gender difference as a risk factor for dementia (Stern et al., 2001). The research objective was to identify risk factors for HAD among 146 HIV-1-seropositive persons (45 of whom developed dementia) and used several factors as independent variables, including age, education, sex, and ethnicity (Caucasian, 52.1%). The study found that neurocognitive deficits, MCMD, and depression might be early manifestations of HAD; among the demographic variables, sex was found to be a strong risk factor. The authors suggested that women might have a higher risk factor for dementia, an observation said to be consistent with "previous reports that HIV-positive women have more rapid progression of neurologic signs and symptoms" (Liu et al., 1996). This neurological study included 38 matched pairs of male and female IDU based on baseline age, education, disease stage, and CD4 count and followed them for 3.5 years. They found that women presented more sensory abnormalities and symptoms at baseline than men; however, over time, men were more prone to develop neurological impairment. The authors suggested that one possible explanation for the gender difference in neurologic progression over time is gender difference in drug and alcohol use, which was more frequent in men.

A neuropsychological battery (HUMANS) for the assessment of HIV-1-infected individuals, with English and Spanish versions, has been developed (Ardila-Ardila et al., 2003; Wilkie et al., 2004). However, studies regarding its validity and reliability are still in progress. A pilot study described the development of a Spanish version of an assessment functional instrument of activities of daily living and explored the functional impact of neurocognitive impairment (Mindt et al., 2003). No significant differences were found regarding age, education, sex, and CD4 cell count. Another study compared the risk of opportunistic infection among HIV-1-infected Latinos born in the United States (71% male) with those for Mexican- (64% male) and Central American-born (28% male) Latinos attending a Los Angeles, CA, clinic (Wohl et al., 2003). Controlling for HAART use, CD4 cell count, and age, U.S.-born Latino men were more likely than Central American-born women to develop an opportunistic infection, while U.S.-born Latino men and women were at greater risk for HIV-1 encephalopathy and Kaposi's sarcoma. Acculturation factors, such as loss of social support and negative lifestyles, were proposed as an explanation for the gender differences found. Racial and ethnic factors in neuropsychological performance were evaluated by Ryan et al., using study participants from the Manhattan HIV

Brain Bank, emphasizing the distinction between education and reading levels. They found that African-Americans and Hispanics showed significantly lower reading and education levels than non-Hispanic Caucasians; interestingly, these minority groups were more likely to have discrepant reading and education levels. These findings are relevant for establishing adequate normative standards and for considering literacy as an important variable (Ryan et al., 2005).

There have been some interesting findings concerning the influence of age in HIV-1 neurocognitive impairment. In a study with the MACS cohort of MSM and bisexual men, a significant effect of age on reaction time and timed neuropsychological measures was revealed, but no interaction between age and serostatus was found (van Gorp et al., 1994). Among other psychosocial factors, age was found to be predictive of HIV-1 disease progression and survival with the MACS longitudinal cohort of HIV-1-seropositive men (Farinpour et al., 2003). Sanchez Rodriguez and Rodriguez Alvarez (2003) compared the levels of neurocognitive performance in three age groups—healthy elderly, young AIDS patients, and healthy children—and found similar neuropsychological performances among the healthy elderly and the young AIDS groups compared to the younger healthy controls. A study of differences in neuropsychological performance (in the domains of language and speed of information processing) as related to ethnicity was conducted with African-American and European-American children (5 to 7 years old) with HIV-1 infection (Llorente et al., 2004). In general, African-American children had lower scores than European-American children, even though there were no group differences in terms of age, immunologic status, intellect, level of maternal education, and CD4 cell count. In a baseline cross-sectional analysis from the Hawaii Aging with HIV Cohort of HIV-1-seropositive individuals grouped into two age groups, older and younger, it was found after adjusting for education, ethnicity, substance dependence, ARV status, viral load, CD4 cell count, and Beck Depression Index score that older age was associated with increased HAD (Valcour et al., 2004a). A longitudinal analysis of this cohort showed a progression of cognitive impairment that was unrelated to the plasma viral load (Valcour et al., 2005). Although aging is a confounding factor for HAD, other factors related to aging must be considered when evaluating HIV-1-infected elderly individuals, since they may present with age-associated comorbidities in addition to the infection (Sacktor et al., 2007).

Recently, there has been increased interest in neuropsychological studies involving gender. A study of African-American women with a history of drug use found no evidence of neurocognitive impairment in early stages of the infection, and individuals with AIDS showed a subcortical pattern of neurocognitive deficits (Mason et al., 1998). Cohen et al. (2001) found that neurocognitive performance was enhanced by HAART in HIV-1-infected women of the HERS cohort compared with those not treated with HAART, but no ethnicity data were reported. A study of the WIHS cohort replicated the finding that working memory was defective in HIV-1-seropositive individuals, as was found previously in men, but the abstract did not include ethnicity or any demographic data (Martin et al., 1999). Studies with women did find significant ethnic differences. A study of the UCLA/Women and Family Project cohort examined predictors of neuropsychological performance in three domains (verbal memory, psychomotor speed, and motor speed) (Durvasula et al., 2001). Despite efforts to achieve demographic equality between groups,

HIV-1-seronegative women were more educated than the other groups. Ethnicity proportions (percentages) were distributed as follows (HIV⁻/HIV⁺ non-AIDS/AIDS): African-American, 32/47/21; European-American, 51/33/17; and Latina, 40/38/22. Controlling for demographic variables, HIV-1 serostatus was associated with slower psychomotor speed. Education, ethnicity, and depressive distress were also associated with neurocognitive performance. African-American women had lower verbal memory and motor speed scores, and Latina women had lower performance on psychomotor speed. Educational levels were not comparable between groups, and a confounding factor among African-American women in their performance on motor tasks might have been long fingernails. Richardson et al. (2002) evaluated neurocognitive performance for 149 HIV-1-seropositive and 82 HIV-1-seronegative women enrolled in the WIHS cohort as related to ARV. Participants were classified either by disease status (HIV⁻/HIV⁺ CD4 > 200/ HIV⁺ CD4 ≤ 200) or by treatment status (HIV⁻/HIV⁺ on ARV/HIV⁺ off ARV). Percentages of ethnic groups by disease status were as follows: African-American, 41.5/63.9/40.5; Caucasian, 19.5/18.5/19.0; and Hispanic, 39.0/17.6/40.5. The risk of abnormal neurocognitive performance was significantly increased for seropositive women not receiving ARV compared with HIV-1-seropositive women on ARV and HIV-1-seronegative women. African-American ethnicity was associated with significantly increased risk of abnormal neurocognitive performance in the univariate analysis, but this finding did not hold in further multivariate analysis. Significant risk factors for obtaining an abnormal neurocognitive protocol by disease status, after controlling by all variables, were older age, lower verbal IQ, and greater depressive Centers for Epidemiological Studies-Depression (CES-D) score. When analyzed by treatment status, the risk factors were absence of ARV, older age, and higher depressive scores. Another finding for the WIHS cohort was that African-American and IDU women with depression were less likely to use HAART; however, once they were treated with antidepressants and mental health therapy, the probability of using HAART was significantly increased (Cook et al., 2005). Coinfection with hepatitis C virus (HCV) was associated with worse neurocognitive performance independent of education or ethnicity; however, with respect to age, this association was maintained only in women younger than 40 years (Richardson et al., 2005).

A study that exemplifies the increasing interest in ethnicity in HIV-1 neurocognitive research (Byrd et al., 2005) compared the prevalence of HIV-1-associated neurocognitive impairments (HAD and MCMD) in 254 HIV-1-seropositive adults (44% African-American, 32% Hispanic, and 24% Caucasian). Two different classification systems, the American Academy of Neurology (AAN) criteria and clinical ratings of the National NeuroAIDS Tissue Consortium, were contrasted. Using the AAN criteria, ethnic minorities were significantly more likely than Caucasians to be diagnosed with HIV-related cognitive impairment (93% versus 79%), in contrast to the clinical-ratings method, which revealed no significant ethnic difference.

Our Experience with the Hispanic Neuro-AIDS Cohort of HIV-1-Infected Women Characterized for Cognitive Function

A cohort of HIV-1-seropositive Hispanic women at risk for cognitive dysfunction (PRNAC) has been followed longitudinally at the University of Puerto Rico Medical Sciences Campus NeuroAIDS Program since 2001. The criteria used to establish this cohort were as follows: Puerto Rican women 18 years old and older, CD4 T lymphocyte counts of <500 cells/mm³, at least a ninth-grade education, and no evidence of either active systemic infection or neurodegenerative disease. This cohort of Spanish-speaking women represented a challenge for the diagnosis of HIV-associated neurocognitive disorders. Neuropsychological testing demanded the establishment of a reference group for identifying appropriate norms and standards. Also, some of the tests and scales had to be translated in a culturally sensitive manner. A modified set of the AAN HAD criteria was used, including an asymptomatic cognitively impaired group. In this cohort, we observed a prevalence of all types of cognitive impairment of 77.6%, divided into asymptomatic (32.7%), MCMD (16.3%), and HAD (28.6%) (Wojna et al., 2006). Recognizing the high prevalence of cognitive impairment in the cohort, there was a need to have an easily administered Spanish screening test for HAD. For this purpose, we translated the HDS scale into Spanish and validated it. We observed an optimum cutoff point of ≤13, with performance characteristics of 87% sensitivity and 46% specificity for HIV-associated cognitive impairment (50% positive predictive value and 85% negative predictive value) in women with HIV-1 infection treated with HAART (Wojna et al., 2007).

In the PRNAC, we also found significant differences among the following parameters: increased CD14⁺/CD16⁺ monocyte phenotype in HIV-1-infected patients compared to seronegative controls (Melendez, 2006) and increased cognitive impairment associated with CSF inflammation (MCP-1) and CSF oxidative stress (mitochondrial membrane potential) (Wojna et al., 2004b). These findings, together with distinct HIV isolates with predominant X4 coreceptor usage (Nieves et al., 2007), a distinct protein macrophage (Luo et al., 2003; Wojna et al., 2004a), and CSF fingerprints observed in HIV-1-infected women with cognitive impairment in the post-HAART era, provide support for (or suggest) a role for gender and/or ethnicity in cognitive dysfunction.

HIV DSP

HIV infection disproportionately affects some ethnic minorities, such as Hispanics and African-Americans, and HIV-associated neuropathy has become the most common neurologic complication in HIV infection since the introduction of HAART (Sacktor, 2002). It is reasonable, then, to infer that HIV-associated peripheral neuropathy is an important problem in these groups. However, there is very limited information about the predominant types and frequency of neuropathy and whether there are other ethnicity-specific factors that modify the expression of this complication in these groups. In addition to the increased number of affected individuals, other factors relevant to ethnic minorities, such as access to health care and treatment, choice of treatment, and increased frequency of comorbid conditions, such as diabetes or hepatitis C, may have a significant impact on how HIV-associated neuropathy affects these groups. These observations and others support the need to focus on specific ethnic groups to achieve a better understanding of ethnicity-specific factors in HIV-associated nervous system complications.

What Do We Know about Ethnicity and HIV Neuropathy?

The question of the prevalence and incidence of peripheral neuropathy in specific ethnic groups in the United States has not been addressed in the post-HAART era. Most studies of HIV neuropathy have concentrated on Caucasian MSM, with very little information about specific ethnic or racial groups. An important issue in the reported values of incidence and prevalence is that the values vary depending on the methods used to identify neuropathy and the diagnostic criteria adopted in the studies. A recent study that included 54% African-American patients reported a prevalence of peripheral neuropathy of 16% (Kilbourne et al., 2001). The study relied on reports from primary-care physicians and may have underdetected cases of neuropathy. Among patients from sub-Saharan Africa, where HIV infection is highly prevalent, the frequency of neurologic complications is largely unknown. The limited available data suggest that peripheral neuropathy is highly prevalent. A recent study of 53 HIV-infected patients from an infectious-disease clinic in Uganda showed that 51% of the patients had symptoms and 38% had signs of peripheral neuropathy (Wong et al., 2004). In one of the few studies that has examined the frequency of neuropathy in a Latino cohort from Sao Paulo, Brazil, Zanetti et al. (2004) found a prevalence of neuropathy of 69% in a sample of 49 patients, with the diagnosis based on clinical grounds. They found more patients with asymptomatic (65%) than symptomatic (35%) neuropathy, with decreased distal sensation being the most common clinical sign. A very high proportion were exposed to toxic dideoxynucleosides or other concomitant neurotoxic medications, such as isoniazid, suggesting a high prevalence of ARV toxic neuropathy (ATN) and other toxic neuropathy. Their study underscores the influence of other ethnicity-specific, highly prevalent conditions, such as tuberculosis, and their treatment as additional modifying factors in the development of neuropathy in some ethnic groups. The apparent high prevalence of asymptomatic (subclinical) neuropathy raises questions about ethnic and cultural differences in the expression of symptoms.

The limited data that have been published about neuro-AIDS complications in sub-Saharan Africa suggest patterns similar to those observed in the pre-HAART era in the United States. In a limited study that relied mainly on electrophysiologic criteria, it was found that inflammatory demyelinating neuropathy occurred in the earlier stages of HIV infection, while DSP was the most common form and occurred more commonly in advanced stages of HIV infection (Parry et al., 1997). They did not find an association between electrophysiologic measures of neuropathy and CD4 cell counts. In at least two series from West Africa, peripheral facial paralysis has figured prominently among the manifestations of HIV infection, in many instances as an initial manifestation (Millogo et al., 2002; Sene-Diouf et al., 2000).

Among the various considerations of how ethnicity may influence the type or frequency of peripheral neuropathy, the disproportionate frequency of certain comorbid conditions that may influence neuropathy has to be taken into account. Type II diabetes and HCV have very high prevalence among Latinos, and particularly among Puerto Ricans, and they may modify both the severity and the expression of HIV-associated neuropathy. However, a recent report that included a large proportion of African-American patients from Baltimore, MD, found that HCV infection was not significantly associated with a greater risk of peripheral neuropathy (McArthur et al., 2004). Longitudinal studies will be needed to fully examine the questions of increased severity and the potential influence of HCV treatments on HIV-associated peripheral neuropathy.

Our Experience with HIV Neuropathy in the Hispanic Cohort

The Puerto Rico HIV Neuropathy Project is one of the studies being conducted under the neuro-AIDS research program at the University of Puerto Rico, addressing questions about the frequency and correlates of HIV-1-associated DSP in pediatric/adolescent and adult Puerto Rican/Latino HIV-1-seropositive patients. For the neuropathy project, patients were recruited from the various clinics in the metropolitan area of San Juan or adjacent towns that provide service to HIV-infected patients or participate in clinical trials. To ensure a more accurate diagnosis of HIV-1-associated DSP, patients with other conditions associated with peripheral neuropathy, such as diabetes, were not included. Peripheral neuropathy was defined as present if the patient had two or more abnormalities on clinical or neurophysiologic examination with symptoms (symptomatic neuropathy) or without symptoms (subclinical neuropathy). Patients with unilateral, proximal, or atypical sensory symptoms were not included as having HIV-1-associated DSP.

The pediatric/adolescent group is currently composed of 28 pediatric patients aged 5.6 to 18.2 years (median, 12.4 years) and is 46% female. Almost all patients (96%) were infected by vertical transmission, with one patient infected by transfusion. The group is relatively immunocompetent, with a median CD4 cell count of 660.5 cells/mm^3 (range, 6.0 to 1,906 cells/mm^3). Viral loads ranged from <50 to 134,425 HIV-1 RNA copies/ml of plasma (median, 1,918.5 copies). Within this pediatric/adolescent group, we identified 9 patients (32%) who fulfilled the criteria for peripheral neuropathy (7 patients with symptomatic peripheral neuropathy and 2 patients with subclinical neuropathy) and 18 patients who did not fulfill the criteria for neuropathy. Most patients had been exposed to stavudine or didanosine at the onset of symptoms, suggesting a large proportion of ATN.

One important diagnostic tool that has been used in the study of HIV DSP has been the assessment of epidermal nerve fibers from punch skin biopsies. It is well accepted that HIV-1-associated DSP predominantly affects small myelinated and unmyelinated axons, making this technique ideal for the assessment of HIV-1-associated DSP. We applied this diagnostic technique to our pediatric/adolescent cohort with some surprising results. The skin biopsy specimens were obtained from the midpoint of the distal third of the lateral leg, anywhere from 6 to 10 cm from the lateral malleolus, depending on the length of the leg. The biopsy specimens were processed using immunohistochemical techniques with antibodies against PGP9.5, a panaxonal marker, and epidermal fibers were counted using an established protocol that has been previously described (McCarthy et al., 1995). Comparing the epidermal nerve fiber densities in the pediatric/adolescent HIV-infected patients and controls, we found a paradoxical increase in fiber densities that was statistically significant (Luciano et al., 2005a). This is contrary to what has been reported in adult HIV-1-seropositive patients, in whom significant decreases in epidermal nerve fiber densities have been observed (Polydefkis et al., 2002). We hypothesize that this may be the result of chronic exposure to neurotoxins (virus-mediated or medications) at an age when there was a heightened capacity for regeneration. Among the pertinent negatives, we have not found any significant differences in median times of exposure to neurotoxic dideoxynucleosides (stavudine or didanosine) between symptomatic, subclinical, and neuropathy-free patients.

At the time of this review, the adult cohort of the Puerto Rican HIV Neuropathy Project was composed of 75 adult subjects aged 20 to 63 years (median, 40 years), 66% females, with the most common mode of infection through heterosexual transmission (61%). Most patients were prescribed HAART, a fact reflected in the median CD4 counts (484.5 cells/mm^3) and viral loads (median, 50 HIV-1 RNA copies/ml of plasma; range, 50 to 428,310 copies/ml). Of the 75 patients, 48 (64%) fulfilled criteria for the diagnosis of HIV-1-associated DSP as previously defined, a very high prevalence resulting from our focus on the study of related markers and mechanisms and a strong referral bias. How do our findings in this cohort compare to those reported in the literature? Our analysis to date has revealed no association between the selected immune markers and the presence or severity of peripheral neuropathy. Using commercially available enzyme-linked immunosorbent assays (Quantikine, Inc.), we measured the concentrations of soluble TNF-α, soluble TNF-α receptor 1, soluble intercellular adhesion molecule 1, matrix metalloproteinase 9, and tissue inhibitor of metalloproteinase 1 from serum or plasma. When we compared the concentrations of these immune activation markers in a subgroup of patients with features of ATN and those with neuropathy but no association with dideoxynucleosides (HIV DSP), we found no significant differences between the two groups (Luciano et al., 2005b). Furthermore, we have not found any significant associations between CD4 cell counts or plasma viral loads and measurements of neuropathy, in agreement with other investigators who have studied patients from the post-HAART era, including a high proportion of African-Americans (Sacktor et al., 2005). These findings suggest that our adult Puerto Rico/Latino cohort behaved similarly to other cohorts on the mainland and imply that HAART has altered the expression of surrogate markers of peripheral neuropathy and perhaps the underlying mechanisms.

Among the various aspects that we have examined to take advantage of our wide age range from the inclusion of pediatric/adolescent patients are various measures of peripheral nerve function as a function of age. Among them, we have used the ratio of amplitudes of the sural and superficial sensory nerve responses as an electrophysiologic measure of length-dependent sensory axon loss, as others have described (Rutkove et al., 1997), and a composite score of clinical and electrophysiologic measures, the total neuropathy score (Cornblath et al., 1999). Correlation analyses of the sural/superficial radial sensory amplitude and the clinical component of the total neuropathy score have shown that there is more distal loss of sensory axons and clinical symptoms of neuropathy are more prominent with advancing age.

In summary, we have found that HIV-1-associated DSP is highly prevalent in both pediatric/adolescent and adult Puerto Rican/Latino patients and that, similar to what has been described in other groups from the mainland United States, the introduction of HAART has altered the association of HIV infection with HIV-1-associated DSP, and we have also shown that aging is a powerful modifying factor in the frequency and severity of neuropathy.

CONCLUSIONS

There is limited literature regarding neuro-AIDS complications in ethnic groups and special populations. Assessing for neurocognitive performance in ethnic groups is critical to establish population-specific normative standards and culturally valid tests. Ethnic, gender, education or literacy, genetic, and age factors may contribute to different manifestations of HIV-1 cognitive impairment; consequently, they should be considered in research design. It is possible that the different scales used for HIV-1 cognitive function (Memorial Sloan Kettering, HDS, and AAN criteria) may fail to correctly identify cognitive impairment in different ethnic groups. Therefore, it is imperative to develop culture-sensitive instruments.

Significant progress has been made toward the identification of protein biomarkers associated with HIV cognitive impairment in macrophages and in CSF from HIV-infected women. However, there is a need to validate these studies in a larger number of samples from different ethnic groups and with both genders to detect possible differences associated with these factors. Studies are needed to confirm the distribution of viral clades in the world and their relation to cognitive impairment. Additional studies are needed for clades other than B, such as C, that circulate in the countries where the epidemic is most devastating. This clade predominantly infects macrophages, which are important reservoirs for HIV and major players in the development of brain inflammation during HAD. In the case of HIV-1-associated distal sensory peripheral neuropathy, age is a contributing factor to the neurological complications in the Puerto Rico cohort. Although no differences regarding ethnicity and sensory peripheral neuropathy were found in the cohort, we conclude that further studies to address this issue are necessary.

REFERENCES

Albright, A. V., J. T. Shieh, T. Itoh, B. Lee, D. Pleasure, M. J. O'Connor, R. W. Doms, and F. Gonzalez-Scarano. 1999. Microglia express CCR5, CXCR4, and CCR3, but of these, CCR5 is the principal coreceptor for human immunodeficiency virus type 1 dementia isolates. *J. Virol.* **73:**205–213.

Anderson, E., W. Zink, H. Xiong, and H. E. Gendelman. 2002. HIV-1-associated dementia: a metabolic encephalopathy perpetrated by virus-infected and immune-competent mononuclear phagocytes. *J. Acquir. Immune Defic. Syndr.* **31** (Suppl 2):S43–S54.

Antinori, A., G. Arendt, J. T. Becker, B. J. Brew, D. A. Byrd, M. Cherner, D. B. Clifford, P. Cinque, L. G. Epstein, K. Goodkin, M. Gisslen, I. Grant, R. K. Heaton, J. Joseph, K. Marder, C. M. Marra, J. C. McArthur, M. Nunn, R. W. Price, L. Pulliam, K. R. Robertson, N. Sacktor, V. Valcour, and V. E. Wojna. 2007. Updated research nosology for HIV-associated neurocognitive disorders. *Neurology* **69:**1789–1799.

Ardila, A., M. Rosselli, and F. Ostrosky-Solis. 1992. Socio-educational, p. 181–192. *In* A. E. Puente and R. J. McCaffrey (ed.), *Handbook of Neuropsychological Assessment. A Biopsychosocial Perspective.* Plenum Press, New York, NY.

Ardila-Ardila, A., K. Goodkin, M. Concha-Bartolini, R. Lecusay-Ruiz, O. Mellan-Fajardo S, P. Suarez-Bustamante, R. Molina-Vasquez, D. Lee, G. Chayeb, and F. L. Wilkie. 2003. HUMANS: a neuropsychological battery for evaluating HIV 1 infected patients. *Rev. Neurol.* **36:**756–762.

Arroyo, M. A., M. Hoelscher, W. Sateren, E. Samky, L. Maboko, O. Hoffmann, G. Kijak, M. Robb, D. L. Birx, and F. E. McCutchan. 2005. HIV-1 diversity and prevalence differ between urban and rural areas in the Mbeya region of Tanzania. *AIDS* **19:**1517–1524.

Avison, M., J. R. Berger, J. C. McArthur, and A. Nath. 2003. HIV meningitis and dementia, p. 251–276. *In* A. Nath and J. R. Berger (ed.), *Clinical Neurovirology.* Marcel Dekker, Inc., New York, NY.

Basso, M. R., and R. A. Bornstein. 2000. Effects of immunosuppression and disease severity upon neuropsychological function in HIV infection. *J. Clin. Exp. Neuropsychol.* **22:**104–114.

Beason-Hazen, S., H. A. Nasrallah, and R. A. Bornstein. 1994. Self-report of symptoms and neuropsychological performance in asymptomatic HIV-positive individuals. *J. Neuropsychiatry Clin. Neurosci.* **6:**43–49.

Becker, J. T., R. Caldararo, O. L. Lopez, M. A. Dew, S. K. Dorst, and G. Banks. 1995. Qualitative features of the memory deficit associated with HIV infection and AIDS: cross-validation of a discriminant function classification scheme. *J. Clin. Exp. Neuropsychol.* **17:**134–142.

Berger, J. R., M. Avison, Y. Mootoor, and C. Beach. 2005. Cerebrospinal fluid proteomics and human immunodeficiency virus dementia: preliminary observations. *J. Neurovirol.* **11:** 557–562.

Boje, K. M. 2004. Nitric oxide neurotoxicity in neurodegenerative diseases. *Front. Biosci.* **9:**763–776.

Boni, J., B. S. Emmerich, S. L. Leib, O. D. Wiestler, J. Schupbach, and P. Kleihues. 1993. PCR identification of HIV-1 DNA sequences in brain tissue of patients with AIDS encephalopathy. *Neurology* **43:**1813–1817.

Bouwman, F. H., R. L. Skolasky, D. Hes, O. A. Selnes, J. D. Glass, T. E. Nance-Sproson, W. Royal, G. J. Dal Pan, and J. C. McArthur. 1998. Variable progression of HIV-associated dementia. *Neurology* **50:**1814–1820.

Burdo, T. H., M. Nonnemacher, B. P. Irish, C. H. Choi, F. C. Krebs, S. Gartner, and B. Wigdahl. 2004. High-affinity interaction between HIV-1 Vpr and specific sequences that span the C/EBP and adjacent NF-kappaB sites within the HIV-1 LTR correlate with HIV-1-associated dementia. *DNA Cell. Biol.* **23:**261–269.

Byrd, D. A., M. Rivera Mindt, E. Ryan, and S. Morgello. 2005. Assessing HIV-related cognitive disorders in U.S. ethnic minorities: effect of classification system, abstr. 60, p. 72. *Central Nervous Syst. Dev. Resource Limited Settings.* Edizioni Internazionali srl, Rome, Italy.

Carey, C. L., S. P. Woods, J. D. Rippeth, R. Gonzalez, D. J. Moore, T. D. Marcotte, I. Grant, and R. K. Heaton. 2004. Initial validation of a screening battery for the detection of HIV-associated cognitive impairment. *Clin. Neuropsychol.* **18:** 234–248.

Carey, C. L., S. P. Woods, J. D. Rippeth, R. K. Heaton, and I. Grant. 2006. Prospective memory in HIV-1 infection. *J. Clin. Exp. Neuropsychol.* **28:**536–548.

Carlson, K. A., P. Ciborowski, C. N. Schellpeper, T. M. Biskup, R. F. Shen, X. Luo, C. J. Destache, and H. E. Gendelman. 2004. Proteomic fingerprinting of HIV-1-infected human monocyte-derived macrophages: a preliminary report. *J. Neuroimmunol.* **147:**35–42.

CDC. 2003. *HIV/AIDS Surveillance Report.* CDC, Atlanta, GA.

CDC. 2004. *HIV/AIDS Surveillance Report.* CDC, Atlanta, GA.

Cherner, M., E. Masliah, R. J. Ellis, T. D. Marcotte, D. J. Moore, I. Grant, and R. K. Heaton. 2002. Neurocognitive dysfunction predicts postmortem findings of HIV encephalitis. *Neurology* **59:**1563–1567.

Ciborowski, P., Y. Enose, A. Mack, M. Fladseth, and H. E. Gendelman. 2004. Diminished matrix metalloproteinase 9 secretion in human immunodeficiency virus-infected mononuclear phagocytes: modulation of innate immunity and implications for neurological disease. *J. Neuroimmunol.* **157:**11–16.

Cohen, M. J., W. B. Braunch, W. G. Willis, L. L. Weyandt, and G. W. Hynd. 1992. Adult development and aging, p. 49–79. *In* A. E. Puente and R. J. McCaffrey (ed.), *Handbook of Neuropsychological Assessment. A Biopsychosocial Perspective.* Plenum Press, New York, NY.

Cohen, R. A., R. Boland, R. Paul, K. T. Tashima, E. E.
Schoenbaum, D. D. Celentano, P. Schuman, D. K. Smith,
and C. C. Carpenter. 2001. Neurocognitive performance
enhanced by highly active antiretroviral therapy in HIV-
infected women. *AIDS* **15:**341–345.

Conant, K., J. C. McArthur, D. E. Griffin, L. Sjulson, L.
M. Wahl, and D. N. Irani. 1999. Cerebrospinal fluid levels
of MMP-2, 7, and 9 are elevated in association with human
immunodeficiency virus dementia. *Ann. Neurol.* **46:**391–
398.

Concha, M., N. M. Graham, A. Munoz, D. Vlahov, W.
D. Royal, et al. 1992. Effect of chronic substance abuse on
the neuropsychological performance of intravenous drug
users with a high prevalence of HIV-1 seropositivity. *Am. J.
Epidemiol.* **136:**1338–1348.

Cook, J. A., M. H. Cohen, J. Burke, D. Grey, K. Anastos,
L. Kirstein, H. Palacio, J. Richardson, T. Wilson, and M.
Young. 2002. Effects of depressive symptoms and mental
health quality of life on use of highly active antiretroviral
therapy among HIV-seropositive women. *J. Acquir. Immune
Defic. Syndr.* **30:**401–409.

Cook, J. A., D. Grey, J. Burke, M. H. Cohen, A. C. Gurtman,
J. L. Richardson, T. E. Wilson, M. A. Young, and N. A.
Hessol. 2004. Depressive symptoms and AIDS-related mor-
tality among a multisite cohort of HIV-positive women. *Am.
J. Public Health* **94:**1133–1140.

Cook, J. E., S. Dasgupta, L. D. Middaugh, E. C. Terry, P.
R. Gorry, S. L. Wesselingh, and W. R. Tyor. 2005. Highly
active antiretroviral therapy and human immunodeficiency
virus encephalitis. *Ann. Neurol.* **57:**795–803.

Corder, E. H., K. Robertson, L. Lannfelt, N. Bogdanovic,
G. Eggertsen, J. Wilkins, and C. Hall. 1998. HIV-infected
subjects with the E4 allele for APOE have excess dementia
and peripheral neuropathy. *Nat. Med.* **4:**1182–1184.

Cornblath, D., V. Chaudhry, K. Carter, D. Lee, M. Seysedadr,
M. Miernicki, and T. Joh. 1999. Total neuropathy score: validation and reliability study. *Neurology* **53:**1660–1664.

Cotter, R., C. Williams, L. Ryan, D. Erichsen, A. Lopez, H.
Peng, and J. Zheng. 2002. Fractalkine (CX3CL1) and brain
inflammation: implications for HIV-1-associated dementia.
J. Neurovirol. **8:**585–598.

Cutler, R. G., N. J. Haughey, A. Tammara, J. C. McArthur,
A. Nath, R. Reid, D. L. Vargas, C. A. Pardo, and M. P.
Mattson. 2004. Dysregulation of sphingolipid and sterol metab-
olism by ApoE4 in HIV dementia. *Neurology* **63:**626–630.

Dana Consortium on Therapy for HIV Dementia and
Related Cognitive Disorders. 1996. Clinical confirmation of
the American Academy of Neurology algorithm for HIV-1-
associated cognitive/motor disorder. *Neurology* **47:**1247–1253.

Davis, H. F., R. L. Skolasky, Jr., O. A. Selnes, D. M. Burgess,
and J. C. McArthur. 2002. Assessing HIV-associated dementia: modified HIV dementia scale versus the Grooved Pegboard.
AIDS Read. **12:**29–31, 38.

Dougherty, R. H., R. L. Skolasky, Jr., and J. C. McArthur.
2002. Progression of HIV-associated dementia treated with
HAART. *AIDS Read.* **12:**69–74.

Durvasula, R. S., E. N. Miller, H. F. Myers, and G. E. Wyatt.
2001. Predictors of neuropsychological performance in HIV
positive women. *J. Clin. Exp. Neuropsychol.* **23:**149–163.

Durvasula, R. S., H. F. Myers, P. Satz, E. N. Miller, H.
Morgenstern, M. A. Richardson, G. Evans, and D. Forney.
2000. HIV-1, cocaine, and neuropsychological performance in
African American men. *J. Int. Neuropsychol. Soc.* **6:**322–335.

Elkabes, S., E. M. DiCicco-Bloom, and I. B. Black. 1996.
Brain microglia/macrophages express neurotrophins that
selectively regulate microglial proliferation and function.
J. Neurosci. **16:**2508–2521.

Enose, Y., C. J. Destache, A. L. Mack, J. R. Anderson,
F. Ullrich, P. S. Ciborowski, and H. E. Gendelman. 2005.
Proteomic fingerprints distinguish microglia, bone marrow,
and spleen macrophage populations. *Glia* **51:**161–172.

Everall, I. P., J. D. Glass, J. McArthur, E. Spargo, and P. Lantos.
1994. Neuronal density in the superior frontal and temporal gyri
does not correlate with the degree of human immunodeficiency
virus-associated dementia. *Acta Neuropathol.* **88:**538–544.

Farinpour, R., E. N. Miller, P. Satz, O. A. Selnes, B. A.
Cohen, J. T. Becker, R. L. Skolasky, Jr., and B. R. Visscher.
2003. Psychosocial risk factors of HIV morbidity and mortality: findings from the Multicenter AIDS Cohort Study
(MACS). *J. Clin. Exp. Neuropsychol.* **25:**654–670.

Fischer-Smith, T., S. Croul, A. E. Sverstiuk, C. Capini,
D. L'Heureux, E. G. Regulier, M. W. Richardson, S. Amini,
S. Morgello, K. Khalili, and J. Rappaport. 2001. CNS
invasion by CD14⁺/CD16⁺ peripheral blood-derived monocytes in HIV dementia: perivascular accumulation and reservoir of HIV infection. *J. Neurovirol.* **7:**528–541.

Flores, I., D. Pieniazek, N. Moran, A. Soler, N. Rodriguez,
M. Alegria, M. Vera, L. M. Janini, C. I. Bandea, A. Ramos,
M. Rayfield, and Y. Yamamura. 1999. HIV-1 subtype F in
single and dual infections in Puerto Rico: a potential senti-
nel site for monitoring novel genetic HIV variants in North
America. *Emerg. Infect. Dis.* **5:**481–483.

Gao, F., E. Bailes, D. L. Robertson, Y. Chen, C. M.
Rodenburg, S. F. Michael, L. B. Cummins, L. O. Arthur,
M. Peeters, G. M. Shaw, P. M. Sharp, and B. H. Hahn.
1999. Origin of HIV-1 in the chimpanzee *Pan troglodytes troglodytes. Nature* **397:**436–441.

Gartner, S. 2000. HIV infection and dementia. *Science* **287:**
602–604.

Gelbard, H. A., H. S. Nottet, S. Swindells, M. Jett, K. A.
Dzenko, P. Genis, R. White, L. Wang, Y. B. Choi, D.
Zhang, et al. 1994. Platelet-activating factor: a candidate
human immunodeficiency virus type 1-induced neurotoxin.
J. Virol. **68:**4628–4635.

Gendelman, H., E. Anderson, L. Melendez, and J. Zheng.
2006. Chemokines and their receptors and the neuropathogenesis of HIV-1 infection, p. 45–80. *In* H. Friedman, S.
Specter, and M. Bendinelli (ed.), *In Vivo Models of HIV Disease
and Control.* Springer-Verlag, New York, NY.

Gendelman, H., J. Zheng, C. Coulter, A. Ghorpade, M. Che,
et al. 1998. The HIV-associated dementia complex: a metabolic encephalopathy reversed by highly active antiretroviral
therapy. *J. Infect. Dis.* **178:**1000–1007.

Gendelman, H. E., Y. Persidsky, A. Ghorpade, J. Limoges,
M. Stins, M. Fiala, and R. Morrisett. 1997. The neuropatho-
genesis of the AIDS dementia complex. *AIDS* **11**(Suppl. A):
S35–S45.

Goldstein, G., and C. H. Shelly. 1972. Statistical and normative studies of the Halstead Neuropsychological Test Battery
relevant to a neuropsychiatric hospital setting. *Percept. Mot.
Skills* **34:**603–620.

Gomez, C. E., E. Iglesias, W. Perdomo, F. Rolo, M. Blanco,
L. Lobaina, A. Martin, and C. A. Duarte. 2001. Isolates
from four different HIV type 1 clades circulating in Cuba
identified by DNA sequence of the C2-V3 region. *AIDS Res.
Hum. Retrovir.* **17:**55–58.

Gonzalez-Scarano, F., and J. Martin-Garcia. 2005. The neuropathogenesis of AIDS. *Nat. Rev. Immunol.* **5:**69–81.

Gonzalez, E., H. Kulkarni, H. Bolivar, A. Mangano, R.
Sanchez, G. Catano, R. J. Nibbs, B. I. Freedman, M. P.
Quinones, M. J. Bamshad, K. K. Murthy, B. H. Rovin, W.
Bradley, R. A. Clark, S. A. Anderson, J. R. O'Connell, B.
K. Agan, S. S. Ahuja, L. Bologna, L. Sen, M. J. Dolan,
and S. K. Ahuja. 2005. The influence of CCL3L1 gene-con-
taining segmental duplications on HIV-1/AIDS susceptibility.
Science **307:**1434–1440.

Gonzalez, E., B. H. Rovin, L. Sen, G. Cooke, R. Dhanda,
S. Mummidi, H. Kulkarni, M. J. Bamshad, V. Telles, S. A.

Anderson, E. A. Walter, K. T. Stephan, M. Deucher, A. Mangano, R. Bologna, S. S. Ahuja, M. J. Dolan, and S. K. Ahuja. 2002. HIV-1 infection and AIDS dementia are influenced by a mutant MCP-1 allele linked to increased monocyte infiltration of tissues and MCP-1 levels. *Proc. Natl. Acad. Sci. USA* **99:**13795–13800.

Goodkin, K., F. L. Wilkie, M. Concha, D. Asthana, P. Shapshak, R. Douyon, R. K. Fujimura, and C. LoPiccolo. 1997. Subtle neuropsychological impairment and minor cognitive-motor disorder in HIV-1 infection. Neuroradiological, neurophysiological, neuroimmunological, and virological correlates. *Neuroimaging Clin. N. Am.* **7:**561–579.

Gorry, P. R., J. Taylor, G. H. Holm, A. Mehle, T. Morgan, M. Cayabyab, M. Farzan, H. Wang, J. E. Bell, K. Kunstman, J. P. Moore, S. M. Wolinsky, and D. Gabuzda. 2002. Increased CCR5 affinity and reduced CCR5/CD4 dependence of a neurovirulent primary human immunodeficiency virus type 1 isolate. *J. Virol.* **76:**6277–6292.

Grant, I., D. Byrd, M. Cherner, D. Clifford, I. Grant, J. Joseph, J. McArthur, M. Nunn, V. Valcour, and V. Wojna. 2005. Towards an updated nosology for HIV-associated neurocognitive disorders, abstr. 38, p. 49. *HIV Infect. Central Nervous Syst. Dev. Resource Limited Settings.* Edizioni Internazionali srl, Rome, Italy.

Gupta, J. D., P. Satishchandra, K. Gopukumar, F. Wilkie, D. Waldrop-Valverde, R. Ellis, R. Ownby, D. K. Subbakrishna, A. Desai, A. Kamat, V. Ravi, B. S. Rao, K. S. Satish, and M. Kumar. 2007. Neuropsychological deficits in human immunodeficiency virus type 1 clade C-seropositive adults from South India. *J. Neurovirol.* **13:**195–202.

Hahn, B. H., G. M. Shaw, K. M. De Cock, and P. M. Sharp. 2000. AIDS as a zoonosis: scientific and public health implications. *Science* **287:**607–614.

Heese, K., C. Hock, and U. Otten. 1998. Inflammatory signals induce neurotrophin expression in human microglial cells. *J. Neurochem.* **70:**699–707.

Heyes, M. P., B. J. Brew, A. Martin, R. W. Price, A. M. Salazar, J. J. Sidtis, J. A. Yergey, M. M. Mouradian, A. E. Sadler, J. Keilp, et al. 1991. Quinolinic acid in cerebrospinal fluid and serum in HIV-1 infection: relationship to clinical and neurological status. *Ann. Neurol.* **29:**202–209.

Ho, D. D., A. U. Neumann, A. S. Perelson, W. Chen, J. M. Leonard, and M. Markowitz. 1995. Rapid turnover of plasma virions and CD4 lymphocytes in HIV-1 infection. *Nature* **373:**123–126.

Janssen, R. S., D. R. Cornblath, and L. G. Epstein. 1991. Nomenclature and research case definitions for neurological manifestations of human immunodeficiency virus type-1 (HIV-1) infection: report of a Working Group of the American Academy of Neurology AIDS Task Force. *Neurology* **41:**778.

Janssen, R. S., A. J. Saykin, L. Cannon, J. Campbell, P. F. Pinsky, N. A. Hessol, P. M. O'Malley, A. R. Lifson, L. S. Doll, G. W. Rutherford, et al. 1989. Neurological and neuropsychological manifestations of HIV-1 infection: association with AIDS-related complex but not asymptomatic HIV-1 infection. *Ann. Neurol.* **26:**592–600.

Jones, D. L., M. Ishii, A. LaPerriere, H. Stanley, M. Antoni, G. Ironson, N. Schneiderman, F. Van Splunteren, A. Cassells, K. Alexander, Y. P. Gousse, A. Vaughn, E. Brondolo, J. N. Tobin, and S. M. Weiss. 2003. Influencing medication adherence among women with AIDS. *AIDS Care* **15:**463–474.

Kaul, M., and S. A. Lipton. 1999. Chemokines and activated macrophages in HIV gp120-induced neuronal apoptosis. *Proc. Natl. Acad. Sci. USA* **96:**8212–8216.

Kelder, W., J. C. McArthur, T. Nance-Sproson, D. McClernon, and D. E. Griffin. 1998. Beta-chemokines MCP-1 and RANTES are selectively increased in cerebrospinal fluid of patients with human immunodeficiency virus-associated dementia. *Ann. Neurol.* **44:**831–835.

Khanna, K. V., X. F. Yu, D. H. Ford, L. Ratner, J. K. Hildreth, and R. B. Markham. 2000. Differences among HIV-1 variants in their ability to elicit secretion of TNF-alpha. *J. Immunol.* **164:**1408–1415.

Kijak, G. H., and F. E. McCutchan. 2005. HIV diversity, molecular epidemiology, and the role of recombination. *Curr. Infect. Dis. Rep.* **7:**480–488.

Kilbourne, A., A. Justice, L. Rabeneck, M. Rodriguez-Barradas, S. Weissman, and V. P. Team. 2001. General medical and psychiatric comorbidity among HIV-Infected veterans in the post-HAART era. *J. Clin. Epidemiol.* **54**(Suppl. 1): S22–S28.

Kim, W. K., S. Corey, X. Alvarez, and K. Williams. 2003. Monocyte/macrophage traffic in HIV and SIV encephalitis. *J. Leukoc. Biol.* **74:**650–656.

La Rue, A. 1992. Adult development and aging, p. 81–119. *In* A. E. Puente and R. J. McCaffrey (ed.), *Handbook of Neuropsychological Assessment. A Biopsychosocial Perspective.* Plenum Press, New York, NY.

Laspiur, J. P., E. R. Anderson, P. Ciborowski, V. Wojna, W. Rozek, F. Duan, R. Mayo, E. Rodriguez, M. Plaud-Valentin, J. Rodriguez-Orengo, H. E. Gendelman, and L. M. Melendez. 2007. CSF proteomic fingerprints for HIV-associated cognitive impairment. *J. Neuroimmunol.* **192:**157–170.

Liner, K. J., II, C. D. Hall, and K. R. Robertson. 2007. Impact of human immunodeficiency virus (HIV) subtypes on HIV-associated neurological disease. *J. Neurovirol.* **13:**291–304.

Liu, X., Y. Stern, K. Bell, J. B. Joseph, Z. Williams, K. Stein, K. Marder, G. Dooneief, G. Todak, W. El Sadr, A. A. Ehrhardt, and R. Mayeux. 1996. Gender differences in HIV-related neurological progression in a cohort of injecting drug users followed for 3.5 years. *J. Neuro-AIDS* **1:**17–30.

Llorente, A. M., M. Turcich, and K. A. Lawrence. 2004. Differences in neuropsychological performance associated with ethnicity in children with HIV-1 infection: preliminary findings. *Appl. Neuropsychol.* **11:**47–53.

Luciano, C., G. Ebenezer, R. L. Skolasky, J. Maldonado, V. Ho-Fung, S. Sanchez, T. Ginebra, E. Castillo, P. Hauer, and J. C. McArthur. 2005a. Increased cutaneous innervation in pediatric/adolescent HIV sensory neuropathy. *5th Annu. Conf. Spec. Neurosci. Res. Progr.*, Adelphi, MD.

Luciano, C., V. Ho-Fung, S. Sanchez, E. Castillo, T. Ginebra, V. Gerena, C. Rivera, and J. C. McArthur. 2005b. A comparison of soluble immune markers in antiretroviral toxic neuropathy and HIV distal sensory neuropathy. *Neurology* **64:**A246.

Luo, X., K. A. Carlson, V. Wojna, R. Mayo, T. M. Biskup, J. Stoner, J. Anderson, H. E. Gendelman, and L. M. Melendez. 2003. Macrophage proteomic fingerprinting predicts HIV-1-associated cognitive impairment. *Neurology* **60:**1931–1937.

Lyketsos, C. G., D. R. Hoover, M. Guccione, W. Senterfitt, M. A. Dew, J. Wesch, M. J. VanRaden, G. J. Treisman, H. Morgenstern, et al. 1993. Depressive symptoms as predictors of medical outcomes in HIV infection. *JAMA* **270:**2563–2567.

Mahadevan, A., S. K. Shankar, P. Satishchandra, U. Ranga, Y. T. Chickabasaviah, V. Santosh, R. Vasanthapuram, C. A. Pardo, A. Nath, and M. C. Zink. 2007. Characterization of human immunodeficiency virus (HIV)-infected cells in infiltrates associated with CNS opportunistic infections in patients with HIV clade C infection. *J. Neuropathol. Exp. Neurol.* **66:**799–808.

Marder, K. S., S. Albert, G. Dooneief, Y. Stern, G. Ramachandran, and L. Epstein. 1996. Clinical confirmation of the American Academy of Neurology algorithm for HIV-1-associated cognitive/motor disorder. *Neurology* **47:**1247.

Martin, E. M., J. A. Cook, M. Chen, V. L. Carson, R. A. Reed, R. Hershow, and J. Burke. 1999. Working memory function in HHIV-seropositive women: the Women's Interagency HIV Study. *J. Int. Neuropsychol. Soc.* **5:**155.

Martin, E. M., T. S. Sullivan, R. A. Reed, T. A. Fletcher, D. L. Pitrak, W. Weddington, and M. Harrow. 2001. Auditory working memory in HIV-1 infection. *J. Int. Neuropsychol. Soc.* **7:**20–6.

Masliah, E., R. M. DeTeresa, M. E. Mallory, and L. A. Hansen. 2000. Changes in pathological findings at autopsy in AIDS cases for the last 15 years. *AIDS* **14:**69–74.

Mason, K. I., A. Campbell, P. Hawkins, S. Madhere, K. Johnson, and R. Takushi-Chinen. 1998. Neuropsychological functioning in HIV-positive African-American women with a history of drug use. *J. Natl. Med. Assoc.* **90:**665–674.

Matthews, J. R. 1992. Sex and gender, p. 121–139. *In* A. E. Puente and R. J. McCaffrey (ed.), *Handbook of Neuropsychological Assessment. A Biopsychological Perspective.* Plenum Press, New York, NY.

Mayeux, R., Y. Stern, M. X. Tang, G. Todak, K. Marder, M. Sano, M. Richards, Z. Stein, A. A. Ehrhardt, and J. M. Gorman. 1993. Mortality risks in gay men with human immunodeficiency virus infection and cognitive impairment. *Neurology* **43:**176–182.

McArthur, J. C. 2004. HIV dementia: an evolving disease. *J. Neuroimmunol.* **157:**3–10.

McArthur, J., J. S. Creighton, L. Lai, R. Moore, K. Carter, S. Wesselingh, and K. Cherry. 2004. Risk factors and determinants for HIV-associated sensory neuropathies: is hepatitis C a modifier? *11th Conf. Retrovir. Opportun. Infect.*, San Francisco, CA.

McCarthy, B. G., S. T. Hsieh, S. Stocks, P. Hauer, C. Macko, D. R. Cornblath, J. W. Griffin, and J. C. McArthur. 1995. Cutaneous innervation in sensory neuropathies: evaluation by skin biopsy. *Neurology* **45:**1848–1855.

Melendez, L. M. 2006. *12th SNIP Meeting*, abstr. SS-7.

Messam, C. A., and E. O. Major. 2000. Stages of restricted HIV-1 infection in astrocyte cultures derived from human fetal brain tissue. *J. Neurovirol.* **6**(Suppl 1)**:**S90–S94.

Miller, E. N., O. A. Selnes, J. C. McArthur, P. Satz, J. T. Becker, B. A. Cohen, K. Sheridan, A. M. Machado, W. G. Van Gorp, and B. Visscher. 1990. Neuropsychological performance in HIV-1-infected homosexual men: The Multicenter AIDS Cohort Study (MACS). *Neurology* **40:**197–203.

Millogo, A., A. B. Sawadogo, A. P. Sawadogo, and D. Lankoande. 2002. Peripheral neuropathies revealing HIV infection at the Hospital Center of Bobo-Dioulasso (Burkina Faso). *Bull. Soc. Pathol. Exot.* **95:**27–30.

Mindt, M. R., M. Cherner, T. D. Marcotte, D. J. Moore, H. Bentley, M. M. Esquivel, Y. Lopez, I. Grant, and R. K. Heaton. 2003. The functional impact of HIV-associated neuropsychological impairment in Spanish-speaking adults: a pilot study. *J. Clin. Exp. Neuropsychol.* **25:**122–132.

Modi, G., K. Hari, M. Modi, and A. Mochan. 2007. The frequency and profile of neurology in black South African HIV infected (clade C) patients—a hospital-based prospective audit. *J. Neurol. Sci.* **254:**60–64.

Morgello, S., R. Mahboob, T. Yakoushina, S. Khan, and K. Hague. 2002. Autopsy findings in a human immunodeficiency virus-infected population over 2 decades: influences of gender, ethnicity, risk factors, and time. *Arch. Pathol. Lab. Med.* **126:**182–190.

Moses, A. V., F. E. Bloom, C. D. Pauza, and J. A. Nelson. 1993. Human immunodeficiency virus infection of human brain capillary endothelial cells occurs via a CD4/galactosylceramide-independent mechanism. *Proc. Natl. Acad. Sci. USA* **90:**10474–10478.

Nath, A., K. Conant, P. Chen, C. Scott, and E. O. Major. 1999. Transient exposure to HIV-1 Tat protein results in cytokine production in macrophages and astrocytes: a hit and run phenomenon. *J. Biol. Chem.* **274:**17098–17102.

Nath, A., V. Hartloper, M. Furer, and K. R. Fowke. 1995. Infection of human fetal astrocytes with HIV-1: viral tropism and the role of cell to cell contact in viral transmission. *J. Neuropathol. Exp. Neurol.* **54:**320–330.

Navia, B. A., E. S. Cho, C. K. Petito, and R. W. Price. 1986a. The AIDS dementia complex: II. Neuropathology. *Ann. Neurol.* **19:**525–535.

Navia, B. A., B. D. Jordan, and R. W. Price. 1986b. The AIDS dementia complex: I. Clinical features. *Ann. Neurol.* **19:**517–524.

Navia, B. A., and K. Rostasy. 2005. The AIDS dementia complex: clinical and basic neuroscience with implications for novel molecular therapies. *Neurotox. Res.* **8:**3–24.

Newman, P. J., and J. J. Sweet. 1986. The effects of clinical depression on the Luria-Nebraska Neuropsychological Battery. *Int. J. Clin. Neuropsychol.* **8:**109–114.

Nieves, D. M., M. Plaud, V. Wojna, R. Skolasky, and L. M. Melendez. 2007. Characterization of peripheral blood human immunodeficiency virus isolates from Hispanic women with cognitive impairment. *J. Neurovirol.* **13:**315–327.

Nottet, H. S. 1999. Interactions between macrophages and brain microvascular endothelial cells: role in pathogenesis of HIV-1 infection and blood-brain barrier function. *J. Neurovirol.* **5:**659–669.

Parry, O., J. Mielke, A. Latif, S. Ray, L. Levy, and S. Siziya. 1997. Peripheral neuropathy in individuals with HIV infection in Zimbabwe. *Acta Neurol. Scand.* **96:**218–222.

Peeters, M., and P. M. Sharp. 2000. Genetic diversity of HIV-1: the moving target. *AIDS* **14**(Suppl. 3)**:**S129–S140.

Polydefkis, M., C. Yiannoutsos, B. Cohen, H. Hollander, G. Schifitto, D. Clifford, D. Simpson, D. Katzenstein, S. Shriver, P. Hauer, A. Brown, A. Haidich, L. Moo, and J. McArthur. 2002. Reduced-intraepidermal nerve fiber density in HIV-associated sensory neuropathy. *Neurology* **58:**115–119.

Power, C., P. A. Kong, T. O. Crawford, S. Wesselingh, J. D. Glass, J. C. McArthur, and B. D. Trapp. 1993. Cerebral white matter changes in acquired immunodeficiency syndrome dementia: alterations of the blood-brain barrier. *Ann. Neurol.* **34:**339–350.

Power, C., J. C. McArthur, A. Nath, K. Wehrly, M. Mayne, J. Nishio, T. Langelier, R. T. Johnson, and B. Chesebro. 1998. Neuronal death induced by brain-derived human immunodeficiency virus type 1 envelope genes differs between demented and nondemented AIDS patients. *J. Virol.* **72:**9045–9053.

Power, C., O. A. Selnes, J. A. Grim, and J. C. McArthur. 1995. HIV Dementia Scale: a rapid screening test. *J. Acquir. Immune Defic. Syndr. Hum. Retrovirol.* **8:**273–278.

Preston, B. D., B. J. Poiesz, and L. A. Loeb. 1988. Fidelity of HIV-1 reverse transcriptase. *Science* **242:**1168–1171.

Price, R. W., and B. J. Brew. 1988. The AIDS dementia complex. *J. Infect. Dis.* **158:**1079–1083.

Price, R. W., C. T. Yiannoutsos, D. B. Clifford, L. Zaborski, A. Tselis, J. J. Sidtis, B. Cohen, C. D. Hall, A. Erice, K. Henry, et al. 1999. Neurological outcomes in late HIV infection: adverse impact of neurological impairment on survival and protective effect of antiviral therapy. *AIDS* **13:**1677–1685.

Pulliam, L., R. Gascon, M. Stubblebine, D. McGuire, and M. S. McGrath. 1997. Unique monocyte subset in patients with AIDS dementia. *Lancet* **349:**692–695.

Pulliam, L., B. Sun, and H. Rempel. 2004. Invasive chronic inflammatory monocyte phenotype in subjects with high HIV-1 viral load. *J. Neuroimmunol.* **157:**93–98.

Quasney, M. W., Q. Zhang, S. Sargent, M. Mynatt, J. Glass, and J. McArthur. 2001. Increased frequency of the tumor necrosis factor-alpha-308 A allele in adults with human immunodeficiency virus dementia. *Ann. Neurol.* **50:**157–162.

Quinn, T. C., and J. Overbaugh. 2005. HIV/AIDS in women: an expanding epidemic. *Science* **308:**1582–1583.

Ranki, A., M. Nyberg, V. Ovod, M. Haltia, I. Elovaara, R. Raininko, H. Haapasalo, and K. Krohn. 1995. Abundant expression of HIV Nef and Rev proteins in brain astrocytes in vivo is associated with dementia. *AIDS* 9:1001–1008.

Ricart, F., M. A. Cohen, C. A. Alfonso, R. G. Hoffman, N. Quinones, A. Cohen, and D. Indyk. 2002. Understanding the psychodynamics of non-adherence to medical treatment in persons with HIV infection. *Gen. Hosp. Psychiatry* 24:176–180.

Richardson, J. L., E. M. Martin, N. Jimenez, K. Danley, M. Cohen, V. L. Carson, B. Sinclair, J. M. Racenstein, R. A. Reed, and A. M. Levine. 2002. Neuropsychological functioning in a cohort of HIV infected women: importance of antiretroviral therapy. *J. Int. Neuropsychol. Soc.* 8:781–793.

Richardson, M. A., E. E. Morgan, M. J. Vielhauer, C. A. Cuevas, L. M. Buondonno, and T. M. Keane. 2005. Utility of the HIV dementia scale in assessing risk for significant HIV-related cognitive-motor deficits in a high-risk urban adult sample. *AIDS Care* 17:1013–1021.

Richardson, M. A., P. F. Satz, H. F. Myers, E. N. Miller, E. G. Bing, F. I. Fawzy, and M. Maj. 1999. Effects of depressed mood versus clinical depression on neuropsychological test performance among African American men impacted by HIV/AIDS. *J. Clin. Exp. Neuropsychol.* 21:769–783.

Riedel, D., M. Ghate, M. Nene, R. Paranjape, S. Mehendale, R. Bollinger, N. Sacktor, J. McArthur, and A. Nath. 2006. Screening for human immunodeficiency virus (HIV) dementia in an HIV clade C-infected population in India. *J. Neurovirol.* 12:34–38.

Rosenberger, P. H., R. A. Bornstein, H. A. Nasrallah, M. F. Para, C. C. Whitaker, R. J. Fass, and R. R. Rice, Jr. 1993. Psychopathology in human immunodeficiency virus infection: lifetime and current assessment. *Compr. Psychiatry* 34:150–158.

Ross, H. L., S. Gartner, J. C. McArthur, J. R. Corboy, J. J. McAllister, S. Millhouse, and B. Wigdahl. 2001. HIV-1 LTR C/EBP binding site sequence configurations preferentially encountered in brain lead to enhanced C/EBP factor binding and increased LTR-specific activity. *J. Neurovirol.* 7:235–249.

Roth, W. W., P. N. Levett, C. P. Hudson, T. C. Roach, C. Womack, and V. C. Bond. 1997. HIV type 1 envelope sequences from seroconverting patients in Barbados. *AIDS Res. Hum. Retrovir.* 13:1443–1446.

Rozek W., M. Ricardo-Dukelow, S. Holloway, V. Wojna, L. M. Melendez, H. E. Gendelman, and P. Ciborowski. 2007. Cerebrospinal fluid Proteomic profiling of HIV-infected patients with cognitive impairment. *J. Proteome Res.* 6:4189–4199.

Rutkove, S., M. Kothari, E. Raynor, M. Levy, R. Fadic, and R. Nardin. 1997. Sural/radial amplitude in the diagnosis of mild axonal polyneuropathy. *Muscle Nerve* 20:1236–1241.

Ryan, E. L., R. Baird, M. R. Mindt, D. Byrd, J. Monzones, and S. M. Bank. 2005. Neuropsychological impairment in racial/ethnic minorities with HIV infection and low literacy levels: effects of education and reading level in participant characterization. *J. Int. Neuropsychol. Soc.* 11:889–898.

Sacktor, N. 2002. The epidemiology of human immunodeficiency virus-associated neurological disease in the era of highly active antiretroviral therapy. *J. Neurovirol.* 8(Suppl. 2):115–121.

Sacktor, N., R. H. Lyles, R. Skolasky, C. Kleeberger, O. A. Selnes, E. N. Miller, J. T. Becker, B. Cohen, and J. C. McArthur. 2001. HIV-associated neurologic disease incidence changes: Multicenter AIDS Cohort Study, 1990–1998. *Neurology* 56:257–260.

Sacktor, N., M. P. McDermott, K. Marder, G. Schifitto, O. A. Selnes, J. C. McArthur, Y. Stern, S. Albert, D. Palumbo, K. Kieburtz, J. A. De Marcaida, B. Cohen, and L. Epstein. 2002. HIV-associated cognitive impairment before and after the advent of combination therapy. *J. Neurovirol.* 8:136–142.

Sacktor, N., R. L. Skolasky, T. Ernst, X. Mao, O. Selnes, M. G. Pomper, L. Chang, K. Zhong, D. C. Shungu, K. Marder, D. Shibata, G. Schifitto, L. Bobo, and P. B. Barker. 2005. A multicenter study of two magnetic resonance spectroscopy techniques in individuals with HIV dementia. *J. Magn. Reson. Imaging* 21:325–333.

Sacktor, N., R. Skolasky, O. A. Selnes, M. Watters, P. Poff, B. Shiramizu, C. Shikuma, and V. Valcour. 2007. Neuropsychological test profile differences between young and old human immunodeficiency virus-positive individuals. *J. Neurovirol.* 13:203–209.

Sacktor, N. C., H. Bacellar, D. R. Hoover, T. E. Nance-Sproson, O. A. Selnes, E. N. Miller, G. J. Dal Pan, C. Kleeberger, A. Brown, A. Saah, and J. C. McArthur. 1996. Psychomotor slowing in HIV infection: a predictor of dementia, AIDS and death. *J. Neurovirol.* 2:404–410.

Saha, R. N., and K. Pahan. 2003. Tumor necrosis factor-alpha at the crossroads of neuronal life and death during HIV-associated dementia. *J. Neurochem.* 86:1057–1071.

Sanchez Rodriguez, J. L., and M. Rodriguez Alvarez. 2003. Normal aging and AIDS. *Arch. Gerontol. Geriatr.* 36:57–65.

Satz, P., H. Morgenstern, E. N. Miller, O. A. Selnes, J. C. McArthur, B. A. Cohen, J. Wesch, J. T. Becker, L. Jacobson, L. F. D'Elia, et al. 1993. Low education as a possible risk factor for cognitive abnormalities in HIV-1: findings from the multicenter AIDS Cohort Study (MACS). *J. Acquir. Immune Defic. Syndr.* 6:503–511.

Saykin, A. J., R. S. Janssen, and G. C. Sprehn. 1988. Neuropsychological dysfunction in HIV-infection: characterization in a lymphadenopathy cohort. *Int. J. Clin. Neuropsychol.* 10:81–95.

Schifitto, G., K. Kieburtz, M. P. McDermott, J. McArthur, K. Marder, N. Sacktor, D. Palumbo, O. Selnes, Y. Stern, L. Epstein, and S. Albert. 2001. Clinical trials in HIV-associated cognitive impairment: cognitive and functional outcomes. *Neurology* 56:415–418.

Selnes, O. A. 2005. Memory loss in persons with HIV/AIDS: assessment and strategies for coping. *AIDS Read.* 15:289–292, 294.

Selnes, O. A., N. Galai, J. C. McArthur, S. Cohn, W. Royal III, et al. 1997. HIV infection and cognition in intravenous drug users: long-term follow-up. *Neurology* 48:223–230.

Selnes, O. A., J. C. McArthur, W. D. Royal, M. L. Updike, T. Nance-Sproson, et al. 1992. HIV-1 infection and intravenous drug use: longitudinal neuropsychological evaluation of asymptomatic subjects. *Neurology* 42:1924–1930.

Selnes, O. A., E. Miller, J. McArthur, B. Gordon, A. Munoz, K. Sheridan, R. Fox, A. J. Saah, et al. 1990. HIV-1 infection: no evidence of cognitive decline during the asymptomatic stages. *Neurology* 40:204–208.

Sene-Diouf, F., M. Ndiaye, A. Diop, A. Thiam, A. Ndao, M. Diagne, M. Ndiaye, and I. Ndiaye. 2000. Epidemiological, clinical and progressive aspects of neurological manifestations associated with retroviral infections: eleven year retrospective study. *Dakar Med.* 45:162–166.

Severe, P. 2005. HIV-associated neurological complications in Haiti, abstr. 7, p. 17. *HIV Infect. Central Nervous Syst. Dev. Resource Limited Settings.* Edizioni Internazionali srl, Rome, Italy.

Sevigny, J. J., S. M. Albert, M. P. McDermott, J. C. McArthur, N. Sacktor, K. Conant, G. Schifitto, O. A. Selnes, Y. Stern, D. R. McClernon, D. Palumbo, K. Kieburtz, G. Riggs, B. Cohen, L. G. Epstein, and K. Marder. 2004. Evaluation of HIV RNA and markers of immune activation as predictors of HIV-associated dementia. *Neurology* 63:2084–2090.

Sevigny, J. J., S. M. Albert, M. P. McDermott, G. Schifitto, J. C. McArthur, N. Sacktor, K. Conant, O. A. Selnes, Y. Stern, D. R. McClernon, D. Palumbo, K. Kieburtz, G. Riggs, B. Cohen, K. Marder, and L. G. Epstein. 2007. An evaluation of neurocognitive status and markers of immune activation as predictors of time to death in advanced HIV infection. *Arch. Neurol.* **64:**97–102.

Silberstein, C. H., F. P. McKegney, M. A. O'Dowd, P. A. Selwyn, E. Schoenbaum, E. Drucker, C. Feiner, C. P. Cox, and G. Friedland. 1987. A prospective longitudinal study of neuropsychological and psychosocial factors in asymptomatic individuals at risk for HTLV-III/LAV infection in a methadone program: preliminary findings. *Int. J. Neurosci.* **32:**669–676.

Singh, K. K., R. J. Ellis, J. Marquie-Beck, S. Letendre, R. K. Heaton, I. Grant, and S. A. Spector. 2004. CCR2 polymorphisms affect neuropsychological impairment in HIV-1-infected adults. *J. Neuroimmunol.* **157:**185–192.

Soontornniyomkij, V., G. Wang, C. A. Pittman, C. A. Wiley, and C. L. Achim. 1998. Expression of brain-derived neurotrophic factor protein in activated microglia of human immunodeficiency virus type 1 encephalitis. *Neuropathol. Appl. Neurobiol.* **24:**453–460.

Stein, D. S., R. H. Lyles, N. M. Graham, C. J. Tassoni, J. B. Margolick, J. P. Phair, C. Rinaldo, R. Detels, A. Saah, J. Bilello, et al. 1997. Predicting clinical progression or death in subjects with early-stage human immunodeficiency virus (HIV) infection: a comparative analysis of quantification of HIV RNA, soluble tumor necrosis factor type II receptors, neopterin, and β2-microglobulin. *J. Infect. Dis.* **176:**1161–1167.

Stern, Y., M. P. McDermott, S. Albert, D. Palumbo, O. A. Selnes, J. McArthur, N. Sacktor, G. Schifitto, K. Kieburtz, L. Epstein, and K. S. Marder. 2001. Factors associated with incident human immunodeficiency virus-dementia. *Arch. Neurol.* **58:**473–479.

Tornatore, C., A. Nath, K. Amemiya, and E. O. Major. 1991. Persistent human immunodeficiency virus type 1 infection in human fetal glial cells reactivated by T-cell factor(s) or by the cytokines tumor necrosis factor alpha and interleukin-1β. *J. Virol.* **65:**6094–6100.

Toro, D. M., J. Perez Laspiur, P. Ciborowski, F. Duan, V. Wojna, H. E. Gendelman, and L. M. Meléndez. Proteomic analysis of HIV-1 infected monocyte-derived macrophage following infection with primary viral strains isolated from Hispanic women with cognitive impairment. *J. Neurovirol.* in press.

Valcour, V., C. Shikuma, B. Shiramizu, M. Watters, P. Poff, O. Selnes, P. Holck, J. Grove, and N. Sacktor. 2004a. Higher frequency of dementia in older HIV-1 individuals: the Hawaii Aging with HIV-1 Cohort. *Neurology* **63:**822–827.

Valcour, V., C. Shikuma, B. Shiramizu, M. Watters, P. Poff, O. A. Selnes, J. Grove, Y. Liu, K. B. Abdul-Majid, S. Gartner, and N. Sacktor. 2004b. Age, apolipoprotein E4, and the risk of HIV dementia: the Hawaii Aging with HIV Cohort. *J. Neuroimmunol.* **157:**197–202.

Valcour, V., C. Shikuma, B. Shiramizu, A. E. Williams, M. Watters, O. Selnes, and N. Sacktor. 2005. Cognitive decline noted in HIV patients with persistently undetetable plasma viremia—The Hawaii Aging with HIV-1 Cohort. *5th Annu. Conf. Spec. Neurosci. Res. Progr.*, Adelphi, MD.

Valdois, S., Y. Joanette, A. Poissant, B. Ska, and F. Dehaut. 1990. Heterogeneity in the cognitive profile of normal elderly. *J. Clin. Exp. Neuropsychol.* **12:**587–596.

van Gorp, W. G., E. N. Miller, T. D. Marcotte, W. Dixon, D. Paz, O. Selnes, J. Wesch, J. T. Becker, C. H. Hinkin, M. Mitrushina, et al. 1994. The relationship between age and cognitive impairment in HIV-1 infection: findings from the Multicenter AIDS Cohort Study and a clinical cohort. *Neurology* **44:**929–935.

Vaughan, H. E., P. Cane, D. Pillay, and R. S. Tedder. 2003. Characterization of HIV type 1 clades in the Caribbean using *pol* gene sequences. *AIDS Res. Hum. Retrovir.* **19:**929–932.

Vedhara, K., G. Schifitto, and M. McDermott, et al. 1999. Disease progression in HIV-positive women with moderate to severe immunosuppression: the role of depression. *Behav. Med.* **25:**43–47.

Vehmas, A., J. Lieu, C. A. Pardo, J. C. McArthur, and S. Gartner. 2004. Amyloid precursor protein expression in circulating monocytes and brain macrophages from patients with HIV-associated cognitive impairment. *J. Neuroimmunol.* **157:**99–110.

von Giesen, H. J., S. Jander, H. Koller, and G. Arendt. 2004. Serum and cerebrospinal fluid levels of interleukin-18 in human immunodeficiency virus type 1-associated central nervous system disease. *J. Neurovirol.* **10:**383–386.

Wiley, C. A., E. Masliah, M. Morey, C. Lemere, R. DeTeresa, M. Grafe, L. Hansen, and R. Terry. 1991. Neocortical damage during HIV infection. *Ann. Neurol.* **29:**651–657.

Wilkie, F. L., K. Goodkin, A. Ardila, M. Concha, D. Lee, R. Lecusay, P. Suarez, M. H. Van Zuilen, R. Molina, and S. O'Mellan. 2004. HUMANS: an English and Spanish neuropsychological test battery for assessing HIV-1-infected individuals—initial report. *Appl. Neuropsychol.* **11:**121–133.

Williams, K. C., S. Corey, S. V. Westmoreland, D. Pauley, H. Knight, C. deBakker, X. Alvarez, and A. A. Lackner. 2001. Perivascular macrophages are the primary cell type productively infected by simian immunodeficiency virus in the brains of macaques: implications for the neuropathogenesis of AIDS. *J. Exp. Med.* **193:**905–915.

Wohl, A. R., S. Lu, J. Turner, A. Kovacs, M. Witt, K. Squires, W. Towner, and V. Beer. 2003. Risk of opportunistic infection in the HAART era among HIV-infected Latinos born in the United States compared to Latinos born in Mexico and Central America. *AIDS Patient Care STDS* **17:**267–275.

Wojna, V., K. A. Carlson, X. Luo, R. Mayo, L. M. Melendez, E. Kraiselburd, and H. E. Gendelman. 2004a. Proteomic fingerprinting of human immunodeficiency virus type 1-associated dementia from patient monocyte-derived macrophages: a case study. *J. Neurovirol.* **10**(Suppl. 1):74–81.

Wojna, V., R. L. Skolasky, J. C. McArthur, E. Maldonado, R. Hechavarria, R. Mayo, O. Selnes, T. Ginebra, T. de la Torre, H. Garcia, E. Kraiselburd, L. M. Melendez, C. D. Zorrilla, and A. Nath. 2007. Spanish Validation of the HIV dementia scale in women. *AIDS Patient Care STDS* **21:**930–941.

Wojna, V., E. Colon, M. Melendez, C. Anderson, J. Turchan, R. Skolasky, A. Hidalgo, R. Mayo, T. Curry, A. Algaze, M. Fernandez, L. Melendez, J. McArthur, and A. Nath. 2004b. American Academy of Neurology **62**(Suppl 5):A408.

Wojna, V., R. Skolasly, R. Hechavarría, R. Mayo, O. Selnes, J. C. McArthur, L. M. Meléndez, E. Maldonado, C. D. Zorrilla, H. García, E. Kraiselburd, and A. Nath. 2006. Prevalence of human immunodeficiency virus-associated cognitive impairment in a group of Hispanic women at risk for neurological impairment. *J. Neurovirol.* **12:**356–364.

Wong, M., P. Hope, K. Robertson, N. Nakasujja, M. Seggane, E. Katabira, J. McArthur, T. Quinn, A. Ronald, and N. Sacktor. 2004. HIV-associated neurological complications among HIV seropositive individuals in Uganda. *Neurology* **62**(Suppl.5):A444.

Wortley, P. M., and P. L. Fleming. 1997. AIDS in women in the United States. Recent trends. *JAMA* **278:**911–916.

Yi, Y., W. Chen, I. Frank, J. Cutilli, A. Singh, L. Starr-Spires, J. Sulcove, D. L. Kolson, and R. G. Collman. 2003. An unusual syncytia-inducing human immunodeficiency virus type 1 primary isolate from the central nervous system that is restricted to CXCR4, replicates efficiently in macrophages, and induces neuronal apoptosis. *J. Neurovirol.* **9:**432–441.

Zanetti, C., G. Manzano, and A. Gabbai. 2004. The frequency of peripheral neuropathy in a group of HIV positive patients from Brazil. *Arq. Neuropsiquiatr.* **62:**253–256.

Zhang, K., G. A. McQuibban, C. Silva, G. S. Butler, J. B. Johnston, J. Holden, I. Clark-Lewis, C. M. Overall, and C. Power. 2003. HIV-induced metalloproteinase processing of the chemokine stromal cell derived factor-1 causes neurodegeneration. *Nat. Neurosci.* **6:**1064–1071.

Zheng, J., M. R. Thylin, A. Ghorpade, H. Xiong, Y. Persidsky, R. Cotter, D. Niemann, M. Che, Y. C. Zeng, H. A. Gelbard, R. B. Shepard, J. M. Swartz, and H. E. Gendelman. 1999. Intracellular CXCR4 signaling, neuronal apoptosis and neuropathogenic mechanisms of HIV-1-associated dementia. *J. Neuroimmunol.* **98:**185–200.

Zheng, J., A. Lopez, Y. Huang, A. Persidsky, J. He, H. Zhang, J. Zhao, and C. Wood. 2007. Comparison of different viral strains from clade B and C on macrophage mediated inflammatory factors and glutamate production and neurotoxicity: a preliminary report, abstr. 354. *14th Conf. Retrov. Opportun. Infect.*

The Spectrum of Neuro-AIDS Disorders:
Pathophysiology, Diagnosis, and Treatment
Edited by K. Goodkin et al.
©2008 ASM Press, Washington, DC

31

Women and Neuro-AIDS Conditions in the Era of HAART

GABRIELE ARENDT, Y. JAEGER, AND TH. NOLTING

In the very beginning, the HIV/AIDS pandemic was a disease of homosexual and bisexual men; in 1985, 35% of all affected individuals were females; now, more than 50% of the HIV carriers worldwide are women (Sabo and Carwein, 1994; Marlink et al., 2001). Thus, the subject of women and HIV has aroused more and more public and scientific interest. It is known that women have a high risk of transvaginal HIV transmission through heterosexual intercourse in the era of highly active antiretroviral therapy (HAART), with another spectrum of medication side effects and often no access to scientific studies (Anastos et al., 2000; Anderson and Garnett, 2000; Antinori et al., 2001). Also with respect to primary prevention, women are often underprivileged (Lichtenstein et al., 2002), which underlines the necessity for education and hygienic training, especially in developing countries (Bazargan et al., 2000; Biber et al., 1999).

All over the world, there are mainly three reasons for initiating HIV tests in both males and females:

1. Symptoms provoking a medical examination and, after different time periods, a blood test for HIV
2. Self-estimated risk of HIV infection in groups with high-risk behavior
3. Individual history of sexually transmitted diseases (Fenton et al., 2002)

Nevertheless, the time when HIV infection was acquired remains unclear in most cases, which increases the risk of females giving birth to an HIV-1-positive child. In developing countries especially, there is a high prevalence of HIV infection in young females compared to males of the same age (Jaffe, 2000), which is due to socioeconomic conditions (Miller et al., 2002). The probability of self-initiated HIV blood tests being performed depends additionally on basic knowledge of transmission pathways, education, occupation,

psychological condition, and sexual identity (Montoya, 2004), as well as on the cultural and religious background (Dunkle et al., 2004). One reason for the younger age of women compared to men at the time of HIV diagnosis is pregnancy; many countries offer HIV tests to every pregnant woman. Furthermore, studies have shown the vaginal mucosa to be especially sensitive to viral attacks (Mahathir, 1997). The viral transmission rate from males to females is 2.3 times higher than that from females to males (Nicolosi et al., 1994; Saul et al., 2001). A study of American adolescents in Kansas City, MO, defined frequent and unprotected sexual intercourse with different partners as a major risk factor for HIV-1 positivity. For young females, early and unprotected sex has been proven to be the only reliable risk factor (Shuter et al., 1999), whereas high numbers of different female partners, high-risk sexual behavior, a history of abuse, and cocaine use have been shown to be predictors for HIV-1 positivity in young males (Gollub et al., 2000; Krantz et al., 2002; Newman and Zimmerman, 2000). Especially in heterosexual virus transmission, gender-specific interaction and power within a relationship, as well as sexual practices, seem to play predominant roles (Wingood and DiClemente, 2000). Many studies have shown that condom use in primary prevention is often a question of dominance in a relationship (Smith, 2003) and thus of female identity (Cornelius et al., 2000; Sanders-Phillips, 2002; Mize et al., 2002). Age plays an important role at this point (Goodkin et al., 2003; Gupta et al., 1995). To insist on condom use, women must be self-confident and ask for what is refused by the male partner. To expect such behavior from young and very young females, who are emotionally and socioeconomically dependent on their partners, demonstrates the discrepancy between theory and reality and could explain not only the younger age of females at diagnosis of HIV-1 positivity, but also their earlier seroconversion. This is underlined by our data from 1,946 women, where Caucasian females (35.18 ± 10.23 years old) are significantly older than non-Caucasians (32.39 ± 8.49 years old) at diagnosis of HIV-1 positivity. Different studies and epidemiological data have shown that HIV transmission in non-Caucasian women takes place in

Gabriele Arendt and TH. Nolting, Department of Neurology, University Hospital of Duesseldorf (UKD), D-40001 Duesseldorf, Germany. **Y. Jaeger,** Department of Surgery, Presbyterian Hospital of Duesseldorf, Duesseldorf, Germany.

their native countries at a very young age. The percentages of non-Caucasian immigrant women who are HIV-1 positive are usually markedly higher than the percentages the groups represent in the total populations of the countries which they have immigrated (Brown et al., 1997).

In previous years, publications reported shorter survival times and a higher relative mortality risk for HIV-1-positive women (Cohen, 1997; Lemp et al., 1992; Melnick et al., 1994; Morlat et al., 1992). These observations could not be confirmed in more recent studies. However, the existence of sex- and gender-specific biological differences is accepted (Gilad et al., 2003), e.g., the influence of female hormones and cycle on the CD4$^+$ cell count and HIV-1 RNA plasma level (Montero et al., 2000; Harlow et al., 2000). According to most studies, women develop AIDS and die with higher CD4$^+$ cell counts and lower HIV-1 RNA levels than men (Foulkes and Deyton, 1999; Hewitt et al., 2001; Junghans et al., 1999a; Levine, 2002; Maini et al., 1996; Prins et al., 1999; Rezza et al., 2000). There are studies that document higher CD4$^+$ cell counts in women over the entire course of HIV-1 disease and others that show initial equality with a more rapid decline of the absolute CD4$^+$ cell count in females (Anastos et al., 2000; Cunningham et al., 2000; Delmas et al., 1997). With respect to the plasma viral load, too, there are sex- and gender-specific differences (Mellors et al., 1995; Coombs et al., 2003; Goodkin et al., 2004; Sterling et al., 2001). Especially in the beginning of HIV-1 disease, even if the data are stratified by age, risk group, CD4$^+$ cell count, and socioeconomic status, the plasma viral load in women is significantly lower than in men (Farzadegan et al., 1998; Gandhi et al., 2002). This is only true at the beginning of infection; later on, with falling CD4$^+$ cell counts, viral plasma levels equalize between males and females; this is due to a more accelerated course in women (Moroni, 1999; Kalish et al., 2000). Farzadegan in 1998 described a 1.6-fold-higher risk for women to progress to AIDS than for men at half the plasma viral load. Therefore, many authors emphasize the necessity for sex- and gender-adapted initiation of therapy (Gasiorowski et al., 2003; Seyler et al., 2003). Other important cofactors for disease progression and duration of HIV-1 disease are therapy benefit and adherence. Generally, HIV-1-positive women start HAART more rarely and later than men (Anderson and Garnett, 2000; McDonald, 2000). This is not due to more difficult or absent access to the health system in different countries but to socioeconomic structures and a low confidence level among women in the benefit of HAART (McDonald, 2000; Mocroft et al., 2000). Once started on HAART, women show higher therapy adherence than men (Anderson and Garnett, 2000; Murphy et al., 2002, 2003; Roca et al., 2000; van Roon et al., 1999). Some studies have reported better therapy response with a more rapid suppression of the plasma viral load and a longer-lasting benefit in females (Jensen-Fangel et al., 2002; Finkel et al., 2003; Mayer et al., 2003; Moore et al., 2001), while others found a less adequate therapy response; however, the majority of the studies did not find greater effectiveness and benefit of HAART in women (Junghans et al., 1999b; Moore et al., 2002; Powderly et al., 1999; Zorrilla, 2000). However, there was definitely a higher frequency of HAART side effects (Currier et al., 2000; Duval et al., 2004; Lucas et al., 1999; Montessori et al., 2004); furthermore, the side effects were more severe than in men, e.g., lipodystrophy (Nolan and Mallal, 2001; Tershakovec et al., 2004), lactic acidosis (Fleischer et al., 2004), rash, elevation of liver enzymes, dyslipidemia, and insulin resistance (Dong et al., 1999; Ofotokun and Pomeroy, 2003; Petit et al., 2002;

Scarsi and Postelnick, 2003). The reasons for these sex differences may include differences between males and females in body mass index, fat composition, and hormonal effects of drug metabolism or the effects of genomic constitutional differences on the levels of various enzymes. Thus, there are studies that propose the hypothesis that women lose part of their natural protection from atherosclerosis during antiretroviral therapy (Pernerstorfer-Schoen et al., 2001). There have also been speculations about pharmacokinetic differences, but these have not been confirmed in well-designed studies (de Maat et al., 2004). All in all, survival rates and HAART benefits are comparable in Africa and in the Western industrialized countries between males and females (Frater et al., 2002). A study by Gantke et al. (1999) even outlined a longer survival time for women under therapy, a result that was confirmed by the analysis of a cohort of 253 women (our unpublished data). This development might be due to an adaptation of care for HIV-1-positive women during the last years, e.g., new drugs, prophylaxis of opportunistic infections, sex- and gender-adapted initiation of HAART, and intensification in providing information and education (Arendt et al., 2001; Box et al., 2003; Wilson, 2001), as well as social support, based on the knowledge that stigma, lack of social support, and depression (Schulte et al., 2000) negatively influence therapy adherence, especially in women (Davidson et al., 1998; Trzynka and Erlen, 2004).

NEURO-AIDS CONDITIONS

HIV can affect the central and peripheral nervous system directly, provoking neurological signs and symptoms, and indirectly by causing immunodeficiency and thus susceptibility to infections with opportunistic infectious bodies. HIV-1 can provoke many neurological diseases, such as HIV-1-associated dementia (HAD), also called AIDS dementia complex, and its precursors, asymptomatic neurocognitive impairment (ANI) and mild neurocognitive disorder (MNCD), and HIV-1-associated myelopathy, as well as different forms of polyneuropathies and myopathies. The opportunistic infections have declined in incidence and prevalence in the era of HAART, whereas directly virus-associated manifestations tend to occur at higher prevalence rates due to patients' longer survival times. This is true for male and female cohorts (Sacktor, 2002).

HAD

HAD commonly develops in parallel with severe immunosuppression (Stern et al., 2001; Stoskopf et al., 2001). Risk factors include high HIV "set points" early during the course of the infection, a low body mass index, age, low CD4$^+$ cell counts, intravenous (i.v.) drug abuse, and female sex (Chiesi et al., 1996). The relevance of the plasma and cerebrospinal fluid (CSF) viral loads for the development of HAD is controversial. Host genetic factors may play a role.

The precursor stages of HAD, ANI and MNCD, occur at about 20% (Janssen et al., 1989; Antinori et al., 2007) in American and at up to 50% in European studies. Different methods for monitoring these deficits, the fact that women were included in the European cohort, and different virus types may account for this difference. MNCD is an important complication of HIV infection, because it reduces adherence and predicts HAD (Arendt et al., 1994). The incidence of HAD has declined in the era of HAART (Bouwman et al., 1998), but in 2002, prevalence rates began to rise again due to the longer survival time of

HIV-1-positive patients (Dore et al., 2003). Severity and progression are attenuated by HAART (Sacktor et al., 2002).

Classical HAD in an untreated patient develops over several months. Patients suffer from cognitive, motor, and emotional deficits, i.e., they present a subcortical form of dementia. Later, they have spastic tetraparesis, incontinence, and mutism. Currently, HAART-treated patients present with milder deficits of mostly cortical origin. Confounding factors with respect to HAD are age, cerebrovascular or infectious disease (hepatitis C), and psychiatric comorbidity.

Neuropsychological tests, including examination of psychomotor speed, are the best tools to detect HIV-1-associated abnormalities in the early stages (Antinori et al., 2007).

It is helpful that screening batteries allowing short-term examination of HIV-1 carriers in clinical practice have been established, because many deficits remain undiagnosed. Neuropsychological tests, like the trail-making or grooved-pegboard test, as well as analysis of fine motor speed (Arendt et al., 1992), are simple tools fulfilling "short and cheap" criteria.

There are subtypes of HAD, such as demyelinating leukoencephalopathy in those patients for whom HAART fails, characterized by extensive white-matter destruction and central nervous system infiltration with infected macrophages, immune reconstitution inflammatory syndrome in patients recovering from high plasma viral loads and low $CD4^+$ cell counts under HAART, and a vacuolar leukoencephalopathy resembling HIV-1-associated vacuolar myelopathy.

The most important diagnostic studies for HAD besides neuropsychological testing are imaging procedures and CSF analysis.

Neuroimaging techniques include routine magnetic resonance tomography showing echointensive spots in the deep grey matter (especially, and early, in the basal ganglia) and cortical and central atrophy, as well as confluent white-matter lesions; the last tend to be reversible under HAART. Magnetic resonance spectroscopy shows increased choline levels as a sign of glial activation in early stages (von Giesen et al., 2001); in later stages of HAD, reductions in N-acetyl-D-aspartate provide hints of neuronal injury.

CSF analysis is not integrated in routine diagnostics of HAD and is performed to exclude cerebral opportunistic infections. Nevertheless, abnormalities are often found in HAD, like slight pleocytosis and elevated protein content and immunoglobulin G, as well as oligoclonal bands, elevated viral loads, and immune activation markers. As more recent studies point out (Arendt et al., 2007), there is a subgroup of HIV-1 carriers with higher CSF than plasma viral loads, often those who are not treated with HAART because of a more or less stable immune status and only a moderate elevation of the plasma viral load. These patients escape diagnosis and often reveal neurological signs and symptoms. Thus, lumbar puncture should be integrated into the routine diagnostic procedures in patients with a good immune status but elevated plasma viral loads (between 20,000 and 50,000 copies/ml) (Towfighi et al., 2004), especially because a decline in the CSF viral load is correlated with clinical improvement of patients. Most of the activated immune markers (neopterin, β_2-microglobulin, quinolinic acid, and Fas ligands) are also correlated with clinical deficits but have not been examined in patients undergoing HAART.

Nothing is known so far about possible differences in CSF viral loads between men and women. On the whole, studies of neuro-AIDS conditions in women and how they possibly differ from men are scarce. Chiesi and coworkers (1996) found that females have a higher risk of developing HAD than men, but these data are based on research before the HAART era. A study published a few years later (Gantke et al., 1999) could not find different outcomes for women and men with respect to neurocognitive deficits. A small study by Stern and coworkers (1998) detected no differences between performances in neurocognitive tests by 17 asymptomatic HIV-1-positive women and 14 seronegative controls, but the authors themselves said that larger sample sizes are necessary to verify these results. The authors also emphasized that in such studies, careful attention must be paid to possible confounding or masking variables, like age, education level, ethnicity, head injury, psychological distress, and drug abuse.

There have been two studies analyzing the effect of HAART on neurocognitive performance in HIV-1-positive women. Richardson and coworkers (2002) emphasized that women under therapy showed less cognitive impairment than those without HAART; a previous study (Cohen et al., 2001) found this beneficial effect only in women with severely impaired immune systems under long-term treatment (longer than 18 months).

Osowiecki and colleagues (2000) pointed out that neurocognitive functioning and emotional status strongly influence the quality of life in women living with HIV/AIDS.

However, it is interesting that there are large cohort studies that analyze neurological disorders in homosexual and bisexual men (e.g., the Multicenter AIDS Cohort Study in the United States), but even large studies like the Women's Interagency HIV Study do not automatically examine neuro-AIDS conditions but leave them to surprisingly small substudies (Hughes, 2002; Richardson et al., 2002).

Thus, a summary article in the *Journal of the American Medical Association* in 2001 (Hader et al., 2001) said that existing knowledge should be used to improve the clinical care of HIV-infected women by enhancing the use of available services, including greater use of antiretroviral therapy options, treating depression and drug abuse, facilitating educational efforts, and providing social support.

HIV-1-Associated Sensory Neuropathies

The peripheral nervous system can be involved in different ways in HIV-1 infection, for example, in mononeuritis, vasculitic neuropathy, inflammatory demyelinating polyneuropathy, motor neuron disease, and polymyositis. One of the most frequently occurring forms is HIV-1-associated sensory neuropathy, which includes two entities, i.e., distal sensory polyneuropathy and toxic neuropathy caused by antiretroviral therapy. Although there are publications indicating a higher rate of side effects in women, prospective studies examining this with respect to toxic polyneuropathy caused by antiretrovirals in females are lacking. Clinically, distal sensory polyneuropathy cannot be distinguished from the toxic form, but the latter may provoke clinical symptoms in cases of a preexisting, silent, virus-associated form. The prevalence of the sensory form is much higher in AIDS-diagnosed patients (Barohn et al., 1993). The risk factors are age, alcohol abuse, nutritional deficits, and a low $CD4^+$ cell count, as well as high viral loads at seroconversion, which make it likely that women could be more frequently and severely affected than men.

Distal sensory neuropathy is characterized by axonal degeneration of sensory fibers (M. Polydefkis, A. Brown, P. Hauer, J. Griffin, and J. McArthur, presented at the 12th

Conference on Retroviruses and Opportunistic Infections, February 2005, Boston, MA). Large myelinated and unmyelinated fibers are affected, so the sensory neuropathy associated with HIV-1 can be differentiated from diseases like diabetes, which predominantly involve small sensory fibers. In HIV-1-associated neuropathy, the rostral gracile tract and the distal axon terminals degenerate. The neuropathological characteristics are inflammatory infiltrates of lymphocytes and macrophages with the presence of proinflammatory cytokines and nitric oxide. The changes in the toxic neuropathy of HIV-1-infected patients have not been intensively studied. It is caused by the so-called D-drugs (dideoxycytosine [ddC], dideoxyinosine [ddI], and stavudine [d4T]), which provoke mitochondrial toxicity by inhibition of the mitochondrial DNA γ-polymerase, limiting the use of these drugs. Therapeutically, tricyclic antidepressants, anticonvulsants, and narcotics are used.

The HIV-1/AIDS-associated neurological manifestations increase with more intensive use of HAART and longer survival of affected people, including women. Thus, it is mandatory to gather more details on women developing neurological complications due to the virus itself or to HAART.

SEX- AND GENDER-SPECIFIC DATA ANALYSIS IN A GERMAN COHORT OF WOMEN LIVING WITH HIV/AIDS

Out of a cohort of 1,926 individuals living with HIV/AIDS, 250 HIV-1-positive women were analyzed for neurological disease and compared to a subgroup of 1,676 men. At first presentation in the neurological outpatient department for individuals living with HIV/AIDS, the average age of the female group was 38.56 ± 9.73 years and the average age at diagnosis of HIV-1-positivity was 35.06 ± 10.20 years. Thus, when they first presented in a neurological department, diagnosis of HIV-1 positivity had been made 1 month to 17 years earlier.

Table 1 shows the average age of the female group compared to the male group. Of the 250 HIV-1-positive women, 84.8% were Caucasian and 15.2% were non-Caucasian; there was no difference in age or in the duration of HIV-1 positivity. Diagnosis of HIV-1 positivity had been made during pregnancy, because in Germany, tests are offered to every pregnant woman. This is one reason why the whole women's cohort (Caucasians and non-Caucasians) was significantly younger than the male group (Caucasians and non-Caucasians). In contrast, the whole non-Caucasian group (38 females and 54 males) showed no male/female

difference with respect to age (Table 1), probably because immigrants are young people regardless of sex.

In the female subcohort, 67.59% had been infected by heterosexual intercourse, 27.27% by i.v. drug abuse, and 4.74% by blood transfusion; in the male subcohort, men having sex with men were the largest group, followed by those infected through heterosexual intercourse, with the latter representing the largest group among non-Caucasian males. When the participants were stratified by risk groups, again, younger age of women infected by heterosexual intercourse could be observed compared to men (Table 1). However, whereas there were no statistically significant differences in age in stratification by risk groups between Caucasian and non-Caucasian women, non-Caucasian men were definitely younger than Caucasians when first diagnosed as HIV-1 carriers (Table 1). The mean age at diagnosis of HIV-1 positivity stratified by all represented risk groups and sex, including Caucasians and non-Caucasians, revealed the oldest age in transfusion patients and the youngest in i.v. drug-abusing individuals for females and the oldest age in bisexual men (Table 1).

The mean duration of HIV disease was defined by the time from diagnosis of HIV-1 positivity until death and did not differ in 48 women and 459 males who died during the observation period (ending on 31 December 2001) or in Caucasians and non-Caucasians, supporting the hypothesis that once integrated into the health system of the receiving country, immigrants had about the same prognosis as non-immigrants (Gantke et al., 1999). However, when stratification was by sex and risk group only, there was a statistically significant difference with respect to the duration of disease between heterosexual females and female i.v. drug abusers and also between female heterosexuals and women who became infected by blood products (Table 2). This might have been due to the fact that heterosexual females are generally diagnosed in more advanced disease stages than those women who obviously belong to risk groups and are integrated early into health programs. There might be other reasons, but this must be subject to further research.

Also among men, heterosexuals died earlier than individuals from other risk groups (Table 2). This might be due to the same reason as for women, i.e., the time to diagnosis of HIV-1 positivity is longer in heterosexuals if they do not obviously belong to one of the known risk groups.

When the risk of death in the whole cohort was analyzed, the data revealed that significantly more men than women died in the same time interval (Table 3). χ^2 analysis underlined the fact that among women, significantly fewer patients actually died than would have been statistically expected ($n = 49$; statistically expected, 66.3; χ^2, 7.035; $P = 0.008$), whereas among men observed deaths corresponded to the statistically expected number ($n = 461$;

TABLE 1 Mean age of HIV-1-positive cohort at diagnosis

Subgroup of cohort	Mean age (yr)	
	Men	Women
All	35.5	32.1
Caucasian[a]	35.59	32.18
Risk groups		
Homosexual	35.19	
Bisexual	40.11	
Heterosexual[a]	39.36	32.76
Transfusion recipients	28.29	40.21
i.v. drug users	30.96	29.14

[a]Mean age at diagnosis of all heterosexual Caucasians, 41.13 years; of all heterosexual non-Caucasians, 32.74 years.

TABLE 2 Mean duration of HIV-1 positivity with respect to risk groups

Risk group	Time from diagnosis to death (yr)	
	Men	Women
Heterosexual	3.15	3.77
Transfusion recipients	7.21	4.55
i.v. drug users	7.71	8.25
Homosexual	5.24	
Bisexual	4.72	

TABLE 3 Death rate over 14 years

Group	Death rate (%) over time of study		
	Men	Women	Overall
Overall	27.2	19.4	
Caucasian	27.7	21.7	27
Non-Caucasian	14.5	7.3	11.5

statistically expected, 443.7). The relative risk of death was 0.676 for HIV-1-positive women and 1.054 for men, i.e., a one-third-lower risk for females to die from HIV/AIDS than for men.

Analysis of the risk of death in Caucasians and non-Caucasians independent of sex revealed that HIV-1-positive non-Caucasians had a 0.364 relative risk of death, while for Caucasians the relative risk was 1.040 (Table 3). This might be due to the fact that the relative risk of death in these patients was multifactorial and was influenced by age, viral set point, and vascular risk profile, among other things. This was also true when stratification by sex was added. Non-Caucasian women (n = 3; expected, n = 7.9) had only one-fourth as high a risk of death as Caucasians (n = 46; expected, n = 41.1) (Table 3). Again, the same was true for men, but to a lesser extent; the relative risk of death from HIV/AIDS was half as high in non-Caucasian as in Caucasian males (Table 3). With respect to sex, death, and age, women generally died at a younger age, especially non-Caucasians (Table 4). There was no such difference between Caucasian and non-Caucasian women, whereas non-Caucasian men died at a younger age than Caucasian males but at an older age than Caucasian females.

Additional stratification for risk groups revealed that heterosexual women died at a younger age than females infected by blood products and i.v. drug abuse (Table 4). Thus, heterosexually infected non-Caucasian women died at the youngest age, followed by heterosexually infected Caucasian females, who died earlier than heterosexually infected men (Table 4).

Other aspects in evaluating the cohort data were the incidence and prevalence of AIDS-defining diseases. During the observation period, AIDS-defining diseases occurred in 42.19% of all patients, i.e., in 821 individuals. The most frequent extracerebral opportunistic infections were as follows:

- *Pneumocystis carinii* pneumonia (PCP)
- Cytomegalovirus retinitis
- Typical and atypical mycobacterial infections
- *Candida* esophagitis

TABLE 4 Age at death

Group	Age (yr) at death			
	Men	Women	All Caucasian	All non-Caucasian
Mean	41.36	38.48	41.26	33.15
Risk groups				
Heterosexual	42.52	33.89		
Transfusion recipient		46.73		
i.v. drug user		39.84		

TABLE 5 Rates of AIDS and neuro-AIDS in HIV-1-positive cohort

Group	% of group with AIDS	% of AIDS group with neuro-AIDS manifestation
Overall		22.9
Men	44.12	22.05
Women	29.25	31.5
Caucasian	42.32	
Non-Caucasian	39.58	

- Wasting syndromes
- Kaposi's sarcoma

When the data were stratified by sex, it became clear that significantly fewer women than expected developed AIDS-defining diseases during the observation period and that the relative risk for getting an AIDS-defining disease was 1.082 for men and only 0.566 for women. Additional stratification for Caucasian and non-Caucasian origin revealed no differences (Table 5).

Neuro-AIDS Manifestations

The cohort was examined with respect to the development of a clinically overt dementia every year from 1987 to December 2001. During the first years, there was no difference between males and females, but from the sixth year on, there was clearly a higher tendency in women to develop HAD (Fig. 1). There was no additional difference between Caucasians and non-Caucasians.

Summarizing the most frequently occurring neurological manifestations in HIV-1 infection (ANI, MNCD, HAD, polyneuropathies, and cerebral opportunistic infections), in the beginning of the observation period, there was a 0.538 relative risk for developing neurological complications for HIV-1-positive women and 1.073 for men, i.e., a 50% lower relative risk for women. Over the years, males continuously tended to have more neurological diseases than females. There was no additional difference for Caucasians versus non-Caucasians. A total of 188 individuals developed a neurological disease manifestation; 165 of these patients were male and 23 female. Table 5 shows the percentage of neuro-AIDS manifestations in the cohort. χ^2 analysis showed 16.7 expected neuro-AIDS cases in men and 17.1 in women, so there was a tendency for developing more neuro-AIDS cases in women but no statistically significant differences in case frequency.

Table 5 compares the neuro-AIDS/AIDS cases in men and women and shows the higher percentage of neuro-AIDS manifestations in women compared to men. When the data were stratified by native countries and risk groups, there were no additional differences.

More generally, it can be derived from the data on this cohort that women have more HIV-1-associated central nervous system complications than men but less frequent polyneuropathies.

With respect to the course and severity of HIV-1-associated neurological disease in men and women, there were no differences; this corresponds to the results of a study by Robertson et al. (2004), who also found similar courses of HIV-1-associated neurological disease in males and females, as European studies had earlier (Gantke et al., 1999). Only Chiesi and colleagues (1996) found a higher dementia rate

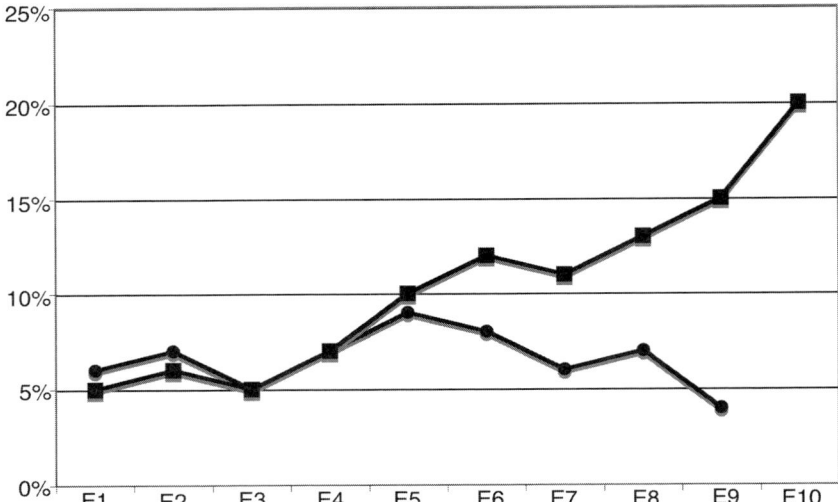

FIGURE 1   Percentages of HIV-1-positive females (squares) and males (circles) with HAD 2 to 10 yrs after diagnosis of HIV-1 positivity.

in women, which might be attributed to the fact that the data were collected in the pre-HAART era.

There is a common consensus that women and HIV disease should be subjected to further research and special care. Data must be analyzed according to ethnicity, as well as special socioeconomic and sociocultural circumstances.

Neuropsychiatric Aspects of the Care of HIV-1-Positive Women

Neurological diagnostic methods should be applied early in the course of HIV-1 infection in order to recognize early brain involvement, which makes initiation of antiretroviral therapy mandatory. Drugs should be able to penetrate into the CSF and have proven central nervous system effectiveness. This means that they should be able to suppress the CSF viral load and improve clinically overt neurological deficits in these patients. The latter is true for zidovudine, lamivudine, emtricitabine, stavudine, efavirenz, nevirapine, amprenavir/r, aztanavir/r, and lopinavir/r (where "r" indicates the drug is boosted by ritonavir). There is some controversy about whether it is really necessary for a drug to be able to penetrate into the CSF in order to effectively suppress the plasma viral load. However, there are subgroups of patients who show a higher viral load in the CSF than in the plasma, and these patients need reliable viral-load suppression in the CSF and, perhaps, additional treatment to protect the brain, which needs to be determined in the near future.

Brain involvement should be diagnosed by short and easily applicable screening methods in clinical practice, such as nonverbal neuropsychological tests (e.g., trail-making, grooved-pegboard, and Wisconsin card-sorting tests), as well as analysis of fine motor speed. These test procedures can be performed in 20 minutes and should be applied every 6 months for immunologically asymptomatic patients and every 3 months for AIDS-defined patients. Thus, HIV-1-related neurological disease could be diagnosed early and affected women could be integrated into special care systems. Here, immigrants could represent an especially problematic group because of cultural differences.

MIGRATION

Migration is a function of complex interactions between economic, social, political, and family factors. Among the most important, according to the international literature, are limited access to educational institutions, a subsequent occupational deficit, unfavorable social and political conditions in the native country, and the disregard of basic human rights. In many countries all over the world, women especially feel they would profit from emigration to other countries with a so-called "open society" with respect to educational and financial opportunities. On the other hand, the social position of a woman in every country in the world is defined by her role within a family and her relationship to a male partner. Thus, migration can place women, especially, in situations that create stress and fear due to loss of their social integration. Educational deficits make social integration into a new environment difficult or even impossible without the support of official institutions (Arendt et al., 2003; Carballo et al., 1996).

Higher vulnerability to sexual violence and abuse (Aday, 1994; McBride et al., 1999), as well as the frequently unavoidable descent into prostitution (Fenton et al., 2002), makes female immigrants one of the major risk groups for sexually transmissible diseases and infection with HIV (Gras et al., 1999; Greenblatt et al., 1999).

Furthermore, for female immigrants, health care procedures and preventive measures are neglected; that is why a high percentage of HIV-1 infections in this population are diagnosed during advanced pregnancy (late in the first trimester).

Generally, female immigrants know little about possible support in the countries to which they have immigrated and usually distrust official authorities (Montoya, 1998).

Heterosexual intercourse is the major source of infection (Robert-Koch-Institut, 2002). Official health authorities are not at all prepared to take care of this specific risk group, whose confidence must be gained in order to establish adequate medical care and prevention procedures. Especially in industrialized and densely populated regions, like the bigger cities, there is an urgent need for specifically trained health workers for female immigrants (Arendt et al., 2003).

In a retrospective study, data on 204 HIV-1-positive female immigrants from seven cities in North Rhine-Westphalia, one of the most populated regions in Germany, were analyzed and compared with those of 282 female German HIV carriers.

The following variables were analyzed: native country, age, duration of HIV-1 positivity, mode of infection, reason for testing, CDC stage, AIDS-defining disease at first presentation, mode of AIDS-defining disease, mode and duration of antiretroviral therapy, number of CD4$^+$ cells, and plasma viral load. All of the women who came to Germany from other European countries or countries outside of Europe and settled in Germany were defined as immigrants.

The majority of the immigrants ($n = 145$) came from equatorial Africa, 19 from Asia, 36 from European countries other than Germany, and 4 from Latin America. The mean age of the immigrants was 32.7 ± 7.7 years; the mean age of the control group was 36.7 ± 10.2 years and thus was significantly higher ($P < 0.0001$).

The risk group profile among the immigrants comprised 189 heterosexuals and 14 i.v. drug addicts; one patient had been infected by a blood transfusion. In the control group, 184 were heterosexual, 83 were i.v. drug addicts, and 15 had been infected by blood transfusions. This distribution was significantly different in a χ^2 table (χ^2 P value < 0.0001).

For more than 55% of the immigrants, the reason for HIV-1 testing was pregnancy; 49 immigrants were AIDS defined at first examination; in the control population, 78 females were AIDS defined (Table 6).

Distribution into the CDC stages did not differ significantly between immigrants and controls (χ^2 P value = 0.3579 in the contingency table). At first examination, 77 of the immigrants were not being treated with antiretroviral medication, 30 were on two-nucleoside combinations, and 97 were receiving HAART. In the control group, 131 women were not being treated, 60 were taking two nucleoside analogues, and 91 were receiving HAART. This distribution was also significantly different in χ^2 tables (P value < 0.0025).

The immigrant cohort was significantly more frequently treated with antiretroviral medication than the controls. This effect was not due to immigrant recruitment later during the course of the disease, as can be concluded from Table 1.

Mean CD4$^+$ cell counts from the last 3 months before the first examination for the present report in the outpatient departments were available for 189 individuals of the

TABLE 7 Mean CD4$^+$ values of migrant and the control groups[a]

CD4$^+$ value/μl	Immigrants [no. (%)][b]	Controls [no. (%)][b]
≥500	51 (27)	70 (27)
200–499	74 (39)	104 (40)
<200	64 (34)	85 (33)

[a]From Arendt et al., 2003.
[b]Means: immigrants, 352 ± 248; controls, 358 ± 273.

immigrant group and for 259 of the controls. Table 7 shows the number of CD4$^+$ cells in both groups.

At first presentation, there were no statistically significant differences in mean values or distribution of CD4$^+$ cells between the groups.

Plasma viral loads were available for 170 immigrants and 168 controls. There were no statistically significant differences between the groups.

Forty-nine immigrants could be assigned to CDC stage C, i.e., they had suffered from an AIDS-defining disease; this was true for 78 individuals of the control group. The AIDS-defining disease was known for 45 immigrants and 75 controls. Table 8 shows the AIDS-defining diseases of both groups.

A comparison of AIDS manifestations in both groups showed that tuberculosis was the most frequent AIDS manifestation in the immigrants, followed by PCP and *Candida* esophagitis, whereas tuberculosis was the AIDS-defining disease in only two members of the control group. Among the controls, PCP was the most frequent AIDS-defining disease, followed by *Candida* esophagitis. There was no high incidence of neurological disease in the migrant group, in contrast to a female cohort in one of the centers (see above).

This data analysis was one of the first that tried to work separately on HIV-1-infected immigrants' characteristics in Germany and thus detected some interesting facts. It must be emphasized that this was a descriptive, retrospective analysis, which accounts for the different patient numbers in the two groups.

As shown in the scarce literature (Robert-Koch-Institut, 2002), the majority of HIV infections in immigrants were

TABLE 6 CDC stages at first examination[a]

CDC stage	Immigrants [no. (%)]	Control group [no. (%)]	Total [no. (%)]
A1	20 (10)	41 (15)	61 (13)
A2	53 (26)	64 (23)	117 (24)
A3	18 (9)	18 (6)	36 (7)
B1	2 (1)	7 (2)	9 (2)
B2	33 (16)	37 (13)	70 (14)
B3	29 (14)	37 (13)	66 (14)
C1	0	2 (1)	2 (<1)
C2	5 (2)	4 (1)	9 (2)
C3	44 (22)	72 (26)	116 (24)
Total	204	282	486

[a]From Arendt et al., 2003.

TABLE 8 Numbers of patients with opportunistic infections in the immigrant and control groups

Infection	No. of immigrants ($n = 45$)	No. of controls ($n = 75$)
Tuberculosis	15	2
Toxoplasmosis	6	8
PCP	7	26
Candida esophagitis	7	19
HIV-associated dementia	2	8
CMV infection	1	2
PML	1	1
MAI	2	2
Carcinoma of the cervix	0	1
Cryptococcosis	2	1
Non-Hodgkin's lymphoma	2	3
Kaposi's sarcoma	1	0
Salmonellosis	1	1
Wasting syndrome	2	8
Zoster vasculitis	0	1

diagnosed during pregnancy and/or were associated with a previous history of sexually transmitted diseases (Fenton et al., 2002; van Haastrecht et al., 1993). Consequently, in this study, immigrants were not as frequently AIDS defined at first examination as in the German control group. Furthermore, the percentage of immigrants treated with antiretroviral medication at first presentation in hospital outpatient departments was considerably higher than in the control group. This could be due to the higher percentage of i.v. drug addicts in the control group, who often do not take antiretroviral drugs regularly, but also to the fact that immigrants were tested because of pregnancy and treated from that time on. In any case, the data did not support the hypothesis that immigrants are primarily not subsequently treated, at least not after having entered the medical care systems (for a pregnancy test or examination).

CD4$^+$ cell counts and plasma viral loads did not differ between the two groups. Obviously, there were no differences between ethnic groups, whereas the gender differences (females get AIDS at higher CD4$^+$ cell counts and lower plasma viral loads than males) have been described in the literature (Farzadegan et al., 1998), as outlined above. On the other hand, there are also hints in the literature that women have an even better outcome than men (Gantke et al., 1999). This might be due to infection with less aggressive virus subtypes, less frequent infections with several virus variants, and better adherence to medication.

The spectrum of AIDS-defining diseases was known only to a certain degree in both groups. Only with respect to tuberculosis was there a statistically significant difference between the groups. The percentage of immigrants ill with tuberculosis was considerably higher than that in the control group, which could be due to social and hygienic conditions in the native countries. The other AIDS-defining diseases were equally distributed in both groups so that obviously there were no group-specific infection patterns.

The data gave some hints that female immigrants are better integrated into health care systems than is generally presumed. However, it has to be taken into account that there might be many undiagnosed HIV infections in this population. Immigrants, regardless of sex, should be integrated not only into health care systems but also into social support structures to minimize the danger of spreading HIV infection.

Furthermore, the importance of prophylactic strategies against the HIV epidemic must be emphasized. Only confidence in health officials and representatives who take cultural aspects into account (McMunn et al., 1998; Nitschke-Ozbay, 1999) will be able to prevent the spread of the virus.

Additionally, it is important to collect and analyze data on immigrant populations in different countries, which should closely cooperate to improve medical care for this subpopulation. It is well known that methodological work is needed to derive standardized definitions of terms. The data in this study are a first attempt to develop uniform standards for evaluating and reporting data on the health status of so-called "vulnerable" populations (Aday, 1994). As stated with respect to other populations (Gras et al., 1999), culturally appropriate AIDS prevention programs are mandatory today in countries with immigrants, especially because there is evidence that perception of AIDS susceptibility may be an important motivator in reducing high-risk behaviors (McBride et al., 1999; McMunn et al., 1998).

The next step should include the design of prospective sex- and gender-matched studies of HIV-1-infected immigrants.

REFERENCES

Aday, L. 1994. Health status of vulnerable populations. *Annu. Rev. Public Health* **15**:487–509.

Anastos, K., S. J. Gange, B. Lau, B. Weiser, R. Detels, J. V. Giorgi, J. B. Margolick, M. Cohen, J. Phair, S. Melnick, C. R. Rinaldo, A. Kovacs, A. Levine, S. Landesman, M. Young, A. Munoz, and R. M. Greenblatt. 2000. Association of race and gender with HIV-1 RNA levels and immunologic progression. *J. Acquir. Immune Defic. Syndr.* **24**:218–26.

Anderson, R. M., and G. P. Garnett. 2000. Mathematical models of the transmission and control of sexually transmitted diseases. *Sex. Transm. Dis.* **27**:636–643.

Antinori, A., F. Baldini, E. Girardi, A. Cingolani, M. Zaccarelli, S. Di Giambenedetto, A. Barracchini, P. De Longis, R. Murri, V. Tozzi, A. Ammassari, M. G. Rizzo, G. Ippolito, and A. De Luca. 2001. Female sex and the use of anti-allergic agents increase the risk of developing cutaneous rash associated with nevirapine therapy. *AIDS* **15**:1579–1581.

Antinori, A., G. Arendt, J. T. Becker, B. J. Brew, D. A. Byrd, M. Cherner, D. B. Clifford, P. Cinque, L. G. Epstein, K. Goodkin, M. Gisslen, I. Grant, R. K. Heaton, J. Joseph, K. Marder, C. M. Marra, J. C. McArthur, M. Nunn, R. W. Price, L. Pulliam, K. R. Robertson, N. Sacktor, V. Valcour, and V. E. Wojna. 2007. Updated research nosology for HIV-associated neurocognitive disorders. *Neurology* **69**:1789–1799.

Arendt, G., TH. Nolting, C. Frisch, I. W. Husstedt, N. Gregor, E. Koutsilieri, M. Maschke, A. Angerer, M. Obermann, E. Neuen-Jacob, O. Adams, S. Loeffert, P. Riederer, V. ter Meulen, S. Sopper, and the Competence-Network HIV/AIDS. 2007. Intrathecal viral replication and cerebral deficits in different stages of human immunodeficiency virus disease. *J. Neurovirol.* **13**:225–232.

Arendt, G., H. J. von Giesen, and the HIV-Women's Forum Northrhine-Westphalia. 2003. HIV-1-positive female migrants in Northrhine-Westphalia—relevant, but unfocussed problem? *Eur. J. Med. Res.* **8**:137–141.

Arendt, G., A. M. Funke, and B. Gantke. 2001. Women and AIDS. HIV-positive patients need special monitoring. *MMW Fortschr. Med.* **143**(Suppl. 1):S68–S71. (In German.)

Arendt, G., H. Hefter, F. Hilperath, H. J. von Giesen, G. Strohmeyer, and H. J. Freund. 1994. Motor analysis predicts progression in HIV-associated brain disease. *J. Neurol. Sci.* **123**:180–185.

Arendt, G., H. Hefter, L. Buescher, F. Hilperath, C. Elsing, and H. J. Freund. 1992. Improvement of motor performance of HIV-positive patients under AZT therapy. *Neurology* **42**:891–896.

Barohn, R. J., G. S. Gronseth, B. R. LeForce, A. L. McVey, S. A. McGuire, C. A. Butzin, and R. B. King. 1993. Peripheral nervous system involvement in a large cohort of human immunodeficiency virus-infected individuals. *Arch. Neurol.* **50**:167–171.

Bazargan, M., E. M. Kelly, J. A. Stein, B. A. Husaini, and S. H. Bazargan. 2000. Correlates of HIV risk-taking behaviors among African-American college students: the effect of HIV knowledge, motivation, and behavioral skills. *J. Natl. Med. Assoc.* **92**:391–404.

Biber, C. L., M. A. Jaker, P. Kloser, S. B. Auerbach, and G. G. Rhoads. 1999. A study of sex differences in presentation for care of HIV. *AIDS Patient Care STDS* **13**:103–110.

Bouwman, F. H., R. L. Skolasky, D. Hes, O. A. Selnes, J. D. Glass, T. E. Nance-Sproson, W. Royal, G. J. Dal Pan, and J. C. McArthur. 1998. Variable progression of HIV-associated dementia. *Neurology* **50**:1814–1820.

Box, T. L., M. Olsen, E. Z. Oddone, and S. A. Keitz. 2003. Healthcare access and utilization by patients infected with human immunodeficiency virus: does gender matter? *J. Womens Health* **12**:391–397.

Brown, A. E., J. D. Malone, S. Y. Zhou, J. R. Lane, and C. A. Hawkes. 1997. Human immunodeficiency virus RNA levels in US adults: a comparison based upon race and ethnicity. *J. Infect. Dis.* **176:**794–797.

Carballo, M., M. Grocutt, and A. Hadzihasanovic. 1996. Women and migration: a public health issue. *World Health Stat. Q.* **49:**158–164.

Chiesi, A., S. Vella, L. G. Dally, C. Pedersen, S. Danner, A. M. Johnson, S. Schwander, F. D. Goebel, M. Glauser, F. Antunes, et al. 1996. Epidemiology of AIDS dementia complex in Europe. *J. Acquir. Immune Defic. Syndr. Hum. Retrovirol.* **11:**39–44.

Cohen, M. 1997. Natural history of HIV infection in women. *Obstet. Gynecol. Clin. N. Am.* **24:**743–758.

Cohen, R. A., R. Boland, R. Paul, K. T. Tashima, E. E. Schoenbaum, D. D. Celentano, P. Schuman, D. K. Smith, and C. C. Carpenter. 2001. Neurocognitive performance enhanced by highly antiretroviral therapy in HIV-infected women. *AIDS* **15:**341–345.

Coombs, R. W., P. S. Reichelderfer, and A. L. Landay. 2003. Recent observations on HIV type-1 infection in the genital tract of men and women. *AIDS* **17:**455–480.

Cornelius, L. J., J. N. Okundaye, and M. C. Manning. 2000. Human immunodeficiency virus-related risk behavior among African-American females. *J. Natl. Med. Assoc.* **92:**183–195.

Cunningham, W. E., D. M. Mosen, L. S. Morales, R. M. Andersen, M. F. Shapiro, and R. D. Hays. 2000. Ethnic and racial differences in long-term survival from hospitalization for HIV infection. *J. Health Care Poor Underserved* **11:**163–178.

Currier, J. S., C. Spino, J. Grimes, C. B. Wofsy, D. A. Katzenstein, M. D. Hughes, S. M. Hammer, D. J. Cotton, et al. 2000. Differences between women and men in adverse events and CD4⁺ responses to nucleoside analogue therapy for HIV infection. *J. Acquir. Immune Defic. Syndr.* **24:**316–324.

Davidson, A. J., S. L. Bertram, D. C. Lezotte, W. M. Marine, C. A. Rietmeijer, B. B. Hagglund, and D. L. Cohn. 1998. Comparison of health status, socioeconomic characteristics, and knowledge and use of HIV-related resources between HIV-infected women and men. *Med. Care* **36:**1676–1684.

Delmas, M. C., C. Jadand, I. De Vincenzi, C. Deveau, A. Persoz, A. Sobel, M. Kazatchkine, J. B. Brunet, L. Meyer, et al. 1997. Gender differences in CD4⁺ cell counts persist after HIV-1 infection. *AIDS* **11:**1071–1073.

de Maat, M. M., J. F. Nellen, A. D. Huitema, F. W. Wit, J. W. Mulder, J. M. Prins, and J. H. Beijnen. 2004. Race is not associated with nevirapine pharmacokinetics. *Ther. Drug Monit.* **26:**456–458.

Dong, K. L., L. L. Bausserman, M. M. Flynn, B. P. Dickinson, T. P. Flanigan, M. D. Mileno, K. T. Tashima, and C. C. Carpenter. 1999. Changes in body habitus and serum lipid abnormalities in HIV-positive women on highly active antiretroviral therapy (HAART). *J. Acquir. Immune Defic. Syndr.* **21:**107–113.

Dore, G. J., A. McDonald, Y. Li, J. M. Kaldor, B. J. Brew, and the National HIV Surveillance Committee. 2003. Marked improvement in survival following AIDS dementia complex in the era of highly active antiretroviral therapy. *AIDS* **17:**1539–1545.

Dunkle, K. L., R. K. Jewkes, H. C. Brown, G. E. Gray, J. A. McIntryre, and S. D. Harlow. 2004. Gender-based violence, relationship power, and risk of HIV infection in women attending antenatal clinics in South Africa. *Lancet* **363:**1415–1421.

Duval, X., V. Journot, C. Leport, G. Chene, M. Dupon, L. Cuzin, T. May, P. Morlat, A. Waldner, R. Salamon, F. Raffi, and the Antiprotease Cohort (APROCO) Study Group. 2004. Incidence of and risk factors for adverse drug reactions in a prospective cohort of HIV-infected adults initiating protease inhibitor-containing therapy. *Clin. Infect. Dis.* **39:**248–255.

Farzadegan, H., D. R. Hoover, J. Astemborski, C. M. Lyles, J. B. Margolick, R. B. Markham, T. C. Quinn, and D. Vlahov. 1998. Sex differences in HIV-1 viral load and progression to AIDS. *Lancet* **352:**1510–1514.

Fenton, K. A., M. Chinouya, O. Davidson, A. Copas, and the MAYISHA Study Team. 2002. HIV testing and high risk sexual behaviour among London's migrant African communities: a participatory research study. *Sex. Transm. Infect.* **78:**241–245.

Finkel, D. G., G. John, B. Holland, J. Slim, and S. M. Smith. 2003. Women have a greater immunological response to effective virological HIV-1 therapy. *AIDS* **17:**2009–2011.

Fleischer, R., D. Boxwell, and K. E. Sherman. 2004. Nucleoside analogues and mitochondrial toxicity. *Clin. Infect. Dis.* **38:**79–80.

Foulkes, M. A., and L. Deyton. 1999. Sex differences in HIV-1 viral load and progression to AIDS. *Lancet* **353:**590–591.

Frater, A. J., D. T. Dunn, A. J. Beardall, K. Ariyoshi, J. R. Clarke, M. O. McClure, and J. N. Weber. 2002. Comparative response of African HIV-1-infected individuals to highly active antiretroviral therapy. *AIDS* **16:**1139–1146.

Gandhi, M., P. Bacchetti, P. Miotti, T. C. Quinn, F. Veronese, and R. M. Greenblatt. 2002. Does patient sex affect human immunodeficiency virus levels? *Clin. Infect. Dis.* **35:**313–322. (Erratum, 35:1455.)

Gantke, B., A. M. Funke, and G. Arendt. 1999. Clinical outcome of a cohort of Caucasian HIV-1-seropositive women under ART/HAART, *7th Eur. Conf. Clin. Aspects Treat. HIV Infect.*, Lisbon, Portugal.

Gasiorowski, J., B. Knysz, and A. Gladysz. 2003. Epidemiological, clinical, immunological and virological characteristics of HIV-1 infected patients at the moment of initiation of antiretroviral therapy. *Przegl Epidemiol.* **57:**449–458.

Gilad, J., A. Walfisch, A. Borer, and F. Schlaeffer. 2003. Gender differences and sex-specific manifestations associated with human immunodeficiency virus infection in women. *Eur. J. Obstet. Gynecol. Reprod. Biol.* **109:**199–205.

Gollub, E. L., D. Rey, Y. Obadia, J. P. Moatti, et al. 2000. Gender differences in risk behaviors among HIV+ persons with an IDU history. The link between partner characteristics and women's higher drug-sex risks. *Sex. Transm. Dis.* **25:**483–488.

Goodkin, K., P. Shapshak, D. Asthana, W. Zheng, M. Concha, F. L. Wilkie, R. Molina, D. Lee, P. Suarez, S. Symes, and I. Khamis. 2004. Older age and plasma viral load in HIV-1 infection. *AIDS* **18**(Suppl. 1):S87–S98.

Goodkin, K., T. Heckman, K. Siegel, N. Linsk, I. Khamis, D. Lee, R. Lecusay, C. C. Poindexter, S. J. Mason, P. Suarez, and C. Eisdorfer. 2003. "Putting a face" on HIV infection/AIDS in older adults: a psychosocial context. *J. Acquir. Immune Defic. Syndr.* **33**(Suppl. 2):S171–S184.

Gras, M. J., J. F. Weide, M. W. Langendam, R. A. Coutinho, and A. van den Hoek. 1999. HIV prevalence, sexual risk behaviour and sexual mixing patterns among migrants in Amsterdam, The Netherlands. *AIDS* **13:**1953–1962.

Greenblatt, R. M., P. Bacchetti, S. Barkan, M. Augenbraun, S. Silver, R. Delapenha, P. Garcia, U. Mathur, P. Miotti, and D. Burns. 1999. Lower genital tract infections among HIV-infected and high-risk uninfected women: findings of the Women's Interagency HIV Study (WIHS). *Sex. Transm. Dis.* **26:**143–151.

Gupta, G. R., E. Weiss, and D. Whelan. 1995. Male-female inequalities result in submission to high-risk sex in many societies. Special report: women and HIV. *AIDS Anal. Afr.* **5:**8–9.

Hader, S. L., D. K. Smith, J. S. Moore, and S. D. Holmberg. 2001. HIV infection in women in the United States: status at the Millennium. *JAMA* **285:**1186–1192.

Harlow, S. D., P. Schuman, M. Cohen, S. E. Ohmit, S. Cu-Uvin, X. Lin, K. Anastos, D. Burns, R. Greenblatt, H. Minkoff, L. Muderspach, A. Rompalo, D. Warren, M. A. Young, and R. S. Klein. 2000. Effect of HIV infection on menstrual cycle length. *J. Acquir. Immune Defic. Syndr.* **24:**68–75.

Hewitt, R. G., N. Parsa, and L. Gugino. 2001. Women's health. The role of gender in HIV progression. *AIDS Read.* **11:**29–33.

Hughes, M. 2002. The Women's Interagency HIV Study (WIHS): research findings. *Surviv. News* **1:**1.

Jaffe, H. 2000. Changing epidemiology of HIV. *Int. J. Clin. Pract. Suppl.* **115:**72–77.

Janssen, R. S., D. R. Cornblath, L. G. Epstein, J. McArthur, and R. W. Price. 1989. Human immunodeficiency virus (HIV) infection and the nervous system: report from the American Academy of Neurology AIDS Task Force. *Neurology* **39:**119–122.

Jensen-Fangel, S., L. Pedersen, C. Pedersen, C. S. Larsen, P. Tauris, A. Moller, H. T. Sorensen, and N. Obel. 2002. The effect of race/ethnicity on the outcome of highly active antiretroviral therapy for human immunodeficiency virus type 1-infected patients. *Clin. Infect. Dis.* **35:**1541–1548.

Junghans, C., B. Ledergerber, P. Chan, R. Weber, M. Egger, et al. 1999a. Sex differences in HIV-1 viral load and progression to AIDS. *Lancet* **353:**589.

Junghans, C., N. Low, P. Chan, A. Witschi, P. Vernazza, and M. Egger. 1999b. Uniform risk of clinical progression despite differences in utilization of highly active antiretroviral therapy: Swiss HIV Cohort Study. *AIDS* **13:**2547–2554.

Kalish, L. A., A. C. Collier, T. P. Flanigan, and P. N. Kumar. 2000. Plasma human immunodeficiency virus (HIV) type 1 RNA load in men and women with advanced HIV-1 disease. *J. Infect. Dis.* **182:**603–606.

Krantz, S. R., D. A. Lynch, and J. M. Russell. 2002. Gender-specific profiles of self-reported adolescent HIV risk behaviors. *J. Assoc. Nurses AIDS Care* **13:**25–33.

Lemp, G. F., A. M. Hirozawa, J. B. Cohen, P. A. Derish, K. C. McKinney, and S. R. Hernandez. 1992. Survival for women and men with AIDS. *J. Infect. Dis.* **166:**74–79.

Levine, A. M. 2002. Evaluation and management of HIV-infected women. *Ann. Intern. Med.* **136:**228–242.

Lichtenstein, B., M. K. Laska, and J. M. Clair. 2002. Chronic sorrow in the HIV-positive patient: issues of race, gender, and social support. *AIDS Patient Care STDS* **16:**27–38.

Lucas, G. M., R. E. Chaisson, and R. D. Moore. 1999. Highly active antiretroviral therapy in a large urban clinic: risk factors for virologic failure and adverse drug reactions. *Ann. Intern. Med.* **131:**81–87.

Mahathir, M. 1997. Women at greater risk of HIV infection. *Arrows Change* **3:**1–2.

Maini, M. K., R. J. Gilson, N. Chavda, S. Gill, A. Fakoya, E. J. Ross, A. N. Phillips, and I. V. Weller. 1996. Reference ranges and sources of variability of CD4 counts in HIV-seronegative women and men. *Genitourin. Med.* **72:**27–31.

Marlink, R., H. Kao, and E. Hsieh. 2001. "Giving Voice to a Silent Epidemic" Working Group. Clinical care issues for women living with HIV and AIDS in the United States. *AIDS Res. Hum. Retrovir.* **17:**1–33.

Mayer, K. H., J. W. Hogan, D. Smith, R. S. Klein, P. Schuman, J. B. Margolick, C. Korkontzelou, H. Farzedegan, D. Vlahov, C. C. Carpenter, and the HIV Epidemiology Research Study (HERS) Group. 2003. Clinical and immunologic progression in HIV-infected US women before and after the introduction of highly active antiretroviral therapy. *J. Acquir. Immune Defic. Syndr.* **33:**614–624.

McBride, D. C., N. L. Weatherby, J. A. Inciardi, and S. A. Gillespie. 1999. AIDS susceptibility in a migrant population: perception and behavior. *Subst. Use Misuse* **34:**633–652.

McDonald, A. 2000. HIV infection, AIDS, hepatitis C, and sexually transmissible infections in Australia: national surveillance results to December 1998. *N. S. W. Public Health Bull.* **11:**58–60.

McMunn, A. M., R. Mwanje, K. Paine, and A. L. Pozniak. 1998. Health service utilization in London's African migrant communities: implications for HIV prevention. *AIDS Care* **10:**453–462.

Mellors, J. W., L. A. Kingsley, C. R. Rinaldo, J. A. Todd, B. S. Hoo, R. P. Kokka, and P. Gupta. 1995. Quantitation of HIV-1 RNA in plasma predicts outcome after seroconversion. *Ann. Intern. Med.* **122:**573–579.

Melnick, S. L., R. Sherer, T. A. Louis, D. Hillman, E. M. Rodriguez, C. Lackman, L. Capps, L. S. Brown, Jr., M. Carlyn, J. A. Korvick, et al. 1994. Survival and disease progression according to gender of patients with HIV infection. *JAMA* **272:**1915–1921.

Miller, C. L., P. M. Spittal, N. LaLiberte, K. Li, M. W. Tyndall, M. V. O'Shaughnessy, and M. T. Schechter. 2002. Females experiencing sexual and drug vulnerabilities are at elevated risk for HIV infection among youth who use injection drugs. *J. Acquir. Immune Defic. Syndr.* **30:**335–341.

Mize, S. J., B. E. Robinson, W. O. Bockting, and K. E. Scheltema. 2002. Meta-analysis of the effectiveness of HIV prevention interventions for women. *AIDS Care* **14:**163–180.

Mocroft, A., M. J. Gill, W. Davidson, and A. N. Phillips. 2000. Are there gender differences in starting protease inhibitors, HAART, and disease progression despite equal access to care? *J. Acquir. Immune Defic. Syndr.* **24:**475–482.

Montero, A., A. G. Giovannoni, and L. Sen. 2000. Hyperprolactinemia is a frequent finding in HIV infection but does not correlate with viral burden. *Medicina* **60:**427–430. (In Spanish.)

Montessori, V., N. Press, M. Harris, L. Akagi, and J. S. Montaner. 2004. Adverse effects of antiretroviral therapy for HIV infection. *Can. Med. Assoc. J.* **170:**229–238.

Montoya, I. D. 1998. Social network ties, self-efficacy, and condom use among women who use crack cocaine: a pilot study. *Subst. Use Misuse* **33:**2049–2073.

Montoya, I. D. 2004. Topography as a contextual variable in infectious disease transmission. *Clin. Lab. Sci.* **17:**95–101.

Moore, A. L., C. A. Sabin, M. A. Johnson, and A. N. Phillips. 2002. Gender and clinical outcomes after starting highly active antiretroviral treatment: a cohort study. *J. Acquir. Immune Defic. Syndr.* **29:**197–202.

Moore, A. L., A. Mocroft, S. Madge, H. Devereux, D. Wilson, A. N. Phillips, and M. Johnson. 2001. Gender differences in virologic response to treatment in an HIV-positive population: a cohort study. *J. Acquir. Immune Defic. Syndr.* **26:**159–163.

Morlat, P., P. Parneix, D. Douard, D. Lacoste, M. Dupon, G. Chene, J. L. Pellegrin, J. M. Ragnaud, F. Dabis, et al. 1992. Women and HIV infection: a cohort study of 483 HIV-infected women in Bordeaux, France, 1985–1991. *AIDS* **6:**1187–1193.

Moroni, M. 1999. Sex differences in HIV-1 viral load and progression to AIDS. ICONA Study Group. Italian cohort of HIV-1 positive individuals. *Lancet* **353:**589–591.

Murphy, D. A., M. Sarr, S. J. Durako, A. B. Moscicki, C. M. Wilson, L. R. Muenz, and the Adolescent Medicine HIV/AIDS Research Network. 2003. Barriers to HAART adherence among human immunodeficiency virus-infected adolescents. *Arch. Pediatr. Adolesc. Med.* **157:**249–255.

Murphy, D. A., L. Greenwell, and D. Hoffman. 2002. Factors associated with antiretroviral adherence among HIV-infected women with children. *Women Health* **36:**97–111.

Newman, P. A., and M. A. Zimmerman. 2000. Gender differences in HIV-related sexual risk behavior among urban

African American youth: a multivariate approach. *AIDS Educ. Prev.* **12:**308–325.

Nicolosi, A., M. L. Correa Leite, M. Musicco, C. Arici, G. Gavazzeni, A. Lazzarin, et al. 1994. The efficiency of male-to-female and female-to-male sexual transmission of the human immunodeficiency virus: a study of 730 stable couples. **5:**570–575.

Nitschke-Ozbay, H. 1999. HIV prevention for migrant prostitutes. *Zentralbl. Gynakol.* **121:**36–41. (In German.)

Nolan, D., and S. Mallal. 2001. Effects of sex and race on lipodystrophy pathogenesis. *J. HIV Ther.* **6:**32–36.

Ofotokun, I., and C. Pomeroy. 2003. Sex differences in adverse reactions to antiretroviral drugs. *Top. HIV Med.* **11:**55–59.

Osowiecki, D. M., R. A. Cohen, K. M. Morrow, R. H. Paul, C. C. Carpenter, T. Flanigan, and R. J. Boland. 2000. Neurocognitive and psychological contributions to quality of life in HIV-1-infected women. *AIDS* **7:**1327–1332.

Pernerstorfer-Schoen, H., B. Jilma, A. Perschler, S. Wichlas, K. Schindler, A. Schindl, A. Rieger, O. F. Wagner, and P. Quehenberger. 2001. Sex differences in HAART-associated dyslipidaemia. *AIDS* **15:**725–734.

Petit, J. M., M. Duong, L. Duvillard, E. Florentin, H. Portier, G. Lizard, J. M. Brun, P. Gambert, and B. Verges. 2002. LDL-receptors expression in HIV-infected patients: relations to antiretroviral therapy, hormonal status, and presence of lipodystrophy. *Eur. J. Clin. Investig.* **32:**354–359.

Powderly, W. G., M. S. Saag, S. Chapman, G. Yu, B. Quart, and N. J. Clendeninn. 1999. Predictors of optimal virological response to potent antiretroviral therapy. *AIDS* **13:**1873–1880.

Prins, M., J. R. Robertson, R. P. Brettle, I. H. Aguado, B. Broers, F. Boufassa, D. J. Goldberg, R. Zangerle, R. A. Coutinho, and A. van den Hoek. 1999. Do gender differences in CD4 cell counts matter? *AIDS* **13:**2361–2364.

Rezza, G., A. C. Lepri, A. d'Arminio Monforte, P. Pezzotti, F. Castelli, F. Dianzani, A. Lazzarin, A. De Luca, M. Arlotti, F. Leoncini, P. E. Manconi, G. Rizzardini, L. Minoli, A. Poggio, G. Ippolito, A. N. Phillips, and M. Moroni, et al. 2000. Plasma viral load concentrations in women and men from different exposure categories and with known duration of HIV infection. *J. Acquir. Immune Defic. Syndr.* **25:** 56–62.

Richardson, J. L., E. M. Martin, N. Jimenez, K. Danley, M. Cohen, V. L. Carson, B. Sinclair, J. M. Racenstein, R. A. Reed, and A. M. Levine. 2002. Neuropsychological functioning in a cohort of HIV infected women: importance of antiretroviral therapy. *J. Int. Neuropsychol. Soc.* **8:**781–793. (Erratum, **11:**120, 2005.)

Robert-Koch-Institut. 2002. HIV-Infektionen und AIDS-Erkrankungen in Deutschland. Aktuelle epidemiologische Daten. *Epidemiol. Bull.* (In German.)

Robertson, K. R., C. Kapoor, W. T. Robertson, S. Fiscus, S. Ford, and C. D. Hall. 2004. No gender differences in the progression of nervous system disease in HIV infection. *J. Acquir. Immune Defic. Syndr.* **36:**817–822.

Roca, B., C. J. Gomez, and A. Arnedo. 2000. Adherence, side effects and efficacy of stavudine plus lamivudine plus nelfinavir in treatment-experienced HIV-infected patients. *J. Infect.* **41:**50–54.

Sabo, C. E., and V. L. Carwein. 1994. Women and HIV/AIDS. *J. Assoc. Nurses AIDS Care* **5:**15–21.

Sacktor, N. 2002. The epidemiology of human immunodeficiency virus-associated neurological disease in the era of highly active antiretroviral therapy. *J. Neurovirol.* **8**(Suppl. 2): S115–S121.

Sacktor, N., M. P. McDermott, K. Marder, G. Schifitto, O. A. Selnes, J. C. McArthur, Y. Stern, S. Albert, D. Palumbo, K. Kieburtz, J. A. De Marcaida, B. Cohen, and L. Epstein. 2002. HIV-associated cognitive impairment before

and after the advent of combination therapy. *J. Neurovirol.* **8:**136–142.

Sanders-Phillips, K. 2002. Factors influencing HIV/AIDS in women of color. *Public Health Rep.* **117**(Suppl. 1):S151–S156.

Saul, J., J. Erwin, C. A. Sabin, R. Kulasegaram, and B. S. Peters. 2001. The relationships between ethnicity, sex, risk group, and virus load in human immunodeficiency virus type 1 antiretroviral-naive patients. *J. Infect. Dis.* **183:** 1518–1521.

Scarsi, K. K., and M. J. Postelnick. 2003. The impact of gender and pregnancy on antiretroviral therapy for HIV: pharmacokinetic and disease-related differences. *J. Gend. Specif. Med.* **6:**7–16.

Schulte, E., C. Claes, T. Korner, J. M. Graf von der Schulenburg, R. E. Schmidt, and M. Stoll. 2000. Deficits in socioeconomic and psychosocial support of HIV-positive women. *Gesundheitswesen* **62:**391–399.

Seyler, C., X. Anglaret, N. Dakoury-Dogbo, E. Messou, S. Toure, C. Danel, N. Diakite, A. Daudie, A. Inwoley, C. Maurice, B. Tonwe-Gold, F. Rouet, T. N'Dri-Yoman, R. Salamon, and the ANRS 1203 Study Group. 2003. Medium-term survival, morbidity and immunovirological evolution in HIV-infected adults receiving antiretroviral therapy, Abidjan, Cote d'Ivoire. *Antivir. Ther.* **8:**385–393.

Shuter, J., P. L. Alpert, M. G. DeShaw, B. Greenberg, C. J. Chang, and R. S. Klein. 1999. Gender differences in HIV risk behaviors in an adult emergency department in New York City. *J. Urban Health* **76:**237–246.

Smith, L. A. 2003. Partner influence on noncondom use: gender and ethnic differences. *J. Sex. Res.* **40:**346–50.

Sterling, T. R., D. Vlahov, J. Astemborski, D. R. Hoover, J. B. Margolick, and T. C. Quinn. 2001. Initial plasma HIV-1 RNA levels and progression to AIDS in women and men. *N. Engl. J. Med.* **344:**720–725.

Stern, R. A., J. E. Arruda, J. A. Somerville, R. A. Cohen, R. J. Boland, M. D. Stein, and E. M. Martin. 1998. Neurobehavioral functioning in asymptomatic HIV-1 infected women. *J. Int. Neuropsychol. Soc.* **4:**172–178.

Stern, Y., M. P. McDermott, S. Albert, D. Palumbo, O. A. Selnes, J. C. McArthur, N. Sacktor, G. Schifitto, K. Kieburtz, L. Epstein, and K. S. Marder, and Dana Consortium on the Therapy of HIV-Dementia and Related Cognitive Disorders. 2001. Factors associated with incident human immunodeficiency virus-dementia. *Arch. Neurol.* **58:**473–479.

Stoskopf, C. H., Y. K. Kim, and S. H. Glover. 2001. Dual diagnosis: HIV and mental illness, a population-based study. *Community Ment. Health J.* **37:**469–479.

Tershakovec, A. M., I. Frank, and D. Rader. 2004. HIV-related lipodystrophy and related factors. *Atherosclerosis* **174:**1–10.

Towfighi, A., R. L. Skolasky, C. StHillaire, K. Conant, and J. C. McArthur. 2004. CSF soluble Fas correlates with the severity of HIV-associated dementia. *Neurology* **62:** 654–656.

Trzynka, S. L., and J. A. Erlen. 2004. HIV disease susceptibility in women and the barriers to adherence. *Medsurg. Nurs.* **13:**97–104.

van Haastrecht, H. J., J. S. Fennema, R. A. Coutinho, T. C. van der Helm, J. A. Kint, and J. A. van den Hoek. 1993. HIV prevalence and risk behaviour among prostitutes and clients in Amsterdam: migrants at increased risk for HIV infection. *Genitourin. Med.* **69:**251–256.

van Roon, E. N., J. M. Verzijl, J. R. Juttmann, A. W. Lenderink, M. J. Blans, and A. C. Egberts. 1999. Incidence of discontinuation of highly active antiretroviral combination therapy (HAART) and its determinants. *J. Acquir. Immune Defic. Syndr. Hum. Retrovirol.* **20:** 290–294.

von Giesen, H. J., H. J. Wittsack, F. Wenserski, H. Koller, H. Hefter, and G. Arendt. 2001. Basal ganglia metabolite abnormalities in minor motor disorders associated with human immunodeficiency virus type 1. *Arch. Neurol.* **58:** 1281–1286.

Wilson, T. E. 2001. Sexual and reproductive behaviour of women with HIV infection. *Clin. Obstet. Gynecol.* **44:**289–299.

Wingood, G. M., and R. J. DiClemente. 2000. Application of the theory of gender and power to examine HIV-related exposures, risk factors, and effective interventions for women. *Health Educ. Behav.* **27:**539–565.

Zorrilla, C. D. 2000. Antiretroviral combination therapy in HIV-1 infected women and men: are their responses different? *Int. J. Fertil. Womens Med.* **45:**195–199.

The Spectrum of Neuro-AIDS Disorders:
Pathophysiology, Diagnosis, and Treatment
Edited by K. Goodkin et al.
©2008 ASM Press, Washington, DC

32

Pediatric Neuro-AIDS

ANITA L. BELMAN

BACKGROUND AND INTRODUCTION

In 1982, four infants with unexplained immunodeficiency and opportunistic infections were reported to the Centers for Disease Control (Centers for Disease Control, 1982). The following year, the clinical and immunological features of pediatric AIDS were described in the literature (Rubinstein et al., 1983; Oleske et al., 1983; Ammann et al., 1983). Shortly thereafter, neurological involvement was recognized as a significant complication. A progressive encephalopathy syndrome was described, as were syndromes with more stable neurological impairments (Belman et al., 1985, 1988; Epstein et al., 1985, 1986, 1988a; Ultmann et al., 1985). It soon became evident that neurological dysfunction was common in infants and children with AIDS, added significantly to the morbidity of the illness, and often had devastating consequences. The numbers of children with HIV/AIDS increased. By the end of the decade, AIDS was reaching epidemic proportions and had become one of the leading causes of childhood morbidity and mortality in this country and worldwide (Chin, 1990).

Since then, much has been learned about the biology of the HIV-1 retrovirus, the cells it infects, and the natural history of pediatric infection with HIV-1. Key studies led to a better understanding of mother-to-infant transmission (Ehrnst et al., 1991; Goedert et al., 1991; Delfraissy et al., 1992; European Collaborative Study, 1992; Fowler et al., 2000) and then to successful strategies to interrupt transmission. Antiretroviral (ARV) therapy for the mother and her infant during the perinatal period proved efficacious and led to a dramatic decrease in maternal-infant viral transmission rates (Connor et al., 1994). More proficient diagnostic techniques, such as PCR, viral culture, and antigen measurements of the HIV-1 "viral load" (Burgard et al., 1992; Rogers et al., 1994; Owens et al., 1996; Papaevangelou et al., 1996; Palumbo, 2000), facilitated the early identification of HIV-1-infected infants and children during asymptomatic or mildly symptomatic disease stages. This, in turn, allowed early institution of prophylactic therapy for life-threatening opportunistic infections (OIs) and treatment of primary HIV-1 infection with highly active ARV therapy (HAART) based upon age, CD4 cell count, and HIV-1 RNA plasma concentrations, resulting in viral suppression, immune reconstitution, and stabilization of disease with a delay in disease progression (U.S. Department of Health and Human Services, 2006). As a result, in countries where these therapies are readily available, there has been a significant decline in the numbers of infants born HIV-1 infected. Survival rates for HIV-1-infected children treated with HAART improved dramatically as well. The incidence and prevalence of HIV-1-associated neurological disorders declined. Children with HIV/AIDS live longer now, and significant and increasing percentages have reached adolescence and young adulthood. In fact, in the United States, of those children who have survived, the majority are now reaching young adulthood (Centers for Disease Control and Prevention, 2005). Pediatric HIV/AIDS has become a chronic disease. With this new status, new concerns have emerged, including, but not limited to, the toxicities related to potential long-term consequences of treatment.

This is not the case worldwide, unfortunately, where access to medical care and to these expensive ARV combination drug therapies remains limited. The World Health Organization (WHO) reports a striking worldwide diversity of HIV-1 prevalence and spread. For example, in nearly 120 countries, the adult HIV-1 prevalence is less than 1%. In contrast, there are some sub-Saharan African countries where the adult rate is reported to be over 30%. Worldwide, heterosexual transmission predominates. Women of childbearing age remain vulnerable, especially those women and girls who live in high HIV-1 prevalence areas. The discrepancy between the epidemiology of pediatric HIV/AIDS in resource-limited versus resource-rich nations is equally striking. For example, in 1990, the CDC estimated about 2,000 babies were born HIV-1 infected, with about 321 born in New York City. In 2003, this number dropped to about 200, with 5 babies born in New York City. This contrasts

Anita L. Belman, Department of Neurology, School of Medicine, Stony Brook University, Stony Brook, NY 11794.

with the estimated 570,000 to 700,000 newly infected children worldwide during the year 2004. Since the epidemiology of pediatric HIV/AIDS parallels the epidemiology of HIV-1 infection in women and since most HIV-1-infected pregnant women in resource-poor regions receive little or no ARV therapy, the potential increase in the numbers of infants born HIV-1 infected and those who will develop neurological disorders remains.

This chapter reviews the clinical, neuroimaging, and neuropathological features of pediatric neuro-AIDS (prior to the use of ARV agents) and the changing neuroepidemiology in the HAART era. Salient features of pediatric HIV/AIDS and its epidemiology are briefly summarized, since there are major differences between adult and pediatric HIV/AIDS, and neurological aspects need to be viewed in the context of this complex and progressive illness for which the epidemiology is diverse and changing, as are treatment protocols and their availabilities.

EPIDEMIOLOGY

Now, in the third decade of the epidemic, WHO/Joint United Nations Program on HIV/AIDS (UNAIDS) estimates that about 60 million people worldwide have been infected with HIV-1. In 2007, the total number of people living with HIV-1 infection was estimated at 33.2 million (30.6 to 36.1 million). Of these, 15.4 million were women and about 2.5 million were children under the age of 15 years (with the vast majority living in sub-Saharan Africa). In the year 2007 alone, 2.5 million persons acquired HIV-1 infection. Of these, about one-half were women and about 420,000 were children. During the same year, 2.1 million people (1.7 million adults and 330,000 children) died of the disease.

Although sub-Saharan Africa continues to be the most affected region, with about 25 million persons infected, the steepest increases during the past few years have occurred in Eastern Europe and Central and East Asia. Between the years 2002 and 2004, the number of people living with HIV-1 in East Asia rose by almost 50%. Compared to the last decade, an ever-increasing proportion of people living with HIV-1 infection are women and girls. In some regions of sub-Saharan Africa, of HIV-infected persons aged 15 to 24 years, 76% are female. Similar trends in female-to-male ratios have been noted in other areas as well (Asia, Latin America, the Caribbean, and Eastern Europe). According to UNAIDS/WHO reports, "most women become infected through their partner's high-risk behaviors (over which they have little control)" (Joint United Nations Program on HIV/AIDS/World Health Organization, 2005). The increase in the number of HIV-1-infected women of childbearing age is paralleled by the potential increase in infants born HIV-1 infected. Although new vertically transmitted infection has now become rare in industrialized countries following the use of ARV therapy, it continues to be rampant in some regions of the world's resource-limited nations.

It is difficult to talk about pediatric AIDS without mention of another tragic sequela of the epidemic, namely, "AIDS orphans." It was estimated a decade ago that 13.2 million children under 15 years of age (HIV-1 infected and uninfected) born to mothers with HIV-1 infection had lost their mother or both parents to AIDS. As grim as these figures are, the total number of children orphaned by the epidemic is forecast to more than double by the year 2010 (Global AIDS Policy Coalition, 1996).

PEDIATRIC HIV/AIDS

Mode of Transmission, Time of Infection, and Risk Factors

Vertically Acquired HIV-1 Infection

Mother-to-child transmission (MTCT) occurs in utero, intrapartum, or postnatally through breast-feeding. At least 90% of infected children acquire infection from their mothers. In the absence of intervention, a 25% rate (13 to 45%) of MTCT is estimated from studies conducted in the United States, Europe, Asia, and Africa (Ryder et al., 1989; Working Group on Mother-to-Child Transmission of HIV, 1995; Lindegren et al., 2000).

Maternal, obstetrical, genetic, and fetal factors modify this transmission rate. Increased transmission risks are associated with high maternal viral loads, advanced maternal HIV-1 disease (low CD4 cell counts, high CD8 cell counts, or AIDS), maternal-fetal HLA concordance, vitamin A deficiency, placental-membrane inflammation, chorioamnionitis, premature rupture of membranes, increased infant exposure to maternal blood or secretions, premature delivery, and breast-feeding (Delfraissy et al., 1992; European Collaborative Study, 1992; St Louis et al., 1993; Boyer et al., 1994; Borkowsky et al., 1994; Semba et al., 1994; Just et al., 1995; Abrams et al., 1995; Mayaux et al., 1995; Fang et al., 1995; Landesman et al., 1996; Dickover et al., 1996; Nduati et al., 1995; Papaevangelou et al., 1996; Thea et al., 1997; Lambert et al., 1997; Pitt et al., 1997; Mofenson et al., 1999; Garcia et al., 1999; International Perinatal HIV Group, 1999; European Mode of Delivery Collaboration, 1999; Fowler et al., 2000; Kuhn et al., 2004; Ioannidis et al., 2004).

The true frequency of in utero versus peripartum transmission is not known. Although HIV-1 has been reported in fetal tissue during the first trimester (Lyman et al., 1990; Sprecher et al., 1985; Jovaisas et al., 1985; Soeiro et al., 1992), current evidence suggests that most viral transmission occurs during or near the time of birth. It appears that a healthy placenta generally protects the in utero fetus from HIV-1 in the maternal blood for most of gestation. The integrity of the placental protection against HIV-1 may, however, be breached by infections and drugs. In a non-breast-feeding population, modeling backward from the earliest detection of HIV-1 in the infant's blood, in utero infection has been operationally defined as detection of HIV-1 by culture, PCR, or HIV-1 genome in the infant's blood within 48 hours of birth. Peripartum infection is defined as negative cultures, or HIV-1 DNA or RNA in the first week of life, followed by a positive test at days 7 to 90 (Auger et al., 1988; Ryder et al., 1989; Ehrnst et al., 1991, 1992; Krivine et al., 1992; Bryson et al., 1992; Rouzioux et al., 1995; Bertolli et al., 1996; Rouet et al., 2003). In utero transmission occurs 26 to 38% and perinatal infection 65 to 74% of the time.

For breast-feeding populations, the risk of postnatal transmission extends beyond delivery and throughout the breast-feeding period. A recent meta-analysis reported that late postnatal transmission may represent up to 24 to 42% of the overall MTCT of HIV-1 and is constant throughout the breast-feeding period, with a longer duration of breast-feeding associated with a greater cumulative risk of late postnatal HIV-1 transmission. Lower maternal CD4 cell counts may also be associated with an increased risk of late postnatal transmission (Bulterys and Goedert, 1996; Coutsoudis et al., 2004). Consequently, in resource-limited regions where safe alternatives to breast-feeding (access to formula milk powder, clean water, and sanitation) are lacking, rates of infection from breast-feeding may offset the benefits of treatment during pregnancy and the perinatal period (Nduati et al., 1995).

Parenterally Acquired HIV-1 Infection

Prior to HIV-1 blood donor screening, recipients of HIV-1-contaminated blood or blood products included children with hemophilia or other coagulation defects, children with illnesses requiring whole blood or blood product transfusions (e.g., leukemia), and sick neonates. Iatrogenic viral transmission also occurred through reuse of contaminated injection equipment in some resource-limited medical settings. Unfortunately, transmission through these routes still occurs in some underdeveloped regions.

Intravenous Drug Use and Sexually Transmitted HIV-1 Infection

Half of all new cases of HIV-1 infection are in persons 15 to 24 years of age. Among adolescents, intravenous drug use and sexual exposure are the most common risk factors for acquiring HIV-1 infection. In 2000, it was estimated that about 65% of adolescents aged 13 to 19 years with AIDS were infected through these routes (Futterman et al., 2000; Centers for Disease Control and Prevention, 2005).

Commercial Sexual Exploitation

It is unknown how many child sex workers there are worldwide due to the clandestine nature of this multibillion dollar world industry. What is known, though, is that most children working in the sex industry are 13- to 18-year-old girls. In one region, about 20% of the estimated 2 million commercial sex workers are 15 years old or younger, and 50% are less than 18 years of age. Estimates from another country reveal that about 30% of commercial sex workers 13 to 19 years of age are HIV-1 infected.

Natural History

Clinical Course

The adverse effects of HIV-1 infection on the immature, developing immune and nervous systems generally result in a more rapid onset of clinical symptoms than with HIV-1 infection acquired in adulthood. Infants and children with vertically acquired infection are separated into two groups based on a bimodal evolution of clinical symptoms and progression to death (Blanche et al., 1990; Scott, 1989; Barnhart et al., 1996). The first group of infants, "rapid progressors" (20 to 25% of cases), have high levels of detectable virus at birth and in early infancy. They present with HIV/AIDS encephalopathy, *Pneumocystis carinii* pneumonia, disseminated cytomegalovirus (CMV) infection, and failure to thrive (wasting syndrome). Disease progression is rapid during the first years of life, and mortality is high.

Children in the second and larger group (75 to 80%) have a form of HIV-1 disease that progresses more slowly ("slow progressors"). Manifestations such as lymphoid interstitial pneumonitis, parotiditis, hepatomegaly, splenomegaly, and lymphadenopathy are common presenting features in this group of youngsters and may result from the immune response to HIV-1 infection.

Recurrent serious bacterial infections with common childhood pathogens, such as *Streptococcus pneumoniae* and *Haemophilus influenzae*, occur in both groups and reflect the B-cell dysfunction noted in pediatric HIV-1 infection (Bernstein et al., 1985; Andiman et al., 1994). Cardiomyopathy, nephropathy, and possibly enteropathy represent

complications related to primary HIV-1 infection (Blanche et al., 1990; Tovo et al., 1992; European Collaborative Study, 1994; Frederick et al., 1994; Vigano et al., 1995; Barnhart et al., 1996; Mayaux et al., 1996; Cooper et al., 1998; Diaz et al., 1998; Abuzaitoun and Hanson, 2000; Gray et al., 2001). The more rapid progression of HIV-1 infection in children may be related in part to HIV-1-mediated effects on the developing thymus (e.g., during periods of active thymopoiesis), as well as the immaturity of the neonatal immune response (Kourtis et al., 1996). For example, neonatal natural killer cells have diminished antibody-mediated recognition and, thus, killing of HIV-1-infected cells; T cells have diminished ability to produce cytokines; and responses of cytotoxic T lymphocytes to HIV-1 Gag protein are detected in a smaller proportion of infants than adults.

A minority of children present in preadolescence (Burger et al., 1990; Persaud et al., 1992; Grubman et al., 1995). As in adults, latency to onset of moderately symptomatic disease in this group may be 10 years or more. What factors underlie the difference between groups and what factors contribute to accelerated disease progression are not entirely clear but may be related to the timing of HIV-1 infection (gestation versus parturition), the stage of maternal HIV-1 disease during pregnancy and delivery, maternal viremia, the neonates' viral load, the virulence of the infecting retrovirus, HLA class I sharing between mother and infant, CCR5 mutations, and other, as-yet-undefined genetic factors (Duliege et al., 1992; Blanche et al., 1994; European Collaborative Study, 1994; Just et al., 1995; Abrams et al., 1995, 1998; Luzuriaga and Sullivan, 2000).

Natural history studies in the United States (prior to ARV availability) showed that about 50% of children were symptomatic by the age of 5 years and that about 75% survived to the mean age. The mean time from birth to severe advanced "AIDS" disease (i.e., CDC clinical stage C) was 6 to 8 years, with an estimated mean survival time of 9.4 years (Barnhart et al., 1996; Lindegren et al., 2000). Children who live in resource-limited countries are at greater risk for early death than are children in resource-rich countries. A recent pooled analysis of mortality data for HIV-1-infected infants showed that by 1 year of age an estimated 35.2% of the children will have died and by the age of 2 years 52.5% will have died (French Pediatric HIV Infection Study Group, 1997; Taha et al., 2000; Newell et al., 2004). Mortality in infants coinfected with tuberculosis, syphilis, or CMV is accelerated (i.e., over 83% die by the age of 9 months).

Viral Parameters, CD4 Cell Counts, and Progression of HIV-1 Disease

Viral parameters and CD4 cell counts in vertically infected infants and young children also differ from those of adults. At the peak, HIV-1 RNA copy numbers are higher and then subsequently decline much more slowly than in newly HIV-1-infected adults. Prospective studies of infants followed from birth show that a peak viremia of 200,000 to over 1 million copies/ml is reached within 4 to 8 weeks of birth, slowly decreasing during the first 2 years of life and requiring several years to decline to a set point (De Rossi et al., 1996; Abrams et al., 1998; Dickover et al., 1996; Palumbo, 2000; U.S. Department of Health and Human Services, 2006). Children with persistently high levels of plasma HIV-1 RNA (especially infants and younger children with RNA values of >750,000 copies/ml) are at risk for rapid clinical disease progression, OIs, and irreversible central nervous system (CNS) disease. In older children, the risk of progression with elevation of the viral load is similar to that seen in adults.

The normal range of CD4 cell counts changes with age. Thus, the assessment of a CD4 cell count in a child must be done in relation to the appropriate count for the child's age. For example, the 50th percentile for CD4 cell counts at the age of 6 months is 3,000/μl, compared to 1,000/μl for a 6-year-old, by which time the CD4 cell count range approaches that of adults (Comans-Bitter et al., 1997). Further, for an individual child, the CD4 cell count varies and is often depressed with intercurrent infections. Therefore, it is recommended that this parameter be measured when the child is in a stable clinical condition. The CD4 cell percentage varies less with age and other factors than the absolute count and is considered a more useful measure of immune function in children. Although the CD4 cell count may be less helpful in infants overall, the baseline CD4 cell count, along with the plasma viral load, is predictive of clinical disease progression (Hughes et al., 1997). The CDC classification of children with HIV-1 infection incorporates both clinical and immunological parameters (Centers for Disease Control and Prevention, 1994).

NEUROLOGICAL DISORDERS

Neurological disorders are classified into two major categories: (i) HIV-1-associated CNS disease, including "progressive encephalopathy" (PE), a syndrome complex with cognitive, motor, and behavioral features related to primary HIV-1 CNS infection (the pediatric counterpart of adult HIV-1-associated dementia, formerly known as "AIDS dementia complex"), and (ii) secondary CNS complications related to immunosuppression or to distinct AIDS-related conditions (CNS neoplasms, CNS infections caused by pathogens other than HIV-1, and cerebrovascular accident [CVA]).

The nervous system can also be adversely affected by complications related to systemic HIV-1 disease (including metabolic and endocrinological derangements associated with systemic HIV-1-related disorders). This can occur by prolonged exposure to the therapies as well (including the toxic and metabolic complications of antimicrobials and/or ARV therapies) (see chapter 1, this volume). These conditions are not mutually exclusive, and coexisting pathologic conditions are common (Belman, 1990).

The child's neurological and neurodevelopmental status can also be affected by HIV-1-related and unrelated conditions. These occur with significant frequency in this population, including those conditions related to maternal high-risk factors during pregnancy, premature birth, complications in the neonatal period, and, postnatally, to factors associated with poverty (such as malnutrition, poor hygiene, and high levels of postnatal psychosocial stressors) (Belman, 1992).

HIV-1-Associated CNS Disease Syndromes

HIV-1-Associated Encephalopathy/Progressive Encephalopathy

The cardinal features of encephalopathy include cognitive impairment, poor brain growth, and abnormalities of motor function and tone (Belman et al., 1985, 1986, 1988; Epstein et al., 1985, 1986). Extrapyramidal signs and movement disorders, usually superimposed upon spasticity, and signs of cerebellar dysfunction do occur, but less frequently (Belman

et al., 1988; Belman, 1990; Mintz et al., 1996). Mood and behavioral problems are common (Brouwers et al., 1994; Havens et al., 1994; Moss et al., 1994; Wolters et al., 1994). HIV-1-associated CNS disease may occur as the AIDS-defining illness or in the context of subsequent disease.

The clinical course of the encephalopathy is highly variable—acute with rapid progression, subacute, or stepwise in decline (i.e., a decline followed by a relatively stable period, which is then followed by further deterioration) (Belman et al., 1985, 1988; Belman, 1990). The severities of motor and cognitive deficits can be discordant. Some children develop progressive and disabling motor deficits yet maintain relatively stable (albeit impaired) cognitive and adaptive social skills, whereas other children have more impaired cognitive than motor function. Finally, some children have relatively stable minor motor and cognitive findings (Belman, 1990). HIV-1-associated CNS disease syndromes present according to the age of onset. This information comes from observational studies conducted during the first 2 decades of the HIV/AIDS epidemic, prior to the advent of HAART regimens (Belman, 1992, 1994; Belman et al., 1985, 1986, 1988, 1996).

Newborns

Clinical signs of HIV-1-associated CNS disease are rare in infected full-term newborns. However, compared to "seroreverters" (non-HIV-1-infected infants born to HIV-1-infected mothers), a greater proportion of HIV-1-infected infants are small for their gestational age or are born prematurely. Premature delivery is often interlinked with high-risk maternal conditions during pregnancy (inadequate prenatal care and nutrition, substance abuse, maternal illness, and infection with pathogens other than HIV-1), as well as with maternal HIV-1 infection and associated illnesses (Volpe, 1995; Belman, 1990). The developing nervous system in HIV-1-infected infants, as in non-HIV-1-infected infants, may be adversely affected by these coexisting factors. Additionally, the premature infant is at risk for developing perinatal CNS complications (e.g., hypoxic-ischemic encephalopathy, periventricular leukomalacia, intracranial hemorrhage, hydrocephalus, and CNS dysfunction related to systemic conditions), which are risk factors for long-term CNS dysfunction and for subsequent neurodevelopmental abnormalities.

Infants

The most clearly recognized, severe, and devastating syndrome is the "early-onset severe infantile" form of HIV-1-associated PE of childhood. CNS signs of this syndrome usually appear within the first year of life but may begin in the second to fifth years. Neurological deterioration results in spastic quadriparesis and mental deficiency (usually by 2 to 3 years of age). The characteristic features are (i) progressive corticospinal tract signs with concomitant loss of previously acquired motor milestones or a markedly deviant rate of acquiring motor skills, (ii) decline in mental development or marked delays in cognitive development, and (iii) acquired microcephaly. Opisthotonic posturing and rigidity may develop and are usually superimposed upon spasticity. Pseudobulbar signs with feeding difficulties are frequent. Play deteriorates; previously acquired language and adaptive skills are lost. The children have a characteristic "mask-like" face (hypomimic, wide-eyed alert appearance with a paucity of spontaneous facial expressions) and other Parkinsonian features (manifestations of basal-ganglia and subcortical pathology), and they are hypophonic (with decreased spontaneous and responsive vocalizations). Serial psychometric assessments show a decline in the composite cognitive score. The end-stage picture is one of an apathetic, withdrawn, often irritable, quadriparetic child with markedly impaired higher cortical function (dementia). Serial head circumference measurements document poor brain growth (acquired microcephaly). Serial neuroimaging studies most often show progressive atrophy with white-matter abnormalities. Progressive basal-ganglion calcification with or without mineralization of the frontal white matter is also commonly observed on computed tomography (CT) scan of the head. Of note, a CT scan of the head obtained during the period of acute clinical neurological deterioration may not show basal-ganglion calcification, but subsequent studies likely will.

Neurological deterioration may be fulminant (over weeks to a few months) (Belman, 1990), slowly progressive (with an insidious decline), or episodic (with periods of deterioration interrupted by periods of relative neurological stability). A less severe neurological syndrome is characterized by hypotonia with marked delays in attainment of motor developmental milestones. For example, unlike most babies, who walk at 12 months of age, these infants may not take independent steps until 19 to 30 months of age. Cognitive development is usually delayed, and concomitant language deficiencies are common. The prognosis is guarded. Some children develop a "diparesis-type syndrome" in early childhood; others remain stable, continuing to acquire new skills (see below), whereas others develop full-blown PE. Neuroimaging studies show mild atrophy with or without basal-ganglion calcification or may be normal. Of note, even when no abnormalities are imaged, poor brain growth, as determined by serial head circumference measurements, is common (Belman, 1990).

Toddlers and Young Children

A change in gait is usually the first sign of HIV-1 motor involvement. Children begin to toe walk, have hyperreflexia, and have increased lower extremity muscle tone. Fine motor ability and dexterity are often compromised. The rate of progression varies. Some children develop a spastic gait yet are able to walk independently, but others require orthotics. Progression in severity in others is rapid; within months, those children are wheelchair bound. Cognitive impairment (low-average or "borderline" intelligence to mild mental retardation) is frequent but not invariable. A subset of children will have a prolonged, stable course. Some continue to gain additional skills; however, the rate of acquisition of these new skills often deviates, not only from the norm but also from the child's own previous rate of developmental progress. Some, however, will ultimately go on to develop full-blown PE. In younger children, poor brain growth (documented by serial head circumference measurements) is common; some will develop acquired microcephaly. Serial neuroimaging studies may or may not show progressive atrophy, white-matter abnormalities, and calcification of the basal ganglia.

School-Age Children

Early signs of HIV-1-associated CNS disease may include loss of interest in school performance, cognitive decline, language-related problems, decreased attention, emotional lability, social withdrawal, and psychomotor slowing. Psychometric testing often documents global involvement (seen by changes in the full-scale IQ [FSIQ] score), as well as specific deficits in selected neurocognitive domains (such as visuomotor skills, psychomotor speed, and expressive language). With advancing disease, psychometric tests show a decline in FSIQ score. Motor involvement of varying severity is common. Hyperreflexia, clumsiness, and poor fine motor ability and dexterity are noted initially. Progressive long-tract signs, movement disorders, cerebellar signs, and myelopathy may develop with advancing disease. At end stage, the child is apathetic and abulic. Progressive cerebral atrophy and white-matter abnormalities are common neuroimaging findings. Some children will also have CT evidence of basal-ganglion calcification, although when present, discrete or punctate lesions are usually observed (Belman et al., 1986).

Neurodevelopmental Deficits

Neurodevelopmental problems are common (Ultmann et al., 1985, 1987; Diamond et al., 1987; Cohen et al., 1991; Condini et al., 1991; Aylward et al., 1992; Wachtel et al., 1993; Chase et al., 1995; Drotar et al., 1997; Nozyce et al., 1994a; Gay et al., 1995). In one study of ARV-naive symptomatic children (Englund et al., 1996; Raskino et al., 1999), about half of the cohort was reported to have abnormal neurodevelopmental findings (abnormal motor function [23%], reflexes [21%], and behavior [13%]). Nearly 50% of the children in the youngest age groups had motor dysfunction. Cognitive deficiencies were present in approximately 21% of the cohort, again with the highest percentages in the youngest age groups: ages 3 to 12 months (33.7%), 12 to 30 months (19%), and 30 months to 6 years (21%). The percentage of these children with documented HIV-1 infection of the CNS was not reported.

HIV-1-Associated Minor Motor and Cognitive Impairment

"Minor" motor impairment, with or without cognitive deficits, is a frequent finding in children, many of whom as infants and toddlers had "delays" in motor and language development. As school-aged children, they are often mildly clumsy, have learning disabilities, and are placed in special-education classes. Several studies have reported selected deficits in visuospatial skills, expressive language, organizational skills, and cognitive flexibility (including children with average or low-average FSIQ scores and children on HAART) (Diamond et al., 1987; Ultmann et al., 1987; Cohen et al., 1991; Condini et al., 1991; Whitt et al., 1993; Brouwers et al., 1995a; Havens et al., 1994; Chase et al., 1995; Levenson et al., 1992; Wolters et al., 1995; Belman, 2002; Jeremy et al., 2005; Foster and Lyall, 2005). These findings (analogous to those observed in adults [see chapter 1, this volume]) suggest that HIV-1 may compromise the normal developmental process and result in "minor motor and cognitive impairment."

Neuropsychiatric Disorders

Psychosis

As in adults, acute psychosis manifested by agitation, mania, and catatonia has been described in children with advanced disease. Changes in mental status may be due to HIV-1 CNS disease but also to complications of nutritional deficiencies, CNS OIs (for example, CMV encephalopathy), or toxic effects of ARV and other therapies.

Mood, Affect, and Depression

The onset of emotional lability, mood swings, extreme impulsiveness, and attentional problems or flattened affect, lack of social responsiveness, and declining interest in the environment that occurs in the advanced disease may be an early sign of HIV-1 CNS disease, OIs, or coexisting HIV/ AIDS-related metabolic disturbances (Brouwers et al., 1995b; Havens et al., 1994; Misdrahi et al., 2004). The effects of chronic disease, frequent hospitalizations, illness and death of family members, changing caretakers, and psychosocial stressors, and the stigma attached to HIV-1 disease itself, may also affect mood and affect and lead to major depressive disorder.

Of note, recent reports show an increased prevalence of the diagnoses of mental disorders. One study found that a major depressive disorder diagnosis was significantly associated with clinical or neuroimaging abnormalities and depressed CD4 cell percentages, suggesting that depressive disorders may be primary manifestations of HIV-1 encephalopathy (Misdrahi et al., 2004). Another study reported increased prevalence rates of psychiatric hospitalization among HIV-1-infected children and adolescents, including those with stable disease on HAART, compared with uninfected control subjects (Gaughan et al., 2004). Depressive and conduct disorders were the most common reasons for psychiatric hospitalization.

Neuropathological Findings

The most common and significant pathological features of pediatric neuro-AIDS conditions include a global reduction in brain tissue volume (cortex, white matter, and subcortical grey matter), basal-ganglion calcification, myelin pathology (diffuse central-hemispheric myelin pallor with striking astrocytosis), and spinal cord pathology (corticospinal tract [CST] "degeneration," not vacuolar myelopathy, as seen in adults) (Belman et al., 1985, 1986, 1988; Dickson et al., 1989a, 1989b; Epstein et al., 1988a; Sharer et al., 1986, 1990; Wiley et al., 1990; Kure et al., 1991; Burns, 1992; Kozlowski et al., 1993, 1997; Vazeux et al., 1992). CST pathology, characterized by prominent myelin pallor, was reported in over two-thirds of the cases in one pediatric AIDS autopsy series (Dickson et al., 1989b). Both axonal and myelin loss were seen in about half of the cases ("axonopathy type"), whereas the other half had disproportionate myelin pallor (poor myelination) with relative preservation of axons ("myelinopathy type"). In general the "axonopathy" cases had marked cerebral pathology (microglial-macrophage infiltrates and immunocytochemical evidence of active CNS infection), suggesting that the CST degeneration was due to Wallerian degeneration (probably secondary to cerebral changes). The insult in the "myelopathy" cases, however, may have been to myelinating glia or newly formed myelin. The investigators hypothesized that HIV-1 may interfere with normal myelination. The last tracts to myelinate may be the most vulnerable to the direct or indirect effects of HIV-1. Myelination may be delayed, newly formed myelin may be injured (cytokine mediated), or myelin-forming glial cells may be affected. It is also possible that proliferating glial precursor cells suffer antenatal HIV-1-mediated injury.

Both adult and pediatric studies show HIV-1 localized primarily in blood-derived macrophages, intrinsic microglia (the resident mononuclear phagocytic system of the brain), and multinucleated giant cells (formed by the fusion of these cell types), found predominantly in the basal ganglia, subthalamic nucleus, substantia nigra, dentate nucleus, and white matter. However, investigators report lower HIV-1 loads in the brains of children than of adults (Wiley et al., 1990; Vazeux et al., 1992; Kure et al., 1990; Brustle et al., 1992). These cells express both CD4 and β-chemokine receptors (CCR5 and CXCR4), which permit cellular entry by HIV-1 and are the primary targets of HIV-1 brain infection. It is these cells that support productive retroviral infection. Although glial cells are capable of harboring HIV-1 infection, it is thought to be limited to restrictive infection (see chapter 12, this volume).

Neuropathophysiological mechanisms underlying pediatric HIV-1-mediated CNS are complex and not fully understood (see chapters 10 to 17, this volume). Current evidence suggests that HIV-1 invades the CNS early in the course of infection (soon after primary infection) in both adults and children. In adults, HIV-1 invades a mature, fully developed, and completely myelinated nervous system. The immune system and CNS elements of the mononuclear-phagocyte system (intrinsic microglia) are also fully developed. In contrast, vertically transmitted HIV-1 infection occurs in an immature, evolving organism (and, as noted above, the point of viral transmission may be in in utero, intrapartum, or postpartum). In adults, HIV-1-associated dementia usually occurs in advanced disease, when the individual is severely immunosuppressed (see chapter 1, this volume). In contrast, "early-onset AIDS encephalopathy" is frequently the AIDS-defining illness in children. The maturational stages of the nervous and immune systems at the time of viral exposure appear to be of crucial importance. Dynamic interactions occur between these two systems during development. It is possible that these complex interactions may, in turn, be affected by HIV-1 infection and its associated changes. The tissue distribution of HIV-1, the maturity of the thymus, the CD4 cell nadir, and bone marrow-derived myelomonocytic cells may be the significant determinants of clinical disease in the immature host. These factors may account for age-specific vulnerabilities and may contribute to age-of-onset differences in clinical manifestations, in disease progression, and in clinical treatment outcomes. Viral factors (e.g., the CNS viral load versus viral strain differences, increased sequence diversity, the high mutation rate of specific HIV-1 genes, the emergence of HIV-1 genotypic variants with altered biological activity [such as high replication rate and cytopathic effects], and the mechanisms underlying viral protein- and cytokine-mediated effects and toxicities) may all be important in affecting the subsequent clinical disease course and outcomes. Of note, it has been shown that cerebrospinal fluid (CSF) HIV-1 RNA copy number correlates significantly with the severity of cortical atrophy but not with intracerebral calcifications in a sample of children 0.5 to 13 years of age with symptomatic HIV-1 disease (Brouwers et al., 2000). Thus, active HIV-1 replication in the CNS may be, at least in part, associated with the severity of brain tissue damage manifested in children. In addition, the lack of correlation of intracerebral calcifications with structural brain abnormalities, as well as with CSF HIV load, suggests that intracerebral calcifications may reflect a different neuropathological process than that accounting for cortical atrophy. Finally, host genetic factors are relevant as well (e.g., CCR5 and CXCR4 polymorphisms, virus-host interactions affecting genes and gene products, and as-yet-undefined virus-host interactions).

The late fetal and postnatal period of brain development is a dynamic time characterized by the ongoing processes of myelination, increase in the size of neuronal cells, developmental elaboration of dendritic and axonal ramifications, establishment of synaptic contacts, selective elimination of neuronal processes and synapses, programmed cell death, and the proliferation of glia and myelination (Volpe, 1995). During this period, astrocytes perform myriad complex and vital neuroendocrine, nutritive, and supportive functions in relation to neuronal homeostasis, as well as in the reaction to metabolic and structural insults. Many of these developmental events are controlled, in part, by neurotrophic factors and amino acid transmitters, which are reflected in receptor ontogeny. In the early postnatal period, there is overexpression of receptors in some regions (e.g., glutamate receptors in the basal ganglia and the thalamus). In the immature brain, it is these regions that appear to be especially vulnerable to various perturbations and insults by HIV-1 (Volpe, 1995). Disturbances in these and other developmental processes may lead to impairment in proliferation, myelination, and neuronal function and cell death (Kozlowski et al., 1997; Epstein and Gelbard, 1999; Epstein and Gendelman, 1993).

As stated above, acquired microcephaly is a characteristic clinical finding. Significant reductions in brain weight and the volume of cortical regions, subcortical gray matter, and cerebral white matter are seen at autopsy. However, there are no gross or microscopic malformations or evidence of disordered neuronal migration, although, as in adult neuropathological studies (Wiley et al., 1991), neuronal loss and damage to the dendritic arbor are observed in some cases. HIV-1 infection of the immature brain may affect brain cell proliferation and account, in part, for acquired microcephaly. It is also tempting to speculate that interference with synaptogenesis, myelination in the brain (similar to the spinal cord), and perturbations or alterations of astrocyte function could explain, at least in part, neurodevelopmental delays and cognitive impairment. Thus, pathologic processes affecting the developing CNS may result in abnormal development (arrested or delayed) and then subsequent regressive changes in some cases (Kozlowski et al., 1997). These issues are the foci of continued investigation.

Secondary CNS Complications

Ultimately, HIV-1 infection culminates in the development of profound immunosuppression. The child becomes susceptible to various infections, neoplasms, and cerebrovascular complications. Secondary CNS complications should be considered in the differential diagnosis of the HIV-1-infected child who presents with new onset of mental status changes, headache, seizures, or focal neurological deficits.

CNS Infections

CNS infections include those caused by common childhood pathogens, such as S. pneumoniae, H. influenzae type b, and Escherischa coli (a reflection of the B-cell dysfunction noted in pediatric AIDS) (Andiman et al., 1994; Bernstein et al., 1985), and OIs. OIs usually occur in advanced disease, when the child is immunosuppressed. CMV encephalopathy and Candida albicans meningitis/microabscesses were the most frequently identified conditions (Belman et al., 1985, 1988; Dickson et al., 1989b; McAbee et al., 1995). Congenital CNS infections (e.g., CNS toxoplasmosis, CMV infection, and neurosyphilis), herpesvirus encephalitis, and measles encephalitis are also described, albeit infrequently (Biggemann et al., 1987; Lacroix et al., 1995; Mitchell et al., 1990; Shanks et al., 1987; Sharer et al., 1994; Taccone et al., 1992). Reactivation of previously acquired infection (e.g., toxoplasmosis and herpes simplex virus and varicella zoster virus [VZV] infections) would not be expected in infants, but as in adults, it does occur in older immunosuppressed children with advanced disease (although less frequently) (Frank et al., 1997; Silliman et al., 1993). Similarly, Cryptococcus neoformans infection, a fairly common complication in

adults, was uncommon in children (Kaur et al., 2003). Progressive multifocal leukoencephalopathy (a rare disease in immunosuppressed children before the HIV/AIDS epidemic [see chapter 26, this volume]) has been the subject of several case reports, including one child who was treated successfully with HAART (Berger et al., 1992; Vandersteenhoven et al., 1992; Robinson et al., 2004). Further, Mycobacterium tuberculosis granulomatous meningitis is now reported as a fairly common complication of HIV-1 infection in infants and children in resource-limited countries.

Neoplasms

As in adults (see chapter 27, this volume), primary CNS lymphoma (PCNSL), followed by systemic lymphoma metastatic to the CNS, is the most frequently reported neoplasm occurring in immunosuppressed children with advanced disease and the most common cause of mass lesions seen at autopsy (Epstein et al., 1988b; Belman et al., 1988; Dickson et al., 1989b; Biggar et al., 2000). PCNSL, predominantly an aggressive B-cell tumor considered to be part of the spectrum of B-cell proliferative disorders associated with pediatric HIV/AIDS, is related to Epstein-Barr virus infection (Andiman et al., 1985). PCNSL is the most frequent cause of mass lesions in pediatric AIDS and can occur either as a single mass lesion or as multicentric lesions.

Characteristics seen in CT scan of the head include hyperdense or isodense mass lesions with variable contrast enhancement, diffusely infiltrating contrast-enhancing lesions, and periventricular contrast-enhancing lesions. The basal ganglia, corpus callosum, and periventricular white matter are the most common locations (Epstein et al., 1988b; Belman, 1992; States et al., 1997). Definitive diagnosis is made by biopsy, although magnetic resonance spectroscopy studies may be able to differentiate lymphoma from other lesions (see chapter 20, this volume). Radiation therapy and steroids have been shown to reduce tumor size (Goldstein et al., 1990), although long-term survival rates have remained grim due to tumor recurrence, as well as to advancing HIV-1 disease. Patients most often succumb to other AIDS-related illnesses, OIs, or both.

Cerebrovascular Complications

Children with HIV/AIDS are at increased risk for transient ischemic attack and CVA. The clinical presentation usually includes new onset of headache, mental status changes, and focal neurological deficits (most commonly hemiparesis), with or without seizures. The clinical presentation is variable, reflecting the severity and location of the insult. CVAs may be catastrophic and fatal or clinically silent (Belman et al., 1988; Park et al., 1990).

Intracerebral hemorrhage occurs in the setting of immune-mediated thrombocytopenia, as hemorrhage into tumor (lymphoma), or as a subarachnoid hemorrhage associated with aneurysmal arteriopathy of major cerebral arteries. Infarctions are usually associated with pathologic changes of cerebral blood vessels, meningeal infections, coagulopathies, or cardiomyopathy (Dickson et al., 1989b). A fibrinoid necrotizing vasculitis of the leptomeningeal vessels associated with multiple hemorrhagic and nonhemorrhagic cerebral infarctions, as well as multiple microscopic infarctions and large areas of encephalomalacia, was described at the autopsy of children with bacterial meningitis (Dickson et al., 1989b). Granulomatous arteritis affecting small and medium-size cerebral vessels has also been described in children with recurrent bouts of cutaneous VZV infection. Autopsy findings in one case included multiple microinfarctions associated with healed arteritis presumed to be due to VZV infection, as Cowdry type A intranuclear inclusions were detected in rare intimal cells (Dickson et al., 1989b). Multiple ischemic infarcts may also result from leptomeningitis associated with other infectious etiologies, such as *M. tuberculosis* and *Treponema pallidum*.

A subacute necrotizing encephalopathy with cystic encephalomalacia appears to be associated with dilated cardiomyopathy and may be related to an acquired mitochondrial cytopathy or hypoxic-ischemic damage in children. A fibrosing inflammatory vasculopathy has been described as well and is thought to be related to primary HIV-1 CNS infection. Pathologic examination showed sclerotic vessels with obliterated or markedly stenosed lumens (Dickson et al., 1989b). Cerebral vascular ectasia and aneurysmal arteriopathy of major cerebral arteries (aneurysmal dilation of the branch vessels of the circle of Willis, diffuse and fusiform or focal and saccular) with thrombosis of these arteries or their vascular territories are increasingly recognized complications of pediatric AIDS and appear to be a more common complication of AIDS in children than in adults (Anders et al., 1986; Mizusawa et al., 1988; Berger et al., 1990; Bell, 2004; Cole et al., 2004; Connor et al., 2000; Evers et al., 2003). The first case of this unusual destructive arteriopathy producing aneurysmal dilation of arteries of the circle of Willis was described in a 6-year-old boy with AIDS who presented with aphasia and hemiparesis. CT scan of the head revealed basal-ganglion infarction. He improved clinically with partial recovery of speech and motor functions. However, within weeks, he developed bihemispheric signs. Multiple areas of infarction were seen on neuroimaging studies. Pathologic studies showed no evidence of infection with typical or opportunistic pathogens. However, there was evidence of demonstrated gp41-positive cells (by immunohistochemical staining in the arterial walls), as well as a positive macrophage marker of leukocyte common antigen, but not with an endothelial cell marker. This suggested that HIV-1 may be directly involved in the vascular pathology associated with pediatric HIV/AIDS (Belman et al., 1988; Kure et al., 1989; Park et al., 1990). Since then, aneurysmal dilation of the branch vessels of the circle of Willis as the cause of subarachnoid hemorrhage, ischemic CVAs, or both has been the subject of numerous case reports and case series (Dubrovsky et al., 1998; Frank et al., 1989; Husson et al., l992; Moriarty et al., 1994; Philippet et al., l994; Shah et al., 1996; States et al., 1997; Picard et al., 1997; Fulmer et al, 1998; Legido et al., 1999; Mazzoni et al., 2000; Bonkowsky et al., 2002; Narayan et al., 2002; Visrutaratna and Oranratanachai, 2002; Patsalides et al., 2002). Some of the children had high plasma HIV-1 RNA viral loads and advanced disease. Viral RNA was undetectable in others with this syndrome receiving ARV therapy. Further, this syndrome occurred in at least one case during immune reconstitution, raising the possibility that it is associated with immune reconstitution inflammatory syndrome as well. The exact mechanism by which HIV-1 causes the arteriopathy remains unclear. Some investigators have suggested direct HIV-1 endothelial invasion and exposure to toxic cytokines may be responsible. Others have hypothesized that other viral agents may play a role, perhaps in synergy with HIV-1 (Park et al., 1990; Kure et al., 1989, 1991; Shah et al., 1996; Visudtibhan et al., 1999).

Cerebrovascular involvement may be a more common complication than has been appreciated. For example, cerebrovascular abnormalities were reported in 52% of cases examined at autopsy. This high incidence probably was secondary to series bias. However, one neuroimaging study of children with HIV/AIDS found a 2.6% incidence in 426 cases evaluated with CT scan or magnetic resonance imaging of the head. The authors of that study felt that the incidence might have been understated, since the majority of children in the cohort were evaluated by CT scan rather than magnetic resonance imaging, which is superior for the detection of cerebrovascular lesions.

Peripheral Nervous System Involvement

In general, peripheral nervous system involvement appears to be a less common complication in children than in adults (perhaps because fewer children have existing peripheral neuropathies that are exacerbated when HIV/AIDS-related peripheral neuropathy becomes superimposed). As in adults, though, complications include distal sensory or sensorimotor axonal neuropathy, demyelinating neuropathy, lumbosacral polyneuropathy, mononeuritis multiplex, inflammatory polyneuropathy, median nerve compression at the carpal tunnel, and toxic neuropathy related to ARV therapy (particularly with the dideoxynucleosides) (Araujo et al., 2000; Raphael et al., 1991; Bakshi et al., 1997; Floeter et al., 1997).

Distal sensory neuropathy (manifesting with pain and burning in the feet and legs) and CMV polyneuropathy occur in the advanced stage of HIV-1 disease, when the child is severely immunocompromised; associated HIV/AIDS CNS disease is common. It is probable that these complications occur more frequently in children than has been appreciated, since they tend to go unrecognized in these very sick, nonverbal youngsters. ARV-associated peripheral neuropathy is thought to be due to mitochondrial toxicity and is seen most commonly in patients receiving the dideoxynucleoside reverse transcriptase inhibitors (i.e., didanosine, zalcitabine, and stavudine). The symptoms include painful dysesthesias, usually on the soles of the feet, and, less often, contact sensitivity or hyperpathia (see chapter 6, this volume).

Neuroepidemiology

Pre-HAART Era

Before the introduction of ARV therapy, the rate of HIV-1-associated encephalopathy for infants and children with symptomatic HIV-1 infection was estimated to be as high as 60% (16 to 60%). The frequency of HIV-1 encephalopathy as the initial AIDS-defining illness in infants was reported at 12 to 67%, much higher than that reported for adults (0.8 to 2.2%) (Berger et al., 1987). Moreover, encephalopathy often manifested before signs and symptoms of immunosuppression (Cooper et al., 1998; Lobato et al., 1995). In older children, as in adults, HIV-1 CNS disease usually paralleled the progression and severity of immunodeficiency and systemic disease, with an overall prevalence estimated at 20 to 40%.

A French study compared children born to HIV-1-infected mothers from the French Perinatal Cohort with adults from the French SEROCO Cohort who had a known date of infection. The incidence of encephalopathy during the first 2 years of infection was also found to be higher than that in adults, 9.9% versus 0.3% and 4.2% versus 0%, in years 1 and 2, respectively. However, this is less than the rate found in U.S. studies. Thereafter, by age, the rates were similar (1% per year) in the two groups. At 7 years postinfection, the cumulative incidence reached rates of 16% in children and 5% in adults (Tardieu et al., 2000).

Changing Neuroepidemiology

Since the advent of HAART, both the incidence and prevalence rates of pediatric HIV-1 encephalopathy have declined markedly. For example, in one well-studied cohort of children, the rate of HIV-1-associated encephalopathy declined from 31% of children in 1992 to less than 2% in 2000 (Chiriboga et al., 2005). In the year 2000, 10% of the cohort had arrested PE. The factors contributing to this dramatic decline, which paralleled the overall decrease in the numbers of infants and children born with and living with HIV/AIDS, include (i) the low rate of infants born HIV-1 infected (due to the successful reduction of MTCT by perinatal ARV therapy), resulting in a decreased incidence of "fast progressors," who are the infants most susceptible to early-onset PE (Centers for Disease Control and Prevention, 2005), and (ii) the early identification and treatment of infected infants and children (resulting in viral suppression, immune reconstitution, stabilization of disease, and delay of disease progression) (De Martino et al., 2000; Gortmaker et al., 2001; Faye et al., 2004). In parallel, it was noted that there was a decreased incidence of secondary CNS complications in the HAART era as well. Of note, many children survived into the HAART era and are now adolescents with motor and cognitive sequelae of early HIV-1 CNS disease in the brain. Many of these children on ARV therapy, including HAART, have "minor cognitive and motor" HIV-1-related disabilities (or "minor cognitive-motor disorder") (see chapter 1, this volume) (Jeremy et al., 2005).

MANAGEMENT AND THERAPY

Probably the most significant advance in the pediatric AIDS epidemic has been the successful reduction of MTCT. HAART prescribed to the mother during pregnancy, labor, and delivery, as well as elective cesarean section to reduce the infant's exposure to blood and secretions, and the continuation of ARV therapy in the neonate can successfully decrease MTCT to 1 to 2% (European Collaborative Study, 2005). Although far from ideal, only a short course of ARV therapy has been shown to decrease MTCT by approximately 40 to 50% (New York State Department of Health AIDS Institute, 2007). ARVs appear to be safe, with severe mitochondrial toxicity associated with nucleoside analogue reverse transcriptase inhibitor (NRTI) use during pregnancy rare. However, possible long-term complications for the exposed fetus are as yet unknown. Studies in France have identified children exposed to ARVs in utero who have developed clinical and neuroimaging features of mitochondrial dysfunction (Blanche et al., 1999; Barret et al., 2003; Tardieu et al., 2005). Follow-up of these and other children with milder forms of possible ARV mitochondrial toxicity will be required to determine if ARV exposure has eventual toxic effects.

Management of the HIV-1-Infected Child

Management of the HIV-1-infected child continues to evolve and is increasingly complex. As for adults, the mainstays of HIV-1 management include early identification of the HIV-1-infected individual, ARV therapy targeted to the specific effects of the retrovirus, prophylaxis and treatment of OIs, and the management of HIV/AIDS-related conditions. Whenever possible, a team approach supervised by an expert is recommended. Management also includes habilitation/rehabilitation programs, special educational programs, attention to pain management, and psychosocial support.

Strategies have expanded greatly from treatment with a single ARV to the use of today's combination therapies. Greater understanding of the biology of HIV-1, factors related to viral entry, virus-host interaction, rates of viral replication, associated fluctuations and progressive CD4 cell depletion, the emergence of viral variants, viral distribution across different cellular compartments, and issues of latency have all been integrated into pathogenesis-based therapeutic strategies. Current recommendations include at least five different classes of ARV agents to target specific components unique to the virus to suppress HIV-1 replication without disrupting normal cellular function, preserving immune function, and reducing the development of resistant organisms. In addition to ARVs, adjunctive neuroprotective therapies are under evaluation (see chapter 1, this volume).

ARV Agents

As of January 2008, 14 ARV drugs had been approved for use in HIV-1-infected children and 25 for adolescents and adults (excluding combination formulations). These drugs fall into five major classes: NRTIs, nonnucleoside analogue reverse transcriptase inhibitors, protease inhibitors, fusion/entry inhibitors, and integrase inhibitors. The fusion/entry inhibitors act at the earliest stage by inhibiting binding or fusion of HIV-1 to target host cells and by preventing viral cell entry. The NRTIs and nonnucleoside analogue reverse transcriptase inhibitors act subsequently, but still in an early stage of viral replication (when HIV-1 reverse transcription of viral RNA into complementary DNA occurs). This is just prior to the step of integration of viral DNA into the host cell genome, when the integrase inhibitors act. Subsequently, the viral protease inhibitors act in a later step of viral integration, before budding.

All available ARVs have significant potential toxicities and side effects, including those affecting the nervous system. In addition, there are possible interactions between ARVs and other drugs used in the treatment of the HIV-1-infected child. Short- and long-term toxicities include headache, peripheral neuropathy, abnormal fat distribution (lipodystrophy syndrome), hyperlipidemia (with possible long-term cerebrovascular effects), mitochondrial toxicity, hypersensitivity reactions, hepatic toxicity, diabetes, renal toxicity, anemia, neutropenia, pancreatitis, and diarrhea.

As mentioned above, the NRTIs can induce mitochondrial dysfunction due to their affinities for mitochondrial gamma DNA polymerase and their interference with mitochondrial replication. This can result in mitochondrial DNA depletion and dysfunction. Toxicity related to mitochondrial dysfunction has been reported in patients receiving long-term treatment with these agents. In general, symptom resolution occurs with discontinuation of the offending agent(s) (see chapters 6 and 7, this volume). Detailed pediatric ARV drug information, mechanisms of action, and toxicities are comprehensively covered and updated by the U.S. Department of Health and Human Services (2006). Because of the need for lifelong treatment and the fact that the impact of long-term ARV therapy on children is unknown, long-term follow-up is crucial.

Issues Unique to Pediatric HIV/AIDS Therapy

Challenges of adherence, toxicities, and drug resistance remain for children, as they do for adults. Additional considerations for the pediatric age group include age-specific pharmacokinetics of drug metabolism and clearance and the need for special formulations of ARV drugs for adherence and tolerance. Prior ARV exposure must also be considered. Incomplete suppression of viral replication and possible selection of resistant viruses can complicate the choice of HAART therapies for infants with ARV exposure in utero and during the perinatal period, as well as for those children who were treated with sequential courses of monotherapy and combination regimens before HAART was introduced. When exactly to initiate therapy in the asymptomatic child, when to consider a "drug holiday" for the child with undetectable viral titers, and when to change therapy, and to which regimen, for the symptomatic child who has evidence of virologic, immunologic, or clinical disease progression, or toxicity, intolerance, or nonadherence to the current drug regimen, continue to be investigated.

Treatment of Neurological Disorders

Treatment with ARV drugs, particularly zidovudine, was reported early on to improve neurobehavioral deficits in some children and in some cases to arrest or even reverse HIV-1 encephalopathy (Pizzo et al., 1988, 1990; Brouwers et al., 1990; DeCarli et al., 1991; Brivio et al., 1991; Wolters et al., 1994). These effects, however, were not always long-lasting, and relapsed occurred (Nozyce et al., 1994b). HAART has been shown to reduce viral loads to low levels (often below the limits of detection) and to increase and normalize CD4 cell counts, as well as delay clinical disease progression (De Martino et al., 2000; Gortmaker et al., 2001; Sanchez-Ramon et al., 2003). For some children who developed HIV-1 encephalopathy prior to this era, HAART was able to halt progression (although for most, significant preexisting neurological impairment persisted) (Chiriboga et al., 2005). HAART has also been shown to reverse HIV-1 encephalopathy (Tepper et al., 1998; Foster and Lyall, 2005). However, some children treated with HAART, who had well-controlled stable disease with undetectable plasma viral loads, showed unexpected declines on serial neurocognitive testing (Tamula et al., 2003) or no change on neurocognitive testing (Jeremy et al., 2005). Possible sequestration (compartmentalization of replicating HIV-1 in the CNS) may explain these results. Changing ARV regimens to agents with greater CNS penetration has proven successful in some cases (Tamula et al., 2003).

HIV-1-Associated CNS Disease

HIV-1-Associated Progressive Encephalopathy

At least one ARV with substantial CNS penetration having CSF/plasma ratios greater than 0.2 (e.g., zidovudine or nevirapine) has been shown to reverse or arrest progressive HIV-1 encephalopathy when treated in the early stage.

HIV-1-Associated Extrapyramidal Symptoms and Signs

Levo-dopa and dopamine agonists may be beneficial for children with "Parkinsonian-like," bradykinetic, rigid syndromes associated with HIV-1 CNS disease (Mintz et al., 1996).

Neuropsychiatric Complications

Neuropsychiatric and neurobehavioral complications are treated with neuroleptics, antidepressants, psychostimulants, and psychotherapy. Neuroleptics are useful in the treatment of acute psychotic episodes and advanced HIV-1 encephalopathy. Major depressive disorder responds to treatment with antidepressant medications. Children with

HIV-1 CNS disease may require doses lower than the usual pediatric doses, and the clinician needs to be keenly aware of the potential for drug-drug interactions.

Psychostimulants may be particularly useful in the early stages of HIV-1 encephalopathy (as well as for major depressive disorder). In particular, methylphenidate may benefit the child with attention deficits due to HIV-1 CNS disease. Behavior modification techniques are recommended and, when possible, should be instituted prior to or in conjunction with a psychostimulant medication trial. Appetite suppression and psychomotor agitation with the psychostimulants can be an undesirable side effect in HIV-1-infected children and require ongoing clinical monitoring (El-Sadr et al., 1994).

Short-term psychotherapy has been recommended to help children cope with the many challenging issues of HIV-1 infection, such as deaths in the family. Long-term therapy in this setting is advocated to help children deal with issues of chronic illness, death, and the social stigmas associated with HIV-1 infection. Psychotherapy should be included in treatment of depressive and psychotic symptoms and disorders.

Pain

Painful medical procedures are frequent, and children may experience pain related to a number of HIV-1-associated conditions (Czarniecki and Oleske, 1993; Schechter et al., 1993; Gaughan et al., 2002; Lolekha et al., 2004). A thorough clinical assessment is required, including the identification and treatment of the underlying cause of pain and an assessment of pain severity. Both pharmacologic and non-pharmacologic therapies for pain control should be considered. The WHO analgesic ladder is a very useful guideline.

SUMMARY

The most effective way to prevent pediatric HIV-1-associated neurological syndromes is to prevent vertically acquired HIV-1 infection. Clearly the most effective strategy to achieve this goal is to prevent HIV-1 infection in all women of childbearing age. Short of that, the next best way is to prevent MTCT. Perhaps the most significant advance in the pediatric AIDS epidemic has been the successful strategies to interrupt MTCT. Unfortunately, this is not the case worldwide, where the epidemic continues, with increasing numbers of women and girls infected every year and access to care remaining limited.

Vertically acquired HIV-1 infection occurs in an immature developing organism. The maturational stage of the nervous and immune systems when exposed to the effects of the retrovirus is of significance and may account for age-specific vulnerabilities and devastating neurological sequelae. The exact mechanisms by which HIV-1 affects the developing brain remain unclear and continue to be investigated.

Major advances in treatment resulting in control of viral replication have altered the course of HIV-1 disease progression. The long-term effects of prenatal exposure to ARVs are not yet fully appreciated and continue to be studied. How HAART ultimately will affect the early signs of HIV-1 CNS disease is also unclear. As some children and adolescents eventually will fail HAART and become immunocompromised, complications secondary to HIV-1, such as CNS OIs, neoplasms, and cerebrovascular disease, may once again become more prevalent. As new ARV agents are still being developed and new combination drug regimens are being instituted, the potential for neurological complications, toxicities, and adverse drug-drug interactions will grow and will need to be further identified and monitored.

REFERENCES

Abrams, E. J., P. B. Matheson, P. A. Thomas, D. M. Thea, K. Krasinski, G. Lambert, N. Shaffer, M. Bamji, D. Hutson, and K. Grimm. 1995. Neonatal predictors of infection status and early death among 332 infants at risk of HIV-1 infection monitored prospectively from birth, New York City Perinatal HIV Transmission Collaborative Study Group. *Pediatrics* **96:**451–458.

Abrams, E. J., J. Weedon, R. W. Steketee, G. Lambert, M. Bamji, T. Brown, M. L. Kalish, E. E. Schoenbaum, P. A. Thomas, D. M. Thea, et al. 1998. Association of human immunodeficiency virus (HIV) load early in life with disease progression among HIV-infected infants. *J. Infect. Dis.* **178:**101–108.

Abuzaitoun, O. R., and I. C. Hanson. 2000. Organ-specific manifestations of HIV disease in children. HIV/AIDS in infants, children, and adolescents. *Pediatr. Clin. N. Am.* **47:**109–125.

Ammann, A. J., M. J. Cowan, D. W. Wara, P. Weintrub, S. Dritz, H. Goldman, and H. A. Perkins. 1983. Acquired immunodeficiency in an infant: possible transmission by means of blood products. *Lancet* **i:**956–958.

Anders, K. H., W. F. Guerra, U Tomiyasu, M. A. Verity, and H. V. Vinters. 1986. The neuropathology of AIDS. UCLA experience and review. *Am. J. Pathol.* **124:**537–556.

Andiman, W. A., J. Mezger, and E. Shapiro. 1994. Invasive bacterial infections in children born to women infected with human immunodeficiency virus type-1. *J. Pediatr.* **124:**846–852.

Andiman, W. A., R. Eastman, K. Martin, B. Z. Katz, A. Rubinstein, J. Pitt, S. Pahwa, and G. Miller. 1985. Opportunistic lymphoproliferation associated with Epstein-Barr viral DNA in infants and children with AIDS. *Lancet* **ii:**1390–1393.

Araujo, A. P., O. J. Nascimento, and O. S. Garcia. 2000. Distal sensory polyneuropathy in a cohort of HIV-infected children over five years of age. *Pediatrics* **106:**e35.

Auger, I., P. Thomas, V. De Gruttola, D. Morse, D. Moore, R. Williams, B. Truman, and C. E. Lawrence. 1988. Incubation periods for paediatric AIDS patients. *Nature* **336:**575–577.

Aylward, E. H., A. M. Butz, N. Hutton, M. L. Joyner, and J. W. Vogelhut. 1992. Cognitive and motor development in infants at risk for human immunodeficiency virus. *Am. J. Dis. Child.* **146:**218–222.

Bakshi, S. S., P. Britto, E. Capparelli, L. Mofenson, M. G. Fowler, S. Rasheed, D. Schoenfeld, B. Zimmer, Y. Frank, R. Yogev, E. Jimenez, M. Salgo, G. Boone, S. G. Pahwa, et al. 1997. Evaluation of pharmacokinetics, safety, tolerance, and activity of combination of zalcitabine and zidovudine in stable, zidovudine-treated pediatric patients with human immunodeficiency virus infection. *J. Infect. Dis.* **175:**1039–1050.

Barnhart, H. X., R. Byers, M. B. Caldwell, H. W. Hsu, Y. Maldonado, L. Mascola, I. Ortiz, R. Parrott, P. Thomas, and J. Schulte. 1996. Natural history of human immunodeficiency virus disease in perinatally infected children: an analysis from the Pediatric Spectrum of Disease Project. *Pediatrics* **97:**710–716.

Barret, B., M. Tardieu, P. Rustin, D. Lacroix, B. Chabrol, I. Desguerre, C. Dollfus, M. J. Mayaux, and S. Blanche for the French Perinatal Cohort Study Group. 2003. Persistent mitochondrial dysfunction in HIV-1-exposed but uninfected infants: clinical screening in a large prospective cohort. *AIDS* **17:**1769–1785.

Bell, J. E. 2004. An update on the neuropathology of HIV in the HAART era. *Histopathology* **45:**549–559.

Belman, A. L. 1992. Acquired immunodeficiency syndrome and the child's central nervous system. *Pediatr. Clin. N. Am.* **39:**691–714.

Belman, A. L. 1990. AIDS and pediatric neurology. *Neurol. Clin.* **8:**571–603.

Belman, A. L. 1994. HIV-1-associated CNS disease in infants and children. *Res. Publ. Assoc. Res. Nerv. Ment. Dis.* **72:**289–310.

Belman, A. L. 2002. HIV-1 infection and AIDS. *Neurol. Clin.* **20:**983–1011.

Belman, A. L., L. R. Muenz, J. C. Marcus, J. J. Goedert, S. Landesman, A. Rubinstein, S. Goodwin, S. Durako, and A. Willoughby. 1996. Neurologic status of human immunodeficiency virus 1-infected infants and their controls: a prospective study from birth to 2 years. Mothers and Infants Cohorts Study. *Pediatrics* **98:**1109–1118.

Belman, A. L., G. Diamond, D. Dickson, D. Horoupian, J. Llena, G. Lantos, and A. Rubinstein. 1988. Pediatric AIDS: neurologic syndromes. *Am. J. Dis. Child.* **142:**29–35.

Belman, A. L., G. Lantos, D. Horoupian, B. E. Novick, M. H. Ultmann, D. W. Dickson, and A. Rubinstein. 1986. AIDS: calcification of the basal ganglia in infants and children. *Neurology* **36:**1192–1199.

Belman, A. L., M. H. Ultmann, D. Horoupian, D. Kurtzberg, B. Novick, B. Cone-Wesson, A. J. Spiro, and A. Rubinstein. 1985. Neurologic complications in infants and children with Acquired immune deficiency syndrome. *Ann. Neurol.* **18:**560–566.

Berger, J., J. Albrecht, A. L. Belman, G. Tornatore, and E. O. Major. 1992. Progressive multifocal leukoencephalopathy in children with HIV infection. *AIDS* **6:**837–841.

Berger, J. R., L. Moskowitz, M. Fischl, and R. E. Kelley. 1987. Neurologic disease as the presenting manifestation of Acquired immunodeficiency syndrome. *S. Med. J.* **80:**683–686.

Berger, J. R., J. O. Harris, J. Gregorios, and M. Norenberg. 1990. Cerebrovascular disease in AIDS: a case-control study. *AIDS* **4:**239–244.

Bernstein, L. J., H. D. Ochs, R. J. Wedgwood, and A. Rubinstein. 1985. Defective humoral immunity in pediatric Acquired immunodeficiency syndrome. *J. Pediatr.* **107:**352–357.

Bertolli, J., M. E. St. Louis, R. J. Simonds, P. Nieburg, M. Kamenga, C. Brown, M. Tarande, T. Quinn, and C. Y. Ou. 1996. Estimating the timing of mother-to-child transmission of human immunodeficiency virus in a breast feeding population in Kinshasa, Zaire. *J. Infect. Dis.* **174:**722–726.

Biggar, R. J., M. Frisch, J. J. Goedert, et al. 2000. Risk of cancer in children with AIDS. *JAMA* **284:**205–209.

Biggemann, B., T. Voit, E. Neuen, W. Wechsler, H. Kramer, R. von Kries, and V. Wahn. 1987. Neurological manifestations in three German children with AIDS. *Hippokrates* **18:**99–106.

Blanche, S., M. Tardieu, A. M. Duliege, C. Rouzioux, F. Le Deist, K. Fukunaga, M. Caniglia, C. Jacomet, A. Messiah, and C. Griscelli. 1990. Longitudinal study of 94 symptomatic infants with materno fetal HIV infection: evidence for a bimodal expression of clinical and biological symptoms. *Am. J. Dis. Child.* **144:**1210–1215.

Blanche, S., M. J. Mayaux, C. Rouzioux, J. P. Teglas, G. Firtion, F. Monpoux, N. Ciraru-Vigneron, F. Meier, J. Tricoire, and C. Courpotin. 1994. Relation of the course of HIV infection in children to the severity of the disease in their mothers at delivery. *N. Engl. J. Med.* **330:**308–312.

Blanche, S., M. Tardieu, P. Rustin, A. Slama, B. Barret, G. Firtion, N. Ciraru-Vigneron, C. Lacroix, C. Rouzioux, L. Mandelbrot, I. Desguerre, A. Rotig, M. J. Mayaux, and J. F. Delfraissy. 1999. Persistent mitochondrial dysfunction and perinatal exposure to antiretroviral nucleoside analogues. *Lancet* **354:**1084–1089.

Bonkowsky, J. L., J. C. Christenson, G. W. Nixon, and A. T. Pavia. 2002. Cerebral aneurysms in a child with acquired immune deficiency syndrome during rapid immune reconstitution. *J. Child. Neurol.* **17:**457–460.

Borkowsky, W., K. Krasinski, Y. Cao, D. Ho, H. Pollack, T. Moore, S. H. Chen, M. Allen, and P. T. Tao. 1994. Correlation of perinatal transmission of human immunodeficiency virus type 1 with maternal viremia and lymphocyte phenotypes. *J. Pediatr.* **125:**345–351.

Boyer, P. J., M. Dillon, M. Navaie, A. Deveikis, M. Keller, S. O'Rourke, and Y. J. Bryson. 1994. Factors predictive of maternal-fetal transmission of HIV-1: preliminary analysis of zidovudine given during pregnancy and/or delivery. *JAMA* **271:**1925–1930.

Brivio, L., R. Tornaghi, L. Musetti, P. Marchisio, and N. Principi. 1991. Improvement of auditory brainstem responses after treatment with zidovudine in a child with AIDS. *Pediatr. Neurol.* **7:**53–55.

Brouwers, P., H. Moss, P. Wolters, J. Eddy, F. Balis, D. G. Poplack, and P. A. Pizzo. 1990. Effect of continuous-infusion zidovudine therapy on neuropsychologic functioning in children with symptomatic human immunodeficiency virus infection. *J. Pediatr.* **117:**980–985.

Brouwers, E., A. L. Belman, and L. Epstein. 1994. Central nervous system involvement: manifestations and evaluation, p. 433–455. *In* P. A. Pizzo and C. M. Wilfert (ed.), *Pediatric AIDS: the Challenge of HIV Infection in Infants, Children and Adolescents*, 2nd ed. Williams & Wilkins, New York, NY.

Brouwers, P., C. DeCarli, A. L. Civitello, H. Moss, P. Wolters, and P. Pizzo. 1995a. Correlation between CT Brain scan abnormalities and neuropsychological function in children with symptomatic HIV disease. *Arch. Neurol.* **52:**39–44.

Brouwers, P., G. Tudor-Williams, C. DeCarli, H. A. Moss, P. L. Wolters, L. A. Civitello, and P. A. Pizzo. 1995b. Relationship between stage of disease and neurobehavioral measures in children with symptomatic disease. *AIDS* **9:**713–720.

Brouwers, P., L. Civitello, C. DeCarli, P. Wolters, and S. Sei. 2000. Cerebrospinal fluid viral load is related to cortical atrophy and not to intracerebral calcifications in children with symptomatic HIV disease. *J. Neurovirol.* **6:**390–397.

Brustle, O., H. Spiegel, S. L. Leib, T. Finn, H. Stein, P. Kleihues, and O. D. Wiestler. 1992. Distribution of HIV in the CNS of children with severe HIV encephalopathy. *Acad. Neuropathol.* **84:**24–31.

Bryson, Y. J., K. Luzuriaga, J. L. Sullivan, and D. W. Wara. 1992. Proposed definitions for *in utero* versus intrapartum transmission of HIV-1. *N. Engl. J. Med.* **327:**1246–1247.

Bulterys, M., and J. J. Goedert. 1996. From biology to sexual behaviour—towards the prevention of mother-to-child transmission of HIV. *AIDS* **10:**1287–1289.

Burgard, M., M. J. Mayaux, S. Blanche, A. Ferroni, M. L. Guihard-Moscato, M. C. Allemon, N. Ciraru-Vigneron, G. Firtion, C. Floch, and F. Guillot. 1992. The use of viral culture and p24 antigen testing to diagnose HIV infection in neonates. *N. Engl. J. Med.* **327:**1192–1197.

Burger, H., A. L. Belman, R. Grimson, A. Kaell, K. Flaherty, J. Gulla, R. A. Gibbs, P. N. Nguyun, and B. Weiser. 1990. Long HIV-1 incubation periods and dynamics of transmission within a family. *Lancet* **336:**134–136.

Burns, D. K. 1992. The neuropathology of pediatric Acquired immunodeficiency syndrome. *J. Child. Neurol.* **7:**332–346.

Centers for Disease Control. 1982. Unexplained immunodeficiency and opportunistic infections in infants-New York, New Jersey, California. *MMWR Morb. Mortal. Wkly. Rep.* **31:**665–667.

Centers for Disease Control and Prevention. 1994. Revised classification system for human immunodeficiency virus infection in children less than 13 years of age. *MMWR Morb. Mortal. Wkly. Rep.* **43**(RR-12):1–10.

Centers for Disease Control and Prevention. 2005. *HIV/AIDS Surveillance Report.* CDC, Atlanta, GA.

Chase, C., M. Vibbert, S. I. Pelton, D. Coulter, and H. Cabral. 1995. Early developmental growth in children with vertically transmitted human immunodeficiency virus infection. *Arch. Pediatr. Adolesc. Med.* **149:**850–855.

Chin, J. 1990. Current and future dimensions of the HIV/AIDS pandemic in women and children. *Lancet* **336:**221–224.

Chiriboga, C. A., S. Fleishman, S. Champion, L. Gaye-Robinson, and E. J. Abrams. 2005. Incidence and prevalence of HIV encephalopathy in children with HIV infection receiving highly active antiretroviral therapy (HAART). *J. Pediatr.* **146:**402–407.

Cohen, S. E., T. Mundy, B. Kaarassik, L. Lieb, D. D. Ludwig, and J. Ward. 1991. Neuropsychological functioning in children with HIV-1 infection through neonatal blood transfusion. *Pediatrics* **88:**58–68.

Cole, J. W., A. N. Pinto, J. R. Hebel, D. W. Buchholz, C. J. Earley, C. J. Johnson, R. F. Macko, T. R. Price, M. A. Sloan, B. J. Stern, R. J. Wityk, M. A. Wozniak, and S. J. Kittner. 2004. Acquired immunodeficiency syndrome and the risk of stroke. *Stroke* **35:**51–56.

Comans-Bitter, W. M., R. de Groot, R. van den Beemd, H. J. Neijens, W. C. Hop, K. Groeneveld, H. Hooijkaas, and J. J. van Dongen. 1997. Immunophenotyping of blood lymphocytes in childhood. Reference values for lymphocyte subpopulations. *J. Pediatr.* **130:**388–393.

Condini, A., G. Axia, C. Cattelan, M. R. D'Urso, A. M. Laverda, F. Viero, and F. Zacchello. 1991. Development of language in 18–30 month old HIV-1 infected but not ill children. *AIDS* **5:**735–739.

Connor, E. M., R. S. Sperling, R. Gelber, P. Kiselev, G. Scott, M. J. O'Sullivan, R. VanDyke, M. Bey, W. Shearer, and R. L. Jacobson. 1994. Reduction of maternal-infant transmission of human immunodeficiency virus type 1 with zidovudine treatment. *N. Engl. J. Med.* **331:**1173–1180.

Connor, M. D., G. A. Lammie, J. E. Bell, C. P. Warlow, P. Simmonds, and R. D. Brettle. 2000. Cerebral infarction in adult AIDS patients. *Stroke* **31:**2117–2126.

Cooper, E. R., C. Hanson, C. Diaz, H. Mendez, R. Abboud, R. Nugent, J. Pitt, K. Rich, E. M. Rodriguez, V. Smeriglio, et al. 1998. Encephalopathy and progression of HIV disease in a cohort of children with perinatally Acquired HIV infection. *J. Pediatr.* **132:**808–905.

Coutsoudis, A., F. Dabis, W. Fawzi, P. Gaillard, G. Haverkamp, D. R. Harris, J. B. Jackson, V. Leroy, N. Meda, P. Msellati, M. L. Newell, R. Nsuati, J. S. Read, S. Wiktor, and the Breastfeeding and HIV International Transmission Study Group. 2004. Late postnatal transmission of HIV-1 in breast-fed children: an individual patient data meta-analysis. *Infect. Dis.* **189:**2154–2166.

Czarniecki, L. M., and J. M. Oleske. 1993. Pain in children with HIV disease. *PAAC Notes* **5:**492–495.

DeCarli, C., L. Fugate, J. Falloon, J. Eddy, D. A. Katz, R. P. Friedland, S. I. Rapoport, P. Brouwers, and P. A. Pizzo. 1991. Brain growth and congnitive improvement in children with HIV induced encephalopathy after 6 months of continous infusion therapy. *AIDS* **4:**585–592.

Delfraissy, J. F., S. Blanche, C. Rouzioux, and M. J. Mayaux. 1992. Perinatal HIV transmission facts and controversies. *Immunodef. Rev.* **3:**305–327.

De Martino, M., P. A. Tovo, M. Balducci, L. Galli, C. Gabiano, G. Rezza, and P. Pezzotti. 2000. Reduction in mortality with availability of antiretroviral therapy for children with perinatal HIV-1 infection. *JAMA* **284:**190–197.

De Rossi, A., S. Masiero, C. GiaQuinto, E. Ruga, M. Comar, M. Giacca, and L. Chieco-Bianchi. 1996. Dynamics of viral replication in infants with vertically Acquired human immunodeficiency virus type 1 infection. *J. Clin. Investig.* **97:**323–330.

Diamond, G. W., J. Kaufman, A. L. Belman, L. Cohen, H. J. Cohen, and A. Rubinstein. 1987. Characterization of cognitive functioning in a subgroup of children with congenital HIV infection. *Arch. Clin. Neuropsych.* **2:**245–256.

Diaz, C., C. Hanson, E. R. Cooper, J. S. Read, J. Watson, H. A. Mendez, J. Pitt, K. Rich, V. Smeriglio, and J. F. Lew. 1998. Disease progression in a cohort of infants with vertically Acquired HIV infection observed from birth: the women and infants transmission study (WITS). *J. Acquir. Immune Defic. Syndr. Hum. Retrovirol.* **18:**221–228.

Dickover, R. E., E. M. Garratty, S. A. Herman, M. S. Sim, S. Plaeger, P. J. Boyer, M. Keller, A. Deveikis, E. R. Stiehm, and Y. J. Bryson. 1996. Identification of levels of maternal HIV RNA associated with risk of perinatal transmission: effect of maternal zidovudine treatment on viral load. *JAMA* **275:**599–605.

Dickson, D. W., A. L. Belman, T. S. Kim, D. Horoupian, and A. Rubinstein. 1989a. Spinal cord pathology in pediatric Acquired immunodeficiency syndrome. *Neurology* **39:**227–235.

Dickson, D. W., A. L. Belman, Y. D. Park, C. Wiley, D. S. Horoupian, J. Llena, K. Kure, W. D. Lyman, R. Morecki, and S. Mitsudo. 1989b. Central nervous system pathology in pediatric AIDS: an autopsy study. *APMIS* **8:**40–57.

Drotar, D., K. Olness, M. Wiznitzer, L. Guay, L. Marum, G. Svilar, D. Hom, J. F. Fagan, C. Ndugwa, and R. Kiziri-Mayengo. 1997. Neurodevelopmental outcome of Ugandan infants with human immunodeficiency virus type 1 infection. *Pediatrics* **100:**e5.

Dubrovsky, T., R. Curless, G. Scott, M. Chaneles, M. J. Post, N. Altman, C. K. Petito, D. Start, and C. Wood. 1998. Cerebral aneurismal arteriopathy in childhood AIDS. *Neurology* **51:**560–565.

Duliege, A. M., A. Messiah, S. Blanche, M. Tardieu, C. Griscelli, and A. Spira. 1992. Natural history of HIV-1 infection in children: prognostic value of the laboratory parameters on the bimodal progression of the disease. *Pediatr. Infect. Dis. J.* **11:**630–635.

Ehrnst, A., S. Lindgren, M. Dictor, B. Johansson, A. Sonnerborg, J. Czajkowski, G. Sundin, and A. B. Bohlin. 1991. HIV in pregnant women and their offspring: evidence for late transmission. *Lancet* **338:**203–207.

Ehrnst, A., S. Lindgren, E. Belfrage, A. Sonnerborg, M. Dictor, B. Johansson, and A. B. Bohlin. 1992. Intrauterine and intrapartum transmission of HIV. *Lancet* **339:**245–246.

El-Sadr, W., J. M. Oleske, B. D. Agins, et al. 1994. *Evaluation and Management of Early HIV Infection.* AHCPR publication no. 94-0572. Agency for Health Care Policy and Research, Public Health Service, U.S. Department of Health and Human Services, Rockville, MD.

Englund, J. A., C. J. Baker, C. Raskino, R. E. McKinney, M. H. Lifschitz, B. Petrie, M. G. Fowler, J. D. Connor, H. Mendez, K. O'Donnell, and D. W. Wara. 1996. Clinical and laboratory characteristics of a large cohort of symptomatic, human immunodeficiency virus-infected infants and children. *Pediatr. Infect. Dis. J.* **15:**1025–1036.

Epstein, L. G., L. R. Sharer, V. V. Joshi, M. M. Fojas, M. R. Koenigsberger, and J. M. Oleske. 1985. Progressive encephalopathy in children with Acquired immune deficiency syndrome. *Ann. Neurol.* **17:**488–496.

Epstein, L. G., L. R. Sharer, J. M. Oleske, E. M. Connor, J. Goudsmit, L. Bagdon, M. Robert-Guroff, and M. R. Koenigsberger. 1986. Neurologic manifestations of human immunodeficiency virus infection in children. *Pediatrics* **78:**678–687.

Epstein, L. G., L. R. Sharer, and J. Goudsmit. 1988a. Neurological and neuropathological features of HIV in children. *Ann. Neurol.* **23**(Suppl.):S19–S23.

Epstein, L. G., F. J. Dicarlo, Jr., V. V. Joshi, E. M. Connor, J. M. Oleske, D. Kay, M. R. Koenigsberger, and L. R. Sharer. 1988b. Primary lymphoma of the central nervous system in

children with Acquired immunodeficiency syndrome. *Pediatrics* **82:**355–363.

Epstein, L. G., and H. E. Gendelman. 1993. Human immunodeficiency virus type 1 infection of the nervous system: pathogenetic mechanisms. *Ann. Neurol.* **33:**429–436.

Epstein, L. G., and H. A. Gelbard. 1999. HIV-1-induced injury in the developing brain. *J. Leukoc. Biol.* **65:**453–457.

European Collaborative Study. 1992. Risk factors for mother-to-child transmission of HIV-1. *Lancet* **339:**1007–1012.

European Collaborative Study. 1994. Natural history of vertically Acquired human immunodeficiency virus-1 infection. *Pediatrics* **94:**815–819.

European Collaborative Study. 2005. Mother-to-child transmission of HIV in the era of highly active antiretroviral therapy. *Clin. Infect. Dis.* **40:**458–465.

European Mode of Delivery Collaboration. 1999. Elective cesarean-section versus vaginal delivery in prevention of vertical HIV-1 transmission: a randomised clinical trial. *Lancet* **353:**1035–1039.

Evers, S., D. Nabavi, A. Rahmann, C. Heese, D. Reichelt, and I. Husstedt. 2003. Ischemic cerebrovascular events in HIV infection. *Cerebrovasc. Dis.* **15:**199–205.

Fang, G., H. Burger, R. Grimson, P. Tropper, S. Nachman, D. Mayers, O. Weislow, R. Moore, C. Reyelt, N. Hutcheon, D. Baker, and B. Weiser. 1995. Maternal plasma human immunodeficiency virus type 1 RNA level: a determinant and projected threshold for mother-to-child transmission. *Proc. Natl. Acad. Sci. USA* **92:**12100–12104.

Faye, A., J. Le Chenadec, C. Dollfus, I. Thuret, D. Douard, G. Firtion, E. Lachassinne, M. Levine, J. Nicolas, F. Monpoux, J. Tricoire, C. Rouzioux, M. Tardieu, M. J. Mayaux, S. Blanche, and the French Perinatal Study Group. 2004. Early versus deferred antiretroviral multidrug therapy in infants infected with HIV type 1. *Clin. Infect. Dis.* **39:**1692–1698.

Floeter, M. K., L. A. Civitello, C. R. Everett, J. Dambrosia, and C. A. Luciano. 1997. Peripheral neuropathy in children with HIV infection. *Neurology* **49:**207–212.

Foster, C., and E. G. Lyall. 2005. Children with HIV: improved mortality and morbidity with combination antiretroviral therapy. *Curr. Opin. Infect. Dis.* **18:**253–259.

Fowler, M. G., R. J. Simonds, and A. Roongpisuthipong. 2000. Update on perinatal HIV transmission. HIV/AIDS in infants, children, and adolescents. *Pediatr. Clin. N. Am.* **47:**21–38.

Frank, Y., W. Lim, E. Kahn, P. Farmer, M. Gorey, and S. Pahwa. 1989. Multiple ischemic infarcts in a child with AIDS, varicella zoster infection and cerebral vasculitis. *Pediatr. Neurol.* **5:**64–67.

Frank, Y., D. Lu, S. Pavlakis, K. Black, P. LaRussa, and R. A. Hyman. 1997. Childhood AIDS, varicella zoster, and cerebral vasculopathy. *J. Child. Neurol.* **12:**464–466.

Frederick, T., L. Mascola, A. Eller, L. O'Neil, and B. Byers. 1994. Progression of human immunodeficiency virus disease among infants and children infected with human immunodeficiency virus or through neonatal blood transfusion. *Pediatr. Infect. Dis. J.* **13:**1091–1097.

French Pediatric HIV Infection Study Group, European Collaborative Study. 1997. Morbidity and mortality in European children vertically infected by HIV-1. *AIDS* **14:**442–450.

Fulmer, B. B., S. C. Dillard, E. M. Musulman, C. A. Palmer, and J. Oakes. 1998. Two cases of cerebral aneurysm in HIV+ children. *Pediatr. Neurosurg.* **28:**31–34.

Futterman, D., B. Chabon, and N. D. Hoffman. 2000. HIV and AIDS in adolescents. HIV/AIDS in infants, children, and adolescents. *Pediatr. Clin. N. Am.* **47:**171–188.

Garcia, P. M., L. A. Kalish, J. Pitt, H. Minkoff, T. C. Quinn, S. K. Burchett, J. Kornegay, B. Jackson, J. Moye, C. Hanson, C. Zorrilla, J. F. Lew, et al. 1999. Maternal levels of plasma human immunodeficiency virus type 1 RNA and the risk of perinatal transmission. *N. Engl. J. Med.* **341**:394–402.

Gaughan, D. M., M. D. Hughes, G. R. Seage III, P. A. Selwyn, V. J. Carey, S. L. Gortmaker, and J. M. Oleske. 2002. The prevalence of pain in pediatric human immunodeficiency virus/Acquired immunodeficiency syndrome as reported by participants in the Pediatric Late Outcomes Study (PACTG 219). *Pediatrics* **109**:1144–1152.

Gaughan, D. M., M. D. Hughes, J. M. Oleske, K. Malee, C. A. Gore, and the Pediatric AIDS Clinical Trials Group 219C Team. 2004. Psychiatric hospitalizations among children and youths with human immunodeficiency virus infection. *Pediatrics* **113**:e544–545.1

Gay, C. L., F. D. Armstrong, D. Cohen, S. Lai, M. D. Hardy, T. P. Swales, C. J. Morrow, and G. B. Scott. 1995. The effects of HIV on cognitive and motor development in children born to HIV-seropositive women with no reported drug use: birth to 24 months. *Pediatrics* **96**:1078–1082.

Global AIDS Policy Coalition. 1996. *AIDS in the World II. Global Dimensions, Social Roots, and Responses.* Oxford University Press, New York, NY.

Goedert, J. J., A. M. Duliege, C. I. Amos, S. Felton, and R. J. Biggar. 1991. High risk of HIV-1 infection for first-born twins: the International Registry of HIV-Exposed Twins. *Lancet* **338**:1471–1475.

Goldstein, J., D. W. Dickson, A. Rubenstein, W. Woods, F. Mincer, A. L. Belman, and L. Davis. 1990. Primary CNS lymphoma in a pediatric patient with Acquired immunodeficiency syndrome treatment with radiation. *Cancer* **66**:2503–2508.

Gortmaker, S. L., M. Hughes, J. Cervia, M. Brady, G. M. Johnson, G. R. Seage III, L. Y. Song, W. M. Dankner, J. M. Oleske, and the Pediatric AIDS Clinical Trials Group Protocol 219 Team. 2001. Effect of combination therapy including protease inhibitors on mortality among children and adolescents infected with HIV-1. *N. Engl. J. Med.* **345**:1522–1528.

Gray, L., M. L. Newell, C. Peckham, J. Levy, and European Collaborative Study. 2001. Fluctuations in symptoms in human deficiency virus-infected children: the first 10 years of life. *Pediatrics* **108**:116–122.

Grubman, S., E. Gross, N. Learner-Weiss, M. Hernandez, G. D. McSherry, L. G. Hoyt, M. Boland, and J. M. Oleske. 1995. Older children and adolescents living with perinatally Acquired human immunodeficiency virus infection. *Pediatrics* **95**:657–663.

Havens, J. F., A. H. Whitaker, J. F. Feldman, and A. A. Ehrhardt. 1994. Psychiatric morbidity in school-aged children with congenital human immunodeficiency virus infection: a pilot study. *J. Dev. Beh. Pediatr.* **15**(Suppl. 3):S18–S25.

Hughes, M. D., V. A. Johnson, M. S. Hirsch, J. W. Bremer, T. Elbeik, A. Erice, D. R. Kuritzkes, W. A. Scott, S. A. Spector, N. Basgoz, M. A. Fischl, and R. T. D'Aquila. 1997. Monitoring plasma HIV-1 RNA levels in addition to CD4[+] lymphocyte count improves assessment of antiretroviral therapeutic response. *Ann. Intern. Med.* **126**:929–938.

Husson, R. N., R. Saini, L. L. Lewis, K. M. Butler, N. Patronas, and P. A. Pizzo. 1992. Cerebral artery aneurysms in children affected with human immunodeficiency virus. *J. Pediatr.* **121**:927–930.

International Perinatal HIV Group. 1999. The mode of delivery and the risk of vertical transmission of human immunodeficiency type-1. *N. Engl. J. Med.* **340**:977–987.

Ioannidis, J. P., A. Tatsioni, E. J. Abrams, M. Bulterys, R. W. Coombs, J. J. Goedert, B. T. Korber, M. J. Mayaux, L. M. Mofenson, J. Moye. Jr., M. L. Newell, D. E. Shapiro, J. P. Teglas, B. Thompson, and J. Wiener. 2004. Maternal viral load and rate of disease progression among vertically HIV-1-infected children: an international meta-analysis. *AIDS* **18**:99–108.

Jeremy, R. J., S. Kim, M. Nozyce, S. Nachman, K. McIntosh, S. I. Pelton, R. Yogev, A. Wiznia, G. M. Johnson, P. Krogstad, K. Stanley, and the Pediatric AIDS Clinical Trials Groups 338 and 377. 2005. Neuropsychological functioning and viral load in stable antiretroviral therapy-experienced HIV-infected children. *Pediatrics* **115**:380–387.

Joint United Nations Program on HIV/AIDS/World Health Organization. 2005. *AIDS Epidemic Update. December, 2005.* UNAIDS/WHO, Geneva, Switzerland.

Jovaisas, E., M. A. Koch, A. Schafer, M. Stauber, and D. Lowenthal. 1985. LAV/HTLV-III in 20-week fetus. *Lancet* **ii**:1129. (Letter.)

Just, J. J., E. Abrams, L. G. Louie, R. Urbano, D. Wara, S. W. Nicholas, Z. Stein, and M. C. King. 1995. Influence of host genotype on progression to Acquired immunodeficiency syndrome among children infected with human immunodeficiency virus type 1. *J. Pediatr.* **127**:544–549.

Kaur, R., D. Rawat, M. Kakkar, R. Monga, and V. K. Sharma. 2003. Cryptococcal meningitis in pediatric AIDS. *J. Trop. Pediatr.* **49**:124–125.

Kourtis, A. P., C. Ibegbu, A. J. Nahmias, F. K. Lee, W. S. Clark, M. K. Sawyer, and S. Nesheim. 1996. Early progression of disease in HIV-infected infants with thymus dysfunction. *N. Engl. J. Med.* **335**:1431–1436.

Kozlowski, P. B., J. H. Sher, C. Rao, P. A. Anzil, M. A. Wrzolek, L. Sharer, E. S. Cho, D. W. Dickson, K. M. Weidenheim, and J. F. Llena. 1993. Central nervous system in pediatric AIDS registry. *Ann. N. Y. Acad. Sci.* **693**:295–296.

Kozlowski, P. B., J. Brudkowska, M. Kraszpulski, E. A. Sersen, M. A. Wrzolek, A. P. Anzil, C. Roa, and H. M. Wisniewski. 1997. Microencephalopathy in children congenitally infected with human immunodeficiency virus—a gross-anatomical morphometric study. *Acta Neuropathol.* **93**:136–145.

Krivine, A., G. Firtion, L. Cao, C. Francoual, R. Henrion, and P. Lebon. 1992. HIV replication during the first few weeks of life. *Lancet* **339**:1187–1189.

Kuhn, L., E. J. Abrams, P. Palumbo, M. Bulterys, R. Aga, L. Louie, T. Hodge, and the Perinatal AIDS Collaborative Transmission Study. 2004. Maternal versus paternal inheritance of HLA class I alleles among HIV-infected children: consequences for clinical disease progression. *AIDS* **18**:1281–1289.

Kure, K., Y. D. Park, T. S. Kim, W. D. Lyman, G. Lantos, S. Lee, S. Cho, A. L. Belman, K. M. Weidenheim, and D. W. Dickson. 1989. Immunohistochemical localization of an HIV epitope in cerebral aneurysmal arteriopathy in pediatric AIDS. *Pediatr. Pathol.* **9**:655–667.

Kure, K., K. M. Weidenheim, W. D. Lyman, and D. W. Dickson. 1990. Morphology and distribution of HIV-1 qp 41 positive microglia in subacute AIDS encephalitis. *Acta Neuropathol.* **80**:393–400.

Kure, K., J. F. Llena, W. D. Lyman, R. Soeiro, K. M. Weidenheim, A. Hirano, and D. W. Dickson. 1991. Human immunodeficiency virus-1 infection of the nervous system: an autopsy study of 268 adult, pediatric and fetal brains. *Hum. Pathol.* **22**:700–710.

Lacroix, C., S. Blanche, E. Dussaix, and M. Tardieu. 1995. Acute necrotizing measles encephalitis in a child with AIDS. *J. Neurol.* **242**:249–251. (Letter.)

Lambert, G., D. M. Thea, V. Pliner, R. W. Steketee, E. J. Abrams, P. Matheson, P. A. Thomas, B. Greenberg, T. M. Brown, M. Bamji, M. L. Kalish, et al. 1997. Effect of maternal CD4[+] cell count, Acquired immunodeficiency syndrome, and viral load on disease progression in infants with perinatally Acquired human immunodeficiency virus type 1 infection. *J. Pediatr.* **130**:890–897.

Landesman, S. H., L. A. Kalish, D. N. Burns, H. Minkoff, H. E. Fox-Zorrilla, C. P. Garcia, M. G. Fowler, L. Mofenson,

R. Tuomala, et al. 1996. Obstetrical factors and the transmission of human immunodeficiency virus type 1 from mother to child. *N. Engl. J. Med.* **334:**1617–1623.

Legido, A., H. W. Lischner, J. P. de Chadarevian, and C. D. Katsetos. 1999. Stroke in pediatric HIV infection. *Pediatr. Neurol.* **21:**588

Levenson, R. L., C. A. Mellins, R. Zawadzki, R. Kairam, and Z. Stein. 1992. Cognitive assessment of human immunodeficiency virus exposed children. *Am. J. Dis. Child.* **146:**1479–1483.

Lindegren, M. L., S. Steinberg, and R. H. Byers. 2000. Epidemiology of HIV/AIDS in children. *Pediatr. Clin. N. Am.* **47:**1–20.

Lobato, M. N., M. B. Caldwell, P. Ng, M. J. Oxtoby, et al. 1995. Encephalopathy in children with perinatally Acquired immunodeficiency syndrome virus infection. *J. Pediatr.* **126:**170–175.

Lolekha, R., P. Chanthavanich, K. Limkittikul, K. Luangxay, T. Chotpitayasunodh, and C. J. Newman. 2004. Pain: a common symptom in human immunodeficiency virus-infected Thai children. *Acta Paediatr.* **93:**891–98.

Luzuriaga, K., and J. L. Sullivan. 2000. Viral and immunopathogenesis of vertical HIV infection. HIV/AIDS in infants, children, and adolescents. *Pediatr. Clin. N. Am.* **47:**65–78.

Lyman, W. D., Y. Kress, K. Kure, W. K. Rashbaum, A. Rubinstein, and R. Soeiro. 1990. Detection of HIV in fetal central nervous system tissue. *AIDS* **4:**917–920.

Mayaux, M. J., M. Burgard, J. P. Teglas, J. Cottalorda, A. Krivine, F. Simon, J. Puel, C. Tamalet, D. Dormont, B. Masquelier, A. Doussin, C. Rouzioux, and S. Blanche. 1996. Neonatal characteristics in rapidly progressive perinatally Acquired HIV-1 disease. *JAMA* **275:**606–610.

Mayaux, M. J., S. Blanche, C. Rouzioux, J. Le Chenadec, V. Chambrin, G. Firtion, M. C. Allemon, E. Vilmer, N. C. Vigneron, J. Tricoire, et al. 1995. Maternal factors associated with perinatal HIV-1 transmission. *J. Acquir. Immune Defic. Syndr.* **8:**188–194.

Mazzoni, P., C. Chiriboga, W. Millar, and A. Rogers. 2000. Intracerebral aneurysms in human immunodeficiency virus infection: case report and literature review. *Pediatr. Neurol.* **23:**252–255.

McAbee, G. N., A. L. Belman, M. Knapik, G. Solitare, P. Ciminera, and D. Dickson. 1995. Rapid and fatal neurological deterioration due to CNS candida infection in an HIV-1 infected child. *J. Child. Neurol.* **10:**405–407.

Mintz, M., B. Tardieu, L. Hoyt, G. McSherry, J. Mendelson, and J. Oleske. 1996. Levodopa therapy improves motor function in HIV infected children with extrapyramidal syndromes. *Neurology* **47:**1583–1585.

Misdrahi, D., G. Vila, I. Furnk-Brenano, M. Tardieu, S. Blanche, and M. C. Mouren-Simeoni. 2004. DSM-IV mental disorders and neurological complications in children and adolescents with human immunodeficiency virus type 1 infection (HIV-1). *Eur. Psychiatry* **19:**182–184.

Mitchell, C. D., S. S. Erlich, M. T. Mastrucci, S. C. Hutto, W. P. Parks, and G. B. Scott. 1990. Congenital toxoplasmosis occurring in infants perinatally infected with HIV-1. *Pediatr. Infect. Dis. J.* **9:**512–518.

Mizusawa, H., A. Hirano, J. F. Llena, and M. Shintaku. 1988. Cerebrovascular lesions in Acquired immunodeficiency syndrome (AIDS). *Acta Neuropathol.* **76:**451–457.

Mofenson, L. M., J. S. Lambert, E. R. Stiehm, J. Bethel, W. A. Meyer III, J. Whitehouse, J. Moye, Jr., P. Reichelderfer, D. R. Harris, M. G. Fowler, B. J. Mathieson, and G. J. Nemo. 1999. Risk factors for perinatal transmission of HIV-type 1 in women treated with zidovudine. *N. Engl. J. Med.* **341:**385–393.

Moriarty, D. M., J. O. Haller, J. P. Loh, and S. Fikrig. 1994. Cerebral infarction in pediatric Acquired immunodeficiency syndrome. *Pediatr. Radiol.* **24:**611–612.

Moss, H. A., P. Brouwers, P. Wolters, L. Wiener, S. Hersh, and P. A. Pizzo. 1994. The development of a Q sort behavioral rating procedure for pediatric HIV patients. *J. Pediatr. Psychol.* **19:**27–46.

Narayan, P., O. B. Samuels, and D. L. Barrow. 2002. Stroke and pediatric human immunodeficiency virus infection. Case report and review of the literature. *Pediatr. Neurosurg.* **37:**158–163.

Nduati, R. W., G. C. John, B. A. Richardson, J. Overbaugh, M. Welch, J. Ndinya-Achola, S. Moses, K. Holmes, F. Onyango, and J. K. Kreiss. 1995. Human immunodeficiency virus type 1-infected cells in breast milk: association with immunosuppression and vitamin A deficiency. *J. Infect. Dis.* **172:**1461–1468.

Newell, M. L., H. Coovadia, M. Cortina-Borja, N. Rollins, P. Gaillard, F. Dabis, and the Ghent International AIDS Society Working Group on HIV Infection in Women and Children. 2004. Mortality of infected and uninfected infants born to HIV-infected mothers in Africa: a pooled analysis. *Lancet* **364:**1236–1243.

New York State Department of Health AIDS Institute. 2007. HIV clinical resource. New York State Department of Health AIDS Institute, New York, NY. http://hivguidelines.org/Content.aspx.

Nozyce, M., J. Hittelman, L. Muenz, S. J. Durako, M. L. Fischer, and A. Willoughby. 1994a. Effect of perinatally Acquired human immunodeficiency virus infection on neurodevelopment in children during the first two years of life. *Pediatrics* **94:**883–891.

Nozyce, M., M. Hoberman, S. Arpadi, A. Wiznia, G. Lambert, J. Dobroszycki, C. J. Chang, and Y. St Louis. 1994b. A twelve month study of the effects of oral zidovudine on neuro developmental functioning in a cohort of vertically injected inner-city children. *AIDS* **8:**635–639.

Oleske, J., A. Minnefor, R. Cooper, K. Thomas, A. dela Cruz, H. Ahdieh, I. Guerrero, V. V. Joshi, and F. Desposito. 1983. Immune deficiency syndrome in children. *JAMA* **249:**2345–2349.

Owens, D. K., M. Holodniy, T. W. McDonald, J. Scott, and S. Sonnad. 1996. A meta-analytic evaluation of the polymerase chain reaction for the diagnosis of HIV infection in infants. *JAMA* **275:**1342–1348.

Palumbo, P. E. 2000. Antiretroviral therapy of HIV infection in children. *Pediatr. Clin. N. Am.* **1:**155–169.

Papaevangelou, V., H. Pollack, M. Riguad, N. Arlievsky, M. L. Lu, G. Rochford, K. Krasinski, and W. Borkowsky. 1996. The amount of early P24 antigenemia and not the time of first detection of virus predicts clinical outcome of infants vertically infected with human immunodeficiency virus. *J. Infect. Dis.* **173:**574–578.

Park, Y. D., A. L. Belman, T. S. Kim, K. Kure, J. F. Llena, G. Lantos, L. Bernstein, and D. W. Dickson. 1990. Stroke in pediatric Acquired immunodeficiency syndrome. *Ann. Neurol.* **28:**303–311.

Patsalides, A. D., L. V. Wood, G. K. Atac, E. Sandifer, J. A. Butman, and N. J. Patronas. 2002. Cerebrovascular disease in HIV-infected pediatric patients: neuroimaging findings. *Am. J. Roentgenol.* **179:**999–1003.

Persaud, D., S. Chandwani, M. Rigaud, E. Leibovitz, A. Kaul, R. Lawrence, H. Pollack, D. DiJohn, K. Krasinski, and W. Borkowsky. 1992. Delayed recognition of human immunodeficiency virus infection in preadolescent children. *Pediatrics* **90:**688–691.

Philippet, P., S. Blanche, G. Sebag, G. Rodesch, C. Griscelli, and M. Tardieu. 1994. Stroke and cerebral infarct in children infected with human immunodeficiency virus. *Arch. Pediatr. Adolesc. Med.* **148:**965–970.

Picard, O., L. Brunereau, B. Pelosse, D. Kerob, J. Cabane, and J. C. Imbert. 1997. Cerebral infarction associated with vasculitis due to varicella zoster virus in patients infected with human immunodeficiency virus. *Biomed. Pharmacother.* **51**:449–454.

Pitt, J., D. Brambilla, P. Reichelderfer, A. Landay, K. McIntosh, D. Burns, G. V. Hillyer, H. Mendez, and M. G. Fowler. 1997. Maternal immunologic and virologic risk factors for infant human immunodeficiency virus type 1 infection: findings from The Women and Infants Transmission Study. *J. Infect. Dis.* **175**:567–575.

Pizzo, P. A., J. Eddy, J. Falloon, F. M. Balis, R. F. Murphy, H. Moss, P. Wolters, P. Brouwers, P. Jarosinski, and M. Rubin. 1988. Effect of continuous intravenous infusion of zidovudine (AZT) in children with symptomatic HIV infection. *N. Engl. J. Med.* **319**:889–896.

Pizzo, P. A., K. Butler, F. Balis, E. Brouwers, M. Hawkins, J. Eddy, M. Einloth, J. Falloon, R. Husson, and P. Jarosinski. 1990. Dideoxycytidine alone and in an alternating schedule with zidovudine in children with symptomatic human immunodeficiency virus infection. *J. Pediatr.* **117**:799–808.

Raphael, S. A., M. L. Price, H. W. Lischner, J. W. Griffin, W. D. Grover, and O. Bagasra. 1991. Inflammatory demyelinating polyneuropathy in a child with symptomatic human immunodeficiency virus infection. *J. Pediatr.* **118**:242–245.

Raskino, C., D. A. Pearson, C. J. Baker, M. H. Lifschitz, K. O'Donnell, M. Mintz, M. Nozyce, P. Brouwers, R. E. McKinney, E. Jimenez, J. A. Englund, et al. 1999. Neurologic, neurocognitve and brain outcomes in human deficiency virus-infected children receiving different nucleoside antiretroviral regimens. *Pediatrics* **104**:e32.

Robinson, L. G., C. A. Chiriboga, S. E. Champion, I. Ainyette, M. DiGrado, and E. J. Abrams. 2004. Progressive multifocal leukoencephalopathy successfully treated with highly active antiretroviral therapy and cidofovir in an adolescent infected with perinatal human immunodeficiency virus. *J. Child. Neurol.* **19**:35–38.

Rogers, M. F., G. Schochetman, and R. Hoff. 1994. Advances in diagnosis of HIV infection, p. 219–240. *In* P. A. Pizzo and C. M. Wilfert (ed.), *Pediatric AIDS: the Challenge of HIV Infection in Infants, Children and Adolescents*, 2nd ed. Williams & Wilkins, New York, NY.

Rouet, F., C. Sakarovitch, P. Msellati, N. Elenga, C. Montcho, I. Viho, S. Blanche, C. Rouzioux, F. Dabis, V. Leroy, and the Abidjan ANRS 049 Ditrame Study Group. 2003. Pediatric viral human immunodeficiency virus type 1 RNA level timing of infection and disease progression in African HIV-1-infected children. *Pediatrics* **112**:e289.

Rouzioux, C., D. Costagliola, M. Burgard, S. Blanche, M. J. Mayaux, C. Griscelli, A. J. Valleron, et al. 1995. Estimated timing of mother to child HIV transmission by use of a Markov model. *Am. J. Epidemiol.* **142**:1330–1337.

Rubinstein, A., M. Sicklick, A. Gupta, L. Bernstein, N. Klein, E. Rubinstein, I. Spigland, L. Fruchter, N. Litman, H. Lee, and M. Hollander. 1983. Acquired immunodeficiency with reversed T4/T8 ratios in infants born to promiscuous and drug addicted mothers. *JAMA* **249**:2350–2356.

Ryder, R. W., W. Nsa, S. E. Hassig, F. Behets, M. Rayfield, B. Ekungola, A. M. Nelson, U. Mulenda, H. Francis, and K. Mwandagalirwa. 1989. Perinatal transmission of the human immunodeficiency virus type 1 to infants of seropositive women in Zaire. *N. Engl. J. Med.* **320**:1637–1642.

Sanchez-Ramon, S., S. Resino, J. M. Bellon Cano, J. T. Ramos, D. Gurbindo, and A. Munoz-Fernandez. 2003. Neuroprotective effects of early antiretrovirals in vertical HIV infection. *Pediatr. Neurol.* **29**:218–221.

Schechter, N. L., C. B. Berde, and M. Yaster (ed). 1993. *Pain in Infants, Children, and Adolescents*. Williams & Wilkins, Baltimore, MD.

Scott, G. B., C. Hutto, R. W. Makuch, M. T. Mastrucci, T. O'Connor, C. D. Mitchell, E. J. Trapido, and W. P. Parks. 1989. Survival in children with perinatally Acquired human immunodeficiency virus type infection. *N. Engl. J. Med.* **321**:1791–1796.

Semba, R. D., P. G. Miotti, J. D. Chiphangwi, A. J. Saah, J. K. Canner, G. A. Dallabetta, and D. R. Hoover. 1994. Maternal vitamin A deficiency and mother-to-child transmission of HIV-1. *Lancet* **343**:1593–1597.

Shah, S. S., R. A. Zimmerman, L. B. Rorke, and L. G. Vezina. 1996. Cerebrovascular complications of HIV in children. *Am. J. Neuroradiol.* **17**:1913–1917.

Shanks, G. D., R. R. Redfield, and G. W. Fischer. 1987. Toxoplasma encephalitis in an infant with Acquired immunodeficiency syndrome. *Pediatr. Infect. Dis.* **6**:70–71.

Sharer, L. R., L. G. Epstein, E. S. Cho, V. V. Joshi, M. F. Meyenhofer, L. F. Rankin, and C. K. Petito. 1986. Pathologic features of AIDS encephalopathy in children: evidence for LAV/HTLV-III infection of the brain. *Hum. Pathol.* **17**:271–284.

Sharer, L. R., P. C. Dowling, J. Michaels, S. D. Cook, J. Menonna, B. M. Blumberg, and L. G. Epstein. 1990. Spinal cord disease in children with HIV-1 infection: a combined molecular and neuropathological study. *Neuropathol. Appl. Neurobiol.* **16**:317–331.

Sharer, L. R., B. Fischer, B. M. Blumberg, and L. G. Epstein. 1994. CNS measles virus infection in AIDS. *J. Neuro-AIDS*.

Silliman, C. C., D. Tedder, J. W. Ogle, J. Simon, B. K. Kleinschmidt-DeMasters, M. Manco-Johnson, and M. J. Levin. 1993. Unsuspected varicella-zoster virus encephalitis in a child with Acquired immunodeficiency syndrome. *J. Pediatr.* **123**:418–422.

Soeiro, R., A. Rubinstein, W. K. Rashbaum, and W. D. Lyman. 1992. Maternofetal transmission of AIDS: frequency of human immunodeficiency virus type-1 nucleic acid sequences in human fetal DNA. *J. Infect. Dis.* **166**:699–703.

Sprecher, S., G. Soumenkoff, F. Puissant, and M. Degueldre. 1985. Vertical transmission of HIV in a 15 week fetus. *Lancet* **ii**:288–289.

States, L. J., R. A. Zimmerman, and R. M. Rutstein. 1997. Imaging of pediatric central nervous system HIV infection. *Neuroimaging Clin. N. Am.* **7**:321–338.

St Louis, M. E., M. Kamenga, C. Brown, A. M. Nelson, T. Manzila, V. Batter, F. Behets, U. Kabagabo, R. W. Ryder, and M. Oxtoby. 1993. Risk for perinatal HIV-1 transmission according to maternal immunologic, virologic, and placental factors. *JAMA* **269**:2853–2859.

Taccone, A., M. P. Fondelli, G. Ferra, and A. Marzoli. 1992. An unusual CT presentation of congenital cerebral toxoplasmosis in an 8 month-old boy with AIDS. *Pediatr. Radiol.* **22**:68–69.

Taha, T. E., S. M. Graham, N. I. Kumwenda, R. L. Broadhead, D. R. Hoover, D. Markakis, L. van Der Hoeven, G. N. Liomba, J. D. Chiphangwi, and P. G. Miotti. 2000. Morbidity among HIV-1 infected and uninfected African children. *Pediatrics* **106**:e77.

Tamula, M. A., P. L. Wolters, C. Walsek, S. Zeichner, and L. Civitello. 2003. Cognitive decline with immunologic and virologic stability in four children with human immunodeficiency virus disease. *Pediatrics* **112**:679–684.

Tardieu, M., J. Le Chenadec, A. Persoz, L. Meyer, S. Blanche, M. J. Mayaux, et al. 2000. HIV-1 related encephalopathy in infants compared with children and adults. *Neurology* **54**:1089–1095.

Tardieu, M., F. Brunelle, C. Raybaud, W. Ball, B. Barret, B. Pautard, E. Lachassine, M. J. Mayaux, and S. Blanche. 2005. Cerebral MR imaging in uninfected children born to HIV-seropositive mothers and perinatally exposed to zidovudine. *Am. J. Neuroradiol.* **26**:695–701.

Tepper, V. J., J. J. Farley, M. I. Rothman, D. L. Houck, K. F. Davis, T. L. Collins-Jones, and R. C. Wachtel. 1998.

Neurodevelopmental/neuroradiologic recovery of a child infected with HIV after treatment with combination antiretroviral therapy using HIV-specific progease inhibitor ritonavir. *Pediatrics* **101:**e7.

Thea, D. M., R. W. Steketee, V. Pliner, K. Bornschlegel, T. Brown, S. Orloff, P. B. Matheson, E. J. Abrams, M. Bamji, G. Lambert, E. A. Schoenbaum, P. A. Thomas, M. Heagarty, and M. L. Kalish. 1997. The effect of maternal viral load on the risk of perinatal transmission of HIV-1. *AIDS* **11:**437–444.

Tovo, P. A., M. de Martino, C. Gabiano, N. Cappello, R. D'Elia, A. Loy, A .Plebani, G. V. Zuccotti, P. Dallacasa, G. Ferraris, et al. 1992. Prognostic factors and survival in children with perinatal HIV-I infection. *Lancet* **339:**1249–1253.

Ultmann, M. H., A. L. Belman, H. A. Ruff, B. E. Novick, B. Cone-Wesson, H. J. Cohen, and A. Rubinstein. 1985. Developmental abnormalities in infants and children with Acquired immune deficiency syndrome (AIDS) and AIDS-related complex. *Dev. Med. Child. Neurol.* **27:**563–571.

Ultmann, M. H., G. Diamond, H. A. Ruff, A. L. Belman, B. E. Novick, A. Rubinstein, and H. J. Cohen. 1987. Developmental abnormalities in infants and children with Acquired immune deficiency syndrome (AIDS): a follow up study. *Int. J. Neurosci.* **32:**661–667.

U.S. Department of Health and Human Services. 2006. Guidelines for the use of antiretroviral agents in pediatric HIV infection. http://www.aidsinfo.nih.gov/guidelines/GuidelineDetail.aspx?MenuItem=Guidelines&Search=Off&GuidelineID=8&ClassID=1.

Vandersteenhoven, J. J., G. Dbaibo, O. B. Boyko, C. M. Hulette, D. C. Anthony, J. F. Kenny, and C. M. Wilfert. 1992. Progressive multifocal leukoencephalopathy in pediatric Acquired immunodeficiency syndrome. *Pediatr. Infect. Dis. J.* **11:**232–237.

Vazeux, R., C. Lacroix-Ciaudo, S. Blanche, M. C. Cumont, D. Henin, F. Gray, L. Boccon-Gibod, and M. Tardieu. 1992. Low levels of human immunodeficiency virus replication in the brain tissue of children with severe Acquired immunodeficiency syndrome encephalopathy. *Am. J. Pathol.* **140:**137–144.

Vigano, A., N. Principi, M. L. Villa, C. Riva, L. Crupi, D. Trabattoni, G. M. Shearer, and M. Clerici. 1995. Immunologic characterization of children vertically infected with human immunodeficiency virus, with slow or rapid disease progression. *J. Pediatr.* **126:**368–374.

Visrutaratna, P., and K. Oranratanachai. 2002. Clinics in diagnostic imaging (75). HIV encephalopathy and cerebral aneurysmal arteriopathy. *Singapore Med. J.* **43:**377–380.

Visudtibhan, A., P. Visudhiphan, and S. Chiemchanya. 1999. Stroke and seizures as the presenting signs of pediatric HIV infection. *Pediatr. Neurol.* **20:**53–56.

Volpe, J. J. 1995. *Neurology of the Newborn*, 3rd ed. W. B. Saunders Co., Philadelphia, PA.

Wachtel, R. C., V. J. Tepper, D. L. Houck, P. Nair, and J. P. Thompson. 1993. Neurodevelopment in pediatric HIV-1 infection: a prospective study. *Pediatric AIDS and HIV Infection: Fetus to Adolescent* **4:**198–203.

Whitt, J. K., S. R. Hooper, M. B. Tennison, W. T. Robertson, S. H. Gold, M. Burchinal, R. Wells, C. McMillan, R. A. Whaley, and J. Combest. 1993. Neuropsychological functioning of human immunodeficiency virus-infected children with hemophilia. *J. Pediatr.* **122:**52–59.

Wiley, C. A., A. L. Belman, D. Dickson, A. Rubinstein, and J. A. Nelson. 1990. Human immunodeficiency virus within the brains of children with AIDS. *Clin. Neuropathol.* **9:**1–6.

Wiley, C. A., E. Masliah, M. Morey, C. Lemere, R. DeTeresa, M. Grafe, L. Hansen, and R. Terry. 1991. Neocortical damage during HIV infection. *Ann. Neurol.* **29:**651–657.

Wolters, P. L., P. Brouwers, H. A. Moss, and P. A. Pizzo. 1995. Differential receptive and expressive language functioning of children with symptomatic HIV disease: comparison with the language of sibling controls and CT scan brain abnormalities. *Pediatrics* **95:**112–119.

Wolters, P. L., P. Brouwers, H. A. Moss, and P. A. Pizzo. 1994. Adaptive behavior of children with symptomatic HIV infection before and after zidovudine therapy. *J. Pediatr. Psych.* **19:**47–61.

Working Group on Mother-to-Child Transmission of HIV. 1995. Rates of mother to child transmission of HIV-1 in Africa, America and Europe: results from 13 perinatal studies. *J. Acquir. Immune Defic. Syndr. Hum. Retrovirol.* **8:**506–510.

The Spectrum of Neuro-AIDS Disorders:
Pathophysiology, Diagnosis, and Treatment
Edited by K. Goodkin et al.
©2008 ASM Press, Washington, DC

33

Interaction of the Aging Process with Neurobehavioral and Neuro-AIDS Conditions in the HAART Era

KARL GOODKIN, MAURICIO CONCHA, BETH D. JAMIESON, ROSA REBECA
MOLINA, ENRIQUE LOPEZ, WENLI ZHENG, DESHRATN ASTHANA, AND
WILLIAM DAVID HARDY

INCIDENCE AND PREVALENCE OF OLDER AGE AND HIV-1 INFECTION

Until the late 1990s, older age and HIV-1 infection were thought to be nonoverlapping health issues. Between 1996 and 1997, newly reported AIDS cases among older persons increased by 12.6%. Currently, the cumulative prevalence estimate is that 11 to 13% of all cases of persons with AIDS (PWAs) defined in the United States are over 50 years of age, the designated cutoff for older age originally promulgated by the Centers for Disease Control and Prevention (CDC, 2007). A widely held misconception about this field is the expectation that the term "older" is consistent with, if not equivalent to, the term "elderly" ($\geq$65 years of age). However, the predominant subgroup over 50 years of age with a diagnosis of AIDS, cumulatively over the epidemic, is in the 50- to 59-year-old age range (74%) (CDC, 2007). An additional 14% are estimated to be in the 60- to 64-year-old

age range. The "true elderly" accounted for only about 2% of AIDS cases in the United States a decade ago but are now estimated to account for a cumulative total of 12% of those living with AIDS (CDC, 2007). It is noteworthy that while the incidence of AIDS among older adults has increased, the incidence among the general population has stabilized (Levy et al., 2003).

The cumulative numbers of people with AIDS over age 50 are higher in Florida (15%) (Florida State Department of Health, 2007), and in Miami-Dade county (16.7%), specifically (Miami-Dade County Health Department, 2007), than at the national level (12.3%). A similarly high rate of older HIV-1-seropositive persons has been noted in Hawaii. This increased concentration of older HIV-1-seropositive persons may be related to the attractiveness of both states to older populations, who may be moving there upon retirement from elsewhere in the United States. With the advent of the cyclic GMP-specific phosphodiesterase type 5 inhibitors (sildenafil [Viagra], tadalafil [Cialis], and vardenafil [Levitra]) and the relative lack of knowledge of safe sex techniques in the older population, the incidence of HIV-1 infection among older persons is expected to continue to grow disproportionately within the population of the newly HIV-1 infected nationwide.

Although newly infected older HIV-1-seropositive individuals have clearly increased in number in recent years, they do not account for the entire shift being observed toward older persons living with HIV/AIDS at the national level. A completely separate cohort of older HIV-1-seropositive persons derives from the successful treatment of HIV-1 infection with highly active antiretroviral (ARV) therapy (HAART). With the introduction of HAART in late 1995, the issue of survival time returned to the forefront of HIV/AIDS studies. The cumulative mortality rate at 12 months after HAART initiation decreased from 15.8% in 1993 to 1995

Karl Goodkin and Enrique Lopez, Dept. of Psychiatry and Behavioral Neurosciences, Cedars-Sinai Medical Center, and Dept. of Psychiatry and Biobehavioral Sciences, David Geffen School of Medicine, UCLA, Los Angeles, CA 90048. **Mauricio Concha,** Intercoastal Medical Group, Sarasota, FL 34232. **Beth D. Jamieson,** UCLA Flow Cytometry Core Facility, Dept. of Medicine/Hematology-Oncology, David Geffen School of Medicine, UCLA, Los Angeles, CA 90048. **Rosa Rebeca Molina,** Sylvester Comprehensive Cancer Center, Fox Cancer Center, University of Miami, Miami, FL 33136. **Wenli Zheng,** Division of Enrollment Management, Market Research & Communications, University of Miami, Coral Gables, FL 33146. **Deshratn Asthana,** Laboratory for Clinical and Biological Studies, Dept. of Psychiatry and Behavioral Sciences, Fox Cancer Center, University of Miami, Miami, FL 33136. **William David Hardy,** Division of Infectious Diseases, Dept. of Internal Medicine, Cedars-Sinai Medical Center, and David Geffen School of Medicine, UCLA, Los Angeles, CA 90048.

to 6.1% in 2002 to 2004, and the life expectancy (at age 20) increased from 9.1 years to 23.6 years during the same period (Lima et al., 2007). However, the mortality of those with HIV-1 infection remains 10 times higher than that of the general population (as estimated by a study of the Australian HIV Observational Database [n= 2,329 patients seen between 1999 and 2004]) (Petoumenos et al., 2006). In accord with this estimate, older HIV-1-seropositive persons have predominantly shown decreased survival time in this (Petoumenos et al., 2006) and other (Skiest et al., 1996; Baillargeon et al., 1999; Butt et al., 2001; Inungu et al., 2001; Welch and Morse, 2002; Darby et al., 2004) studies, with few exceptions (Keller et al., 1999). Of additional concern in the recent Australian database study (Petoumenos et al., 2006) is the fact that more deaths were non-HIV-1 related (52%) than HIV-1 related (40%) (the remainder had an "unknown" HIV-1 relationship). Older HIV-1-seropositive persons have also been found to have greater decrements across activities of daily living than younger HIV-1-seropositive persons (Goodkin et al., 2004). These data raise concerns that HIV-1-associated morbidity and mortality remain significant and that the causes may be merging with those for the general population as the HIV-1-infected patient population ages.

In regard to HIV-1-associated neurocognitive impairment (NCI)/disorder status and mortality, HIV-1-associated dementia (HAD) has long been appreciated to carry a poor prognosis, estimated to carry a median survival time pre-HAART of approximately 6 months (McArthur et al., 1993) but now estimated at 44 months. Mayeux et al. (1993) reported that HIV-1-associated NCI in HIV-1-infected individuals prior to the development of AIDS was correlated significantly with an increased relative risk (4.1) of mortality. Later, Ellis et al. (1997) reported that HIV-1-associated minor cognitive-motor disorder (MCMD) was associated with increased relative risk (2.2) for mortality. Subsequently, Wilkie et al. (1998) reported that for otherwise-asymptomatic HIV-1-seropositive individuals the specific cognitive domains of information-processing speed and verbal memory were also associated with an elevated risk for mortality of 6.4 and 3.5, respectively. Hence, the association of older age with early mortality in HIV-1 infection might prove to be compounded by that of HIV-1-associated NCI/disorder with mortality (including mild levels of impairment well prior to the diagnosis of HAD).

THE EPIDEMIOLOGIES OF TWO OLDER HIV-1-SEROPOSITIVE POPULATIONS

The foregoing introduction to the epidemiology of aging in HIV-1 infection leads us to an important preliminary conclusion. That is, the study of older age in HIV-1 infection is more properly considered as (i) the study of a population of newly infected older individuals and (ii) the study of a separate group of long-term HIV-1-infected patients successfully treated with HAART. There are many reasons to expect that these two populations may be significantly different from one another. Newly diagnosed older persons are comprised of a group of newly infected older persons and another group of those infected for a longer period who were not given HIV antibody testing due to a low index of suspicion among their primary care providers for HIV-1 in older persons. The newly infected subgroup of older patients is more likely to be suffering stigma due their HIV/AIDS diagnosis than those older but diagnosed long term and those who are younger. In association with this fact, it might be expected that the prevalence of psychological distress (specifically, depressed mood), high stressful-life-event burden, lack of social support, and passive, maladaptive coping strategies might be higher in the newly infected subgroup. This deleterious psychosocial constellation would be expected to increase the likelihood of a less active and effective pursuit of access to treatment, as well as adherence once treatment is obtained.

The group of long-term HIV-1-infected older persons represents a different point of view regarding psychosocial factors. These patients have survived through the changes in ARV therapies prior to the introduction of HAART and are more likely to have become assertive in addressing their treatment needs. In association with this, a different psychosocial constellation is anticipated in which the patient is expected to have more positive life events, greater access to social support (from involvement in patient support groups, for example), and more active, adaptive coping strategies (associated with understanding the changes in their treatment over time and the need for high levels of ARV adherence). Studies predominantly reflecting this subgroup of older, long-term HIV-1-infected individuals have confirmed that this might be the case (Goodkin et al., 2003). Ultimately, these two subgroups must be routinely separated and studied individually in order to successfully elucidate the relationships between aging and HIV-1 infection.

DESCRIPTIVE ASPECTS OF THE OLDER HIV-1-SEROPOSITIVE POPULATION

A significant change has occurred since 1990 in the demography of older patients with HIV-1 infection. In that year, most male patients 50 years of age or over diagnosed with AIDS were men who had sex with men (65.8% of those aged 50 to 59), with heterosexual contact at <10% and hemophilia or blood transfusion still accounting for significant percentages (blood transfusion, 13.1% of those over 60) (Mack and Ory, 2003). However, of older males diagnosed with AIDS in 1999, men who had sex with men accounted for fewer cases (35.6% of those aged 50 to 59) and the hemophilia and blood transfusion risk factors were greatly reduced (e.g., blood transfusion, 1.9% of those over 60). However, the heterosexual route among men increased from 3.5% to 11.5% for those aged 50 to 59 and from 7.8% to 16.4% for those aged 60 and older. Though females represented only 13% and 24% of the total number of AIDS cases aged 50 or over in 1990 and 1999, respectively, they were persistently predominantly infected by heterosexual contact (44.2% in 1990 and 41.3% in 1999 of those aged 50 to 59). Likewise, the injection substance use route was relatively stable in incidence among older men and women during this period. Thus, the sociodemographic profile of older HIV-1-seropositive individuals in the United States has come to resemble that of the larger HIV-1-seropositive population in regard to the increased rates of heterosexual transmission documented over the last decade.

A shift in the overall demographic pattern of the older HIV-1-seropositive patient population has also occurred in regard to ethnicity. In 1990, Caucasians accounted for 57.8% of those aged 50 to 59 diagnosed with AIDS, while in 1999, they accounted for only 35.5%. In contrast, in 1990, African-Americans accounted for only 27.0% of those aged 50 to 59, whereas in 1999, they accounted for 44.9%. Similar changes were seen for Hispanic-Americans, but less so than African-Americans; they accounted for 14.3% of patients aged 50 to 59 diagnosed with AIDS in 1990, increasing to 18.0% in 1999.

Issues related to ethnicity and symptom burden may account for discrepancies in the research on survival time with older age in HIV-1 infection. Zingmond et al. (2001) studied a nationally representative sample of HIV-1-infected adults under care in the United States from the HIV Cost and Service Utilization Study. They reported that non-Caucasian older persons reported fewer symptoms and were less likely to have AIDS than Caucasians but nevertheless showed a trend toward shorter survival time (Zingmond et al., 2001). Potential explanations offered for this confusing finding were that non-Caucasian older persons might show decreased survival time after developing AIDS or that older non-Caucasians receive less effective treatment. Support for the latter interpretation has been reported in the literature. While Ghani et al. (2003) found that HAART had become the standard of care in 1999, with 84% beginning ARV therapy with HAART, African-Americans were reported to be significantly less likely to begin ARV therapy with HAART (odds ratio, 0.59). Lower ARV adherence could further extend the deleterious health impact of the relationship of limited HAART access among African-Americans. In a follow-up study, Zingmond et al. (2003) compared the previously reported HIV Cost and Service Utilization Study sample to the Veterans Aging Cohort 3 Site Study sample, showing a still stronger effect of non-Caucasian older persons reporting fewer HIV/AIDS symptoms than older Caucasians or younger non-Caucasians or Caucasians. Of note, older Veterans Aging Cohort 3 Site Study participants were less likely to report depressive symptoms specifically, in line with a report by Goodkin et al. (2003), but were more likely to report peripheral neuropathy, in line with a report by Simpson et al. (1998), as well as weight loss. Hence, it might be concluded that ethnicity is a potentially confounding factor in examining disease progression and survival time in the field of older age and HIV-1 infection.

VIROLOGIC ISSUES IN AGING AND HIV-1 INFECTION

Early studies of older persons with HIV-1 infection suggested that older persons have a higher plasma viral load than younger persons among the recently diagnosed (Operskalski et al., 1997). However, this could have been the result of a longer delay in HIV antibody testing among older individuals due to a lower index of suspicion for HIV-1 infection in this age group. Alternatively, such results could be due to immunosenescence (see "Immunologic Issues in Aging and HIV-1 Infection" below) or, possibly, to decreased ARV adherence among older individuals, potentially related to a higher frequency of ARV toxicities and/or a higher total symptom burden (owing to higher concurrent medical comorbidities). In contrast, higher ARV medication adherence reported in some samples of older HIV-1-seropositive persons might confer the likelihood of a lower plasma viral load in this patient group.

Our own work among those with longer-term HIV-1 infection treated with HAART indicated that a lower plasma viral load may be observed in this subgroup of older HIV-1-seropositive persons. Such an association was documented, controlling for ARV therapy usage, disease stage, ARV adherence, HIV-1 serostatus duration, alcohol and substance use, recent sexually transmitted disease, and sociodemographics (except income) (Goodkin et al., 2004). Thus, we did not find that these results were mediated by higher ARV adherence in our older sample. However, despite a lower plasma viral load, older HIV-1-infected individuals

are disposed to a higher frequency of HIV-1-associated neurocognitive disorders. It is relevant that HIV-1 sequences are known to diverge or increase their sequence heterogeneity over the course of infection. While it is true that mutations that reduce viral replication capacity emerge under chronic selection pressure (Prado et al., 2005) and that increased transmission of attenuated HIV-1 strains has been documented as well (Arien et al., 2007), an alternative explanation presents itself that is more specific to the observed increase in frequency of HIV-1-associated neurocognitive disorder in the subgroup of long-term HIV-1-infected older patients. HIV-1 has been shown to evolve differently in the plasma, cerebrospinal fluid, and brain tissue; further, in brain tissue, HIV-1 has been shown to exhibit strain variation (in gp120) by brain region (Shapshak et al., 1999). Thus, a difference in viral evolution within brain tissue (a viral reservoir) might occur that is specific to long-term HIV-1-infected older individuals, in whom a more central nervous system (CNS)-tropic and/or neurovirulent strain is favored. This could explain the increased frequency of HIV-1-associated neurocognitive disorder in the face of a lower plasma viral load.

Another potential explanation is that a substantial amount of viral-protein production may continue in the face of a lower plasma viral load. Most HAART regimens combine two nucleoside reverse transcriptase inhibitors (nRTIs) with a protease inhibitor (PI). While the nRTIs act prior to the translational stage, it is known from the dual-nRTI era that control of viral replication with such combinations was suboptimal. The addition of a PI in HAART regimens was shown to substantially add to the control of viral replication. However, the PIs discontinue viral replication at a late stage, after the virion has been largely assembled, leaving viral remains (referred to as "viral ghosts"). Selected viral-protein remains, such as gp120 (glycoprotein coat) and Tat (a regulatory protein), have been shown to be neurotoxic, independently of the presence of whole virions. It should be noted that patients treated with HAART have been shown to have cell-associated Tat (Zhang and Crumpacker, 2001), that circulating levels of Tat have been demonstrated (Wu and Schlossman, 1997), and that Tat has been associated with disruption of the blood-brain barrier (Banks et al., 2005). Thus, this process also generates a context in which the long-term use of the PIs among older patients may increase the risk for HIV-1-associated neurotoxicity in the face of consistently undetectable viral-load results in the plasma.

IMMUNOLOGIC ISSUES IN AGING AND HIV-1 INFECTION

The possibility that older HIV-1-infected patients might well be expected to be vulnerable to a higher overall "viral burden" (including viral products as well as whole virions) due to immunosenescence must also be considered (Murasko et al., 1988; Franceschi et al., 1996). While the process of "immunosenescence" might generally be expected to refer to those over age 65, it varies considerably based on the specific immune measures examined and may begin as early as 45 years of age. Thus, in general, it applies to our focus on HIV-1-seropositive persons who are 50 years old and older; however, the extent to which it potentially contributes to an increased likelihood of clinical disease progression and decreased survival time has not yet been elucidated.

Apropos of this point, while studies of older age and immunity have sometimes demonstrated a lower CD4 cell count (Olsson et al., 2000), this finding has been inconsistent (Jackola et al., 1994) and may be dependent upon differential immunological differences occurring within subgroups in the older age range. As older HIV-1-infected patients are typically in the younger range of "old age" (i.e., 50 to 59 years old), an aging effect directly on their CD4 cell count may be a less prominent, clinically relevant immunologic association.

This may be different for subsets of the CD4 cell population. In untreated HIV-1 infection, aging has been associated with a CD4 cell loss disproportionate to the naive subset (Saule et al., 2006). While older patients ultimately have shown a response to HAART similar to that of younger patients, older patients tend to show CD4 cell increments that occur more slowly and with a smaller maximum extent than those in younger patients (Nogueras et al., 2006). An age-related decline in the CD4 cell count with HAART may be sample specific, e.g., due to a shorter duration of viral-load suppression to undetectable levels and/or a lower CD4 nadir prior to HAART initiation among older HIV-1-seropositive patients.

Decreased thymic function and thymic involution associated with aging may account for the delayed recovery of the CD4 cell count in older patients post-HAART. However, recent data suggest that the output of CD4 cells may be maintained in older age despite decreased thymic function. One measure of thymic function is the number of circulating T-cell receptor excision circles (TRECs). Circulating TREC levels have been correlated inversely with age, plasma viral load, and activated T-cell counts in the peripheral blood. Early after the initiation of HAART, TRECs and naive CD4 cell counts increase in the peripheral blood, suggesting a process by which recent thymic emigrants are sequestered in lymphoid tissues during untreated HIV-1 infection but are selectively released into the peripheral circulation upon treatment (Diaz et al., 2003). Further documentation of the thymic contribution to the immunologic response to HAART may lead to specific immunotherapies that may be targeted to older HIV-1-seropositive patients.

Another aspect of the immune response to HIV-1 infection is its monitoring by $CD8^+$ T lymphocytes. Effective CD8 cell control over HIV-1 infection is a complex issue, one aspect of which may be an intrinsic, genetically programmed barrier to proliferation characteristic of all normal human somatic cells. What is termed "replicative senescence" comprises irreversible cell cycle arrest and striking changes in cellular functions (Effros, 2003). Senescent CD8 cells may show the absence of CD28 expression and an inability to proliferate, among other changes. These cells are known to increase progressively during the normal aging process, as well as with the clinical progression of HIV-1 infection. Thus, this particular type of immunosenescence may be critical to the deleterious interaction of HIV-1 infection and aging.

OLDER AGE AND NEURO-AIDS CONDITIONS

Older Age and HIV-1-Associated Neurocognitive Status

Old age has been studied with respect to HIV-1-associated neurocognitive status in three respects: HAD, MCMD, and HIV-1-associated NCI independent of disorder status. For the most part, studies have been conducted on HAD and NCI (regardless of disorder) as the outcomes, with studies of MCMD being less frequent. Studies reported to date have been in accord with the American Academy of Neurology (1991) definitions of HAD and MCMD; however, these criteria have recently been revised (Antinori et al., 2007). Moreover, no standard definition of HIV-associated NCI per se has been accepted in the literature. Hence, progress in the field has been hampered by the limited research at levels of disorder less severe than dementia and—for NCI—by the use of variable definitions of the term.

Older Age and HAD

Some time ago, older age was associated with a linear increase in the diagnosis of HIV encephalopathy (consonant with a diagnosis of HAD) by decade of life (Janssen et al., 1992). Of 144,184 PWAs, 10,553 (7.3%) were reported to have HIV encephalopathy. In PWAs 15 years old or older, the proportion progressively increased with age, from 6% in PWAs 15 to 34 years old to 19% in PWAs 75 years old or older. This study was limited by the fact that it was based upon national AIDS case data reported to the CDC, which monitors only initial AIDS-defining illnesses (ADIs). However, HAD is estimated to present as the ADI in only 10 to 15% of cases. This work was soon complemented by McArthur et al. (1993), who showed that during the first 2 years after AIDS, HAD developed at an annual rate of 7%. Overall, 15% of the cohort followed through death developed HAD. Older age at AIDS onset was a risk factor for more rapid development of HAD (relative hazard, 1.60 per decade older). This work was supported by the results of an epidemiological study performed on patients' clinical records from 52 clinical centers in 17 countries across Europe pre-HAART ($n = 6,548$ adults) (Chiesi et al., 1996). HAD was reported in 4.5% of patients at the time of AIDS diagnosis and during follow-up in an additional 7.8% of patients sustaining another ADI. The HAD risk was greater in older patients (14 and 19% greater at AIDS diagnosis and after, respectively, for a 5-year difference in age). A post-HAART study has also documented the persistent association of older age with the prevalence of HAD. HAD was more frequent in older (25.2%) than younger (13.7%) individuals, corresponding to an odds ratio of 2.13 for the older (50 years old or older; $n = 106$) versus the younger (20 to 39 years old; $n = 96$) group (Valcour et al., 2004a). Control variables were employed and showed that, adjusting for education, race, substance dependence, ARV medication status, viral load, CD4 cell count, and Beck Depression Inventory score, the odds of HAD in the older group increased to 3.26 times that of the younger group, further verifying the association reported. Of note, Larussa et al. (2006) reported another study in which the impact of HAART was examined with respect to the incidence of HAD. The prior results relating older age to HAD were replicated among ARV-naive, but not among ARV-experienced, participants. It was concluded that HAART may show a neuroprotective effect on HAD, although this was apparently not the case in another HAART era cohort (Valcour et al., 2004a). Hence, further study of the relationship between aging and HAD in HIV infection related to ARV treatment history may be required to better define the relationship.

Older Age and MCMD

As mentioned above, the relationship of aging to MCMD has been much less studied than that of aging to HAD. However, older age in HIV-1-infected persons has been associated with a mean MCMD symptom frequency higher than that among younger HIV-1-infected persons

(Goodkin et al., 2001). In addition, older age in HIV-1-seronegative persons was associated with a higher MCMD symptom frequency than among younger HIV-1-seronegative persons. We observed a similar effect of older age and MCMD symptom frequency in a study of older versus younger HIV-1-seropositive and -seronegative primary Spanish speakers. We used a generalized linear models approach with age category, HIV-1 disease category (HIV-1 seronegative, CDC stage B/early symptomatic HIV-1 infection, and CDC stage C/AIDS), and their interaction as predictors of the total number of MCMD symptoms (zero to six) defined by the American Academy of Neurology (1991). The model we used controlled for the CD4 cell count ($n = 136$) and showed a significant age category effect and an interaction of HIV disease category with age category. Older HIV-1-seronegative individuals showed a higher MCMD symptom mean (adjusted for control variables) than younger HIV-1-seronegative individuals, documenting an effect of age, while persons with CDC stage C/AIDS showed a larger MCMD symptom difference by age. However, a significant difference by age was not seen at CDC stage B (the early symptomatic stage). From these studies, overall, we have concluded that the aging process itself may be independently associated with the occurrence of MCMD symptoms, which are nonspecific for HIV-1 infection. Further, the impact of aging on cognitive-motor disorder in HIV-1 infection may vary by ethnicity and may apply to the less severe disorder (MCMD), as well as to the more severe disorder (HAD). However, Larussa et al. (2006) did not observe a relationship between aging and the diagnosis of MCMD. Of note, in this study, age was defined in three categories (20 to 39, 40 to 49, and ≥50 years of age). This definition could dilute the potential for finding a relationship compared to defining age as a continuous variable; in addition, a report of the MCMD diagnosis to a central registry was relied upon as the source of MCMD data, and an analysis of MCMD symptom frequency was not conducted. Thus, a diagnostic bias could have been operating. Nevertheless, this study supports the need for future research to account for a number of cofactors occurring in the relationship of aging to MCMD.

Older Age and NCI

Most studies of the neurocognitive performance of older HIV-1-infected individuals have been performed without concomitant definition of neurocognitive-disorder status (i.e., the presence or absence of MCMD and HAD). In one of the first studies to address the aging issue and NCI, van Gorp et al. (1994) showed no significant effects associated with age. However, very few of his sample were over 50 years of age, and therefore, they did not qualify as "older" according to the definition of the CDC. Likewise, Hardy et al. (1999) reported on a sample of 257 men in which older HIV-1-infected individuals (mean age, 44.5 years; all were ≥37 years old) performed worse than younger individuals (mean = 31.5 years) on a number of tests. Those with AIDS, as expected, performed more poorly than those pre-AIDS. Significant differences were found on the trail-making test B (referable to frontal-lobe function) and the grooved-pegboard test (referable to motor function), with older adults with AIDS showing the lowest levels of performance. However, their results supported large interindividual variation in these associations within the group of older HIV-1-infected individuals. Hence, it might be concluded that control variables are especially important to utilize in the future of this work, as has been pointed out previously (Wilkie et al., 2003). In addition, as with van Gorp et al. (1994), the import

of a truly "older" group of HIV-1-seropositive individuals is highlighted. More recently, Hinkin et al. (2001) reported an investigation of the interaction between age (<40, 40 to 49, and ≥50 years of age) and HIV-1 disease status (HIV-1 seronegative, HIV-1 seropositive/pre-AIDS, and HIV-1 seropositive/AIDS). In this study, older age did appear to act as a significant risk factor for a subgroup in the development of HIV-1-associated NCI. Patients ≥50 years old who had progressed to AIDS had a greater rate of NCI than did those in the other groups; however, again, use of appropriate control variables was not possible in order to fully evaluate these results as specifically due to the aging process.

Working memory (WM) is a particularly important neurocognitive domain to examine. It is highly dependent on prefrontal-cortical processes and is required in the temporary maintenance of information on-line for the purpose of rehearsal and manipulation (Baddeley, 1992). WM is required for many higher-order tasks, such as recalling newly learned information (episodic memory), language comprehension, and strategies to maintain and manipulate information in problem-solving and reasoning tasks, and WM may represent a "gateway" to subsequent deficits in other neurocognitive domains. Deficits in WM tasks have been observed in HIV-1-infected individuals, particularly with disease progression (Stout et al., 1995; Wood et al., 1998), as well as with aging. Hence, this neurocognitive domain may be particularly important for future research.

It might be concluded that the area of older age and NCI suffers from several methodological issues, including a predominant lack of specificity in the definition of concurrent neurocognitive-disorder status. Studies of NCI have predominantly not reported concomitant criteria for MCMD and HAD. Given that NCI is being studied without a neurocognitive-disorder clinical referent (i.e., participants with NCI may have HAD, MCMD, or subclinical ["asymptomatic"] NCI), this reduces the utility of the results obtained. While controls for educational level and HIV-1 clinical disease stage were common, controls for other factors influencing NCI were not (e.g., ethnicity, gender, HIV risk factor, CNS penetration of ARV regimen used, adherence level, depressed mood level, and substance use). Another issue in the area has been a variation in the neurocognitive domains assessed and a relative lack of focus upon WM. Finally, this area has been negatively impacted by variation among studies in the definition of older age and to what extent the older age range was well represented. Given the recent addition of the condition of "asymptomatic neuropsychological impairment" to the neurocognitive disorders previously identified as associated with HIV-1 infection (Antinori et al., 2007), a specific focus on aging and this condition would be of special interest.

Mechanisms of the Association between Older Age and HIV-1-Associated NCI and Disorder

The interaction of the older population and the HIV-1-infected population is of greater import than ever before. In approaching a discussion of the mechanisms by which aging and HIV-1 infection could interact to cause NCI and disorder, it is helpful to begin by defining the populations to be examined. NCI occurs with increased frequency compared to the general population in both the older and the HIV-1-infected populations. Hence, the interaction of these two populations with a third population of those with NCI in the United States would also be expected to be disproportionately large compared to either group alone (Fig. 1). Moreover, we expect that a true synergism may

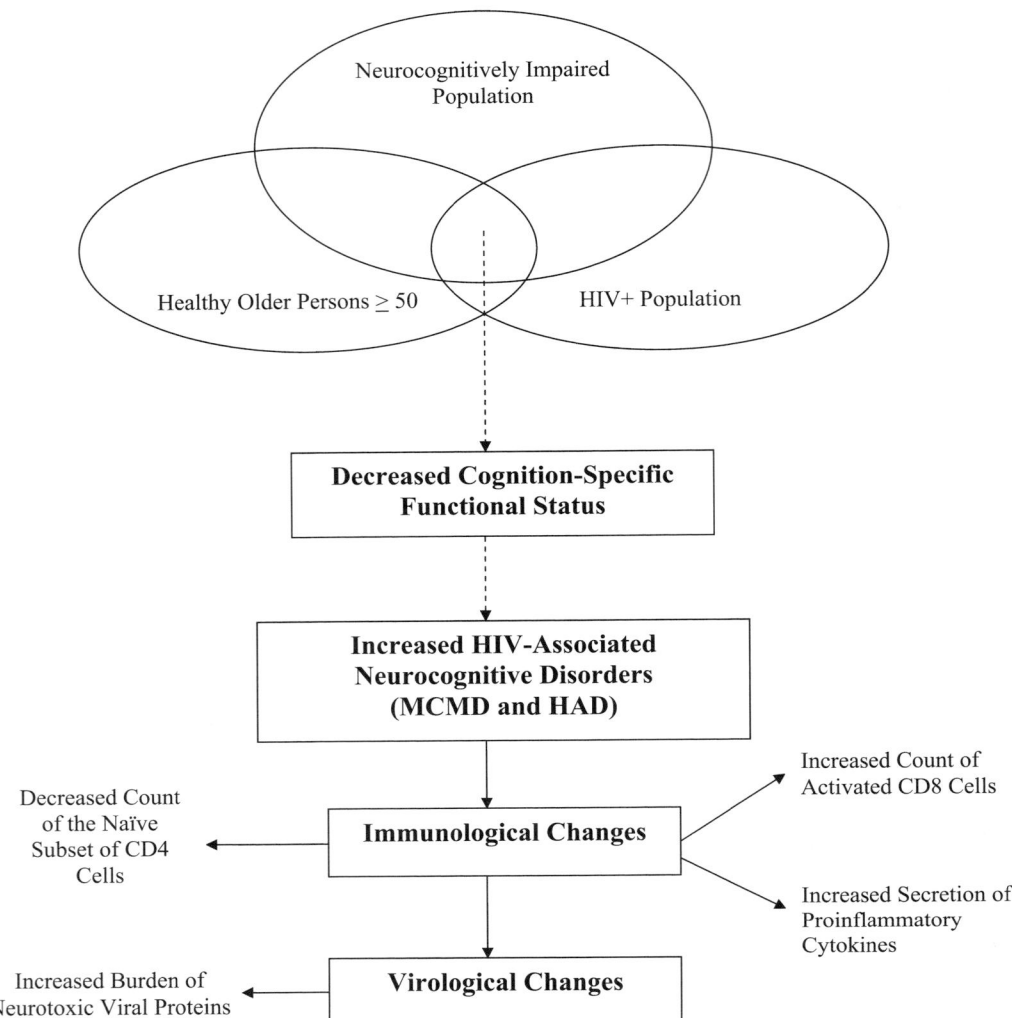

FIGURE 1 The overlap of two populations, older persons and the HIV-1 infected, has been increasing in recent years. A third population, those with NCI, normally significantly overlaps each of these populations independently. In the intersection of those with older age and those with HIV infection, the area of such overlap is expected to be proportionately greater. In association with this overlap, it is expected that there will be a high rate of decrements of functional status in the activities of daily living that are most closely related to NCI. In turn, it is expected that there will be proportionately higher rates of the HIV-1-associated neurocognitive disorders (MCMD and HAD). These disorders relate particularly well to anticipated immunological changes occurring in this overlap group—decreases in naive CD4 cell counts and increases in the activation state of CD8 cells, as well as in the secretion of proinflammatory cytokines (TNF-α, IL-1, and IL-6). These immunological changes are expected to be associated with virologic changes characterized by an increase in the elaboration of neurotoxic viral proteins (gp120 and Tat).

be operating, in which the actual overlap that exists may outweigh the sum of the independent impacts of both aging and HIV-1 infection as etiological factors. In this triple-overlap population of the aged, the HIV-1 infected, and the neurocognitively impaired, we expect that there will be an association with significantly decreased functional status in activities of daily living (Knippels et al., 2002), an increased frequency of unemployment (Heaton et al., 1994), and an increased frequency of the diagnosis of neurocognitive disorders. It is, therefore, of interest to consider how this triple-overlap group specifically relates to mechanisms that might

be observed within both the older and the HIV-1-infected patient populations.

Several pathophysiological sources exist for a synergism in CNS tissue damage in the overlap of aging and HIV-1 infection. For example, increases in oxidative stress (oxidative free radical formation) are associated with neurotoxicity in both aging and HIV-1 infection, as well as specifically with NCI in HIV-1 infection. Quinolinic acid, a neurotoxin and convulsant activating N-methyl D-aspartate receptor-induced excitotoxicity, represents another source for such an interaction in that aging and HIV-1 infection are both associated with the increased elaboration of quinolinic acid. Moreover, neuronal apoptosis is a process that co-occurs with aging and HIV-1 infection that is more likely to occur in this triple-overlap population with NCI. The compounded impacts across these putative mechanisms may be greater than the simple sums of the independent negative impacts, since there is evidence for shared pathophysiology.

The extent of such potentially shared neuropathophysiology is unclear. HIV-1-associated NCI should not be confused with the definition of "mild cognitive impairment" (MCI) in the general population. The latter has been supported as a transition between the milder age-associated memory impairment and the more severe Alzheimer's disease (AD) in the general population. Most research on MCI has focused on memory deficits. Though deficits can occur in other neurocognitive domains, only MCI with memory impairment has been linked to AD. As with HIV-1-associated MCMD, some patients with MCI progress to dementia, others remain stable, and still others revert to normal. (With HIV-1-associated NCI, reversion to normal is more common with subclinical HIV-1-associated NCI than with MCMD.)

In addition to the effects of the aging process itself, the age-associated increase in risk for cerebrovascular accident (CVA) might also be linked to increased risk for HIV-1-associated NCI and neurocognitive disorder. Increased CVA risk has been documented to occur in HIV-1-infected patients, in part due to the dyslipidemia now known to result from the long-term use of the PIs (as well as, to a lesser extent, the nRTIs). While NCI has also been associated with the short-term side effects of the nonnucleoside RTI (NNRTI) efavirenz, the NNRTIs as a class are least likely to be involved in the etiology of HIV-1-associated NCI and neurocognitive disorder; moreover, efavirenz itself may yet prove to be salutary in its neurocognitive effect over long-term use (Clifford et al., 2005). The occurrence of the aforementioned dyslipidemia in HIV-1-associated lipodystrophy syndrome may exert a novel contribution to the pathophysiology of the HIV-1-associated neurocognitive disorders specific to the HAART era (Goodkin, 2002). A vascular component of pathogenesis related to neuronal cell death by ischemia (without transient ischemic attack [TIA] or CVA) may now be expected to be "layered upon" the pre-HAART era causes of neuronal cell death, i.e., primary virologic effects (mediated by neurovirulence and/or macrophage tropism), as well as neuroinflammatory effects (mediated by bystander effects due to secretion of proinflammatory cytokines, such as tumor necrosis factor alpha (TNF-α), from activated macrophages in brain tissue). In addition, the existence of hepatitis C virus (HCV) coinfection may cause CNS tissue damage by primary virologic effects of HCV in brain tissue, as well as by indirect, metabolic effects exerted through the accelerated destructive effects of HCV on the liver that take place in HIV-1-coinfected patients. Further, a history of prior alcohol and substance abuse or dependence (particularly on cocaine and methamphetamine) in older HIV-1-infected persons may further increase the risk for HIV-1-associated NCI and disorder.

Of note, neuroanatomically, the impact of HIV-1 infection has been most consistently related to the frontal lobes and the basal ganglia. Nevertheless, other brain regions may frequently be involved with this heterogeneous infection of the brain as well, including the hippocampus. The expression of CD4 receptor glycoprotein has been demonstrated in the human brain; HIV-1 enters macrophages and microglia by CD4 receptors, as well as an HIV-1 coreceptor, predominantly CCR5 (Kramer-Hammerle et al., 2005). The frontal lobes and perilimbic cortex show high concentrations of CD4 receptor glycoprotein, with the greatest density in the hippocampus. One neuroimaging study suggested a specificity of HAD for high-signal lesions in the splenium of the corpus callosum and in the crura of the fornices (Kieburtz et al., 1990); the fornix provides reciprocal innervation for the hippocampus and the mammillary bodies. While the basal ganglia are more frequently affected than the hippocampi, the latter are more frequently involved than previously noted, with the expected relationship to verbal memory impairment (particularly with emotion-focused memories) (Wiley et al., 1998). Histopathologically, HIV-1 encephalitis is associated with gross cerebral, as well as hippocampal, atrophy; microglial nodules; and syncytium formation (multinucleate giant cells). Significant cellular atrophy (without cell death) has been reported in the hippocampus, characterized by dendritic pruning (Sa et al., 2000, 2004; Korbo and West, 2000). The CA3 hippocampal subregion has been shown to be most susceptible to HIV-1 infection in association with an increased expression of the chemokine coreceptors for HIV-1 locally; HIV-1 encephalitis cases were associated with increased expression of CXCR4 and decreased expression of CCR5 in this subregion (Petito et al., 2001). Both neuroimaging (Archibald et al., 2004) and neurocognitive testing (Moore et al., 2006) support this subregional specificity of hippocampal susceptibility to cellular dysfunction. Moreover, the aging process appears to predominantly affect the subiculum and dentate gyrus subregions of the hippocampus (Small et al., 2002); given the predominant effect on the CA3 hippocampal subregion by HIV-1, the interaction may represent a source for a potential mechanistic synergism at the subregional brain level.

Aging, chronic stressors, and major depressive disorder are each known to exert neurotoxic effects on the hippocampus. Chronic stressors and major depressive disorder, in particular, are thought to cause neuronal destruction due to neurotoxic levels of glucocorticoids and a high glucocorticoid receptor density in the hippocampus. Chronic psychosocial stressors have in fact been independently associated with hippocampal neuronal loss resulting in disinhibition of the hypothalamic-pituitary-adrenal axis and hypercortisolemia (Sapolsky and Scavone, 2006). In regard to major depressive disorder, one study divided the total time each of 38 female outpatients had been in a depressive episode by days in which antidepressant medication was and was not received; longer durations without treatment were associated with reduced hippocampal volume (Sheline et al., 2003). Given the hypercortisolemia-induced neuronal cellular toxicity associated with major depressive disorder and with chronic stressor exposure, both of these conditions may enhance the likelihood of NCI and neurocognitive disorder when superimposed upon the above-mentioned toxicities associated with the aging process and HIV-1 infection of the brain.

A possible overlap in the neuropathogenesis of HIV-1 with that of AD has also been considered for some time. One object of focus on this overlap has been the proinflammatory cytokines. In regard to HAD, TNF-α has been associated with both demyelination and the up-regulation of HIV-1 replication (Wilt et al., 1995). Related to the putative overlap with AD, TNF-related apoptosis-inducing ligand (TRAIL) has been shown to be involved in apoptosis. Recent data show that TRAIL is unregulated in activated, HIV-1-infected macrophages—a link with apoptosis known to occur in HAD (Petito and Roberts, 1995). TRAIL is also induced on neurons by Aβ protein (Huang et al., 2005).

Interleukin-1 (IL-1) is another proinflammatory cytokine released by activated, HIV-1-infected macrophages in the brain. IL-1 may cause cytotoxicity either in its membrane-bound (α) or in its secreted (β) form and could play a role in the pathogenesis of HIV-1-associated NCI and disorder. The associated neurotoxic effects may be due to chronic overexpression of IL-1α and/or the β isoform of S100, a small (10-kDa), soluble calcium-binding protein that is synthesized and released by astrocytes. S100β activates the transcription factors Sp1 and NF-κB, which is followed by an increase in IL-1β mRNA levels. Both S100β and IL-1 are elevated in AD, and each has been implicated in AD-associated neuropathology (Liu et al., 2005); IL-1 stimulates the synthesis and processing of the β-amyloid precursor proteins in vitro. In regard to HAD, IL-1 is known to up-regulate HIV-1 replication, as well as TNF-α (Poli and Fauci, 1992). S100β increases intraneuronal free calcium levels (Barger and van Eldik, 1992), which in turn have been implicated in the pathogenesis of neuronal cell death and dementia in both AD and HAD. AD and HAD may also be interrelated by the increased production of IL-6, a third proinflammatory cytokine released by activated, HIV-1-infected macrophages in the brain that also up-regulates HIV-1 replication (Poli and Fauci, 1992). Increased IL-6 expression occurs during normal brain aging, suggesting a direct link of this overlap mechanism to the normal aging process. IL-6 blood levels are also associated with higher risk of AD and with neurocognitive decline in older age. Hence, the proinflammatory cytokines TNF-α, IL-1, and IL-6 may each be involved in the potential overlap and interaction of HAD neuropathogenesis with that of AD.

The ApoE 4 allele is well known for its effect on accelerating the age at onset of AD and may increase the risk for HAD as well (Finch and Morgan, 2007). The genotype at greatest risk for AD (and at an earlier age than normal) is the homozygous ApoE 4,4. The heterozygous ApoE 3,4 genotype is at increased risk, though less so than ApoE 4,4. While 40 to 65% of AD patients have at least one copy of the 4 allele, ApoE 4 is not a determinant of the disease—at least a third of AD patients are ApoE 4 negative. In regard to HAD, however, discrepant findings have been reported on the relationship of ApoE 4 to HAD. One study has shown that the relationship of ApoE 4 to increased risk for HAD was specific to older patients (Valcour et al., 2004b). Hence, this relationship may merit further investigation.

Aging is a known risk factor for Aβ accumulation. Aβ is degraded in the brain by neprilysin, a neuronal endopeptidase. Of note in regard to the issue of aging and HAD, HIV-1 Tat has been shown to inhibit neprilysin activity by 80% (Rempel and Pulliam, 2005). In fact, recombinant HIV-1 Tat added directly to brain cultures has been shown to result in a 125% increase in soluble Aβ. Further supporting this relationship, postmortem human brain sections from patients with HIV-1 infection demonstrated a significant increase in Aβ compared to controls, and the Aβ load was significantly correlated with the duration of positive HIV-1 serostatus.

In contrast, another recent study examining the presence of Aβ in HIV-1 infection found no evidence of significant premature Aβ deposition (Anthony et al., 2006). Of note regarding the specific susceptibility of the hippocampus in this overlap, elevated levels of hyperphosphorylated Tau were found in the hippocampi of many HIV-1-infected subjects in this study (compared to age-matched controls), with the highest levels noted in those treated with HAART. Of additional interest, ARVs have recently been preliminarily demonstrated to increase Aβ generation (50 to 200%) in

murine N2a cells and to markedly inhibit microglial phagocytosis of Aβ1-42 peptide in murine microglia (Shytle et al., 2006). This suggests the intriguing possibility that the CNS-penetrating ARVs themselves may actually contribute to the long-term likelihood of HIV-1-associated neurocognitive disorder, although they are now largely agreed to be associated with improvement in HIV-1-associated NCI in the short term. The clinical relevance of these findings for HIV-1-associated NCI and disorder remains to be determined. Thus, it might be concluded that the pathogenic mechanisms relevant to the overlap between aging and HIV-1-associated neurocognitive impairment and disorders involve a number of putative foci requiring further investigation, including proinflammatory cytokine secretion in the brain, atherogenic profiles associated with long-term HAART use, the specific vulnerability of the hippocampus, the presence of the ApoE 4 allele, and neprilysin activity level.

Aging and Other Neuro-AIDS Conditions

Age and HIV-1-Associated Peripheral Neuropathy

Although HAD remains better studied, HIV-1-associated peripheral neuropathy is now considered to be the most common neuro-AIDS condition in the HAART era. Distal sensory polyneuropathy (DSP) is the most common type of peripheral neuropathy occurring in the HIV-1 infected and most commonly occurs in late-stage disease. Inflammatory demyelinating polyneuropathies, acute and chronic, also occur (and may be seen in the earlier stages of HIV-1 disease). In regard to DSP, there are two major types observed in HIV-1 infection, that due to HIV-1 infection itself and that due to the toxicity of the ARVs, most prominently, the dideoxynucleosides (dideoxyinosine, dideoxycytosine, and stavudine); however, data have implicated the PIs as well (Lichtenstein et al., 2005). ARV-induced mitochondrial toxicity has been suggested as a mechanism; in addition, ARV-induced dyslipidemia may also play a role, particularly in the older patient. The clinical features of DSP involve pain, numbness, and dysesthesias. These first appear in the soles of the feet and gradually ascend; symptoms may also occur in the fingertips. Ankle reflexes are absent or reduced, and motor symptoms are minimal. The symptoms frequently plateau eventually but tend to persist regardless of treatment efforts. In the past, laboratory evaluation has been of little value; however, quantification of epidermal nerve fiber density by skin biopsy has more recently been used successfully for confirmation of the diagnosis and has been suggested for the assessment of disease progression and treatment response as well (Cornblath and Hoke, 2006; Zhou et al., 2007). Neuropathologically, there is loss of unmyelinated axons in the distal regions of sensory nerves and later Wallerian degeneration of the distal myelinated fibers (see chapter 6, this volume, for more details).

Aging is associated with deterioration in light touch sensation in the foot in both soft and calloused skin (Mitchell and Mitchell, 2000). One pre-HAART electrophysiological study of patients with AIDS without clinical evidence of peripheral neuropathy showed changes similar to those in normal aging (Fuller et al., 1991). A clinical association of aging with DSP in HIV-1 infection has now been documented in several studies (Simpson et al., 1998; Lopez et al., 2004; Morgello et al., 2004; Watters et al., 2004). Of further clinical relevance for older persons with HIV-1 infection, peripheral neuropathy has been demonstrated to be a true risk factor for falls in the elderly (Munhoz et al., 1995) and to be associated with neurocognitive disorder. In addition, the pain associated with peripheral neuropathy may cause suboptimal ARV adherence, which could have implications for systemic disease progression as well. Hence, older patients should be considered at high risk for HIV-1-associated peripheral neuropathy and screened regularly for this condition. Furthermore, evaluations for other causes of DSP commonly found in the older population, such as B_{12} deficiency and abnormal glucose metabolism, need to be executed thoroughly.

Those diagnosed with peripheral neuropathy should receive specific attention to the ARVs used (e.g., the dideoxynucleosides and PIs), maximal pain control, and regular reviews of ARV adherence.

Age and PML

Progressive multifocal leukoencephalopathy (PML) is a severe neurological disease estimated to arise in 2 to 7% of all HIV-1-infected individuals due to a lytic infection of oligodendrocytes by John Cunningham virus (JCV). The clinical presentation is one of focal neurological disease associated with radiographic evidence of white-matter disease in the absence of mass effect. The most common presentations include focal weakness and sensory disturbances, visual deficits, and cognitive abnormalities. Visual deficits, such as quadrantanopsia (most common), homonymous hemianopsia, and cortical blindness, occur in 50% of patients with PML (Berger and Concha, 1995). Cognitive decline in PML is generally rapid and focal, with memory impairment, dyslexia, dyscalculia, and aphasia; dysarthria also occurs. Lesions range in size from 1 mm to several centimeters and have a predilection for the parieto-occipital regions, but they may involve any area of white matter. Neuropathologically, PML is characterized by the triad of multifocal demyelination; hyperchromatic, enlarged oligodendroglial nuclei; and enlarged, bizarre astrocytes with lobulated hyperchromatic nuclei (Major et al., 1992). Prior to HAART, PML usually progressed to death within a mean of 4 months, with >80% succumbing within 1 year from the time of diagnosis (Berger and Concha, 1995). Post-HAART, the median survival time has increased to 10.5 months (Clifford et al., 1999).

In regard to aging, PML is a disease of reactivation. De novo infection is found in 10% of children aged 1 to 5, 40 to 60% by age 10, and 80 to 90% by middle adulthood. Hence, PML is a disease predominantly seen in adulthood. PML is seen in the setting of cellular immunodeficiency, with the AIDS epidemic having contributed to a large rise in incidence. In regard to a greater risk in older adulthood, immunosenescence might well be a contributing factor to determining the small percentage of those with cellular immunodeficiency who eventually develop the disease. JCV may be frequently present in the brains of immunocompetent older patients and is transactivated by HIV-1. Hence, it might be reactivated relatively early in systemic HIV-1 disease progression. This would have a greater impact among older HIV-1-infected patients, who are more likely to have JCV resident in their brain tissue (Mori et al., 1992). While HAART has improved the survival time of PML patients, the improvement in many patients is still limited, and a variety of JCV-specific therapies (Ara-C, cidofovir, and topotecan) have failed. Thus, research and developmental efforts in this area are still sorely needed. Related to research contributions, for example, the cellular receptor for JCV has been defined as the 5HT2a receptor (Elphick et al., 2004), and drugs binding 5HT2a receptors block JCV infection of glial cells in vitro; thus, the atypical antipsychotics (such as zisprasidone and risperidone) are potent 5HT2a receptor antagonists, and it is possible that they may prove to be useful treatments for PML.

Age and Risk for TIA and CVA

While a small but elevated CVA risk was noted pre-HAART, in the HAART era, preventive management of CVA has been a more prominent focus. Related to the increased likelihood of insulin resistance, glucose intolerance, and dyslipidemia in long-term treatment with the PIs and, to a lesser extent, with the nRTIs, studies evaluating vascular neurotoxicities in HIV-1 infection have increased. Despite a number of articles initially focusing exclusively upon elevated risk for myocardial infarction, research on vascular toxicity in the cerebrovascular tree has steadily increased. An increased prevalence of premature carotid atherosclerosis was found in HIV-1-infected individuals treated with PI-containing regimens for at least 12 months (Maggi et al., 2000). One study focused upon clinical events and showed a total prevalence of TIA and CVA of 1.9% (TIA, 0.8%; CVA, 1.2%) (n = 772) (Evers et al., 2003). The clinical import of the cerebrovascular risk issue in the HIV-1-infected population generally has been described as a "clockwork bomb that will explode" (Maggi et al., 2002). Older age would be expected to further enhance this risk, although this specific issue has not yet received systematic study. Aggressive CVA risk screening is warranted for older HIV-1-infected patients (Sacco et al., 2006).

Age and PCNSL

The incidence of non-Hodgkin's lymphoma is greatly increased in HIV-1-infected persons. The vast majority are clinically aggressive B-cell-derived tumors. Approximately 80% arise systemically (nodal and/or extranodal); the remaining 20% arise as primary CNS lymphomas (PCNSLs). PCNSL occurs in 1 to 4% of HIV-1-infected persons, and AIDS is the most common disease associated with the tumor. PCNSL is often associated with severe immunosuppression. After CNS toxoplasmosis, PCNSL is the most common cause of CNS mass lesions among the HIV-1 infected. An epidemiological study in Australia documented that the overall incidence of non-Hodgkin's lymphoma decreased (by 37.5%) in the HAART era. Nevertheless, this was less of a decrement than for other AIDS-associated illnesses (which decreased by 55%) (Grulich, 1999).

One post-HAART study of all French hospital wards involved in managing HIV-1 infection in the year 2000 prospectively examined the cause of death in all patients (Bonnet et al., 2004). Of a total of 964 deaths, 269 (28%) were due to cancer. Malignancies defined as AIDS related were the cause of death in 149 cases (15%), with non-Hodgkin's lymphoma causing 11% (systemic, n = 78, with a median CD4 cell count of 86 cells/mm³; PCNSL, n = 27, with a median CD4 cell count of 20 cells/mm³). Kaposi's sarcoma was associated with 40 deaths (4%), and cervical carcinoma was associated with 5 deaths (0.5%). Interestingly, cancers not defined as AIDS related were the cause of 120 deaths (13%), including 103 solid tumors (50 respiratory, 19 hepatic, 9 gastrointestinal, and 6 anorectal) and 17 hematologic tumors (12 Hodgkin's lymphomas, 4 myeloid leukemias, and 1 myeloma). Of special note here, patients who died from cancer were more likely to be older and to have higher CD4 cell counts.

Data from the U.S. AIDS-Cancer Registry Match study on risk for Kaposi's sarcoma and lung cancer among PWAs have been presented. For 132,346 homosexual men with AIDS, the Kaposi's sarcoma incidence was highest for men

30 to 39 years old (5.0 cases/100 person-years) and declined with age, related to a decreased likelihood of human herpesvirus 8 infection with age (Engels, 2001). Generally, younger age has been associated with the incidence of PCNSL (Obrams and Grufferman, 1991), with most patients reported as being in their fourth decade. However, the incidence appears to be increasing across a wider age range. Older age is associated with decreased survival time in PCNSL. Given the short survival time of PCNSL, limited treatment efficacy, and unlikely patient candidacy for combined chemotherapy and radiation therapy due to toxicity, older HIV-1-infected patients with suspected PCNSL should be considered early for brain biopsy (rather than after empirical treatment for CNS toxoplasmosis).

Lung cancer and malignant melanoma incidence have now also been documented to increase with HIV-1 infection, and these tumors may metastasize to the brain. As HIV-1-infected persons age, new patterns in cancer incidence may emerge, potentially involving the brain as a primary or a metastatic site. Hence, assertive prevention strategies are needed to address the increasing concern for non-AIDS-defining cancers that may affect the brain in the older HIV-1-infected patient, in addition to PCNSL.

AGE, HIV-1 INFECTION, AND COMORBIDITIES

In addition to the consideration of how aging might interact with HIV-1 infection in specific neuro-AIDS conditions, an overarching issue exists. That issue is related to how an increased frequency of medical comorbidities might interact with aging in the likelihood of expression of neuro-AIDS conditions. One report from the Multicenter AIDS Cohort Study regarding survival time after AIDS showed the impact of aging (>37 years, relative hazard = 1.28) and "multiple medical diagnoses" (relative hazard = 1.64) on survival (n = 886) (Saah et al., 1994). Skiest et al. (1996) published a report on the explicit impact of medical comorbidity among the HIV infected using the Charleston comorbidity index and showed an impact of increased medical comorbidity upon survival as well. Another issue related to medical comorbidity in older HIV-1-infected patients involves the delay known to occur in identifying HIV-1 infection in older people. Symptom ambiguity due to the presence of increased medical comorbidities could account for a delay in the attribution of symptoms as possibly due to de novo HIV-1 infection (rather than to previously existing conditions associated with aging) (Siegel et al., 1999). This is particularly likely when the presenting symptoms of HIV-1 infection are constitutional symptoms. Regarding the increased diagnosis of comorbid medical conditions with neuro-AIDS conditions, the common medical comorbidities of type 2 diabetes mellitus and hypertension are of major import. Type 2 diabetes mellitus may also be caused or exacerbated by the length of ARV treatment, increasing the cerebrovascular risk (as well as that of DSP) associated with aging. Also of relevance is the growing aforementioned problem of non-AIDS-defining malignancies among the HIV-1 infected (Pantanowitz et al., 2006).

In addition to the presence of medical comorbidities, neuropsychiatric comorbidities may be of special concern in the older age group as well. One study has suggested that older HIV-1-infected individuals may show a higher rate of major depressive disorder than older and younger HIV-1-seronegative individuals, as well as their younger seropositive counterparts (Rabkin et al., 2004). However, the specific comparison of older to younger HIV-1-seropositive individuals was not statistically significant. Goodkin et al. (2003) have reported that high clinically rated anxiety and depressed mood levels were not more common in the subgroup of older HIV-1-seropositive persons aging in the setting of long-term, successful HAART. In addition, one recent study in Australia confirmed that older patients living with HIV/AIDS were less likely to describe good or excellent physical health and more likely to have a higher percentage of general medical comorbidities; however, neuropsychiatric comorbidities showed no significant differences (Pitts et al., 2005). Hence, the issue of a possible contribution to neuro-AIDS conditions by neuropsychiatric comorbidities specifically more common in older patients is not yet supported by the evidence and requires further investigation.

Outside of medical and neuropsychiatric comorbidities, the issue of ARV toxicity is of great relevance in older persons. There is little evidence to date to suggest that older persons have increased neurotoxicity with the NNRTI efavirenz or with alpha-interferon (used in the treatment of HCV coinfection). In regard to ARV toxicities overall, however, ARV-associated adverse events are more likely among older patients with metabolic (glucose and lipids), hematologic (absolute neutrophils and hemoglobin), and renal (creatinine) abnormalities in high profile (Silverberg et al., 2007). Another study specifically evaluating the modulating effects of age on changes in plasma lipid levels in the response to HAART showed that total cholesterol levels increased in all patients, with the greatest increases in older, PI-treated patients (Leitner et al., 2006). In addition, the concern for drug-drug interactions is elevated among older HIV-1-infected patients due to decrements in hepatic and renal clearance and a tendency toward polypharmacy in this patient population. Specific guidelines for the use of ARVs (and concomitant medications) in older HIV-1-seropositive patients may be forthcoming in the near future.

REFERENCES

American Academy of Neurology. 1991. Nomenclature and research case definitions for neurological manifestations of human immunodeficiency virus type-1 (HIV-1) infection. *Neurology* **41**:778–785.

Anthony, I. C., S. N. Ramage, F. W. Carnie, P. Simmonds, and J. E. Bell. 2006. Accelerated Tau deposition in the brains of individuals infected with human immunodeficiency virus-1 before and after the advent of highly active anti-retroviral therapy. *Acta Neuropathologica* **111**:529–538.

Antinori, A., G. Arendt, J. T. Becker, B. J. Brew, D. A. Byrd, M. Cherner, D. B. Clifford, P. Cinque, L. G. Epstein, K. Goodkin, M. Gisslen, I. Grant, R. K. Heaton, J. Joseph, K. Marder, C. M. Marra, J. C. McArthur, M. Nunn, R. W. Price, L. Pulliam, K. R. Robertson, N. Sacktor, V. Valcour, and V. E. Wojna. 2007. Updated research nosology for HIV-associated neurocognitive disorders. *Neurology* **69**:1789–1799.

Archibald, S. L., E. Masliah, C. Fennema-Notestine, T. D. Marcotte, R. J. Ellis, J. A. McCutchan, R. K. Heaton, I. Grant, M. Mallory, A. Miller, and T. L. Jernigan. 2004. Correlation of in vivo neuroimaging abnormalities with postmortem human immunodeficiency virus encephalitis and dendritic loss. *Arch. Neurol.* **61**:369–376.

Arien, K. K., G. Vanham, and E. J. Arts. 2007. Is HIV-1 evolving to a less virulent form in humans? *Nat. Rev. Microbiol.* **5**:141–151.

Baddeley A. 1992. Working memory. *Science* **255**:556–559.

Baillargeon, J., M. Borucki, S. A. Black, and K. Dunn. 1999. Determinants of survival in HIV-positive patients. *Int. J. STD AIDS* **10**:22–27.

Banks, W. A., S. M. Robinson, and A. Nath. 2005. Permeability of the blood-brain barrier to HIV-1 Tat. *Exp. Neurol.* **193:**218–227.

Barger, S. W., and L. J. van Eldik. 1992. S100β stimulates calcium fluxes in glial and neuronal cells. *J. Biol. Chem.* **267:**9689–9694.

Berger, J. R., and M. Concha. 1995. Progressive multifocal leukoencephalopathy: the evolution of a disease once considered rare. *J. Neurovirol.* **1:**5–18.

Bonnet, F., C. Lewden, T. May, L. Heripret, E. Jougla, S. Bevilacqua, D. Costagliola, D. Salmon, G. Chene, and P. Morlat. 2004. Malignancy-related causes of death in human immunodeficiency virus-infected patients in the era of highly active antiretroviral therapy. *Cancer* **101:**317–324.

Butt, A. A., K. K. Dascomb, K. B. DeSalvo, L. Bazzano, P. J. Kissinger, and H. M. Szerlip. 2001. Human immunodeficiency virus infection in elderly patients. *South. Med. J.* **94:**397–400.

Centers for Disease Control and Prevention. 2007. Cases of HIV infection and AIDS in the United States and dependent areas, 2005. *HIV/AIDS Surveillance Report* vol. 17, revised ed.

Chiesi, A., S. Vella, L. G. Dally, C. Pedersen, S. Danner, A. M. Johnson, S. Schwander, F. D. Goebel, M. Glauser, F. Antunes, and J. D. Lundgren for the AIDS in Europe Study Group. 1996. Epidemiology of AIDS dementia complex in Europe. *J. AIDS Hum. Retrovirol.* **11:**39–44.

Clifford, D. B., S. Evans, Y. Yang, E. P. Acosta, K. Goodkin, K. Tashima, D. Simpson, D. Dorfman, H. Ribaudo, and R. M. Gulick for the A5097s Study Team. 2005. Impact of efavirenz on neuropsychological performance and symptoms in HIV-infected individuals. *Ann. Intern. Med.* **143:**714–721.

Clifford, D. B., C. Yiannoutsos, M. Glicksman, D. M. Simpson, E. J. Singer, P. J. Piliero, C. M. Marra, G. S. Francis, J. C. McArthur, K. L. Tyler, A. C. Tselis, and N. E. Hyslop. 1999. HAART improves prognosis in HIV-associated progressive multifocal leukoencephalopathy. *Neurology* **52:**623–625.

Cornblath, D. R., and A. Hoke. 2006. Recent advances in HIV neuropathy. *Curr. Opin. Neurol.* **19:**446–450.

Darby, S. C., S. W. Kan, R. J. Spooner, P. L. Giangrande, C. A. Lee, M. Makris, C. A. Sabin, H. G. Watson, J. T. Wilde, M. Winter, and the UK Haemophilia Centre Doctors' Organisation. 2004. The impact of HIV on mortality rates in the complete UK haemophilia population. *AIDS* **18:**525–533.

Diaz, M., D. C. Douek, H. Valdez, B. J. Hill, D. Peterson, I. Sanne, P. J. Piliero, R. A. Koup, S. B. Green, S. Schnittman, and M. M. Lederman. 2003. T cells containing T cell receptor excision circles are inversely related to HIV replication and are selectively and rapidly released into circulation with antiretroviral treatment. *AIDS* **17:**1145–1149.

Effros, R. B. 2003. Replicative senescence: the final stage of memory T cell differentiation? *Curr. HIV Res.* **1:**153–165.

Ellis, R. J., R. Deutsch, R. K. Heaton, T. Marcotte, J. A. McCutchan, J. Nelson, I. Abramson, L. J. Thal, J. H. Atkinson, M. R. Wallace, I. Grant, and the HIV Neurobehavioral Research Center Group. 1997. Neurocognitive impairment is an independent risk factor for death in HIV infection. *Arch. Neurol.* **54:**416–424.

Elphick, G. F., W. Querbes, J. A. Jordan, G. V. Gee, S. Eash, K. Manley, A. Dugan, M. Stanifer, A. Bhatnagar, W. K. Kroeze, B. L. Roth, and W. J. Atwood. 2004. The human polyomavirus, JCV, uses serotonin receptors to infect cells. *Science* **306:**1380–1383.

Engels, E. A. 2001. Human immunodeficiency virus infection, aging, and cancer. *J. Clin. Epidemiol.* **54**(Suppl. 1):S29–S34.

Evers, S., D. Nabavi, A. Rahmann, C. Heese, D. Reichelt, and I. W. Husstedt. 2003. Ischaemic cerebrovascular events in HIV infection: a cohort study. *Cerebrovasc. Dis.* **15:**199–205.

Finch, C. E., and T. E. Morgan. 2007. Systemic inflammation, infection, ApoE alleles, and Alzheimer disease: a position paper. *Curr. Alzheimer Res.* **4:**185–189.

Florida State Department of Health. 2007. *Florida Division of Disease Control Surveillance Report* no. 272, p. 28, Table 5. Florida State Department of Health, Tallahassee, FL.

Franceschi, C., D. Monti, D. Barbieri, S. Salvioli, E. Grassilli, M. Capri, L. Troiano, M. Guido, M. Bonafè, F. Tropea, P. Salomoni, F. Benatti, E. Bellesia, S. Macchioni, R. Anderlini, P. Sansoni, S. Mariotti, M.L. Wratten, C. Tetta, and A. Cossarizza. 1996. Successful immunosenescence and the remodelling of immune responses with ageing. *Nephrol. Dial. Transplant.* **11**(Suppl. 9):18–25.

Fuller, G. N., J. M. Jacobs, and R. J. Guiloff. 1991. Subclinical peripheral nerve involvement in AIDS: an electrophysiological and pathological study. *J. Neurol. Neurosurg. Psychiatry* **54:**318–324.

Ghani, A. C., C. A. Donnelly, and R. M. Anderson. 2003. Patterns of antiretroviral use in the United States of America: analysis of three observational databases. *HIV Med.* **4:**24–32.

Goodkin, K., F. L. Wilkie, A. Ardila, D. Lee, R. R. Molina, D. Asthana, P. Shapshak, A. Frasca, S. O'Mellan, W. Zheng, and I. Khamis. 2004. Older age and functional status in HIV+ and HIV− primary Spanish speakers in the USA (#MoPeB3368), p. 57. *In* CONGREX Sweden AB (ed.), *Abstr. XVth Int. Conf. AIDS,* 11–16 July 2004, Bangkok, Thailand. International AIDS Society, Stockholm, Sweden.

Goodkin, K., T. Heckman, K. Siegel, N. Linsk, I. Khamis, D. Lee, R. Lecusay, C. C. Poindexter, S. J. Mason, P. Suarez, and C. Eisdorfer. 2003. "Putting a face" on HIV infection/AIDS in older adults: a psychosocial context. *J. AIDS* **33**(Suppl. 2):S171–S184.

Goodkin, K. 2002. Evolution of neuro-AIDS during the HAART era. *J. Neuro-AIDS* **2:**1–17.

Goodkin, K., F. L. Wilkie, M. Concha, C. H. Hinkin, S. Symes, T. T. Baldewicz, D. Asthana, R. K. Fujimura, D. Lee, M. H. van Zuilen, I. Khamis, P. Shapshak, and C. Eisdorfer. 2001. Aging and neuro-AIDS conditions: a potential interaction with the changing spectrum of HIV-1 associated morbidity and mortality in the era of HAART? *J. Clin. Epidemiol.* **54**(Suppl. 1):S35–S43.

Grulich, A. E. 1999. AIDS-associated non-Hodgkins lymphoma in the era of highly active antiretroviral therapy. *J. Acquir. Immun. Defic. Syndr.* **21**(Suppl. 1):S27–S30.

Hardy, D. J., C. H. Hinkin, P. K. Stenquist, W. G. van Gorp, L. Moore, and P. Satz. 1999. Age differences and neurocognitive performance in HIV-infected adults. *N. Z. J. Psychol.* **28:**94–101.

Heaton, R. K., R. A. Velin, J. A. McCutchan, S. J. Gulevich, J. H. Atkinson, M. R. Wallace, H. P. Godfrey, D. A. Kirson, and I. Grant. 1994. Neuropsychological impairment in human immunodeficiency virus-infection: implications for employment. *Psychosomat. Med.* **56:**8–17.

Hinkin, C. H., S. A. Castellon, J. H. Atkinson, and K. Goodkin. 2001. Neuropsychiatric aspects of HIV infection older adults. *J. Clin. Epidemiol.* **54**(Suppl. 1):S44–S52.

Huang, Y., N. Erdmann, H. Peng, Y. Zhao, and J. Zheng. 2005. The role of TNF related apoptosis-inducing ligand in neurodegenerative diseases. *Cell. Mol. Immunol.* **2:**113–122.

Inungu, J. N., E. D. Mokotoff, and J. B. Kent. 2001. Characteristics of HIV infection in patients fifty years or older in Michigan. *AIDS Patient Care STDs* **15:**567–573.

Jackola, D. R., J. K. Ruger, and R. A. Miller. 1994. Age-associated changes in human T cell phenotype and function. *Aging Clin. Exp. Res.* **6:**25–34.

Janssen, R. S., O. C. Nwanyanwu, R. M. Selik, and J. K. Stehr-Green. 1992. Epidemiology of human immunodeficiency virus encephalopathy in the United States. *Neurology* **42:**1472–1476.

Keller, M. J., J. M. Hausdorff, L. Kyne, and J. Y. Wei. 1999. Is age a negative prognostic indicator in HIV infection or AIDS? *Aging* **11:**35–38.

Kieburtz, K. D., L. Ketonen, A. E. Zettelmaier, D. Kido, E. D. Caine, and J. H. Simon. 1990. Magnetic resonance imaging findings in HIV cognitive impairment. *Arch. Neurol.* **47:**643–645.

Knippels, H. M. A., K. Goodkin, J. J. Weiss, F. L. Wilkie, and M. H. Antoni. 2002. The importance of cognitive self-report in early HIV-1 infection: validation of a cognitive functional status subscale. *AIDS* **16:**259–267.

Korbo, L., and M. West. 2000. No loss of hippocampal neurons in AIDS patients. *Acta Neuropathol.* **99:**529–533.

Kramer-Hammerle, S., I. Rothenaigner, H. Wolff, J. E. Bell, and R. Brack-Werner. 2005. Cells of the central nervous system as targets and reservoirs of the human immunodeficiency virus. *Virus Res.* **111:**194–213.

Larussa, D., P. Lorenzini, A. Cingolani, S. Bossolasco, S. Grisetti, M. Bongiovanni, F. Moretti, I. Uccella, P. Zannoni, S. Foresti, G. Mazzarello, M. I. Arcidiacono, R. Pedale, A. Ammassari, V. Tozzi, C. F. Perno, A. D. Monforte, P. Cinque, A. Antinori, and the Italian Registry Investigative Neuro AIDS (IRINA). 2006. Highly active antiretroviral therapy reduces the age-associated risk of dementia in a cohort of older HIV-1-infected patients. *AIDS Res. Hum. Retrovir.* **22:**386–392.

Leitner, J. M., H. Pernerstorfer-Schoen, A. Weiss, K. Schindler, A. Rieger, and B. Jilma. 2006. Age and sex modulate metabolic and cardiovascular risk markers of patients after 1 year of highly active antiretroviral therapy (HAART). *Atherosclerosis* **187:**177–185.

Levy, J. A., M. G. Ory, and S. Crystal. 2003. HIV/AIDS interventions for midlife and older adults: current status and challenges. *J. Acquir. Immune Defic. Syndr.* **33**(Suppl. 2)**:**S59–S67.

Lichtenstein, K. A., C. Armon, A. Baron, A. C. Moorman, K. C. Wood, S. D. Holmberg, and the HIV Outpatient Study Investigators. 2005. Modification of the incidence of drug-associated symmetrical peripheral neuropathy by host and disease factors in the HIV outpatient study cohort. *Clin. Infect. Dis.* **40:**148–157.

Lima, V. D., R. S. Hogg, P. R. Harrigan, D. Moore, B. Yip, E. Wood, and J. S. Montaner. 2007. Continued improvement in survival among HIV-infected individuals with newer forms of highly active antiretroviral therapy. *AIDS* **21:**685–692.

Liu, L., Y. Li, L. J. Van Eldik, W. S. Griffin, and S. W. Barger. 2005. S100B-induced microglial and neuronal IL-1 expression is mediated by cell type-specific transcription factors. *J. Neurochem.* **92:**546–553.

Lopez, O. L., J. T. Becker, M. A. Dew, and R. Caldararo. 2004. Risk modifiers for peripheral sensory neuropathy in HIV infection/AIDS. *Eur. J. Neurol.* **11:**97–102.

Mack, K. A., and M. G. Ory. 2003. AIDS and older Americans at the end of the twentieth century. *J. Acquir. Immune Defic. Syndr.* **33**(Suppl. 2)**:**S168–S175.

Maggi, P., G. Fiorentino, G. Epifani, N. Ladisa, A. Lillo, F. Perilli, G. Impedovo, S. Ferraro, M. Gargiulo, G. Angarano, A. Chirianni, and G. Pastore. 2002. Premature vascular lesions in HIV-positive patients: a clockwork bomb that will explode? *AIDS* **16:**947–948.

Maggi, P., G. Serio, G. Epifani, G. Fiorentino, A. Saracino, C. Fico, F. Perilli, A. Lillo, S. Ferraro, M. Gargiulo, A. Chirianni, G. Angarano, G. Regina, and G. Pastore. 2000. Premature lesions of the carotid vessels in HIV-1-infected patients treated with protease inhibitors. *AIDS* **14:**F123–F128.

Major, E. O., K. Amemiya, C. Tornatore, S. Houff, and J. R. Berger. 1992. Pathogenesis and molecular biology of progressive multifocal leukoencephalopathy, the JC virus-induced demyelinating disease of the human brain. *Clin. Microbiol. Rev.* **5:**49–73.

Mayeux, R., Y. Stern, M. X. Tang, G. Todak, K. Marder, M. Sano, M. Richards, Z. Stein, A. A. Ehrhardt, and J. M. Gorman. 1993. Mortality risks in gay men with human immunodeficiency virus infection and cognitive impairment. *Neurology* **43:**176–182.

McArthur, J. C., D. R. Hoover, H. Bacellar, E. N. Miller, B. A. Cohen, J. T. Becker, N. M. Graham, J. H. McArthur, O. A. Selnes, L. P. Jacobson, et al. 1993. Dementia in AIDS patients: incidence and risk factors. *Neurology* **43:**2245–2252.

Miami-Dade County Health Department. 2007. *Monthly AIDS Surveillance Report,* p. 1–11. Miami-Dade Health Dept., Miami, FL.

Mitchell, P. D., and T. N. Mitchell. 2000. The age-dependent deterioration in light touch sensation on the plantar aspect of the foot in a rural community in India: implications when screening for sensory impairment. *Leprosy Rev.* **71:**169–178.

Moore, D. J., E. Masliah, J. D. Rippeth, R. Gonzalez, C. L. Carey, M. Cherner, R. J. Ellis, C. L. Achim, T. D. Marcotte, R. K. Heaton, I. Grant, and the HNRC Group. 2006. Cortical and subcortical neurodegeneration is associated with HIV neurocognitive impairment. *AIDS* **20:**879–887.

Morgello, S., L. Estanislao, D. Simpson, A. Geraci, A. DiRocco, P. Gerits, E. Ryan, T. Yakoushina, S. Khan, R. Mahboob, M. Naseer, D. Dorfman, V. Sharp, and the Manhattan HIV Brain Bank. 2004. HIV-associated distal sensory polyneuropathy in the era of highly active antiretroviral therapy: the Manhattan HIV Brain Bank. *Arch. Neurol.* **61:**546–551.

Mori, M., N. Aoki, H. Shimada, M. Tajima, and K. Kato. 1992. Detection of JC virus in the brains of aged patients without progressive multifocal leukoencephalopathy by the polymerase chain reaction and Southern hybridization analysis. *Neurosci. Lett.* **141:**151–155.

Munhoz, C. D., L. B. Lepsch, E. M. Kawamoto, M. B. Malta, L. de Sá Lima, M. C. Avellar, J. K. Richardson, and E. A. Hurvitz. 1995. Peripheral neuropathy: a true risk factor for falls. *J. Gerontol.* **50:**M211–M215.

Murasko, D. W., P. Weiner, and D. Kaye. 1988. Association of lack of mitogen-induced lymphocyte proliferation with increased mortality in the elderly. *Aging Immunol. Infect. Dis.* **1:**1–6.

Nogueras, M., G. Navarro, E. Antón, M. Sala, M. Cervantes, M. Mengual, and F. Segura. 2006. Epidemiological and clinical features, response to HAART, and survival in HIV-infected patients diagnosed at the age of 50 or more. *BMC Infect. Dis.* **6:**159.

Obrams, G. I., and S. Grufferman. 1991. Epidemiology of HIV associated non-Hodgkin lymphoma. *Cancer Surv.* **10:**91–102.

Olsson, J., A. Wikby, B. Johansson, S. Lofgren, B. O. Nilsson, and F. G. Ferguson. 2000. Age-related changes in peripheral blood T-lymphocyte subpopulations and cytomegalovirus infection in the very old: the Swedish longitudinal OCTO immune study. *Mech. Ageing Dev.* **121:**187–201.

Operskalski, E. A., J. W. Mosley, M. P. Busch, and D. O. Stram. 1997. Influences of age, viral load and CD4⁺ count on the rate of progression of HIV-1 infection to AIDS. *J. AIDS. Hum. Retrovirol.* **15:**243–244.

Pantanowitz, L., H. P. Schlecht, and B. J. Dezube. 2006. The growing problem of non-AIDS-defining malignancies in HIV. *Curr. Opin. Oncol.* **18:**469–478.

Petito, C. K., B. Roberts, J. D. Cantando, A. Rabinstein, and R. Duncan. 2001. Hippocampal injury and alterations in neuronal chemokine co-receptor expression in patients with AIDS. *J. Neuropathol. Exp. Neurol.* **60:**377–385.

Petito, C. K., and B. Roberts. 1995. Evidence of apoptotic cell death in HIV encephalitis. *Am. J. Pathol.* **146:**1121–1130.

Petoumenos, K., M. G. Law, and the Australian HIV Observational Database. 2006. Risk factors and causes of death in the Australian HIV Observational Database. *Sex. Health* 3:103–112.

Pitts, M., J. Grierson, and S. Misson. 2005. Growing older with HIV: a study of health, social and economic circumstances for people living with HIV in Australia over the age of 50 years. *AIDS Patient Care STDs* 19:460–465.

Poli, G., and A. S. Fauci. 1992. The effect of cytokines and pharmacologic agents on chronic HIV infection. *AIDS Res. Hum. Retrovir.* 8:191–197.

Prado, J. G., N. T. Parkin, B. Clotet, L. Ruiz, and J. Martinez-Picado. 2005. HIV type 1 fitness evolution in antiretroviral-experienced patients with sustained CD4$^+$ T cell counts but persistent virologic failure. *Clin. Infect. Dis* 41:729–737.

Rabkin, J. G., M. C. McElhiney, and S. J. Ferrando. 2004. Mood and substance use disorders in older adults with HIV/AIDS: methodological issues and preliminary evidence. *AIDS* 18(Suppl. 1):S43–S48.

Rempel, H. C., and L. Pulliam. 2005. HIV-1 Tat inhibits neprilysin and elevates amyloid beta. *AIDS* 19:127–135.

Sa, M. J., M. D. Madeira, C. Ruela, B. Volk, A. Mota-Miranda, and M. M. Paula-Barbosa. 2004. Dendritic changes in the hippocampal formation of AIDS patients: a quantitative Golgi study. *Acta Neuropathol.* 107:97–110.

Sa, M. J., M. D. Madeira, C. Ruela, B. Volk, A. Mota-Miranda, H. Lecour, V. Goncalves, and M. M. Paula-Barbosa. 2000. AIDS does not alter the total number of neurons in the hippocampal formation but induces cell atrophy: a stereological study. *Acta Neuropathol.* 99:643–653.

Saah, A. J., D. R. Hoover, Y. He, L. A. Kingsley, and J. P. Phair. 1994. Factors influencing survival after AIDS: report from the Multicenter AIDS Cohort Study (MACS). *J. Acquir. Immune Defic. Syndr.* 7:287–295.

Sacco, R. L., R. Adams, G. Albers, M. J. Alberts, O. Benavente, K. Furie, L. B. Goldstein, P. Gorelick, J. Halperin, R. Harbaugh, S. C. Johnston, I. Katzan, M. Kelly-Hayes, E. J. Kenton, M. Marks, L. H. Schwamm, T. Tomsick, American Heart Association, American Stroke Association Council on Stroke, Council on Cardiovascular Radiology and Intervention, and the American Academy of Neurology. 2006. AHA/ASA Guidelines. Guidelines for prevention of stroke in patients with ischemic stroke or transient ischemic attack. A statement for healthcare professionals from the American Heart Association/American Stroke Association Council on Stroke. *Stroke* 37:577–617.

Sapolsky, R. M., and C. Scavone. 2006. Chronic unpredictable stress exacerbates lipopolysaccharide-induced activation of nuclear factor-κB in the frontal cortex and hippocampus via glucocorticoid secretion. *J. Neurosci.* 26:3813–3820.

Saule, P., J. Trauet, V. Dutriez, V. Lekeux, J. P. Dessaint, and M. Labalette. 2006. Accumulation of memory T cells from childhood to old age: central and effector memory cells in CD4$^+$ versus effector memory and terminally differentiated memory cells in CD8$^+$ compartment. *Mech. Ageing Dev.* 127:274–281.

Shapshak, P., S. M. Segal, K. A. Crandall, R. K. Fujimura, B.-T. Zhang, K.-Q. Xin, K. Okuda, C. K. Petito, C. Eisdorfer, and K. Goodkin. 1999. Independent evolution of HIV type 1 in different brain regions. *AIDS Res. Hum. Retrovir.* 15:811–820.

Sheline, Y. I., M. H. Gado, and H. C. Kraemer. 2003. Untreated depression and hippocampal volume loss. *Am. J. Psychiatry* 160:1516–1518.

Shytle, R. D., D. Obregon, J. Ehrhart, F. Fernandez, and J. Tan. 2006. Antiretrovirals increase neuronal production and disrupt microglial phagocytosis of β-amyloid. *In* CONGREX Sweden AB (ed.), *Abstr. XVIth Int. Conf. AIDS*, 13–18

August 2006, Toronto, Canada. International AIDS Society, Stockholm, Sweden.

Siegel, K., E. W. Schrimshaw, and L. Dean. 1999. Symptom interpretation: implications for delay in HIV testing and care among HIV-infected late middle-aged and older adults. *AIDS Care* 11:525–535.

Silverberg, M. J., W. Leyden, M. A. Horberg, G. N. DeLorenze, D. Klein, and C. P. Quesenberry, Jr. 2007. Older age and the response to and tolerability of antiretroviral therapy. *Arch. Int. Med.* 167:684–691.

Simpson, D. M., D. A. Katzenstein, M. D. Hughes, S. M. Hammer, D. L. Williamson, Q. Jiang, J. T. Pi, et al. 1998. Neuromuscular function in HIV infection: analysis of a placebo-controlled combination antiretroviral trial. *AIDS* 12:2425–2432.

Skiest, D. J., E. Rubinstein, N. Carley, L. Gioiella, and R. Lyons. 1996. The importance of comorbidity in HIV-infected patients over 55. A retrospective case-control study. *Am. J. Med.* 101:605–611.

Small, S. A., W. Y. Tsai, R. DeLaPaz, R. Mayeux, and Y. Stern. 2002. Imaging hippocampal function across the human life span: is memory decline normal or not? *Ann. Neurol.* 51:290–295.

Stout, J. C., D. P. Salmon, N. Butters, M. Taylor, G. Peavy, W. C. Heindel, D. C. Delis, L. Ryan, J. H. Atkinson, J. L. Chandler, and I. Grant. 1995. Progressive cerebral volume loss in human immunodeficiency virus infection. *Arch. Neurol.* 55:161–168.

Valcour, V., C. Shikuma, B. Shiramizu, M. Watters, P. Poff, O. Selnes, P. Holck, J. Grove, and N. Sacktor. 2004a. Higher frequency of dementia in older HIV-1 individuals: the Hawaii Aging with HIV-1 Cohort. *Neurology* 63:822–827.

Valcour, V., C. Shikuma, B. Shiramizu, M. Watters, P. Poff, O. A. Selnes, J. Grove, Y. Liu, K. B. Abdul-Majid, S. Gartner, and N. Sacktor. 2004b. Age, apolipoprotein E4, and the risk of HIV dementia: the Hawaii Aging with HIV Cohort. *J. Neuroimmunol.* 157:197–202.

van Gorp, W. G., E. N. Miller, T. D. Marcotte, W. Dixon, D. Paz, O. Selnes, J. Wesch, J. T. Becker, C. H. Hinkin, M. Mitrushina, et al. 1994. The relationship between age and cognitive impairment in HIV-1 infection: findings from Multicenter AIDS Cohort Study and clinical cohort. *Neurology* 44:929–935.

Watters, M. R., P. W. Poff, B. T. Shiramizu, P. S. Holck, K. M. Fast, C. M. Shikuma, and V. G. Valcour. 2004. Symptomatic distal sensory polyneuropathy in HIV after age 50. *Neurology* 62:1378–1383.

Welch, K., and A. Morse. 2002. Predictors of survival in older men with AIDS. *Geriatric Nursing* 23:62–68.

Wiley, C. A., V. Soontornniyomkij, L. Radhakrishnan, E. Masliah, J. Mellors, S.A. Hermann, P. Dailey, and C. L. Achim. 1998. Distribution of brain HIV load in AIDS. *Brain Pathol.* 8:277–284.

Wilkie, F. L., K. Goodkin, I. Khamis, M. H. van Zuilen, D. Lee, R. Lecusay, M. Concha, S. Symes, P. Suarez, and C. Eisdorfer. 2003. Cognitive functioning in younger and older HIV-1 infected adults. *J. Acquir. Immune Defic. Syndr.* 33(Suppl. 2):S93–S105.

Wilkie, F. L., K. Goodkin, R. Morgan, D. Feaster, M. A. Fletcher, N. Blaney, M. Baum, J. Szapocznik, and C. Eisdorfer. 1998. Mild cognitive impairment and risk of mortality in HIV-1 infection. *J. Neuropsychiatry Clin. Neurosci.* 10:125–132.

Wilt, S. G., E. Milward, J. M. Zhou, K. Nagasato, H. Patton, R. Rusten, D. E. Griffin, M. O'Connor, and M. Dubois-Dalcq. 1995. In vitro evidence for a dual role of tumor necrosis factor-α in human immunodeficiency virus type 1 encephalopathy. *Ann. Neurol.* 37:381–394.

Wood, S., C. Hinkin, S. Castellon, and K. Yarema. 1998. Working memory deficits in HIV-1 infection. *Brain Cognition* **37**:163–166.

Wu, M. X., and S. F. Schlossman. 1997. Decreased ability of HIV-1 Tat protein-treated accessory cells to organize cellular clusters is associated with partial activation of T cells. *Proc. Natl. Acad. Sci. USA* **94**:13832–13837.

Zhang, J., and C. S. Crumpacker. 2001. Human immunodeficiency virus type 1 RNA in peripheral blood mononuclear cells of patients receiving prolonged highly active antiretroviral therapy. *J. Infect. Dis.* **184**:1341–1344.

Zhou, L., D. W. Kitch, S. R. Evans, P. Hauer, S. Raman, G. J. Ebenezer, M. Gerschenson, C. M. Marra, V. Valcour, R. Diaz-Arrastia, K. Goodkin, L. Millar, S. Shriver, D. M. Asmuth, D. B. Clifford, D. M. Simpson, J. C. McArthur, NARC and the ACTG A5117 Study Group. 2007. Correlates of epidermal nerve fiber densities in HIV-associated distal sensory polyneuropathy. *Neurology* **68**:2113–2119.

Zingmond, D. S., N. S. Wenger, S. Crystal, G. F. Joyce, H. Liu, U. Sambamoorthi, L. A. Lillard, A. A. Leibowitz, M. F. Shapiro, and S. A. Bozzette. 2001. HCSUS Consortium. Circumstances at HIV diagnosis and progression of disease in older HIV-infected Americans. *Am. J. Public Health* **91**:1117–1120.

Zingmond, D. S., A. M. Kilbourne, A. C. Justice, N. S. Wenger, M. Rodriguez-Barradas, L. Rabeneck, D. Taub, S. Weissman, J. Briggs, J. Wagner, S. Smola, and S. A. Bozzette. 2003. Differences in symptom expression in older HIV-positive patients: the Veterans Aging Cohort 3 Site Study and HIV Cost and Service Utilization Study experience. *J. Acquir. Immune Defic. Syndr.* **33**(Suppl. 2):S84–S92.

SPECIAL HEALTH
CARE ISSUES AND
NEURO-AIDS

VI

34

Neurologic Aspects of Palliative Care for HIV/AIDS

PETER A. SELWYN AND JOHN BOOSS

In the first decade of the AIDS epidemic in the United States and other developed countries, AIDS care was essentially palliative care. While there was little that could be done to alter or reverse the course of the underlying illness, there was much to be done to help patients and their loved ones navigate the devastating effects of the disease. Provision of pain and symptom management, helping those affected cope physically and emotionally with the burden of this disease, addressing goals of care at the end of life, and being committed to the dignity and well-being of patients even as they were dying—these are all hallmarks of the clinical discipline that is now called more explicitly palliative care.

With the advent of highly active antiretroviral therapy (HAART) and the ability now to impact on the course of the illness and help patients live with what has been dramatically transformed into more of a manageable chronic disease, much of the focus of care has now shifted away from this original palliative framework and more towards an infectious disease subspecialty model of care. While this may offer some benefits in terms of the growing complexity of antiretroviral therapy management, there is a risk that the heightened attention to the virus may in fact lead us to lose sight of the patient and his or her total care needs.

The World Health Organization defines palliative care as follows:

> ... the study and management of patients with active, progressive, far advanced disease for whom the prognosis is limited and the focus of care is the quality of life. [It is] the active total care of patients whose disease is not responsive to curative treatment. Control of pain, of other symptoms, and of psychological, social, and spiritual problems, is paramount. The goal of palliative care is achievement of the best quality of life for patients and their families.
>
> World Health Organization, 1990

This orientation—which stresses comprehensive care, attending to the multiple dimensions of patients' needs, not simply the cure of an infectious disease—is certainly a useful one in which to consider the current care of patients with HIV/AIDS, even in the era of HAART. This chapter attempts to address the palliative-care issues that currently affect patients with HIV/AIDS and neurologic disease in many developed countries that have moved into the chronic-disease phase of the epidemic.

MORTALITY TRENDS

As discussed below, the spectrum of morbidity and mortality in patients with AIDS has changed dramatically in recent years, following the advent of HAART in the mid-1990s. However, several themes are worth noting at the outset.

- While the rates of mortality from AIDS did indeed fall by more than 50% in 1996–1997 in most populations who then had access to the new therapies, death rates have since moved toward a plateau, although there has been a continuing decline in mortality rates in the United States through 2004 (Centers for Disease Control, 1997; Centers for Disease Control and Prevention, 2000; Chiasson et al., 1999; Egger et al., 1997; Hellinger, 2007; Palella et al., 1998). Because HIV incidence rates have not substantially decreased over the same time period, the net result is an increase in the prevalence of people living with HIV/AIDS, and in fact it is currently estimated that there may be more people living with HIV than at any other time in the epidemic (Hellinger, 2007).

- Current causes of death include both traditional AIDS-related opportunistic infections and, of increasing importance, other causes such as end-stage liver disease/cirrhosis (from chronic hepatitis B or C and/or alcohol-related liver disease), non-AIDS-defining cancers, miscellaneous infections, and other end-organ diseases, e.g., cardiac, pulmonary, and renal (Kravcik et al., 1997; Mayor et al., 2006; Puoti et al., 2000; Sansone and Frengley, 2000; Selwyn et al., 2000; Valdez et al., 2001).

Peter A. Selwyn, Department of Family and Social Medicine, Montefiore Medical Center, Albert Einstein College of Medicine, Bronx, NY 10467. **John Booss,** Yale University School of Medicine, Virology Laboratories, VA Connecticut, New Haven, CT 06510.

- While neurologic causes of death are not increasing in frequency, the prevalence of certain chronic neurologic conditions and symptoms, as discussed below, has in fact become of growing importance, given the growing number of patients living with HIV as a chronic disease. Thus, the need for palliative care as defined above, i.e., pain and symptom management, attention to functional status, and focus on quality of life and goals of care, becomes even more pronounced for patients with symptomatic neurologic disease, even if this not a source of increased mortality in the current era.

- With the advent of effective therapy for HIV, there have been growing disparities in outcome among different subpopulations of patients with AIDS, such that drug users, minorities, and women have been less likely to experience the benefits of the new therapies on a population basis. This appears to reflect differences in access and other underlying inequities in health care distribution, but it also raises important challenges for patient care. The ideal goal is not to promote "HAART for the rich and palliative care for the poor"—a tension which has also played out recently on a global scale with the relative lack of access to HAART in many heavily affected developing countries—but rather to provide comprehensive, integrated care at all stages of the disease process, so that patients receive the benefits of both disease-specific and palliative interventions.

We discuss these issues and the importance of incorporating a palliative care approach with respect to specific HIV-related neurologic conditions and symptoms, while recognizing that we do not wish to revisit many of the more general aspects of neurologic disease management in HIV/AIDS, which are covered in extensive detail in other chapters in this volume.

NEUROLOGICAL CONDITIONS ASSOCIATED WITH DEATH OR PROGRESSIVE DISABILITY IN THE HAART ERA

The clinical changes in the epidemic noted above were also associated with a major shift in emphasis on conditions affecting the nervous system and its care. The reader is referred to preceding chapters in this volume for in-depth coverage of the specific conditions. Our purpose here is to briefly summarize the trends in the specific HIV-associated neurological illnesses and the consequent shift in the responsibilities for the care provider. We follow this section on specific conditions with a section on pain and symptom management.

Louie et al. examined the causes of death among all persons over the age of 12 years who died with a diagnosis of AIDS in San Francisco from January 1994 until December 1998 (Louie et al., 2002). This time period straddled the 1996 introduction of HAART. There was a statistically significant decline in deaths attributed to nontuberculous mycobacteria, wasting syndrome, cytomegalovirus, *Pneumocystis carinii* pneumonia, Kaposi's sarcoma, progressive multifocal leukoencephalitis, toxoplasmosis, and cryptosporidiosis. Sacktor et al. reviewed the epidemiology of neurological conditions associated with HIV infection following the introduction of HAART (Sacktor et al., 2000). Examining data from the Multi-Center AIDS Cohort Study and the Johns Hopkins HIV Clinic, declines in cryptococcal meningitis and central nervous system (CNS) toxoplasmosis were found. Trends toward a slight decrease in progressive multifocal

leukoencephalitis were found in these data sets, as was a trend toward reduction in the incidence of primary CNS lymphoma. Among chronic conditions of the CNS, the incidence of AIDS dementia was found to drop significantly. After 1996, there was a tendency for an increased number of cases to develop with CD4$^+$ T-lymphocyte counts of >200 cells/mm^3. Furthermore, HIV dementia in comparison to other AIDS-defining illnesses increased in proportion. McArthur et al. reported an increased cumulative prevalence of HIV dementia in the Johns Hopkins University Clinic from 1994 until 2001 (McArthur et al., 2003). They hypothesized that after the introduction of HAART three types of HIV-associated dementia existed: first, a subacute progressive dementia in patients not receiving HAART; second, a chronic active dementia in patients with poor adherence to antiretroviral regimens or viral resistance; and third, a chronic inactive dementia in patients under treatment with good virologic suppression. The second category of patient was at risk for progression, whereas some recovery and stability were possible for patients in the third category. Also, as HIV-infected individuals age they may be at significantly greater risk of HIV-related cognitive decline than younger individuals (Valcour et al., 2004).

Among distal symmetric sensory neuropathies, Sacktor reported a reduction in the incidence of the HIV-associated neuropathy but an increase in the antiretroviral-associated toxic neuropathy (Sacktor, 2002). With the enhanced survival of AIDS patients in the HAART era, the sensory neuropathies in HIV infection have demonstrated a rising prevalence and now constitute the most common complication of HIV in the nervous system (McArthur et al., 2003). Increased symptomatic distal sensory neuropathy has been found after the age of 50 in comparison to younger age groups (Watters et al., 2004). Although accurate figures on the incidence and prevalence of the HIV-associated vacuolar myelopathy are difficult to collect because of the absence of a widely accepted case definition, there does not appear to have been a significant decline in prevalence.

NEUROLOGIC SYMPTOMS REQUIRING PALLIATIVE CARE

The clinician is often presented with symptom complexes in the HAART era, which, although possibly resulting from a single etiology, are often the result of combinations of HIV-associated processes. Hence, we address three major symptom complexes: cognitive impairment, pain syndromes, and gait impairment.

Cognitive Impairment

Cognitive impairment reduces the capacity of an individual to fend for oneself and to participate in those activities which are most distinctly human. The most common forms of cognitive impairment in HIV, the minor cognitive motor complex and the AIDS dementia complex, characterized as subcortical, are associated with mental slowing and affective blunting. These features reduce the ability to succeed in competitive environments. For example, one of the first patients seen by us was a man with AIDS who had been working as an art dealer in New York City and had given up his work when he realized that he had lost his edge to succeed in a highly competitive field. In other circumstances, homeless people living on the streets need a certain mental agility to avoid danger and obtain food and shelter, however primitive, to survive. In the latter circumstance, the functional capacity of individuals may have been further compromised by mental illness and/or substance abuse.

When feasible, it is important in all types of dementia/cognitive impairment to attend to a number of legal matters before an individual becomes mentally incompetent. Although the illness itself, as well as complicating conditions such as mental illness and substance use, may impoverish an individual, the drawing up of a will remains important, regardless of financial status. Assignment of durable power of attorney status to a trusted individual ensures that decisions will be made in patients' best interests when they can no longer look out for themselves. Cognitive impairment is of course not the only rationale to establish a durable power of attorney. Serious mental illness and substance use sometimes present insurmountable barriers to decision making in the patients' own best interests. Legal assignment of a health proxy is necessary for all individuals. It is particularly so for those individuals suffering a chronic illness such as HIV/AIDS, which can be punctuated by severe acute illness in which decision-making capacity may become blunted. The individual may also suffer from the intrusions of serious mental illness and the self-destructive effects of substance use. Similarly, it has become progressively clear in this society that written formal expressions of end-of-life decisions should be articulated. Serious disagreement arises in our society about the use of technology to prolong life and about what represents appropriate, or futile, interventions as an individual approaches the end of life. The evolution of dementia may compromise the validity of decision-making capacity. Hence, it is advisable to have a person's wishes formally established in writing so that no ambiguity exists for health care providers or legal guardians.

There are no clinical or laboratory markers to predict the course of cognitive impairment in HIV. Hence, it is important, in several respects, to establish a baseline and to perform follow-up assessments of cognitive capacities. At a most fundamental level, such evaluations buttress clinical impressions about the capacity for independent living. Decisions about the degree of health care and personal assistance required are facilitated by cognitive assessments over time. For certain HIV-infected individuals, the loss of cognitive capacity is relatively mild and nonprogressive. Case management to assist home or community living is sufficient in such circumstances. Therapeutic trials for the treatment and prevention of cognitive decline continue to be undertaken in cases of HIV infection. A related topic, fatigue in HIV infection, is highly complex with multiple potential causes. Once reversible conditions have been sought and treated, pharmacologic intervention with agents such as modafinil (Rabkin et al., 2004) may offer some enhancement of alertness, thereby improving the quality of life (see below for further discussion of palliative symptom management). However, progression of cognitive loss, either continuously or after a period of relative stability, may point toward the need for admission to a long-term care facility. Intermediate decisions include the decision to seek day care facility attendance. In optimal circumstances too, formal cognitive testing allows some assessment and prediction of the types of activities of which the affected individual remains capable. As the illness progresses or is seriously compromised by an acute disease or worsening of a complicating illness such as liver failure or renal failure, regular assessment of the capacity to perform activities of daily living should be instituted to supplement cognitive assessments.

There are models for dementia care that can be adapted to the care of persons with HIV cognitive impairment. The most common, of course, is the management of Alzheimer's dementia. These care models are structured for the elderly and often fall under federal Medicaid programs for funding. Important home- and community-based Medicaid waivers exist in some states, which facilitate maintenance of services in the home for affected individuals. Adaptation of such models of care to HIV-infected persons has proven cost-effective, as well as being more acceptable to patients, in certain states which have adopted such waivers (Anderson and Mitchell, 2004). However, state legislators are often reluctant to initiate such programs, despite the likely long-term savings, because of the "up front" costs of initiating them. Provision of long-term care facilities with daily rates specific to the HIV-infected population also falls prey to start-up cost concerns. The resultant lack of appropriate services falls hardest on those who cannot fend for themselves, particularly those with compromised cognition.

Chronic Pain

In contradistinction to cognitive decline, in which the burden of awareness falls mainly on loved ones, chronic pain inflicts on its sufferers a moment-to-moment experience of life's burden. Pain must be assigned priority among those conditions that impair the quality of life. The causes of pain in patients with HIV/AIDS are multiple, including specifically neuropathic forms. Yet the treatment of pain in HIV/AIDS is often inadequate. Particularly difficult for care providers are assessing and managing pain in substance abusers.

Many of the difficulties in the treatment of chronic pain in HIV/AIDS center on the use of narcotics. There is evidence that regimens including a narcotic are effective in treating neuropathic pain (Gilron et al., 2005). However, drug-seeking behavior on the part of certain patients serves to make some providers conservative in their prescribing practices. This is abetted by a medical culture that seeks to avoid establishing or sustaining narcotic addiction, and a political-social culture that emphasizes punishment rather than providing sufficient rehabilitation resources. The situation is made more complex by the potential sale of prescription drugs "on the street" by impoverished patients. Hence, it is clear that hospitals, clinics, and offices with individual providers serving a chronic-pain-suffering population need well-established and well-implemented guidelines for narcotics-prescribing practices. Absent such prescribing guidelines, chronic-pain sufferers will be subjected to inconsistent management practices.

While management of chronic pain in an HIV-infected chronic substance-abusing patient represents a severe challenge, it should not be forgotten that patients with HIV/AIDS suffer from acute pain syndromes, as well as the more common varieties of pain which afflict the general population. Acute opportunistic infections, with associated pain, still occur in the HAART era. Examples include the subacute meningitis of cryptococcosis and visceral pain with *Mycobacterium avium* complex (Selwyn and Rivard, 2003). When analyzed by site of pain, Norval found that limbs, mouth, head, throat, and chest (in descending order) were the most common sites (Norval, 2004). The abrupt or recent appearance of headache, or a change in the pattern of headache, merits prompt evaluation for life-threatening causes such as meningitis or the intracranial mass effect of infection or tumor. More commonly one is presented with chronic head pain refractory to common headache remedies.

It is worthwhile to consider the several potential causes of headache and head pain. Often neglected is the role of cervical spine disease as a trigger to headache in the absence of cervical pain radiating into the shoulders and arms. Examination of the cervical musculature for contraction, restriction of cervical mobility, and tenderness of the muscle attachment sites at the base of the skull provides physical examination clues. Sinus disease, particularly acute sinusitis, can masquerade as an intracranial process. The physical exam may identify the site of pain, and the infection can be identified in neuroimaging studies done primarily for intracranial disease. Gum and dental hygiene is compromised by oral cavity infection. A gloved digital examination of gums and teeth may turn up a focal offending cause of headache. Chronic infections of the throat can radiate as if primarily a headache. Careful examination of the ears, mastoids, and tympanic membranes is, of course, obligatory. While intraorbital and visual accommodation defects have not proven to be in excess in our experience in the HIV/AIDS population, they merit consideration. With respect to conserving vision, however, a headache exam should include palpation of the superficial temporal arteries and consideration of temporal arteritis. Those physical examinations considered, one is often left with management of migraine headache, muscle tension headache, or mixed headaches. Considerations of these common entities are beyond the scope of this chapter.

The pain associated with the distal symmetric sensory peripheral neuropathy (DSSPN) of HIV and/or toxic neuropathy of dideoxynucleoside analog antiretroviral therapy (i.e., didanosine, stavudine, and dideoxycytidine) has emerged as a significant cause of pain in the HAART era (Selwyn and Rivard, 2003). This has resulted from the relative insensitivity of the HIV-associated neuropathy to therapeutic intervention, combined with the longer survival of HIV-infected persons in the HAART era.

Pharmacologic management of HIV-associated neuropathic pain is similar to the approach to neuropathic pain in non-HIV-infected patients. It is recommended that clinicians use the WHO "analgesic ladder" approach, which categorizes pain into mild, moderate, or severe on a 10-point scale. Each level of pain corresponds to a recommended type of analgesic, e.g., nonopioids such as acetaminophen, ibuprofen, or ketorolac for mild pain, weak opioids such as codeine or hydrocodone for moderate pain, and strong opioids such as oxycodone, morphine, hydromorphone, methadone, or fentanyl for severe pain (Fig. 1) (Jacox et al., 1994; World Health Organization, 1990).

For neuropathic pain, regardless of the severity, it is recommended often to try an adjuvant medication in addition to the analgesic, such as an antidepressant (amitriptyline or imipramine), an anticonvulsant (gabapentin or lamotrigine), or other options (clonazepam, prolixin, or dronabinol).

While it is often possible to achieve effective relief of neuropathic pain with a combination of analgesic and adjuvant medications, it should be noted that there are some possible drug interactions that should be anticipated between some of the HIV-specific medications (such as the nonnucleoside reverse transcriptase inhibitors and the protease inhibitors) and certain anticonvulsants (such as phenytoin, carbamazepine, and others), due to their combined metabolism through the cytochrome P450 hepatic enzyme system (U.S. Department of Health and Human Services, 2006; Ogbuokiri, 2003; Piscitelli and Gallicano, 2001).

For more detailed discussion of diagnosis and management of HIV-related neuropathic pain, we refer the reader to the contribution of Simpson and colleagues elsewhere in this volume. The pain associated with DSSPN, particularly

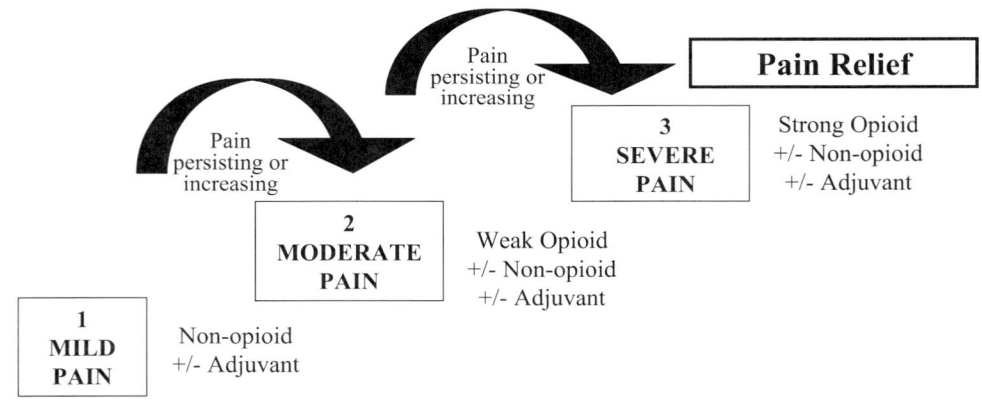

FIGURE 1 Treatment of pain: the WHO analgesic ladder. The guidelines for pain management are as follows:

- Use the WHO analgesic "ladder" for mild, moderate, and severe pain.
- Adjuvant medications (e.g., amtriptyline, gabapentin, lamotrogine, carbamazepine) are particularly helpful for neuropathic pain.
- Mild pain (1–3 on 0–10 scale): non-opioid analgesics (ibuprofen, indomethicin, acetylsalicylic acid, acetaminophen) with or without adjuvants.
- Moderate pain (4–6 on 0–10 scale): weak opioids (codeine, hydrocodone) with or without adjuvants.
- Severe pain (7–10 on 0–10 scale): strong opioids (morphine, oxycodone, methadone, hydromorphone, fentanyl) with or without adjuvants.

(Adapted from WHO, 1990.)

a burning sensation in the feet, is one of the complex causes of gait impairment, considered next.

GAIT IMPAIRMENT

Gait impairment is socially isolating. As the impairment worsens, the individual becomes less autonomous and more dependent on the assistance of friends, family, and social services. For individuals living in buildings without an elevator in apartments above the first floor, trips out for food, medical care, and social contact become more difficult and more infrequent. Visits by social workers, visiting nurses, care providers, or case managers become essential for maintenance of vital functions. Individuals with a progressive loss of independent ambulation may become fearful and resist attempts to have them admitted to long-term care facilities. Community, religious, or health institution-based home care becomes essential to sustain an acceptable quality of life and life itself. Tragically, just as an individual's needs for assistance become greater, the reduction in social contact may result in less spontaneous assistance by friends and social contacts. Persons in remote rural settings are at enhanced risk because such municipalities may not be able to provide the necessary outreach services. Homeless persons with gait impairment are uniquely at risk for the loss of vital services and the incapacity to avoid the harms associated with life on the street.

The causes of gait impairment in persons living chronically with HIV are manifold and may be cumulative in any one individual. This includes the residua from treated acute infections of the CNS or incomplete recovery from inflammatory disorders of the peripheral nervous system such as the Guillain-Barré syndrome.

More insidious, however, are the gradual losses of motor dexterity, motor strength, balance, and sensory perception necessary for gait caused by any of several chronic HIV-associated disorders. Most common is the DSSPN of HIV, compounded on occasion by the antiretroviral-related toxic neuropathy. The loss of proprioception confers instability to gait, which may be compounded by pain in the feet. Loss of proprioception, loss of motor strength, and a spastic component can result from a myelopathy. Most commonly seen in combination with cognitive impairment, the vacuolar myelopathy of HIV has proven frustratingly difficult to pin down diagnostically and is resistant to treatment. Furthermore, the signature findings of brisk deep tendon reflexes present at the knees while absent at the ankles suggest that it is often found in combination with DSSPN. Other causes of myelopathy should be sought including the subacute combined degeneration of vitamin B_{12} deficiency, other infections of the spinal cord, and compressive lesions such as infection, tumor, or herniated disk. Other spinal cord infections can include those caused by herpes simplex virus, varicella-zoster virus, cytomegalovirus, human herpesvirus 6, and syphilis. Dual infection with human T-cell virus-1 (HTLV-1) or HTLV-2 can also occur in HIV-infected drug users. A study among Brazilians with myelopathy found that coinfection with HIV and HTLV-1 was strongly associated with myelopathy (Harrison et al., 1997). Added to the mix of peripheral nerve and/or spinal cord pathology can be the minor cognitive motor complex or the AIDS dementia complex. These disorders include a reduction in motor speed and agility, progressing in severe cases to motor weakness. Separately, or in its aggregate, these disorders of neural function may be overlaid in advanced AIDS by the fatigue and weakness of the wasting syndrome or generalized systemic opportunistic infections such as Mycobacterium avium complex.

Regrettably, the DSSNP of HIV and the vacuolar myelopathy of HIV are not amenable to antiretroviral therapy. On occasion, progression of the cognitive motor disorders associated with HIV infection can be halted and partially reversed by such therapy. More commonly, however, a stable deficit or a gradually progressive loss of function occurs. Hence, in the aggregate, gait disorders may worsen for some patients, even in the face of antiretroviral treatment.

There is a useful model for the evaluation and management of gait disorders in HIV, namely multiple sclerosis. Gait disorder is common in multiple sclerosis. It may result from involvement of corticospinal tracts in the spinal cord or brain and is commonly complicated by ataxia of cerebellar/brain stem or sensory origin. While peripheral neuropathy is not a feature of multiple sclerosis, the evaluation and management strategies for multiple sclerosis can be applied to the gait disorders of HIV. Thus, clinical evaluation of progression of multiple sclerosis is heavily dependent on gait independence progressing through the need for a series of ambulation aids. Assessment is undertaken for the need for a cane for balance or to compensate for weakness and progression to the use of a walker, to a wheelchair, and to a motorized scooter. Focusing on ambulation capacities and the need for ambulation assistance at once provides an assessment of progression of disability, the need for prosthetics and gait instruction, and the nature and timing of community-based services or long-term care facility admission. Multiple sclerosis also provides a useful guide to the management of spasticity in HIV-infected individuals. One must judiciously treat spasticity so as to retain weight-bearing capacity. Baclofen and tizanidine are commonly used pharmacologic interventions in multiple sclerosis. However, installation of a catheter to facilitate intrathecal baclofen delivery, as has been used in multiple sclerosis, may pose a significant risk of opportunistic infection in the HIV-infected population. Botulinum toxin injections may deserve consideration to reduce spasticity in some cases. In more severe cases, passive range of motion exercises should be regularly performed to reduce the development of contractures and the breakdown of skin integrity. Additionally, amelioration of spasticity at most stages reduces the associated pain.

ORGANIZATION OF CARE SERVICES

As is evident from the preceding discussion, the evolution of neurological symptoms and syndromes among HIV-infected patients in the HAART era has posed new challenges for clinical management. An ironic situation has developed whereby some patients are now surviving longer during a relatively stable chronic disease phase of the illness, during which their HIV-specific problems are generally not acute, and instead what is required is long-term, comprehensive care of these secondary comorbidities, symptoms, and functional disabilities, including the neurological conditions we have discussed.

This current environment thus requires not only individual clinicians' sensitivity and expertise in dealing with these chronic symptom syndromes but also the institutional and programmatic response of the care delivery system in order to meet these needs effectively. Acute-care hospitals are not appropriate venues for chronic disease management. One area of growing need for this subpopulation is in-home care services, which can help patients maintain as high a level of function as possible and remain at home as long as possible. It should be clear from this discussion that some of these chronic care needs and the options to address them may be similar to those necessitated for the care of elderly patients with Alzheimer's disease, multiple sclerosis, cerebrovascular disease, amyotrophic lateral sclerosis, and other neurological conditions. The reader is referred to an excellent text on palliative care for neurologic disease, which provides much useful information pertinent to these other conditions, which also have some relevance for the chronic disease phase of HIV/AIDS (Voltz et al., 2004).

Home care services may include home health attendants for personal care needs, skilled nursing visits for clinical assessment, with physician collaboration as needed, physical therapy, and potentially other rehabilitative care services as well. Case management to coordinate these services and enhance adherence with important medications is of particular importance for those members of the HIV-infected population who are often unsuccessful in negotiating routine processes of care; this need is made even more critical as HIV care becomes more complex and chronic in nature.

For patients who are unable to be maintained at home, long-term care is another option, either in AIDS-dedicated or other nursing homes or other facilities, although it is important for any such facility caring for patients with HIV/AIDS to be able to provide adequate HIV specialty input as well as chronic disease and rehabilitative care (Selwyn et al., 2000). Moreover, due to the nature of the population affected by HIV/AIDS in the United States, with a high prevalence of substance use, such facilities must also be prepared to address the behavioral and mental health issues associated with drug and alcohol misuse both within and outside the facility.

In addition to home-based and institutional care, in some settings it may also become necessary to develop supervised housing options, including group homes, or independent units with enhanced on-site case management services, or other variations to help provide for the ongoing nonacute care needs of this long-term population that is neither ill enough to require institutional care nor functional enough to be cared for at home. This will necessitate not only case management, administrative coordination, and program development but also thoughtful attention to financing health services issues, since this new type of structure will not fit readily within one of the existing "silo-like" frameworks in which care has historically been delivered and financed.

PALLIATIVE CARE AT THE END OF LIFE

While we have been focusing on the palliative and supportive management of patients with HIV/AIDS with chronic neurologic disabilities and symptoms, it is important also to focus on care needs at the end of life for patients who die either of AIDS-related causes, of incurable comorbidities, or of other etiologies. For more detailed information on palliative care principles and management, the reader is referred to the *Oxford Textbook of Palliative Care* (Doyle et al., 1998); to the U.S. Department of Health and Human Services Health Resources and Services Administration's guidebook, *Palliative and Supportive Care for HIV/AIDS* (O'Neill et al., 2003); and to several web-based resources (End-of-Life Physician Education Resource Center [EPERC] [http://www.eperc.mcw.edu]; Center to Advance Palliative Care [CAPC] [http://www.capc.org/support-from-capc]; Education in Palliative and End-of-life Care [EPEC] [http://epec.net/EPEC/Webpages/resources.cfm]).

As noted above, much of the logic of palliative care needs to be anticipatory. For patients with HIV-related dementias—or, increasingly, for intractable hepatic encephalopathy due to end-stage cirrhosis from hepatitis C—it is important to address goals of care, identify a health care agent, and generate the documents required to define and help articulate patients' advance directives (e.g., living will, designation of health care agent, durable power of attorney, etc.) before an emergency or crisis situation. These directives can address specific health care-related issues, e.g., wishes concerning resuscitation, rehospitalization, initiation of withdrawal of specific or general care interventions, the use of artificial nutrition and hydration, as well as important other personal and legal matters, e.g., special wishes, preferences, or other concerns regarding funeral preparations, legacy arrangements, custody of children, etc.

Lastly, it should be mentioned that there are important cultural and social issues involved in advance care planning for patients with HIV/AIDS. AIDS is a disease that affects young adults primarily, so decisions to "limit" care by definition may make patients, families, and caregivers more uneasy than in situations where elderly patients are dying at a more expected time in their life cycle. In addition, there is a concentration of AIDS cases in the United States among racial-ethnic minorities, and issues of cross-cultural communication are important and need to be acknowledged, especially when dealing with what is still a highly stigmatized illness affecting potentially vulnerable populations. It has also been observed that patients with AIDS have been relatively unlikely, compared with other patient populations, to speak with their physicians about end of life and advance care planning issues and that this discrepancy was even more pronounced in drug users and racial-ethnic minority patients (Curtis and Patrick, 1997; Curtis et al., 1999, 2000; Wenger et al., 2001). All of these factors highlight both the difficulty and the importance for providers to raise and appropriately discuss these issues to make sure that patients' wishes are understood, articulated, documented, and respected. Some authors have advocated the use of a "disease-specific" advance directive instrument for HIV/AIDS, as well as for other specific diseases, to help formulate and frame the issues that are particularly relevant for this condition (Singer et al., 1997, 1998).

In addition to advance care planning, palliative care interventions for dying patients include continuing pain management, which may be facilitated by the use of a continuous subcutaneous infusion pump, and treatment of common symptoms such as delirium, fatigue, dyspnea, nausea/vomiting, and diarrhea or constipation. Again, the reader is referred to more in-depth texts of palliative medicine (Doyle et al., 1998; O'Neill et al., 2003), but it is helpful to highlight the many possible existing interventions that can improve patients' comfort and quality of life and can help families in coping with the difficult burden of a dying loved one, made somewhat less overwhelming when the patient is not suffering. There is a growing body of evidence-based practice in palliative medicine which provides many specific pharmacologic interventions that can significantly help reduce symptom burden for all of the symptoms indicated above and more, not only for dying patients but across the continuum of care (Table 1). The key is to recognize that even when disease-modifying therapy may not be available, there is still much that can be done to improve quality of life, relieve suffering, and enhance functional status.

Many patients with dementia, encephalopathy, and/or cerebrovascular disease eventually lose the ability to

TABLE 1 Medications used for palliative treatment of common symptoms in HIV/AIDS

Symptoms	Palliative medication	Usual starting dose
Nausea, vomiting	Haloperidol	0.5–2 mg p.o. or i.m.; tid-qid
	Prochlorperazine	5–10 mg p.o., i.m./i.v., or p.r.; tid
	Promethazine	12.5–25 mg p.o. or i.m./i.v.; tid
	Metoclopramide	5–10 mg p.o. or i.m./i.v.; tid
	Ondansetron	4–8 mg p.o. or i.m./i.v.; bid
	Granisetron	1 mg p.o. or i.m./i.v.; bid
	Meclizine	12.5–25 mg p.o.; tid
	Scopolamine	1 mg by transdermal patch q72h
	Lorazepam	0.5–2 mg p.o.; up to tid
	Dexamethasone (or equivalent corticosteroid)	1–4 mg p.o.; qid
	Dronabinol	2.5–5 mg p.o.; tid
Fatigue, weakness	Prednisone	10–40 mg p.o.; qd
	Dexamethasone	4–16 mg p.o.; qd
	Methylphenidate	5–10 mg p.o.; bid
	Dextroamphetamine	5–10 mg p.o.; bid
	Modafinil	100–200 mg p.o.; qd
Anorexia, weight loss	Megestrol acetate	400–800 mg p.o. (liquid form); qd
	Prednisone	10–40 mg p.o.; qd
	Oxandrolone	10–20 mg; qd
	Growth hormone	0.1 mg/kg s.c.; qd
	Dronabinol	2.5–5 mg p.o.; tid
	Testosterone	Transdermal (2.5–5 mg qd), topical gel (5 mg qd), i.m. (200 mg q2wks)
Dyspnea ("death rattle")	Morphine (or other opioid)	5–10 mg p.o. or i.m./i.v.
	Lorazepam	
	Scopolamine	0.5–1 mg p.o. or i.m./i.v.
		0.2–0.4 s.c.; q6–8h (or 1 mg transdermal patch q72h)
Fever	Acetaminophen	650–1,000 mg p.o./p.r.; q6h
	Ibuprofen	200–600 mg p.o.; q6h
	Dexamethasone	4–16 mg p.o.; qd (or divided doses)
Sweats	Indomethicin	10–25 mg p.o.; tid or qhs
	Cimetidine	400–800 mg p.o.; bid or qhs
	Hyoscine	0.125–0.25 mg p.o.; q4h or qhs
Agitation, delirium	Haloperidol	0.5–2 mg p.o./i.m.; up to qid
	Chlorpromazine	25–50 mg p.o./i.m.; up to qid
	Risperidone	0.5–2 mg p.o.; bid

[a] qd, once per day; bid, twice per day; tid, three times per day; qid, four times per day; q[n]h, every n hours; qhs, at bedtime; p.o., orally; p.r., per rectum; i.m., intramuscularly; i.v., intravenously; s.c., subcutaneously.

swallow, and so the use of artificial hydration and nutrition needs to be addressed ideally as part of discussions about goals of care and advance care planning while patients are still cognitively intact. The current literature suggests that when patients stop eating as a result of advanced dementia or other progressive illness, it is not necessarily beneficial to provide artificial feeding or hydration and that the underlying disease course results in death, with artificial feedings exerting little impact on survival (Finucane et al., 1999; Gillick, 2000). Moreover, such interventions can be noxious—such as nasogastric tubes, especially for demented or disoriented patients—and do not even necessarily protect against the putative adverse events for which they are sometimes employed (e.g., percutaneous enterogastrostomy tubes for tube feedings, which do not demonstrably reduce risk of aspiration). In addition, it has long been the observation

of palliative care and hospice clinicians that as part of the dying process, the natural tendency to decrease oral intake does not appear to be associated with symptom distress in dying patients, for whom the major identifiable symptom of dry mouth and occasional thirst can readily be managed by careful oral care, the use of ice chips and sucking candy, and other simple measures that do not involve artificial hydration, which in itself can also cause problems due to incontinence, skin maceration and breakdown, increased respiratory secretions, and volume overload. Notwithstanding all of these medical considerations, however, it should be noted that there are often strong cultural issues regarding food and fluids, and care providers need to address these issues sensitively and appropriately with patients and families as needed.

Other considerations for dying patients include decisions to discontinue certain disease-specific therapies; in the case of AIDS, most commonly this involves HAART and/or opportunistic infection prophylaxis, and here as well these questions are best addressed in the context of the previously discussed goals of care, and what the potential risks, benefits, and implications of continuing therapy might be. This might even apply further, as for patients with advanced Alzheimer's disease, to considerations of withholding antibiotic treatment for a new acute infection—aspiration pneumonia is a common example—in a patient whose cognitive and functional status is so diminished as to be inconsistent with the patient's previously stated goals of care and important personal values and preferences. Clinicians can be very helpful in these situations in providing palliative care and literally accompanying patients through the course of an ultimately fatal illness. This is regrettably often a time when physicians, accustomed to "curing" and perhaps uncomfortable when confronted by their inability to "rescue" patients from death, may unconsciously tend to withdraw from patients and families, as if they are no longer sure what their role should be. It is crucial in the care of patients with advanced AIDS that their care providers do not abandon them, and this time is replete with opportunities to make meaningful palliative interventions which will not only relieve patients' suffering and allow them to ultimately die with dignity and in accordance with their wishes but also help families cope with the dying process and the important process of grief and bereavement beyond. This opportunity to provide expert care and support throughout the dying process is important for neurologists as well as primary care providers, and one would hope that the benefit of an ongoing relationship with neurologic consultants would be as valuable as that of patients' primary physicians, even in primarily the "palliative" phase of the illness.

In closing, we must mention that the stresses and cumulative burden of caring for patients with AIDS in this chronic disease phase of the epidemic are also different from what they were earlier, when patients did not survive as long and there was a shorter shared history with their caregivers than is now the case. In whatever the setting where medical and associated care providers give care to patients with chronic, progressive illness, it is very important to provide opportunities for mutual support, identification, and prevention of "burnout" and otherwise to help support these professional caregivers in the very demanding work that they do. Otherwise we risk providing excellent care to our patients at the expense of ourselves, which ultimately serves neither of our needs.

We acknowledge the expert assistance of Tami Rivera with manuscript preparation.

REFERENCES

Anderson, K., and J. Mitchell. 2004. AIDS home- and community-based waivers: effects on use of services, expenditures, and survival. *South. Econ. J.* **71**:60–77.

Centers for Disease Control. 1997. Update: trends in AIDS incidence, deaths, and prevalence--United States, 1996. *Morb. Mortal. Wkly. Rep.* **46**:165–173.

Centers for Disease Control and Prevention. 2000. US HIV and AIDS cases reported through June 2000. *HIV/AIDS Surv. Rep.* **12**(2):1–44.

Chiasson, M. A., L. Berenson, W. Li, S. Schwartz, T. Singh, S. Forlenza, B. A. Mojica, and M. A. Hamburg. 1999. Declining HIV/AIDS mortality in New York City. *J. Acquir. Immune Defic. Syndr.* **21**:59–64.

Curtis, J. R., and D. L. Patrick. 1997. Barriers to communication about end-of-life care in AIDS patients. *J. Gen. Intern. Med.* **12**:736–741.

Curtis, J. R., D. L. Patrick, E. Caldwell, H. Greenlee, and A. C. Collier. 1999. The quality of patient-doctor communication about end-of-life care: a study of patients with advanced AIDS and their primary care clinicians. *AIDS* **13**:1123–1131.

Curtis, J. R., D. L. Patrick, E. S. Caldwell, and A. C. Collier. 2000. Why don't patients and physicians talk about end-of-life care? *Arch. Intern. Med.* **160**:1690–1696.

Doyle, D., G. W. C. Hanks, and N. MacDonald (ed.). 1998. *Oxford Textbook of Palliative Medicine*, 2nd ed. Oxford University Press, New York, NY.

Egger, M., B. Hirschel, P. Francioli, P. Sudre, M. Wirz, M. Flepp, M. Rickenbach, R. Malinverni, P. Vernazza, and M. Battegay. 1997. Impact of new antiretroviral combination therapies on HIV-infected patients in Switzerland: prospective multicentre study. *BMJ* **315**:1194–1199.

Finucane, T. E., C. Christmas, and K. Travis. 1999. Tube feeding in patients with advanced dementia: a review of the evidence. *JAMA* **282**:1365–1370.

Gillick, M. R. 2000. Rethinking the role of tube feeding in patients with advanced dementia. *N. Engl. J. Med.* **342**:206–210.

Gilron, I., J. M. Bailey, D. Tu, R. R. Holden, D. F. Weaver, and R. L. Houlden. 2005. Morphine, gabapentin, or their combination for neuropathic pain. *N. Engl. J. Med.* **352**:1324–1334.

Harrison, L. H., B. Vaz, D. M. Taveira, T. C. Quinn, C. J. Gibbs, S. H. de Souza, J. C. McArthur, and M. Schechter. 1997. Myelopathy among Brazilians coinfected with human T-cell lymphotropic virus type 1 and HIV. *Neurology* **48**:13–18.

Hellinger, F. J. 2007. The changing pattern of hospital care for persons living with HIV: 2000 through 2004. *J. Acquir. Immune Defic. Syndr.* **45**:239–246.

Jacox, A., D. B. Carr, and R. Payne. 1994. *Clinical Practice Guideline: Management of Cancer Pain.* AHCPR Publication no. 93-0595. Agency for Health Care Policy and Research, U.S. Department of Health and Human Services, Public Health Service, Rockville, MD.

Kravcik, S., N. Hawley-Foss, G. Victor, J. B. Angel, G. E. M. Garver, S. Page, N. Denomme, L. O'Reilly, and D. W. Cameron. 1997. Causes of death in HIV-infected persons in Ottawa, Ontario, 1984-1995. *Arch. Intern. Med.* **157**:2069–2073.

Louie, J. K., L. C. Hsu, D. H. Osmond, M. H. Katz, and S. K. Schwarcz. 2002. Trends in causes of death among persons with acquired immunodeficiency syndrome in the era of highly active antiretroviral therapy, San Francisco, 1994-1998. *J. Infect. Dis.* **186**:1023–1027.

Mayor, A. M., M. A. Gomez, D. M. Fernandez, E. Rios-Olivares, J. C. Thomas, and R. F. Hunter. 2006. Morbidity and mortality profile of human immunodeficiency virus-infected patients with and without hepatitis C co-infection. *Am. J. Trop. Med. Hyg.* **74**:239–245.

McArthur, J. C., N. Haughey, S. Gartner, K. Conant, C. Pardo, A. Nath, and N. Sacktor. 2003. Human immunodeficiency virus-associated dementia: an evolving disease. *J. Neurovirol.* **9**:205–221.

Norval, D. A. 2004. Symptoms and sites of pain experienced by AIDS patients. *S. Afr. Med. J.* **94**:450–454.

Ogbuokiri, J. 2003. Pharmacologic interactions of HIV and palliative medications, p. 549–586. *In* J. F. O'Neill, P. A. Selwyn, and H. Scheitinger (ed.), *A Clinical Guide to Supportive and Palliative Care for HIV/AIDS.* Health Resources and Services Administration, Rockville, MD.

O'Neill, J. F., P. A. Selwyn, and H. Scheitinger (ed.). 2003. *A Clinical Guide to Supportive & Palliative Care for HIV/AIDS.* Health Resources and Services Administration, Rockville, MD.

Palella, F. A., Jr., K. M. Delaney, A. C. Moorman, M. O. Loveless, J. Fuhrer, G. A. Satten, D. J. Aschman, and S. D. Holmberg. 1998. Declining morbidity and mortality among patients with advanced human immunodeficiency virus infection. *N. Engl. J. Med.* **338:**853–860.

Piscitelli, S. C., and K. D. Gallicano. 2001. Drug therapy: interactions among drugs for HIV and opportunistic infections. *N. Engl. J. Med.* **344:**984–996.

Puoti, M., A. Spinetti, A. Ghezzi, F. Donato, S. Zaltron, V. Putzolu, E. Quiros-Roldan, B. Zanini, S. Casari, and G. Carosi. 2000. Mortality from liver disease in patients with HIV infection: a cohort study. *J. Acquir. Immune Defic. Syndr.* **24:**211–217.

Rabkin, J. G., M. McElhiney, R. Rabkin, and S. J. Ferrando. 2004. Modafinil treatment for fatigue in HIV+ patients: a pilot study. *J. Clin. Psychiatry* **65:**1688–1695.

Sacktor, N. 2002. The epidemiology of human immunodeficiency virus-associated neurological disease in the era of highly active antiretroviral therapy. *J. Neurovirol.* **8**(Suppl. 2)**:**S115–S121.

Sacktor, N. C., R. L. Skolasky, R. H. Lyles, D. Esposito, O. A. Selnes, and J. C. McArthur. 2000. Improvement in HIV-associated motor slowing after antiretroviral therapy. *J. Neurovirol.* **6:**84–88.

Sansone, R. G., and J. D. Frengley. 2000. Impact of HAART on causes for death of persons with late-stage AIDS. *J. Urban Health* **77:**166–175.

Selwyn, P. A., J. L. Goulet, S. Molde, J. Constantino, K. P. Fennie, P. Wetherill, D. M. Gaughan, H. Brett-Smith, and C. Kennedy. 2000. HIV as a chronic disease: long-term care for patients with HIV at a dedicated skilled nursing facility. *J. Urban Health* **77:**187–203.

Selwyn, P. A., and M. Rivard. 2003. Palliative care for AIDS: challenges and opportunities in the era of highly active anti-retroviral therapy. *J. Palliat. Med.* **6:**475–487.

Singer, P. A., D. K. Martin, J. V. Lavery, E. C. Thiel, M. Kelner, and D. C. Mendelssohn. 1998. Reconceptualizing advance care planning from the patient's perspective. *Arch. Intern. Med.* **158:**879–884.

Singer, P. A., E. C. Thiel, I. Salit, W. Flanagan, and D. Naylor. 1997. The HIV-specific advance directive. *J. Gen. Intern. Med.* **12:**729–735.

U.S. Department of Health and Human Services. 10 October 2006. *Guidelines for the Use of Antiretroviral Agents in HIV-1 Infected Adults and Adolescents.* U.S. Department of Health and Human Services, Washington, DC.

Valcour, V., C. Shikuma, B. Shiramizu, M. Watters, P. Poff, O. Selnes, P. Holck, J. Grove, and N. Sacktor. 2004. Higher frequency of dementia in older HIV-1 individuals: the Hawaii Aging with HIV-1 Cohort. *Neurology* **63:**822–827.

Valdez, H., T. K. Chowdhry, R. Asaad, I. J. Woolley, T. Davis, R. Davidson, N. Beinker, B. M. Gripshover, R. A. Salata, G. McComsey, S. E. Weissman, and M. M. Lederman. 2001. Changing spectrum of mortality due to HIV: analysis of 260 deaths during 1995-1999. *Clin. Infect. Dis.* **32:**1487–1493.

Voltz, R., J. D. Bernat, G. D. Borasio, I. Maddocks, D. Oliver, and R. K. Portenoy. 2004. *Palliative Care in Neurology.* Oxford University Press, London, United Kingdom.

Watters, M. R., P. W. Poff, B. T. Shiramizu, P. S. Holck, K. M. Fast, C. M. Shikuma, and V. G. Valcour. 2004. Symptomatic distal sensory polyneuropathy in HIV after age 50. *Neurology* **62:**1378–1383.

Wenger, N. S., D. E. Kanouse, R. L. Collins, H. Liu, M. A. Schuster, A. L. Gifford, S. A. Bozzette, and M. F. Shapiro. 2001. End-of-life discussions and preferences among persons with HIV. *JAMA* **285:**2880–2887.

World Health Organization. 1990. *Cancer Pain Relief and Palliative Care. Report of a WHO Expert Committee.* Publication 1100804. World Health Organization, Geneva, Switzerland.

The Spectrum of Neuro-AIDS Disorders:
Pathophysiology, Diagnosis, and Treatment
Edited by K. Goodkin et al.
©2008 ASM Press, Washington, DC

35

Medico-Legal Issues in HIV/AIDS in the 21st Century

SOMA SAHAI-SRIVASTAVA

AIDS was first identified in 1981 and has reached pandemic proportions in the last 2 decades. It is truly a public health challenge like none other known to mankind. AIDS carries with it a huge stigma and prejudice; hence, patients already infected with the human immunodeficiency virus (HIV), those who are at greatest risk of HIV infection (men who have sex with men and injection drug users [IDUs]), and even those working with these specific populations are vulnerable to discrimination. The challenge of the 21st century lawmakers is to balance public safety and containment of this pandemic, while preserving basic human rights to privacy and autonomy. The medico-legal and ethical issues surrounding this disease are complex and interdisciplinary. In this chapter, we focus on some of the key legal elements relating to HIV infection and AIDS.

HIV ANTIBODY TESTING

Following the licensing of the first HIV antibody test (enzyme-linked immunosorbent assay) by the Food and Drug Administration in 1985, there was a wave of legislation adopted both by individual states and by the federal government defining the parameters of HIV antibody testing (Schochetman and George, 1994). In the United States, HIV antibody testing is not a mandatory procedure, nor can it be considered an emergency procedure. Informed consent prior to HIV antibody testing should be obtained under almost all circumstances (Terl, 1993). If the patient is mentally incapacitated, then consent of a parent, guardian, or conservator can be obtained prior to HIV antibody testing. It is of importance to note that any person 12 years of age or older is considered legally competent, unless proven otherwise in court.

Under federal regulations, HIV antibody testing is mandatory only for the armed forces, foreign service, and certain federal programs like the Job Corps and the Peace Corps (Buss et al., 1987). In 1987 the U.S. Public Health Service added AIDS to the list of seven other "dangerous contagious

diseases" for immigration purposes. Federal regulations also require mandatory HIV antibody testing for people applying for immigration to the United States. Any alien who has a positive test for HIV infection will not be allowed to immigrate to this country. In the public sector, mandatory HIV antibody testing is required only when applying for life or disability insurance policies.

Involuntary HIV antibody testing can be court mandated for certain criminal suspects, defendants, and convicts. Victims of sexual acts may request HIV antibody testing of the person convicted of the said crime. However, some state statutes also authorize involuntary HIV antibody testing of persons who are arrested or charged.

Any individual who consents to HIV antibody testing should preferably receive pretest and posttest counseling. One of the goals of pretest counseling sessions is behavior modification regarding safer sexual practices. The purpose of the test and its potential uses and limitations—including false-positive and -negative results—should be explained prior to testing. The psychological, social, and medical implications of the HIV antibody test should also be discussed. Posttest counseling varies depending on the test result. If the test is negative for HIV, a typical session should include reinforcement of knowledge gained in the pretest session including safer sex practices. If it is a positive HIV result, then more extensive and in-depth counseling sessions, including crisis intervention, may be necessary. The physician then needs to offer advice regarding further medical and psychosocial treatment of the patient and also to educate the patient regarding the risk of HIV transmission. Federally funded and state-funded counseling and testing programs to which such individuals can be referred are readily available. The Ryan White AIDS Resources Emergency (CARE) Act of 1990 established an HIV Health Care Services program to provide emergency assistance to those who are disproportionately affected and to fund states and other public or private organizations in developing delivery systems for essential services to HIV-infected patients (Fee and Fox, 1992).

The presidential commission on the HIV epidemic recommended that all correctional systems offer counseling and voluntary HIV antibody testing to prison inmates. Some states require all prison inmates to be tested for

Soma Sahai-Srivastava, Department of Neurology, University of Southern California, 1200 N. State St., Los Angeles, CA 90033.

HIV. Several other states require mandatory HIV antibody testing of only high-risk prisoners, e.g., IDUs.

Rapid HIV Antibody Testing

There have been some exciting advancements in the field of HIV antibody testing. Self-testing (with the person collecting his or her own specimen at home) and rapid HIV test kits are now commercially available in several countries including Canada (Weir, 2000; Spielberg et al., 2004). An HIV self-test is a simple test like a pregnancy test and can be performed by individuals in the privacy of their own homes. Results are read as positive or negative by the patient himself or herself within 15 to 30 min. In the United States, self-tests are not considered legal and the FDA has not approved any of them for commercial use. There are four FDA-approved rapid HIV antibody test kits available in the United States for use by health care personnel.

In developing countries, rapid HIV antibody testing is often a less expensive and more acceptable option, especially for developing countries and particularly for women. Self-testing can be done privately at home and eliminates some of the stigma attached to an office visit for an HIV antibody test. On the other hand, the dangers of self-testing include the possibility that a person may not understand or follow instructions (or may be illiterate) and, therefore, may perform or interpret the test incorrectly. A false-negative test may lead to a delay in treatment and partner notification. Moreover, there is no provision for pretest counseling regarding false-positive results and a need for confirmatory testing and posttest counseling in positive cases. There should be further research into the feasibility of self-testing and situations in which testing, counseling, and early treatment can be tightly linked together in a chain. This could prove to be a powerful tool to prevent HIV transmission.

Charting and Disclosure of HIV Antibody Test Results

HIV antibody test results may be documented in the medical records without prior authorization. The HIV Antibody Testing Confidentiality Act of 1988 was amended in January 1989 to allow physicians who ordered the test to include HIV antibody test results in a patient's medical record without prior authorization. This act also allows disclosure of HIV antibody test results to another health care provider without authorization, if necessary for diagnosis, care, or treatment. Other practitioners including psychiatrists, licensed psychologists, clinical social workers, school psychologists, and licensed marriage, family, and child counselors may also be given this information without prior consent from patients, if they are directly involved in the care of the patient (Scott, 1993). HIV antibody test results can also be disclosed to the patient's legal representative if the patient is a child less than 12 years of age. This does not apply to insurance companies, health maintenance organizations, or anyone not directly involved in the care of the patient. Insurers and the workman's compensation act require a separate HIV-specific release before this information can be given.

It is required by state and federal regulation to report every AIDS case to the Centers for Disease Control and Prevention (CDC). Disclosure to public health agencies mandated by law includes the CDC and public health agencies designated by the state. These reports do not require authorization by the patient.

Duty To Warn Third Parties

There are exceptions to the physician's duty of confidentiality with regard to a patient's HIV antibody test status. The antibody testing confidentiality act was amended in January 1989 to allow medical doctors, including psychiatrists, to disclose their patients' HIV antibody test results to those persons who they reasonably believe to be the sexual partner(s) or needle-sharing partner(s) of the patients.

Practitioners have a duty to educate HIV-infected patients regarding activities that may increase risk of transmission of the disease to their sexual or needle-sharing partner(s). Patients should agree to indulge only in safer sexual practices and to abstain from needle sharing, and their compliance with this advice should be monitored. If a physician is satisfied that the HIV-infected patient will not willfully engage in behavior that will transmit HIV infection, the physician does not have any further responsibility to third parties. However, if the physician believes that the patient is noncompliant and is putting another person at high risk for infection with the virus by his/her behavior, then the physician has a duty to warn this third party (Glantz, 1996). The physician must first try to obtain voluntary consent for disclosure and to document this effort. The physician needs to inform the patient of his/her intention to warn their significant other at risk of being infected with HIV if the patient refuses to do so. The physician can then make the disclosures in good faith but should not include identifying information about individual patients. The individual notified must then be referred for treatment and counseling. The doctor may choose not to directly take on this responsibility and may simply notify the local public health authority, which will then alert the partner. A physician working with any population of patients needs to follow some simple guidelines from the medico-legal aspect (Table 1).

AIDS IN THE WORKPLACE

Individuals with AIDS face some major challenges, like discrimination in the workplace. The Americans with Disabilities Act of 1990 (ADA) protects such individuals from discrimination in the workplace (Webber, 1997). This act provides for protection against discrimination of individuals with disabilities in job applications, hiring, and

TABLE 1 Do's and don'ts of HIV law

Do
  Obtain and document informed consent before testing
  Pretest counseling
  Posttest counseling
  Document result in chart without requiring consent
  Release test result to public health agency and CDC without requiring consent
  Warn sexual or needle-sharing partner of HIV seropositivity
  Refer for HIV antibody test counseling and testing
  Document all related efforts

Don't
  Disclose HIV antibody test results to insurance or workman's compensation without specific release on informed consent form
  Disclose identifying information of patient when warning a significant other
  Disclose HIV antibody test results even to parents of a minor over 12 years of age

firing. The rehabilitation act defines a handicapped or disabled individual as a person satisfying one of three criteria:

1. A person with mental or physical impairments that substantially limit one or more of the person's major life activities. Major life activities include walking, talking, seeing, taking care of oneself, and working.
2. A person who has a record of such impairment.
3. A person who is regarded and treated by others as if that person has such impairment.

An individual with AIDS who is symptomatic and has significant impairment due to his condition qualifies as disabled under the first or second criterion. However, even an asymptomatic person infected with HIV without any disabling impairment may qualify as handicapped under the third criterion.

In order to be nondiscriminatory, an employer should make reasonable accommodations to the known physical or mental limitations of an otherwise qualified individual with a disability who is an applicant or employee, unless it causes undue hardship on the business or employer. Mandatory medical testing by employers may include HIV antibody testing, provided that the result of the test is not used against the individual to exclude him or her from the job. The employer cannot require a person applying for employment to reveal the results of his/her HIV antibody test. The exceptions to this rule are certain federal jobs, such as the foreign services, which have mandatory HIV antibody testing. Employers cannot discriminate against employees in terms of offering health care insurance on the basis of HIV serostatus. Employees can choose to continue participation in the health care plan of their former employer for a period of 29 months after they lose their job secondary to disability.

While lawmakers want to protect HIV-infected persons against discrimination in the workplace, they also want to ensure that public safety is not jeopardized. An individual with a contagious disease such as AIDS is protected from discrimination only if his/her disease does not pose a significant risk of harm to others. The Chapman amendment to the ADA allows employers to reassign employees from food-handling positions if they have a communicable disease, including HIV infection.

Employers with 15 or more employees are covered under the ADA. In 1991, the U.S. Congress amended this legislation to include U.S. citizens employed in foreign countries. The nondiscrimination standards of ADA have been extended to include people who work with AIDS or HIV-infected patients (Banta, 1993).

DISABILITY BENEFITS FOR HIV INFECTION

HIV-infected patients may be eligible for disability benefits based on the Social Security Administration regulations of 1993, which set forth the criteria for such individuals (Bartlett and Finkbeiner, 1996). A person may qualify for disability based upon the diagnosis of any one of 41 stand-alone conditions associated with HIV infection (Table 2). An HIV-infected person with any opportunistic infection or AIDS indicator conditions, even without functional impairment, can qualify as a disabled individual. If one does not have an AIDS indicator condition, then a series of repeated manifestations of HIV infection with functional impairment is a qualifying factor.

AIDS PREVENTION AND TREATMENT

Since the introduction of the protease inhibitors as treatment for HIV infection in 1996, there has been a dramatic improvement in the mortality rate of HIV-infected patients. Highly active antiretroviral therapy (HAART), using three or more drugs in HIV-infected patients, leads to a substantial reduction in plasma HIV RNA levels, a decreased incidence of opportunistic infections, and lower mortality rates. However, the cost of providing HIV treatment to all those who need it is often a limiting factor. The cost of antiretroviral treatment is over $12,000 per annum, which is well beyond the reach of low-income individuals and/or uninsured patients. Government programs are, therefore, critical to ensuring access to these medications. The AIDS Drug Assistance Program is one of the key government-funded programs that provide AIDS-related drugs to those who could otherwise not afford them.

A recent study (Porco et al., 2004) found that HIV therapies reduce infectivity by 60%. Access to HIV therapies reduces the viral load (or the amount of HIV present in a person's bloodstream)—a key factor in curbing infectivity and in reducing the ability to transmit HIV. Lawmakers are finally recognizing the need to address this issue of adequate and early treatment as another effective preventive tool. The Early Treatment for HIV Act (ETHA) was introduced in the U.S. Senate in February of 2005 and is an important step in recognizing the issues of cost in HIV treatment. ETHA gives states the option to change Medicaid eligibility requirements to include previously disabled low-socioeconomic-status patients living with HIV infection. Early access to HIV therapies as provided under ETHA is important not only for early treatment but also for HIV prevention.

HIV-Associated Dementia

There is now evidence that AIDS, if untreated, affects the cognitive functioning of patients, sometimes quite early in the disease process. The spectrum of HIV-associated neurocognitive impairment is broad and can start with very mild, subclinical cognitive difficulties. Formal neuropsychological testing can help to determine the extent and nature of cognitive difficulties. If a patient with HIV infection presents with features of a possible dementia (or mild neurocognitive disorder), it is very important on the part of the physician to do a reasonable investigation to exclude common and especially treatable causes of neurocognitive disorder other than HIV itself. HIV-associated dementia and mild neurocognitive disorder are diagnoses of exclusion, and there is no definitive in vivo laboratory test that can prove that the dementia is due to HIV alone (Sahai and Jones, 2001).

AIDS patients should be educated about the common neurological complications of HIV infection, including peripheral neuropathy as well as neurocognitive disorder. It is very important for a health care provider to discuss issues like a living will and durable power of attorney in managing health care for the HIV-infected patient. Patients should be strongly encouraged to prepare a living will or to assign power of attorney early in their disease process. In a case where HIV-associated dementia is established, it is also important to address issues of competence to make medical decisions.

There are several issues of critical importance with regard to a neurocognitively impaired patient with HIV infection that health care providers need to address, the first being the matter of consent and the right to refusal of treatment. A patient may, at times, reject treatment offered by a physician—even at the risk of remaining ill. A person's right

TABLE 2   Stand-alone disabling HIV conditions for adults

Bacterial infections
  Mycobacterial infection
  Pulmonary tuberculosis resistant to treatment
  Nocardiosis
  Salmonella bacteremia, recurrent nontyphoid
  Syphilis or neurosyphilis resulting in neurological or other sequelae
  Multiple or recurrent bacterial infections requiring hospitalization or intravenous antibiotic treatment three or more times in 1 year

Fungal infections
  Aspergillosis
  Candidiasis, at a site other than the skin, urinary tract, intestinal tract, or oral or vulvovaginal mucous membranes; or candidiasis
    involving the esophagus, trachea, bronchi, or lung
  Coccidioidomycosis, at a site other than the lungs or lymph nodes
  Cryptococcosis, at a site other than the lungs (e.g., cryptococcal meningitis)
  Histoplasmosis, at a site other than the lungs or lymph nodes
  Mucormycosis

Protozoan or helminthic infections
  Cryptosporidiosis, isosporiasis, or microsporidiosis
  Pneumocystis carinii pneumonia or extrapulmonary *P. carinii* infections
  Strongyloidosis
  Toxoplasmosis

Viral infections
  Cytomegalovirus disease, at a site other than liver, spleen, or lymph node
  Herpes simplex virus causing mucocutaneous infection or disseminated infection
  Herpes zoster
  Progressive multifocal leukoencephalopathy
  Hepatitis

Malignant neoplasms
  Carcinoma of the cervix
  Kaposi's sarcoma, with extensive oral lesions; or involvement of the gastrointestinal tract, lungs, or other visceral organs; or
    involvement of the skin or mucous membranes with extensive fungating or ulcerating lesions not responding to treatment
  Lymphoma of any type
  Squamous cell carcinoma of the anus

Skin or mucous membranes
  Conditions of the skin or mucous membranes, with extensive fungating or ulcerating lesions not responding to treatment
    (e.g., dermatological conditions such as eczema or psoriasis, vulvovaginal or other mucosal candidiasis, condylomata caused by
    human papillomavirus, genital ulcerative disease)
  Anemia
  Granulocytopenia
  Thrombocytopenia

Neurological abnormalities
  HIV encephalopathy, characterized by cognitive or motor dysfunction that limits function and progresses
  Other neurological manifestations of HIV infection (e.g., peripheral neuropathy) with significant and persistent disorganization of
    motor function in two extremities, resulting in sustained disturbance of gross and dextrous movements, or gait and station

HIV wasting syndrome
  Characterized by involuntary weight loss of 10% or more of baseline (or other significant involuntary weight loss) in the absence of
    a concurrent illness that could explain these findings, involving chronic weakness and documented fever greater than 38°C for
    majority of 1 month or longer

Diarrhea
  Lasting for 1 month or longer, resistant to treatment, and requiring intravenous hydration, intravenous alimentation, or tube
    feeding

Cardiomyopathy (chronic heart failure, or cor pulmonale, or other severe cardiac abnormality not responsive to treatment)

Nephropathy
  Results in chronic renal failure

Infections resistant to treatment or requiring hospitalization or intravenous treatment three or more times in 1 year
  Sepsis
  Meningitis
  Pneumonia (non-*Pneumocystis carinii* pneumonia)
  Septic arthritis
  Endocarditis
  Sinusitis

to autonomy cannot be challenged, provided that he/she has the competence to understand the risks and benefits of the treatment offered (Smith, 1998). Competence to consent to medical treatment is defined as the "mental capacity necessary to comprehend the risks and benefits of a proposed medical treatment and its alternatives." The only exception to this situation would be a medical emergency in which the hospital or physician may obtain consent from a surrogate, a close family member, or a spouse. The health care provider may then render care to the patient in his/her best interest and treat the medical emergency.

In a psychiatric setting, competence is considered as "the ability to understand and appreciate those duties to society owed by an ordinary citizen of reasonable prudence and care" (Wood et al., 1990). This is pertinent for the HIV-associated dementia patients who, due to their severe neurocognitive impairment, may be unable to provide for themselves and may endanger themselves or others. California's Welfare and Institutions Code, Section 5150, allows the custodial detention and involuntary hospitalization of a person believed to be disabled due to his or her mental condition such that he/she poses a grave danger to himself or herself or to others.

Involuntary hospitalization can be authorized only by a county mental health professional, psychiatric crisis team, state-designated mental health professional, or peace officer. Within a 72-h period, the patient has to be evaluated for mental capacity and grave disability. "Grave disability" is determined by the ability of a person to provide basic food, clothing, and shelter for himself or herself. If it is determined that the patient is "gravely disabled," the hold can be extended for 14 days and the superior court can be petitioned for appointment of a conservator.

In late-stage HIV-associated dementia, and earlier as well, the ability to safely operate a motor vehicle may be jeopardized. The clinician has a duty to advise both the patient and the Department of Motor Vehicles that it is unsafe for the patient to drive. Some patients may have severe sensory loss related to HIV-associated peripheral neuropathy and thus may be unsafe drivers on that basis as well. It is the direct responsibility of the health care provider to report such patients to the Department of Motor Vehicles as potentially unsafe to be driving.

AIDS IN HEALTH CARE

The American Medical Association has stated that physicians have an ethical obligation to provide care for patients with HIV infection and AIDS. In most circumstances, individual physicians or health care facilities cannot decline to take care of such patients unless they can prove that they do not have the expertise to treat them. In case of an emergency, all hospitals must provide adequate care to HIV/AIDS patients. In dealing with this disease, from the point of view of a health care worker, universal (and simple) precautions (Table 2) should be assimilated into routine practice, not solely for the HIV/AIDS patient but also in the context of provision of sound medical services.

The other side of the coin is the health care workers' need to be protected from becoming HIV infected at the workplace. The Occupational Safety and Health Administration (OSHA) has defined the employer's responsibility to protect against exposure to blood-borne infections in the workplace. OSHA has also set up what is called the blood-borne pathogen standards; the employer must assess the risk of a possible exposure to blood-borne pathogens, protect

against such an event, and have specific protocols in place if such an exposure were to occur. There should be written exposure control plans; methods of compliance detailed; appropriate training given; and postexposure treatment and counseling provided (Chhetri et al., 2002).

There is a small but real risk of contracting HIV infection in an occupational setting. The risk of infection with HIV following a needlestick is 0.3% and from mucous membrane exposure is 0.09%. In about 10 years of working with HIV-infected patients, there were 37 documented cases of HIV infection by occupational transmission. There have been 14 such cases among laboratory workers, mostly phlebotomists, with occupational transmission of HIV. Health care workers who have been exposed to blood from a patient can request testing of the patient in question. Some states have specific statutes allowing testing of such patients without their consent, whereas others do require informed consent (Johnson and Soskolne, 1986).

An area of concern is whether an HIV-infected health care worker increases the risk of HIV transmission. After almost 2 decades of dealing with the HIV/AIDS epidemic, public health officials have identified only one instance of HIV transmission from a health care worker, that of a dentist with AIDS who infected six of his patients through a means of transmission that was not clear. The issue of whether physicians performing surgical or other invasive procedures have a duty to reveal their HIV antibody status to their employer and whether they can continue with their jobs if testing seropositive has been not infrequently litigated.

In July 1991, the CDC issued guidelines for physicians and health care workers to prevent transmission of HIV in the health care setting. CDC advised the following.

1. Infected health care workers who adhere to universal precautions and who do not perform certain invasive procedures pose no risk for transmitting HIV or hepatitis B virus (HBV) to patients.
2. Infected health care workers who adhere to universal precautions and who do perform invasive procedures pose a small risk for transmitting HIV or HBV to patients. HIV is transmitted much less readily than HBV.

The guidelines recommended that HIV-infected individuals who perform invasive procedures should know about their HIV antibody status and should not perform such procedures unless they have sought counsel from an expert panel. Congress adopted the Dole Amendment in 1992 mandating states to issue their own guidelines (or to concur with CDC's guidelines). Employers who have used the risk of HIV transmission as justification to terminate residencies and jobs of HIV-infected dentists, surgeons, or similar health care professionals have generally won court cases in their favor. It appears that the burden to prove that he or she poses no risk of transmission falls upon the physician or health care worker.

AIDS IN THE FAMILY

AIDS has affected all aspects of family life. The matter most discussed and legislated is whether a person has a duty to disclose his or her HIV antibody test result to his/her sexual partner. As with other fatal contagious diseases, a person with HIV/AIDS is deemed responsible to either avoid sexual activity or take reasonable precautions to prevent the transmission of HIV to his or her partner. If a person with HIV/AIDS conceals his/her test results from his/her partner and continues with his/her sexual relationship, it is a criminal offense, even though the partner may never become HIV infected (Jarvis et al., 1991). Illinois and Louisiana had previously imposed mandatory HIV antibody testing as part of their required premarital testing. These statutes have been repealed. The states of West Virginia and California require that marriage applicants should receive an offer of HIV antibody testing and counseling by the physician conducting the premarital examination prior to issuing a marriage license.

Routine HIV prenatal counseling and voluntary antibody testing programs should be offered to all pregnant women and should be the standard of care. Congress mandated that the CDC, in collaboration with health care officials in all states, develop a reporting system to determine any new prenatal transmission. Certain states also have mandatory HIV antibody testing of all newborns.

HIV transmission by donor semen was reported in 12 cases of women who underwent artificial donor insemination before 1985. In 1988, the American Society of Reproductive Medicine issued guidelines mandating the use of frozen thawed semen in donor insemination (Lyerly and Anderson, 2001). According to these guidelines, a potential donor should be tested for HIV with a repeat antibody test after 6 months; only when both tests are seronegative can he then donate sperm. Arguments have been made recently that women should have the option of choosing fresh semen without the required 6-month waiting period for an HIV antibody test from the donor to be seronegative, since the rate of successful pregnancies is much higher with fresh than with frozen semen (Payne and Lamb, 2004).

AIDS AT SCHOOL

A child with HIV/AIDS cannot be excluded from the classroom unless there is evidence that he or she poses a high risk of HIV transmission to other children. If a child with HIV/AIDS has a significant mental or physical impairment, the school needs to accommodate that child with a special education program. Confidentiality regarding the results of HIV antibody testing applies to a child as well as an adult. Teachers with HIV/AIDS also cannot be discriminated against and can continue to teach since their risk of HIV transmission to children is negligible. Several states have introduced legislation mandating HIV/AIDS prevention education at the school level, since awareness and education are critical to preventing disease dissemination.

AIDS IN HIGH-RISK GROUPS

Injection Drug Use

Injection drug use is responsible for over 30% of the transmission of HIV/AIDS in certain parts of this country, like New York City (Coffin et al., 2004). This is due to sharing of injection drug equipment, including syringes, needles, cookers, cotton, and rinse water. The National Commission on AIDS over a decade ago had recommended removal of legal barriers to the purchase and possession of injection equipment in order to decrease HIV transmission. Syringe exchange programs (whereby a user receives a sterile syringe and needle in exchange for returning a used one) are very effective and dramatically reduce this mode of transmission. In spite of this solid evidence, the federal government has withheld support for syringe exchange programs. Sale of syringes and needles without a prescription is criminal

under federal law and a few state laws. Possession of injection equipment without a prescription is also prohibited by some states. Despite the overall negative view of syringe exchange programs by lawmakers, several states with legislative approval have started syringe exchange programs at local levels. In Connecticut, purchase and possession of up to 10 needles and syringes without a prescription are permitted.

In 2000 the New York legislature passed the Expanded Syringe Access Demonstration Program to increase accessibility to sterile syringes for IDUs. The state of New York legally allows health care providers to prescribe syringes to IDUs. However, there is still unwillingness among health care providers, either because of lack of knowledge or due to legal and ethical concerns (Burris et al., 2002).

Recent legislation signed by the governor of California in September 2004 permits cities and counties to authorize local pharmacies to sell up to 10 syringes to adults without a prescription and permits individuals to possess up to 10 syringes obtained from authorized sources. HIV/AIDS advocates have called the bill essential to further reducing the transmission of HIV, hepatitis, and other blood-borne diseases. California was one of only five remaining states that prohibited the sale of syringes without a prescription. Expansion of these programs is yet another important preventive step to help contain the HIV/AIDS pandemic.

CSWs

Commercial sex workers (CSWs) previously known under the term "prostitution" are another high-risk group for the spread of HIV. In general, HIV infection among female CSWs is highly associated with injection drug use. The model penal code that defines prostitution as a criminal offense has not deterred this profession, only driving it "underground" and making it more difficult to educate this population regarding safer sexual practices. Only the state of Nevada has licensed CSWs and requires that CSWs be HIV antibody tested when they start working and monthly thereafter. State regulations also require this population to wear latex condoms. Thus far, this regulation of CSWs has had a positive impact to the extent that there have been no reported cases of CSWs in Nevada testing seropositive for HIV. State laws in Nevada state that a CSW with known HIV infection who continues to work will face imprisonment.

From the experience of the state of Nevada, it appears that legalizing and regulating CSWs have had better outcome with regard to change of sexual practices and limitation of the spread of HIV/AIDS than outlawing commercial sex. In this era of rapid globalization, identification of the HIV-infected CSWs in geographically separate parts of the world, like Africa, Southeast Asia, and Europe, can be instrumental in deterring the further spread of HIV infection across the globe.

Another less well known but high-risk group for HIV infection is the adult film industry. An epidemiological study done to study the extent of infection in this group reported transmission of HIV by an adult worker to three other workers (Taylor et al., 2007). Many of these workers participate in monthly testing programs, but unless a more comprehensive safety program is offered, it will not prevent HIV infection in this high-risk group.

Tattooing and Body Piercing

Tattooing and body piercing have become very popular in recent years, especially among teens and young adults.

Fifteen to 20% of young adults in this country have tattoos. Tattooing is also often performed in prison among jail inmates with nonsterile equipment. A Canadian survey found that 45% of jail inmates had been tattooed behind bars. Tattooing and body piercing are known potential sources of transmission of HIV. The CDC has issued recommendations for all personal service workers (hair dressers, barbers, etc.); these state that all instruments used to penetrate the skin should be either disposed of after each use or thoroughly sterilized prior to reuse. Only 13 states in the United States have regulatory policies in effect for tattooing facilities. The state of Oklahoma has outlawed tattooing altogether. Regulatory policies for body-piercing facilities are yet less frequent, and only four states (Maine, Ohio, Oregon, and Wisconsin) have such regulations to date (Braithwaite et al., 1999).

HIV- AND AIDS-RELATED RESEARCH

The issue of confidentiality has far-reaching implications for individuals who test antibody positive for HIV. A person participating in an HIV drug trial may face discrimination when the individual applies for the armed services or is an alien applying for immigration. Since 1985, the U.S. Army has had mandatory screening of all active and reserve personnel, as well as new recruits, on a regular basis. Test results could result in detention or deportation if the individual is in the United States illegally. U.S. immigration law excludes aliens with HIV seropositivity and with high-risk behaviors like injection drug use, addiction, and commercial sex. Besides HIV information, other demographic data that many research studies may collect, like sexual behavior, may put the participant at a higher risk for discrimination, if the information were to be revealed.

The HIV/AIDS Research Confidentiality Act was passed in 1985 with other HIV confidentiality legislation. Under this act, all documentation relating to HIV/AIDS research is confidential and may not be disclosed, even to an attorney in a civil action or to an audit team (Loue, 1995). An investigator may, however, be forced to disclose patient-identifying information if a subpoena is received. Only a few states have specific protections for HIV/AIDS-related research documents and release of public health information in court. Since U.S. law mandates reporting of HIV-seropositive results to public health officials, researchers can disclose information to CDC regarding diagnosed cases of AIDS without prior consent from the participant (Loue, 1995).

The principles of human research are based on beneficence and autonomy. Mass mandatory HIV antibody screening programs are enforced in correctional facilities, and the rate of seropositivity is estimated to be 1% of the population. Federal law allows no discrimination against prisoners and gives them the same opportunity to participate in clinical trials as others. However, there are some real practical implications which may prevent patients from having the same opportunities to participate in a clinical trial as for those not in jail. Yet another related dilemma for the researcher regards partner notification.

INTERNATIONAL AIDS LAW

In 1988 the London Declaration on AIDS Prevention, which evolved from a conference including over 148 delegates, for the first time addressed the global need for HIV/AIDS prevention programs. It emphasized the need to protect human rights and human dignity in the context of the HIV/AIDS pandemic. The United Nations General Assembly finally, in 1991, declared that member countries should protect the human dignity and human rights of persons infected with HIV.

In 1995, a nongovernmental organization based in India, the Indian Law Institute, had a conference from which the New Delhi Declaration was made with regard to global HIV/AIDS legislation. The four major points made were as follows:

1. Law must protect human rights and empower individuals so that by their cooperation, the spread of HIV infection is contained.
2. Law must promote voluntary behavior, which will protect the health of individuals throughout the world.
3. Law must prevent coercive and punitive action against persons with demonstrated or suspected HIV infection or AIDS.
4. Law must protect society and promote a sense of responsibility in the face of an epidemic which poses a serious threat.

According to the World Health Organization data, of 191 member countries, only 121 have legislation addressing reporting requirements. Only 24 countries explicitly require confidentiality (Hamers and Downs, 2004). Certain countries have legislation on specific HIV high-risk groups like CSWs, men who have sex with men, IDUs, and multiple-transfusion recipients (Harrington, 2002). Most countries do not have specific legislation to protect against discrimination in jobs or access to public places and services or other social activities by HIV-infected persons (Raffaele et al., 2001).

In September 2003, President Bush introduced "the Emergency Plan for AIDS Relief," which commits the United States to providing $15 billion over the next 5 years for HIV prevention, treatment, and care programs in the developing world. The plan hopes to focus on 14 of the most HIV-affected countries in Africa and the Caribbean, including Botswana, Cote d'Ivoire, Ethiopia, Guyana, Haiti, Kenya, Mozambique, Namibia, Nigeria, Rwanda, South Africa, Tanzania, Uganda, and Zambia. This contribution significantly increases the U.S. contribution to the Global Fund to Fight AIDS and is another step forward in fighting the global pandemic of AIDS.

The Jean Chretien Pledge to Africa Act was approved by the Canadian legislature in 2004 to provide developing countries with cheaper drugs to treat AIDS and also to allow these countries to import less expensive generic versions of patented drugs. These are important steps that Western countries are taking, as a global AIDS initiative is critical to the containment and ultimate cure of this pandemic.

CONCLUSIONS

Public health and human rights have historically been at odds with each other in deciding whether the rights of the public to regulate infectious disease should prevail over the rights of the individual to privacy, autonomy, and confidentiality. The AIDS epidemic has forced us as citizens and lawmakers to seek a middle ground. In developed countries, policymakers (especially in the areas of HIV testing and disclosure) have reinforced the individual's right to autonomy. Federal laws also have extensive regulations to protect the individual infected by HIV from discrimination at work or in public places. HIV-infected individuals now have better access to public assistance and health care than a decade ago.

Efforts to prevent the spread of HIV have helped decrease the transmission in developed countries. We have learned from experience that coercion in the form of threats, penalty, and discrimination is not an effective tool to prevent the spread of an epidemic such as AIDS. The more effective approach is to provide access to information and to encourage voluntary measures and cooperation, while ensuring the individual's right to privacy. It is hoped and anticipated that individuals should choose to reduce the risk of HIV infection based on the knowledge gained.

Much remains to be done in the developing world in terms of regulations, policies, and legislation to protect the rights of the HIV-seropositive individual and to prevent discrimination. The stigma attached to HIV infection remains strong in the developing world, and there is much that needs to be done by the developed nations to influence policymakers worldwide. HIV transmission knows no geographical boundaries, and in fact, the epicenter of this disease has shifted back to Africa and Asia because of the lack of education and of measures to decrease disease transmission in those parts of the world. Only a truly international effort with consensus among different countries will have a long-term impact on the natural history of AIDS.

REFERENCES

Banta, W. F. 1993. *AIDS in the Workplace: Legal Questions and Practical Answers*, p. 30–71. Lexington Books, New York, NY.

Bartlett, J. G., and A. K. Finkbeiner. 1996. *The Guide to Living with HIV Infection*, p. 254–280. Johns Hopkins University Press, Baltimore, MD.

Braithwaite, R. L., S. Stephens, and K. Braithwaite. 1999. Risks associated with tattooing and body piercing. *J. Public Health Policy* **20:**459–470.

Burris, S., J. S. Vernick, A. Ditzler, and S. Strathdee. 2002. The legality of selling or giving syringes to injection drug users. *J. Am. Pharm. Assoc.* **42**(6 Suppl. 2)**:**S13–S18.

Buss, W., W. Dornett, L. Gasarch, L. Hoyt, K. Kelly, D. Leifer, A. Macher, R. O'Brien, M. Rhodes, D. Robinson, T. Schuck, P. Stano, and D. Webber. 1987. *AIDS and the Law*, p. 1–50. Wiley Law Publications, New York, NY.

Chhetri, D., P. Mukhopaddhaya, and S. Gupta. 2002. AIDS and the medico-legal experts. *J. Indian Med. Assoc.* **100:**698–699.

Coffin, P. O., C. Fuller, S. Blaney, L. Vadnai, S. Miller, and D. Vlahov. 2004. Syringe distribution to injection drug users for prevention of HIV infection: opinions and practices of health care providers in New York City. *Clin. Infect. Dis.* **38:**438–441.

Fee, E., and D. Fox. 1992. *AIDS: The Making of a Chronic Disease*, p. 50–104. University of California Press, Berkeley.

Glantz, L. H. 1996. *Legal Issues Regarding HIV Infection*, p. 663–674. *In* H. Libman and R. A. Witzburg (ed.), *HIV Infection*. Little, Brown, and Company, Boston, MA.

Hamers, F. F., and A. M. Downs. 2004. The changing face of the HIV epidemic in Western Europe: what are the implications for public health policies? *Lancet* **364:**83–94.

Harrington, J. A. 2002. The instrumental uses of autonomy: a review of AIDS law and policy in Europe. *Soc. Sci. Med.* **55:**1425–1434.

Jarvis, R., M. Closen, D. Hermann, and A. Leonard. 1991. *AIDS Law in a Nutshell*. West Publishing Company, Saint Paul, MN.

Johnson, B., and C. Soskolne. 1986. AIDS: medico legal considerations for Canadian hospitals. *Can. Med. Assoc. J.* **135:**1091–1096.

Loue, S. 1995. *Legal and Ethical Aspects of HIV-Related Research*, p. 145–148. Plenum Press, New York, NY.

Lyerly, A. D., and J. Anderson. 2001. Human immunodeficiency virus and assisted reproduction: reconsidering evidence, reframing ethics. *Fertil. Steril.* **75:**843–858.

Payne, M. A., and E. J. Lamb. 2004. Use of frozen semen to avoid human immunodeficiency virus type 1 transmission by donor insemination: a cost-effectiveness analysis. *Fertil. Steril.* **81:**80–91.

Porco, T. C., J. N. Martin, K. A. Page-Shafer, A. Cheng, E. Charlebois, R. M. Grant, and D. H. Osmond. 2004. Decline in HIV infectivity following the introduction of highly active antiretroviral therapy. *AIDS* **18:**81–88.

Raffaele, D., T. Emmanuelle, P. Olga, B. Roberto, N. Sergio, and K. A. Stuart. 2001. Global review of legislation on HIV/AIDS: the issue of HIV testing. *J. Acquir. Immune Defic. Syndr.* **28:**173–179.

Sahai, S., and B. Jones. 2001. *HIV-Associated Dementia*. Online Medical Textbook. http://www.emedicine.com.

Schochetman, J., and J. R. George. 1994. *AIDS Testing*, 2nd ed., p. 25–50. Springer-Verlag, New York, NY.

Scott, B. 1993. Testing, disclosure, and the right to privacy, p. 115–149. *In* B. Scott, H. Dalton, J. Miller, and the Yale AIDS Law project (ed.), *AIDS Law Today*. Yale University Press, New Haven, CT.

Smith, W. S. 1998. *Legal & Ethical Issues of HIV-Induced Dementia*, p. 565–568. *In* H. E. Gendelman, S. A. Lipton, L. Epstein, and S. Swindells (ed.), *The Neurology of AIDS*. International Thomas Publishing, New York, NY.

Spielberg, F., R. O. Levine, and M. Weaver. 2004. Self-testing for HIV: a new option for HIV prevention. *Lancet Infect. Dis.* **4:**640–646.

Taylor, M. M., H. Rotblatt, J. T. Brooks, J. Montoya, G. Aynalem, L. Smith, K. Kenney, L. Laubacher, T. Bustamante, R. Kim-Farley, J. Fielding, B. Bernard, E. Daar, and P. R. Kerndt. 2007. Epidemiologic investigation of a cluster of workplace HIV infections in the adult film industry: Los Angeles, California, 2004. *Clin. Infect. Dis.* **44:**301–305.

Terl, A. H. 1993. *AIDS and the Law. A Basic Guide for the Nonlawyer*, p. 15–22. Hemisphere Publishing Corp., Washington, DC.

Webber, D. W. 1997. *AIDS and the Law*, 3rd ed., p. 97–175. Wiley Law Publications, Somerset, NJ.

Weir, E. 2000. Rapid HIV testing. *Can. Med. Assoc. J.* **162:**1605.

Wood, G., R. Marks, and J. Dilley. 1990. *AIDS Law for Mental Health Professionals*. University of California at San Francisco AIDS Health Project, San Francisco.

The Spectrum of Neuro-AIDS Disorders:
Pathophysiology, Diagnosis, and Treatment
Edited by K. Goodkin et al.
©2008 ASM Press, Washington, DC

36

Global Issues in Neuro-AIDS and Their Evolution over the Future of the HAART Era

BRUCE J. BREW

The neurological complications of HIV were originally defined in patients from developed countries. Now that the epidemic is entering its third decade, there is an increasing awareness of the possible differences in the complications that occur in the developing world, not just those relating to geographically specific opportunistic conditions but also the direct complications such as dementia and neuropathy. With the 3 by 5 WHO program, increasing numbers of developing countries have access to antiretroviral drugs, thereby making highly active antiretroviral therapy (HAART) regimens possible. In developed countries the effect of HAART on the neurological complications in the short term has been well described, but the long-term effects are only just starting to be clarified. Similar data need to be addressed in developing countries.

These issues are best discussed within a framework that structures the complications according to whether they are direct (related to HIV per se) or indirect (when another pathogen or process is directly involved in the disease). Within this framework this review deals briefly with the more significant aspects of nervous system involvement in HIV infection emphasizing three points: possible new complications in developing countries, new complications in HAART-treated patients as well as complications such as progressive multifocal leukoencephalopathy (PML) that have only marginally changed with HAART, and future directions.

DIRECT COMPLICATIONS

In this section the direct complications are organized according to the degree of advancement of HIV disease and anatomical region involved.

Bruce J. Brew, Departments of Neurology, HIV Medicine, Centre for Immunology, and National Centre in HIV Epidemiology and Clinical Research, St. Vincent's Hospital, University of New South Wales, Sydney 2010, Australia.

Early HIV Disease: PHI

Symptomatic primary HIV infection illness (PHI) occurs in up to 90% of patients (Kahn and Walker, 1998; Clark et al., 1991), but neurological manifestations vary widely, from 8 to 60% (Clark et al., 1991; Pedersen et al., 1989; Boufassa et al., 1995; Schacker et al., 1996), largely as a result of some studies including headache even if it is the sole neurological manifestation.

The systemic illness typically is acute with a median duration of 18 days (Kaufman et al., 1998; Gaines et al., 1988; Quinn, 1997) consisting of fever, adenopathy, headache, rash, myalgia or arthralgia, and mucocutaneous ulceration.

The neurological complications are varied and most often occur within a week or two of the systemic illness. Meningoencephalitis (Carne et al., 1985; Ho et al., 1985b) may be fulminant but more often is mild with generalized or focal symptomatology (Carne et al., 1985; Ho et al., 1985b; Biggar et al., 1986; Hardy et al., 1991; Brew et al., 1989). Seizures may be a feature of the encephalitis (Carne et al., 1985). A transverse myelitis has also been described (Gaines et al., 1988; Denning et al., 1987; Zeman and Donaghy, 1991; Silver et al., 1997). A facial nerve palsy closely resembling a Bell's palsy may occur (Paton et al., 1990; Piette et al., 1986; Wiselka et al., 1987). Rarely, there may be a Guillain-Barré syndrome, a sensory neuropathy, an acute brachial neuritis, or a lumbosacral polyradiculoneuropathy (Paton et al., 1990; Piette et al., 1986; Hagberg et al., 1986; Steiner et al., 1999; Elder et al., 1986; Castellanos et al., 1994). There have been occasional reports of rhabdomyolysis (McDonagh and Holman, 2003).

At present there is no evidence that the neurological complications of PHI are any different in patients from developing countries.

Investigations are directed according to the clinical syndrome, but almost always the cerebrospinal fluid (CSF) shows a mild to moderate mononuclear pleocytosis (Carne et al., 1985; Ho et al., 1985a, 1985b), with raised protein levels and HIV RNA concentrations (Tambussi et al., 2000).

Specific therapy in terms of antiretroviral drugs with or without immunomodulatory treatments for the neurological complications of PHI is debatable. This is an area that deserves further rigorous research. Theoretically, there is the opportunity to lower the viral set point and possibly to limit the dissemination of HIV to the central nervous system (CNS). However, there are no good clinical data: the single randomized study that has been done used zidovudine monotherapy, and this showed short-term benefits only (Kinloch-de Loes and Perneger, 1997). Other studies have been observational and have not shown benefit despite the use of HAART (Desquilibet et al., 2004; Kaufman et al., 2004; Smith et al., 2004). But no study has examined neurological outcome. Patients with neurological complications of PHI may benefit because they are associated with a worse prognosis for subsequent AIDS development, as well as more rapid development of cognitive impairment. Thus, at present, most would use HAART (Apoola et al., 2002), preferably using drugs that reach efficacious concentrations in the CNS (Cysique et al., 2004a) but avoiding a triple-nucleoside combination (Kassutto and Rosenberg, 2004). Specifically a combination of the following drugs is recommended: zidovudine, stavudine (but not zidovudine and stavudine together), abacavir, lamivudine, nevirapine, efavirenz, indinavir, and possibly ritonavir-boosted lopinavir (Brew, 2001a; M. Gisslen, personal communication). The duration of therapy is contentious, but most would treat for at least 6 months. The utility of immunomodulatory therapies such as mycophenolate mofetil, cyclosporine, or interleukin-2 (IL-2) (Kassutto and Rosenberg, 2004; Rizzardi et al., 2002) alone or in combination with antiretroviral drugs is currently under assessment.

Early and Moderately Advanced HIV Disease

In the pre-HAART era, early and moderately advanced HIV disease was characterized as the phase in which the CD4 cell count was either normal, >500 cells/μl, or between 200 and 500 cells/μl. In therapy-naïve patients this is still the case, but in HAART-treated patients it is less certain whether CD4 cell counts can adequately define this phase of the disease. HAART can return CD4 cell counts to normal or near-normal from levels that in the pre-HAART era would have been consistent with advanced HIV disease. Is the risk of direct neurological complications in such patients related to their nadir CD4 cell count or to their current count? Early and moderately advanced HIV disease phases were noted for the occasional occurrence of complications that were considered to be autoimmune, such as immune thrombocytopenic purpura, Guillain-Barré syndrome, and so on. Indeed, there is much evidence for the presence of increased antibody production against various components of the nervous system even in patients without neurological symptoms (Schutzer et al., 2003).

In the past this tended to be dismissed, but in HAART-treated patients it may assume clinical significance given that they are living longer and that HAART only partly restores immune function (Azzoni et al., 2002). More work in this area is needed.

Cognitive Impairment

The issue of neuropsychological impairment in otherwise healthy HIV-positive individuals is complex. In the pre-HAART era, large studies had not shown any significant impairment. Indeed, in this group of patients subjective cognitive complaints alone most often relate to the effects of depression (Wilkins et al., 1991). However, there was some

evidence for neuropsychological dysfunction in a subgroup of patients with advanced HIV disease that has no clinical correlate and no impact on functioning (Cysique et al., 2004b). The issue is different in HAART-treated patients. Although the prevalence of deficits has not significantly declined (in contradistinction to the decline in AIDS dementia complex [ADC] in the HAART era versus pre-HAART era), the pattern of neuropsychological impairment has changed, with a reduction in attention and visuoconstruction deficits but a deterioration of learning efficiency and some aspects of complex attention. This change remained even in patients with an undetectable plasma viral load (Cysique et al., 2004b). Moreover, these abnormalities occurred in patients with only mildly depressed CD4 cell counts.

Aseptic Meningitis

Aseptic meningitis occurs quite commonly in patients who are otherwise well in relation to HIV disease. It usually occurs in patients with a normal or only mildly depressed CD4 cell count. Its relationship, however, to the plasma HIV RNA level is unknown. Hollander and Stringari (Hollander and Stringari, 1987) classified patients into those with acute symptoms and those with chronic symptoms. The acute-symptoms patients usually had fever and headache with meningeal signs, while the chronic-symptoms patients had headache sometimes with a cranial neuropathy, especially a seventh nerve palsy. Meningeal signs were not present.

The significance of aseptic meningitis in terms of increased susceptibility to the development of ADC is unknown. Similarly, no one has examined the role of HAART in this complication.

Neuropathies

Occasionally, patients at this stage of HIV disease develop an illness consistent with Guillain-Barré syndrome or chronic inflammatory demyelinating neuropathy. The only unusual aspect is that the CSF shows a mild mononuclear pleocytosis instead of the more classical finding of no cells and raised protein. The response of either of these complications to HAART has not been rigorously studied.

A variant of Guillain-Barré syndrome, acute axonal motor neuropathy, is peculiarly common in northern China (Wu et al., 1997; Monos et al., 1997). It is unknown whether its incidence is increased in the context of HIV disease and whether it might respond to HAART.

Some patients also develop various mononeuropathies, especially of the seventh cranial nerve, that seem to be directly related to HIV. The response to HAART is unknown.

Diffuse infiltrative lymphocytosis syndrome is an unusual systemic disease associated with a painful distal sensory neuropathy, which is usually axonal and more often symmetric. It seems to be peculiarly more prevalent in Europe, especially France. The systemic features are those of a Sjögren's-like syndrome with a CD8 hyperlymphocytosis. It does respond to HAART (Moulignier et al., 1997).

Advanced HIV Disease

In the pre-HAART era, advanced HIV disease was defined as the stage occurring when the CD4 cell count was <200 cells/μl. In HAART-treated patients it may be defined by the nadir CD4 cell count, but the duration of HIV disease may also be important. These issues too require rigorous evaluation.

ADC

ADC is classically defined as the subacute onset of a sub-cortical type of dementia in an HIV patient usually with advanced HIV disease. As delineated below, this definition may no longer be adequate. Indeed, a working party was convened by the National Institutes of Health in the United States to reexamine this very issue (Antinori et al., 2007).

Epidemiological Features

Pre-HAART, the prevalence of ADC was approximately 20 to 30% of patients with advanced HIV disease (McArthur et al., 1993), while the incidence was approximately 7% per year (McArthur et al., 1993; Dore et al., 1997). In the HAART era, the prevalence has approximately doubled because of an increased life span, while the incidence has halved (Dore et al., 1999; Maschke et al., 2000). These and other data (Bacellar et al., 1994; Brew et al., 1996) now strongly suggest that ADC only occurs in some patients because of both host and viral factors (see "Pathogenesis" below).

Clinical Features

As mentioned above, ADC is a subcortical dementia: aphasia, alexia, and agraphia are absent, and motor disturbance is prominent (Navia et al., 1986). However, when it is severe, these differentiating features are lost and there is global impairment. Pre-HAART, ADC symptomatology developed over several weeks to months. ADC in HAART-treated patients now appears to unfold over a much longer time period, but rigorous data are needed. Classically, ADC has three areas of abnormality: cognition, motor function, and behavior. Typical symptoms include decreased concentration, forgetfulness, gait unsteadiness, clumsiness, and apathy. Often on examination primitive reflexes, slowing of fine finger movements, and impairment of tandem gait are found.

The myelopathy that sometimes accompanies ADC is characterized by a spastic paraparesis usually without a definite sensory level (Petito et al., 1985; Dal Pan et al., 1994). Diminished proprioception and vibration sense are dominant over pinprick or light touch deficits. Changes are largely confined to the legs, and the onset is usually over weeks to months.

ADC occurring in HAART-treated patients appears to be different; however, much work needs to be done. It seems that ADC can now be either active or inactive, the latter meaning that the deficit is fixed and represents past injury (Brew, 2004). For those patients with active ADC, a classification system has yet to be agreed upon, but one that is potentially useful and intuitive is outlined in Table 1. In general, active ADC appears to be milder. While there are changes to the tempo and severity of ADC in HAART-treated patients, are there any changes to the disorder itself? In other words, are there any "phenotypic" changes? A definitive answer to this is not possible at present, and indeed it may not be possible for some years. Some clinical features may be starting to change in view of the differences seen with neuropsychological assessment (see below). Furthermore there is neurovirological evidence of different resistance patterns to antiretroviral drugs in brain regions that are not classically involved in productive brain infection (Smit et al., 2004). Additionally, there may be more cortical features developing as a result of an interaction with the effects of aging, Alzheimer's disease, and cerebrovascular disease (Brew, 2004).

The potential relationship to Alzheimer's disease (AD) is particularly interesting and important. ADC patients and

TABLE 1 A preliminary classification of ADC

Inactive
- The disorder has not changed clinically or neuropsychologically for more than 6 months, and
- The CSF has no evidence of viral or immunological activity, and
- MR spectroscopy does not show evidence of increased glial turnover

Active
- Progressive: the disorder is worsening clinically or neuropsychologically
- Stable: the disorder has not changed in more than 6 months but there is activity in the CSF (viral or immunological) or by MRS
- Regressive: the disorder is improving

clearly HIV patients in general may be at an increased risk of AD because of increased life span, hypercholesterolemia, and common mechanisms of toxicity. More than 10% of all AIDS cases in the United States are currently patients over the age of 50 years (Centers for Disease Control and Prevention, 2001). The numbers of HIV-infected patients with raised cholesterol and triglycerides are increasing for a variety of reasons: increased age, HIV disease itself, and HAART use, especially the protease inhibitor drugs. Raised cholesterol concentrations have been repeatedly shown to be a risk factor for AD (Kivipelto et al., 2002). Also of importance is the finding, in neuroasymptomatic HIV-infected patients, of increased amyloid precursor protein expression, a marker of axonal injury, in neurons (Adle-Biassette et al., 1999; Nebuloni, 2001). The latter has also been found in head injury patients who are at an increased risk of AD, making it likely therefore that HIV-infected patients may similarly be at increased risk. The mechanism of increased amyloid precursor protein expression is probably related to the direct effects of raised IL-1 production on neurons and glia (Forloni et al., 1992). Finally, the HIV regulatory protein tat is probably important. Rempel and Pulliam (Rempel and Pulliam, 2005) found in vitro that tat inhibits the activity of the amyloid β (Aβ)-degrading enzyme, neprilysin. Given that there are reasons for suspicion, is there any evidence? tau-like structures have been identified in the brains of some HIV-infected patients (Stanley et al., 1994; Anthony et al., 2004). Moreover, Esiri and colleagues (Esiri et al., 1998) have found Aβ-rich neuritic plaques more commonly in HIV-infected patients than in controls. It is important to note that while the last study found neuritic plaques only very occasionally, these are the type of plaques associated with AD. Furthermore, the study found that 18% of the patients who were in their fourth decade had plaques (usually of the diffuse type, which most investigators consider to be the forerunner of the neuritic plaque) while none of the controls for that age had plaques. Additionally, Achim and colleagues (Achim et al., 2004) have observed diffuse Aβ plaques in HIV-infected patients as well. Finally, Brew and colleagues (Brew et al., 2005) have found lowered concentrations of CSF amyloid β1-42 and raised concentrations of tau, each of the same magnitude as found in patients with AD.

Natural History

Pre-HAART the mean time to death for patients with ADC was approximately 6 months (median, 3.8 months)

(Bouwman et al., 1998): 10 months for stage 1, 4.6 months for stage 2, and 1.4 months for stages 3 and 4 combined (Dore et al., 2003). Pre-HAART, ADC occurred usually in advanced disease, with mean CD4 cell count of 109/μl (Portegies et al., 1993), while the median CD4 cell count was 50/μl (Dore et al., 1999). With HAART, a normal or near-normal CD4 cell count is found (Cysique et al., 2005; McArthur et al., 2004). The reason for this change is not clear. It may be that some of the patients have inactive ADC, reflecting damage from a time when their CD4 cell count was low prior to the introduction of HAART. Alternately or in addition, it may mean that the duration of HIV disease is important and that there has been a change to a more R5 type viral strain (see below) as a consequence of HAART. The latter in the simian immunodeficiency virus model has been shown to cause encephalitis in the absence of immunodeficiency as assessed by CD4 cell count (O. Narayan, personal communication). There is increasing evidence that HAART does lead to a shift to R5 strains.

Investigations

It should be remembered that no investigation is diagnostic of ADC; it remains a disorder of exclusion in conjunction with supportive test results (Table 2). With the introduction of HAART, some aspects of investigations have changed; however, this is an evolving area that still needs clarification (Brew, 2004). In assessing more recent investigations for their diagnostic utility in ADC, the activity of ADC in the patients that were studied is of fundamental significance. Unfortunately, this concept has not been appreciated. If the study population has a mix of active and inactive ADC, the results will be diluted possibly to the point of nonsignificance, while a cleaner study of active ADC patients may find strong correlative results. A marker of the activity of ADC is urgently needed to underpin future studies. In this regard CSF HIV RNA measurement down to 10 copies/ml may be of some use (Cysique et al., 2005).

The usual metabolic investigations that are performed as part of a dementia workup should also be performed in this situation: vitamin B_{12}, red cell folate concentrations, and thyroid function tests.

Either computed tomographic (CT) scanning or magnetic resonance imaging (MRI) of the brain should be performed to exclude a mass lesion such as toxoplasmosis or lymphoma, as well as to address the likelihood of disorders such as cytomegalovirus (CMV) encephalitis and PML.

MRI is, however, superior to CT generally and especially for the delineation of the last two entities.

The following findings that are supportive of ADC were defined in patients who were either naïve to antiretroviral therapy or who were studied in the pre-HAART era. The abnormalities presumably are still relevant to those patients developing ADC on HAART.

The supportive imaging findings for an ADC diagnosis are as follows. CT scanning of the brain usually demonstrates general cerebral atrophy especially of the caudate nuclei (Dal Pan et al., 1992). MRI additionally often has T_2 weighted patchy or diffuse periventricular abnormalities (Jarvik et al., 1988).

Similarly, single-photon emission computed tomography (SPECT) often shows multifocal cortical and subcortical areas of hypoperfusion, although the changes are very nonspecific (Schielke et al., 1990). Positron emission tomography, on the other hand, has been found to show areas of hypometabolism in the basal ganglia that are relatively specific for ADC (Rottenberg et al., 1987).

Magnetic resonance spectroscopy (MRS) appears to be helpful in ADC. There are reduced levels of N-acetyl aspartate, a marker of neuronal function, in the deep frontal white matter and basal ganglia along with elevated levels of myoinositol (found only in glial cells) and choline, a marker that is present in higher concentrations in glial cells, reflecting changes in cell membrane injury, turnover, or glial cell activation (Chang et al., 1999). Other MRI techniques such as magnetization transfer ratio and diffusion tensor imaging are beginning to be explored and hold promise in the identification and quantification of fixed damage, that is, inactive ADC (Ragin et al., 2004).

CSF analysis may reveal background abnormalities that can occur in asymptomatic HIV-infected individuals: a mild mononuclear pleocytosis, a mildly raised CSF protein, intrathecal immunoglobulin G synthesis, and oligoclonal bands (Marshall et al., 1988). Again, the influence of HAART on these abnormalities has not been fully addressed. CSF analyses primarily serve the purpose of excluding other illnesses. In the pre-HAART era, the number of HIV RNA copies in the CSF was helpful. It was the best correlate of severity (Brew et al., 1997; McArthur et al., 1997) in patients with advanced HIV disease. There are several caveats to the interpretation of CSF HIV RNA, as for other tests, though it is often abnormal for patients who are systemically well and naïve to antiretroviral agents. CNS infections such as

TABLE 2 Investigations for the diagnosis of ADC

Investigation	Result
CT brain scan	Cerebral atrophy Exclude mass lesion, PML
MRI brain scan	Cerebral atrophy Exclude mass lesion, PML (MRI more sensitive than CT) Possibly diffuse periventricular T2 abnormalities
MRS	Reduced levels of N-acetyl aspartate Increased levels of choline, myoinositol
CSF	Increased concentrations of immune activation markers Increased HIV RNA load Antiretroviral drug resistance Exclude Cryptococcus, CMV, syphilis
Neuropsychological assessment	Psychomotor slowing and decreased mental flexibility

cryptococcal meningitis can lead to significant elevations. Other virological markers, such as p24, HIV antibodies, and HIV culture, have little clinical utility (Brew et al., 1994). Measures of immune activation within the CSF may be helpful as adjuncts to the diagnosis of ADC in patients naïve to antiretroviral drugs or unexposed to HAART. Elevated CSF concentrations of β_2 microglobulin (Brew et al., 1992), neopterin (Brew et al., 1990), quinolinic acid (Heyes et al., 1991), and monocyte chemotactic protein-1 (MCP-1) (Cinque et al., 1998) parallel the severity of ADC in patients without other confounding neurological illnesses. The matrix metalloproteinases (MMPs) 2, 7, and 9 are raised in approximately one-half of ADC patients (Conant et al., 1999), indicating blood-brain barrier disruption. CSF analysis is useful for antiretroviral therapy decisions. The patterns of resistance to antiretroviral drugs in the CSF and blood are discordant in either direction in up to one-third of patients (Cunningham et al., 2000).

Neuropsychological testing is important, as it can validate the history of cognitive decline by comparing performance with estimates of premorbid intellect and assist ADC diagnosis by the pattern of deficits that is found. Neuropsychological tests can be used to monitor response to therapy. The disturbances are characterized by subcortical deficits suggestive of ADC: impaired attention, slowing of intellectual processes, especially motor based, deficits of executive or frontal lobe type function (for example, mental flexibility), only relatively mild disturbances of memory with frequent sparing of recognition memory, and less commonly visuospatial abnormalities (Maruff et al., 1994). For patients who develop ADC on HAART there is emerging evidence that there is a change to the pattern of abnormalities with fewer deficits in motor-based tests (Cysique et al., personal communication). While there is some controversy over which tests should be used, most agree that the following are useful: timed gait, Trail Making Tests A and B, finger tapping dominant and nondominant, grooved pegboard dominant and nondominant, digit symbol test, the Rey Auditory Verbal Learning Test, Rey-Osterreith Complex Figure, symbol digit modalities test, simple and choice reaction times, and California computerized assessment package (CAL-CAP).

Neuropathology

Macroscopically, there is cerebral atrophy in virtually all patients (Brew et al., 1995), dominantly involving the frontal lobes (Gelman and Guinto, 1992). Leptomeningeal fibrosis occurs in approximately one-third of patients. Histopathological changes of perivascular mononuclear infiltrates are predominant in the deeper parts of the brain, especially the basal ganglia (Brew et al., 1995). Microglial cells are frequently activated, forming microglial nodules or multinucleated giant cells (Glass et al., 1993). HIV encephalitis is the term used for the combination of infiltrating mononuclear cells and multinucleated giant cells. Astrocytes are commonly increased in number, and in patients who rapidly progress there is increased apoptosis (Thompson et al., 2001). Oligodendrocyte numbers are occasionally increased (Esiri and Morris, 1996). White-matter pallor is common and is more probably related to blood-brain barrier-induced myelin damage than demyelination (Power et al., 1993). Rarely, there may be vacuolation throughout the white matter that has been termed vacuolar leukoencephalopathy (Budka et al., 1991). Finally, there may be neuronal loss: the large pyramidal neurons and interneurons in the cortex, spiny neurons in the putamen, medium-size neurons in the globus pallidus, and occasionally the interneurons in

the CA3 region of the hippocampus (Masliah et al., 1997; Giometto et al., 1997). There are also frequent alterations in ultrastructure, again mainly in the frontal lobes and the basal ganglia. There is dendritic pruning and simplification of synaptic contacts and axonal damage with the accumulation of beta amyloid precursor protein (Giometto et al., 1997).

The aforementioned neuropathological features relate to the pre-HAART era. The few studies that have been performed in the HAART era have usually shown a decrease in ADC frequency but with four additional findings. There is attenuation of the inflammatory response in most; in some patients, however, there can be a fulminant inflammatory leukoencephalopathy perhaps related to HAART-induced immune reconstitution (Gray et al., 2003); there is early evidence for more prominent involvement of the hippocampus (Anthony et al., 2004); and finally there is increased cerebral atherosclerosis (Morgello et al., 2002). It is likely that the neuropathological features will continue to evolve over the next few years as patients who have been on HAART for extended periods of time come to autopsy.

In the pre-HAART era, the best neuropathological correlate of ADC was the presence of activated microglia. White-matter pallor and multinucleated giant cells are found in only one-half of the patients, and HIV encephalitis is found in only one-quarter to one-half (Glass et al., 1993; Brew et al., 1995). Importantly, neuronal loss is more a feature of severe ADC (Gray et al., 2001). Neither beta amyloid precursor protein accumulation nor the degree of dendritic change correlates with ADC severity.

Some of these neuropathological changes may also occur in the absence of ADC. Cerebral atrophy, leptomeningeal fibrosis, white-matter pallor, microgliosis, and microglial nodules occur in approximately one-third to one-half of patients with advanced HIV disease (Glass et al., 1993; Bell et al., 1993; Gelman, 1993; Brew et al., 1995). Astrocytosis is very common in advanced HIV disease. Conversely, mononuclear infiltrates in the meninges, choroid plexus, and perivascular spaces in the brain have been found in HIV-infected patients but not in ADC patients (Glass et al., 1993; Bell et al., 1993; Gelman, 1993; Brew et al., 1995).

In approximately one-half of ADC patients there is evidence of vacuolar myelopathy and varying degrees of multinucleated giant cell myelitis (Petito et al., 1985; Dal Pan et al., 1994). Vacuolar myelopathy is characterized by multiple non-tract-associated vacuoles in the white matter of the posterior and lateral columns, especially in the thoracic area, infrequent lipid-laden macrophages, and separation of the myelin lamellae on electron microscopy. Axonal damage occurs only in more severe forms (Rottnek et al., 2002). Multinucleated cell myelitis is characterized by multinucleated cell infiltrates without a predilection for any particular part of the cord (Rosenblum et al., 1989).

Neurovirology

The only intrinsic neural cell that can consistently support productive HIV infection is the microglial cell (Brew et al., 1995). Endothelial cells may also be able to support productive infection, but this seems to be uncommon and its significance is unknown (Moses et al., 1996). Astrocytes can support only restricted infection, in which the production of viral particles stops at the stage of regulatory proteins (especially nef) and whole virions are not produced. This is especially important in children (Takahashi et al., 1996; Tornatore et al., 1994). Oligodendrocytes and neurons cannot support productive or restricted infection (Esiri and

Morris, 1996). Latent infection on the other hand, whereby the viral RNA has been reverse transcribed into the host DNA, has been described in neurons and not unexpectedly in microglial cells (Bagasra et al., 1996).

Although there is still controversy as to what constitutes neurotropism and neurovirulence as they pertain to HIV, the dominant viral strain that can be isolated from the brain is R5. This relates to the dichotomous classification of HIV into R5 (that is, it utilizes the CCR5 receptor and is almost always macrophage tropic) and X4 (that is, it utilizes the CXCR4 receptor and is almost always T-cell tropic). It is not surprising that the dominant viral strain is R5, given that the only intrinsic neural cell that can be productively infected is the microglial cell. The X4 strain seems to be important in astrocyte infection. What this means in the HAART era, where there is a shift to R5 strains as mentioned above, is unclear. Perhaps astrocytic infection will be much less common in HAART-treated patients.

Neuroimmunology

ADC brains have diffused upregulation of expression of major histocompatibility complex classes I and II on both the infiltrating inflammatory cells and intrinsic neural elements. As well, there is increased expression of tumor necrosis factor alpha (TNF-α) and decreased levels of IL-4 in the brain parenchyma, which correlate with the severity of ADC (Wesselingh et al., 1993). The latter findings strongly suggest that there is a degree of immune dysregulation within the brain leading to unchecked immune activation.

As mentioned in the previous section, the chemokine receptors CCR5 and CXCR4 are important. CCR5 is localized to macrophages, microglia, astrocytes, and neurons. CXCR4 is expressed on astrocytes and hippocampal neurons. Chemokines have been found to be elevated in the brain parenchyma, predominantly in areas of inflammatory infiltrates but also in brain tissue with normal appearance: MIP-1α, MIP-1β, RANTES, IL-8, and IP-10 (Sanders et al., 1998). These probably amplify HIV and associated inflammatory changes by recruiting mononuclear cells into the brain.

Pathogenesis

HIV probably enters the brain by crossing the blood-brain barrier in infected mononuclear cells either because the barrier is disturbed by HIV infection of the endothelial cells or because activated and infected lymphocytes traffic through the brain as part of their normal immune surveillance function (Brew, 2001a). Additionally, monocytes derived from the bone marrow are probably important in the turnover of brain perivascular macrophages and so may provide another mechanism of entry (Gartner, 2000). This would explain the perivascular distribution of the neuropathology of ADC. It should also be mentioned that there is some evidence for HIV brain entry through the CSF compartment, which in turn is involved by infection of the choroid plexus and the meningeal macrophages (Brew, 2001a). This would partly explain the dominance of the pathological changes in the deeper parts of the brain. Clearly, these potential modes of entry are not exclusionary, and most likely they act together in some dynamic way.

HIV probably enters the brain soon after seroconversion but probably not in everyone. This is based on patient anecdotes and the fact that latent infection of the brain has not been consistently found in those with moderately advanced HIV disease (Sinclair et al., 1994). The most convincing data

come from the macaque model infected with a hyperneurovirulent strain of simian immunodeficiency virus: there is universal brain involvement at seroconversion, which is then quelled by the immune system, leaving only evidence of latent infection. Later, in the course of immunodeficiency there is resurgence of productive intracerebral infection (Zink and Clements, 2002). This would suggest that immunodeficiency is important in the recrudescence of cerebral infection, but another model advanced by Narayan has demonstrated that encephalitis can occur with R5 strains in the absence of immunodeficiency (Narayan, personal communication). Perhaps immunodeficiency acts only as an accelerant to the expression of brain damage and is not an absolute requirement.

HIV damages the brain by a variety of toxins elaborated by both the host and the virus itself: quinolinic acid, TNF-α, platelet activating factor, nitric oxide, neopterins, peroxynitrite, Ntox, chemokines, gp120, tat, and nef (Brew, 2001a). Interestingly, the viral toxins largely mediate their toxicity through secondarily activating the production of some of the last-mentioned host toxins. Most host and viral toxins affect neuronal death and dysfunction by activation of the N-methyl-D-aspartate (NMDA) receptor (Lipton and Gendelman, 1995). Once neurons are killed, it seems likely that neurotransmitters such as glutamate are released in concentrations that initially are not neurotoxic, but because of HIV- and TNF-α-induced astrocyte dysfunction (Fine et al., 1996) they cannot be cleared from the microenvironment and so accumulate, leading to further neuronal death. Chemokines may damage neurons directly or may do so indirectly through activation of microglia (Cartier et al., 2005). Perhaps one of the most interesting chemokines is SDF1, which is overproduced by astrocytes in HIV infection and which can be cleaved to a highly neurotoxic fragment by MMP2, one of the matrix metalloproteinases (Zhang et al., 2003). Furthermore, there is some evidence that they may lead to neurodegeneration through inhibition of neural stem cell proliferation (Krathwohl and Kaiser, 2004). It should not be thought that all chemokines have neurotoxic potential. There is increasing evidence that fractalkine may be neuroprotective and capable of antagonizing the neurotoxicity of some chemokines (Mizuno et al., 2003). Moreover, other factors such as brain-derived neurotrophic factor may also have similar potential (Bachis et al., 2003). Finally, Gelman has advanced a novel aspect to pathogenesis, namely, that to some extent ADC is a channelopathy (Gelman et al., 2004). The concept is supported by gene expression profiling data from ADC brains in which perturbations in 13 such channels were identified. Moreover, it is known that vpr, a component of HIV, can induce ion channel formation (Piller, 1999).

The most important principle of ADC pathogenesis is the discordance between productive viral burden in the brain and clinical deficit (Brew et al., 1995). ADC is not simply correlated with the amount of virus in the brain parenchyma. There is, however, a relationship between cytokine excess in the brain and CSF and the severity of ADC (Tyor et al., 1992). These data reinforce the idea that indirect mechanisms are important.

There are aspects of pathogenesis that may vary according to region and possibly ethnicity. Chemokines and chemokine receptor polymorphisms seem to have some importance in children, and these data are similar for adults. Singh and companions (Singh et al., 2003) found that children who were CCR5Δ32 heterozygous had less cognitive impairment and those who were SDF1 3A homozygous had more rapid progression of cognitive deficit. In a smaller series of adults similar results have been found (my unpublished data). An MCP-1 mutation is associated with more rapid onset of ADC probably by increased levels of MCP-1, thereby enhancing macrophage brain infiltration (Gonzalez et al., 2002). Cytokine polymorphisms may also be important: TNF receptor mutations correlate with the presence of dementia (Quasney et al., 2001). ApoE4 homozygosity is also related to ADC perhaps through increased vulnerability to oxidative stress (Cutler et al., 2004). There is also some evidence that changes in HIV according to the clade may confer less neuropathogenicity. Ranga and colleagues (Ranga et al., 2004) demonstrated that clade C is associated with a less chemotactic form of tat that is thought to lead to diminished monocyte attraction to the brain and therefore less HIV. These data have been advanced as the biological basis for the diminished incidence of ADC in India. However, the epidemiological data supporting a reduced incidence compared to other parts of the world where clade B is prevalent are controversial.

The pathogenesis of HIV-related vacuolar myelopathy is controversial. In vitro TNF-α is associated with changes similar to those of vacuolar myelopathy, but it is not clear if the association is causal (Weidenheim et al., 1996). A metabolic pathogenesis such as a methylation defect has been identified in HIV infection, leading to the hypothesis that there is reduced production of S-adenosylmethionine, perhaps because of macrophage-derived nitric oxide. This in turn inhibits methionine synthase and increases consumption of S-adenosylmethionine in an attempt to repair cytokine and free-radical-induced myelin damage. A recent trial, however, with S-adenosylmethionine did not lead to any improvement (Di Rocco et al., 2004), suggesting either that the drug does not work or that the trial may have been compromised by including patients with fixed damage. Finally, there is evidence for HIV playing a direct role: nef seemed causally related to the disease in a mouse model (Radja et al., 2003). Multinucleated cell myelitis is essentially the spinal cord equivalent of HIV encephalitis.

Management

The management of the ADC patient is evolving. The following is a suggested approach (Table 1). The first step is to determine whether the disorder is active or inactive as discussed previously. The chief tool by which this is assessed is the history from the patient, loved ones, and family. The second step in management then hinges on the nature of the activity: it should be possible to assess whether it is progressive, regressive, or stable. However, at present better tools are needed to distinguish between inactive ADC and stable ADC; the latter seems to be characterized by evidence of CSF viral and immunological activities that presumably are just keeping each other in check, while the former has no evidence of viral or immunological activity in the CSF. Active progressive and stable ADC patients should have their antiretroviral regimen altered if possible.

ADC treatment at present is centered on antiretroviral drugs. Adjunctive therapy in the form of NMDA receptor and cytokine antagonists as well as inhibitors of apoptosis is yet to have a well-defined and proven role. Evidence for efficacy of individual antiretroviral agents is checkered, and despite the current proven practice of combination therapy in systemic disease the relative neurological potencies (either additive or synergistic) of different combinations of antiretroviral drugs are unknown. Antiretroviral drugs can be divided into the following classes: nucleoside reverse

transcriptase inhibitors (NRTIs), ribonucleotide reductase inhibitors, nucleotide reverse transcriptase inhibitors, nonnucleoside reverse transcriptase inhibitors (NNRTIs), protease inhibitors, and entry inhibitors. There are three characteristics of an antiretroviral drug that theoretically at least should make it likely to be effective in ADC: (i) it should be able to enter the brain in efficacious concentrations; (ii) it should be effective against HIV infection in the infiltrating cells, i.e., the lymphocytes and monocytes; and (iii) it should be effective against the intrinsic brain cells, the perivascular macrophages and microglia. The significance of astrocytic infection and therefore the need for a drug to be able to work in astrocytes are under evaluation. Currently, the CSF concentration of a particular drug is the only practical method of addressing the first criterion. There are standard features of a drug that make it more likely to be able to enter the brain: small size, increased lipophilicity, and more acidic composition. But in relation to antiretroviral drugs, there are active transporter systems that pump drugs out of the brain that must be considered. Of special importance are the multiple-resistance-associated transporters and the P-glycoprotein system: the first is important for zidovudine and possibly other nucleosides, while the second is important for the protease inhibitors (Konig et al., 1999; Kim et al., 1998). Ritonavir, a protease inhibitor, is not only a substrate but also a potent inhibitor of the P-glycoprotein system. Consequently, combining ritonavir with another protease inhibitor may facilitate brain entry, but definitive data are needed. The fact that there is neuropathological evidence of increased P-glycoprotein expression in HIV encephalitis further supports the importance of adding ritonavir to a protease inhibitor (Langford et al., 2004). The ability of a particular drug to be effective in lymphocytes, macrophages, and microglia is critical to ADC efficacy and involves two important types of infection: acute (in lymphocytes) and chronic (in monocytes, macrophages, and microglia). All antiretroviral drugs are effective against acute infection, but only some (abacavir, lamivudine, didanosine, dideoxycytidine, and possibly the NNRTIs and protease inhibitors) are effective against chronic infection. Comparative efficacy data are limited (Aquaro et al., 1997; Saavedra-Lozano et al., 2004).

Most of the NRTIs are useful in ADC. Zidovudine is the only antiretroviral medication with proven efficacy in ADC (Sidtis et al., 1993), but higher-than-usual doses are required with the resultant risk of hematological intolerance manifesting as anemia. Thus, the highest tolerable dose of zidovudine should be given. Didanosine (ddI), another NRTI, does not appear to be effective in adults (Gisslen et al., 1997). Zalcitabine (ddC) probably has no role in ADC (Brew, 2001a). Stavudine (d4T) appears to be effective in ADC based on its ability to penetrate into the CSF in efficacious concentrations and to clear CSF viral load in a small number of patients (Foudraine et al., 1998). Lamivudine can also reach efficacious steady-state concentrations in the CSF and may be useful (Foudraine et al., 1998). Abacavir, a relatively new NRTI with CSF penetration comparable to that of zidovudine, should be beneficial, although a large randomized double-blind placebo-controlled trial did not show this, despite superior CSF viral load clearance. The failure may have been related to background combination therapy efficacy as well as resistance to abacavir and the fact that some patients had inactive disease (Brew, 2001a).

Hydroxyurea is a ribonucleotide reductase inhibitor that effectively inhibits HIV replication (Lori et al., 1994), especially in combination with d4T and ddI. The drug has good brain penetration, but firm evidence for ADC efficacy is lacking. Recently, it has fallen out of fashion because of the risk of myelosuppression and, when used with d4T or ddI, neuropathy.

The only nucleotide reverse transcriptase inhibitor currently available is tenofovir. Data on its potential neurological efficacy are lacking.

The NNRTIs nevirapine and efavirenz are likely to be effective in ADC because of potentially efficacious steady-state CSF concentrations. Neurologists, however, should be aware of the side effects of efavirenz that may occur in the first few weeks of treatment, especially mild confusion and somnolence (Brew, 2001a). Usually these settle spontaneously.

The only protease inhibitor with the potential for ADC efficacy is indinavir because of favorable CSF steady-state concentrations (Martin et al., 1999). This is probably improved by the addition of ritonavir through its inhibition of the P-glycoprotein efflux transporter system. There is also preliminary evidence of the efficacy of lopinavir when used in combination with ritonavir (Gisslen, personal communication).

The entry inhibitors are a new class of antiretroviral drug. Their mode of action is the inhibition of entry of HIV into the cell either by stopping fusion of HIV with the cell membrane (T20, also known as fuzeon) or by blocking one of the chemokine receptors (either CCR5 or CXCR4). At present neurological efficacy data for this class are lacking, but given the large molecular weight of T20 it is unlikely to be able to penetrate into the brain.

In clinical practice, ADC patients should have their blood and CSF analyzed for any evidence of resistance mutations to the latter-mentioned antiretroviral drugs. The results of the resistance testing can then be used to guide which antiretrovirals would be appropriate to use. At present, however, it is still not apparent how many and which should be used; nonetheless, the guiding principles are that at least three of the following drugs should be used: the neurologically active NRTIs (zidovudine, stavudine, abacavir, and lamivudine) (but not zidovudine and stavudine together) along with one of the NNRTIs (nevirapine or efavirenz) and the protease inhibitor indinavir, possibly lopinavir preferably boosted by ritonavir to aid in brain penetration and compliance.

The recommendations given above are based upon evolving evidence of the need for three neuroactive drugs in the regimen (Cysique et al., 2004a). However, there are some clinicians who hold that it does not matter whether the antiretroviral regimen has neuroactive drugs in it or not. This complex issue is critically reviewed by Cysique and colleagues (Cysique et al., 2004a).

The potential toxicity of these regimens should not be forgotten. NRTIs can be associated with tissue-specific mitochondrial toxicity, for example, zidovudine with myopathy and didanosine with peripheral neuropathy. There is also the potential for additive and perhaps synergistic mitochondrial toxicity when several NRTIs are used together.

Memantine, an open-channel NMDA antagonist, holds some promise as adjunctive therapy, while pentoxifylline, nimodipine, and lexipafant appear to be less helpful. Recently, the monoamine oxidase inhibitor deprenyl showed promise, probably through its antiapoptotic effect (Brew, 2001a). Minocycline is effective in inhibiting HIV infection of microglia in vitro and has antiapoptotic and immunoregulating properties, thereby making it an attractive candidate for adjunctive therapy in ADC (Si et al., 2004).

DSPN

Distal sensory polyneuropathy (DSPN) is a symmetrical sensory neuropathy that in the pre-HAART era developed in approximately 30% of patients with advanced HIV disease (Levy et al., 1985). The annual incidence in such advanced patients was approximately 7%. The epidemiological features in the HAART era are different, although precise data are difficult because studies often combine such patients with those whose neuropathy is related to toxicity from antiretroviral drugs. Nonetheless, Lichtenstein and colleagues (Lichtenstein et al., 2005) have shown that neuropathy in general and probably DSPN in particular have decreased in incidence, similar to that which has occurred in relation to ADC. However, data from neurologists in a smaller cohort of patients show that the incidence of neuropathy is increasing (Schifitto et al., 2005). In the pre-HAART era risk factors included age, nutritional deficiencies, alcohol exposure, HIV "set-point," and low CD4 count (Childs et al., 1999). With HAART, Schifitto and colleagues (Schifitto et al., 2005) have found these to be no longer important, but Lichtenstein and colleagues (Lichtenstein et al., 2005) have found that CD4 cell count and HIV RNA are still important and indeed have observed that a nadir CD4 cell count of <50 copies/ml was a risk factor. The reason for the discrepancies between the two studies is not entirely apparent, but in part it may be related to the severity of the neuropathy: it would seem probable that nonneurologists would be unlikely to diagnose mild neuropathy.

Clinical Features

DSPN develops subacutely over weeks to months beginning symmetrically in the feet and sometimes spreading to involve the lower legs. There is reduction in pinprick and temperature sensation and diminished vibration sense but preserved proprioception. Arm involvement is very uncommon, and weakness is almost always confined to the small muscles of the feet. DSPN is often associated with painful parasthesias. Nerve conduction studies reveal changes of an axonal neuropathy, although they may be normal in up to 20% of DSPN patients (Brew, 2003).

There are no investigations that are diagnostic of DSPN. As with ADC, the chief role of tests is to exclude other causes in a patient for whom the clinical picture is compatible with HIV DSPN. Nerve conduction studies may be helpful. Testing for coinfection with hepatitis B or C should be considered as they may also cause a neuropathy. In HAART-treated patients the clinician should exclude the development of diabetes as a consequence of the protease inhibitor component of HAART. The clinician should also consider d4T and ddI as a cause of DSPN; the latter is especially important for those patients also taking tenofovir. Punch skin biopsy is sometimes helpful when there are few signs (McArthur and Griffin, 2005). Quantitative sensory testing is a research tool and not widely available for clinical use.

Pathology

DSPN is a length-dependent axonal degeneration of sensory fibers, with minimal evidence of nerve fiber regeneration (Brew, 2003). Unmyelinated and, less often, large myelinated fibers are affected, frequently with prominent involvement of small fibers. The latter changes are easily demonstrated by punch skin biopsies. There are some inflammatory infiltrates of lymphocytes and activated macrophages along with decreased numbers of dorsal root ganglion neurons and increased frequency of nodules of Nageotte (Pardo et al., 2001).

Pathogenesis

Clinicopathological correlation reveals parallels with ADC: immune activation is prominent, and it is this rather than productive viral burden that is important. The degree of macrophage activation within the dorsal root ganglion best correlates with the clinical findings (Pardo et al., 2001). Only one study has shown HIV infection of dorsal root ganglion neurons (Brannagan et al., 1997). Indeed, HIV can be isolated from the peripheral nerve perivascular macrophages and the nodules of Nageotte in only 50% of patients (Brew and Tomlinson, 2004), whereas all patients have prominent activation of macrophages and release of proinflammatory cytokines including IL-6 and adhesion molecules such as ICAM-1 especially around the dorsal root ganglion (Brew and Tomlinson, 2004). This local immune activation appears to be driven by HIV. The envelope glycoprotein of HIV gp120 has been shown to bind to sensory neurons, resulting in inflammation and the induction of pain (Herzberg and Sagen, 2001). As well, in vitro studies have suggested that gp120 can induce apoptosis in cultures of dorsal root ganglion cells (Keswani et al., 2003). Not only may DSPN be driven by excess gp120-induced inflammation, but it may also be related at least in part by lack of normal neuroprotective strategies. Keswani and colleagues (Keswani et al., 2004) have shown that erythropoietin in animal models of DSPN can stop the development and possibly progression of neuropathy. It seems plausible therefore that DSPN patients may have low concentrations of erythropoietin in serum or that such low levels may mark patients who are at risk of DSPN.

The painful parasthesias may be the result of upregulation of sodium channels within the dorsal root ganglia with consequent neuronal hyperexcitability (Waxman, 1999). Alternately or additionally, the loss of unmyelinated input into lamina II of the substantia gelatinosa and ingrowth of A fibers may lead to the aberrant processing of sensory input (Baba et al., 1999).

Treatment

Treatment of DSPN essentially consists of therapy directed towards the painful component. There are no regenerative therapies: nerve growth factor trials have been disappointing (McArthur et al., 2000). Given the likely prominent pathogenetic role played by HIV, it would seem reasonable to expect that HAART would minimize or even reverse the neuropathy. However, it is critically important that such therapies, including any further regenerative treatments, include patient groups that are homogeneous, either with active or inactive disease; otherwise there will be false-negative results (Brew and Tomlinson, 2004). Unfortunately no proper trials to address the potential for HAART efficacy in DSPN have been done. However, there are some data from Martin and colleagues (Martin et al., 2000) and anecdotal cases (Markus and Brew, 1998) that provide support for the concept. The component drugs should exclude those associated with a neuropathy (d4T, ddI, and ddC). Whether drugs that can cross the blood-nerve barrier (zidovudine, lamivudine, indinavir, nevirapine, and efavirenz) are required is unknown.

Clonazepam or carbamazepine may be useful for the dysasthesias. Pain has been shown to respond to lamotrigine (Simpson et al., 2003), but despite promising initial results topical lidocaine has been shown to be ineffective (Estanislao et al., 2004). In clinical practice, low doses of one of the tricyclic antidepressants, such as amitriptyline or nortriptyline, seem to be effective despite the lack of

efficacy from one clinical trial (Kieburtz et al., 1998). The latter was probably stopped prematurely and was probably underpowered. Other agents that are helpful in clinical practice but for which there are no randomized controlled trial data are valproic acid, gabapentin, and topical capsaicin, especially when used in very high dose. Carnitine and prouridine require further formal assessment, as do the neuroimmunophilin ligands and prosaposin. Occasionally, patients require narcotic analgesics.

NN or Antiretroviral Toxic Neuropathy

Some of the current antiretroviral drugs can be associated with the development of a neuropathy that clinically is indistinguishable from DSPN. The terminology has not been formally agreed upon, but the two most common terms are nucleoside neuropathy (NN) or antiretroviral toxic neuropathy. The drugs that are associated with this neuropathy are commonly known as the "d" drugs, namely, ddC (zacitabline), ddI (didanosine), and d4T (stavudine) (Brew, 2003). The evidence linking lamivudine to neuropathy is weak. Some recent investigators (Lichtenstein et al., 2005) have raised the possibility that some of the protease inhibitors may also be associated with neuropathy. The evidence here too is unconvincing: there was no standardized definition of neuropathy, and the diagnosis of neuropathy was made by nonneurologists. It is commonly known that ritonavir and some other protease inhibitors can be associated with a tingling sensation in the limbs and sometimes lips. Some nonneurologist clinicians have interpreted this as indicating neuropathy when in fact the pathogenesis is entirely unclear.

The risk of developing NN depends on the individual drug, the dose, the duration of exposure, and the presence of other factors associated with neuropathy. Of the "d" drugs, ddC is the most neurotoxic while ddI is the least. Combinations of the latter set of drugs definitely increase the risk; the most commonly used combination is d4T and ddI. Until recently, hydroxyurea was often used with d4T or ddI; this too increased the risk (Cherry et al., 2003). Currently, a popular combination is ddI and tenofovir; the dose of ddI has to be reduced because of increased intracellular phosphorylation, but there is still probably an increased risk of NN.

Clinical Features

As mentioned above, the clinical features of NN and DSPN are essentially indistinguishable. Both lead to a distal symmetrical sensory neuropathy that is often painful. The mean time to the development of NN is between 16 and 23 weeks from the commencement of the drug, depending on the drug that is used.

Pathology

Sural nerve biopsies have shown severe axonal destruction, prominent in unmyelinated fibers.

Pathogenesis

The most widely accepted theory at present is that the disorder is the result of mitochondrial toxicity from the particular drugs. There are several lines of evidence in support of this. In vivo, raised serum lactate levels (Brew et al., 2003) and reduced serum levels of acetyl-carnitine (Famularo et al., 1997) have been found in NN. In vitro, there are models of NN in which the clinical degree of neurotoxicity matches the degree of inhibition of gamma DNA polymerase (Martin et al., 1994) as well as the inhibition of neurite outgrowth

(Keswani et al., 2003). Moreover, there is a reduction in the copy numbers of mtDNA. The mechanism of the neurotoxicity appears to be through necrosis (Keswani et al., 2003).

Treatment

The diagnosis is made usually by the temporal association between the development of the neuropathy and the commencement of the drug as well as by ancillary investigation results such as raised lactate concentrations. Treatment first and foremost is the discontinuation of the offending drug with revision of the regimen in which the drug was incorporated so that a new HAART regimen can be constructed. It should be remembered that one drug of a HAART regimen should not be stopped in isolation, as this will leave the virological efficacy of the remaining drugs in the regimen suboptimal. Consequently viral load will increase and there will be the rapid development of resistance to the remaining drugs. If it is not possible to stop the drug because there is no other HAART regimen that can be constructed, then the patient will have to remain on the offending drug and the symptoms will have to be controlled by other drugs as discussed above for DSPN.

Disorders Not Linked to Disease Advancement

Myopathies

There are several myopathies that have been linked to HIV disease. The association seems to be at least in part causal rather than just associative. The two most important are polymyositis and inclusion body myositis.

Polymyositis

This is a rare complication of HIV disease, and consequently little is known of its natural history. The clinical features of HIV-related polymyositis are no different from those occurring in the absence of HIV infection (Dalakas and Pezeshkpour, 1998). Differential diagnosis should include human T-cell leukemia virus type 1 (HTLV-1) infection, microsporidia, and a statin-related myopathy. Treatment is along standard lines with the use of prednisone and possibly intravenous gamma globulin. It is unknown whether HAART has any role.

Inclusion Body Myositis

Inclusion body myositis has been associated with HIV infection (Cupler et al., 1996). It seems different from the more classical disease because of an earlier age of onset and higher elevation of creatinine kinase. Treatment with intravenous gamma globulin may be worthwhile. The utility of HAART is unknown.

Epilepsy

Approximately 10% of patients may develop epilepsy in the absence of any definable cause apart from HIV. It would seem that HIV lowers seizure threshold, but this has yet to be proven conclusively. The influence of HAART on HIV-related epilepsy is unknown. Clinicians, however, should be aware of the potential for interaction between protease inhibitor drugs and anticonvulsants (Romanelli et al., 2000).

Stroke

Cerebrovascular disease occurs relatively infrequently in HIV disease. The usual causes relate to opportunistic conditions, cardiac diseases, HIV per se, and accelerated atherosclerosis. Any of the classical opportunistic infections can be complicated by the development of stroke, but perhaps the most important from a global perspective is tuberculosis, through an obliterative arteritis secondary to meningitis or an endarteritis related to tuberculosis per se. The other significant cause is varicella-zoster vasculopathy. Cardiac disease may occur through endocarditis in intravenous drug users, and marantic endocarditis can occur in the context of malignancy and Kaposi's sarcoma. The mechanism by which HIV directly leads to stroke is unclear. It seems to be related to active HIV disease. As such it is likely that HAART may make a significant impact. Accelerated atherosclerosis is beginning to be observed in patients on HAART. Although this is manifesting at present as ischemic heart disease, it is anticipated that accelerated atherosclerotic cerebrovascular disease will also become important in the near future (Brew, 2001b).

INDIRECT NEUROLOGICAL COMPLICATIONS

The indirect neurological complications related to HIV disease are many. Only the more important are discussed here. The most significant aspects of these disorders in the era of HAART are that the incidence of opportunistic infections has significantly declined with HAART and that HAART may induce the clinical expression of previously subclinical disease through the immune reconstitution syndrome. Furthermore, if HAART leads to a sustained rise in CD4 cell count so that it is above the usual level associated with risk of that particular opportunistic infection, then maintenance therapy can probably be ceased.

HTLV-1 and -2

Both HTLV-1 and HTLV-2 may occur in the context of HIV infection. HTLV-1 coinfection occurs more commonly in Brazil and parts of the Caribbean. HTLV-2 is endemic in American Indian and pygmy tribes. It has now spread to injecting drug users in the United States and Europe (Roucoux and Murphy, 2004). HTLV-1 is associated with myelopathy, neuropathy, and myopathy. Coinfected patients have a higher incidence of myelopathy (Harrison and Schechter, 1998) and peripheral neuropathy (Harrison et al., 1997). Additionally, they seem to have a higher CD4 cell count. The clinical features of HTLV-2 infection as it affects the nervous system are still incompletely defined. Nonetheless, it does appear to cause an illness indistinguishable from HTLV-1-associated myelopathy. Whether it has other neurological manifestations is unclear (Araujo and Hall, 2004). HAART does not appear to have any effect on HTLV-1 in coinfected patients, but it paradoxically increases HTLV-2 proviral load.

Cryptococcal Disease

Cryptococcal disease may affect the nervous system through cryptococcal meningitis or cryptococcomas. In advanced HIV disease this is still one of the most common complications regardless of the country. Cryptococcal meningitis is far more common than cryptococcomas; the latter may occur in the absence of cryptococcal meningitis. The typical presentation is one of headache sometimes associated with fever. Patients with cryptococcomas present with the relevant focal neurological disturbance. Serum cryptococcal antigen is almost always positive in meningitis, but it can often be negative in cryptococcomas. Treatment with fluconazole or amphotericin is often effective (Brew, 2001c).

Tuberculosis

Tuberculosis is commonly associated with HIV disease in developing countries and intravenous drug users in developed countries. CNS involvement is similarly common and has three forms: meningitis, tuberculoma, and tuberculous abscess (Whiteman et al., 1995). In clinical practice the chief problem is deciding which empirical treatment should be used for a patient presenting with a CNS mass lesion. In developed countries the first empirical treatment would be for CNS toxoplasmosis. It is controversial as to whether this is also true for developing countries. Only a few epidemiological studies have been performed in such settings, and they have shown that CNS toxoplasmosis is still more likely to be a cause of a cerebral mass lesion than tuberculosis is (Lanjewar et al., 1998). Nonetheless, data are limited and local experience should guide the clinician as to what is more likely. Additionally, there may be clues. Concomitant respiratory disease would make tuberculosis more likely, while the absence of positive serology for toxoplasmosis and the patient's having taken cotrimoxazole argue against CNS toxoplasmosis. An empirical trial of antituberculosis therapy can be undertaken, but clinicians should be aware of two problems: the response time may be of the order of weeks to months, and there may be an initial deterioration. Definitive diagnosis requires brain biopsy, which is not always available especially in resource-limited situations. Antituberculous therapy may interact with the protease inhibitor drugs used in HAART regimens.

Toxoplasmosis

As discussed above in the section on tuberculosis, the principal issue is whether to empirically treat a cerebral mass lesion as toxoplasmosis or tuberculosis. Development of such a lesion in a patient taking cotrimoxazole for *Pneumocystis carinii* prophylaxis and who is serologically negative for toxoplasmosis renders toxoplasmosis unlikely. An empirical trial of antitoxoplasmosis therapy usually leads to some clinical response within 1 to 2 weeks. It is probably best to delay the institution of HAART for several months to minimize the risk of immune restoration leading to clinical deterioration. However, the issue has not been rigorously studied. Induction doses of antitoxoplasmosis drugs should be continued for several months according to clinical and radiological response: there should be no enhancement of any residual lesions on imaging. Maintenance doses can then be continued until the CD4 cell count is sustained at >200 cells/µl (Brew, 2001d).

CMV

CMV may lead to several types of nervous system disease: CMV encephalitis, CMV mass lesion, polyradiculopathy, and mononeuritis multiplex. These are complications of very advanced HIV disease, usually occurring when the CD4 cell count is 50 cells/µl or less. Diagnosis is by detection of CMV DNA in the CSF; the clue to CMV being a likely explanation for the clinical presentation is the finding of a polymorphonuclear pleocytosis in the CSF. Treatment is with intravenous ganciclovir or foscarnet, although both together are recommended for CMV encephalitis. As with other opportunistic complications HAART should be delayed to avoid immune reconstitution-induced deterioration. Maintenance therapy can be ceased once the CD4 cell count is sustainably increased to >200 cells/µl (Brew, 2001e).

Primary CNS Lymphoma

Primary CNS lymphoma usually occurs in advanced HIV disease. Where possible, amplification of Epstein-Barr virus DNA from the CSF is supportive but not necessarily diagnostic. Brain biopsy is the only certain means of diagnosis. Standard therapy involves radiation treatment, but there is some evidence for the adjunctive efficacy of HAART.

PML

PML is the only opportunistic infection whose incidence does not appear to have significantly fallen with the introduction of HAART. Clinically it is characterized by the subacute onset over weeks of a focal neurological deficit in the absence of fever or obtundation in a patient with a CD4 cell count usually <100 cells/µl. Diagnosis is by the characteristic MRI appearance and the amplification of JC virus DNA from the CSF, although the latter occurs in only at most 60% of patients. There is no proven therapy for PML apart from HAART (Brew, 2001f).

Cerebral Malaria

Unfortunately, few data are available at present to address the issue of how HIV might interact with malaria and, in particular, cerebral malaria. Nonetheless, it does appear that earlier thinking on the topic was incorrect and that there is an increased risk of cerebral malaria in HIV-positive patients (Chirenda and Murugasampillay, 2003). The effect of HAART is unknown.

Leprosy

Similarly, data on the interaction between HIV and leprosy are sparse. Inasmuch as the few studies allow, HIV-positive patients appear to have more advanced manifestations of leprosy (Moses et al., 2001). The effect of HAART has not been studied yet.

Hepatitis C

There is preliminary evidence of increased frequency and perhaps severity of cognitive deficits in hepatitis C coinfected patients (Ryan et al., 2004). The effect of HAART on this interaction has not yet been reported.

Statin Myopathy

With the increasing awareness of hyperlipidemia in HIV-positive patients and especially those on HAART, more patients are being treated with cholesterol-lowering drugs. Any of these can be associated with a myopathy, but the statins are particularly important. In the non-HIV-infected population the complication is rare but well recognized. At present it is not clear whether HIV-infected patients have an increased risk of myopathy when they are treated with one of the statins.

REFERENCES

Achim, C. L., D. A. Green, M. Avramut, J. Schindelar, D. Knight, and E. Masliah. 2004. Axonal degeneration in the HIV brain. *J. Neurovirol.* 10(Suppl. 3):S60.

Adle-Biassette, H., F. Chretien, L. Wingertsmann, C. Hery, T. Ereau, F. Scaravilli, M. Tardieu, and F. Gray. 1999. Neuronal apoptosis does not correlate with dementia in HIV infection but is related to microglial activation and axonal damage. *Neuropathol. Appl. Neurobiol.* 25:123–133.

Anthony, I. C., S. Ramage, F. W. Brannan, and J. E. Bell. 2004. Premature neurodegeneration, inflammation and opiate misuse in HIV/AIDS before and after HAART. *J. Neurovirol.* 10(Suppl. 3):S52.

Antinori, A., G. Arendt, J. T. Becker, B. J. Brew, D. A. Byrd, M. Cherner, D. B. Clifford, P. Cinque, L. G. Epstein, K. Goodkin, M. Gisslen, I. Grant, R. K. Heaton, J. Joseph, K. Marder, C. M. Marra, J. C. McArthur, M. Nunn, R. W. Price, L. Pulliam, K. R. Robertson, N. Sacktor, V. Valcour, and V. E. Wojna. 2007. Updated research nosology for HIV-associated neurocognitive disorders. *Neurology* 69:1789–1799.

Apoola, A., S. Ahmad, and K. Radcliffe. 2002. Primary HIV infection. *Int. J. STD AIDS* 13:71–78.

Aquaro, S., C. F. Perno, E. Balestra, J. Balzarini, A. Cenci, M. Francesconi, S. Panti, F. Serra, N. Villani, and R. Calio. 1997. Inhibition of replication of HIV in primary monocyte/macrophages by different antiviral drugs and comparative efficacy in lymphocytes. *J. Leukoc. Biol.* 62:138–143.

Araujo, A., and W. W. Hall. 2004. Human T-lymphotropic virus type II and neurological disease. *Ann. Neurol.* 56:10–19.

Azzoni, L., E. Papasavvas, J. Chehimi, J. R. Kostman, K. Mounzer, J. Ondercin, B. Perussia, and L. J. Montaner. 2002. Sustained impairment of IFN-gamma secretion in suppressed HIV-infected patients despite mature NK cell recovery: evidence for a defective reconstitution of innate immunity. *J. Immunol.* 168:5764–5770.

Baba, H., T. P. Doubell, and C. J. Woolf. 1999. Peripheral inflammation facilitates Abeta fiber-mediated synaptic input to the substantia gelatinosa of the adult rat spinal cord. *J. Neurosci.* 19:859–867.

Bacellar, H., A. Munoz, E. N. Miller, B. A. Cohen, D. Besley, O. A. Selnes, J. T. Becker, and J. C. McArthur. 1994. Temporal trends in the incidence of HIV-1-related neurologic diseases: Multicenter AIDS Cohort Study 1985–1992. *Neurology* 44:1892–1900.

Bachis, A., E. O. Major, and I. Mocchetti. 2003. Brain-derived neurotrophic factor inhibits human immunodeficiency virus-1/gp120-mediated cerebellar granule cell death by preventing gp120 internalization. *J. Neurosci.* 23:5715–5722.

Bagasra, O., E. Lavi, L. Bobroski, K. Khalili, J. P. Pestaner, R. Tawadros, and R. J. Pomerantz. 1996. Cellular reservoirs of HIV-1 in the central nervous system of infected individuals: identification by the combination of in situ polymerase chain reaction and immunochemistry. *AIDS* 10:573–586.

Bell, J. E., A. Busuttil, J. W. Ironside, S. Rebus, Y. K. Donaldson, P. Simmonds, and J. F. Peutherer. 1993. Human immunodeficiency virus and the brain: investigation of virus load and neuropathologic changes in pre-AIDS subjects. *J. Infect. Dis.* 168:818–824.

Biggar, R. J., B. K. Johnson, S. S. Musoke, J. B. Masembe, D. M. Silverstein, M. M. Warshow, and S. Alexander. 1986. Severe illness associated with the appearance of antibody to human immunodeficiency virus in an African. *Br. Med. J.* 293:1210–1211.

Boufassa, F., C. Bachmeyer, C. Carne, C. Deveau, A. Persoz, C. Jadand, D. Sereni, D. Bucquet, et al. 1995. Influence of neurologic manifestations of primary human immunodeficiency virus infection on disease progression. *J. Infect. Dis.* 171:1190–1195.

Bouwman, F. H., R. Skolasky, D. Hes, O. A. Selnes, J. D. Glass, T. E. Nance-Sproson, W. Royal, G. J. Dal Pan, and J. C. McArthur. 1998. Variable progression of HIV-associated dementia. *Neurology* 50:1814–1820.

Brannagan, T. H., G. J. Nuovo, A. P. Hays, and N. Latov. 1997. Human immunodeficiency virus infection of dorsal root ganglion neurons detected by polymerase chain reaction in situ hybridization. *Ann. Neurol.* 42:368–372.

Brew, B. J. 2001a. AIDS dementia complex, p. 74–77. In B. J. Brew (ed.), *HIV Neurology*. Oxford University Press, New York, NY.

Brew, B. J. 2001b. Cerebrovascular complications and transient neurologic deficits, p. 146–151. In B. J. Brew (ed.), *HIV Neurology*. Oxford University Press, New York, NY.

Brew, B. J. 2001c. Cryptococcal meningitis, p. 91–96. In B. J. Brew (ed.), *HIV Neurology*. Oxford University Press, New York, NY.

Brew, B. J. 2001d. Toxoplasmosis, p. 117–123. In B. J. Brew (ed.), *HIV Neurology*. Oxford University Press, New York, NY.

Brew, B. J. 2001e. Uncommon causes of nonfocal brain disorders in advanced HIV disease, p. 101–104. In B. J. Brew (ed.), *HIV Neurology*. Oxford University Press, New York, NY.

Brew, B. J. 2001f. Progressive multifocal leukoencephalopathy, p. 132–141. In B. J. Brew (ed.), *HIV Neurology*. Oxford University Press, New York, NY.

Brew, B. J. 2003. The peripheral nerve complications of human immunodeficiency virus (HIV) infection. *Muscle Nerve* 28:542–552.

Brew, B. J. 2004. Evidence for a change in AIDS dementia complex (ADC) in the era of highly active antiretroviral therapy and the possibility of new forms of ADC. *AIDS* 18(Suppl. 1): S75–S78.

Brew, B. J., R. B. Bhalla, M. Paul, H. Gallardo, J. C. McArthur, M. K. Schwartz, and R. W. Price. 1990. Cerebrospinal fluid concentrations of neopterin in human immunodeficiency virus infection. *Ann. Neurol.* 28:556–560.

Brew, B. J., R. B. Bhalla, M. Paul, J. J. Sidtis, J. J. Keilp, A. E. Sadler, H. Gallardo, J. C. McArthur, M. K. Schwartz, and R. W. Price. 1992. Cerebrospinal fluid β₂ microglobulin in patients with AIDS dementia complex: an expanded series including response to zidovudine treatment. *AIDS* 6:461–465.

Brew, B. J., L. Evans, C. Byrne, L. Pemberton, and L. Hurren. 1996. The relationship between AIDS dementia complex and the presence of macrophage tropic and non syncytium inducing isolates of human immunodeficiency virus type 1 in the cerebrospinal fluid. *J. Neurovirol.* 2:152–157.

Brew, B. J., M. Paul, A. Khan, M. Gallardo, and R. W. Price. 1994. Cerebrospinal fluid HIV-1 p24 antigen and culture: sensitivity and specificity for AIDS dementia complex. *J. Neurol. Neurosurg. Psychiatry* 57:784–789.

Brew, B. J., L. Pemberton, K. Blennow, A. Wallin, and L. Hagberg. 2005. CSF amyloid beta42 and tau levels correlate with AIDS dementia complex. *Neurology* 65:1490–1492.

Brew, B. J., L. Pemberton, P. Cunningham, and M. Law. 1997. Levels of HIV-1 RNA correlate with AIDS dementia. *J. Infect. Dis.* 175:963–966.

Brew, B. J., M. Perdices, P. Darveniza, P. Edwards, B. Whyte, W. J. Burke, R. Garrick, D. O'Sullivan, R. Penny, and D. A. Cooper. 1989. Neurological complications of HIV infection in the absence of immunodeficiency. *Aust. N. Z. J. Med.* 19:700–705.

Brew, B. J., M. Rosenblum, K. Cronin, and R. W. Price. 1995. The AIDS dementia complex and human immunodeficiency virus type 1 brain infection: clinical-virological correlations. *Ann. Neurol.* 38:563–570.

Brew, B. J., S. Tisch, and M. Law. 2003. HIV nucleoside neuropathy and HIV distal symmetrical neuropathy: relationships to serum lactate and plasma HIV viral load. *AIDS* 17:1094–1096.

Brew, B. J., and S. E. Tomlinson. 2004. HIV neuropathy: time for new therapies. *Drug Discov. Today Dis. Models* 1:171–176.

Budka, H., C. A. Wiley, P. Kleihues, J. Artigas, A. K. Asbury, E. S. Cho, D. R. Cornblath, M. C. Dal Canto, U. DeGirolami, and D. Dickson. 1991. HIV-associated disease of the nervous system: review of nomenclature and proposal for neuropathology based terminology. *Brain Pathol.* 1:143–152.

Carne, C. A., R. S. Tedder, A. Smith, S. Sutherland, S. G. Elkington, H. M. Daly, F. E. Preston, and J. Craske. 1985. Acute encephalopathy coincident with seroconversion for anti-HTLV-III. *Lancet* ii:1206–1208.

Cartier, L., O. Hartley, M. Dubois-Dauphin, and K. H. Krause. 2005. Chemokine receptors in the central nervous system: role in brain inflammation and neurodegenerative diseases. *Brain Res. Brain Res. Rev.* **48:**16–42.

Castellanos, F., J. Mallada, C. Ricart, and J. A. Zabala. 1994. Ataxic neuropathy associated with human immunodeficiency virus infection. *Arch. Neurol.* **51:**236.

Centers for Disease Control and Prevention. 2001. U.S. HIV and AIDS cases reported through June 2001. *HIV/AIDS Surv. Rep.* **13:**1–44.

Chang, L., T. Ernst, M. Leonido-Yee, I. Walot, and E. Singer. 1999. Cerebral metabolites correlate with clinical severity of HIV-cognitive motor complex. *Neurology* **52:**100–108.

Cherry, C. L., J. C. McArthur, J. F. Hoy, and S. L. Wesselingh. 2003. Nucleoside analogues and neuropathy in the era of HAART. *J. Clin. Virol.* **26:**195–207.

Childs, E. A., R. H. Lyles, O. A. Selnes, B. Chen, E. N. Miller, B. A. Cohen, J. T. Becker, J. Mellors, and J. C. McArthur. 1999. Plasma viral load and CD4 lymphocytes predict HIV-associated dementia and sensory neuropathy. *Neurology* **52:**607–613.

Chirenda, J., and S. Murugasampillay. 2003. Malaria and HIV co-infection: available evidence, gaps and possible interventions. *Cent. Afr. J. Med.* **49:**66–71.

Cinque, P., L. Vago, M. Mengozzi, V. Torri, D. Ceresa, E. Vicenzi, P. Transidico, A. Vagani, S. Sozzani, A. Mantovani, A. Lazzarin, and G. Poli. 1998. Elevated cerebrospinal fluid levels of monocyte chemotactic protein-1 correlate with HIV-1 encephalitis and local viral replication. *AIDS* **12:**1327–1332.

Clark, S. J., M. S. Saag, W. D. Decker, S. Campbell-Hill, J. L. Roberson, P. J. Veldkamp, J. C. Kappes, B. H. Hahn, and G. M. Shaw. 1991. High titers of cytopathic virus in plasma of patients with symptomatic primary HIV-1 infection. *N. Engl. J. Med.* **324:**954–960.

Conant, K., J. C. McArthur, D. E. Griffin, L. Sjulson, L. M. Wahl, and D. N. Irani. 1999. Cerebrospinal fluid levels of MMP-2, 7 and 9 are elevated in association with human immunodeficiency virus dementia. *Ann. Neurol.* **46:**391–398.

Cunningham, P., D. Smith, C. Satchell, D. A. Cooper, and B. J. Brew. 2000. Evidence for independent development of reverse transcriptase inhibitor resistance patterns in the cerebrospinal fluid. *AIDS* **14:**1949–1954.

Cupler, E. J., M. Leon-Monzon, J. Miller, C. Semino-Mora, T. L. Anderson, and M. C. Dalakas. 1996. Inclusion body myositis in HIV-1 and HTLV-1 infected patients. *Brain* **119(**Pt. 6**):**1887–1893.

Cutler, R. G., N. J. Haughey, A. Tammara, J. C. McArthur, A. Nath, R. Reid, D. L. Vargas, C. A. Pardo, and M. P. Mattson. 2004. Dysregulation of sphingolipid and sterol metabolism by ApoE4 in HIV dementia. *Neurology* **63:**626–630.

Cysique, L. A., B. J. Brew, M. Halman, J. Catalan, N. Sacktor, R. W. Price, S. Brown, J. H. Atkinson, D. B. Clifford, D. Simpson, G. Torres, C. Hall, C. Power, K. Marder, J. C. McArthur, W. Symonds, and C. Romero. 2005. Undetectable cerebrospinal fluid HIV RNA and beta-2 microglobulin do not indicate inactive AIDS dementia complex in highly active antiretroviral therapy-treated patients. *J. Acquir. Immune Defic. Syndr.* **39:**426–429.

Cysique, L. A., P. Maruff, and B. J. Brew. 2004a. Antiretroviral therapy in HIV infection: are neurologically active drugs important? *Arch. Neurol.* **61:**1699–1704.

Cysique, L. A., P. Maruff, and B. J. Brew. 2004b. Prevalence and pattern of neuropsychological impairment in human immunodeficiency virus-infected/acquired immunodeficiency syndrome (HIV/AIDS) patients across pre- and post-highly active antiretroviral therapy eras: a combined study of two cohorts. *J. Neurovirol.* **10:**350–357.

Dalakas, M. C., and G. H. Pezeshkpour. 1998. Neuromuscular diseases associated with human immunodeficiency virus infection. *Ann. Neurol.* **23:**S38–S48.

Dal Pan, G. J., J. H. McArthur, E. Aylward, O. A. Selnes, T. E. Nance-Sproson, A. J. Kumar, E. D. Mellits, and J. C. McArthur. 1992. Patterns of cerebral atrophy in HIV-1-infected individuals: results of a quantitative MRI analysis. *Neurology* **42:**2125–2130.

Dal Pan, G. J., J. D. Glass, and J. C. McArthur. 1994. Clinicopathological correlations of HIV-1 associated vacuolar myelopathy: an autopsy based case control study. *Neurology* **44:**2159–2164.

Denning, D. W., J. Anderson, P. Rudge, and H. Smith. 1987. Acute myelopathy associated with primary infection with human immunodeficiency virus. *Br. Med. J.* **294:**143–144.

Desquilbet, L., C. Goujard, C. Rouzioux, M. Sinet, C. Deveau, M.-L. Chaix, D. Sereni, F. Boufassa, J.-F. Delfraissy, L. Meyer, and the PRIMO and SEROCO study groups. 2004. Does transient HAART during primary HIV-1 infection lower the virological set-point? *AIDS* **18:**2361–2369.

Di Rocco, A., P. Werner, T. Bottiglieri, J. Godbold, M. Liu, M. Tagliati, A. Scarano, and D. Simpson. 2004. Treatment of AIDS-associated myelopathy with L-methionine: a placebo-controlled study. *Neurology* **63:**1270–1275.

Dore, G., P. Correll, J. Kaldor, and B. J. Brew. 1999. Changes to the natural history of AIDS dementia complex in the era of HAART. *AIDS* **13:**1249–1253.

Dore, G. J., J. F. Hoy, S. A. Mallal, Y. Li, A. M. Mijch, M. A. French, D. A. Cooper, and J. M. Kaldor. 1997. Trends in incidence of AIDS illnesses in Australia from 1983 to 1994: The Australian AIDS Cohort. *J. Acquir. Immune Defic. Syndr.* **6:**39–43.

Dore, G. J., A. McDonald, Y. Li, J. Kaldor, and B. J. Brew. 2003. Marked improvement in survival following AIDS dementia complex in the era of highly active antiretroviral therapy. *AIDS* **17:**1539–1545.

Elder, G., M. Dalakas, G. Pezeshkpour, and J. Sever. 1986. Ataxic neuropathy due to ganglioneuritis after probable acute human immunodeficiency virus infection. *Lancet* **ii:**1275–1276.

Esiri, M. M., S. C. Biddolph, and C. S. Morris. 1998. Prevalence of Alzheimer plaques in AIDS. *J. Neurol. Neurosurg. Psychiatry* **65:**29–33.

Esiri, M. M., and C. S. Morris. 1996. The cellular basis of HIV infection of the CNS and the AIDS dementia complex: oligodendrocyte, p. 133–160. *In* R. W. Price and J. J. Sidtis (ed.), *The Cellular Basis of Central Nervous System HIV-1 Infection and the AIDS Dementia Complex.* Haworth Press, Philadelphia, PA.

Estanislao, L., K. Carter, J. McArthur, R. Olney, D. Simpson, and the Lidoderm-HIV Neuropathy Group. 2004. A randomized controlled trial of 5% lidocaine gel for HIV-associated distal symmetric polyneuropathy. *J. Acquir. Immune Defic. Syndr.* **37:**1584–1586.

Famularo, G., S. Moretti, S. Marcellini, V. Trinchieri, S. Tzantzoglou, G. Santini, A. Longo, and C. de Simone. 1997. Acetyl-carnitine deficiency in AIDS patients with neurotoxicity on treatment with antiretroviral nucleoside analogues. *AIDS* **11:**185–190.

Fine, S. M., R. A. Angel, S. W. Perry, L. G. Epstein, J. D. Rothstein, S. Dewhurst, and H. A. Gelbard. 1996. Tumor necrosis factor α inhibits glutamate uptake by primary human astrocytes: implications for pathogenesis of HIV-1 dementia. *J. Biol. Chem.* **271:**15303–15306.

Forloni, G., F. Demicheli, S. Giorgi, C. Bendotti, and N. Angeretti. 1992. Expression of amyloid precursor protein mRNAs in endothelial, neuronal, and glial cells: modulation by interleukin-1. *Brain Res.* **16:**128–134.

Foudraine, N. A., R. M. Hoetelmans, J. M. Lange, F. de Wolf, B. H. van Benthem, J. J. Maas, I. P. Keet, and P. Portegies. 1998. Cerebrospinal-fluid HIV-1 RNA and drug concentrations after treatment with lamivudine plus zidovudine or stavudine. *Lancet* **351:**1547–1551.

Gaines, H., M. von Sydow, P. O. Pehrson, and P. Lundbergh. 1988. Clinical picture of primary HIV-1 infection presenting as a glandular-fever-like illness. *Lancet* 297:1363–1368.

Gartner, S. 2000. HIV infection and dementia. *Science* 287: 602–604.

Gelman, B. B. 1993. Diffuse microgliosis associated with cerebral atrophy in the acquired immunodeficiency syndrome. *Ann. Neurol.* 34:65–70.

Gelman, B. B., and F. C. Guinto. 1992. Morphometry, histopathology and tomography of cerebral atrophy in the acquired immunodeficiency syndrome. *Ann. Neurol.* 32:31–40.

Gelman, B. B., V. M. Soukup, K. W. Schuenke, M. J. Keherly, C. Holzer III, F. J. Richey, and C. J. Lahart. 2004. Acquired neuronal channelopathies in HIV-associated dementia. *Neuroimmunology* 157:111–119.

Giometto, B., S. F. An, M. Groves, T. Scaravilli, J. F. Geddes, R. Miller, B. Tavolato, A. A. Beckett, and F. Scaravilli. 1997. Accumulation of β amyloid precursor protein in HIV encephalitis: relationship with neuropsychological abnormalities. *Ann. Neurol.* 42:34–40.

Gisslen, M., G. Norkrans, B. Svennerholm, and L. Hagberg. 1997. The effect on human immunodeficiency virus type 1 RNA levels in the cerebrospinal fluid after initiation of zidovudine or didanosine. *J. Infect. Dis.* 175:434–437.

Glass, J. D., S. L. Wesselingh, O. A. Selnes, and J. C. McArthur. 1993. Clinical-neuropathologic correlation in HIV-associated dementia. *Neurology* 43:2230–2237.

Gonzalez, E., B. H. Rovin, L. Sen, G. Cooke, R. Dhanda, S. Mummidi, H. Kulkarni, M. J. Bamshad, V. Telles, S. A. Anderson, E. A. Walter, K. T. Stephan, M. Deucher, A. Mangano, R. Bologna, S. S. Ahuja, M. J. Dolan, and S. K. Ahuja. 2002. HIV-1 infection and AIDS dementia are influenced by a mutant MCP-1 allele linked to increased monocyte infiltration of tissues and MCP-1 levels. *Proc. Natl. Acad. Sci. USA* 99:13795–13800.

Gray, F., H. Adle-Biassette, F. Chretien, G. Lorin de la Grandmaison, G. Force, and C. Keohane. 2001. Neuropathology and neurodegeneration in human immunodeficiency virus infection. Pathogenesis of HIV-induced lesions of the brain, correlations with HIV-associated disorders and modifications according to treatments. *Clin. Neuropathol.* 20: 146–155.

Gray, F., F. Chretien, A. V. Vallat-Decouvelaere, and F. Scaravilli. 2003. The changing pattern of HIV neuropathology in the HAART era. *J. Neuropathol. Exp. Neurol.* 62:429–440.

Hagberg, L., B.-E. Malmvall, L. Svennerholm, K. Alestig, and G. Norkrans. 1986. Guillain-Barre syndrome as an early manifestation of HIV-1 central nervous system infection. *Scand. J. Infect. Dis.* 18:591–592.

Hardy, W. D., E. S. Daar, R. T. Sokolov, Jr., and D. D. Ho. 1991. Acute neurologic deterioration in a young man. *Rev. Infect. Dis.* 13:745–750.

Harrison, L. H., and M. Schechter. 1998. Coinfection with HTLV-I and HIV: increase in HTLV-I-related outcomes but not accelerated HIV disease progression? *AIDS Patient Care STDs* 12:619–623.

Harrison, L. H., B. Vaz, D. M. Taveira, T. C. Quinn, C. J. Gibbs, S. H. de Souza, J. C. McArthur, and M. Schechter. 1997. Myelopathy among Brazilians coinfected with human T-cell lymphotropic virus type I and HIV. *Neurology* 48:13–18.

Herzberg, U., and J. Sagen. 2001. Peripheral nerve exposure to HIV viral envelope protein gp120 induces neuropathic pain and spinal gliosis. *J. Neuroimmunol.* 116:29–39.

Heyes, M. P., B. J. Brew, A. Martin, R. W. Price, A. M. Salazar, J. J. Sidtis, J. A. Yergey, M. M. Mouradian, A. E. Sadler, and J. Keilp. 1991. Cerebrospinal fluid quinolinic acid concentrations are increased in acquired immune deficiency syndrome. *Ann. Neurol.* 29:202–209.

Ho, D. D., T. R. Rota, R. T. Schooley, J. C. Kaplan, J. D. Allan, J. E. Groopman, L. Resnick, D. Felsenstein, C. A. Andrews, and M. S. Hirsch. 1985a. Isolation of HTLV-III from cerebrospinal fluid and neural tissues of patients with neurologic syndromes related to the acquired immunodeficiency syndrome. *N. Engl. J. Med.* 313:1493–1497.

Ho, D. D., M. G. Sarngadharan, L. Resnick, F. Dimarzo-Veronese, T. R. Rota, and M. S. Hirsch. 1985b. Primary human T-lymphotropic virus type III infection. *Ann. Intern. Med.* 103:880–883.

Hollander, H., and S. Stringari. 1987. Human immunodeficiency virus-associated meningitis. Clinical course and correlations. *Am. J. Med.* 83:813–816.

Jarvik, J. G., J. R. Hesselink, C. Kennedy, R. Teschke, C. Wiley, S. Spector, D. Richman, and J. A. McCutchan. 1988. Acquired immunodeficiency syndrome. Magnetic resonance patterns of brain involvement with pathologic correlation. *Arch. Neurol.* 45:731–736.

Kahn, J. O., and B. D. Walker. 1998. Acute human immunodeficiency virus type 1 infection. *N. Engl. J. Med.* 339:33–39.

Kassutto, S., and E. S. Rosenberg. 2004. Primary HIV type 1 infection. *Clin. Infect. Dis.* 38:1447–1453.

Kaufman, D. E., M. Lichterfeld, M. Altfield, M. M. Addo, M. N. Johnston, P. K. Lee, B. S. Wagner, E. T. Kalife, D. Strick, E. S. Rosenberg, and B. D. Walker. 2004. Limited durability of viral control following treated acute HIV infection. *PLoS Med.* 1:1–12.

Kaufman, G., C. Duncombe, J. Zaunders, P. Cunningham, and D. Cooper. 1998. Primary HIV-1 infection: a review of clinical manifestations, immunologic and virologic changes. *AIDS Patient Care STDs* 12:759–767.

Keswani, S. C., G. J. Leitz, and A. Hoke. 2004. Erythropoietin is neuroprotective in models of HIV sensory neuropathy. *Neurosci. Lett.* 371:102–105.

Keswani, S. C., M. Polley, C. A. Pardo, J. W. Griffin, J. C. McArthur, and A. Hoke. 2003. Schwann cell chemokine receptors mediate HIV-1 gp120 toxicity to sensory neurons. *Ann. Neurol.* 54:287–296.

Kieburtz, K., D. Simpson, C. Yiannoutsos, M. B. Max, C. D. Hall, R. J. Ellis, C. M. Marra, R. McKendall, E. Singer, G. J. Dal Pan, D. B. Clifford, T. Tucker, T. Cohen, et al. 1998. A randomized trial of amitriptyline and mexiletine for painful neuropathy in HIV infection. *Neurology* 51:1682–1688.

Kim, R. B., M. F. Fromm, C. Wandel, B. Leake, A. J. Wood, D. M. Roden, and G. R. Wilkinson. 1998. The drug transporter P glycoprotein limits oral absorption and brain entry of the HIV-1 protease inhibitors. *J. Clin. Investig.* 101:289–294.

Kinloch-de Loes, S., and T. V. Perneger. 1997. Primary HIV infection: follow up of patients initially randomized to zidovudine or placebo. *J. Infect.* 333:408–413.

Kivipelto, M., E. L. Helkala, M. P. Laakso, T. Hanninen, M. Hallikainen, S. Alhainen, S. Iivonen, A. Mannermaa, J. Tuomilehto, A. Nissinen, and H. Soininen. 2002. Apolipoprotein E epsilon4 allele, elevated midlife total cholesterol level, and high midlife systolic blood pressure are independent risk factors for late-life Alzheimer disease. *Ann. Intern. Med.* 137:149–155.

Konig, J., A. T. Nies, Y. Cui, I. Leier, and D. Keppler. 1999. Conjugate export pumps of the multidrug resistance protein (MRP) family: localization, substrate specificity, and MRP2-mediated drug resistance. *Biochim. Biophys. Acta* 1461:377–394.

Krathwohl, M. D., and J. L. Kaiser. 2004. HIV-1 promotes quiescence in human neural progenitor cells. *J. Infect. Dis.* 190:216–226.

Langford, D., A. Grigorian, R. Hurford, A. Adame, R. J. Ellis, L. Hansen, and E. Masliah. 2004. Altered P-glycoprotein expression in AIDS patients with HIV encephalitis. *J. Neuropathol. Exp. Neurol.* 63:1038–1047.

Lanjewar, D. N., P. P. Jain, and C. R. Shetty. 1998. Profile of central nervous system pathology in patients with AIDS: an autopsy study from India. *AIDS* 12:309–313.

Levy, R. M., D. E. Bredesen, and M. L. Rosenblum. 1985. Neurological manifestations of the acquired immunodeficiency syndrome (AIDS): experience at UCSF and review of the literature. *J. Neurosurg.* 62:475–495.

Lichtenstein, K. A., C. Armon, A. Baron, A. C. Moorman, K. C. Wood, S. D. Holmberg, and the HIV Outpatient Study Investigators. 2005. Modification of the incidence of drug-associated symmetrical peripheral neuropathy by host and disease factors in the HIV outpatient study cohort. *Clin. Infect. Dis.* 40:148–157.

Lipton, S. A., and H. E. Gendelman. 1995. Dementia associated with the Acquired Immunodeficiency Syndrome. *N. Engl. J. Med.* 332:934–940.

Lori, F., A. Malykh, A. Cara, D. Sun, J. N. Weinstein, J. Lisziewicz, and R. C. Gallo. 1994. Hydroxyurea as an inhibitor of human immunodeficiency virus type 1 replication. *Science* 266:801–805.

Markus, R., and B. J. Brew. 1998. HIV-1 peripheral neuropathy and combination antiretroviral therapy. *Lancet* 352:1906–1907.

Marshall, D. W., R. L. Brey, W. T. Cahill, R. W. Houk, R. A. Zajac, and R. N. Boswell. 1988. Spectrum of cerebrospinal fluid findings in various stages of human immunodeficiency virus infection. *Arch. Neurol.* 45:954–958.

Martin, C., G. Solders, A. Sönnerborg, and P. Hansson. 2000. Antiretroviral therapy may improve sensory function in HIV-infected patients: a pilot study. *Neurology* 54:2120–2127.

Martin, C., A. Sonnerborg, J. O. Svensson, and L. Stahle. 1999. Indinavir-based treatment of HIV-1 infected patients: efficacy in the central nervous system. *AIDS* 13:1227–1232.

Martin, J. L., C. E. Brown, N. Matthews-Davis, and J. E. Reardon. 1994. Effects of antiviral nucleoside analogs on human DNA polymerases and mitochondrial DNA synthesis. *Antimicrob. Agents Chemother.* 38:2743–2749.

Maruff, P., J. Currie, V. Malone, C. McArthur-Jackson, B. Mulhall, and E. Benson. 1994. Neuropsychological characterisation of the AIDS dementia complex and rationalisation of a test battery. *Arch. Neurol.* 51:689–695.

Maschke, M., O. Kastrup, S. Esser, B. Ross, U. Hengge, and A. Hufnagel. 2000. Incidence and prevalence of HIV-associated neurological disorders since the introduction of highly active antiretroviral therapy (HAART). *J. Neurol. Neurosurg. Psychiatry* 69:376–380.

Masliah, E., R. K. Heaton, T. D. Marcotte, R. J. Ellis, C. A. Wiley, M. Mallory, C. L. Achim, J. A. McCutchan, J. A. Nelson, J. H. Atkinson, and I. Grant. 1997. Dendritic injury is a pathological substrate for human immunodeficiency virus related cognitive disorders. *Ann. Neurol.* 42:963–972.

McArthur, J. C., and J. W. Griffin. 2005. Another tool for the neurologist's toolbox. *Ann. Neurol.* 57:163–167.

McArthur, J. C., D. R. Hoover, H. Bacellar, E. N. Miller, B. A. Cohen, J. T. Becker, N. M. Graham, J. H. McArthur, O. A. Selnes, and L. P. Jacobson. 1993. Dementia in AIDS patients: incidence and risk factors. Multicenter AIDS Cohort Study. *Neurology* 43:2245–2252.

McArthur, J. C., D. R. McClernon, M. F. Cronin, T. E. Nance-Sproson, A. J. Saah, M. St Clair, and E. R. Lanier. 1997. Relationship between human immunodeficiency virus-associated dementia and viral load in cerebrospinal fluid and brain. *Ann. Neurol.* 42:689–698.

McArthur, J. C., M. P. McDermott, D. McClernon, C. St Hillaire, K. Conant, K. Marder, G. Schifitto, O. A. Selnes, N. Sacktor, Y. Stern, S. M. Albert, K. Kieburtz, J. A. deMarcaida, B. Cohen, and L. G. Epstein. 2004. Attenuated central nervous system infection in advanced HIV/AIDS with combination antiretroviral therapy. *Arch. Neurol.* 61:1687–1696.

McArthur, J. C., C. Yiannoutsos, D. M. Simpson, B. T. Adornato, E. J. Singer, H. Hollander, C. Marra, M. Rubin, B. A. Cohen, T. Tucker, B. A. Navia, G. Schifitto, D. Katzenstein, C. Rask, L. Zaborski, M. E. Smith, S. Shrivers, L. Millar, D. B. Clifford, I. J. Karalnik, et al. 2000. A phase II trial of nerve growth factor for sensory neuropathy associated with HIV infection. *Neurology* 54:1080–1088.

McDonagh, C. A., and R. P. Holman. 2003. Primary human immunodeficiency virus type 1 infection in a patient with acute rhabdomyolysis. *South. Med. J.* 96:1027–1030.

Mizuno, T., J. Kawanokuchi, K. Numata, and A. Suzumura. 2003. Production and neuroprotective functions of fractalkine in the central nervous system. *Brain Res.* 979:65–70.

Monos, D. S., M. Papaioakim, T. W. Ho, C. Y. Li, and G. M. McKhann. 1997. Differential distribution of HLA alleles in two forms of Guillain-Barre syndrome. *J. Infect. Dis.* 176 (Suppl. 2):S180–S182.

Morgello, S., R. Mahboob, T. Yakoushina, S. Khan, and K. Hague. 2002. Autopsy findings in a human immunodeficiency virus-infected population over 2 decades: influences of gender, ethnicity, risk factors, and time. *Arch. Pathol. Lab. Med.* 126:182–190.

Moses, A. E., K. A. Adelowo, and E. A. Nwankwo. 2001. Effect of HIV infection on the clinical spectrum of leprosy in Maiduguri. *Niger. Postgrad. Med. J.* 8:74–77.

Moses, A. V., S. G. Stenglein, and J. A. Nelson. 1996. HIV infection of the brain microvasculature and its contribution to the AIDS dementia complex. *J. NeuroAIDS* 1:85–100.

Moulignier, A., F. J. Authier, M. Baudrimont, G. Pialoux, L. Belec, M. Polivka, B. Clair, F. Gray, J. Mikol, and R. K. Gherardi. 1997. Peripheral neuropathy in human immunodeficiency virus-infected patients with the diffuse infiltrative lymphocytosis syndrome. *Ann. Neurol.* 41:438–445.

Navia, B. A., B. D. Jordan, and R. W. Price. 1986. The AIDS dementia complex. I. Clinical features. *Ann. Neurol.* 19:517–524.

Nebuloni, M., A. Pellegrinelli, A. Ferri, S. Bonetto, R. Boldorini, L. Vago, M. P. Grassi, and G. Costanzi. 2001. Beta amyloid precursor protein and patterns of HIV p24 immunohistochemistry in different brain areas of AIDS patients. *AIDS* 15:571–575.

Pardo, C. A., J. C. McArthur, and J. W. Griffin. 2001. HIV neuropathy: insights in the pathology of HIV peripheral nerve disease. *J. Peripher. Nerv. Syst.* 6:21–27.

Paton, P., H. Poly, P.-M. Gonnaud, J. C. Tardy, J. Fontana, K. Kindbeiter, R. Tete, and J. J. Madjar. 1990. Acute meningoradiculitis concomitant with seroconversion to human immunodeficiency virus type 1. *Res. Virol.* 141:427–433.

Pedersen, C., B. Lindhardt, B. L. Jensen, E. Lauritzen, J. Gerstoft, E. Dickmeiss, J. Gaub, E. Scheibel, and T. Karlsmark. 1989. Clinical course of primary HIV-1 infection: consequences for subsequent course of infection. *Br. Med. J.* 299:154–157.

Petito, C. K., B. A. Navia, E. S. Cho, B. D. Jordan, D. C. George, and R. W. Price. 1985. Vacuolar myelopathy pathologically resembling subacute combined degeneration in patients with acquired immunodeficiency syndrome. *N. Engl. J. Med.* 312:874–879.

Piette, A. M., F. Tusseau, D. Vignon, A. Chapman, G. Parrot, J. Leibowitch, and L. Montagnier. 1986. Acute neuropathy coincident with seroconversion for anti-LAV/HTLV-III. *Lancet* i:852.

Piller, S. C., G. D. Ewart, D. A. Jans, P. W. Gage, and G. B. Cox. 1999. The amino-terminal region of Vpr from human immunodeficiency virus type 1 forms ion channels and kills neurons. *J. Virol.* 73:4230–4238.

Portegies, P., R. H. Enting, J. de Gans, P. R. Algra, M. M. Derix, J. M. Lange, and J. Goudsmit. 1993. Presentation and course of AIDS dementia complex: 10 years of follow-up in Amsterdam, The Netherlands. *AIDS* 7:669–775.

Power, C., P. A. Kong, T. O. Crawford, S. Wesselingh, J. D. Glass, J. C. McArthur, and B. D. Trapp. 1993. Cerebral white matter changes in acquired immunodeficiency syndrome dementia: alterations of the blood brain barrier. *Ann. Neurol.* **34**:339–359.

Quasney, M. W., Q. Zhang, S. Sargent, M. Mynatt, J. Glass, and J. McArthur. 2001. Increased frequency of the tumor necrosis factor-alpha-308 A allele in adults with human immunodeficiency virus dementia. *Ann. Neurol.* **50**:157–162.

Quinn, T. C. 1997. Acute primary HIV infection. *JAMA* **278**:58–62.

Radja, F., D. G. Kay, S. Albrecht, and P. Jolicoeur. 2003. Oligodendrocyte-specific expression of human immunodeficiency virus type 1 Nef in transgenic mice leads to vacuolar myelopathy and alters oligodendrocyte phenotype in vitro. *J. Virol.* **77**:11745–11753.

Ragin, A. B., P. Storey, B. A. Cohen, R. R. Edelman, and L. G. Epstein. 2004. Disease burden in HIV-associated cognitive impairment: a study of whole-brain imaging measures. *Neurology* **63**:2293–2297.

Ranga, U., R. Shankarappa, N. B. Siddappa, L. Ramakrishna, R. Nagendran, M. Mahalingam, A. Mahadevan, N. Jayasuryan, P. Satishchandra, S. K. Shankar, and V. R. Prasad. 2004. Tat protein of human immunodeficiency virus type 1 subtype C strains is a defective chemokine. *J. Virol.* **78**:2586–2590.

Rempel, H. C., and L. Pulliam. 2005. HIV-1 Tat inhibits neprilysin and elevates amyloid beta. *AIDS* **19**:127–135.

Rizzardi, G. P., A. Harari, B. Capiluppi, G. Tambussi, K. Ellefsen, D. Ciuffreda, P. Champagne, P. A. Bart, J. P. Chave, A. Lazzarin, and G. Pantaleo. 2002. Treatment of primary HIV-1 infection with cyclosporine A coupled with highly active antiretroviral therapy. *J. Clin. Investig.* **109**:681–688.

Romanelli, F., H. R. Jennings, A. Nath, M. Ryan, and J. Berger. 2000. Therapeutic dilemma: the use of anticonvulsants in HIV-positive individuals. *Neurology* **54**:1404–1407.

Rosenblum, M., A. C. Scheck, K. Cronin, B. J. Brew, A. Khan, M. Paul, and R. W. Price. 1989. Dissociation of AIDS related vacuolar myelopathy and productive HIV-1 infection of the spinal cord. *Neurology* **39**:892–896.

Rottenberg, D. A., J. R. Moeller, S. C. Strother, J. J. Sidtis, B. A. Navia, V. Dhawan, J. Z. Ginos, and R. W. Price. 1987. The metabolic pathology of the AIDS dementia complex. *Ann. Neurol.* **22**:700–706.

Rottnek, M., A. Di Rocco, D. Laudier, and S. Morgello. 2002. Axonal damage is a late component of vacuolar myelopathy. *Neurology* **58**:479–481.

Roucoux, D. F., and E. L. Murphy. 2004. The epidemiology and disease outcomes of human T-lymphotropic virus type II. *AIDS Rev.* **6**:144–154.

Ryan, E. L., S. Morgello, K. Isaacs, M. Naseer, and P. Gerits. 2004. Neuropsychiatric impact of hepatitis C on advanced HIV. *Neurology* **62**:957–962.

Saavedra-Lozano, J., C. C. McCoig, Y. Cao, E. S. Vitetta, and O. Ramilo. 2004. Zidovudine, lamivudine, and abacavir have different effects on resting cells infected with human immunodeficiency virus in vitro. *Antimicrob. Agents Chemother.* **48**:2825–2830.

Sanders, V. J., C. A. Pittman, M. G. White, G. Wang, C. A. Wiley, and C. L. Achim. 1998. Chemokines and receptors in HIV encephalitis. *AIDS* **12**:1021–1026.

Schacker, T., A. C. Collier, J. Hughes, T. Shea, and L. Corey. 1996. Clinical and epidemiologic features of primary HIV infection. *Ann. Intern. Med.* **125**:257–264.

Schielke, E., K. Tatsch, H. W. Pfister, C. Trenkwalder, G. Leinsinger, C. M. Kirsch, A. Matuschke, and K. M. Einhaupl. 1990. Reduced cerebral blood flow in early stages of human immunodeficiency virus infection. *Arch. Neurol.* **47**:1342–1345.

Schifitto, G., M. P. McDermott, J. C. McArthur, K. Marder, N. Sacktor, D. R. McClernon, K. Conant, B. Cohen, L. G. Epstein, K. Kieburtz, and the NEAD Consortium. 2005. Markers of immune activation and viral load in HIV-associated sensory neuropathy. *Neurology* **64**:842–848.

Schutzer, S. E., M. Brunner, H. M. Fillit, and J. R. Berger. 2003. Autoimmune markers in HIV-associated dementia. *J. Neuroimmunol.* **138**:156–161.

Si, Q., M. Cosenza, M. O. Kim, M. L. Zhao, M. Brownlee, H. Goldstein, and S. Lee. 2004. A novel action of minocycline: inhibition of human immunodeficiency virus type 1 infection in microglia. *J. Neurovirol.* **10**:284–292.

Sidtis, J. J., C. Gatsonis, R. W. Price, E. J. Singer, A. C. Collier, D. D. Richman, M. S. Hirsch, F. W. Schaerf, M. A. Fischl, K. Kieburtz, et al. 1993. Zidovudine treatment of the AIDS dementia complex: results of a placebo controlled trial. *Ann. Neurol.* **33**:343–349.

Silver, B., K. McAvoy, S. Mikesell, and T. W. Smith. 1997. Fulminating encephalopathy with perivenular demyelination and vacuolar myelopathy as the initial presentation of human immunodeficiency virus infection. *Arch. Neurol.* **54**:647–650.

Simpson, D. M., J. C. McArthur, R. Olney, D. Clifford, Y. So, D. Ross, B. J. Baird, P. Barrett, A. E. Hammer, and the Lamotrigine HIV Neuropathy Study Team. 2003. Lamotrigine for HIV-associated painful sensory neuropathies: a placebo-controlled trial. *Neurology* **60**:1508–1514.

Sinclair, E., F. Gray, A. Giardi, and F. Scaravilli. 1994. Immunohistochemical changes and PCR detection of HIV provirus DNA in brains of asymptomatic HIV positive patients. *J. Neuropathol. Exp. Neurol.* **53**:43–50.

Singh, K. K., C. F. Barroga, M. D. Hughes, J. Chen, C. Raskino, R. E. McKinney, and S. A. Spector. 2003. Genetic influence of CCR5, CCR2, and SDF1 variants on human immunodeficiency virus 1 (HIV-1)-related disease progression and neurological impairment, in children with symptomatic HIV-1 infection. *J. Infect. Dis.* **188**:1461–1472.

Smit, T. K., B. J. Brew, W. Tourtellotte, S. Morgello, B. B. Gelman, and N. K. Saksena. 2004. Independent evolution of human immunodeficiency virus (HIV) drug resistance mutations in diverse areas of the brain in HIV-infected patients, with and without dementia, on antiretroviral treatment. *J. Virol.* **78**:10133–10148.

Smith, D. E., B. D. Walker, D. A. Cooper, E. S. Rosenberg, and J. M. Kaldor. 2004. Is antiretroviral treatment of primary HIV infection clinically justified on the basis of current evidence? *AIDS* **18**:709–718.

Stanley, L. C., R. E. Mrak, R. C. Woody, L. J. Perrot, S. Zhang, D. R. Marshak, S. J. Nelson, and W. S. Griffin. 1994. Glial cytokines as neuropathogenic factors in HIV infection: pathogenic similarities to Alzheimer's disease. *J. Neuropathol. Exp. Neurol.* **53**:231–238.

Steiner, I., O. Cohen, R. R. Leker, B. Rubinovitch, R. Handsher, S. Hassin-Baer, D. H. Gilden, and M. Sadeh. 1999. Subacute painful lumbosacral polyradiculoneuropathy in immunocompromised patients. *J. Neurol. Sci.* **162**:91–93.

Takahashi, K., S. L. Wesselingh, D. E. Griffin, J. C. McArthur, R. T. Johnson, and J. D. Glass. 1996. Localization of HIV-1 in human brain using polymerase chain reaction/in situ hybridization and immunohistochemistry. *Ann. Neurol.* **39**:705–711.

Tambussi, G., A. Gori, B. Capiluppi, C. Balotta, L. Papagno, B. Morandini, M. Di Pietro, D. Ciuffreda, A. Saracco, and A. Lazzarin. 2000. Neurological symptoms during primary human immunodeficiency virus (HIV) infection correlate with high levels of HIV RNA in cerebrospinal fluid. *Clin. Infect. Dis.* **30**:962–965.

Thompson, K. A., J. C. McArthur, and S. L. Wesselingh. 2001. Correlation between neurological progression and astrocyte apoptosis in HIV-associated dementia. *Ann. Neurol.* **49**:745–752.

Tornatore, C., R. Chandra, J. R. Berger, and E. O. Major. 1994. HIV-1 infection of subcortical astrocytes in the pediatric central nervous system. *Neurology* **44:**481–487.

Tyor, W. R., J. D. Glass, J. W. Griffin, P. S. Becker, J. C. McArthur, L. Bezman, and D. E. Griffin. 1992. Cytokine expression in the brain during the acquired immune deficiency syndrome. *Ann. Neurol.* **31:**349–360.

Waxman, S. G. 1999. The molecular pathophysiology of pain: abnormal expression of sodium channel genes and its contributions to hyperexcitability of primary sensory neurons. *Pain* **1999**(Suppl. 6)**:**S133–S140.

Weidenheim, K. M., M. Ausubel, and W. D. Lyman. 1996. Quantification of microglia in vacuolar myelopathy is a more sensitive measure of pathology than changes in myelin protein immunoreactivity. *J. Neuropathol. Exp. Neurol.* **55:**660.

Wesselingh, S. L., C. Power, J. D. Glass, W. R. Tyor, J. C. McArthur, J. M. Farber, J. W. Griffin, and D. E. Griffin. 1993. Intracerebral cytokine messenger RNA expression in acquired immunodeficiency syndrome dementia. *Ann. Neurol.* **33:**576–582.

Whiteman, M., L. Espinoza, M. J. Post, M. D. Bell, and S. Falcone. 1995. Central nervous system tuberculosis in HIV-infected patients: clinical and radiographic findings. *Am. J. Neuroradiol.* **16:**1319–1327.

Wilkins, J. W., K. R. Robertson, C. R. Snyder, W. K. Robertson, C. van der Horst, and C. D. Hall. 1991. Implications of self reported cognitive and motor dysfunction in HIV positive patients. *Am. J. Psychiatry* **148:**641–643.

Wiselka, M. J., K. G. Nicholson, S. C. Ward, and A. J. E. Flower. 1987. Acute infection with human immunodeficiency virus associated with facial nerve palsy and neuralgia. *J. Infect.* **15:**189–194.

Wu, H. S., T. C. Liu, Z. L. Lu, L. P. Zou, W. C. Zhang, G. Zhaori, and J. Zhang. 1997. A prospective clinical and electrophysiologic survey of acute flaccid paralysis in Chinese children. *Neurology* **49:**1723–1725.

Zeman, A., and M. Donaghy. 1991. Acute infection with human immunodeficiency virus presenting with neurogenic urinary retention. *Genitourin. Med.* **67:**345–347.

Zhang, K., G. A. McQuibban, C. Silva, G. S. Butler, J. B. Johnston, J. Holden, I. Clark-Lewis, C. M. Overall, and C. Power. 2003. HIV-induced metalloproteinase processing of the chemokine stromal cell derived factor-1 causes neurodegeneration. *Nat. Neurosci.* **6:**1064–1071.

Zink, M. C., and J. E. Clements. 2002. A novel simian immunodeficiency virus model that provides insight into mechanisms of human immunodeficiency virus central nervous system disease. *J. Neurovirol.* **8**(Suppl. 2)**:**S42–S48.

Index